Advanced Concepts in Clinical Nursing

Contributors

Curtis P. Artz, M.D., F.A.C.S.
Professor of Surgery and Chairman of Department
Medical University of South Carolina
Charleston, South Carolina

Elizabeth W. Bayley, R.N., M.S.
Nurse Coordinator
Burn Treatment Center
Crozer Chester Medical Center
Chester, Pennsylvania

Donna R. Beshear
Medical Writer
Literary Research Consultant

Elizabeth M. Cameron, R.N.
Formerly Head Nurse, Dialysis and Transplant Unit,
Hospital of the University of Pennsylvania
Philadelphia, Pennsylvania

Elizabeth Moir Carmelite, R.N., B.S.N.
Formerly Supervisor for ICU-Surgery Units,
Department of Nursing,
Hospital of the University of Pennsylvania
Philadelphia, Pennsylvania

Gloria Ferraro Donnelly, R.N., M.S.N.
Instructor, Mental Health
Community Health Nursing
College of Nursing, Villanova University
Villanova, Pennsylvania

Mary Early, R.N., M.S.
Associate Professor, College of Nursing
University of Delaware
Newark, Delaware

Lawrence J. Hourany, Ph.D.
Assistant Professor of Psychology
Cedar Crest College
Allentown, Pennsylvania

JoAnn Shafer Jamann, M.S.N., Ed.D.
Assistant Dean
Rush University College of Nursing
Chicago, Illinois

Clara H. Jordan, B.S.N.Ed., M.S.N.
Associate Professor and Director
Graduate Program in Maternity Nursing
School of Nursing
University of Pennsylvania
Philadelphia, Pennsylvania

Anne Keane, R.N., M.S.N.
Associate Professor Nursing, Graduate Division, School
of Nursing
University of Pennsylvania
Philadelphia, Pennsylvania

Nancy Perpall Kelly, R.N., B.S.
Formerly, Instructor, Greater Delaware Valley Regional
Medical Program
Allentown, Pennsylvania

James E. Kintzel, M.D.
Chairman of Nephrology Section and Hemodialysis Unit
Allentown General Hospital
Allentown, Pennsylvania

Patricia A. Lawrence, R.N., M.A.
Associate Professor
Continuing Education Program
School of Nursing
University of North Carolina
Chapel Hill, North Carolina

Deborah Lindell, M.S.N.
Instructor in Medical-Surgical Nursing
College of Nursing, University of Delaware
Newark, Delaware

Barbara Lowery, B.S.N., M.S.N., Ed.D
Associate Professor of Nursing
Graduate Division, School of Nursing
University of Pennsylvania
Philadelphia, Pennsylvania

Wealtha Collins McGurn, R.N., M.S.N., Ph.D.
Lecturer, University of Pennsylvania School of Nursing
Director, Health Professions Advisory Board
University of Pennsylvania
Philadelphia, Pennsylvania

Mary Evans Melick, R.N., B.S.Ed., M.S.N., Ph.D
Assistant Professor of Nursing
State University of New York at Albany

Donna Nativio, R.N., B.S.N., M.S.
Pediatric Nurse Practitioner,
Childrens Hospital of Pittsburgh
Clinical Instructor, University of Pittsburgh
Pittsburgh, Pennsylvania

Mary Rieser, R.N., M.S.
Assistant Director of Nursing for Staff Development
Hospital of the University of Pennsylvania
Philadelphia, Pennsylvania

Richard Schwarz, M.D.
Professor of Obstetrics and Gynecology
University of Pennsylvania School of Medicine
Philadelphia, Pennsylvania

Howard Silberman, M.D.
Assistant Professor of Surgery
University of Southern California
Formerly Chief, General Surgery Service
USAF Medical Center, Scott AFB, Illinois
and Associate in Surgery, University of Pennsylvania
Philadelphia, Pennsylvania

Marianne Costopoulos Slater, R.N., M.N.
Clinical Nurse Specialist
Neurological-Neurosurgical Nursing
Havertown, Pennsylvania

W. D. Snively, Jr., M.D., F.A.C.P.
Professor of Life Sciences
University of Evansville
Evansville, Indiana

Doris Cook Sutterley, R.N., M.S.N.
Assistant Professor
Project Director Continuing Education
Trenton State College
Trenton, New Jersey

Dolores Lake Taylor, R.N., M.S.N.
Associate Professor of Nursing
Bucks County Community College
Newtown, Pennsylvania

Martha Taylor, R.N., B.S.N.
Evening Supervisor, Hospital of University of
Pennsylvania
Formerly, Supervisor, ICU-Surgery Units, Department
of Nursing,
Hospital of the University of Pennsylvania
Philadelphia, Pennsylvania

Judith Diegnan Worrell, B.S.N., M.S.N.
Formerly Senior Program Coordinator,
Medical-Surgical Nursing,
School of Nursing
Hospital of the University of Pennsylvania
Philadelphia, Pennsylvania

Advanced Concepts
in Clinical Nursing *Second Edition*

Edited by

KAY CORMAN KINTZEL, R.N., M.S.N.

Formerly Instructor in Nursing Research
School of Nursing, Graduate Division
University of Pennsylvania
Instructor in Medical-Surgical Nursing
Duke University, Durham, North Carolina

J. B. LIPPINCOTT COMPANY   *Philadelphia*

New York   San Jose   Toronto

Copyright © 1977 by J. B. Lippincott Company

This book is fully protected by copyright and, with the exception of brief excerpts for review, no part of it may be reproduced in any form by print, photoprint, microfilm, or by any other means without the written permission of the publishers.

Distributed in Great Britain by
Blackwell Scientific Publications
London   Oxford   Edinburgh

ISBN 0-397-54191-0

Library of Congress Catalog Card Number 77-8375

Printed in the United States of America

2 4 6 8 9 7 5 3 1

Library of Congress Cataloging in Publication Data
Main entry under title:

Advanced concepts in clinical nursing.

Bibliography: p.
Includes index.
1. Nursing.   I. Kintzel, Kay Corman.
RT41.A36 1977   610.73   77-8375
ISBN 0-397-54191-0

Preface

Nothing endures except change. While this observation is neither new nor startling, surely none can better attest to the truth of the sentiment than editors of textbooks. This editor, at least, has found change to be so characteristic of contemporary nursing as to require that a text called *Advanced Concepts in Clinical Nursing* must be extensively revised within a very few years merely to remain true to its title. However, having duly noted this sense of necessity, I must go on to say that the task of revision has been both exciting and enjoyable. The reception of the previous edition of this text has been gratifying to me and to the contributing authors, and we present this second volume with enthusiasm.

In this edition we intend to continue to serve professional undergraduate students of nursing, as well as graduate students and nurse practitioners. We provide advanced content, designed to supplement more basic texts, concerning selected concepts relevant to the nursing process and to health care. We assume that the reader has already mastered those concepts of the arts and sciences which serve as the foundation for nursing, as well as those procedures and activities detailed in basic nursing texts. Physiological, psychological, and sociological processes in health and disease are strongly emphasized and woven throughout the fabric of the book. As before, this book derives its real strength and breadth from the collective knowledge of contributing authors with personal experience in the health care arenas. Although each chapter reflects the unique point of view of its author or authors, collaborative emphasis is placed on mechanisms which produce both actual and potential health problems or affect their course; manifestations of these problems in relation to the mechanisms generating them; and information relevant to the activities of nursing process—assessment or diagnosis of a problem, formulation of a plan of action, appropriate intervention, and evaluation.

More than ever before, the discipline of contemporary nursing encompasses a myriad of activities concerning the promotion and maintenance of health and the treatment of illness. The scope of nursing practice includes a concern for the well-being of all segments of the population, wherever they may be—in the hospital or any other care facility, at home, in school, or at work. Though nursing needs of individuals range from the simple to the highly complex and may be met by persons with various kinds or levels of education and experience, I consider the professional nurse to be the fulcrum upon which the total practice of nursing is balanced. Of course, all professional nurses are not alike in terms of either abilities or education. Considering the broad scope of health care required for clients of all ages, I believe we must have professional nurses who are prepared to function within ambiguous or unstructured situations, as well as within existing patterns of practice.

The material in this text has been expanded to keep pace with the needs of the student or practitioner who must cope with societal changes which are having a significant impact on the knowledge and skills required for professional nursing practice. As I see it, some of these significant trends include rapidly evolving technological advances and increased use of automation; the increasing value placed by society on higher education for all American youth; upgraded nursing education, producing more competent nursing personnel who are better equipped for responsible, independent decision making; a patient population which is developing more sophisticated expectations of health care; augmentation of the consumer's role in providing and financing health services; the expansion of federal and state legislative health programs aimed at making the best care available for all segments of the population; and a continuing emphasis on specialization for health personnel which leads to the necessity for a coordinated multidisciplinary approach to health problems.

Of particular importance, I believe, is evidence of a readiness, both within and without the sick-treatment system, to further develop and emphasize the concept of health. Currently the goals of nursing care center on the maintenance and restoration of health, with care of the sick included within this health-centered orientation. Selected nurses should be ready to act as the principal care providers in community-based activities directed toward health maintenance, prevention of disease and disability, and services to the chronically ill and elderly. At the same time, while the physician is the principal care practitioner in acute care settings, professional nurses must continue to provide competent contributing and/or supportive services. Thus the total scope of nursing functions should include such activities as diagnostic assessment, case finding, detailed health teaching and counseling for individuals and for families, and therapeutic or restorative intervention for physiological and psychological illness or disability.

The professional nurse must also cultivate an acute awareness of the interpersonal nature of the nursing process. Every patient is a composite of interdependent physiological and psychological systems, a factor that deserves consideration in each shared nurse-client encounter. Thus the nurse profits from an understanding of the nature of man in health and in illness as an individual and as a member of a family within a community that is part of a larger society. Recognition of all the foregoing prompts my belief, shared with all the contributors to this book, that effective nursing activities may be regarded as those which 1) help patients and families to attain and maintain optimum well-being by coping constructively with health problems; 2) help those who are ill to mobilize mechanisms that will foster a return to optimum health; and 3) help those whose health problems cannot be resolved to achieve and maintain such optimum adaptation to circumstances as is possible for them.

With this philosophical framework in mind, we have expanded and revised all the pre-existing chapters in this text. In addition, we have included an appreciable amount of new content. Although I will not attempt to discuss all these revisions here, a summary of major changes in content and format is in order. Speaking first of new material, we have added chapters concerning the following: 1) delivery of health care, 2) psychological concepts of health-related behavior, 3) the diagnostic assessment of health status, 4) the pediatric nurse practitioner's role in providing care for the growing child, 5) health needs during adolescence, and 6) health problems and the aging individual.

Extensive revisions have been made in chapters previously found in the text. The chapter concerning nursing needs throughout the life cycle has been completely rewritten and retitled. It is now "Nursing Process and Human Development: A Systems View," and, as Chapter 1, sets a tone for the text as a whole. It includes examples and references taken from material in chapters throughout the book. Additional material relevant to the problems and needs of those undergoing abortion has been included in Chapter 5, "Family Planning". Chapter 6, which focuses on care and health requirements of those with hereditary health problems, has a wealth of new content, including entirely new sections on genetic counseling, prenatal diagnosis, and care of the fetus. Chapter 17, "The Insulted Kidney," incorporates so much new material, particularly concerning long-term health problems of those undergoing chronic hemodialysis in the home or in centers, that it has been reorganized into three sections. Part 1 deals with management and care of patients with acute renal failure, Part 2 with chronic renal failure, and Part 3 with renal homotransplantation. The previous discussion of the immune process and care of allergic patients has been expanded into a triad of chapters, each concerning different aspects of immunity and health. These include, "Inflammation and Repair: Non-Specific Mechanisms of Immunity," "The Immune Response," and "Nursing Intervention for Patients with Allergic Disorders."

The chapters centering on mechanisms of shock, intensive care nursing, nursing intervention for patients with central nervous system dysfunction, and management of the burned patient have been rewritten to incorporate much new data and additional case examples. Other chapters found in the previous edition of this text (e.g., the discussion of health maintenance, and the material on dysfunctional problems related to the heart, the gaseous exchange process, diabetes mellitus, sensory deprivation, corticosteroid therapy, and water and electrolytes) have also been revised to include more material on current concepts of nursing assessment and management, as well as relevant aspects of health maintenance.

Kay Corman Kintzel
April 1977

Acknowledgments

As editor, I'd like to acknowledge all those who contributed to the completion of this project. Special thanks are due to all who used the first edition—particularly those who offered valuable advice, as well as investing time and energy in the construction of this revision. In this category I would certainly place all the previous contributing authors, in addition to those whose chapters appear here for the first time.

As before, David Miller of J. B. Lippincott Company provided continuous help in all phases of the job at hand, a contribution which I've come to regard as characteristic of the man. Mary Morgan, senior editor at Lippincott, devoted many hours of thought and energy to the task of turning a chaotic bundle of manuscript into an orderly text.

As one who has never fully mastered the challenge of the typewriter, I extend my personal thanks to Mrs. Barbara Caliendo, for prompt and able typing assistance.

Finally my gratitude goes to my family—husband Jim and sons Timothy, Jeffrey, and Christopher. My husband has given his unflagging support and the time necessary to enlarge his original contribution to the chapter concerning health problems and renal failure, and my sons have cheerfully adapted to the requisites of sharing me with a textbook.

Kay Corman Kintzel

Contents

1

Nursing Process and Human Development: a systems view

DORIS COOK SUTTERLEY and GLORIA FERRARO DONNELLY

The Growth Process ● *The Organizing Process* ● *The Communication Process*
● *The Sexuality Process* ● *The Learning Process* ● *The Creative Process*
● *The Stabilizing Process* ● *The Evolutionary Process* ● *The Nursing Process*

General systems theory, which has been called a "science of sciences" or a "perspective philosophy," is being increasingly utilized as a frame of reference in considering human development and concomitant implications for the nursing process. Nursing literature is replete with references to and descriptions of the principles of general systems theory as well as its direct application in clinical situations. But why systems? Is it really a useful theory, a practical one? Can nursing legitimate its use as a frame of reference for clinical practice? To answer these questions, we must consider systems theory in the context of three issues: first, its usefulness as an interdisciplinary, theoretical framework; second, its application to the human organism; and third, its relevance to the nursing process within a network of social systems.

Systems theory has become the conceptual framework for physiologists, astronomers, communication specialists, sociologists, and economists, as well as for other disciplines. Systems orientation represents to each a body of concepts, models, and a philosophy that treats the whole and considers the synergistic interplay of multiple factors both from within and outside the system. The notion of "wholeness" is fundamental to the concept of systems. Holism, which purports to convey the nonsummativity of human nature, may serve the nurse as a "methodological caveat to be on the watch constantly for overlooked factors and relations which affect the complex event of illness and health in humans. . . ."[1]

Systems theorists believe that it is possible to represent all forms of matter as systems which may be expressed in different forms but which have common properties. Universal laws can be found which describe the structure of these systems and their manner of functioning. Thus, general systems theory aims at discovering how this "wholeness" functioning is operational in the widest varieties of systems.

Models are often utilized to symbolize systems (Fig. 1-1). These often differ in metaphor and level of abstractness. Depending upon their characteristics, there are two models of systems, closed systems and open systems.

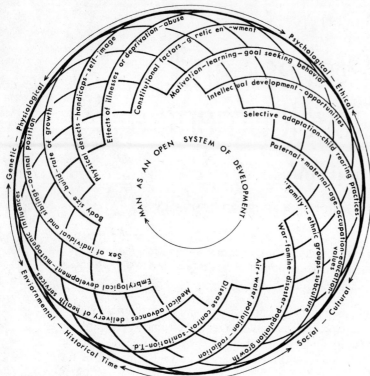

FIGURE 1-1.
Man as an open system of development.

The essential difference is that open systems are related to and exchange matter and energy with their environment while closed systems do not.

All the characteristics of systems in general also apply to organismic open systems. An open system, like the human organism, has subsystems, for example, body systems and value systems. It is part of many supra-systems, the family and the community. But each of these has a boundary. There are systems variables and environmental parameters. Systems exist in both proximal and distal environments. Living open systems also exchange energy and information with their environments to maintain themselves in a steady state. All this is managed through the operation of self-regulating processes. Process is an attribute of all systems, for the functions or characteristic activities inherent in a system are mediated via process. Currently, the open, self-maintaining and self-regulating biological system is the dominant model in many fields. This is in contrast to the medical model which is based on mechanistic rather than organismic theory.

Has the mechanistic tradition with its cause and effect orientation served the person well? Perhaps, for a time, when medical and nursing care were simpler matters; however, it has also fragmented the care of the person in a health care delivery system which must still be considered an illness-centered delivery system. The changing focus on maintaining health and wholeness lends itself to systems orientation. Systems theory, which permits us to consider all the components of the system in dynamic interaction, has raised the nurse's "complexity-consciousness."[2]

The study of individual development from the vantage point of general systems theory is a rather recent innovation in the sciences, even though von Bertalanffy referred to the concept of systems as early as 1933. He defined open systems as ones "maintained in exchange of matter and energy with environment by import and ex-

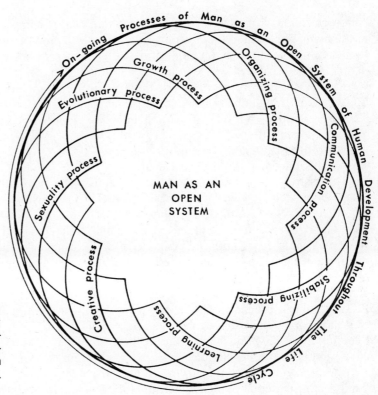

FIGURE 1-2.
Ongoing processes of man as an open system of development. For a fuller discussion of life processes, see Sutterley, D. and Donnelly, G.: Perspectives in Human Development. Philadelphia, J. B. Lippincott, 1973.

port and building up and breaking down of components.''[3] More recently, Lawrence Frank described the human being as an open system:

The living, growing, developing, maturing, aging organism is an open system . . . with continual inputs and outputs. It is compelled as an organism to maintain continuous intercourse with the environment and . . . to learn as a personality, to live in a symbolic cultural world, exhibiting purposive, goal-seeking conduct. Moreover, each individual is a unique organism, with his unique heredity, his own body size, shape, rates of growth and development and aging, and his own individual experience that has shaped his idiomatic relations to the world of events and to other persons and to himself.[4]

Studying the individual as an open system throughout the life cycle permits the nurse to simultaneously consider factors from both the internal and external environment of the individual, including stress, functional limitations, adaptation, and the interaction of the life processes.

The individual interacts with the environment via dynamic life processes as he or she ''grows, develops, matures, ages and contributes to the future of other men throughout the life cycle.''[5] These processes are that of growth, organization, communication, sexuality, learning, creativity, stabilization, and evolution. The nurse needs to perceive each of these processes in dynamic interaction with the other and ultimately to develop skills in managing the interaction between the various systems that interface (Fig. 1-2).

The Growth Process

The process of growth is basic to any living system and is taking place on every level of complexity, from the molecular to the evolutionary. The complexity of growth is exquisitely revealed as living organisms grow and acquire specialized parts and functions, going through phenomenal combinations of simultaneously ongoing processes. Growth takes place at all levels of biological organization, from the microscopic structure of the living organism to the diversity of cell and tissue architecture, to the functions of tissue and organs, to an organized whole in a sociocultural world. The human organism grows, both quantitatively and qualitatively, in uneven tempos. There are critical periods in growth and development and differing rates of growth. The growth process ultimately results in an expression of the uniqueness of the individual.

To illustrate the growth process, let us consider Wayne and Debbie, the siblings with PKU (see Chapter 6). While the growth process is affected by both the internal and the external environments, early recognition of inborn errors of metabolism can be mediated by altering external influences, such as the nutritional intake of the child. Although both children were victims of PKU, Debbie's prognosis was encouraging because the condition was recognized early enough to modify potential brain damage during the critical period of neural development.

The problems incurred in trying to alter the family eating pattern also created tensions affecting the social and behavioral climate in which Wayne and Debbie were developing. Both children began with the same genetic potential, or in this case, handicap. However, their growth and development would be vastly different due not only to the early medical intervention, but to the differences in parental attitudes and expectations, the different ordinal positions of the children in the family, and the differences in their gender roles.

The independent practice of nursing rests upon the ability of the nurse to assess developmental parameters from which the health status can be determined. Monitoring the normal growth process has become one of the primary functions of the pediatric nurse practitioner. Case examples in Chapter 7 are particularly illustrative of how one begins to use systems theory. In case example 2, the pediatric nurse practitioner was constantly assessing all of the parameters that might affect the growth and development of Mary and Sara Lane. Her approach was to the whole family and how they interacted with one another. The parents' divorce was hav-

ing its impact on the children. The nurse considered divorce a process that might continue to affect the healthy development of the Lane children. Because she had considered the family system with its history and its stresses, the nurse was better able to anticipate developmental outcomes in caring for the Lane children.

The Organizing Process

The incredible process of growth suggests the operation of still another process—that of organization—for growth in all of the organism's dimensions is beautifully coordinated. An organizing control is apparent not only in the complex development of the human organism, but in the activities by which life is maintained. Thus, the human being as an open system is not only part of larger organizations, such as family and society, but also an organizer of the environment. We can better appreciate the organizing process in living systems if we consider the concept of hierarchy (patterns of wholes, subwholes, environments, feedback, and values). We can consider the relationships between the biological level of organization of the nervous and endocrine systems which could include such things as biological rhythms and circadian cycles, and the psychosocial level of organization throughout a person's life cycle. These subwholes can also be viewed with respect to their relationships to the larger cultural-temporal level of organization in which the human organism is affected by the phenomena of rapid change, alienation, or the impact of changing family and social values.

The case of the young mother of twins who had just undergone a kidney transplant illustrates the organizing process (see Chapter 17). While facing possible death from a transplant rejection, her life was organized around multiple roles of wife and mother at this stage in her life cycle. Resuming her role as the mother of twins legitimated for her the risk incurred in renal transplant. In order to organize her environment around her selected roles within the family system, this woman chose to prolong and/or insure her biophysical integrity at some risk. This situation, however, is not always the case, especially when the person's life is not so firmly organized around roles within a family or even a community system. In contrast, a 62-year-old widower had successfully been maintained on a home dialysis program for three years. Several months after his wife died, the man began to slowly deteriorate. He was no longer motivated to maintain himself on a home program. The patient was not successful at reorganizing his life style and reintegrating himself into his son's family system. Despite the best efforts of those who cared for him, the patient declined further treatment and died.

The Communication Process

Communication is essentially an organizing process which makes social living possible. The process of human communication is very difficult to describe because there are so many complex behavioral events that occur simultaneously and are interrelated to make up even one small bit of communication. If we utilize Birdwhistell's systems orientation to the study of the communication process, we can conceive of it as being a complex, multisensory system rather than the sum of information that passes between people.[6] We can view it as a continuous and ordered system rather than exclusively a verbal process. Communication also affords a structural system of meaningful symbols, both verbal and nonverbal, that permits human interaction rather than simply a mechanical process of action-reaction.

The communication process is rooted in cultural and family systems. Because of this, the nurse must often look beyond the individual relationship with the patient in order to understand more effectively the person's needs. The human organism is compelled to communicate with every blink of the eye and unconscious gesture. Human attempts at noncommunication, such as catatonia, can be most revealing of the person's perspective on living.

There are many cases in the following chapters in which the communication process can be cited. The case of Karen, a critically injured adolescent, portrays the awareness of the nursing staff in making every attempt to facilitate the communication process (see Chapter 10). From the moment of her admission Karen was given brief, clear explanations for what she was experiencing. The staff provided her with several means of communication because she could not speak. Particular attention was given to calling equipment by its proper name instead of by the abbreviated jargon critical care personnel often utilize. Such measures reduce the stress experienced by a critically ill patient.

The communication process is often affected when a patient simultaneously experiences sensory overload (see Chapter 19) and sensory deprivation in an alien environment, such as a critical care or coronary care unit. As the person attempts to cope and to find meaning in the environment, psychotic expressions of behavior may be temporarily manifested. When nurses must concentrate so intensely on maintaining the physical integrity of the critically ill person, communicational needs are often given low priority. The systems orientation with its holistic perspective will assist the nurse in integrating and maintaining the communication process with any patient or client in any setting.

The Sexuality Process

Sexuality can be viewed as one of the dynamic life processes when we consider the complexities and the intricate relationships of an individual's developing sexuality, all of which create separate sexual roles within a particular historical time, place, and culture. Sexuality in its broadest sense might be defined as a deep and pervasive aspect of the total personality, the sum total of an individual's feelings and behavior not only as a sexual being, but as a male or female. Throughout the life cycle physiological, emotional, social, and cultural forces condition sexuality. The expression of sexuality goes beyond purely genital responses and is constantly modified as a result of sexual experiences and social learning. Thus, sexuality is a process that demands and finds expression at all age levels throughout the life cycle.

An obvious example of the sexuality process as an integral part of all the other life processes is the case study of Mr. R. (see Chapter 20). This 24-year-old guidance counselor developed symptoms of multiple sclerosis which raised doubts about the wisdom of his plans to marry.

Because the expression of a person's sexuality is such an integral part of all development, it will follow the overall pattern of health and physical performance. Any alteration in psychophysiological functioning will have concomitant effects upon the process of human sexuality. The proliferation of publications and courses in human sexuality for health professionals is testimony to the fact that we have begun to acknowledge the relationship between sexuality and physical and mental well-being; a step toward the holistic approach to health care. Beyond this is the emerging concept of "sexual health care,"* an essential part of total health care to which everyone is entitled and for which provision must be made in comprehensive health care planning. The Sex Information and Education Council of the United States (SIECUS) predicts that "the physical, mental and social components of sexual health care must, and in time will, become integrated into total health care, preventive as well as therapeutic, and subject to the same financial support systems as other forms of health care."[7]

The Learning Process

Learning is an integral part of all the other life processes. We learn to organize our lives around certain patterns of experience. We learn a system of communication common to our culture that is both digital (verbal) and analogic (nonverbal). We learn to learn, and through this process creativity often emerges. Stabilizing each of the life processes on the health-illness continuum in-

*Sexual health care as defined by SIECUS: (SIECUS Report, Vol. III, September, 1974) Preventive aspects include

"a) the influence of parents upon the sexuality of their children from early infancy through adolescence;

b) the prevention or amelioration of the effects of sexual trauma, i.e., molestation, exhibition, incest and rape;

c) peer group influences during adolescence; and

d) interpersonal relationships during adolescence and adult life."

volves learning. Although we do not learn to grow or evolve in the physical sense, continued cognitive and social learning are interdependent with growth and evolution.

There is often much for a person to learn as he or she adjusts or adapts to critical or chronic illness. A knowledge of the learning process and its operation in the individual and the family system is often crucial in nursing care planning. The case of Ken emphasizes the importance of the health care team's understanding the learning process and its relationship to Ken's emotional problems encountered in adjusting to diabetes mellitus (see Chapter 15).

The case of Gregg in Chapter 8 also illustrates how the learning process is integrated with and dependent upon other vital life processes. Gregg who had exceptional ability could not learn effectively because of his poor self-image. He had been diagnosed schizophrenic which some theorists believe to be one of the outcomes of a disturbed family system. By focusing on the learning process, the nurse achieved some therapeutic success with Gregg. As his self-confidence increased he was able to teach his peers. Through positive feedback his self-image was strengthened.

The Creative Process

Of all the life processes, the creative process alone is distinctly human. Other species grow, communicate, engage in sexual activity, and learn, at least on an instinctual level, but only humans engage in the creative experience. The creative urge is part of the human evolutionary heritage. It is universal and exists in all individuals but "biological, historical, psychological and sociological determinants serve either to enhance or to constrain the realization of these urges."[8]

Creativity cannot be localized in one person and thus described. It is a fluid, dynamic, and highly individual process. Since creativity is most often viewed in terms of the novel productions of the person, we tend to overlook the many spheres of life in which creativity exists. As Maslow points out, the word "creative" must be applied not only to products, but to individuals in a characteristic way and to processes, activities, and attitudes.[9]

Creative expression is often therapeutic as in the case of Gregg (see Chapter 8). Through "creative work" that he was able to share with the nurse, he began to view himself as a person with unique abilities. In this case, creativity enhanced identity.

The Stabilizing Process

The stabilizing process is a self-regulatory process that is characteristic of living open systems. All living systems tend to maintain steady states among many variables, seeking a balance between many finely adjusted, interlocking processes or subsystems which process matter, energy, or information. The steady state is not static. Parts and processes of open systems are in constant flux. The human organism makes adaptive changes congruent with its environment. All through the life cycle the stabilizing process works to maintain a steady biophysical and psychosocial state in the developing individual.

An example of the stabilizing process is the physiological mechanism of shock as defined in Chapter 13. When effective circulating blood volume is reduced, resulting in poor tissue perfusion, there are two specific compensatory mechanisms: 1) generalized vasoconstriction; 2) increased cardiac output and respiratory rate. The negative feedback mechanism tends to decrease or cancel the initiating stimulus which augments compensation and the restoration of homeostasis. Positive feedback mechanisms all serve to augment the initiating stimulus, resulting in progressive shock and the irreversible stage of refractory shock as illustrated in the case of Mr. Malone, who went into shock following an appendectomy (see Chapter 13). By Saturday morning (D) Mr. Malone's condition had begun to deteriorate so that there was either no response or merely a transient one to all the therapeutic measures and attempts to reestablish homeostatic balance between the various body systems.

In the case of Mr. R., the 70-year-old gentleman with emphysema (see Chapter 14), the health professionals were able to intervene therapeutically to relieve his hypoxia and reestablish homeostasis, or in systems terminology, a "steady state." All of the nursing measures were directed toward altering any of the interferences with the various parameters of the breathing process.

To maintain a steady state in the presence of altered physiology, such as occurs with chronic emphysema, the individual is forced to modify his or her life style and adopt health practices that will permit optimal functioning within the limitations of his or her physical condition. This is illustrated most effectively by the case of Mr. O. This father of a large family was forced to change his occupation to maintain his position as provider for his family without a loss of self-esteem because of his inability to function as he did when in good health.

Many other examples of the stabilizing process can be found in Chapter 3. Particularly interesting is the multiproblem family whose style and pattern of living seemed to revolve around crises and chaos. Maloney's description of such families as "crisis generators" seems a paradox in light of the stabilizing process. Such families and individuals seem to thrive or structure their existence in an unsteady state. The nurse often becomes absorbed into the family system as he or she attempts to help the family deal with succeeding crises. The whole concept of crisis intervention is based upon the need to identify strengths and provide situational support for the adequate resolution of the problem so that equilibrium or stabilization can be regained.

The Evolutionary Process

The human system and the larger systems to which it belongs are the outcomes of evolution. Evolution is an adjustive process through which systems develop and are modified in relation to specific environments. Evolution does not insure continued survival unless the human organism learns to build a world suited to its nature. Although it is adaptive, there are limits to its adaptive powers. There is no doubt that the human organism has the skill and the imagination to create a world more suited to its nature. Through the growth of evolutionary biology and through increased understanding of the mechanisms of heredity, adaptation, and the evolutionary process, human beings have a renewed perspective of their place in the world of living things and their responsibility to preserve the continuance of the total system.

Until recently there was little recourse families could take if they believed their offspring might be affected with genetic disease. The availability of genetic counseling and prenatal diagnosis has brightened the futures of many families who have feared reproduction. The case of the Goldbergs, a middle-aged couple heterozygous for Tay-Sachs disease, illustrates the health team in action through the counseling process (see Chapter 6).

The field of genetic counseling and the conscious application of selective forces has and will raise many philosophical and ethical questions. As technology becomes sophisticated enough to select out those who are defective or diseased, who shall determine defect in situations that are not as clear-cut as that of Tay-Sachs? Should the health team be composed of only medical, nursing, and biomedical professionals? Is there not a place for the clergy, an ethical specialist, a philosopher, or an anthropologist on such a team? As the human organism attempts to control the conditions around itself and the future of the species, ethical issues need to be discussed with those families and individuals seeking professional counsel.

> The pattern of human life is not based upon communities composed of identical individuals. Rather, we depend upon the presence of varied capacities, motivations, satisfactions, and hence opinions. . . . To recognize the importance of variety for homeostasis is fundamental for human welfare.[10]

Since we have focused on systems as a point of reference and on the human organism as an open system, we must consider the nursing process within the systems framework.

The Nursing Process

Nursing process essentially began as a problem-solving approach with an assessment or diagnosis of the problem or problems, appropriate intervention or a plan of action, followed by evaluation and reevaluation. Nursing process has been defined and refined in many ways.[11] Fundamental to this process is the nurse's ability to assess the person's needs through the establishment of a broad data base in order to formulate a nursing diagnosis and a plan of intervention. (Tools such as the nursing history, see Chapter 20, facilitate the process. See Chapter 4 for physical assessment.) The systems approach permits the nurse to see relationships between identified parameters as he or she enters the person's system for intervention. "All laymen know that a uterus or a red cell or an eyeball or a depressed feeling doesn't come into the office all alone. Nor does the abnormality begin and end with a visit to the physician. In spite of specialization by members of the profession, patients see the interrelatedness of problems in their own lives."[12]

What is paramount is that the nursing process begin with the PERSON, his or her level of wellness, problems or potential problems, as the target system. The process must not begin with the nurse, nor the physician, nor a segment of the health care system. For example, in the assessment of the patient/client health status, the nurse elicits data concerning how the patient perceives the illness or health-related problem. THE PATIENT'S PERCEPTION OF HIS HEALTH STATUS MAY NOT PARALLEL THAT OF THE NURSE OR THE PHYSICIAN IF WE CONCUR THAT HEALTH IS A STATE RELATIVE TO THE GOALS THAT THE INDIVIDUAL FORMULATES FOR HIMSELF. The assessment of the patient's health status should reflect the nurse's concern for more than just the preservation of life or death with dignity. It must concern itself with the quality of personal existence or the person's state of health and well-being as experienced and perceived by the person throughout his or her life cycle. PRIMARY RESPONSIBILITY FOR HEALTH IS SHIFTED FROM THE HEALTH PROVIDER TO THE INDIVIDUAL. Weed, originator of the problem-oriented medical rec-

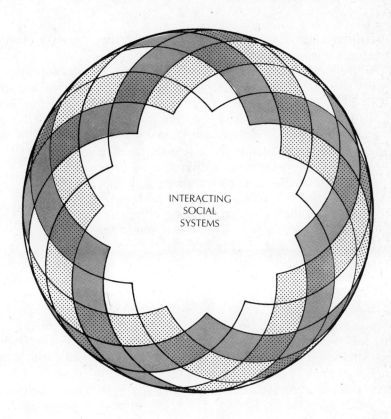

FIGURE 1-3.
Interacting social systems. White—A social-cultural-political system—norms, values, for example, health care delivery. Black—A social unit, such as family, peers, colleagues. Dots—An individual, such as a client, patient, nurse, other health professional

ord, urges consumers to become involved in the management of their own health care by keeping their own medical record.[13] He has published a book that provides consumers with the philosophy and the tools with which to manage health problems and the health care system that is often unresponsive to their needs. The individual receiving care or services needs to be involved in all phases of this care from the collection of data and the planning to the evaluation of that care. This philosophy is strongly reflected in the ANA Revised Standards of Nursing Practice.[14]

Because the practice of nursing is changing its focus, nursing process will permit us to find more effective approaches to some of the philosophical dualisms inherent in nursing. For example, the nurse must seek to maintain a balance between the scientific-technological and the humanistic-ethical components of care, as in the case of the Goldbergs. A process model permits the nurse to unify subjective and objective experience and create a synthesis. Folta reminds us that "it is of

no value to be a humanist and watch a man die for lack of technology nor is it of any value to be rich in technology only to watch man live and die without dignity."[15]

Nurses have learned the fallacy of trying to use the normal-abnormal dichotomy as a criterion of psychosocial and physiological functioning. What may be perceived as abnormal or unhealthy behavior in one culture or subculture or time span may be perfectly normal or healthy in another. Likewise, according to Jahoda (who developed criteria for judging positive mental health), if we consider health and disease as being qualitatively different and not as opposite ends of a continuum, we can allow everyone to have simultaneously healthy or sick aspects with one or the other predominating.[16] With this outlook, the nurse draws attention to the healthy potential in sick patients and the sick potential in healthy persons.

Finally, nurses are continually confronted with the mind-body dualism. Despite what is written today about "holism," much of health care is fragmented according to primary concern with either the physical or psychological aspects of care. Often, it is the nurse alone that attempts to give complete or holistic care in spite of the setting, that is if the focus is on the process of nursing the person and not on the goals of the agency or the institution. A basic understanding of human development within the systems framework would facilitate the meshing of some of these dualisms within the nursing process.

Another dimension that can be considered within the systems framework is the interaction between social systems, in particular, the patient as a system, and the nurse as a system within the particular health care system (Fig. 1-3, p. 9).

The nurse often encounters conflict and frustration attempting to nurse the whole person in an environment, such as a hospital or agency system, the structure of which is not compatible with the nursing process as we have described it. For example, Leininger points out that our present health care system is essentially a system which permits only limited, if any, exchange of varied health manpower resources and potentials with community demands.[17] There is inadequate exchange. Instead, inputs of skills and services from other health personnel are largely controlled, regulated, and overshadowed both socially and professionally by one group, physicians. A health care system modeled on an open system that is client-centered, focuses primarily on the client and his or her community, with emphasis on the roles of various health disciplines and community groups within the system. An open health care system would offer the client a choice of services from several health disciplines and not limit the client to only the physician's services as a point of entry into the system. An open system would be responsive to change, encouraging an exchange of ideas among all health disciplines, constantly looking for feedback from individuals and the community to modify and improve the system. This open system model for health care is able to give full consideration to health and wellness because of its emphasis on the use of cultural, social, and community data, the criteria by which wellness states are defined.

The nurse is also a target system within a su-

prasystem and a subsystem, with all the systems properties and characteristics of the living open system, influencing and being influenced by its environment. A nurse researcher described the nurse's evolution in this way:

> Nurses are born into and undergo primary socialization within family and social systems which differ widely in their values and cultural imperatives. Then they undergo a secondary socialization in nursing schools which results in their being much more alike than different in their professional behaviors. Then nurses proceed to undergo still another resocialization when they become employees in hospitals and other agencies because even though the systems in which they work have varied compositions and structures the functional requirements are the same in all systems.[18]

Nursing on the larger scale is becoming increasingly aware not only of itself, but of its relationships with the other social-political systems with which it interfaces. As nursing asserts its rights and responsibilities to independent practice based on systems principles, the health system should become more responsive to the needs of the clients it serves. The following chapters find the nurse practicing in a variety of settings and in a variety of roles. Patients and families encountered present a wide range of health problems. Although certain chapters focus in depth on specific problem areas, the human system adapting needs to be the nurse's focus. A knowledge of human development and its variety will add an often missing dimension to the care of a person and his or her family in any setting.

If we can view nursing as a living open system in dynamic interchange with the human open system and social systems, it might be possible for the nursing profession to develop simultaneously in many urgently needed directions in response to the health needs of society while meeting its responsibilities to the even larger family of humanity.

References

1. Walker, L. O.: Toward a clearer understanding of the concept of nursing theory. Nurs. Research 20, 5:431, Sept.-Oct. 1971.
2. Livesey, L. J.: Noetic planning: the need to know,

but what? *In* E. Laszlo (ed.): The Relevance of General Systems Theory. New York, Braziller, 1972, p. 160.

3. von Bertalanffy, L.: General system theory and psychiatry. *In* S. Arieti (ed.): American Handbook of Psychiatry, Vol. III. New York, Basic Books, 1966, pp. 705-721.

4. Frank, L.: Human development an emerging scientific discipline. *In* A. Solnit and S. Provence (eds.): Modern Perspectives in Child Development. New York, International Universities Press, 1963, pp. 10-36.

5. Sutterley, D. and Donnelly, G.: Perspectives in Human Development. Philadelphia, J. B. Lippincott, 1973, p.13.

6. Birdwhistell, R.: Kinesics and Context. Philadelphia, University of Pennsylvania Press, 1970.

7. Long, R.: Sexual health care. SIECUS Report III, 1, Sept. 1974.

8. Rosner, S. and Abt, L. E.: The Creative Experience. New York, Grossman Publishers, 1970, p. 379.

9. Maslow, A.: Creativity in self-actualizing people. *In* H. H. Anderson (ed.): Creativity and Its Cultivation. New York, Harper, 1959, pp. 83-95.

10. Young, J. Z.: An Introduction to the Study of Man. New York and Oxford, Oxford University Press, 1971, p. 543.

11. Yura, H. and Walsh, M.: The Nursing Process. New York, Appleton-Century Crofts, 1973.

12. Weed, L.: Your Health Care and How to Manage It. Essex Junction, Vermont, Essex Publishing Co., 1975.

13. *Ibid.*

14. American Nurses Association: Standards of Nursing Practice. Kansas City, Missouri, 1974.

15. Folta J.: The humanization of health services. Sigma Theta Tau Lecture, Philadelphia, Dec. 14, 1973.

16. Jahoda, M.: Current Concepts of Positive Mental Health. New York, Basic Books, 1958.

17. Leininger, M.: An open health care system model. Nurs. Outlook 21, 3:171-175, March 1973.

18. Smoyak, S.: Toward understanding nursing situations: a transaction paradigm. Nurs. Research 18, 5:405, Sept.-Oct. 1969.

2
Providing for the Maintenance of Health

JOANN SHAFER JAMANN

Concepts of Health Maintenance • Maintenance Versus Restoration • Health and Illness • Factors Affecting Health • Principles of Health Maintenance • Nursing Intervention • Delivery of Health Care

Concepts of Health Maintenance

Health is a provisory state which can be maintained only through constant effort. This effort must be made independently and collectively by the individual, society, and all of the health professions. A coordinated vigilance is necessary to preserve an acceptable level of health. The individual must accept responsibility for society as well as for his or her own health. Society, in turn, has an obligation to maintain the integrity and dignity of each of its citizens. Finally, the health professions, particularly medicine, nursing, and social work, must seek to share their specialized knowledge and skills with individuals and communities.

Maintenance Versus Restoration

For as long as the human race has been aware that it could manipulate the status of its health, it has oscillated between placing emphasis on health maintenance and on health restoration. A study of the classic civilization of the Greeks reveals that they first worshiped and followed the precepts of the goddess Hygeia. Hygeia was the guardian of health, and symbolized the belief that people would maintain their health if they would live according to reason. Although Hygeia was identified with health, she was never associated with the treatment of the ill. About the 5th century B.C., the emphasis moved to the healing god, Asclepius, who, according to Greek legend, was the first physician. Asclepius was revered because of his skill in restoring health, and Hygeia soon became subservient to him. A look at the history of Eastern civilizations shows that Oriental peoples also shared this vacillating philosophy of health care—health maintenance and disease prevention versus the treatment of imperfections. It seems that these two philosophical bases for the practice of the health professions have contested for primacy in all civilization; however, it must be remembered that they have existed simultaneously.

In addition to the philosophical basis for health care practices, the pursuit of and techniques for scientific knowledge have also had an influence. Particularly influential have been theories of disease causation. These have fluctuated between the complex concept of a multiplicity of interrelated causative factors and the relatively simple concept of a specific cause for a given state of illness. In general, when the philosophy of health maintenance was in vogue, the scientific search for knowledge and techniques encompassed a variety of causative factors, such as environment, physiology, spiritual influences, and so on. It may be assumed that there was reciprocal reinforcement of the health maintenance philosophy as the complexity of influential health factors was uncovered.

Similarly, as isolated or specific causative health factors were discovered, impetus was added to the acceptance of the philosophical primacy of health restoration. Most influential for modern health care practices was the discovery of the germ theory of disease. This scientific breakthrough generated a powerful force to pursue research and develop skills and techniques related to the specificity of disease. Thus came the rapid acceptance of nutritional deficiencies, congenital anomalies, biochemical and genetic disorders as specific etiologies of disease, and like acceptance of surgery and drugs as therapy. Since the discovery of the germ theory about 150 years ago, and the rather universal acceptance by the health professions of the specificity of disease etiology, the emphasis of health care practices has been on health restoration.

Maintenance of health has always been one of the goals of nursing; however, only cursory attention has been given to it. Florence Nightingale, generally accepted as the founder of modern nursing, declared the need to teach people how to live:

> The very elements of what constitutes good nursing are as little understood for the well as for the sick. The same laws of health or of nursing, for they are in reality the same, obtain among the well as among the sick. The breaking of them produces only a less violent consequence among the former than among the latter—and this sometimes, not always.[1]

She also indicated that the symptoms and suffering of the ill are not always "inevitable and incident to the disease." Nursing has been slow in following the leadership of Miss Nightingale in the area of health maintenance; however, there is a growing awareness that pathological states and manifestations are the consequence of multiple determinants operating simultaneously. Also, recent emergence of systems analysis as an acceptable research methodology has led nursing and the other health care professions to orient their practices toward the complexity of disease causation. Hopefully, health care that emphasizes health maintenance will follow.

The work of Hans Selye on the General Adaptation Syndrome gave cognizance to the interrelationship of specificity and complexity both in causation and manifestations of disease. He perceived that stress is not necessarily detrimental, since it is also the spice of life, and that a specific stressor for one person can make that person sick at a given time and yet be an invigorating experience at another time. These perceptions signified that individuality is extremely important in both health care maintenance and restoration.

Health and Illness

What then is health? Is it a state in which a person has no physical, psychological, or social pathology present? Is it a sense of well-being or an absence of disease (dis-ease)? Is it that a person is in equilibrium with his environment? It may be all, part, or none of these suggested states. Each individual has his or her own concept of health, as well as of what constitutes illness, which is the only legitimate definition of health for that individual. An individual's criteria of health are largely tempered by the aspirations and values that give direction to his or her life. Indeed, the standards of health in many parts of the world include a considerable amount of disease. The term "health" is meaningful only when defined in terms of a given person functioning in a given physical and social environment.

Perhaps a universally useful description of health is that of a state in which a person may live a satisfying life which makes a contribution to society. Such a definition implies that health is more than mere existence free of disease or disability. It is more than a state in which the person has maintained an internal equilibrium—homeostasis—and more than a state in which he has adapted to his surroundings. Such a definition highlights that a healthy person is one who with his or her human variabilities is capable of expressing creativity within a self-defined social context. Living certainly implies responding and functioning. To be "healthy," an individual must be able to respond to regulatory mechanisms in society, such as pressures for conformity, value systems, social organization, and so on, while retaining his or her integrity. Thus health is a dynamic process in which the individual must draw upon all his or her biological, economic, educational, psychological, philosophical, spiritual, and social resources to respond adaptively to life situations while retaining his or her individual integrity.

Likewise illness is also a dynamic state, defined by each individual within his or her social context, that lies between the antithetical states of health and death. There is a wide variety of interpretations of illness, and a person's interpretation may wax and wane with fluctuations in any of the numerous factors that influence one's state of health. Since this book is largely devoted to various illnesses on the health-illness-death continuum, it is sufficient to state here that illness is a condition in which the individual is conscious of symptoms or disability, or someone else has decided that disease, which cannot be ignored without danger to self or to the community, is present.

Factors Affecting Health

There are numerous ways of classifying illness, for example, by etiology, manifestations, or treatment. Likewise, there are a variety of ways in which health factors can be classified, including: external-internal milieu; genotypic-phenotypic factors and mechanisms; psychological-biological or psychosomatic-somato-psychic; genetic, historic, and environmental factors. Certainly each classification has its merits; however, it is doubtful whether any classification, in and of itself, sheds much light on that extremely complex state known as health. Therefore, the factors affecting health isolated here are not classified or presented in any significant order. Nor is this list of factors all-

inclusive. The reader is reminded that, although these factors are isolated for the purpose of closer examination, none of them functions in isolation; rather all are interrelated as they affect the health of an individual and the environment in which he or she lives.

In reality the human being is an integrated entity and each health factor plays a simultaneously influential part, to a greater or lesser degree, in the process of health. These biological, psychological, and socioeconomic processes are affected by a person's individual and collective past, present, and future. For example, his or her responses are predetermined not only by genetic factors, but also by past personal life—from acquired behavior to allergies. Thus, the state of health is multidimensional and there are no simple solutions to the problem of maintaining or restoring this state.

ENVIRONMENT

Our relations with our environment are the keystone to health maintenance; however, these relationships are extremely complex. The worldwide energy crisis of 1973 served to increase the individual's awareness of these complexities. No longer are only ecology and conservation groups discussing the relationship of such energy sources as nuclear power and the source of food supply. While relatively few communities have experienced "fish kills" from the heated water discharged from nuclear plants, the question of natural life being affected by the nuclear energy industry has become an important one for many groups and individuals. There is a delicate balance between our needs and desires in using the environment to maintain health. Environmental resources and their relatedness to the human ecosystem must be considered.

The very air we breathe has as great an influence on our state of health as does any other factor or group of factors. Certainly life cannot be sustained if its quality continues to deteriorate. Even those of us who are well on the healthy side of the illness continuum are aware of variations in the temperature and humidity of the atmosphere around us and the effects these have on our feelings of comfort and well-being. Unfortunately we are less cognizant of another quality of atmosphere on our state of health. The purity, or chemical composition, of the air rarely concerns us unless the impurities are sufficient to be visible, odoriferous, or physically irritating. As with our other natural resources, there needs to be a balance between what we take and what we return. When more wastes are discharged into the atmosphere than can be dissipated, the result is air pollution.

Air pollution is a major threat to the health of the people in most of the industrialized countries, and it is growing with the increase in urbanization nationally and the trend toward industrialization internationally. Air pollution is especially severe in many cities of the United States, such as Chicago, Los Angeles, or New York, and has been for almost a decade. Unfortunately, personal experiences have revealed that rapidly developing countries have not taken preventive measures to maintain their air quality. Mexico City, for example, was relatively free of air contamination in 1968; however, by 1973 a UNESCO expert reported that the level of contamination was 100 times the tolerable level.[2] Indeed, those nurses who attended the International Congress of Nursing witnessed the effects of this rapidly deteriorating quality of air—an essential health factor.

Many governments, like those of the United States and Mexico, have recognized the problem of maintaining the air quality and have established special departments to focus on the environment. For example, governmental action can provide a framework for maintaining a reasonably healthful environment by enforcing laws governing industrial pollution. Although industries contribute substantial amounts of the pollutants, the automobile is considered the chief culprit. Such measures as increasing the utilization of mass transit systems, particularly trains; antipollution devices on cars; use of smaller cars, and so on, would significantly reduce the pollution of our air, thereby increasing the quality of one factor in maintaining health. Ultimately, it is each individual in society who must voluntarily make these efforts to increase the quality of the air we all breathe.

Similarly we have ignored the quality of our water, another essential ingredient for health. Pollution of water is a major threat to our well-being. The primary sources of water pollution are found in urban-industrial areas. Considerable quantities of organic wastes are dumped into our rivers, thus decreasing the amount of dissolved oxygen which is necessary to support life in the food chain—plankton to fish. Inorganic substances, such as detergents, pesticides, and industrial wastes, also threaten the food chain which indirectly affects man's reliance on water to maintain his life. More obvious is the threat of polluted drinking water.

The recreational uses of water are also important to our health. Man uses water in his recreative processes—swimming, boating, fishing. More subtle, but no less important, is the aesthetic and spiritual significance of streams, lakes, and oceans. In fact, it becomes apparent that different activities require differing degrees of purity—for example, a lake considered to be both safe and desirable for boating activities would not necessarily be suitable for swimming. Certainly man needs to demonstrate a greater concern for controlling the pollution of water to meet his biological, psychological, and aesthetic health needs. An essential element in his consideration must be the hidden structure of culture.

FOOD AND NUTRITION

Generally, customs and mores are as important as physiological needs in determining the dietary habits of people. Until recently, it would have been difficult for an American mother to understand how her child could want hamburgers for breakfast instead of cereal. Why? Because traditionally, cereal is to be eaten in the morning, not meat—even though farmhands and cowboys have always eaten large quantities of meat for breakfast. Food selection is far more often influenced by psychosocial criteria than by deep concern with nutritive value of foods, nutritional requirements, and adequate performance of biochemical processes. Fortunately our tastes and habits have helped us make good use of available resources. Through empirical learning we have taken advantage of a great variety of natural resources in our environment, thereby managing a fairly complete and balanced diet even under conditions of scarcity. For example, Puerto Ricans use a mixture of beans and Mexicans use juice from cactus in a variety of ways in preparing their meals, with the biochemical end result being complete proteins.

It would seem easy to apply nutritional knowledge, but faulty nutrition is the largest single cause of disease in the world today. Most of us are quite aware of the problem of supplying sufficient food to the world's rapidly increasing population. But the real problem is not undernutrition but malnutrition, particularly shortage of good quality protein, and overnutrition. In prosperous countries, obesity is an increasing health problem. Obesity has been associated with changes in various normal body functions, increased risk of developing certain diseases, exacerbation of established diseases (see Chapter 15; concerning diabetes mellitus), and adverse psychological reactions. It would seem a simple matter for an obese person to decrease his food intake below that required for energy expenditure; however, the mechanisms that regulate food intake and utilization are complex and not fully understood.

On the other hand, malnutrition is a problem in most "developing nations" as well as for most of the poor in prosperous countries. There is little doubt that a poorly nourished cell cannot function optimally and, in fact, may not function at all. We cannot expect a child who has not eaten to be attentive and learn as quickly as the well-nourished child; nor can we expect a poorly nourished man to be inventive, productive, and able to help his "developing" country become self-sufficient. How we make use of our genetic endowment and adapt to our environment greatly depends upon our nutrition. For example, our nutritional state can affect the response of the body to infection. Antibody production depends upon the amount of nutrients available, and in profound deficiencies, the serum levels of antibodies are appreciably lowered. Likewise, the metabolism of macrophages depends upon available nutrients, thereby lowering the malnourished person's defenses to the numerous microbes found in the environment.

MAN-MICROBE INTERACTION

Microbes are not necessarily good or bad in themselves. It is their relationship with other living things, influenced by circumstances like those just discussed, that determines their detrimental or beneficial effects. Certain microbes play an essential role in the normal development and physiological activities of man. Types of indigenous microbes increase resistance to pathogens and influence the efficiency of food utilization. This is a highly integrated system, and anything that disturbs or interferes with one of the components necessarily disrupts the equilibrium of the whole system. Thus, man-microbe interaction must be considered as a factor affecting health. We must be concerned not only with sanitary conditions of our surroundings, but also with the wise use of antibiotics and disinfectants.

An excellent example of this complex relationship of man and microbe is the well-known fact that certain acquired bacteria in the intestinal flora of man synthesize vitamin K. Treatment of patients with sulfonamides or certain antibiotics reduces and may even abolish intestinal synthesis of vitamin K_2.[3] Thus, precautions must be taken in the administration of drugs to maintain this delicate physiological balance, just as cautious use of insecticides in protecting plant life must be observed to maintain the immensely important food chain of birds, animals, and man. Dubos points out, "Whether the method of treatment affects the animal predators in the wilderness or the bacteria in the gut, it is always risky to tamper with the natural balances of forces in nature."[4]

DRUGS

Self-administration of drugs is a great hazard to man's delicate biological system. Clear relationships have been demonstrated between the use of aspirin and gastrointestinal ulcers, phenacetin and hemolytic anemia, and numerous drug and allergic reactions. Such drug-induced diseases are increasing. This increase may be due in part to society's increasing dependence upon drugs to cope with the complexities and discomforts of living (i.e., with the increasing availability of drugs, many individuals may be less willing to experience the vicissitudes of daily living without them). In these instances, psychobiological manifestations, such as headache, insomnia, uneasiness, dissatisfaction or lack of energy, are not utilized as guideposts for examination of an individual's status of health and pattern of living, but rather are dulled or eliminated by simply taking a pill. Such dependence upon or misuse of drugs has even led to accidental suicides. Drug dependence does not foster attempts to determine the etiology of psychobiological manifestations.

It is apparent, of course, that wise use of drugs facilitates restoration of health and in some instances, such as in the use of insulin by diabetics, helps to maintain our health. The danger lies in developing an attitude that pill-taking in and of itself is good and therefore acceptable as a solution to the problems of living. The increase in drug-induced illness is clear evidence that the utilization of drugs is a health factor which must be considered seriously in maintaining the health of an individual or a society. One need only observe the parade of drugs across our television screens, or the array of nonprescription drugs in our stores, or the numerous young drug addicts who reveal that their drug habit started by taking the parent's pills, to realize that ours is a drug-oriented society. Drugs often seem to be used to counteract the normal manifestations of living. For example, the well-known cycle of "pep pills—sleeping pills" is substituted for physiological rest when one has the feeling of tiredness, and activity when one is psychobiologically alert. Short-term gratifications often seem to take precedence over long-range effects. However, in many instances, long-range results of drug ingestion are equally as important as immediate effects—for example, in using the "pill" to control the worldwide problem of population expansion.

POPULATION EXPANSION

Population expansion, in relation to food supply and other natural resources, housing and territorial limitations, and cultural and economic development, is undoubtedly another influential factor in the maintenance of health. And it seems likely that this expansion will need controls, but it is still uncertain whether "the pill" is the best way. It is also uncertain whether control through the female is the most efficient and healthy avenue to population control. Much is written and communicated about the use of female contraceptives, chemical and mechanical sterilization, and legalized abortion. Less has been mentioned about male contraception, for example, vasectomy, which is a relatively simple procedure and very rarely affects potency. Contraception through the male may indeed be the more effective control in the sense that the male's ability to procreate is considerably greater than the female's ability. Society's double standards have inhibited such a movement, but with the current changing attitudes, men may find it increasingly acceptable.

Intricately related to population expansion are the factors of adequate housing and space for healthful living. Most of us take for granted the conveniences of a safe and plentiful water supply, sufficient waste disposal systems, comfortable heating systems, clean and pleasant surroundings, and adequate space to afford privacy when desired. Unfortunately, this description does not exemplify many of the homes of the world. In many countries, the majority of the population lacks all of the housing characteristics mentioned. In some countries, it is not uncommon to find people sleeping in the streets because they are unable to crowd into a place with walls and a roof. Little needs to be said about the relationship of such housing conditions to health. (To gain an appreciation of such unfamiliar housing conditions read Oscar Lewis's book, *The Children of Sanchez.*)

It should be kept in mind that the urban and rural United States is not free of such poor housing. Although the problem is less acute here than in most parts of the world, many of our citizens live in dilapidated, overcrowded dwellings. The poor in the Appalachian mountains have difficulty in keeping warm as the wintry winds blow through their meager homes. The Navajo's hogans generally afford them little protection from the ravages of the elements and disease. Citizens of the urban slums must fight the battle of rat infestation. The housing problem seems to speak for itself, but we should be mindful that in our cities we should consider the total complex of streets, services and the like, as extensions of our homes.

Another aspect of space as a health factor is less clear-cut. There is reason to question how much congestion man can tolerate. Animal studies indicate that severe congestion tends to lead to an increase in aggressive behavior, abnormal mating and nesting and maternal activity, and the rates of illness and death. Some say our urban populations are also exhibiting such symptoms. There needs to be sufficient open space for access to sunlight, fresh air, recreational facilities and for some, at least, areas of privacy where they can observe nature. How the individual adapts to hordes of human beings and responds to crowding depends, partially at least, upon past experiences. For example, social distance may be one way to compensate for lack of territorial distance.

SENSORY STIMULATION

Psychological and physiological development depends upon a multiplicity of environmental stimuli. Sensory stimulation is essential for complete and orderly development. The quantity and quality of sensory stimulation are directly related to the status of a person's physical health. One type of sensory stimulation that has been given considerable attention is sound. The consequences of sound deprivation on a person's health are fairly obvious (see Chapter 19 for discussion of the patient experiencing sensory deprivation). Sound overload can also be detrimental to a person's health. Hearing loss as an occupational hazard has long been realized. Studies on tolerable noise levels in industry have been conducted and recommendations implemented. It is only recently, however, that noise levels in other areas of our environment have come under investigation. Several years ago, studies reported on national television indicated a causal relationship between current

levels of electronic amplification of music and temporary impairment of hearing. With increased crowding, electronic amplification, greater household and industrial use of machines, increased numbers of jet airplanes, and so on, sensory stimulation is becoming an increasingly important health factor.

CREATIVITY AND LIFE STYLE

Just as sensory stimulation is important to a person's development, so is creative expression. An individual's reaction to his or her work or occupation is an essential ingredient of that person's health. Work can ennoble and give meaning to a person's life, make him or her economically healthy, enhance his or her dignity and be an integral part of his or her life goals. Life goals are necessary, since the human organism is a goal-seeking animal and without goals his or her strength is dissipated in irregular pursuits or is exhausted from listlessness. On the other hand, work that is uncreative drudgery can be both quantitatively and qualitatively harmful to a person's health. Hence, work is a powerful health factor. It helps to balance daily life and to determine its rhythm.

The balance and rhythm of our lives are not only an expression of the state of our health, but our own life style also affects our health status. We have biological rhythms that assist in the regulation of our physiological systems. These rhythms seem to be adapted to nature's periodicities, such as light and dark or the 24-hour period (circadian rhythms), and persist for long periods even in the absence of environmental change. We seem to have little awareness of the influence of our biological rhythms, which probably accounts for the little conscious utilization of at least the gross rhythm periods for our benefit. For example, knowledge about the circadian temperature rhythm could readily be used for promoting more healthful living.

With almost clocklike regularity the body temperature rises and falls each 24 hours. The highest temperature is likely to coincide with a person's "best hours" of wakefulness, his favorite time of day, the time when he feels most alive and alert. The nadir generally occurs in the late hours of sleep. If a person happens to be awake during the low-temperature period, he may sense a slump in his vitality and may feel chilled . . . Whatever its origins, the circadian temperature cycle appears to be quite hard to alter in the normal adult.[5]

Few of us consciously plan our work, play, or rest in accordance with our circadian temperature cycle. Industry has given this cycle little consideration, with work schedules fixed by the clock. Today, as our modern technology increasingly modifies our environment to obliterate nature's periodicities, with windowless air-conditioned buildings and jet travel, further study of individual reactions to environment and rhythms is needed.

There are numerous other biological rhythms that influence our lives; for example, the 28-day menstrual cycle has been utilized as a basis for birth control. The life cycle itself has been insufficiently studied, however. Much attention has been given to the beginning of the cycle—infancy, childhood, and adolescence. Only recently have we studied (and implemented programs based on the findings) the remainder of this cycle, and even here the emphasis has been on the other end of the cycle—old age. Greater study certainly should be given to young adulthood and middle age and, perhaps, study of the interrelations of all phases of development would yield beneficial information.

Wittingly or unwittingly we develop life styles and tastes. Our genetic endowment and past life experiences, as well as intellectual considerations and future goals, influence the balance we reach between work, play, rest, and sleep. As Selye suggests, we need deviation of stress from one part to another or to the whole, thereby equalizing the stress.[6] "The human body—like the tires on a car or the rug on a floor—wears longest when it wears evenly."[7] We are all aware of the need to balance exercise and rest. It is obvious that an extreme of either can be detrimental to the body as a whole, or to any organ-system within the body. Some of each is necessary to sustain life and a moderated balance is required to attain a healthy life. Similarly, we need to acquire a balance between work and play. What might be work for one person may be play for another and vice versa. The commercial fisherman may relax with a book; the college professor with a rod and reel. What one considers work the other considers play. These personal definitions of work and play, along with the individual's biological rhythms, develop into the individual's pattern of life—his life style.

Equally as important as the pattern of our life style is "the stuff it's made of." All the aforementioned factors which affect health, and admittedly many others, certainly help to construct the quality of life and thus the quality of health. But there is another rather elusive characteristic of healthful living: a zest for life. We all know a few people who seem to radiate *joie de vivre*. They seem to have a talent for pure enjoyment of life. For some this distinctive quality seems to be rooted in their spiritual beliefs; for others, their capacity to contemplate. Whatever the nature of this quality that embellishes a person's life style, it is evident that it promotes a state of health.

Principles of Health Maintenance

Sound analysis and reflective contemplation of the principles involved in maintaining health may increase the probability that health maintenance can become a reality for a greater proportion of the world's population. Health professionals should periodically reflect on their personal understanding of the importance of principles of health maintenance in everyday living. These include principles regarding health education, environmental control, accident prevention, life style, and health surveillance.

HEALTH EDUCATION
It is essential that each individual have a basic awareness of the factors affecting his health status. Likewise, to have a healthy society it is necessary to have an informed public. Granted, these are very simple and basic principles with which few would disagree. What is not so simple, and wherein many disagree, is the application of these principles. Who is responsible for health education? How should "health" be taught?

What are the best methods of making people aware of the factors affecting their health? The answers to these questions vary with the interests of the respondent. Physicians refer to the many pamphlets and public service announcements on TV sponsored by the American Medical Association. Educators proudly talk of their health education classes. Nurses defend their teaching of patients in hospitals, clinics, and homes. What seems to emerge is that educators and all health professionals readily accept only isolated responsibility for health education, and thus all have made only fragmentary efforts and progress.

Surely if the human being is an integrated entity, and each health factor plays a simultaneously influential part, the approach to increasing an individual's awareness of health should be integrated in all of his or her experiences. An example of such integration was given by Dr. Delbert Obertueffer, who aptly said:

> We simply must disabuse ourselves of the notion that the school exists solely for purposes of training the mind. It doesn't—because there is no such thing as a mind to be trained all by itself, sitting on a desk top. There is a child—a child who comes to school all in one piece—brain, thyroid, ovaries, retina, feet, stomach, spleen, fears, anxieties, and sensitivities. There is no process in the world whereby the teacher can say "Now thyroid, you remain quiet while I teach this brain that $\frac{a + b - C_2}{y}$ = the square root of Z." The thyroid may, because of reasons unknown to the teacher say "The hell with it" and motivate the owner thereof to join the dropouts.[8]

Not only must education include the study of the human being and that which is relevant to his or her existence, but we all must make a concerted effort to communicate with each other—teacher with child, child with nurse, nurse with teacher—as integrated human beings. Second, we must attempt to reduce fragmentation by combining our efforts to increase public awareness. Many artificial boundaries of medicine, nursing, and education should be done away with. An individual begins by having confidence in his or her own knowledge and skills, respect

for the dignity of the other (professional or lay person), and a desire and willingness to take the first step.

ENVIRONMENTAL CONTROL

The second principle of health maintenance is to work toward effective environmental control. The form these controls take should vary with changes in technology, cultural attitudes, and societal trends. They run the gamut from antiemission devices on automobiles to provisions for natural settings in our cities. They encompass such areas as family planning, city planning, natural resources conservation, food distribution, disease prevention, and antipoverty legislation. Thus, implementation of the principle of environment control is multidimensional and complex. Such complexity is nevertheless desirable to meet the ever-changing multiplicity of needs with the required flexibility of solutions.

ACCIDENT PREVENTION

Environmental control may encompass the principle of accident prevention, but probably not totally. In implementing environmental control, we are dealing with what is known and foreseeable. In working toward effective accident prevention, this is not the case. An accident, by its very nature, takes place without individual foresight or expectation and in relation to health maintenance is often catastrophic. In addition to environmental controls, it therefore seems imperative that other approaches be utilized to reduce the probability of the occurrence of certain accidents. The fatalities that take place on U.S. highways each year appear to be due largely to ineffective environmental control. That is, much of what causes these "accidents" is known and foreseeable. The same can be said for "accidental shootings," toddlers ingesting poisons, and some "industrial accidents." On the other hand, what is suggested here is that systematic methods should be employed to uncover lesser-known causative factors. The techniques reviewed by Herman Kahn in his book, *Thinking About the Unthinkable*, might prove useful in delineating methods of accident prevention. In addition to techniques of operations research and

systems analysis, Kahn suggests and describes some unconventional thinking aids, namely abstract models, scenarios, games, historical examples, and novels.[9] With such methods, we might "accidentally" uncover new knowledge and techniques to apply in health maintenance.

LIFE STYLE

As mentioned earlier, life style is a pattern of living which is consciously or unconsciously developed. One of the principles of health maintenance involves *consciously* choosing a uniquely personal, healthy way of living. To obtain such individuality, considerable self-insight is necessary, consisting of a knowledge of one's strengths and limitations and the ability to accept them gracefully. Though it is no easy task to recognize and understand one's personal, physical, psychosocial, and spiritual needs, it is essential if one would develop a healthful life style. In addition to self-insight, a given individual's knowledge of health practices, as well as his or her determination and persistence in pursuing the goal of health, are vital ingredients in the achievement of a life style which embodies healthful living.

HEALTH SURVEILLANCE

To achieve or maintain health requires thoughtful vigilance. This means being alert to what could be dangerous or detrimental to one's health as well as recognizing signs or symptoms of impending illness. It does not require a constant preoccupation with one's health status, for this is frequently detrimental in itself. Rather, it requires a sensible plan for periodic review. In relation to maintaining physical health, this includes such measures as routine medical examinations, regular dental examinations, and periodic multiphasic screening procedures. Unfortunately, knowledge of these practices of health maintenance is taken for granted, so that in reality few people have the opportunity, or at least take the opportunity, to utilize these practices. Even fewer have sufficient knowledge and motivation to institute any form of self-examination. (Although efforts have been made, for example, to have women routinely perform breast self-examinations, these

practices are not widespread.) Pla[...]
flection or analysis is given small co[...]
the training of health professionals,[...]
a practice would be advantageous i[...]
choosing life goals and patter[...]
Another little-known health surve[...]
dure is the periodic economic revi[...]
systematic assessment by an indi[...]
her personal economic resource[...]
or her to consider distributing [...]
phasis on maintaining health as [...]
ing it should illness occur.

Some health surveillance m[...]
does for himself; others require[...]
professionals. Such assistance [...]
and encouraged from appropr[...]
persons in whom the individ[...]
confidence. These may be pro[...]
verse knowledge and skills and[...]
agents, ministers, marriage c[...]
on, as well as physicians and [...]
tent professional will make re[...]
sultation when he does not p[...]
knowledge or skill to assist a[...]
taining health. To have the [...]
referrals presupposes not [...]
the contribution of the par[...]
own field of practice, but [...]
standing of the contributio[...]
the maintenance of health[...]

EARLY TREATMENT

Early treatment is not [...]
health maintenance, for t[...]
however, it is only one [...]
on the health-illness-d[...]
think of health in its b[...]
earlier, there are instan[...]
this inf[...]
a society can be mainta[...]
als who have no manif[...]
lation programs, such [...]
cine to eradicate po[...]
examples of such i[...]
perhaps, are measure[...]
payment insurance [...]
may call these meas[...]
health maintenance; [...]
kind are based on [...]

strength, will or knowledge. And to do this in such a way as to help him gain independence as rapidly as possible.[10]

Naturally each nurse interprets this definition differently as an individual practitioner. However, there is a common thread that unites the practices of nurses. It is the natural relationship they have with those who seek or need their services. They have an empathetic understanding of the person's living and the association is mutually advantageous. The advantage for the person is maintaining or recovering health, or having a peaceful death as the case may be, while nurses gain deep satisfaction and dignity from this work, which usually is an integral part of their life goals.

The nurse who functions with this philosophical base is the patient's advocate in regaining his health. Similarly, the nurse must be the healthy person's advocate in maintaining his health. Like a lawyer, the nurse might intervene for a single individual or may plead the case for many individuals through legislation.

Nursing intervention in providing for the maintenance of health is concerned with assisting the well individual to perform the activities that contribute to retaining his healthy state. This requires the same depth and breadth of knowledge and intellectual skill as the nursing process in caring for the ill. Perhaps the nurse must have keener observational skills, since the signs and symptoms are more obscure. Clarification of the problems threatening health may require greater utilization of multidisciplinary groups, including members not traditionally thought of as health professionals, such as police and community leaders. The evaluation of health intervention necessitates a vigilant nurse with reasonable knowledge of fields other than nursing. Nursing intervention can be planned and effected for the individual either singly or as a member of a group.

Nursing intervention for the maintenance of health can be categorized as the four "C's"— case finding, community resources, counseling, and care. There is nothing magical about this categorization, nor is there any pretense of comprehensiveness. The reader is invited to exercise

his or her imagination and expand this list of possible nursing interventions. There is no doubt that the extent of nursing intervention in health maintenance is limited only by a given nurse's knowledge, skill, desire, and creativity.

Case finding in health maintenance is the identification of factors and situations with the potential of producing illness. This type of intervention applies the principles of health surveillance, early treatment, accident prevention, and environmental control which were discussed previously in this chapter. Each nurse must exercise personal judgment and creativity in her specific application and be cautious not to restrict her contribution in case finding by limiting her application to the employment situation or the traditional roles of nursing.

For many years, the area of community resources was almost exclusively the tool of the community health nurse in nursing intervention. The social worker also utilized community resources, mainly as a restorative measure, but more often than other health professionals for health maintenance. Therefore, this colleague should be fully utilized for consultation and referral. Nursing intervention requires a thorough knowledge of the available resources in the community in which the nurse works and lives. Knowing the so-called health resources available to assist the ill is not enough for the nurse involved in health maintenance. Social, recreational, and educational resources may also be employed. Health professionals have the specialized knowledge to make such determinations; however, health professionals need to be mindful that the community's or individual's *needs* as they identified them are not necessarily the *wants* of the community or individual. Often it is imperative to fulfill the wants before the needs can be met. This is particularly true in areas where the educational, cultural, and economic resources are limited or poorly developed. Thus, nursing intervention is utilizing a variety of means to secure the needed community resources to maintain health.

The nurse involved in health maintenance also has a responsibility to contribute to community resources. This contribution may be in the form of political action or as a member of an organization or a community group.

The third mode of nursing intervention, health maintenance counseling, encompasses a wide diversification of knowledge and skills. The nurse who engages in such counseling must have, or acquire command of, several effective counseling techniques to be of assistance to individuals, families, and groups, as well as a reservoir of up-to-date knowledge and a *reasonable* understanding of multiple areas of study. In addition to counseling persons in such familiar areas as elementary hygiene measures and normal pregnancy, counseling in certain specialized fields of knowledge assumes fundamental importance, including such seemingly esoteric areas as genetics, bioclimatological factors, biological rhythms, nutrition, and economics. Further, specific knowledge of the beliefs and customs of individuals and families receiving counseling facilitates and smoothes the way for change in health practices.

Chapter 6 exemplifies the depth of knowledge that must be mastered for the nurse specialist to participate in effective genetic counseling. Likewise, a basic understanding of the changing needs of individuals during the life cycle is necessary if the nurse is to be of aid in the genetic counseling of all members of the family.

Bioclimatological factors are associated with an individual's response to climatic stresses. Little has been done in this area of health counseling because the fundamental mechanisms have been poorly understood. Recent basic research is beginning to shed light on some of these mechanisms. The effect of extreme heat or cold on an individual's physical, and often mental, well-being is readily expressed. (Try to remember your own feelings the last time the temperature was in the 90's and the humidity over 70 percent.) Other bioclimatological factors that warrant consideration are atmospheric pressure, radiation, and possibly space charges of small ions. There is increasing evidence from epidemiological, clinical, and experimental studies indicating that sudden atmospheric changes may have ill effects or may cause exacerbations where illness or disease is present (see Chapter

22.) Until more definitive research findings are available, those involved in bioclimatological health counseling must be prepared to utilize the few isolated facts that they have. For example, the relationship between the sun's ionizing radiation and the occurrence of certain skin cancers has clearly been demonstrated. A systematic assessment of bioclimatological factors and an individual's state of health would be most useful in counseling him. Therefore, one would need to be aware of personal biases in this area and the findings of recent research and be able to apply skill in nursing assessment and research techniques in order to offer bioclimatological health counseling.

Implications for health counseling in relation to biological rhythms have already been suggested. The importance of an adequate nursing assessment from which a baseline for counseling could be drawn must be stressed. Few individuals wish to undergo the complicated laboratory tests necessary to determine their individual biological rhythms. Thus, it is necessary for the nurse counselor to gain useful information by direct observation and counselee recall. Here again, the counselor needs to be cognizant of recent basic research findings and be sufficiently involved with counselees in order to render beneficial counseling.

The human race is highly adaptable with regard to nutrition, and much has been written elsewhere about nutritional needs and nutritional counseling. However, customs and taboos, as well as physiological needs, are important in determining dietary habits. Generally, we have learned, through empirical experience, to take advantage of a great variety of natural food resources and, thereby, to achieve a fairly well-balanced diet even under conditions of scarcity. Therefore, the nurse's nutritional counseling should begin with a sound knowledge of the dietary habits of the counselees. From this base, the nutritive value of their dietary patterns can be determined. The changes needed for optimal nutrition can then be planned without injecting the nurse's personal dietary biases. Nutritional counseling should blend scientific knowledge of nutrition with a sound understanding of the dietary habits of the counselees. Certainly all the counseling in the world is to no avail if the suggested changes are not acceptable to the counselees, thereby making no persistent changes in their dietary habits.

One thread that is continuously interwoven within health counseling is economics. Traditionally, nursing has been reluctant to establish economics as a discreet area of health counseling, but the important influence of economics on health matters cannot be denied. In the United States, for example, health statistics indicate that poor people have higher mortality and morbidity rates and suffer more chronic conditions than the rest of the population.[11] Thus, it seems that nurses should be prepared to assist the poor, at least, in setting economic priorities in relation to health factors. Less obvious perhaps is the role the nurse could assume in economic counseling in relation to insurance coverage. Individual counseling based on a sound knowledge of health insurance practices, or reliable consultation from health insurance experts, can be of particular assistance to the poor, who have significantly less health insurance coverage. Second, the prepared nurse can counsel employers on the benefits of health insurance or insurance groups about the need to expand "health" insurance to cover such health measures as multiphasic screening. On an even wider scale, the nurse can counsel legislators, and those who influence legislators, on the economic priorities essential to promote the fulfillment of the highest level of health attainable to all citizens. The nursing profession needs to recognize its responsibility for economic health counseling. Individual nurses must fortify themselves with a reasonable knowledge of health economics and be willing to talk dollars and cents with individuals without sacrificing any individual's dignity, and with groups and legislators without personal embarrassment.

The last aspect of nursing intervention to be emphasized in providing for health maintenance is the care function of nursing. Although nursing care includes the laying on of hands, for instance with the disabled-well or infants, the main force in this type of caring is a sense of broad responsi-

bility. To be involved in another's health care implies interest in the total health of the other. It connotes a thoughtfulness for the other's welfare and an attentiveness to his desires and needs. It requires watchfulness to assist him in maintaining his equilibrium of health. It means that the nurse involved in health maintenance must frequently derive satisfaction from mental rather than physical activities, from the overt achievement of others rather than directly from personal achievement, and from accomplishments that may not be dramatic or concrete in nature.

The extent of expressing care is limited only by the individual nurse's abilities and attitudes. It is within the reach of every nurse, for example, to actively participate in the American Nurses Association and to support legislative action beneficial to the maintenance of health. Some nurses might utilize more specific talents, by writing or serving as consultants in communication media. Whether the selected method is directly or indirectly expressed is of little import; whether the impact of the act is felt by an individual, by a local community, or worldwide is not of primary significance; whether it is of large or small proportion is of small consequence. In the final analysis, the expression of care by acting is the acme of caring.

Delivery of Health Care

For many professionals and lay persons, health care and medical care are synonymous. At midcentury, the limitations of knowledge, technology, and socioeconomic influences restricted the utilization of health resources primarily to the delivery of medical care. Medical care focuses on the diagnosis and treatment of disease or pathology and is delivered by relatively few professionals—for example, dentists, physicians, podiatrists, and their assistants. Medical care is only one aspect of health care, albeit a vital component. In the delivery of health care today, medical professionals are complemented by a wide array of other professionals.

Health care is primarily oriented toward promoting and maintaining health. Emphasis is on prevention of disease. American society recognizes health as a positive value and considers high-level wellness a right for all individuals. Recent advances in the behavioral sciences, as well as medical technology, have facilitated the evolution of health care to include comprehensive services rendered by many different and diverse disciplines. Indeed, isolated practitioners are incapable of offering essential comprehensive services for the delivery of health care. Health care systems must organize the multidisciplinary health professionals available to meet the needs of defined societal groups.

As one of the health professions, nursing has an integral role in the present health care systems. It is acknowledged that multidisciplinary contributions, in both thought and action, are essential to health care decisions. Therefore, nursing must accept responsibility and be accountable for the nursing aspects of health care and join with other disciplines in defining health care delivery systems. This health care planning combines the resources of specific populations to provide defined services and health care benefits.

Fundamental to the development of health care systems are societal attitudes, expectations, and demands. The increasing affluence of Americans has enabled a greater sophistication in understanding health matters by the average citizen. There is a concomitant resentment of the paternalistic, patronizing services offered in the past. Likewise, with the prolongation of life, a result of technological advances, there is an increasing emphasis on health. Society is becoming more and more concerned about the quality of life.

Individuals and community groups expect to share decision-making power with health professionals. There is greater recognition of areas of competence. No longer is economic power the only leverage in changing the decision-making process in health care. There is greater acceptance that the knowledge of consumers, as well as that of a greater variety of providers, should be integrated in health care decisions and delivery.

The mode of consumer compliance exemplifies the changing composition of health care decisions. Formerly, individuals were expected to conform to regimens outlined by health pro-

fessionals. Failure to comply generally resulted in removal of the health service. The consumer was given the choice of taking what the health professional offered or doing without. As consumers have become more knowledgeable, they have increased their competence in making decisions concerning their own health care. Blind conformity is giving way to individual compliance through commitment which synthesizes the competencies of both consumer and provider of health care services.

Similarly, the adversary relationship was exemplified by American society through rapid increase in lawsuits brought against an ever greater variety of health professionals. The increase in lawsuits was reflected in the increased costs for health care necessitated by expanded insurance coverage. This spiraling aspect of health care costs is reversible by replacing the antagonistic decision-making process with collaborative mechanisms for planning and implementing individual and community health programs.

Governmental forces are being exercised to bring about changes to meet the present societal demands and for redefining goals. Some states have legislated community involvement in health care planning and evaluation. For example, in 1970 New York provided for some hospitals to have an ''advisory board composed of at least 51% community representation.''[12] Similarly, the federal government has increased community involvement through such legislation as Comprehensive Health Planning. Comprehensive Health Planning boards are charged with the responsibility of setting local and state priorities. Generally, these priorities are based on the health care principle that the greater investments must go where they serve the greatest need.

Financial investments in health care exert a major influence on health care delivery systems. Illustrative of the inflation of health care was the 204 percent increase in hospital expenses from 1960 to 1970. Hospital care amounted to 38 percent of the health care expenditures in the United States.[13] Hospital costs rose disproportionately to the general inflationary trend of the 1960's because increased technology required more and better educated staff, and hospital personnel demanded more appropriate pay. The financial burden for illness care has led to demands for expanded and extended health care. As consumers have infiltrated such financing programs as Blue Cross, the coverage for diagnostic, preventive, and home care is more readily available. Consumers have recognized, and are providing for, the economics of health maintenance.

Society limits the financial investment it is willing to make for health care. It demands the greatest value from its finite resources. In general, this is interpreted to mean the greatest benefit for the most people. Decisions of whether to invest in research or care programs are based on this premise. Likewise, decisions concerning preventive or therapy care programs are carefully weighed. Through participation in the decision-making process, consumers realize that medical care is only a part of health care; therefore, those served by the health care system are moving from participation into control of health care decisions.

PARAMETERS OF HEALTH CARE SYSTEMS

The parameters of health care systems are determined by the potential users of the system. In the evaluative process, health professionals may have a tendency toward quantitative measures. However, full evaluation of a health care system must go beyond functional values and include the potentials of the system. The parameters determined by consumers incorporate the traditional evaluative measures into these potentials. At least four parameters of health care systems (which could be called the 4 A's of health care delivery systems) can be identified: accessibility, availability, acceptability, and accountability.

Accessibility means that health care services are easily approachable and accessible. This parameter has both time and space dimensions. Does the health care system of a given society have intake facilities open when the users of the system need them? The work patterns of the users should be taken into consideration. Family structures also dictate some of the time factors to be considered in determining access to the system. Can family problems be admitted all at once? Or must each family member seek individual admission? Can any problem be presented at any time, or must the user conform to the system's timing for consideration of specific health problems?

The second dimension of accessibility is the location of the intake structure and the mechanisms of the system. Must the user travel long distances to gain access to the system? What kind of transportation is available? For example, many older individuals may require public transportation. In rural areas, it might be necessary to bring the service to the users by mobile clinics. Another aspect of the space dimension is safety. Many urban users may need assurance that the location of the intake component of the health system is safe for them to travel in during the hours they can, or will, seek health care.

In general, accessibility is met if the primary facilities of the health care system are neighborhood-based and -oriented. Since health care is rarely high on the priority lists of individuals, entry into the system must be competitive with other interests and desires. In other words, the primary facilities must be convenient to use and encourage repeated and extended utilization.

The available services of the primary unit should have a broad scope of interest for the individual being served. It must be to the advantage of the consumer to seek the services offered by a health care system. To accomplish the appropriate constellation of services requires a breadth of understanding of the health problems, including environmental, social, and cultural variables experienced by the specific population. The entry unit should be virtually limitless. That is, it should be flexible enough to meet changing health needs and to offer a variety of health care guidance and supervision.

The health care system might also have mechanisms designed and functioning well that go beyond the usual problems presented on entry. For example, formal linkage with other agencies, or even another system, could make services available to the relative few within the system who may require these services. These linkages should be horizontal, such as to other primary units, as well as vertical which would make available services more complicated or acute in nature.

The parameter of availability is met if the health care system meets the purposes determined by its potential users. It should be noted that participating health professionals may have the responsibility to expand the population's notion of the purposes of the health care system. Indeed, although health education may not readily be recognized as an important part of any health care system, it certainly should be an integral part.

The third parameter, acceptability, determines the consumers compliance with the system. Many factors affect any one individual's approval. These factors may range from the cost of service to understanding the expected behavior for maintaining or regaining health. Again, there must be a basic understanding of socioeconomic and cultural variables within the population to be served. With this understanding, an appropriate environmental context with effective communicative and financial mechanisms can be developed.

Modification or changing of the traditional health care system may be seen as a threat to the traditional values of consumers. Therefore, consumer input into the development of a health care system can be most helpful in assuring the acceptability of the system. It is not uncommon for this solicited input to slow down the progress of developing a system, but such input can increase the probability for long-range progress. Likewise, consumer participation in the delivery of care can increase the acceptability of the system—particularly when the cultures of the providers and consumers are different.

Accountability, the last parameter identified, means that the health professional is answerable to the person receiving care, and/or the health care system is responsible to the specified population. Until recently, most health professionals have not had to experience being accountable to consumers. Accountability requires the collaborative relationship referred to earlier. There is a give and take between the participants which leads to mutually agreed upon health care plans—individual or community. The health professional encourages the consumer's development and independence. (This relationship is consistent with Henderson's definition of nursing, p. 22.) Each accepts responsibility for his or her area of expertise; the health care professional for knowledge and skill in health maintenance or restoration strategies and the consumer for knowledge of self and/or community and ability to comply with the health plan.

Accountability in health care systems implies that there are evaluative mechanisms in the system to monitor its effectiveness. Does the system do what it purports to do? Are the objectives of a health care system being met? If so, to what degree? A reporting system devised to assist managerial control and program planning is essential. Generally these reporting systems include basic population, utilization, and financial data. Consumers are always interested in cost-benefits. It is obvious that evaluative mechanisms are considered and constructed during the developmental phase of a health care system.

Individual accountability is also an essential of the health care system. Consumers who have entered into a contractual relationship with a health care system to receive specific benefits or services must have assurance of receiving these services when they need them. Health professionals must accept responsibility for their individual professional competence and for monitoring the competence of their colleagues through such activities as peer review and comprehensive patient conferences, including the patient when possible. Second, staffing must be adequate to be accessible and available when needed. Just as the reporting system evaluates the pattern of health care offered and the health of the population, the individual's care plan should be evaluated periodically with the individual to determine his or her state of health and the cost-effectiveness of the individual plan.

Systematic accounting for a health care system's objectives, practices, and costs enables identification of needed changes. In addition, it fosters improvement in management procedures. Productivity of a system is given as much emphasis as inputs, which were the traditional measures of the quality of a health care service. Many traditions in health care delivery are being modified and the parameters must keep pace.

It must be emphasized that health care systems serve local populations; therefore, there will be variations in the identified parameters. As suggested previously, these parameters will be interpreted and evaluated differently by various groups, resulting in cultural and/or socioeconomic variations.

Culture is how members of a particular group eat, work, play, sleep, and relate to each other. It is determined by the group's values and beliefs. All cultural factors have a direct influence on a specific population's perception and interpretation of what health is, as well as its health practices and relationships with health care providers. Frequently, health professionals are inclined to consider only cultures that differ dramatically from their own. However, the United States has many cultures and subcultures. There are significant cultural differences among Americans which influence their evaluation of any health care system, hence, their utilization of and compliance with the system.

The health practices of an individual are largely determined by his cultural background. For example, folk beliefs influence whether the person will seek assistance from the scientifically oriented health professional or from the culturally defined healer. Help may be sought from folk healers, such as the curanderos of the Mexican-Americans, the pow-wows of the Pennsylvania Dutch, or the local spiritualists of many ethnic groups. These folk healers generally are not used exclusively, but rather share the delivery of health care with modern health professionals. It is the individual who determines which offers the appropriate service at a price he can pay for his self-defined problems.

Communication patterns are also culturally determined. Differences in these patterns are more subtle than those in language. Different subcultures may speak the same language, but the words have different meanings. Personal experiences of moving from a rural mountain area to an urban area, caring for individuals from many American subcultures, and traveling in several Latin American countries have verified these differences in word meanings. There are also differences in verbal style and nonverbal forms of communication as witnessed by the work of Ray Birdwhistell, Erving Goffman, and Edward T. Hall.

It is imperative that the planning and implementation of health care systems be predicated on a sound knowledge and understanding of the value, belief, and communication systems of the specific population to be served. To be deemed relevant and valuable, the structure and process of the health care delivery system must be congruent with the consumers' culturally based constructs of health care and health services.

Likewise, the health care system must reflect a deep comprehension and concern for the socioeconomic factors that impinge upon the consumers' ability or desire to participate. The obvious factors—ability to pay, associated dignity—need no comment. Less obvious, but certainly as important for examples, are variables associated with socioeconomic status, such as self-image and significant others.

It is not uncommon for individuals from low-income families to have a low or poor self-image when encountering health care professionals. With this understanding, the health care professional should strive to become a sensitive, exceptionally good listener, and by manner and presence to convey respect. Condescension has no place in a health care system designed to meet the needs of low-income populations.

The significant others in low-income families are frequently quite different from those identified by middle-class families whence come most health professionals. Low-income families are frequently extended families and a significant person for a child might very well be a grandmother or godmother, rather than the mother. In such instances, the system must be patterned after the social structure of the specified population to render effective health care.

The cultural and socioeconomic variations on the identified parameters further highlight the usefulness of consumer participation in all aspects of the health care delivery system. The efficiency of the system can be measured in economic terms, that is, a comparison of the product (health care) with the cost in time, money, and so on, of the input by health care workers. The identified parameters take into consideration not only efficiency, but also effectiveness. Effectiveness measures the desired outcomes of health care—mainly high-level wellness and improved quality of life for the population served.

Whether or not the health care system is proceeding toward the identified goals at optimal speed is determined by regulatory mechanisms within the system. These mechanisms include autofeedback mechanisms and peripheral review. Both are essential for determining progress toward long-term organizational goals and for modifying current practices in order to immediately increase the system's effectiveness.

Autofeedback mechanisms encompass such procedures as periodic utilization review, regular consumer evaluations, and cost-benefit analysis. Periodic utilization reviews, both intradisciplinary and interdisciplinary, serve as monitors of the strengths and weaknesses of a given unit or service within the system, of the competence of individual practitioners, and of the articulation of the various units or subsystems with the total system. Systematic consumer evaluation of the system complements the benefits of utilization review and renders parallel benefits. As mentioned earlier, cost-benefit analysis does not measure the effectiveness of a system, but can contribute invaluable information. Such analysis highlights the relationship between the various elements and/or subsystems and the productivity of the subsystem and/or system. Input costs are related to output and serve as the economic barometer of the system. The information yield from autofeedback mechanisms can identify needed adjustments or modifications and guide the system toward its goals.

The other regulatory mechanism, peripheral review, permits broad inspection and perception. It attempts to evaluate a total health care system, taking into account its dynamics and effectiveness. Generally, this type of review is done by governing boards and advisory committees. These peripheral units determine the course and goals of a health care system. Ideally they are composed of a representative sample of the population to be served and sufficient health professionals to give expert information. The governing boards require individuals with experience in decision making, while the advisory boards require individuals with expert knowledge of the population. Together, these units identify consumer needs by such procedures as community surveys, epidemiological studies, and the like, and make the policies which set the objectives and mode of operation for the system. Their systematic review and decisions keep the system relevant to changing health needs.

Obviously output analysis is an essential component, not only as an autofeedback mechanism, in the determination of the system's effectiveness. Outputs, such as service utilization, regulate the system through modification of services. Measures that determine the relationship between the pattern of health care services and the health of the population are useful in policy determinations. The most valuable, and perhaps the most difficult to ascertain, is health status of individuals served by the health care system.

Theoretically, the effective health care system meets the needs of individuals of a specific population. Their health is improved. They are able to function more successfully. Ultimately their quality of life is improved. These outputs are extremely difficult to determine, but necessary to determine effectiveness of health care and reallocation of community resources. The effective system should eventually require less of the community's resources and be able to maintain high-level wellness using a minimum of these resources.

MODELS OF HEALTH CARE DELIVERY SYSTEMS

There are many ways to organize the delivery of health care, and several models are worth further consideration, including exploration and/or experimentation. Organization may be simple, such as the traditional sole practitioner, or complex and multilevel. In addition to the traditional medical model of the sole practitioner, the most ac-

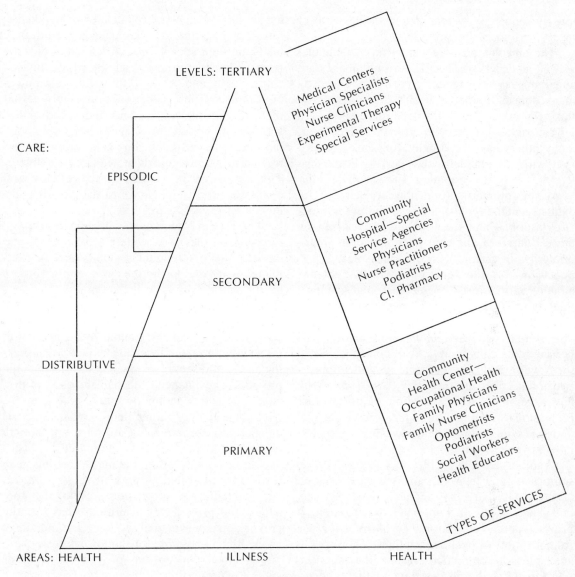

LEVELS: TERTIARY

CARE:

EPISODIC

SECONDARY

DISTRIBUTIVE

PRIMARY

Medical Centers
Physician Specialists
Nurse Clinicians
Experimental Therapy
Special Services

Community
Hospital—Special
Service Agencies
Physicians
Nurse Practitioners
Podiatrists
Cl. Pharmacy

Community
Health Center—
Occupational Health
Family Physicians
Family Nurse Clinicians
Optometrists
Podiatrists
Social Workers
Health Educators

TYPES OF SERVICES

AREAS: HEALTH   ILLNESS   HEALTH

FIGURE 2-1.
Health care delivery resources.

cepted model is that of group medical practice. Group models are being adopted by a greater variety and number of health care professionals, thereby increasing the availability of entry sites in the total system of health resources (Fig. 2-1). Nevertheless there still remains the fragmentary arrangement of health services.

Fragmentation of singular practice can be reduced by established horizontal and vertical communication and referral mechanisms. The singular practice is the simplest organization, that is, one provider to one consumer, and may represent any aspect of care along the continuum of health-illness and any level of care from primary to tertiary. The health care worker in individual practice may be a physician, a family nurse clinician, a dentist, or any of the numerous (approximately 400) different types of health care workers. If there is easy access to a sufficient array of other health care professionals, this loosely connected system may meet the needs of many consumers and providers.

The singular practice model has advantages as well as disadvantages. The disadvantages are apparent and have recently been denounced by many demanding better health care. Generally, this negative criticism has been directed toward physicians as private entrepreneurs. However, many others have been delivering care successfully within the model with relatively little negative criticism. An example is the vision care delivered by optometrists or dental care delivered by dentists and their assistants. The health service is circumscribed and their limitations realized by most. Therefore, the consumer seeks the appropriate health care professional, has realistic expectations for the service, generally receives humane care at a reasonable cost, and is appropriately referred if his or her needs are not met. With these inherent characteristics, the advantage is that services *can be* more widely dispersed in the community. Also, consumer's cost for travel is reduced. Personal identification between consumer and provider *is possible*. With few exceptions, maldistribution of health care professionals and lack of mutual knowledge and understanding among them have prevented this model from exploiting its advantages.

Another model for the organization of resources on any level of care is group services. Group health care may include illness service, but generally it is a horizontal organization. It brings together comparable levels of expertise from a variety of health disciplines. The services available are comprehensive and the organization facilitates the accessibility of the services. The scope of the grouped health resources may vary widely.

The Philadelphia Interdisciplinary Health Education Project* (PHIHEP) is one example of the efforts currently being made to facilitate the development of group health services. Educational experiences are provided for interdisciplinary teams to gain clinical skills in a variety of primary entry settings. The disciplines participat-

ing in this particular project include medicine, nursing, optometry, pharmacy, podiatric medicine, and social work. After initial didactic study, students of these disciplines function as a clinical team and rotate to three different outpatient clinics. These experiences not only permit them to gain the mutual knowledge and understanding to exploit the singular practice model, but enable them to develop skills to function effectively in group models of health care delivery. The extension of PHIHEP is to develop and evaluate interdisciplinary health care delivery models of primary care.

The Health Maintenance Organization (HMO) is probably the most widely publicized group model. The HMO model assumes that marketplace economic principles are applicable to health care delivery. A defined population is offered full utilization of a wide range of multilevel health care services. This comprehensive health care, including but not limited to medical care, offers greater resources than any individual seeking care could secure or any one physician could provide. The financial mechanism used is prepayment. The economic incentive is to keep the individual healthy rather than to wait for crisis diagnosis and treatment. Care most appropriate to each individual's needs, unlimited by insurance policies that often dictate the setting, may readily by extended to preventive, restorative, and rehabilitative dimensions. Thus, the consumer and provider of health care have a congruent objective—namely to keep the individual as healthy as possible for the lowest cost.

The HMO concept has proven successful in such long-standing plans as the well-known Kaiser-Permanente program. Recent government financing (HMO Act of 1973) has encouraged the establishment of several new HMOs to facilitate appropriate modification of the prototype for a number of quite different populations. Experimentation and evaluation of modified HMO models should lead to improved health care at reasonable cost for effective, as well as efficient, systems tailored to the unique needs of each population served.

The more complex organizations of health care are the multilevel comprehensive organiza-

*The author has participated in the planning and implementation of this project.

tions. These may be comprised of several subsystems, such as comprehensive neighborhood centers, community hospitals, and medical centers. The resources of multilevel organizations are broad in scope, that is they cover both health and illness areas, and the depth of many services are components of this model. The formal linkages are contractual agreements which increase the accessibility and availability of the services of any subsystem and facilitate the communication of valuable information.

The inherent advantages of the loosely organized multilevel health care system are directly related to the flexibility of this system for the consumer. The attractive elements of the one-to-one relationship can be maintained. At the same time, the individual has the reassurance that the latest knowledge and skill available will be used if necessary. This type of structure accommodates multiple portals of entry into the system and referral mechanisms quickly guide the individual to the most appropriate care. If HMOs are an integral part of a particular multilevel system, the focus on health is maintained. Both distributive and episodic care are blended in this model of health care delivery (see Fig. 2-1).

The complexity of the multilevel system may also create disadvantages. An individual requiring the services of several different components of the system could experience the fragmentation effects of isolated specialty services. Careful consideration of structure and process of the multilevel organization can, to a large degree, prevent or alleviate these problems. Each consumer should have a focal health professional who functions as his advocate-coordinator regardless of the subunits or subsystems in which he is receiving care. Patient-oriented record keeping with easy retrieval for all subunits facilitates integration of care, decreases deleterious interaction effects, and permits a comprehensive health history. A communications matrix for client information and professional education maximizes full utilization of multidisciplinary health care services.

Each model of health care delivery has inherent advantages and disadvantages; however, in-

herent superiority of any one model has not been demonstrated. Health care can be considered as an industrial-business complex composed of a multitude of direct care providers supported by a vast array of technological and economic providers. In general, the health care complex must reflect the pluralistic health care needs of society; therefore, a variety of health care delivery models is required. Insofar as possible, the individual, in determining the quality of his life, must have the freedom to choose a health care delivery model best suited to his wants, needs, and economic resources.

MAJOR CHALLENGES FOR NURSING

As indicated earlier, nursing has an integral role in health care delivery. In addition to having the largest number of health care professionals, nursing has vital dependent and independent functions, within a comprehensive health care system. The unique biosocial syntax of the nursing discipline offers a health care delivery system a cohesive force. Nurses functioning as patient advocates can generally make primary entry decisions as well as coordinate and facilitate the individual's participation in any health care system. Interdependent functions in delivering particular diagnostic, restorative, and rehabilitation services are shared with other health care professionals. Relatively few nursing functions are solely dependent on the knowledge and skill of another health professional. Currently, the major challenges for nursing in health care delivery are colleague participation, preparation and maintenance of expanding roles, and self-renewal.

Perhaps the most difficult challenge in effecting change in the structure and function of health care delivery is that of establishing and maintaining colleague relationships of the various health professions. Current structures and functions are generally founded in past knowledge and traditional professional attitude. There is little common understanding and appreciation among health professionals of the educational foundation and functional skills of health disciplines other than their own. This situation perpetuates archaic attitudes and inhibits transition to more appropriate constellations of health care professionals. Likewise, responsibility for various areas of health care remain inappropriately placed. Redistribution of responsibility and rewards among the health professionals is essential to deliver comprehensive health care for today's society.

Nursing is one of the health professions that has traditionally been considered, particularly by the medical profession, to have few independent functions and analytic judgments. Therefore, the establishing of colleague relationships with other health professions is an arduous task that requires patience and perseverance. Nursing leaders must take the initiative to alter old hierarchical structures of organization and to enlighten other health professionals as to the invaluable contributions nursing makes in comprehensive health care. Traditional attitudes and power structures are neither easily nor quickly changed. Thus, nurses must maintain their resilience and versatility to direct their efforts for effecting these changes where there is high probability for success and the resultant ramifications of the change will be widespread.

Colleague relationships are built on mutual understanding and respect. To establish these relationships requires nursing professionals to be as eager to learn about other health professions as to share the virtues of nursing. Once initiated, the colleague relationship must be strengthened and maintained. In many ways this nurturing process is easier because it is done in the concrete world of work. Nevertheless, the participants must recognize that these relationships will evidence the signs and symptoms of growth and development. Building mutual trust, teaching each other skills, and appropriately rotating team leadership is stressful to even the most mature of health professionals. This mutual sharing and development necessitates self-confident, knowledgeable, skillful participants. Only those possessing these qualities and having sincere commitment to changing the health care system should embark upon this challenge.

Interrelated with establishing and maintaining colleague relationships is the challenge of preparing and maintaining the expanding roles of nursing. The central contribution of nursing to com-

prehensive health care delivery does not change. It remains essentially the patient advocacy role. The expansion comes in developing peripheral skills and frequently results in role blurring with other disciplines. Increasing numbers of nurses are needed with these additional skills and abilities.

Nurse educators, having analyzed the past, and taken the pulse of the present, must direct their vision to the future. Prediction always has a degree of failure; however, nursing must be willing to take this risk to keep pace with the rapidly changing demands for nursing services. Innovative educational programs must anticipate the skills needed by their graduates to practice effectively in multidisciplinary situations. And as far as possible supply should keep pace with demand for nurses to function in developing health care delivery systems. One way to meet this challenge is to develop and/or participate in demonstration projects attempting to improve the quality of health care.

To discuss the specific preparation for any given role today would be relatively superfluous for tomorrow. The preparation of the nurse clinician requires constant curriculum revision. It should be noted that nurse clinicians, as do teachers, administrators, and researchers, require knowledge and skills derived from experiencing graduate study. Their skill in self-directed and disciplined learning should enable them to maintain their positions on the edge of expansion. Nurse practitioners functioning in newly developed roles, such as the pediatric or adult nurse practitioner, generally have a specific, short-term educational experience for that particular role. Therefore, it is unreasonable to expect most nurse practitioners to function beyond the presently developed roles.

Nursing education must accept the responsibility of providing learning opportunities to fill the needs for nurses to function in expanded roles. Three levels of students are readily identified: teachers, practicing nurses, and nursing students. Because changes occur with such rapidity and demands for personnel to function in these new roles are immediate, simultaneous learning must take place on these three levels. In the past, this has generally been accomplished by faculty inservice or development programs (and not infrequently by independent action), continuing education programs, such as the Primex program, and, finally, integration into basic nursing education programs. Perhaps this aspect of the educational challenge could be better met by more innovative learning experiences for all these students. At least the possibilities should be explored, such as an undergraduate nursing student and teacher learning newly developing roles together.

Along with the continued, individual self-renewal suggested above, nursing needs to provide opportunities for parallel development and research with other health professions. Self-renewal of the discipline and profession of nursing is essential to the improvement of the delivery of health care. Historically, nurses themselves have provided the greatest resistance to meeting this challenge. However, antiintellectualism and fear of new responsibility and accountability of the past are fading. New attitudes of acceptance and respect for nurse researchers and innovators are gaining strength in the profession. Like the individual, a professional group must also have self-respect and confidence to have a colleague relationship with other professions. It allows for interdisciplinary search for new ways of delivering health care to the American people and in some instances beyond.

A growing number of nurses now possess comparable research knowledge and skill to fully participate in interdisciplinary research and demonstration projects. Indeed nurses should be primary investigators on some projects. Again the responsibility for dispelling the traditional attitudes of other disciplines toward nursing's research capabilities rests with the nursing profession itself. As the profession gives greater recognition to the value of the nurse researcher, so too will the other professions and finally society. Then the doors will be clearly opened to the complemental definition of health care delivery systems.

It seems quite obvious to this writer that the challenges presented in health care delivery offer nursing the circumstantial factors to emerge with its mature stature. The intrinsic elements of the nursing discipline (art and science) are fundamental to the development of high quality health care delivery systems. What remains then is for nursing to seize these opportunities—to fulfill its long-held aspiration for humane, health-oriented delivery systems of care.

References

1. Nightingale, F.: Notes on Nursing. London, Harrison and Sons. 1860, p. 6.
2. Darkness at noon. Newsweek, Aug. 27, 1973, p. 88.
3. Best, C. H. and Taylor, N. B. (eds.): The Physiological Basis of Medical Practice, ed. 8. Baltimore, Williams & Wilkins, 1966, p. 1443.
4. Dubos, R.: Man Adapting. New Haven, Yale University Press, 1965, p. 68.
5. U.S. Department of Health, Education and Welfare: Current Research on Sleep and Dreams. Washington, D.C., U.S. Government Printing Office, 1966, p. 5.
6. Selye, H.: The Stress of Life. New York, McGraw-Hill, 1956, pp. 226-277.
7. *Ibid.*, p. 277
8. Speech given by Dr. Delbert Oberteuffer, at the 22nd National Conference on Rural Health, Philadelphia, Mar. 21, 1969.
9. Kahn, H.: Thinking About the Unthinkable. New York, Avon Books, 1962, pp. 133-185.
10. Henderson, V.: The nature of nursing. Am. J. Nurs. 64:62-68, Aug. 1964.
11. U.S. Department of Health, Education and Welfare: Services for the Poor. Washington, D.C., U.S. Government Printing Office, 1967.
12. The surge of community involvement. Medical World News May 19, 1972, p. 37.
13. The staggering cost of applying our knowledge. Medical World News June, 2, 1972, p. 40.

Bibliography

Bennis, W., Benne, K. and Chin, R.: The Planning of Change, ed. 2. New York, Holt, Rinehart and Winston, 1969.
Birdwhistell, R. L.: Kinesics and Content. Philadelphia, University of Pennsylvania Press, 1970.

Brockington, F.: World Health, ed. 2. Boston, Little, Brown, 1968.

Bush, V.: Science Is Not Enough. New York, William Morrow, 1967.

Changing Patterns of Nursing Practice: New Needs, New Roles. New York, Am. J. Nurs. Company, 1971.

Culclasure, D. F.: Medical benefits from space research. Am. J. Nurs. 74:275-278, Feb. 1974.

DeChow, R.: Research + primex = improved health service. Internat. Nurs. Review 19:319-27, 1972.

Dubos: Mirage of Health. New York, Doubleday, 1959.

Ehrlich, G. E.: Health challenges of the future. Annals Am. Acad. Pol. and Soc. Sci. 408:70-82, Jul. 1973.

Gardner, J. W.: Self-Renewal. New York, Harper Colophon Books, 1965.

Garfield, S.: The delivery of medical care. Sci. Am. 222, 4:15-23, Apr. 1970.

Goffman, E.: Strategic Interaction. Philadelphia, University of Pennsylvania Press, 1970.

Gordon, G.: Role Theory and Illness. New Haven, College and University Press, 1966.

Hall, E. T.: The Hidden Dimension. Garden City, New York, Anchor Books, 1969.

————: The Silent Language. New York, Doubleday, 1959.

Health Care Needs—Basis for Change. New York, National League for Nursing, 1968.

Hymovich, D. P. and Barnard, M. U. (eds.): Family Health Care. New York, McGraw-Hill, 1973.

Ingelfinger, F. J.: Haves and have-nots in the world of disease. New Eng. J. Med. 287:1198-1199, Dec. 7, 1972.

Mayeroff, M.: On Caring. New York, Harper & Row, 1971.

Miller, D. L.: A mythologist looks at the realities of comprehensive health planning. Nurs. Outlook 17:24-27, Jul. 1969.

National Advisory Commission on Health Facilities: A Report to the President. Washington, D.C., U.S. Government Printing Office, 1968.

Saward, E. W.: The organization of medical care. Sci. Am. 229:169-175, Sept. 1973.

Sigerist, H. E.: Civilization and Disease. Chicago, University of Chicago Press, 1943.

Taylor, C.: In Horizontal Orbit: Hospitals and the Cult of Efficiency. New York, Holt, Rinehart and Winston, 1970.

The Fitness of Man's Environment. Smithsonian Annual II. New York, Harper & Row, 1968.

U.S. Department of Health, Education and Welfare: Toward a Social Report. Washington, D.C., U.S. Government Printing Office, 1969.

Vaillot, Sister Madeleine Clemence: Existentialism: a philosophy of commitment. Am. J. Nurs. 66:500-505, Mar. 1966.

Vickers, G.: Value Systems and Social Process. Middlesex, England, Penguin Books, 1970.

Williams, R. J.: Free and Unequal. New York, John Wiley & Sons, Science Editions, 1964.

3

Some Psychological Concepts of Health-Related Behavior

BARBARA LOWERY

Mental Health • *Psyche-Soma Dualism* • *Crisis Intervention* • *Multiproblem Families* • *Locus of Control* • *Psychological Reactance* • *Compliance with the Treatment Regimen*

What is it that we are striving for? Why is it that we desire the "best" (however we define that term) in family life, in the school, in the university, in the community? It is, I believe, because we hope to develop the "best" of human beings. But rarely do we give explicit thought to the exact meaning of this goal. What sort of human being do we wish to grow?[1]

For the past twenty years, the United States has been focusing increasing attention on the mental health of its citizens. The provisions of the Mental Health Study Act of 1955 established a Joint Commission on Mental Illness and Health. This commission focused its efforts on two general areas: the current care of the mentally ill and the current concepts of mental health. In its final report, *Action for Mental Health*, the Commission summarized the results of its work and offered an outline for change. Pointing to the ineffectiveness of the existing treatment-oriented programs, it suggested that concerned groups turn their attention to the promotion of mental health, as well as to the treatment and rehabilitation of existing illness. As federal funding became available in the early 1960s, community mental health centers developed. Those professional groups traditionally associated with the treatment of the mentally ill—psychiatrists, psychologists, nurses, and social workers—began to move into the community with a commitment to mental health maintenance as well as to mental health restoration.

Other groups also began to indicate their concern for mental health. Human relations training with its encounter, sensitivity, and T-group experiences became common occurrences in industries, schools, and church organizations. While psychoanalysis still remained available for the affluent upper class, couples groups and transactional analysis groups were introduced to the suburban middle class. To be a more effective member of a group, to become more sensitive to one's own and others' feelings, to allow yourself to be more open to the potentials that life holds, all became the legitimate goals of the day.

But what sort of human beings are we growing? Do the above goals eventuate in mental health? The youth who says he has reached these goals through drug use might be defined by many as mentally ill. Efforts to evaluate the new mental health programs are just beginning. The reader has already been introduced to the idea that health should be defined as more than just the absence of disease (see Chapter 2). Thus, evaluation of mental health programs must include more than determining whether the incidence of diagnosed mental illness has decreased. But as was true when the Joint Commission began its study in 1955, there is still no clearly delineated concept of mental health to guide evaluation efforts. In the first of the Commission's monographs, Jahoda called for extensive research to delineate criteria of mental health and the conditions affecting its acquisition and maintenance.[2] Unfortunately, the need for this research still exists today.

Just what is mental health? Perhaps the average citizen would be satisfied with the criterion of absence of mental illness. But if it is more than this, is it being "average," or "normal," or "happy?" As the next section will show, there is no clear and concise definition of mental health that is broadly accepted. Thus, the nurse who is assessing a patient's response to his or her current situation in terms of whether it is mentally healthy or unhealthy may find it difficult to get consensual validation for whichever judgment she makes.

This chapter cannot hope to fill the major gap in research noted by Jahoda. Instead, it will attempt to focus on providing a broadened understanding of a patient's or family's psychological response to the health situation in which each finds himself. There will be no attempt to review what the reader has already learned in basic psychology or psychiatric nursing courses. Hopefully, the concepts discussed will add to the knowledge already gained.

After a brief discussion of the current state of the concept "mental health," the chapter will turn to the psyche-soma dualism, basic issues in crisis intervention, and a view of the multiproblem family. Later sections will deal largely with two of the more recently delineated psychological variables which may shed more light on the conditions affecting the patient's response to the health situation and his or her subsequent compliance with the prescribed regimen.

Mental Health

It may surprise the reader to know that there is only about one chance in 6,500 that he individually has a medium size stomach, a heart with medium pumping capacity, a thyroid gland of medium activity, a medium number of islets of Langerhans in his pancreas, a medium calcium requirement and a medium Vitamin A requirement. If we make the number of categories larger, and even if we enlarge the median group to include much more than the middle one-third, the chance that any individual will be in the median group in all respects is so small as to be negligible.[3]

Williams's statement highlights one of the many difficulties one encounters when attempting to define what is "normal," "average," or "healthy." Does variation from the statistical norm signify abnormality? If it does, according to Williams's figures, most of us are biologically abnormal in one sense or another, and few, if any, individuals can be considered "normal" in all respects. But if variation, even in the biological sense, is expected, the question becomes: How much variation is "normal," "average," or "healthy"? At what point does variation become "abnormal" or "unhealthy"? And who has the right to specify this point: the individual? his family? physicians? the state? society?

Definitions of mental health are similarly divided. According to some views, mental health, like being medium in all respects biologically, is an ideal which is seldom, if ever, reached.

Offer and Sabshin review much of the psychoanalytical literature related to normality (mental health). They summarize their review as follows:

In our opinion, the underlying and pervasive philosophical premise is that all men are at least part-neurotic. According to the dominant psychoanalytic motif, the normal man is the near-perfect man and perfection is an ideal that living men can never reach, albeit a few select individuals have, at times, come close to the ideal.[4]

Another definition of mental health as an ideal state is offered by Carl Rogers. He describes the ultimate goal which actual clients approach but never fully reach—the fully functioning person. Among other characteristics:

He is able to live fully in and with each and all of his feelings and reactions. He is making use of all his organic equipment to sense, as accurately as possible, the existential situation within and without. . . . He is able to permit his total organism to function in all its complexity in selecting, from the multitude of possibilities, that behavior which in this moment of time will be most generally and genuinely satisfying. . . . He is able to experience all of his feelings; he is his own sifter of evidence, but is open to evidence from all sources; he is completely engaged in the process of being and becoming himself, and thus discovers that he is soundly and realistically social. . . . He is a fully functioning organism, and because of the awareness of himself which flows freely in and through his experiences, he is a fully functioning person.[5]

Melanie Kline, who describes the integrated personality as one which is mentally healthy, states: "Complete integration never exists, but the more it has succeeded, and the more the individual is able to have insight into his anxieties and impulses . . . the greater will be his mental balance."[6]

Clearly, according to this theoretical view, few, if any, individuals whom the nurse encounters in practice will be mentally healthy. Further, concern with the maintenance of a mentally healthy state, which the nurse is not likely to encounter, would seem a somewhat illogical goal. Treatment of existing mental illness or prevention of further disabling symptoms might be the more logical focus of nursing efforts.

Other definitions stated that health or normality is an attainable goal. Sociological definitions, which generally depict the mentally healthy person as one whose behavior or functioning is within the limits set by the culture, fall within this group. Parsons for example, states that "Health may be defined as the state of optimum *capacity* of an individual for the effective performance of the roles and tasks for which he has been socialized."[7]

Erich Fromm sees the mentally healthy person as

. . . the productive and unalienated person: the person who relates himself to the world lovingly, and who uses his reason to grasp reality objectively; who experiences himself as a unique individual entity, and at the same time feels one with his fellow man; who is not subject to irrational authority, and accepts willingly the rational authority of conscience and reason; who is in the process of being born as long as he is alive, and considers the gift of life the most precious chance he has.[8]

Karl Menninger also views mental health as an attainable goal:

. . . the adjustment of human beings to the world and to each other with a maximum of effectiveness and happiness. Not just efficiency, or just contentment—or the grace of obeying the rules of the game cheerfully. It is all of these together. It is the ability to maintain an even temper, an alert intelligence, socially considerate behavior, and a happy disposition.[9]

Saul describes mental and emotional health as

. . . the adequate achievement of emotional maturity, which means the growth from helplessness and need for love to the capacity to love, to be a good, responsible spouse, parent, and citizen; and this depends upon good human reactions in the earliest years, for the pattern of these feelings and relationships continue on through adult life.[10]

While all of these definitions clearly imply that mental health is attainable, one major problem in using them as guides for assessment of the mental health of an individual is obvious. The problem is one of values. For example, who is to define what is "productive," "objective," "rational," "good," "responsible," "loving," "happy," "even-tempered," and "considerate"? Although such definitions provide a logical base for the discussion of mental health maintenance, their value-laden descriptions of the mentally healthy person pose practical problems when delineation of specific maintaining activities is attempted.

While suggesting strongly that much research is necessary before mental health can be adequately described, Jahoda provides some direction for practice. She points out that mental health might be defined in at least one of two ways:

> . . . as a *relatively constant and enduring function of personality*, leading to predictable differences in behavior and feelings depending on the stresses and strains of the situations in which a person finds himself; or as a *momentary function of personality and situation*. Looking at mental health in the first way will lead to a classification of individuals as more or less healthy; looking at it in the second way, will lead to a classification of actions as more or less healthy.[11]

She further clarifies this distinction:

> Take a strong man with a bad cold. According to the first, he is healthy; according to the second he is sick. Both statements are justifiable and useful. But utter confusion will result if either of these correct diagnoses are made in the wrong context—that is, if he is regarded as a permanently sick person or as one who is functioning healthily. Much of the confusion in the area of mental health stems from the failure to establish whether one is talking about mental health as an enduring attribute of a person or as a momentary attribute of functioning.[12]

While speaking from a different framework, Maslow describes the problem similarly:

> The classical approach to personality problems considers them to be problems in an undesirable sense. Struggle, conflict, guilt, bad conscience, anxiety, depression, frustration, tension, shame, self-punishment, feelings of inferiority or unworthiness—they all cause psychic pain, they disturb efficiency of performance, and they are uncontrollable. They are therefore automatically regarded as sick and undesirable and they get "cured" away as soon as possible.
>
> But all of these symptoms are found in healthy people, or in people who are growing toward health. . . . In essence I am deliberately rejecting our present easy distinction between sickness and health, at least as far as surface symptoms are concerned. Does sickness mean having symptoms? I maintain now that sickness might consist of not having symptoms when you should. Does health mean being symptom free? I deny it.[13]

The above statements seem extremely relevant to nursing practice. According to both views, the presence of psychological conflicts should not lead to the identification of the individual as mentally ill. Nor should a statement identifying an individual as mentally healthy (or as free from mental illness) lead the nurse to believe that he or she will not have psychic conflicts. The more recent theory of and research in crisis intervention follow these views. While staying fairly clear of classifying individuals as mentally ill or healthy, proponents of crisis intervention direct themselves to the study of psychic conflict, crises, and their resolution. (See pp. 42 to 45 for a review of some of the basic concepts in crisis theory and intervention).

In summary, the above problems of conceptualizing mental health are only a few of those that are outlined in current literature. Their presentation here is not an effort to induce the nurse to accept one theoretical framework or another, but rather to emphasize the need for further research toward a more broadly acceptable conceptualization of mental health.

Psyche-Soma Dualism

Before discussing psychic conflict and other psychological responses to illness, a brief review of mind-body dualism seems warranted. The reader has already been introduced to the concept of the individual as an integrated entity (see Chapter 1). Consideration of the "whole patient" and "nursing the psyche as well as the soma" are but two of the phrases found in current nursing literature which deals with this concept.

In their educational programs, modern nurses may have learned of the age-old philosophical arguments about the mind and body as separate entities. But after introduction to the work of Hans Selye and current literature on psychophysiological disorders, they probably agree that the mind and body are not separate, but integrated. Selye's work provides extensive descriptions of the physiological changes which occur with stress. Moreover, diseases such as peptic ulcer, asthma, and ulcerative colitis are commonly accepted as having stress as a major etiological base. Many nurses might think that the dualistic approach has long-since been rejected by health professionals. However, a few examples will illustrate that dualism is still present in today's nursing practice.

For example, the nurse who encounters a patient in pain, and asks, "How much of this patient's pain is physical and how much is psychological?" asks a dualistic question. She apparently sees the psyche and soma not only as separate entities, but as entities which are somehow additive.

Consider the nurse in an emergency room or a critical care unit who emphatically states, "My first task is to keep the patient alive; I will worry about his psychological problems later." This nurse is attempting to practice in a dualistic manner. Moreover, she fails to recognize that the existing physical problems may become even more grave as physiological stress (psychologically termed anxiety) overtaxes vital organs.

Nurses who contend that they are much too busy on their unit or in their agency to deal with psychological matters, and psychiatric nurses who fail to consider obvious physical problems are further examples. With all due respect to nurses who do not practice in this way, it seems that the view of the psyche and soma as separate entities is still prevalent in nursing today.

Nurses who recognize some of their own practices in the above examples might consider the following statement by Rotter:

> The alternative to . . . dualism is to consider that events take place in space time and that descriptions of these events or constructions from these events may be made from many different points of view. The psychological and physiological represent points of view regarding an event. . . . There are also biological, biochemical, sociological, and economic points of view. . . .[14]

For example, every event of human pain the nurse encounters can be described from both physiological and psychological viewpoints. The nurse who elects to view the event from only a physiological framework necessarily limits her *planned* intervention to physiological solutions. That physical intervention is planned does not limit the nurse's intervention to physical means. Someone viewing the whole event from the psychological framework will see the nurse's entrance into the event as effecting a psychological change, whether planned or unplanned.

The nurse in the emergency situation provides an even better example of the problem. Carrying out what is described as excellent physical care based on assessment of the patient's physical status is obviously extremely important. But if one is describing the whole event of the emergency from a psychological framework, the impact of the nurse's entrance into the event and each interaction thereafter will be considered in terms of its positive or negative effects on the patient. The fallacy, of course, is in the nurse's belief that psychological intervention will occur at some later time. It may be true that *planned* intervention occurs later, but the nurse at that point must realize that a great deal of unplanned psychological intervention has gone before.

In the case of the psychiatric patient who has attempted suicide by slashing her wrists, much of the immediate care on the psychiatric unit will center on preventing further attempts and establishing an interpersonal bond. If concern about nursing care of a patient with possible tendon or nerve injury does not occur immediately, the result can be loss of the use of an extremity for the patient. Someone viewing this event from the physiological framework may see the nursing care of this patient as contributing to an already grave problem.

On the other hand, when the nurse believes that each event she encounters might be described from a physical, emotional, social, spiritual, or economic viewpoint, planned intervention to deal with problems gleaned from each view is possible. When the nurse judges that the problem as viewed from one or more of these areas is beyond her skill in that area, she should call upon the appropriate person to intervene.

The alternative to this kind of nursing activity is to provide someone who will view each of the nurse's encounters with the patient from those viewpoints the nurse fails to consider. Caplan, in speaking of this problem in relation to primary prevention of mental illness, states:

> It must be recognized that, although the caregiving professions are the agents of the community in fostering the well-being of a citizen and in

helping him deal with unfavorable circumstances, their functioning is not traditionally designated in regard to its effect on the mental health of their clients.[15]

He further suggests that, in the case of some professions, the alternative to changing their characteristic "professional *persona*," which may not consider their own or the patient's psychological reaction to an event, is the addition of another person to the group. Using obstetricians as an example he states: "This person would not attempt to persuade the obstetrician to change his ways, but only to permit someone else to have collaborative access to his patients."[16]

If, on the other hand, the profession believes that it must consider the "whole patient," as nursing professes to do, adding another worker to assess the psychological impact of the situation should be unnecessary. For, as is further noted by Caplan, if the addition of another worker is necessary in too many professions, ". . . the program of primary prevention (of mental illness) would inevitably fail because of lack of human resources."[17]

Nursing education has long believed that some knowledge of the skill in the psychology and sociology of the patient are essential. One can only hope that each nurse also develops a personal commitment to the use of what she has learned, regardless of the situations in which she encounters the patient.

Crisis Intervention

The current emphasis on mental health is evidenced by the use of such terms as mental health professionals, mental health centers, mental health legislation, and so on. But the fact is that most so-called mental health efforts are still directed toward individuals who are diagnosed mentally ill. The major exception is crisis intervention. Parad and Caplan, two of the earlier proponents of crisis intervention, recognize that ". . . conflict and unhappiness are not synonymous with mental ill health; in fact, at the appropriate time and place the presence of conflict and unhappiness is a criterion of mental health."[18] However, the unsuccessful resolution of conflict can result in diagnosed mental illness.

Throughout this text, the reader will be reminded that psychic conflict is likely to be a part of any of the nursing situations described. In family planning, for example, a woman ". . . may be confronted with severe conflict because of discord between the values she holds and those to which she is exposed" (Ch. 5). In the critical care setting: "The typical patient remains oriented and rational, but demonstrates verbally or nonverbally the nerve-racking effect of pain, anxiety about the future or death itself, and loss of positive body- and/or self-image" (Ch. 10). The cardiac patient "suffers greater problems than most from stress related to his own welfare, the everyday concerns he has been removed from, and his environment" (Ch. 12). The severely burned patient faces ". . . threat to survival, fear of disfigurement . . ., feelings of inadequacy and rejection, emotional overtones associated with the accident, possible effect of injury on future plans, and conflict engendered by a state of utter dependency" (Ch. 11). And in the diagnosis of a hereditary disorder in medical genetics, "The far-reaching effects of guilt and sorrow disrupt individual and family life, sometimes to catastrophic proportions" (Ch. 6).

Examples of psychic conflict could be extended to human situations the nurse encounters in whatever setting she works. Thus, the theory of and research in crisis intervention are most appropriately included in any discussion related to the nurse's concern with the mental health of her patients. Understanding of the techniques of crisis intervention might also enhance nursing assessment, planning, and intervention with patients, regardless of the degree of conflict present.

Crisis theory suggests that when conflict arises, the individual attempts to reduce the resultant anxiety by using problem-solving mechanisms that have helped him in the past. For some individuals this may involve immediate attempts to identify the problem, collect the facts associated with it, generate possible solutions, and begin testing these solutions. For others, there may be initial denial that any problem exists and a later, gradual recognition of the problem and a working through of possible solutions. (Individual differences related to problem solving in crisis and other situations will be discussed in a later section.) The use of other mechanisms, such as regression, anger, depression, and projection of blame for the problem, might also be part of the eventual resolution.* Thus, the personality of the individual and his past history of other conflict-solving methods are important variables for the nurse to consider.

Another major variable in conflict resolution is the nature of the problem itself. Obviously, a situation that the individual views as an everyday problem of living or one which he or she has previously resolved successfully will evoke less anxiety than one which he or she views as a major threat to his or her existing equilibrium. A number of conflicts arising simultaneously might also lessen the individual's ability to deal with one or all effectively.

The nature of the social relationships to which the individual can turn for help in resolving conflict is also of major importance. In the usual health-related situation, the individual's family is the primary social field in which conflict resolution occurs. Other helping sources, such as friends, neighbors, or clergy, may also be part of the usual interpersonal problem-solving resources.

Conflict becomes crisis when, as Caplan notes:

> The usual homeostatic, direct problem-solving mechanisms do not work, and the problem is such that other methods which might be used to sidestep it also cannot be used. In other words, the problem is one where the individual is faced by stimuli which signal danger to a fundamental need satisfaction or evoke major need appetite, and the circumstances are such that habitual problem-solving methods are unsuccessful within the time span of past expectations of success.[19]

In addition to symptoms of severe anxiety and obvious acute emotional upset, the individual in crisis may also evidence feelings of helplessness and inability to cope with his current life situation. The acute episode may last several weeks. Whether the individual emerges from the crisis psychologically stronger or weaker depends, according to Caplan, on the kind of help received during the crisis as well as upon the factors described above.[20]

Situations which may evoke crises are also described by Caplan:

> Such problems have usually consisted of novel situations that the individual has not been able to handle . . . The problems have been both serious and unavoidable, such as the death of a loved person; loss or change of a job; a threat to bodily integrity by illness, accident, or surgical operation; or change of role due to developmental or sociocultural transitions, such as going to college, getting married, and becoming a parent.[21]

While such situations might be defined by helping professionals as *potential* crisis situations, the actual event of crisis must be defined by the individual. "Crisis must be looked at through an individual, or perhaps, a group's definition of it: what is a crisis to one person is an episode in zestful living to another."[22]

When a potential crisis situation exists, and when the patient gives the nurse indications that he is becoming increasingly unable to cope with the current conflict, it becomes vitally important that the patient receive help. The nurse who feels inadequate to deal with the situation should refer the patient to the psychiatric nurse consultant of her unit or agency. However, it is also important that the nurse understand the major elements of crisis intervention which must be considered when planning any nursing care during the time of crisis.

While several paradigms for crisis intervention have been described in the literature, the following steps are basic to most crisis intervention efforts.

1. The patient and his family must be helped to identify the problem that confronts them. They must be encouraged to realize and talk about the facts of the situation they face. Cadden points out that the facts of even the most difficult situations are often much less painful than the fantasies that are generated in the absence of facts. She further

---

*The concepts of anxiety and the defense mechanisms commonly seen in patients with physical illness have been discussed extensively in other nursing literature and thus will not be reviewed here. The nurse who is not familiar with these concepts might find the work of Francis and Munjas or that of Carlson most valuable. (Francis, A. and Munjas, B.: Promoting Psychological Comfort. Iowa, Wm. C. Brown, 1968. Carlson, C. (coordinator): Behavioral Concepts and Nursing Intervention. Philadelphia, J. B. Lippincott, 1970.)

cautions, however, that these facts must be confronted in manageable doses—that is, the individual may need time in which to direct his thinking away from the crisis.[23]

Unfortunately, the medical situation for patients in crisis and for those whose conflicts are not of crisis proportions may present blocks to their usual problem-solving efforts. The patient may be unable to get enough facts to define the problem which confronts him. While his whole being may sense that something is drastically wrong, and while this feeling may be enhanced by his interaction with evasive persons who are caring for him, his questions directed toward defining the problem often go unanswered. It seems that in these instances, the interference may be responsible for precipitating crises. In their research with mothers of extremely premature babies, Kaplan and Mason found that while many mothers actively sought information about the possibilities of life or death for their babies, "In general, there seems to be no prompt and frank discussion about the prognosis or cause of prematurity, and a state of suspense is encouraged."[24] Yet without this information the mothers were unable to begin the psychological tasks related to solving the problem.

The problem of data gathering has been further specified by the research of Dodge.[25] Her results indicate that patients were most concerned about the seriousness of their situations. They were interested in hearing about the chances of recovery, the possibilities of recurrence of their problem, the results of surgical or diagnostic procedures, and the complexity of their cases. However, Dodge found that none of this information was rated as highly important by the nurses. They felt that information to prepare the patient for present or future care was highly important. Patients saw these data as less important than answers to the previously listed questions.

While there may be patients who do not wish to gather this kind of information, Dodge's research suggests that many patients do want to clarify what is happening to them relative to their health. The responsibility for answering certain of the patient's questions is said by many nurses to belong only to the physician. This does not relieve the nurse of the responsibility of communicating to the patient's physician that the patient is actively seeking this kind of information. Frequently, even when the patient has heard some facts about his or her problem, questions will remain that the nurse should attempt to answer.

2. Another major step in crisis intervention is to encourage the individual or family to accept help from other helping sources close to them—clergy, extended family members, neighbors, and so on—or relevant health professional in the situation. Frequently, while these helpers may not provide direct solutions to the problem, their entrance into the situation relieves some of the everyday worries and may reduce anxiety enough that problem solving can move forward. As noted earlier, one of the major variables in crisis is the social field in which it occurs. The family is generally the interpersonal resource which is most effective in assisting with the working through of the problem. In the view of many writers, crisis is a family phenomenon and not limited to an individual. That particular view will be discussed further in the next section.

Unfortunately, the medical situation may create a shortage of interpersonal help instead of supplying it. While the resources of the family are generally mobilized immediately to help a member who is facing a conflict, the medical situation frequently interferes with this process. All too often the patient's family is asked to absent itself from the patient during his most stressful periods. Perhaps this practice could be justified if nursing or other medical personnel were capable and willing to fill the gap. However, as noted earlier many nurses admit to having very little time to concern themselves with psychological problems. When the family is excluded, and this gap is not filled, the patient is left, virtually isolated, to solve the problem. While there do seem to be a few situations in which the presence of the patient's family might aggravate the situation, these are far too few to warrant the widespread practice of sending the family away while nursing care is being given. Instead of encouraging the gathering of facts and the mobilization of resources, this practice may aggravate the problem.

3. Another factor of major importance in crisis in-

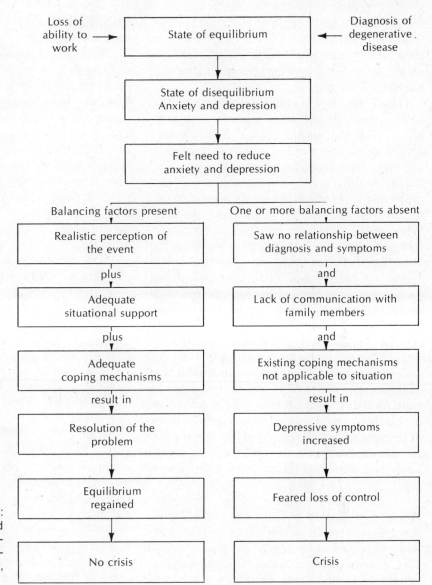

FIGURE 3-1.
Crisis intervention. Source:
Aguilera, D., Messick, J. and
Farrell, M.: Crisis Intervention: Theory and Methodology. St. Louis, C. V. Mosby,
1970.

tervention is the determination with the individual and family, of the strengths which they
have in their own individual or social systems
which can be brought to bear on the problem.
Both need to believe that they are strong enough
to cope with the present conflict, and focusing on
current strengths and past successful coping efforts can reinforce this belief. Where gaps seem
to exist, suggestions of other coping mechanisms
or helping agents may assist resolution.

While the paradigm has elements that differ
from those presented above, a summary of the

crisis situation of a patient faced with the diagnosis of a degenerative disease may further
clarify the crisis intervention process. Fig. 3-1
presents the situation as outlined by Aguilera, *et
al.*[26]

Multiproblem Families

Community health nurses have long been confronted with the task of working with multiproblem families. However, it has been only in recent
years that research in and literature on family

therapy have been directed toward such families. While the nurse who has encountered these families may need no description of them, the multiproblem family can best be characterized by examples.

The T. family was referred to the community health agency by the physician who discharged Mr. T. from the hospital. Mr. T. had suffered a severe stroke and was still unable to walk without help. During the first few weeks, the community health nurse encountered the following problems: 1) No one in the family wanted to care for Mr. T. in the intervals between nursing visits. While he still lived in the house, most family relationships with Mr. T. had apparently been broken off years before the stroke occurred. 2) Mrs. T. lost her job in a local factory because of seasonal layoffs. 3) The adolescent daughter who was living in the household ran away and was not located by police for eight days. 4) Upon her return, she confided to the community health nurse that she was three-months pregnant and had sought no antepartal care. 5) Another adolescent daughter was about to be discharged from the state mental hospital adolescent unit, and no one in the family felt she could be managed at home. 6) Because of the sudden loss of income, the family was unable to pay the rent for their present home and was being forced to seek other housing.

The A. family was referred for therapy to a mental health center because one of the family's three adolescent daughters ran away from home and was picked up by police. The authorities felt Mrs. A. needed help in controlling this daughter. Within six weeks of their entry into therapy, the following events (along with several others) occurred: 1) The youngest child (a male) was diagnosed as retarded educable (RE) and was being changed to an RE class in the city school system against the wishes of the mother. 2) The two other daughters were harassed by a girls' gang on their way home from school, and one of the A. girls stabbed a gang member with a small penknife. Police and the courts became involved in this episode. 3) The father of the male child was found dead in a distant city. 4) Another of the mother's male friends, who had been living in the household and providing some financial support, left suddenly.

From the previous discussion on crisis, it can be seen that each of the episodes in the above examples might have been viewed as a crisis. However, while the therapist and the community health nurse were both tempted to view each event as a crisis and were frantically trying to provide substantial support, neither family seemed to view any of these events as crises. They apparently saw the problems as the kinds which typically confront families such as their own. Moreover, they seemed to feel little pressure to focus on and resolve each problem as it occurred.

Maloney terms such families "crisis generators." Of their life style she states:

> A relatively simple question can be asked: what makes this person or family feel alive? From whence comes the zest for the battle?. . . If, in early life, a subtle or overt pattern of moving from one emergency state to another is given value, then it may become a way of life for selected offspring. . . . The symptoms in later life can be identified as relating to people whose finest hours are when they are fighting (a) the system, (b) someone they love, (c) absolute strangers, and (d) passing acquaintances.[27]

In both of the above cases, the nurse who attempts to find solutions to each problem will eventually become exhausted. Again, in relation to "crisis generators," Maloney makes the point that "Those in the helping occupations patch up each new emergency only to find another looming; finally, panting in the rear, the professionals consign the individual or family to a category known as hard-core cases."[28]

Referral of this kind of family to a community mental health center is probably not too common. Moreover, since it may be the professional and not the family who sees the situation as crisis prone, some commitment by the family to become involved in therapy may be difficult to get. While no ready answers are available, some points may help guide the nurse who encounters the multiproblem family. First, the nurse should assess who is in crisis, she or the family. She should try to get some picture of how the family members seem to be responding to each event. She may determine that they respond with much less anxiety than she does, regardless of the apparent dire nature of the event. She may also find that they believe that most, if not all, of life's successes will come to them through someone else's efforts. The likelihood is that this kind of family will see little need for gathering facts and attempting to generate solutions for each problem that arises. (The concept of feelings of control versus feelings of noncontrol will be discussed in the next section.)

On the other hand, the nurse may find that the family members have a strong need to reestablish some control over life's events and that they do have some problem-solving resources to do so. Encouraging them to review and utilize their own strengths is of utmost importance. The professional who attempts to do the problem solving herself does the family a disservice.

As is true with all of the other concepts discussed in this chapter, much more research on multiproblem families and those approaches which are found effective with them is necessary. Since nursing often bears the major burden of confronting such families, research by those nurses involved would probably be most effective.

Locus of Control

It has been suggested throughout this chapter that the kind and amount of information a patient or family members desire about the illness situation and their overall behavior in response to it may be related to their psychological makeup as well as to the nature of the situation. No doubt the reader accepts this view to some degree. While there will be no attempt to review here what has been presented in the reader's basic psychology course, there are at least two recently delineated psychological variables which may further enhance the health team's understanding of a patient's or a family's response to a particular situation. Locus of control, the first variable to be discussed, has been studied extensively by social learning theorists for the past ten years. However, only recently have health pro-

fessionals begun to see its broad applicability to health situations.

As delineated by Rotter, the basic concept of locus of control is that a person's expectancy that reinforcement will occur in a given situation is likely to be based on past experiences in situations which he perceives as the same or similar.[29] Generalization of expectancies might then be predicted from knowledge of an individual's past reinforcement history. Each time an individual's behavior is followed by the expected reinforcement, the individual increases his or her expectancy that reinforcement is related to his or her own behavior. A history of reinforcements which have not necessarily been related to the individual's own efforts results in an expectancy that reinforcements are not contingent upon one's own behavior but are dependent upon an outside source.

These two different reinforcement patterns lead to different expectancies for control of rewards. An individual with an *internal* locus of control believes that rewards are contingent upon his own internal resources or skill. An individual with an *external* locus of control expects rewards to be externally related—that is, rewards are related to luck, chance, fate, or powerful others. Rotter states:

> From social learning theory one would anticipate that the more clearly and uniformly a situation is labeled as skill or luck determined in a given culture, the lesser the role such a generalized expectancy would play in determining individual differences in behavior.[30]

The situation of illness, hospitalization, and treatment is not clear-cut in terms of the source of reinforcement. There are many factors about the patient's return to health in which the patient is under the control of "powerful" medical others. The patient may view other aspects of the illness, treatment, and return to an optimum health level as more dependent upon his or her behavior. Thus, a person's feelings of control might play a rather strong role in the health situation.

For example, in the case of chronic disease there is frequently a need for the patient to control his or her own therapy following hospitalization. With diabetics, for example, Bondy states that

> . . . the physician merely acts as consultant, and the actual control of therapy lies in the hands of the patient. Education of the patient is therefore of paramount importance. He must learn the tools by which his disease is controlled and how to use them.[31]

However, a recent investigation by Lowery indicates that the learning of diabetics and the control of their disease is mediated to an extent, by the locus of control variable.[32] Other research also indicates that the variable should receive stronger consideration by health professionals.

Using the terms "powerlessness" and "alienation" with regard to degree of external feelings, Seeman and Evans studied learning in hospitalized white male tuberculosis patients.[33] With a primary focus of determining the amount of objective knowledge which a patient had about his illness, the investigation secondarily considered how this knowledge was reflected in the patient's behavior. The hypothesis was that patients who were high in alienation (external feelings of control) would know less about their illness than those who were less alienated (internal feelings of control). Using a true-false patient information test and a questionnaire for staff to answer, the investigators found, as predicted, that the more alienated patients knew less about their illness than those with some feelings of internal control. Staff questionnaires also indicated that the more "internal" patients seemed to evidence greater knowledge of their illness.

In another study, the defensive adoption of an external attitude and subsequent difficulties with hemodialysis patients' involvement in their treatment regimen was investigated. The hypothesis was that:

> . . . as an attempt to cope with the continuous responsibility and anxiety of keeping one's self alive by following a rigid treatment regimen, the hemodialysis patient adopts an external locus of control, with the result that his behavior is no longer perceived as life sustaining and a threatening area of responsibility is avoided.[34]

Twenty-two male hemodialysis patients who had been on the program for four months or longer were compared with a control group of 24 male patients in the convalescent stage of a minor medical condition. The groups were matched for age, race, socioeconomic level, and length of hospitalization. The significantly greater externality of hemodialysis patients over control patients, as measured by Rotter's I-E Scale, supported the hypothesis.

The obvious dangers inherent in external behavior on the part of patients who must be involved in their treatment regimen were noted by the authors.

> . . . In a chronically ill patient, external locus of control can produce disastrous consequences whenever his cooperation in his treatment is essential for him to remain alive. If the chronically ill patient perceives his behavior as being unrelated to his condition, the likelihood of his rejecting his role in the treatment program increases.[35]

For the hemodialysis patient, this rejection of his role in treatment takes the form of abandoning his prescribed dietary regimen.

Kilpatrick, Miller, and Williams attempted to replicate the above findings and to evaluate whether the dialysis process itself increases externality.[36] They also attempted to determine whether individuals who were more internal demonstrated better adjustment to their treatment regimen (as rated by their physician). They suggested that their results gave indirect evidence that length of time in dialysis and locus of control are related. However, they noted that as the sample's mean length of time in dialysis increased, sample composition changed due to the death of those unable to follow the treatment—the group predicted to be external personalities. They suggested that the relationship might be clarified by a longitudinal study obtaining repeated locus of control measures as patients progress through dialysis treatments.

Another medically related study using locus of control as a variable was conducted by Johnson, *et al.*[37] Studying 62 female patients' adaptive responses to surgery, they found, among other results, that internal subjects had significantly more influence over their time of discharge from the hospital and obtained more needed analgesics than external subjects.

Thus, while medically related research on the locus of control variable is limited, it does suggest that a patient's generalized feelings of control should be considered at several points on the nursing care continuum. Since it is most often the nurse who attempts health teaching, the nurse should be aware of the possibility that the patient who feels that control of life's rewards is in the hands of others, may feel little need to learn information related to control of the illness. On the other hand, the patient who constantly seeks information related to the illness and who seems motivated to carry out any activity which would hasten return to health may be attempting to gain control over a situation which was temporarily out of his or her control.

In a learning-related investigation, Seeman reported that internal prison inmates learned more control-related information about their prison life than did those with external feelings of control.[38] Other kinds of factual data, e.g., things not related to control of their life situation, were learned to the same degree by both the internal and external prisoners. In a test of a similar hypothesis with diabetic patients, Lowery found that essentially the same phenomenon occurred. Diabetics who were internal on the Rotter I-E Scale scored significantly higher on control-related items about their diabetes and other health data than did external diabetics. However, there were no significant differences between internal and external diabetic scores on factual (noncontrol) kinds of questions. The same investigation suggested that differences in problems of control of diabetes may also be related to the locus of control variable. While the results were not as clear-cut as those on learning, they did indicate that relatively new diabetics who were internal in outlook had fewer diabetes control problems than their external counterparts.

Rotter points out that individuals with emotional problems tend to be at either extreme of internal or external behavior. Thus, it should not be assumed that an internal outlook is always synonymous with health and externality with ill health. The likelihood is that, to a large extent, the nature of the situation determines which behavior is most functional. In health situations where dependency is essential, for example, a coronary patient who is being encouraged to be completely dependent for even a short time, perhaps an external outlook is better. While the specific health situation has not been investigated, it may be the case that an external person would have less anxiety about being so dependent and would feel quite comfortable leaving control of his or her life in the hands of others. Clearly, more research on this and other related health situations is essential.

Psychological Reactance

Psychological reactance is another variable which has recently been introduced to psychological literature. The variable has apparently not been investigated in relation to health matters, but a brief review should show its possible relevance to understanding patients' responses to health-related situations. Brehm describes psychological reactance as follows:

> . . . if a person's behavioral freedom is reduced or threatened with reduction, he will become motivationally aroused. This arousal would presumably be directed toward the re-establishment of whatever freedom had already been lost or threatened.[39]

Brehm cites several hypothetical examples of psychological reactance and its reduction through recovery of freedom. One example follows:

> Picture first Mr. Smith, who normally plays golf on Sunday afternoons, although occasionally he spends Sunday afternoon watching television or puttering around his workshop. The important point is that Smith always spends Sunday afternoon doing whichever of these three things he prefers; he is free to choose which he will do. Now consider a specific Sunday morning on which Smith's wife announces that Smith will have to play golf that afternoon since she has invited several of her ladyfriends to the house for a party. Mr. Smith's freedom is threatened with reduction in several ways: (1) he cannot watch television, (2) he cannot putter in his workshop, and (3) he must (Mrs. Smith says) play golf. According to the present view, Smith would be motivationally aroused to re-establish

these threatened freedoms. We therefore might expect to hear him protest that there was an important television program that he wanted to watch and that he had planned to do some special work in his shop. We might also expect to hear him say that he is tired of golf, that the course is not in good condition, and so forth. If the amount of reactance aroused were great, we might indeed expect Smith to spend the afternoon watching television, perhaps with the volume turned unusually high.[40]

One might develop an extensive list of illness situations which either immediately or progressively limit the freedoms that an individual has previously enjoyed. The reader could probably also cite numerous examples of patients who, realizing the damaging effects of their actions, consciously decide to default on their prescribed treatment regimen. Perhaps these are attempts to reduce the anxiety associated with psychological reactance.

Brehm also proposes that the proportion of behaviors involved will affect the magnitude of the reactance. Thus, as a patient gradually loses more and more prior freedoms because of a chronic illness, the likelihood that reactance might occur would seem to increase. Brehm further notes that the individual, though perhaps not aware of reactance,

> . . . will feel an increased amount of self-direction in regard to his own behavior. That is, he will feel that he can do what he wants, that he does not have to do what he doesn't want, and that at least in regard to the freedom in question, he is the sole director of his own behavior.[41]

The reader may already have concluded that there should be some relationship between the psychological reactance variable and the locus of control variable. Several investigations have found that the two are related. The research of Ritchie and Phares,[42] MacDonald and Hall,[43] Julian and Katz,[44] and especially that of Biondo and MacDonald[45] give strong evidence that the behavior of individuals with an internal locus of control in response to attempts of overt influence fits that of psychological reactance. On the other hand, external individuals did not attempt to reestablish their own freedom in order to decide

the issue at hand. Thus, in illness situations where freedoms must be limited, one might expect to see individuals with an internal locus of control putting forth stronger attempts to reestablish their freedoms. Obviously, research alone can determine whether and to what extent the reactance phenomenon does mediate the patient's response to illness.

Compliance with the Treatment Regimen

There have been many attempts in recent medical research and literature to determine what factors mediate the patient's compliance with the medical or nursing regimen prescribed for the patient. Medical teams often find it difficult to comprehend why patients would fail to carry out activities which would probably hasten their return to health or perhaps even prevent their deaths. In the research on hemodialysis patients cited earlier, Goldstein and Reznikoff termed noncompliance in the patients they studied "suicidal behavior." While it seems obvious that not all instances of a patient's failure to take his medicine, to return for clinic appointments, to follow a prescribed diet, and so on can be labeled suicidal behavior, the problem is widespread enough (and at times dangerous enough) that a more extensive look at some possible psychological causes might prove fruitful.

In a recent review of the literature on compliance, Marston reported that wide variations in operational definitions of compliance make it difficult to compare various studies and reach definite conclusions about compliance rates.[46] She noted studies which showed variations from 4 to 100 percent in the extent to which patients default (Fox, 1958; Luntz and Austin, 1960) and another review estimating that 30 to 35 percent of patients failed to follow their physicians orders (Davis, 1966).

Reported measures used to assess compliance included blood testing, drug excretion tests, pill counts, patient self-report, observation of the patient, or a combination of these methods. Follow-through medical supervision also provided a combination of indices that have been used to indicate compliance. Actual physical condition of the patient was rarely used as a compliance measure. As noted earlier, physiological changes may occur even in the patient who is following the prescribed regimen.

Marston's extensive review yielded several important conclusions regarding the variables associated with compliance. The studies indicated that neither age, socioeconomic status, education, or race are significantly related to compliance. It seemed likely that length of illness was related to compliance, with patients who were ill longer complying less. (Perhaps psychological reactance is a factor here.) The review also indicated that the relationship between knowledge about illness and compliance was not clear.

One of the compliance studies used a measure related to feelings of control as one of a group of possible motivational predictors of health behaviors.[47] In a general approach to the variable, they asked two agree-disagree questions of the subjects. One question suggested that one cannot do much about health, the other that one cannot do much to prevent accidents. Their results indicated that the feelings of control, at least as they had measured them, were not related to a mother's compliance behavior of giving medications and keeping medical appointments for her child.

An extensive study of the compliance behavior of diabetics was carried out by Williams *et al.*[48] Using only patients who were receiving insulin, their samples were 46 patients from a university medical clinic, 40 patients from a similar source, 84 patients from the private practice of an internist, and 43 from a city health insurance program group. The samples included patients with juvenile and adult onset diabetes.

The dependent variable which was assessed was control of the diabetes. Criteria for assessing control included information about insulin reactions, blood sugars, urine sugars, episodes of diabetic acidosis, and body weight. The independent variables were intelligence, socioeconomic resources, motivation to comply, and knowledge of how to carry out the recommendations.

The knowledge score, derived from an interview which included true-false and situational questions related to diabetes, was compared with the patient's performance of the treatment regimen. In this study, performance was measured by the placement of nurse-observers in the home. The investigators found a positive correlation between the knowledge score and the performance of the prescribed treatment. However, they found no correlation between performance of the prescribed regimen and actual control of the disease. Moreover, they found a negative correlation between patient's knowledge about the disease and the control factors. For each separate sample and for the combined groups, the greater the knowledge about diabetes, the more control problems were noted.

One explanation given for this finding was that patients who are in poor control may get more attention from medical people and thus learn more. This reasoning, however, does not speak to the finding that following the regimen was not related to control of the disease either. The other more plausible explanation given by the writers was that ". . . the major features of the disease process itself and its treatment are still too poorly understood to permit adequate therapeutic recommendations for many patients."[49] (See Chapter 15.)

Along with other motivational variables in this study, an attempt was made during the interview to determine patients' feelings of fate versus self-control. The feelings of control as measured were apparently not correlated with diabetic control and so, along with several other measures, were not discussed in the report. The relationship between this control score and either the knowledge or performance scores was apparently not examined.

Thus, there is no doubt that many questions are still unanswered in the area of patient's compliance and control over his treatment. Whether the previously described psychological variables, locus of control and psychological reactance, will provide answers upon further research is not clear. There seems little doubt that answers to the compliance problem could lead to more effective treatment for illness and to more effective performance of preventive or health maintenance measures.

Summary

While the review of the concept of mental health attempted to show that the term "mental health" has no broadly accepted definition, some understanding of the psychological reaction of an individual and/or family to the health situation can still be seen as an essential part of the professional *persona* of the nurse. Without identifying responses as either mentally healthy or mentally ill, the concepts reviewed in this chapter—crisis intervention, multiproblem families, locus of control, and psychological reactance—may enhance this understanding. The concepts chosen for review, however, are obviously only a minor portion of those which can help the nurse to better understand and intervene in the total health care situation. References to other concepts which may further the reader's learning have been included throughout the chapter. The need for more research in each area discussed has also been emphasized throughout. It is the writer's hope that each nurse who begins to consider these concepts in her everyday practice will realize the need to evaluate their applicability to the situation in which she works and will also see the need to share her perceptions with other nurses and health professionals with whom she functions.

References

1. Rogers, C.: Freedom to Learn. Columbus, Charles E. Merrill, 1969.
2. Jahoda, M.: Current Concepts of Positive Mental Health. New York, Basic Books, 1958.
3. Williams, R.: Sigma Xi National Lecture (1956-57). *In* D. Offer and M. Sabshin: Normality. New York, Basic Books, 1966.
4. Offer, D. and Sabshin, M.: Normality, New York, Basic Books, 1966, p. 46.
5. Rogers, *op. cit.*, p. 288.
6. Klein, M.: On mental health. Brit. J. Med. Psych. 33, 237-241, 1960.
7. Offer and Sabshin, *op. cit.*, p. 230.
8. Fromm, E.: The Sane Society. New York, Holy, 1959, p. 275.
9. Menninger, K.: The Human Mind, ed. 3. New York, Knopf, 1945, p. 2.
10. Saul, L.: Emotional Maturity. Philadelphia, J. B. Lippincott, 1960, p. 343.
11. Jahoda, *op. cit.*, p. 8.
12. *Ibid.*
13. Maslow, A.: Toward a Psychology of Being. New York, Van Nostrand Reinhold, 1968, pp. 6-7.
14. Rotter, J.: Social Learning and Clinical Psychology. New Jersey, Prentice Hall, 1954, p. 42.
15. Caplan, G.: Principles of Preventive Psychiatry. New York, Basic Books, 1964, p. 50.
16. *Ibid.*, p. 72.
17. *Ibid.*
18. Parad, H. and Caplan, G.: A framework for studying families in crisis. *In* H. Parad (ed.): Crisis Intervention: Selected Readings. New York, Family Service Association of America, 1965, p. 56.
19. Caplan, *op. cit.*, p. 40.
20. *Ibid.*, p. 53.
21. *Ibid.*, p. 35.
22. Maloney, E.: The subjective and objective definition of crisis. Perspec. Psych. Care 258, 1971.
23. Cadden, V.: Crisis in the family. *In* G. Caplan: Principles of Preventive Psychiatry. New York, Basic Books, 1964, pp. 293-294.
24. Kaplan, D. and Mason, E.: Maternal reactions to premature birth viewed as acute emotional disorder. *In* H. Parad (ed.): Crisis Intervention: Selected Readings. New York, Family Service Association of America, 1965, p. 121.
25. Dodge, J.: What patients should be told: patients' and nurses' beliefs. Am. J. Nurs. 72, 1852-1854, 1972.
26. Aguilera, D., Messick, J. and Farrell, M.: Crisis Intervention: Theory and Methodology. St. Louis, C. V. Mosby, 1970, p. 76.
27. Maloney, *op. cit.*, pp. 263-264.
28. *Ibid.*, p. 263.
29. Rotter, J.: Generalized expectancy for internal versus external control of reinforcement. Psych. Monograph 609:80, 1966.
30. *Ibid.*, p. 20.
31. Bondy, P.: Diabetes mellitus. *In* P. Beeson and W. McDermott (eds.): Cecil-Loeb Textbook of Medicine, ed. 13. Philadelphia, W. B. Saunders, 1971, p. 1649.
32. Lowery, B.: Disease-related learning and disease control in diabetics as a function of locus of control. Unpublished doctoral dissertation, Temple University, 1973.
33. Seeman, M. and Evans, J.: Alienation and learning in a hospital setting. Am. Soc. Review, 27, 772-783, 1962.
34. Goldstein, M. and Reznikoff, M.: Suicide in chronic hemodialysis patients from an external locus of control framework. Am. J. Psych. 1205, 1971.
35. *Ibid.*, p. 1206.
36. Kilpatrick, D., Miller, W. and Williams, A.: Locus of control and adjustment to long-term hemodialysis. Proceedings of the Annual Convention of the American Psychological Association 1972, 7, 727-728.
37. Johnson, J., Leventhal, J. and Dabbs, J.: Contribution of emotional and instrumental response processes in adaptation to surgery. Soc. Psych. 20, 55-64, 1971.
38. Seeman, M.: Alienation: a map. Psych. Today 83-4, 94-5, Aug. 1971.
39. Brehm, J.: A Theory of Psychological Reactance. New York, Academic Press, 1966, p. 2.
40. *Ibid.*, p. 40.
41. *Ibid.*, p. 9.
42. Ritchie, E. and Phares, E. J.: Attitude ch function of internal-external control municator status. J. Person. 37, 429-4
43. MacDonald, A. and Hall, J.: Internal-locus of control and perception of disa Consult. and Clin. Psych. 36, 338-343,
44. Julian, J. and Katz, S.: Internal versus control and the value of reinforcement. son. and Soc. Psych. 8, 89-94, 1968.
45. Biondo, J. and MacDonald, A. P.: Int external locus of control and respon influence attempts. J. Person. 39, 407-419,
46. Marston, M.: Compliance with medical regir a review of the literature. Nurs. Researc 312, 323, 1971.
47. Becker, M., Drachman, R., and Kirscht, J.: N vations as predictors of health behavior. He Serv. Reports 87, 852-862, 1972.
48. Williams, F., Martin, D., Hogan, M., Watkins and Ellis, E.: The clinical picture of diabe control studied in four settings. Am. J. P Health 57, 441-451, 1967.
49. *Ibid.*, p. 445.

cal condition of the patient was rarely used as a compliance measure. As noted earlier, physiological changes may occur even in the patient who is following the prescribed regimen.

Marston's extensive review yielded several important conclusions regarding the variables associated with compliance. The studies indicated that neither age, socioeconomic status, education, or race are significantly related to compliance. It seemed likely that length of illness was related to compliance, with patients who were ill longer complying less. (Perhaps psychological reactance is a factor here.) The review also indicated that the relationship between knowledge about illness and compliance was not clear.

One of the compliance studies used a measure related to feelings of control as one of a group of possible motivational predictors of health behaviors.[47] In a general approach to the variable, they asked two agree-disagree questions of the subjects. One question suggested that one cannot do much about health, the other that one cannot do much to prevent accidents. Their results indicated that the feelings of control, at least as they had measured them, were not related to a mother's compliance behavior of giving medications and keeping medical appointments for her child.

An extensive study of the compliance behavior of diabetics was carried out by Williams *et al.*[48] Using only patients who were receiving insulin, their samples were 46 patients from a university medical clinic, 40 patients from a similar source, 84 patients from the private practice of an internist, and 43 from a city health insurance program group. The samples included patients with juvenile and adult onset diabetes.

The dependent variable which was assessed was control of the diabetes. Criteria for assessing control included information about insulin reactions, blood sugars, urine sugars, episodes of diabetic acidosis, and body weight. The independent variables were intelligence, socioeconomic resources, motivation to comply, and knowledge of how to carry out the recommendations.

The knowledge score, derived from an interview which included true-false and situational questions related to diabetes, was compared with the patient's performance of the treatment regimen. In this study, performance was measured by the placement of nurse-observers in the home. The investigators found a positive correlation between the knowledge score and the performance of the prescribed treatment. However, they found no correlation between performance of the prescribed regimen and actual control of the disease. Moreover, they found a negative correlation between patient's knowledge about the disease and the control factors. For each separate sample and for the combined groups, the greater the knowledge about diabetes, the more control problems were noted.

One explanation given for this finding was that patients who are in poor control may get more attention from medical people and thus learn more. This reasoning, however, does not speak to the finding that following the regimen was not related to control of the disease either. The other more plausible explanation given by the writers was that ". . . the major features of the disease process itself and its treatment are still too poorly understood to permit adequate therapeutic recommendations for many patients."[49] (See Chapter 15.)

Along with other motivational variables in this study, an attempt was made during the interview to determine patients' feelings of fate versus self-control. The feelings of control as measured were apparently not correlated with diabetic control and so, along with several other measures, were not discussed in the report. The relationship between this control score and either the knowledge or performance scores was apparently not examined.

Thus, there is no doubt that many questions are still unanswered in the area of patient's compliance and control over his treatment. Whether the previously described psychological variables, locus of control and psychological reactance, will provide answers upon further research is not clear. There seems little doubt that answers to the compliance problem could lead to more effective treatment for illness and to more effective performance of preventive or health maintenance measures.

Summary

While the review of the concept of mental health attempted to show that the term "mental health" has no broadly accepted definition, some understanding of the psychological reaction of an individual and/or family to the health situation can still be seen as an essential part of the professional *persona* of the nurse. Without identifying responses as either mentally healthy or mentally ill, the concepts reviewed in this chapter—crisis intervention, multiproblem families, locus of control, and psychological reactance—may enhance this understanding. The concepts chosen for review, however, are obviously only a minor portion of those which can help the nurse to better understand and intervene in the total health care situation. References to other concepts which may further the reader's learning have been included throughout the chapter. The need for more research in each area discussed has also been emphasized throughout. It is the writer's hope that each nurse who begins to consider these concepts in her everyday practice will realize the need to evaluate their applicability to the situation in which she works and will also see the need to share her perceptions with other nurses and health professionals with whom she functions.

References

1. Rogers, C.: Freedom to Learn. Columbus, Charles E. Merrill, 1969.
2. Jahoda, M.: Current Concepts of Positive Mental Health. New York, Basic Books, 1958.
3. Williams, R.: Sigma Xi National Lecture (1956-57). *In* D. Offer and M. Sabshin: Normality. New York, Basic Books, 1966.
4. Offer, D. and Sabshin, M.: Normality, New York, Basic Books, 1966, p. 46.
5. Rogers, *op. cit.*, p. 288.
6. Klein, M.: On mental health. Brit. J. Med. Psych. 33, 237-241, 1960.
7. Offer and Sabshin, *op. cit.*, p. 230.
8. Fromm, E.: The Sane Society. New York, Holy, 1959, p. 275.
9. Menninger, K.: The Human Mind, ed. 3. New York, Knopf, 1945, p. 2.
10. Saul, L.: Emotional Maturity. Philadelphia, J. B. Lippincott, 1960, p. 343.
11. Jahoda, *op. cit.*, p. 8.
12. *Ibid.*
13. Maslow, A.: Toward a Psychology of Being. New York, Van Nostrand Reinhold, 1968, pp. 6-7.
14. Rotter, J.: Social Learning and Clinical Psychology. New Jersey, Prentice Hall, 1954, p. 42.
15. Caplan, G.: Principles of Preventive Psychiatry. New York, Basic Books, 1964, p. 50.
16. *Ibid.*, p. 72.
17. *Ibid.*
18. Parad, H. and Caplan, G.: A framework for studying families in crisis. *In* H. Parad (ed.): Crisis Intervention: Selected Readings. New York, Family Service Association of America, 1965, p. 56.
19. Caplan, *op. cit.*, p. 40.
20. *Ibid.*, p. 53.
21. *Ibid.*, p. 35.
22. Maloney, E.: The subjective and objective definition of crisis. Perspec. Psych. Care 258, 1971.
23. Cadden, V.: Crisis in the family. *In* G. Caplan: Principles of Preventive Psychiatry. New York, Basic Books, 1964, pp. 293-294.
24. Kaplan, D. and Mason, E.: Maternal reactions to premature birth viewed as acute emotional disorder. *In* H. Parad (ed.): Crisis Intervention: Selected Readings. New York, Family Service Association of America, 1965, p. 121.
25. Dodge, J.: What patients should be told: patients' and nurses' beliefs. Am. J. Nurs. 72, 1852-1854, 1972.
26. Aguilera, D., Messick, J. and Farrell, M.: Crisis Intervention: Theory and Methodology. St. Louis, C. V. Mosby, 1970, p. 76.
27. Maloney, *op. cit.*, pp. 263-264.
28. *Ibid.*, p. 263.
29. Rotter, J.: Generalized expectancy for internal versus external control of reinforcement. Psych. Monograph 609:80, 1966.
30. *Ibid.*, p. 20.
31. Bondy, P.: Diabetes mellitus. *In* P. Beeson and W. McDermott (eds.): Cecil-Loeb Textbook of Medicine, ed. 13. Philadelphia, W. B. Saunders, 1971, p. 1649.
32. Lowery, B.: Disease-related learning and disease control in diabetics as a function of locus of

She concludes that professional nursing must accept broader and more significant responsibilities if the future health needs of people are to be met.

Along with increased education, one must also consider the effects of changes in the woman's role within society in general. This is particularly relevant since the nurse is still the major female health professional. Broader role definitions and boundaries are now possible for women, and there is, perhaps, greater sanction for nurses who advocate major role revisions. The social climate for women favors their assumption of the increased responsibilities of which Mereness spoke.

Role Revision

However, Shetland cautions that role structure and function which are defined by the system are frequently based on the cultural role rather than individual or group competencies.[2] In her view, it is not especially difficult for nursing to assume new functions or responsibilities if these are subordinated to the traditionally defined medical leadership model. Difficulties arise when the nurse is seen as using new skills in a basically independent manner. In this sense, the nurse who is competent to perform physical assessment skills is more likely to be accepted if seen as functioning within the general framework of the traditional medical model. Acceptance of a more independent function then may lag behind the development of role competencies and may be viewed as a type of "cultural lag" which will change slowly as more nurses demonstrate competence in the area.

An important issue to be considered is whether nurses believe that they should become involved in providing an assessment of the patient's health status. Is this a logical, timely extension of function, or does it represent a thoughtless response of nurses attempting to be all things to all people? McCormack and Crawford investigated the receptivity of baccalaureate nurses toward the provision of primary ambulatory care to patients.[3] They found that a majority of nurses considered such a role extension to be highly desirable and felt that it would enhance professional nursing's image and encourage recruitment.

Rather than a possible increase in status, the Secretary's Committee to Study Extended Roles for Nurses holds that the important question here is "the need to assure every person access to health services when and where they are needed at a cost that society can afford."[4] Attitudinal barriers of nurses were not viewed as nonexistent or minor, but the potential pool of more than one million active and inactive nurses was seen as one possible solution to needed improvement in the health delivery system. If it is true that the public believes nurses could do more or different things in an effort to meet its health care needs, nursing has to respond, for it is also a social institution which must be responsive to the changing demands of society.

Obtaining the History

DEFINITION AND OBJECTIVES

Obtaining the history is usually the first step in evaluating a person's health status. It can be defined as an account of current and past events which are relevant to an individual's mental and physical health.[5] The history is reported by the patient, or, if necessary, by another informed person, through a guided interview. In obtaining a history, the nurse is interested in gaining a clear understanding of the patient's current health status, factors which may affect the patient's health, reasons for seeking health care, and expectations regarding the outcome of care.

Collecting a history can be thought of as one step in a problem-solving approach, that of accumulating a data base. As pertinent details are elicited, the examiner is primed to stress certain parts of the physical examination which will follow. Some authors note that sufficient information for diagnosis of internal ailments can be obtained from studying the history at least 50 percent of the time, while another 20 percent of diagnosis can be recognized by physical examination and an additional 20 percent require laboratory tests.[6,7] Apparently the remaining 10 percent presents great difficulty in arriving at a diagnosis. If the history is to act as such a helpful tool, the nurse must develop the ability to listen carefully, to logically sort out pertinent facts, and to constantly develop an awareness of the natural history of illnesses.

TALKING WITH THE PATIENT

To obtain the information required in the history it is necessary for the nurse to participate in a guided interview with the patient. While acquisition of pertinent information is one objective of such an interview, the nurse is also interested in establishing at least a beginning rapport with the patient and in conveying the feeling of personal interest in his health. A calm attentive manner is helpful as many patients are quite anxious about the possible outcome of their illnesses or the meaning of certain symptoms. Any interview of this kind should start with a personal introduction and a brief statement about the purpose of the session. This introduction is particularly important if the patient is not prepared for the physical assessment to be done by the nurse.

Throughout the interview it is wise not to assume a knowledge of what ___ ng to say. Many common words ___ ctly used and have widely different connotations. For example, a "pain in the stomach" could mean a pain in the epigastric region or one in the left, lower quadrant of the abdomen. Similarly, a report from the patient that he is a "social drinker" is not as helpful as one which indicates the amount and type of alcoholic intake per week. On the other hand, the patient must be able to understand what he is being asked if he is to answer accurately. For example, asking a patient about the presence of tarry stools may not mean as much as asking him to describe the color, consistency, and amount of his bowel movements. Further, if a patient does not understand the question he may be embarrassed at his lack and attempt an answer. It is helpful to learn the specific terms commonly used by groups of patients when describing symptoms or past illnesses. For example a past complaint of "high blood" may refer to hypertension, while one of "bad blood" may refer to syphilis. In these examples, of course, it is even more helpful to have the patient describe the symptoms that accompanied his illness.

Thoughtful use of questioning can add critical information to the history. In general, patients are willing to cooperate but sometimes dismiss symptoms as minor or as unconnected with their current problem. Questioning in this instance can jar their memory. However, some subjects can be particularly sensitive and care should be exercised to avoid offending the patient or increasing his tension. Sex, alcoholism, mental illness, epilepsy, and venereal disease are common examples of such sensitive areas.[8] Others may include a history of drug usage or abortion. If it is suspected that a particularly sensitive subject is pertinent to the patient's health problem, tactful persistence and an explanation of the importance of the information is necessary. However, the nurse may chose to return to this area of questioning later in the interview when more rapport has been established. Frequently, successful questioning in sensitive areas depends upon the degree of comfort and the lack of moral judgment evidenced by the nurse.

Time spent in wording a question more specifically can help the patient understand exactly what information is needed, and this kind of direct question has its place. However, care must be taken to avoid over use of questions which do not encourage discussion by the patient. "Do you have any pain?" is not as likely to elicit a description as "Can you tell me about the pain?" Also, a more general or neutral question such as "Tell me about it" is less likely to influence the patient's answer than one which asks if the pain radiates down the arm.

Organizing the Data

THE CHIEF COMPLAINT (CC)

Much information is collected in the history and a certain orderliness in noting the information is helpful to insure that no areas are missed and also to provide organization later when studying the history. If a patient is seeking help for a specific problem rather than an interval health evaluation, it makes sense to start the interview at that point. This area is commonly called the chief complaint(s) (CC). Usually a brief quote from the patient is recorded in answer to a general question of "What has been troubling you?"

or "How have you been feeling?" When quoting the patient, it is helpful to elicit a report of symptoms rather than a diagnosis. Some authors feel, however, that the patient's complaint is not necessarily the best expression of the problem and urge that the complaint be translated into precise medical language.[9] This criticism is frequently true because the examiner can, perhaps, state the problem more precisely than many patients. The advantage in recording the patient's words is that it offers insight into how the patient is currently defining his problem.

HISTORY OF THE PRESENT ILLNESS (HPI)

In this section, a historical account of the current illness is presented. It should include a chronological narrative of symptoms experienced by the patient and any factors which either relieve or worsen his symptoms. In seeking this information, it is wise to encourage the patient to discuss his illness and to proceed with specific questions which serve to bring important symptoms or precipitating factors into focus. Frequently the questions "When did you first start feeling ill?" or "How long have you been feeling this way?" are sufficient to direct the patient into a discussion of his illness. In this part of the discussion the examiner collects the leads or clues concerning the nature of the patient's illness. Skill in discussing the history of the current illness depends upon both interviewing skill and a knowledge of the natural history of diseases.

When a specific symptom is identified, it is important to obtain a precise description of its characteristics. For instance, if the patient complains of a cough, the nurse must determine if it is a chronic cough, if it is more bothersome at certain times of the day or year, if it is productive and if productive, the appearance and amount of sputum produced, and whether it was affected by physical activity. The nurse would also check for the presence of other respiratory complaints such as wheezes or dyspnea. Along with this questioning, the nurse should also consider possibly related areas such as fatigue, weight loss, smoking, industrial inhalants, or the presence of allergies, fever, or night sweats. The patient's response to these questions generally determines the areas of further questioning to be pursued, but it is also wise to consider areas not apparently related. A more complete picture is presented when important negatives are recorded. In the above example, the absence of chest pain in general and more specifically chest pain upon inspiration is significant.

When collecting this history a helpful learning tool is the sketching of a diagram of the progression describing symptoms and important findings. This visual account can alert the nurse to areas of information not yet obtained. For example, the following diagram shows a steady progression of respiratory symptoms.

If weight loss or fatigue were problems, they too could be noted on the diagram. Certainly an important part of this diagram would be the notation of whether any changes in work pattern or activities of daily living were necessitated by the current symptoms. The following criteria are helpful in determining whether information elicited is adequate for the history of the present illness, whether it conveys a clear picture of the patient's suffering amid his own surroundings, how the illness affected him and his family, how it interfered with his work, and how his finances were affected.[10]

THE PAST MEDICAL HISTORY (PMH)

Information obtained in this area may not have direct relevance to the patient's current health situation. In fact, if it does, it would be more appropriate to include it in the history of the current illness. However, obtaining a past medical

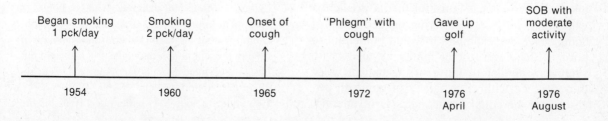

Began smoking 1 pck/day	Smoking 2 pck/day	Onset of cough	"Phlegm" with cough	Gave up golf	SOB with moderate activity
1954	1960	1965	1972	1976 April	1976 August

history is important since the nurse can gain an appreciation of the patient's overall health status. As health care moves from an episodic approach to illness toward a broader approach of preventive care, data obtained here may have added importance for their predictive value. Current work is being conducted in an ongoing effort to identify and quantify significant health care risks.[11] Data from these studies could be used by the nurse as a basis for health counseling.

Information obtained in this area should include dates and known complications and be presented in a chronological sequence. It could be grouped as follows:

1. A statement of general past health. Include the patient's height and current weight. Past weights may be helpful in order to detect significant changes.
2. An account of infectious diseases including childhood diseases. Question the patient about measles, mumps, chicken pox, diphtheria, whooping cough, polio, scarlet fever, rheumatic fever (include joint pains, murmurs, "strep" throats, and kidney problems), chorea, pneumonia, bronchitis, tuberculosis, venereal disease, and hepatitis.
3. An account of other major illnesses. If the patient required hospitalization or surgery, note this. Also include a history of accidents or trauma, including violent traumas such as gunshot wounds or stabbings.
4. An account of past pregnancies, deliveries and abortion.
5. A known history of allergies. Include the allergen and the type of reaction.
6. Transfusions.
7. Medications. In addition to prescription drugs, include over-the-counter preparations. State amount and frequency of drug ingestion.

THE FAMILY HISTORY (FH)

Data obtained in the family history may also contain information that is useful for its predictive value or helpful in identifying needed areas of counseling. For example, it would be helpful to know if there were other family members with symptoms similar to those of the patient. Also the presence within the family of common diseases with hereditary tendencies is of interest,

including diabetes, hypertension, heart disease, stroke, kidney disease, cancer, allergies, tuberculosis, mental illness, bleeding tendencies, or other chronic debilitating diseases. If appropriate, a family pedigree could be sketched indicating which family members are affected by a particular disease. Finally, if chronic illness is present in the family, this fact could have relevance to the patient as a potential influence on his adjustment to illness or on his expectations for a full recovery.

When collecting this information obtain the age and health status of parents and siblings. If any are deceased, include their age at death as well as the cause of death if known.

THE PERSONAL OR SOCIAL HISTORY (SH)

Data of a personal nature are needed so that the patient can be evaluated on an individual basis. As is commonly known, many physical complaints have their basis in life's situations. Additionally, many symptoms can be greatly aggravated by factors in the environment. Systematic evaluation of the patient's total status can be the basis for identifying positive factors or strengths which could aid the patient in adjusting to a change in health status or to a return to health. Similarly, potential problem areas can be identified which do not favor an adequate adjustment by the patient. In collecting this information, the following organization may be used:

1. Birthplace and position in the family.
2. Education. Identify grade completed.
3. Source of income and health insurance coverage.
4. Occupation. Describe responsibilities and general conditions, question if work includes exposures to industrial inhalants, toxic metals, solvents or other hazards.
5. Marital status. If married, rate adjustment, if single, identify living arrangement and adjustment.
6. Living conditions. Describe significant items in living conditions, for example, whether house or apartment, number of stairs, location of bathroom, number of persons in household, length of time in present home; may question if the patient has always lived in same geographical area; include description of diet.
7. Life style. Include how patient describes his life

style and personality, what he does with leisure time, whether he has traveled to areas where diseases not commonly found in current location predominate, how he would rate his adjustment to life, excluding family and job.

8. Use of tobacco and alcohol. Identify type and amount smoked and period of time; indicate how long patient has smoked or has stopped smoking; identify amount and type of alcoholic intake per day or week; avoid terms such as "moderate social drinker" or "occasional smoker."

THE REVIEW OF SYSTEMS (ROS)

In this part of the history, questions are asked regarding symptoms related to major anatomic areas of the body. Purposes of this review are to identify symptoms related to the present illness that have remained undetected and to identify symptoms related to conditions other than those considered in the history of the present illness. Generally, the review of systems proceeds in a head to toe manner, and such an order is presented below with common symptoms included. DeGowin and DeGowin suggest that the examiner conduct the review of systems while examining that part of the body to which the questions pertain.[12] This is ideal, but the beginning student will probably have to direct attention to developing skill with both questioning and with the techniques of physical examination. Combining these two tasks represents more than beginning skill in the area.

1. Skin. Color changes, temperature, moisture, infections, rashes, scaling, pruritus, tumors, hair changes, nail changes.
2. Head. History of headaches (including a description of type, location, duration, known precipitating events, and time of occurrence), trauma to head (include loss of consciousness if known), vertigo, syncope, convulsive seizures.
3. Eyes. Patient's impression of vision, glasses or corrective lenses, date of last refraction, diplopia, blurring, scotomas, hemianopsia, loss of vision, trauma, inflammation, discharge, tearing, pain, photophobia, swelling of lids.
4. Ears. Patient's impression of hearing, deafness, tinnitus, discharge, inflammation, pain, vertigo.
5. Nose. Patient's impression of sense of smell, frequency of colds, discharge, postnasal drip, obstruction, epistaxis, sinusitis, pain over nasal sinus area.
6. Mouth and throat. Patient's impression of sense of taste, soreness of mouth or tongue, ulcers of mouth or tongue, bleeding or receding gums, presence and state of teeth, date of last dental examination, sore throats, tonsillitis, hoarseness or voice change, difficulty in swallowing or chewing.
7. Neck. History of goiter, stiffness, limitation of movement, enlargement of nodes.
8. Hematopoietic system. Anemia, fatigue, weakness, abnormal bleeding, excessive bruising, enlarged nodes or organs.
9. Breasts. Lumps or masses, change in size or shape, pain or soreness, discharge from nipples, gynecomastia.
10. Respiratory system. Dyspnea at rest or upon exertion, nocturnal dyspnea or orthopnea, sputum or expectoration (include description), hemoptysis, night sweats, fever, pain in chest, history of frequent colds, wheezing, asthma, pneumonia, bronchitis, tuberculosis, date and result of last x-ray examination of the chest or PPD.
11. Cardiovascular system. Palpitations, tachycardia, irregular rhythms, bradycardia, fainting spells, exertional dyspnea, paroxysmal nocturnal dyspnea, orthopnea, cough, cyanosis, pain, discomfort or tightness, knowledge of murmurs, ascites or dependent edema, leg cramps, cold extremities, phlebitis, varicose veins.
12. Gastrointestinal system. Changes in appetite or weight, dysphagia, early satiety, food intolerances, heart burn, pain or bloating related to eating, eructation, nausea, vomiting, hematemesis, regularity, change in bowel habits, diarrhea or constipation, jaundice, clay or tarry stools, fresh blood in stools, hemorrhoids, pain related to bowel movement, flatulence.
13. Genitourinary system. Color of urine, change in amount or frequency of normal voiding pattern, polyuria, oliguria, nocturia, dysuria, hematuria, pyuria, retention, frequency, incontinence, history of stones or infections, change in character or force of stream, urgency, difficulty starting stream, dribbling.
14. Genitoreproductive system. (Male) history of infection, ulceration or penile discharge, known positive serology, type of treatment, testicular

pain or mass, change in libido, infertility, impotence, ability to maintain erection. (Female) age of onset of menses, frequency of period, regularity, duration, amount of flow, dates of last normal period and of preceding period, number of pads or tampons used, presence of clotting or gushing, dysmenorrhea or leukorrhea, if postmenopausal, age at last period, presence of hot flashes, presence of vaginal discharge, pruritis, history of ulceration or infection, type of treatment, known positive serology, change in libido; number of pregnancies, abortions, full-term deliveries of living children; complications of pregnancies, infertility, type of contraceptives, if used.

15. Musculoskeletal system. Pain, stiffness, swelling, redness, deformity, limitation of function in joint, muscle or bone; relationship of symptoms to activity, rest, or position; weakness, wasting or atrophy of muscle or muscle groups; history of fractures, sprains or dislocations.

16. Neuromuscular system. Numbness, paresthesia, paralysis, dysarthria, aphasia, memory change or loss, gait disturbances or difficulty with coordination, fasciculations, involuntary movement, convulsions, decreased awareness of pain, temperature, and touch.

17. Endocrine system. Weakness, sweating, nervousness, tachycardia, polyphagia, polydipsia, polyuria, glycosuria, dryness of hair or skin, change in tolerance to heat or cold, tremors, change in emotional stability, exophthalmus, history of goiter, history of growth, body configuration, or weight changes during adulthood (especially in hands, feet, or head size); change in hair distribution or in skin pigmentation, weakness, postural hypotension.

The Physical Examination

The following section presents an approach to the physical examination. Findings which fall within the range of normal are stressed. Much of the assessment described has probably been used by the nurse at some time in her practice, while other parts have not. The nurse will probably have to direct attention to aquiring skill with the use of an ophthalmoscope or with percussion and will have to increase skill with the use of the

stethoscope or with palpation. In addition, experience is required to gain an appreciation of the range of normal findings that will be observed. Supervised practice with direct feedback is essential if the nurse is to gain the confidence necessary for deciding that observations noted fall within the range of normal and do not reflect pathology.

The physical examination is presented in a head to toe order. Specialized examinations such as that of the nervous system or the gynecological examination are not included. (See Chapter 20, Nursing Intervention for the Patient with Central Nervous System Dysfunction, for material on assessment of neurological status.) Remember that it is necessary to provide privacy for the patient during the examination. Adequate covering, avoidance of undue exposure, and comfortably heated surroundings are appreciated by most patients. In addition, good lighting is required to note subtle findings.

EXAMINATION OF THE HEAD

Examination of the head starts with general inspection and palpation of the scalp for masses or lesions. The character and distribution of hair is observed, and unusual hair loss or thinning is noted. Remember that normal adult male hair distribution includes temporal recession while female distribution does not. The general symmetry of the face is noted along with a check for unusual facial expressions or lack of expression.

EXAMINATION OF THE EYE

Examination of the eyes can be divided into the following parts: measurement of visual acuity, assessment of ocular movements, inspection of external structures, testing of pupillary reactions, evaluation of the ocular fundus, and estimation of intraocular pressure.[13]

MEASURING VISUAL ACUITY. This can be done with the use of the standard Snellen charts. Measurement requires adequate lighting and is a function of the size of the letters and their distance from the eye. Near and far vision can be rated, and the vision in each eye is independently assessed. If glasses are worn during the test, this should be noted. Results are recorded as a frac-

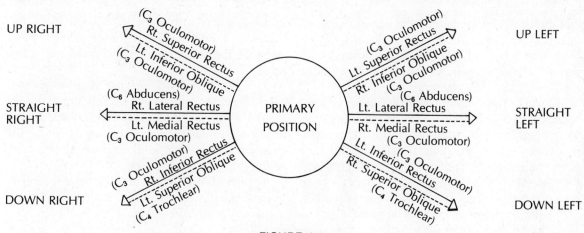

FIGURE 4-1.
Positions of gaze with muscles and nerve innervation.

tion, the numerator indicating the distance of the patient from the chart and the denominator indicating the distance at which the line of letters should be read by a normal eye. Normal visual acuity is 20/20 meaning the patient read the proper line at 20 feet.

Frequently this part of the eye examination is not included in the routine physical assessment and a more gross estimate of acuity is made with the use of newspaper print for both near and far vision. However, if trauma to the eye or head is suspected, a careful check of acuity is required if the examiner is to note subtle changes. If the patient is unable to see newspaper print, the examiner usually holds up several fingers to determine if the number can be identified. If this fails, the examiner should determine whether the motion of her hand or the flashing of a light into the patient's eye can be perceived.

The examiner can also evaluate the patient for gross defects in his peripheral visual fields by standing in front of the patient, instructing him to look ahead and close one eye, and moving a wiggling finger or a flickering light in from the periphery. This manuever can test horizontal, vertical, and oblique planes temporally and nasally on each eye. The patient's beginning awareness of the stimuli is evaluated against that of the examiner's.

ASSESSMENT OF OCULAR MOVEMENT. The examiner must determine whether the alignment of the two eyes is parallel. To do this, the reflection of a light beam directed onto the pupils is observed to see if it is in parallel position in both eyes. One eye is then covered while the patient is still looking at the light. The examiner should note whether the covered eye moves in an attempt to regain fixation on the light when the eye is quickly uncovered. Drifting of the eye while it was covered can be an indication of muscle imbalance.[14] Evaluation of the range of movements of the eye is then done to identify possible weakness of the individual extraocular muscles. Range of motion includes abduction and adduction, elevation and depression, and intorsion and extorsion, with six cardinal muscles being responsible for these movements. Figure 4-1 indicates the six positions of gaze with the muscles responsible for these positions and their cranial nerves innervation.

The patient is asked to follow a beam of light directed in these successive positions, while the examiner observes the position of the corneal light reflexes to determine if they are parallel. If the light reflex goes out of parallel position, the muscle and nerves involved can be identified. If the light reflex remains parallel, the results are recorded as "extraocular muscles intact."

INSPECTION OF EXTERNAL STRUCTURES. The examiner should systematically inspect the general appearance of the eyes, lids, conjunctiva, cornea, anterior chamber, iris, pupils, and lacrimal ducts. When evaluating the general appearance of the eyes, the examiner checks for an alert, startled or dull expression and observes for prominence or recession of one or both eyes on the frontal and side position.

Eyelids. The eyelids are observed for edema, redness, styes, ptosis, changes in the skin, such as raised yellow plaques (Xanthelasma—associated with hypercholestremia). Differences in the height of the palpebral fissures (the space between the eyelids) are noted. The examiner tests for the presence of lid lag (whether the lids are noted to follow the iris in downward gaze). With lid lag, part of the white sclera remains exposed. The examiner checks whether the lids are inverted or everted.

Conjunctiva. The conjunctiva is the thin, transparent mucous membrane inner lining of the eyelids which continues over the front of the eyeball. The lids must be everted to examine the palpebral conjunctiva, while the bulbar conjunctiva, along with the normally white sclera, is readily observed. The examiner looks for vascular congestion or the presence of foreign bodies. Some discharge in the inner canthus is normal. The examiner looks for the smooth pink appearance of the palpebral conjunctive versus the pallor seen with anemia.

Cornea. Along with the sclera, the cornea is part of the fibrous coat of the eyeball. It is normally avascular and transparent and reflects brightly the light from a flashlight. If scarring or other breaks of continuity are present, dullness of reflected light shone from an oblique angle may be noted. If abrasions of the cornea are suspected, an aqueous preparation of fluoresein dye can be instilled into the eye, or a fluorescein-impregnated tape can be touched to the eye sac. When the excess fluorescein solution has been removed, a green stain will be noted at the site of an abrasion. A white ring or partial ring (arcus senilis) at the outer margin of the cornea is commonly seen in older patients and has no pathological significance but represents a degenerative change of aging.

Anterior Chamber. The anterior chamber is the space in front of the lens, bounded by the lens and the iris behind and by the cornea in front, which is filled with clear aqueous humor. The examiner should note that the chamber is clear and that the iris does not appear to bulge forward.

Iris. The iris is a circular diaphragm suspended between the cornea and the lens, attached at its peripheral circumference to the ciliary body. The color and consistency of the iris should be noted and the size, shape, and equality of the two pupils compared.

Pupils. Shining a light into the pupil will result in contraction of the pupil (direct light reaction), and also constriction of the other pupil (consensual light reaction). To check this, the patient should be directed to fix his gaze on a distant object, while the light is shone quickly in his eyes. To test the accommodation reflex, the patient is asked to focus on the examiner's finger which is brought toward the patient's nose. At this time the pupils should constrict. Commonly, results within the normal range are recorded as PERLA, meaning pupils equal, react to light and accommodation.

Lacrimal Ducts. Tears normally drain off through the lacrimal canals. Pressure on the inner edge of each lid should be applied. Normally no fluid can be expressed.

EVALUATION OF THE OCULAR FUNDUS. Direct information about the blood vessels, the status of the optic disc, and changes common in hypertension and diabetes can be identified through an examination of the ocular fundus with an ophthalmoscope. In a routine physical examination, the pupils are generally not dilated, as the optic disc and surrounding area can usually be adequately visualized for screening purposes. The examiner should first focus the light onto the patient's pupil at a distance of 10 to 12 inches with a lens setting of +8 or +10.* The red reflex should be observed when looking through the ophthalmoscope at this distance. If opacities are present in either the lens or the vitreous, black spots may be seen against the red reflex. If the spots move upward when the patient is asked to

*The number on each lens corresponds with its focal length expressed in diopters. One diopter is the strength of a lens whose focal length is one meter. Plus numbers are convex, minus numbers are concave.[15]

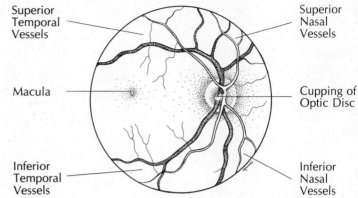

Superior Temporal Vessels

Superior Nasal Vessels

Macula

Cupping of Optic Disc

FIGURE 4-2.
The right optic disc. Veins darker red, one fourth wider than arteries. Arteries with light reflex strip along length.

Inferior Temporal Vessels

Inferior Nasal Vessels

look up, the spots are on the cornea or anterior part of the lens; if near the center of the lens little movement will be noted. If noted to move downward with a downward gaze, the opacities are located in the posterior lens or in the vitreous.[16] The examiner should then move to a distance of approximately 3 inches from the patient's eye, using her right eye to examine the patient's right eye and holding the ophthalmoscope in her right hand. At this distance a lens setting of 0 should provide the best view of the retina if neither refractive error nor accommodation in either the patient or the examiner have to be taken into account. The correct setting can be found by turning the lens slowly in an attempt to focus on the optic disc. Remember that a minus lens is required for a myopic eye and a plus lens for a hypermetropic eye,[17] while a setting of approximately +10 is required for an eye with an extracted cataract.[18] If the patient is highly astigmatic, he may have to wear his own glasses for the examination.

Just as in examining the external structures, it is wise to follow a routine when examining the fundus. The optic disc should be examined first, then the arteries and veins, the appearance of the retina as a whole, and finally the macula and its surroundings.[19]

The Optic Disc. The optic disc is the round or oval area where the optic nerve exits from the eyeball (Fig. 4-2). It is a weak spot since it is not covered by the sclera, and because of this its appearance will reflect an increase in either intraocular or intracranial pressure. If the disc is not seen immediately, the examiner can follow an artery or vein toward it. The disc is normally lighter orange in color than the rest of the retina, its borders are sharply defined, a darker pigmented area is common on some parts of the circumference, and the nasal upper or inferior margins may be less defined than the temporal margins.[20] The optic cup is white or pale yellow in color and deeper than the rest of the disc. Its size and depth is variable and as much as two diopters change in the lens setting may be necessary to focus on the base of the cup, the lamina cribrosa.[21]

Blood Vessels. The blood vessels emerge from and enter the optic disc in four main pairs of arteries and veins: the superior nasal, the inferior nasal, the superior temporal, and the inferior temporal.[22] Each pair should be examined to note if it appears straight or tortuous. The veins are usually one-fourth wider than the arteries and darker in color; the arteries can be further identified by their brighter red color and by the light reflex strip running along their length. At the site of arteriovenous crossings, the vessels share their media and adentitia. These areas should be observed carefully for signs of nicking, deviation, humping, or banking.[23] Finally the veins should be observed to note their normal pulsations.

The Retina. The appearance of the retina as a whole should be noted to detect any evidence of hemorrhages or exudate. Pigmentation which corresponds to the patient's complexion, may be noted on the retina. While the retina is red-

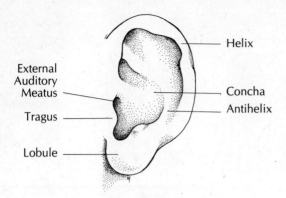

FIGURE 4-3.
External structure of the left ear.

orange in color, it is thinner and therefore lighter toward the nasal area.[24]

The Macula. The macula, the area of most acute vision and its surroundings should be examined last, since shining light on this area will produce discomfort, and the patient will probably look away. The macular area is located approximately two disc widths temporally from the optic disc. It is a darker red than the rest of the retina. The fovea centralis in the center of the macula can be noted to reflect light.

ESTIMATION OF INTRAOCULAR PRESSURE can be assessed grossly by tactile tension or more precisely by the use of a tonometer. Palpation is used in tactile tension when both forefingers are placed on the patient's closed upper lid. The examiner applies gentle pressure with one finger and senses the amount of pressure required to move the other finger outward.[25] Judgment concerning increases or decreases in pressure comes with practice, but if any increase in intraocular pressure is suspected a more precise measurement with a tonometer must be done.

EXAMINATION OF THE EAR

The examiner should first observe the structures of the external ear, the auricle (pinna), and the external acoustic meatus (Fig. 4-3). There is normally wide variation in size, shape, and detail. The major components of the auricle, which is composed of fibroelastic cartilage, are as follows: the helix, antihelix, lobule, tragus and concha. The external acoustic meatus extends as a canal from the auricle to the tympanic membrane, a distance of approximately 1 inch.

Inspection may reveal the presence of congenital anomalies such as the absence of parts of the auricle or the presence of tophi (sodium biurate crystals found in gout) deposited on the cartilage. Palpation of the external ear should not cause pain.

THE TYMPANIC MEMBRANE. The tympanic membrane should be examined with the use of an otoscope. The auricle must be pulled upward and backward in adults to properly view the tympanic membrane. Since the outer third of the external acoustic canal contains hair follicles, sebaceous glands, and cerumen glands, it may be necessary to clean the canal in order to adequately visualize the membrane.

The normal landmarks of the membrane are the manubrium of the malleus radiating upward and forward from the umbo or center, the two malleolar folds diverging from the nob of the periphery, the light reflex, a bright wedge of light with apex at the umbo and tail at 5 o'clock, and often the shadow of the incus shining through in the upper posterior quadrant.[26] (Fig. 4-4.)

Blurring of the landmarks is associated with bulging of the membrane, while accentuation of the landmarks is associated with retraction of the membrane.[27]

Normally the membrane is shiny and pearly grey, while serum in the middle ear produces a yellow or amber color; pus, a chalky white color; blood, a blue color; a dull appearance indicates fibrosis.[28] Occasionally air bubbles or a fluid level may be seen. The entire surface of the

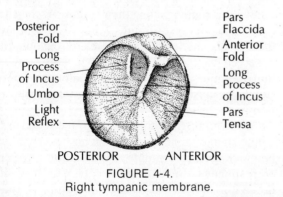

FIGURE 4-4.
Right tympanic membrane.

membrane should be carefully inspected for the presence of perforations.

ASSESSMENT OF PERCEPTIVE AND CONDUCTIVE HEARING LOSS. If the patient's hearing is to be tested, several methods are available, such as the whispered voice, the ticking of a watch, the use of tuning forks, and audiometers. If a hearing loss is suspected, generally a distinction between perceptive and conductive hearing loss is attempted. With conductive loss, there is a disturbance of sound conduction as the sound passes through the ear canal, tympanic membrane, middle ear, or ossicular chain to the stapes.[29] With perceptive hearing loss, there is disturbance from the cochlear, auditory nerve, or hearing center in the cerebral cortex.[30] The Weber's test is used to distinguish between perceptive and conductive hearing loss.[31] A vibrating tuning fork with a frequency of 512 to 1024 cycles per second placed against the midline of the patient's skull can be used to determine if the sound is equal in both ears. With normal perceptive hearing and no conductive hearing loss, the sounds are equal in both ears. If there is a conductive hearing loss, the sound will lateralize to the side of the loss. If there is perceptive loss on one side, the sounds appear louder on the other side.

The Rinne test compares the duration of air conduction with that of bone conduction. Normally the patient will hear air conduction twice as long as bone conduction.[32] In this test, a vibrating tuning fork is placed first against the patient's mastoid process, with the opposite ear covered, until he no longer hears the sound. The still vibrating fork is then held next to his ear without touching him until the sound is no longer heard.

EXAMINATION OF THE NOSE

In the routine nasal examination, the external structure of the nose should be observed for any abnormalities such as a deviated septum. The patency of each naris should then be tested by gently occluding one naris, and having the patient inspire through the other with his mouth closed. Deviations, perforations, and masses can be observed through one naris if the nasal tip is pushed up and a penlight flashlight is shone into the other naris.[33] Finally the area over the nasal sinuses should be palpated to detect possible tenderness.

EXAMINATION OF THE THROAT

This examination includes an assessment of the lips, teeth, gums, salivary duct orifices, salivary glands, palate, floor of the mouth, tongue, tonsils, and breath.

LIPS. The lips are observed for normal color or evidence of cyanosis, for fissures, cracking, or presence of ulcers. The examiner notes if the patient can purse his lips.

TEETH. There are normally 32 teeth in the permanent set, but the four wisdom teeth—last molars in each jaw—may not erupt. The examiner observes for discoloration, caries, missing teeth, or unusual notching.

GUMS. The gums are observed for bleeding, retraction, and for narrow lines of inflammation, or of discoloration or exudate.

SALIVARY DUCT ORIFICES. These orifices include the parotid duct openings on the buccal mucosa opposite the second upper molar teeth, the submaxillary duct openings on the floor of the mouth beside the root of the frenulum of the tongue, and the sublingual duct openings, at least

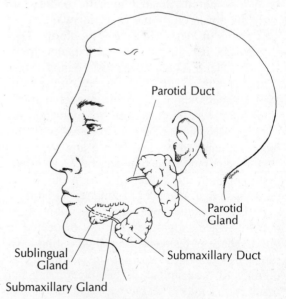

FIGURE 4-5.
Salivary glands and ducts.

ten, in the floor of the mouth (Fig. 4-5) [34] These areas can be readily identified if a flow of saliva is provoked. They should be palpated to determine if calculi are present.

SALIVARY GLANDS. These include the parotid glands located below and in front of the ear between the mastoid processes of the temporal bone and the rami of the mandible.[35] Normally they cannot be palpated. The submaxillary glands lie medial to the inner surface of the mandible. The lower portion can be palpated from beneath the inferior mandibular border anterior to the angle of the jaw.[36] The sublingual glands lie beneath the floor of the mouth but cannot normally be palpated.

PALATE. The anterior two thirds of the palate is the hard palate. Its appearance and shape should be noted. The posterior one third of the palate is the soft palate or uvula. Its position in the midline should be noted. The examiner also notes whether the uvula is drawn upward in the midline when the patient says "eh." The tongue may have to be depressed to observe this. Behind the tonsillar fossae and the soft palate, the oropharynx is continuous with the nasopharynx. It can be observed if the tongue is depressed and a good light is used. Evidence of mucous or pus should be noted. Small lymphatic nodules are normally observed on the posterior wall.[37]

FLOOR OF THE MOUTH. The floor of the mouth should be inspected and palpated for lesions or calculi. The tongue must be moved from side to side to do this. The mucosa on the inside of the cheeks should also be inspected for lesions, ulcers, vesicles, or areas of pigmentation.

TONGUE. The patient should be asked to stick out his tongue. Its size, shape, and symmetry should be noted. The examiner checks whether a tight frenulum interferes with the protrusion of the tongue and whether the tongue can be maintained in a midline position. The anterior and dorsal surface should be carefully inspected for the presence of lesions. Color and coating of the tongue should be noted, but this may vary according to food intake. Excessive furring may result from a milky diet but may also reflect fever or dehydration. Any areas of tenderness should be carefully palpated to detect lesions.

TONSILS. The tonsils are masses of lymphoid tissue located between the pillars of the fauces. If present, their size should be noted, as well as evidence of inflammation such as redness, swelling, exudate, or membranes.

BREATH. The breath may be evaluated for the presence of acetone, ammonia, fetor.

EXAMINATION OF THE NECK

Examination of the neck includes an assessment of the cervical muscles and bones, the cervical lymph nodes, and the thyroid gland. The examiner begins by inspecting the neck for deformities, asymmetry, spasm of the muscles, or unusual anterior or posterior pulsations. Any unusual position or limitation of movement of the neck is noted. The examiner evaluates the range of movement of the neck in flexion, extension, lateral bending, and rotation. Remember such movement may be decreased in the elderly, and some positions may temporarily occlude the vertebral artery yielding symptoms ranging from giddiness to unconsciousness. This would occur in patients with some blockage of the arterial circulation. Care should be taken with this procedure. The cervical vertebrae and muscles should then be palpated to identify any masses or areas of tenderness.

THE CERVICAL LYMPH NODES. Systematic inspection and palpation of the cervical lymph

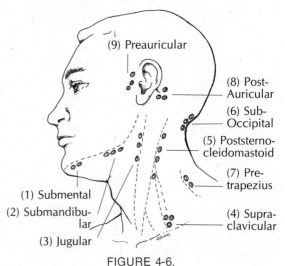

FIGURE 4-6.
Superficial lymph nodes of the head and neck.

nodes are done next. If small nodes are to be sensed by the fingertips, palpation must be light. If nodes are felt, their location, size, degree of fixation and consistency or texture must be recorded. Figure 4-6 identifies the superficial lymph nodes of the neck and a suggested order for their examination. Normally these nodes are not palpable.

THE THYROID GLAND. The thyroid gland consists of two lateral lobes connected by an isthmus. The lobes are located below the larynx on either side of the trachea, while the isthmus passes anteriorly just below the cricoid cartilage. It is firmly fixed to the trachea, and this is important in observation for it moves up with the trachea during swallowing. In some thin people, the isthmus may be palpated over the tracheal rings, but usually the adult thyroid cannot be palpated.

The lower part of the neck should be inspected and the patient directed to swallow. Normally the thyroid is not visible. The examiner should then attempt to palpate the thyroid. Standing behind the patient the examiner should place two or three fingertips of both hands on either side of the trachea below the level of the thyroid cartilage.[38] In this way, both lobes can be simultaneously assessed when the patient swal-

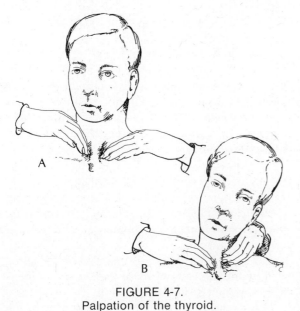

FIGURE 4-7.
Palpation of the thyroid.

lows (Fig. 4-7,A). Each lobe can be assessed separately. The patient should incline his head slightly toward the side being palpated, as this will relax the sternocleidomastoid muscle. Two fingers of one hand are used to palpate a lobe, while the other hand is placed behind the sternocleidomastoid muscle to evert the gland (Fig. 4-7, B).[39]

EXAMINATION OF THE CHEST

Examination of the chest includes an assessment of the breasts, the lungs, the heart, and the thoracic spine.

THE BREASTS. Both male and female breasts should be routinely examined. Examination of the female breast will be described, but the approach is also useful when assessing the male breast. First, the examiner inspects the breasts for symmetry and for evidence of swelling or retraction of the breast tissue. Inspection should be done with the patient seated. Her arms should first be at her sides, then raised over her head. Then the patient should lean over, and finally she should tense her pectoralis muscles by firmly pushing the palms of her hands together. This combination of positions will help demonstrate retraction, evidenced by dimpling, if it is present. Remember that the size of normal breasts varies widely and is influenced by heredity, age, sex, obesity, time of menstrual cycle, parity, lactation, and pregnancy.

The nipples should be inspected for evidence of retraction, bleeding, discharge, fissures, scaling or excoriation. Remember that inverted nipples are a common developmental anomaly. Therefore, if the nipple appears inverted, the patient should be questioned whether the inversion is recent. The pigmentation of the nipple and areola is darker in the pregnant woman than in the nonpregnant woman, but, in general, it varies from pink to brown depending upon the person's complexion.

Palpation of the breast is then systematically carried out. Consistency of the breast tissue will be influenced by the same variables which influence breast size. The palmar aspects of the fingers held together are used to apply a gentle pressure to the breast tissue. With palpation, the

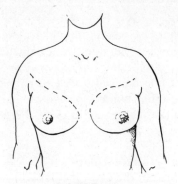

FIGURE 4-8.
Breasts with axillary tails.

breast tissue is gently flattened out against the chest wall while the patient is seated and supine. When the patient is supine, a small pillow or rolled towel should be placed under the back on the side being examined.

The breast tissue is generally circular in distribution, but there is also an axillary tail projecting laterally toward the axilla. (Fig. 4-8). If a routine is established for palpation, there is less chance that an area of the breast tissue will be omitted. The examiner begins at 12 o'clock on the left breast, palpates clockwise around the breast, and finally palpates the axillary tail. This routine is carried out in the erect and supine positions with the arms at the sides and over the head. The nipple is then palpated, and gentle pressure applied toward the nipple in a stripping action to determine if any secretions can be ex-

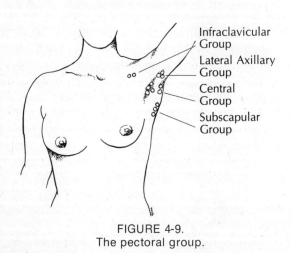

FIGURE 4-9.
The pectoral group.

Infraclavicular Group

Lateral Axillary Group

Central Group

Subscapular Group

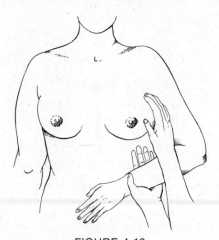

FIGURE 4-10.
Palpation of axilla with cupped hand while supporting the patient's arm.

pressed. Unless the patient is lactating, no secretion should be expressed. The procedure is repeated on the right breast.

The axillary, pectoral, infraclavicular and subscapular areas on both sides should then be palpated (Fig. 4-9). Supporting the patient's arm on the side being examined, the examiner palpates the apex of the axilla with a cupped hand, and then draws the hand down over the chest wall and finally down over the inner aspect of the arm (Fig. 4-10).

THE LUNGS. To assess the lungs, the examiner uses inspection, palpation, percussion, and auscultation. It is suggested that they be used in the order listed and that the lung fields be examined in a definite apices to bases direction, in the anterior, axillary, and posterior position. In this way, a routine will be established which will help decrease the chances of omitting the examination of a critical area.

To know what to look for and where to find it, the examiner must know the important anatomic surface landmarks and the location of underlying structures. This understanding aids in reporting findings and in deciding whether an elicited sign reflects pathology or the expected underlying presence of bone or nonresonant tissue. Figures 4-11 and 4-12 show views of the chest and identify important structures.

First, the chest should be inspected with the

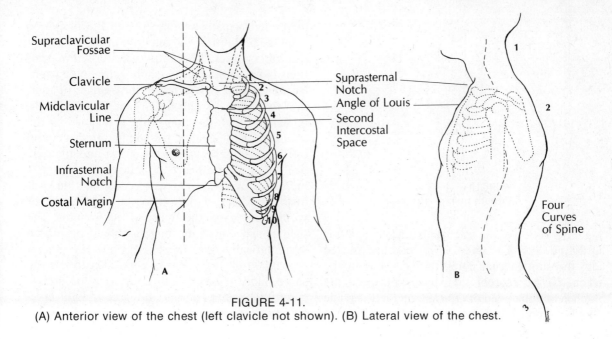

FIGURE 4-11.
(A) Anterior view of the chest (left clavicle not shown). (B) Lateral view of the chest.

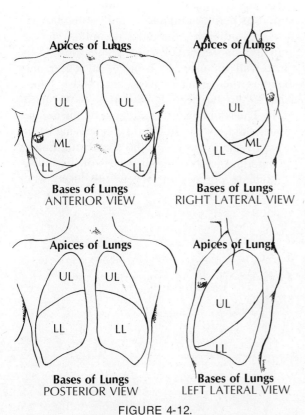

FIGURE 4-12.
Location of the lobes of the lungs. (UL) upper middle lobe; (ML) middle lobe; (LL) lower lobe.

patient in the sitting position. The general structure of the chest is evaluated. It is normally symmetrical and broader from side to side than from front to back. The examiner checks for the presence of kyphosis (anterior-posterior spinal deviation) or of scoliosis (lateral spinal deviation), or for a combination of the two. Respiratory rate and rhythm are noted while the patient is breathing normally. The examiner checks whether there is any distress associated with respiration, any preferred position, or any retraction or bulging of the intercostal spaces or neck muscles. Respiratory movement can be evaluated by having the patient breathe a little deeper than normal through his mouth. Chest movement is normally lateral and upward with inspiration. The amplitude of respiratory movements can be evaluated by comparing the excursion of the upper, anterior middle, and posterior thorax. The examiner's hands are placed successively over these areas so that the thumbs approximate in the midline. The patient is then instructed to breathe deeply and the examiner's hands are allowed to move over the chest wall. The speed and distance traveled by the thumbs are noted.

Palpation continues with the examiner check-

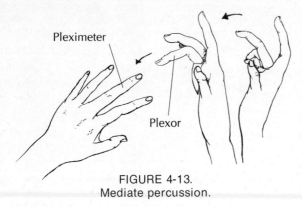

FIGURE 4-13.
Mediate percussion.

ing the position of the trachea to determine if it is in the midline. The index finger can be inserted into the suprasternal notch on each side of the trachea. The size of the spaces between the trachea and the head of the right and left clavicle should be compared.

Palpation is continued systematically over the anterior, axillary, and posterior chest wall to identify masses or areas of tenderness, and to evaluate musculoskeletal status. The ribs and vertebral bodies should be carefully palpated. For convenience, flexibility and range of motion of the thoracic and lumbar spine can be evaluated later during assessment of the lower extremities.

The chest should then be carefully palpated for the presence of tactile fremitus (a palpable vibration reflecting a nonvascular state).[40] Movement of air in and out of the lungs is not normally palpable, but, if sound is produced by

the patient usually saying 99 or 1, 2, 3, it can be palpated and reflect the integrity of the lungs and respiratory tract.[41] Fremitus is better felt in positions close to the larynx, such as the interscapular area, and less well felt in the axillae. In addition to distance from the larynx, fremitus is diminished by obstruction of the bronchus, by the presence of air or fluid in the pleural space, and by tissue lying between the lungs and thoracic wall such as the heart or breasts,[42] while it is increased over other areas of consolidation. Additionally, the higher pitch in the voices of women decreases the ability to feel fremitus. The palmar aspects of the fingers should be placed systematically over the chest while the patient repeats 99 or 1, 2, 3. It is good idea to use the same hand when palpating for fremitus and to carefully exert a consistent degree of light pressure with the fingers.

Percussion of the chest is then done to determine the resonance of the underlying tissue (sonorous percussion) and to outline the borders of tissues adjoining the lungs (definitive percussion). Percussion involves striking a blow to the chest wall in order to produce a sound. The sound is then evaluated in light of the sounds expected to be heard in different parts of the chest. The sound heard is affected by the amount of air, fluid, or solids in the underlying structures, by the thickness of the chest wall, and by the amount of force and briskness of the blow.

Mediate percussion is generally used when

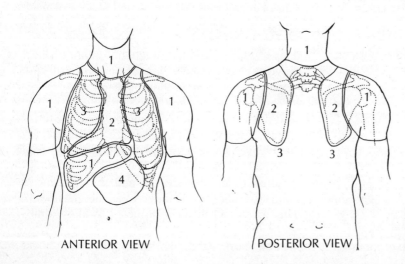

ANTERIOR VIEW

POSTERIOR VIEW

FIGURE 4-14.
Normal percussion outlines. (1) flat; (2) dull; (3) resonant; (4) tympanic.

evaluating the chest. The middle finger of one hand (the pleximeter), placed firmly against the chest wall in an intercostal space, is struck sharply on the distal interphalangeal joint by the tip of the middle finger of the other hand (the plexor). The action of the striking motion is made by the wrist, while the forearm is held steady (Fig. 4-13). It should be rhythmical and quickly removed. If it's not sharp and brisk, the sound will be dampened.

The anterior chest is percussed with the patient in the supine position. The examiner should start under the clavicles and work her way down on each side while comparing the sound on the contralateral side. On the right, the chest is resonant to the fourth intercostal space where the underlying lung and liver combine to yield a relatively dull sound. By the sixth intercostal space, the flatness of underlying liver can be heard. On the left side, resonance will be decreased over that portion of the lung covered by the heart and flat when just over the heart. Finally, the resonant sound of the left lower border of the lung melds into the tympanic sound heard over the stomach. The sounds heard in percussion should be compared to those heard on the contralateral side, keeping in mind the expected differences (Fig. 4-14).

The patient should be sitting for percussion of the apices, the axillae, and the posterior chest. The upper edges of the lungs, or apices, may extend anteriorly 3 to 4 centimeters above the upper margins of the clavicles and posteriorly to the seventh cervical vertebra (that spinous prominence felt with the head bent forward).[43] The sound elicited when percussing this area is higher in pitch than that heard in the lower parts of the lungs, and it may normally be higher in pitch on the right than on the left.[44] The axillae can be percussed with the patient's hands resting on his hips. A resonant sound is elicited until about the eighth rib inferiorly.

The posterior chest wall should be examined while the patient is sitting with his arms, and therefore his scapulae, pulled forward. Again, percussion should proceed from apices to bases comparing the sound on the contralateral side. The presence of the scapulae and their muscles decreases the resonance of the sound heard. The sound produced when percussing the posterior chest wall will be less resonant than that heard anteriorly due to the thicker musculature. Percussion of the lower borders of the lungs should be done with the patient holding his breath after an inspiration and again, holding his breath after an expiration. With inspiration, the lung bases should be about 5 to 6 centimeters lower than with expiration. During quiet respirations the posterior-inferior lung edges are located at about the ninth rib on the left and the eighth interspace on the right,[45] while the dullness below the lung bases begins at about the tenth rib.[46]

The examiner can then auscultate the lungs to listen to breath sounds and voice sounds. This is done with the use of a stethoscope. Many stethoscopes now come equipped with both a bell and a diaphragm chestpiece. The diaphragm is used for general screening purposes and is especially good for detecting high-pitched sounds, while the bell is used for detecting low-pitched sounds.[47] Littmann notes that all normal, and with rare exceptions, abnormal pulmonary sounds are relatively high pitched and are well heard with the diaphragm pickup.[48]

Attention to the environment is necessary when auscultating the lungs. The room has to be quiet so that the sounds can be heard. It must also be warm enough to avoid shivering as these muscle sounds could be mistaken for râles. Another extraneous source of sound comes from the hair on the patient's chest which resembles the sound of fine râles. Finally, when the examiner listens to lung sounds she must learn to filter out sounds coming from the heart.

The procedure used with auscultation is similar to that used with percussion. The patient is examined in the sitting position and is instructed to breathe a little deeper than normal through his open mouth. It is helpful for the examiner to demonstrate this to the patient. The lung fields are systematically assessed with the stethoscope, beginning at the apices and proceeding to the bases. Contralateral areas are compared before moving to a lower area. The examiner should note where the breath sounds disappear and compare this to her findings with percussion.

Sounds heard during auscultation are evaluated to determine the type of breath sound which they represent, and the areas where they were heard. Vesicular breath sounds are heard over most of the lung fields, except in the upper interscapular area and the area of the manubrium sterni. They are soft, swishy high-pitched sounds with the inspiratory phase longer than the expiratory phase. Bronchial breath sounds are usually higher pitched and louder than vesicular sounds with an expiratory phase longer than the inspiratory phase. These sounds are not normally heard in the lung and reflect consolidation or compression of lung tissue. Bronchovesicular breath sounds are a combination of the above two types and have approximately an equal inspiratory and expiratory phase. They are normally heard in the upper interscapular area and in the area of the manubrium sterni. They may also be heard over areas of early or incomplete lung consolidation.

Other sounds which may be heard during auscultation are called adventitious sounds, and are abnormal. They may result from the passage of air through fluid (râles) or from the loss of lubricating fluid between the pleural surfaces (friction rubs). Râles are variously classified according to pitch (high, medium, or low),[49] or as moist, with thin secretions or dry, with thick secretions.[50] Another distinction is that if these gurgling or crackling sounds are discontinuous they are called râles, while if continuous, they are termed rhonchi.[51] Travers notes that fine râles are heard at the very end of inspiration, medium râles are usually heard about halfway through inspiration, coarse râles are heard at the very beginning of inspiration, and rhonchi, while continuous, are frequently more audible during expiration.[52] On the other hand, friction rubs can be heard during both inspiration and expiration but may be more audible during inspiration. The sound of a friction rub has been described as the sound of two pieces of dry leather rubbing together.

The examiner may be confused about the type of adventitious sound heard as it requires experience to familiarize oneself with the various sounds. However, the examiner can note the presence of an adventitious sound, identify its location and its timing in the respiratory cycle, and decide whether the sound clears when the patient is directed to cough after an expiration.

After the lung fields have been thoroughly evaluated for the type of breath sounds and for the presence of adventitious sounds, the lungs should be auscultated for voice sounds. The patient is instructed to whisper and to say 99 or 1, 2, 3 while the examiner systematically auscultates contralateral areas of the chest. Normally voice sounds are indistinctly heard with the stethoscope, but with areas of atelectasis, consolidation, or tumor, the sounds may be louder, clearer, or more distinct. Whispered sounds, if heard clearly, are called whispered pectoriloquy while spoken words heard more clearly are called bronchophony. Bronchophony can be normally expected over the trachea or posteriorly in the right upper lobe.

THE HEART. Evaluation of cardiac status includes an assessment of the precordium, the neck vessels, and the extremities. Examination of the extremities will be discussed later. Again, it is wise to establish a routine approach so that subtle changes are not missed. Inspection, palpation, percussion, and auscultation are used to assess cardiac status although in some instances percussion is omitted.

The heart lies between the lungs but about two thirds of it is located to the left of the mid-

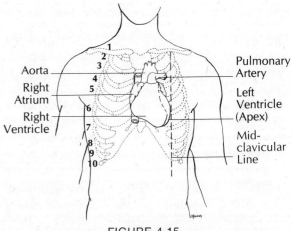

FIGURE 4-15.
Anterior view of the heart.

line. Unlike the lungs, the base of the heart is directed upward and to the right while the apex points downward and to the left where it rests on the diaphragm.[53] The precordium, that area of the chest which lies over the heart, normally extends from the second to the fifth intercostal spaces vertically and from the right sternal border to the left midclavical line in the fifth and sixth interspaces transversely.[54]

Figure 4-15 illustrates an anterior view of the heart. Note that most of the central portion of the heart in this position is taken up by the right ventricle while only the apex of the heart and a thin lateral strip on the left represents the left ventricle. The right border of the heart is located to the right of the sternum in the third to fifth interspaces and is composed of the right atrium.

The precordium, is first inspected while the patient is supine. Adequate lighting is required while the examiner looks for the presence of pulsations originating from the heart. Pulsations are caused by the forward and rightward rotation of the heart against the chest wall at the beginning of systole. The area in which the pulsations are seen is the point of maximum impulse (PMI) or the point of ventricular impulse (PVI). This area is usually located in the fifth interspace in the left midclavicular line, but, if the patient is lying on his left side, it may be noted 2 to 3 centimeters to the left.

Pulsations are seen in this area in about one fifth of all normal persons[55] but obesity, the presence of marked development of chest musculature, or the presence of emphysema may interfere with their visualization. Instructing the patient to hold his breath after an expiration may accentuate the pulsations. Holding either a tongue blade or a pencil lightly to the chest wall over the apex may result in the mechanical amplification of the pulsations at the free end of the blade or pencil.

Pulsations noted medially to those seen in the apex should be considered abnormal, and the rest of the precordium should be carefully inspected to note their presence or the presence of marked precordial heaves. On the other hand, pulsations are normally seen in the epigastric area especially in thin people, and in others after exercise. These pulsations reflect the normal activity of the abdominal aorta, while in some instances such pulsations are seen in the emphysematous patient with a displaced heart. Finally, in some normal patients, a systolic retraction may be noted in the fifth interspace near the apex and does not necessarily signify pathology.[56]

The precordium should then be carefully palpated using the palmar bases of the fingers while the patient is still in the supine position. The examiner can first palpate over the apex, where the impulse can be felt as a tap against the fingers, although the same factors which interfered with visualization of the pulsation may also interfere with palpation. A marked increase in the force of the impulse is associated with left ventricular hypertrophy, but recognition of the strength or force of the normal impulse is something which must be learned.

The examiner should then carefully palpate over the left sternal border and over the pulmonic and aortic areas. Normally pulsations are not felt in these areas when the patient is resting.

The palmar base of the hand should be used to determine the presence of thrills which are palpable murmurs, or of ventricular thrusts. When doing this, the fingers of the hand should be curved up so that they do not touch the chest wall. Thrills have been described as feeling like the purring of a cat. If a thrill is felt, its location and timing should be identified. To identify timing, the examiner notes whether it is systolic, synchronous with the apical beat, or diastolic.

The neck vessels are then inspected to estimate jugular venous pressure and to determine the presence and quality of the carotid pulses. The carotid pulse is palpated medially to the sternocleidomastoid muscle just below the angle of the jaw. Its rate, rhythm, and volume should be noted, and compared side to side.

The base of the neck should then be observed for venous pulsations. They are seen normally in most adults when in the supine position. Venous pulsations on the lateral aspect of the sternocleidomastoid muscle seem to move toward the head with expiration and application of moderate pressure with the finger above the level of the clavicle will obliterate the venous pulse. The head of the bed or examining table should then be gradually elevated to a 45° angle to determine if the external jugular veins can still be visualized. Normally they can not be visualized in this position, and, if visible, an increase in jugular venous pressure is suspected.

With the patient returned to the supine position, the precordium may be percussed to determine the cardiac borders. Since the ear can detect a change from resonance to dullness fairly easily, it is recommended that percussion always begin near the axilla and proceed medially toward the sternum. The fifth, fourth, and third interspaces can be percussed in this manner, while the examiner records the area of relative dullness at each level and its relationship to the midclavicular line. This is called the left border of cardiac dullness (LBCD), and normally it is located inside the midclavicular line and at, or slightly medial to, the point of maximum impulse. The right border of cardiac dullness (RBCD) cannot normally be clearly identified. Obesity, thick chest musculature, or a large breast may interfere with percussion of the cardiac borders. Common variations in body build may also influence the location of the cardiac borders, as will a change in the patient's position. Remember, if the patient is lying on either side, there will be a slight shift in the cardiac border in that direction.

The heart is then auscultated. This part of the cardiac assessment requires a knowledge of the sounds expected to be heard and an adherence to an examining schedule. The examiner should listen for one specific event at a time. In this way, the beginning examiner can organize what may seem to be a hopelessly complex task. The room should be quiet and the examiner should carefully attend to each aspect of the examination in sequence. The patient may be examined in the sitting position as sounds from the base are more easily heard when the patient is sitting or leaning forward. However, there are some events, such as the third or fourth heart sound or the sound of mitral stenosis, which may only be heard when the patient is lying on his left side. Therefore, it is wise to include both positions in a routine examination. The following sequence can be used.

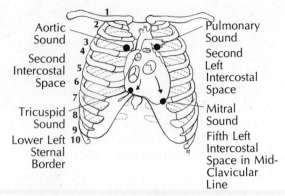

FIGURE 4-16.
Location of heart valves and areas where valve sounds are best heard.

1. The apical rate is counted and recorded. When doing this, the examiner must remember that each pair of heart sounds is counted as one beat. The lub-dub heard at the apex represents one heartbeat. After the heart rate is counted, the examiner should identify the rhythm noting whether it is regular or irregular. If it is irregular, the examiner should note whether there is any regularity to the irregular beat. If so, it is classified regularly irregular; if not, it is classified irregularly irregular.

2. The examiner listens next to the first and second heart sounds, the lub-dub. The first heart sound, S_1, is thought to be caused by mitral and tricuspid valve closure while the second heart sound, S_2, is the result of vibrations produced by aortic and pulmonic valve closure.[57] The sounds from the valves are not heard right over their anatomical locations but are usually loudest in that part of the precordium nearest their point of origin. The sounds from the pulmonic and tricuspid valves are best heard quite near their anatomic location, while the sounds from the aortic and mitral valves, which are deep in the chest, are best heard when they are transmitted to points closer to the chest wall. Figure 4-16 identifies the location of the heart valves and the areas where their sounds are best heard.

The examiner should then listen to just the first heart sound, S_1. There are several ways to identify this:

1. S_1 is synchronous with a visible or palpable apical pulse.

2. S_1 is almost synchronous with the carotid pulse wave.

3. If the heart rate is less than 100 beats per minute, the diastolic interval is longer than the systolic interval. Therefore, S_1 is heard first.

$$\text{LUB} \quad \text{DUB} \quad \text{LUB} \quad \text{DUB}$$
$$S_1 \qquad S_2 \qquad S_1 \qquad S_2$$

4. S_2 is usually louder at the base than S_1.[58]

In the first two examples, the examiner can palpate either the apex or the carotid beat and at the same time listen to the heart sounds. The sound which is heard at the same time the impulse is palpated is S_1. Once the examiner has identified this sound, she should try to screen out all other sounds and listen just to it. Using the diaphragm, she should then systematically auscultate the chest beginning at the base and slowly move toward the apex. This should be repeated listening only to S_2. Remember that S_1 is louder at the apex than at the base, while S_2 is louder or more prominent at the base. Diagrammatically the sounds at the base could be shown as follows:

☐ ☐ and heard lub DUP. The sounds at the
S_1 S_2
apex could be shown as follows: ☐ ☐ and heard
$\qquad\qquad\qquad\qquad\qquad\qquad S_1$ S_2

LUB dup. When the examiner has identified S_1 and S_2, she should compare their changing sounds as she moves slowly from the base toward the apex.

3. The heart sounds should be evaluated for the presence of physiological splitting. The valve closures which make up S_1 and S_2 are almost, but not quite simultaneous in this action. The left-sided events in the heart occur slightly before those of the right side and therefore the sounds can be split into two components. S_1 is composed of the mitral, M_1, and tricuspid, T_1, sounds while S_2 is composed of the aortic, A_2, and pulmonic, P_2, sounds. In S_1, the mitral component is of higher intensity and frequency than the tricuspid sound. Because of this, splitting of S_1 can only be heard with the closed diaphragm chestpiece at the lower left sternal border. Here the louder M_1 is followed by the soft T_1 which is then followed by S_2.[59] If a delay in the contraction time between the two ventricles occurs, the time between the two components of S_1 increases; if the

mitral valve were delayed in closing, the soft sound of tricuspid closure might be heard before the loud mitral closure.[60]

Since right ventricular ejection time is slightly longer than left ventricular ejection time, the louder aortic component of S_2 is heard before the softer pulmonic component. Splitting of S_2 is best heard in the second left intercostal space, since the pulmonic closure is poorly transmitted elsewhere. The splitting of S_2 is heard with the closed diaphragm chestpiece during inspiration. It is wider than the splitting of S_1. Normally the louder sound of A_2 is followed by the softer sound of P_2.[61] If the splitting sound is markedly widened, this is abnormal. Splitting should disappear during expiration. If it does not, a delay in aortic closure is suspected, and, in this instance, the soft pulmonic sound may be heard before the loud aortic sound.[62] If splitting is heard with equal intensity during inspiration and expiration, it is called fixed splitting and is abnormal.

4. The examiner should listen for the presence of extra sounds, such as high-pitched or clicking snaps associated with mitral stenosis or for ejection sounds associated with the opening of atrioventricular and semilunar valves. To do this, the examiner should again auscultate systematically with the diaphragm. The high-pitched clicking sounds of an opening snap are best heard along a line between the apex and the lower left sternal edge while ejection sounds, which are heard at the onset of a murmur, are heard in the same place as the murmur.[63]

The extra sound of the third heart sound may be heard normally in children and in young adults with thin chest walls. It is thought to be caused by sudden stretching of the ventricular walls during filling.[64] It is normally not heard in older adults and may indicate pathology if it is heard. The bell chestpiece lightly applied is needed to hear this sound, and the patient must be supine or lying on his left side. It occurs early in diastole and is best heard at the beginning of expiration and may be accentuated by exercise.

The fourth heart sound is due to ventricular filling as a result of atrial contraction and indicates atrial hypertrophy. It occurs late in diastole. It is necessary to use the bell chestpiece and to listen in the apical area with the patient supine,

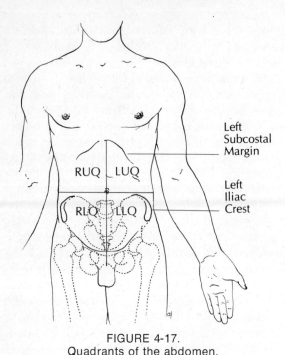

FIGURE 4-17.
Quadrants of the abdomen.

from turbulent blood flow and tend to be heard in the direction of their flow.[65] The examiner should first listen for the presence of murmurs during the systolic interval, that period after the first heart sound but before the second heart sound

LUB	DUB,	LUB	DUB,
Systole	Diastole	Systole	Diastole

When doing this, each valve area must be examined with both the diaphragm and the bell chestpieces. The examiner starts at the base and proceeds slowly toward the apex, with the patient sitting and lying on his left side. The same routine should be repeated during the diastolic interval. If a murmur is heard, the following characteristics must be recorded:

1. Timing—whether systolic or diastolic.
2. Duration—whether early, middle, or late or continuous during this period.
3. Location—where it is heard the loudest in terms of anatomic landmarks, whether it radiates, and where.
4. Loudness—generally reported on a six point scale with one over six barely audible with a stethoscope, proceeding to grade five over six which is loudest with a stethoscope, and finally to six over six which can be heard without a stethoscope.
5. Pitch—described as low (heard best with the bell),

but the sound is of such low intensity that it cannot usually be heard.

5. The examiner should listen for the presence of murmurs. Unlike heart sounds which have an abrupt beginning and ending, murmurs have gradual beginnings and endings. They result

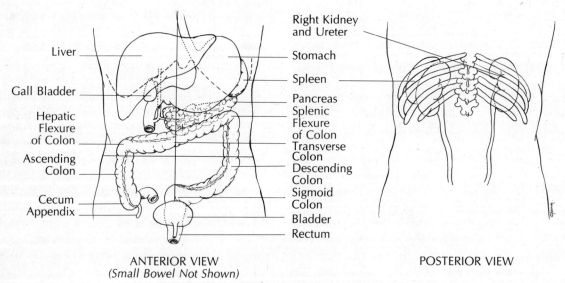

ANTERIOR VIEW
(Small Bowel Not Shown)

POSTERIOR VIEW

FIGURE 4-18.
Quadrants of the abdomen with partial contents shown.

medium and high (heard best with the diaphragm).

6. Quality—whether the pattern or configuration of the sound increases in loudness (crescendo) or decrease in loudness (decrescendo) or whether it could be described as blowing, harsh, rumbling, or musical.[66]

EXAMINATION OF THE ABDOMEN

The abdomen is examined using inspection, auscultation, percussion, and palpation in that order. The abdomen is generally divided into four quadrants in order that findings can be located (Fig. 4-17). In addition to the quadrants, other prominent landmarks are the subcostal margins, the umbilicus at the level of the fourth lumbar vertebra, the pubic bone, and the anterior spines of the right and left iliac bones.[67] The examiner must understand the location of the abdominal contents and their relation to various anatomic landmarks (Fig. 4-18). These structures are as follows:[68,69]

Right Upper Quadrant (RUQ)
liver
gallbladder
duodenum
head of the pancreas
part of right kidney
right adrenal gland
hepatic flexure of the colon
portions of the ascending colon and transverse colon
loops of small bowel

Left Upper Quadrant (LUQ)
stomach
spleen
left lobe of liver
part of left kidney
left adrenal
body of pancreas
spenic flexure of colon
portions of transverse and descending colon
loops of small bowel

Right Lower Quadrant (RLQ)
lower right kidney
cecum and appendix
portions of ascending colon
right ovary and tube
uterus if enlarged
right spermatic cord
right ureter
bladder if enlarged
loops of small bowel

Left Lower Quadrant (LLQ)
lower left kidney
sigmoid colon
portions of descending colon
left ovary and tube
uterus if enlarged
left spermatic cord
left ureter
bladder if enlarged
loops of small bowel

The abdomen is first inspected. The patient should be in the supine position with the examiner sitting to his right. The examiner observes general characteristics of the skin to note elasticity and smoothness. Scars, striae, or lesions are noted. Normally the venous pattern is barely visible but is more prominent in older people. The examiner observes the hair distribution, keeping in mind that pubic hair in the male normally extends upward toward the umbilicus in a triangular pattern. However, the pattern in the female has a horizontal border at the upper edge of the pubic area which does not extend upward toward the umbilicus, although some dark hairs are commonly found on the abdomen and around the areolae. The examiner looks for the presence of visible peristalsis which can be seen as slow undulations in people with thin abdominal walls. If seen in people with walls of normal thickness, the waves may be increased in amplitude and strength. The examiner then looks for abdominal pulsations normally seen in the epigastric area, and for any other pulsations.

Next, the abdomen is observed for its general contour which may be described as flat, rounded, or scaphoid (depressed). The examiner judges whether there is normal symmetry with no localized bulging, swelling, distention or prominences. She notes whether the umbilicus is located in the midline. The examiner instructs the patient to cough and inspects for bulges and prominences as he does so. She asks the patient to lift his head up off the table and inspects the abdomen in the midline for separation of the abdominal rectus muscles. Normally, separation does not occur.

Abdominal movement is seen in the male during respiration with the abdominal wall moving outward during inspiration. On the other hand, respiration in the female is costal and little abdominal movement is seen.

The abdomen is then auscultated before percussion or palpation so that it is not disturbed and the sounds of peristalsis and murmurs can be more readily heard. Peristaltic sounds reflect the movement of the bowel's contents, and, because of this, they are affected by the time of day, by food intake, and by the amount of fluid and gas in the intestinal tract. The bubbling and gurgling of peristalsis is normally present and varies in frequency, intensity, and pitch. The examiner should place her stethoscope below and to the right of the umbilicus and listen to peristaltic sounds. Since frequency of peristaltic sound varies, the examiner may have to listen for at least five minutes. If sounds are still not heard, flicking the abdominal wall with a finger may stimulate them. All four quadrants should be auscultated before concluding that no peristalsis can be heard. While peristaltic sounds normally vary in frequency, intensity, and pitch, the examiner should note whether the sounds appear decreased, suggesting inhibited bowel motility or whether they appear increased suggesting hyperactivity of the bowel. The rush of hyperactive bowel sounds, borborygmus, is normally heard in the right lower quadrant four to six hours after a meal.[70]

The examiner should then attempt to filter out the sound of bowel activity and listen just for the sound of murmurs which are heard as soft systolic bruit. She places the stethoscope over the aorta (in the midline above the umbilicus) and listens carefully. Normally abdominal murmurs are not present.

The abdomen can then be percussed to determine the outline of air containing organs, the hollow viscera, or to identify the borders of the solid viscera. Percussion may also serve as a method of relaxing the abdominal muscles and may help in identifying areas of tenderness.

The four quadrants should be systematically percussed noting the amount of resonance in the abdominal cavity. If the urinary bladder or the uterus are distended, dullness may be heard in the suprapubic area. The area over the stomach in the left upper quadrant will yield a high-pitched tympanic sound which varies with the amount of air in the stomach. The area occupied by the spleen, in the left posterior axilla, along the ninth, tenth, and eleventh ribs with a width of 7 centimeters should then be routinely percussed. Finally, the liver should be percussed to identify its borders. Remember that the ear can readily detect a change from resonance to dullness. Therefore the examiner percusses from lung resonance downward in the right midclavicular line to note the upper border of liver dullness, usually beginning in the fourth intercostal space. Then she percusses upward in the midclavicular line from well below the costal margin until the flat sound of the liver is heard. This distance is measured in centimeters. The upper and lower borders of the liver should not be more than 10 centimeters apart. However, gas in the overlying bowel may obliterate the dullness heard at the lower edge. This will make the liver size appear smaller.

The abdomen is palpated, first with light then deep palpation. This is done to identify areas of tenderness, resistance, or of organ enlargement.

With light palpation, the palms of the hands are placed on the abdomen and the approximated fingers are gently pressed into the abdomen for a distance of about 1 centimeter. Areas of resistance, tenderness, or guarding are noted. If the examiner's hands are cold or if the patient is anxious or ticklish, muscular tone may appear increased. The abdomen should be systematically palpated in all four quadrants with light palpation. Remember to lift the hand when moving from place to place to avoid inducing muscle spasm.

With deep palpation, the examiner presses more deeply into the abdomen. Care is taken to apply a gradual pressure and to avoid causing discomfort to the patient. The same technique of

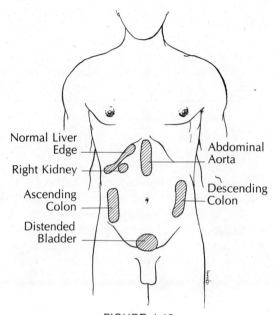

FIGURE 4-19.
Normally palpable abdominal structures.

Normal Liver Edge
Right Kidney
Ascending Colon
Distended Bladder
Abdominal Aorta
Descending Colon

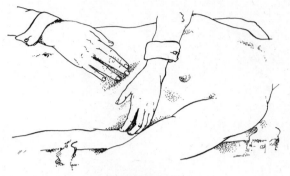

FIGURE 4-20.
Bimanual palpation of the left upper quadrant.

placing the palm on the abdomen and pressing in with the fingertips can be used. In addition to pressing inward, the fingertips should also glide back and forth over the abdominal contents for a distance of 4 to 5 centimeters. If resistance to palpation is particularly strong, reinforced palpation can be used. With this technique, the examining hand is placed on the abdomen with the fingers approximated but the depressing force is applied by the fingers of the other hand. The right hand receives the sensations from the abdomen while the left hand applies the pressure.

A systematic approach to deep palpation is necessary rotating through all four quadrants. What is felt on deep palpation will be affected by normal abdominal tone and the amount of subcutaneous fat. If the abdominal wall is quite muscular or if there are thick fat layers, palpation will be more difficult. If there is decreased abdominal tone or if the patient is quite thin, palpation is more likely to be successful in identifying the abdominal contents (Fig. 4-19).

In the relaxed, thin patient, the examiner may identify the abdominal aorta pulsating in the midline above the umbilicus, the ropelike descending colon in the lower left quadrant, the ascending colon in the lower right quadrant, and the edge of the liver and the lower pole of the right kidney in the upper right quadrant. If any other masses are palpated, their location, size, shape, mobility, consistency, and surface characteristics must be recorded. Additionally, the examiner should note whether the mass pulsates or is tender to palpation. If the urinary bladder or uterus is distended, it may be palpated in the midline above the pubic bone.

Bimanual palpation is necessary when examining the liver, kidneys, and spleen. The examiner begins with the left upper quadrant while standing at the patient's right side. The left hand is used to elevate the patient's left flank by supporting the thoracic wall at the eleventh and twelfth ribs. The right hand with the fingers approximated is placed below the costal margin in the left anterior axillary line. When the patient inspires, the tip of the spleen is displaced downward. The patient should be instructed to take a deep breath through his open mouth. As he does this, the left hand should lift the thoracic wall while the right hand gently pushes posteriorly and upward behind the costal margin (Fig. 4-20). If the spleen is enlarged about three times its normal size, the lower border will be felt to push against the fingers of the right hand during inspiration. The kidney should be palpated in the same manner. To do this the examiner must palpate deeper and slightly more to the midline. Normally the spleen and the left kidney cannot be palpated.

In the upper right quadrant, the liver is pal-

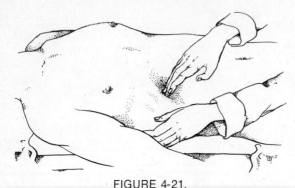

FIGURE 4-21.
Bimanual palpation of the right upper quadrant.

pated in the same manner. The examiner should stand at the patient's right side and place the left hand under the thorax at the eleventh and twelfth ribs. The right hand is placed under the right costal margins with the fingers pointing parallel to the abdominal rectus muscles and not parallel to the costal margin.[71] As the patient inspires deeply through his open mouth, the right hand presses posteriorly and upward (Fig. 4-21). At the same time, the left hand lifts the thoracic wall upward. The liver edge can normally be felt with this maneuver. Keep in mind that the right hand must be placed below the level of percussed liver dullness or the edge will be missed.

Again the technique for palpating the right kidney is similar, but it is necessary to palpate more deeply. The right kidney, since lower than the left, may be palpable in thin patients.

The groin can be palpated to identify the presence and character of the femoral pulses, and superficial inguinal and femoral lymph nodes by applying a light rotary pressure with the fingertips. If nodes are found, their location, size, degree of fixation, and consistency or texture should be recorded. The examiner also observes for bulges in the femoral region, medial to the femoral artery which transmits an impulse upon coughing. This may indicate a femoral hernia, the most common hernia in women.

A rectal examination is then done with the patient on his left side with knees flexed. With the buttocks separated, the skin around the anus should be inspected for signs of inflammation or excoriation. The gloved, lubricated, index finger

should be inserted pointing toward the umbilicus. This should be done gradually and gently while the patient strains down. When the patient relaxes, the finger is gradually advanced further into the anal canal. Sphincter tone is evaluated and all walls systematically palpated, to identify masses, nodules, or areas of tenderness. In the male, the anterior wall is palpated carefully to evaluate the condition of the prostate. The upper edges, lateral lobes and median sulcus should be palpated for any irregularities.[72] Normally the prostate feels smooth and rubbery and is not tender. Size varies but usually increases with age. The examiner should gently withdraw her finger and test any feces on her glove for occult blood.

The penis and scrotum of the male should then be inspected and the testicles, epididymes, and spermatic cords should be carefully palpated. The examiner first inspects the penis while the patient is supine. If the foreskin is present, the patient should retract it from the glans penis. Normally this is easily done. The examiner inspects the glans and the urethral meatus for any ulcers or discharge, and palpates the shaft of the penis for any nodules, plaques, induration, or cords.

The scrotum is inspected next. The left side normally hangs lower than the right. The walls of the scrotum should be inspected by spreading its layers between the fingers. The examiner checks for any unusual swelling, and palpates the scrotum to identify each testis, epididymis, and spermatic cord (Fig. 4-22). The testes are felt as

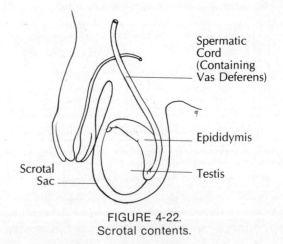

Spermatic
Cord
(Containing
Vas Deferens)

Epididymis

Testis

Scrotal
Sac

FIGURE 4-22.
Scrotal contents.

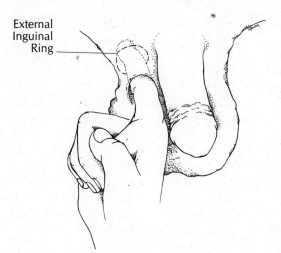

External
Inguinal
Ring

FIGURE 4-23.
Examining the inguinal canal in the male.

solid ovoid structures, suspended by the spermatic cord. The epididymis is felt as a comma-shaped bulge on the posterolateral surface of each testis. If swelling of the testes is noted, transillumination of the scrotal sac with a penlight flashlight may help distinguish scrotal contents.

With the patient standing and the examiner sitting, the femoral and inguinal areas can be examined for the presence of hernia. The examiner instructs the patient to strain down or cough and observes and palpates the area for bulges. Then she inserts an examining finger into the most dependent loose part of the scrotal sac and gently invaginates it upward into the external inguinal ring (Fig. 4-23). The examiner asks the patient to strain down or cough and notes if any mass which would indicate a hernia can be felt with the fingertip. Normally a mass is not palpated. The procedure is repeated on the other side.

EXAMINATION OF THE EXTREMITIES

This examination includes assessment of the status of the peripheral vascular and musculoskeletal systems. Inspection and palpation are used to conduct the assessment.

First, the upper extremities are inspected. The examiner judges whether both arms and hands seem equal in muscular development,

length, size, and shape. She looks for any sign of hypertrophy or atrophy of the muscles or for fasciculations, which are isolated contractions of portions of the muscle fibers. She looks for evidence of deformity, such as swelling or redness of joints or presence of nodules. Then, she determines if the color of both arms and hands appears similar. She looks for areas of blanching or bruising and carefully inspects the fingernails for their color, for any evidence of clubbing, or for the presence of small splinter hemorrhages.

The examiner compares the temperature of both hands and arms, then systematically palpates the pulses of the upper extremities. These include: the subclavian artery in the supraclavicular fossa, the brachial artery in the groove between the biceps and the triceps muscle medially above the elbow, the radial artery on the flexor surface of the wrist medial to the distal end of the radius, and the ulnar artery on the flexor surface of the wrist lateral to the lower end of the ulna.[73] The volume of these pulses are noted and compared to those of the other arm.

With the patient's elbows flexed 90 degrees, the examiner palpates each arm medially above the elbow for the presence of an epitrochlear node. If present, she notes its size, consistency, and whether it is tender to palpation.

The joints of the upper extremities are palpated systematically for areas of tenderness, nodularity, or bogginess. Normally the synovial membrane surrounding joints is not palpable. The examiner begins at the shoulder and proceeds to the fingers so that joints are not missed.

Next the examiner checks active and passive range of motion of the upper extremities. This includes the following:[74]

finger. flexion, extension, abduction, adduction opposition of the thumbs

wrists. extension, flexion, ulnar-radial deviation

forearm. supination, pronation

elbow. flexion, extension

upper arm and shoulder joint. elevation, elevation with abduction, or elevation with adduction

Then, flexibility and range of motion of the thoracic and lumbar spine can be evaluated. The standing patient bends forward and touches his toes. The examiner instructs him to lean forward, extend, and laterally bend his spine. Then, the patient rotates his upper trunk from side to side while keeping his hips and legs stationary. These movements should be performed with ease. While the patient is still standing, the examiner observes all four curves of the spine from a lateral and posterior view to determine the presence of the curves and to look for deviation of the spine from the midline. The examiner palpates the spine to determine areas of tenderness.

The lower extremities are evaluated, using a similar approach. The examiner begins at the groin and buttocks and proceeds to the feet. She judges whether both legs seem equal in muscular development, length, size, and shape, and checks for symmetry of the buttocks. Signs of hypertrophy or atrophy of the muscles or of fasciculations are noted. Joint shape is checked for swelling, nodes, deformities, or unusual position, and the skin inspected for the presence of rashes, pigmentation, ulcers, or venous distention. The examiner looks for signs of edema or for loss of hair over the anterior part of the lower legs. She determines if the color of the lower extremities appears similar and looks for blanching or bruising. The toenails are observed for their color or for unusual ridges. The presence of corns, calluses or other signs of pressure are noted.

The temperatures of both legs are compared. The examiner systematically palpates the pulses of each of the lower extremities, including: the femoral pulse below the inguinal ligament midway between the anterior-superior iliac spine and the pubic tubercles, the popliteal pulse in the popliteal fossa behind the patella, the posterior tibial pulse in the groove between the medial malleolus and the Achilles tendon, and the dorsalis pedis pulse on the dorsum of the foot lateral to the extensor tendon of the big toe.[75] The patient should be supine when palpating these pulses. Of the pulses of the lower extremities, the popliteal pulse may be the most difficult to identify. To palpate it the examiner places both hands around the knee and presses the fingers firmly into the popliteal space. She notes the character of all of the pulses of the lower extremities and compares them with those of the other extremity.

The lower extremities should be palpated to identify areas of tenderness, bogginess or swelling of joints, or edema. The examiner begins at the hip and proceeds to the toes when palpating for joint tenderness. Then she firmly palpates and squeezes the calf to identify any deep calf tenderness associated with phlebitis, and presses over the tibia, the medial malleolus, and the dorsum of the foot to identify edema. These results are compared with those of the other leg and foot.

Then active and passive range of motion should be evaluated and compared with the opposite side. Range of motion in the lower extremities includes the following:[76]

hip. rotation with extension of the knee
      rotation with flexion of the knee
      abduction-adduction
      flexion - extension
knee. flexion - extension
      (lateral mobility of the joint is an abnormal motion)
ankle. dorsiflexion - plantar flexion
foot. dorsiflexion, plantar flexion
      eversion, inversion

Finally, the patient is asked to walk across the room. The examiner observes the posture and ease of gait and notes any awkwardness or discomfort.

Evaluating the Data

The particular way in which data are used will depend upon their significance and upon the setting in which they were collected. For example, if the setting is an outpatient clinic, there will probably be a protocol or schedule which sets guidelines for the nurse's activity. Even if the nurse is functioning alone in a primary care setting, in addition to her independent problem solving, she will probably also have to be responsive to established guidelines which identify the manner of the patient's admission into the health system.

Some of the techniques used in physical assessment will gradually be incorporated into most nurses' practice. For example, in some acute care settings, nurses are already evaluating the fresh postoperative's respiratory status to determine whether râles are present in the lung bases. Because they are useful to the nurse, other aspects of physical assessment will be incorporated into her practice over time. Such changes will require curriculum revisions in schools of nursing and in organized continuing education departments.

References

1. Mereness, D.: Recent trends in expanding the role of the nurse. Nurs. Outlook 18, 5: 33, 1970.
2. Shetland, M.: An approach to role expansion: the elaborate network. Am. J. Pub. Health 61, 10: 1959, 1971.
3. McCormack, R. and Crawford, R.: Attitudes of professional nurses toward primary care. Nurs. Research 18, 6: 542-544, 1969.
4. Extending the Scope of Nursing Practice. A Report of the Secretary's Committee to Study Extended Roles for Nurses. Washington, D.C.: Department of Health, Education and Welfare, Nov. 1971, p. 2.
5. DeGowin, E. and DeGowin, R.: Bedside Diagnostic Examination, ed. 2. New York, Macmillan, 1969, p. 11.
6. Delp, M. and Manning, R.: Major's Physical Diagnosis, ed. 7. Philadelphia, W. B. Saunders, 1968, p. 13.
7. MacBryde, C. (ed.): Signs and Symptoms, ed. 4. Philadelphia, J. B. Lippincott, 1964, p. 11.
8. Judge, R. and Zuidema, G. (ed.): Methods of Clinical Examination: A Physiologic Approach, ed. 3. Boston, Little, Brown, 1974, p. 17.
9. DeGowin and DeGowin, *op. cit.*, p. 17.
10. *Ibid.*, p. 18.
11. Robbins, L. and Hall, J.: How to Practice Prospective Medicine. Indianapolis, Methodist Hospital of Indiana, 1970.
12. DeGowin and DeGowin, *op. cit.*, p. 23.
13. Judge and Zuidema, *op. cit.*, p. 76.
14. *Ibid.*, p. 78.
15. Macleod, J. (ed.): Clinical Examination, ed. 2. Edinburgh, Livingstone, 1967, p. 494.
16. DeGowin and DeGowin, *op. cit.*, p. 103.
17. Macleod, *op. cit.*, p. 497.
18. DeGowin and DeGowin, *op. cit.*, p. 104.
19. Macleod, *op. cit.*, p. 500.
20. *Ibid.*, p. 502.
21. *Ibid.*, p. 503.
22. Judge and Zuidema, *op. cit.*, p. 85.
23. DeGowin and DeGowin, *op. cit.*, p. 106.
24. *Ibid.*, p. 106.
25. *Ibid.*, p. 103.
26. *Ibid.*, p. 176.
27. Judge and Zuidema, *op. cit.*, pp. 124-125.
28. DeGowin and DeGowin, *op. cit.*, pp. 176-177.
29. Judge and Zuidema, *op. cit.*, p. 125.
30. *Ibid.*
31. DeGowin and DeGowin, *op. cit.*, p. 184.
32. Judge and Zuidema, *op. cit.*, p. 128.
33. DeGowin and DeGowin, *op. cit.*, p. 120.
34. Chaffee, E. and Grisheimer, E.: Basic Physiology and Anatomy. Philadelphia, J. B. Lippincott, 1964, p. 472.
35. *Ibid.*
36. DeGowin and DeGowin, *op. cit.*, p. 168-169.
37. Macleod, *op. cit.*, p. 88.
38. Judge and Zuidema, *op. cit.*, p. 47.
39. *Ibid.*
40. *Ibid.*, p. 132.
41. Seedor, M.: The Physical Assessment. New York, Teachers College Press, 1974, p. 137.
42. *Ibid.*
43. Delp and Manning, *op. cit.*, p. 103.
44. *Ibid.*
45. DeGowin and DeGowin, *op. cit.*, p. 294.
46. *Ibid.*, p. 292.
47. Littmann, D.: Stethoscopes and auscultation. Am. J. Nurs. 72, 7: 1240, 1972.
48. *Ibid.*, p. 1241.
49. Delp and Manning, *op. cit.*, p. 113.
50. DeGowin and DeGowin, *op. cit.*, p. 300.
51. Traver, G.: Assessment of thorax and lungs. Am. J. Nurs. 73, 3: 470, 1973.
52. *Ibid.*
53. Chaffee and Greisheimer, *op. cit.*, p. 328.
54. DeGowin and DeGowin, *op. cit.*, p. 326.
55. *Ibid.*, p. 329.
56. *Ibid.*, p. 330.
57. Lehman, Sr. J.: Auscultation of heart sounds. Am. J. Nurs. 72, 7: 1243 and 1245, 1972.
58. DeGowin and DeGowin, *op. cit.*, p. 353.
59. Lehman, *op. cit.*, p. 1244.
60. *Ibid.*
61. *Ibid.*

62. *Ibid.*, p. 1245.
63. Macleod, *op. cit.*, p. 148-149.
64. *Ibid.*, p. 147.
65. *Ibid.*, p. 150.
66. Judge and Zuidema, *op. cit.*, p. 214.
67. Seedor, *op. cit.*, p. 226.
68. Judge and Zuidema, *op. cit.*, p. 231.
69. Seedor, *op. cit.*, p. 224 and 226.
70. *Ibid.*, p. 261.
71. Judge and Zuidema, *op. cit.*, p. 234.
72. Judge and Zuidema, *op. cit.*, p. 283.
73. DeGowin and DeGowin, *op. cit.*, p. 401.
74. *Ibid.*, pp. 636-37, 655, 659, 662, 673.
75. *Ibid.*, p. 403.
76. *Ibid.*, pp. 698, 712, 728, 729.

Bibliography

Billings, G.: NHSC carries health care to the community. Am. J. Nurs. 72: 1836-1838, Oct. 1972.

Edwards, J., et al.: The Cambridge-council concept or two nurse practitioners make good. Am. J. Nurs. 72: 460-465, Mar. 1972.

Freemon, B.: How do nurses expand their role in well child care. Am. J. Nurs. 72: 1866-1871, Oct. 1972.

Gelfand, M.: The four techniques of physical diagnosis. Philadelphia, Smith, Kline and French, 1964.

Kelly, D.: One town's nurse service. Am. J. Nurs. 73: 1536-1538, Sept. 1973.

Kelly, L.: Nursing practice acts. Am. J. Nurs. 74: 1310-1319, July 1974.

Keough, G. and Niebel, H.: Oral cancer detection—a nursing responsibility. Am. J. Nurs. 73: 684-686, Apr. 1973.

Leininger, M., et al.: Primex. Am. J. Nurs. 72: 1274-1277, July 1972.

Lynaugh, J. and Bates, B.: The two languages of nursing and medicine. Am. J. Nurs. 73: 66-69, Jan. 1973.

Noonan, B.: Eight years in a medical nurse clinic. Am. J. Nurs. 72: 1128-1130, June 1972.

Porter, C.: Without standing orders. Am. J. Nurs. 73: 1559-1561, Sept. 1973.

Preston, T.: More people like Ruth Murphy. Am. J. Nurs. 72: 672-675, Apr. 1972.

Schutt, B.: Frontier's family nurses. Am. J. Nurs. 72: 903-909, May 1972.

———: Spot check of primary care nursing. Am. J. Nurs. 72: 1996-2003, Nov. 1973.

Schwab, Sr. M.: Caring for the aged. Am. J. Nurs. 73: 2049-2066, Dec. 1973.

Sheedy, S.: Medical nurse practitioner in a neighborhood center. Am. J. Nurs. 72: 1416-1419, Aug. 1972.

Tests of Mental Function in the Elderly. New York, Ives Lab., 1972.

Wagner, M.: Assessment of patients with multiple injuries. Am. J. Nurs. 72: 1822-1827, Oct. 1972.

Willacker, J.: Bowel sounds. Am. J. Nurs. 73: 2100-2101, Dec. 1973.

5

Family Planning: a vital family health service

CLARA H. JORDAN

Scanning the Past ● Present Population Trends ● Control of Fertility–Female ● Other Means of Fertility Regulation–Female ● Control of Fertility–Male ● Other Means of Fertility Regulation–Male ● Nursing Implications ● Psychological and Social Factors in Family Planning ● Nursing Implications for the Woman who Chooses to have an Abortion ● Summary of Nursing Management

Family planning may be thought of as a premeditated method of postponing a pregnancy, of spacing between pregnancies, or of avoiding pregnancy altogether. It includes the utilization of modern methods of conception control for regulating pregnancies, for establishing adequate intervals between births, for assuring that every pregnancy is a wanted pregnancy, and for treating infertility. Parents have the freedom to space and to limit their children to the number that can be adequately cared for. In an atmosphere in which every child is a "wanted" child, the concepts of responsible parenthood and a loving family environment are likely to be apparent. In addition to the use of contraceptive devices by an individual family unit, contraceptive practices may be advocated by a society or national group as a means of controlling and limiting population increases.

There is no universal definition of family planning. In the broadest sense family planning suggests voluntary control of family size or child spacing by contraception. Frequently the emphasis is on child spacing rather than limitation. However, the reader may be interested in a sampling of the various definitions or descriptions given by authorities in this area of health practice.

Family planning is an integral part of the overall effort to reduce poverty, raise educational levels, improve health and general welfare and thus make possible a greater freedom of individual choice. . . . family planning should no longer be the privilege of the middle and upper classes but should be available to all citizens.[1]

Family planning, utilizing modern methods of conception control, enables parents to have their babies as they want and can afford them.[2]

Family planning is preventive medicine—a preventive against personal, family, and social ills.[3]

Family planning represents, on the individual family basis, the voluntary choice of parents as to the number of children they want and can provide for.[4]

Current family planning programs and methods are designed to enable each individual or couple to make a decision regarding reproduction. This freedom of choice may be based on health factors, conscience or desire alone.

While family planning is variously defined, it is readily apparent that, although the definitions may differ, the concept remains the same.

The World Health Organization has defined health as a "state of complete physical, mental and social well-being—not only the absence of disease or illness." The planned family has a real contribution to make to health as defined. Medical evaluation may indicate that the health or even life of a woman may be endangered by an additional pregnancy. Further, the health of the prospective mother, the unborn child, present family members, and children not yet conceived deserves consideration. As health educators who recognize that family planning is an integral part of family-centered care, nurses are in a unique position to provide family-planning services.

During the last decade, the need for improved and more effective methods for the control of population, whether in individual families or nations, has become more apparent. Because of this increased awareness and concern, research has been intensified in an effort to develop methods that will not only be effective, but will also meet the widely varying needs of individuals according to their religious beliefs, cultural mores, socioeconomic backgrounds, and intellectual and emotional motivations. The concept of family planning, including within it such factors as health, fertility, social economics, and conception control as desired, necessarily involves the total physical and emotional relationship between man and woman.

Scanning the Past

How far have we advanced in contraceptive practices? Family planning is not a modern concern; birth control has presumably been practiced since long before recorded time. Techniques designed to prevent pregnancy go back almost to the beginning of the human race. Although until recently there was no true understanding of the process of conception and pregnancy, the idea of contraception is believed to be 4,000 or 5,000 years old. Because of the lack of knowledge concerning the reproductive system, the efficacy of any technique or method utilized was due to pure chance rather than to scientific rationale.

The Ebers Papyrus, a collection of seven medical records set down more than 1,000 years before the birth of Christ, deals with many of the same problems facing medicine today. Of these seven records, three are concerned with gynecological matters: how to prevent conception or produce abortion, how to cure infertility, and how to promote lactation. The Egyptian papyri, the earliest medical records in existence, reveal that contraception was a serious concern of the priest-physician of the pharaohs 4,000 years ago. These papers describe a medicated lint tampon to prevent a woman from conceiving for more than a year. Even before this time, there were written prescriptions for a contraceptive agent consisting of crocodile or elephant fat mixed with pastelike substances such as honey. Any effectiveness of this method was due to clogging action rather than to a spermicidal effect. These instructions appeared in writings for almost 3,000 years and were mentioned in Arab manuscripts as late as the 11th century. In the Greek and Roman eras, similar unguents were made of oily substances, such as honey and cedar wood oil, mixed with pomegranate pulp or the inside of figs.[5] References to contraception can be found in all types of literature, including the Bible. The story of Onan in Genesis, Chapter 38, is an example.

> And Judah said unto Onan, Go in unto thy brother's wife, and marry her, and raise up seed to thy brother.
> And Onan knew that the seed should not be his; and it came to pass, when he went in unto his brother's wife, that he spilled it on the ground, lest that he should give seed to his brother.[6]

The Sumatrans used a contraceptive agent made primarily from local plants and containing a large proportion of tannic acid. A Persian manuscript believed to have been written in the 10th century advised mixing rock salt with oily or pastelike materials. Table salt is known to be an effective spermaticide; therefore, a strong rock salt solution would almost certainly destroy sperm. Spermaticidal materials to be placed in the vagina prior to intercourse became available commercially in the late 1800s, when an English pharmacist concocted an unguent containing quinine. Despite the lack of advanced communication media, the news spread rapidly by word of mouth and the product was in great demand.

An Egyptian papyrus of 1850 B.C. recommended fumigation before intercourse and douching after intercourse. Fumigation was achieved by sitting astride an elaborate form of burner, which permitted vapor or medicated steam to enter the vagina. Douches of wine and garlic with fennel were recommended for use immediately after intercourse. The same technique of fumigation and douching was mentioned in Indian writings of the 1st century B.C. It is thought that perhaps the effervescent or foaming tablet available for birth control today is an historical descendant of this earlier type of fumigation of the vagina, since it forms a froth of gas which carries the spermaticidal agent into the folds of the vaginal mucosa.[7]

The first reference to the use of intrauterine devices for contraceptive purposes has been found in *Diseases of Women,* Hippocratic writings of over 2,000 years ago.[8] The device was inserted into the uterus through a hollow lead sound passed through the cervix. For centuries Arabian and Turkish camel drivers inserted a small round stone into the uterus of their saddle animals prior to a desert trip.[9]

Early in the 20th century a German physician, Richter of Waldenburg, described the insertion of two or three strands of silkworm gut into the uterus for contraceptive purposes;[10] and in 1930 Grafenberg reported on the use of silkworm and silver rings in over 2,000 women.[11] The modern intrauterine devices (loop, coil, and bow) were developed in 1959.

The varieties of mechanical barriers that have been recommended as contraceptives through the ages stagger the imagination. In India and parts of Asia, it was a frequent practice to plug the back of the vagina with wads of feathers or other bulky materials. In Biblical times, a sponge was commonly inserted. (The sponge method, with and without a spermaticidal agent, is in use today.) Other recommended mechanical barriers have included leaves of plants coated with honey; tampons made of wool soaked in wine or smeared with pitch; a pomegranate cut in half with the inside removed; and chopped grass or chopped rags wadded into a mass.[12]

In ancient China and Japan, strips of very fine paper were made into a ball and placed in the vagina to form a cervical barrier. Other nations recommended beeswax discs which were inserted in the vagina and forced over the entrance to the cervix. This technique proved fairly efficient since beeswax does not liquefy at the temperature of the human body. The concept of occluding the cervix by methods such as the cervical cap and the diaphragm developed from such techniques.[13]

The use of the condom, or sheath, can be traced back to primitive peoples. Prehistoric cave sketches portray intercourse with the male seemingly using some form of sheath. It is believed that the sheath was developed as a protection against disease. Bladders of animals were used for this purpose in ancient Rome. The Chinese used sheaths of oiled silk paper and the Japanese developed a device of tortoise shell or leather. Italian writings of the 16th century describe a linen sheath. The condom itself was probably invented in the 17th century by a physician at the court of Charies II.[14]

One of the most ancient techniques for preventing pregnancy is coitus interruptus. Mention of this practice can be found in the oldest books written about this topic.[15] The concept of a safe period also goes back many years. One common belief was that pregnancy was connected with a particular season of the year, and that if intercourse was avoided during that season there would be no conception. Another belief was that the period of menstruation was related to the period of ovulation, and that, therefore, pregnancy would not occur if intercourse were avoided just prior to and after menstruation. The relationship between ovulation and menstruation became clear in time and the dimensions of what might be termed a safe period could be determined. Because it was impossible for authorities to recommend a "safe period" for every woman, an elaborate tradition grew up in some cultures about abstention. Indian writings warned that coitus was not to take place during sunset, or from the first to the fourteenth day after the beginning of menstruation, or on the eighth or fourteenth day of each fortnight, on the anniversary days of dead parents, or on the nights prior to those days, or at midday during an eclipse![16]

Prescriptions for oral contraceptives, today considered a contemporary development, can be found in early history. A prescription in a Chinese book dated 2700 B.C. reads, "take some quicksilver, fry it for a whole day in oil, take a piece about the size of a lozenge and swallow it on an empty stomach—the taker will never become pregnant."[17] Writings of the ancient Greeks and Romans suggest drinking a mixture of water containing rust and willow leaves. Solutions of iron and copper sulfates were also recommended.

During the Middle Ages the ingestion of lead, arsenic, strychnine, and iodine preparations became popular methods of killing the sperm internally. During this same period, the castor oil plant and its beans were popular means of preventing conception throughout Europe and the Middle East. The belief prevailed that a mother, desiring no more children, would be free from childbirth for one year if she were to eat a single seed of the castor oil plant.[18]

With the advent of the Industrial Revolution and the emergence of a middle class in society, contraceptive practices became more in demand because of the economic benefits derived from smaller families. Beginning with World War I, the more liberal sexual attitudes that prevail following wars provided further impetus for demanding prevention of pregnancy.

Margaret Sanger, a nurse, after marrying and bearing several children, worked with mothers in the slums of Manhattan and devoted much of her life to bringing birth control information to the poor. It was she who opened the first birth control clinic in Brooklyn on October 16, 1916. In 1969, 53 years later, Planned Parenthood-World Population was operating birth control clinics in approximately 134 cities throughout the United States. Of the 350,000 women seen in the 500 clinics in operation, 275,000 are in the poverty group. In addition, this organization stimulates local hospitals and health departments to operate clinics.

Although it has only been since January, 1969, that the UN Fund for Population Activities began its population and family-planning program, this organization, along with various agencies of the United Nations, has assumed world leadership in coping with population problems. In 1973 the International Planned Parenthood Federation had a budget of over $30,000,000, whereas in 1965 the worldwide budget was less than $1,000,000.

Man's effort to prevent conception has a long history and reveals a wide range of imagination and ingenuity. Present-day concepts of contraceptive techniques will be considered later in this chapter.

Present Population Trends

Concern with population problems and action toward their solution have become matters of world interest. In the United States, Europeans and their descendants have achieved what they could not achieve in Europe. A common language, an expanding frontier, rich and plentiful natural resources in a temperate climate, a cultural heritage of literacy and skills were advantages destined to create a nation of wealth, power, and prestige. It is not possible to accurately determine the population of the world, but it is possible to make reasonable estimates. The UN estimates are generally accepted as the most reliable and have reported the population of the world to be in excess of 3.7 billion in midyear 1971, and in 1975 in excess of 4 billion. From information available we know that the world population is greater than it has ever been and that it is increasing at a high rate. The rate of increase in a population is the reflection of the extent to which births exceed deaths. Currently the United Nations estimates that there are 1.9 births for every one death. A continuation of this rate would result in a doubling of the world population in 35 years.[19]

The growing interest in population problems is focusing on specific appraisals of the situation in various parts of the world. Many people in the developed nations have learned to control their reproduction whereas many people in the underdeveloped nations have not had the opportunity to learn to do so. In the developed countries a decline in fertility has generally followed a decline in mortality. Experts have projected that from 1975 to the year 2000 the less developed countries will be the source of more than 90 percent of the world's population growth.[20] The most rapid increases in population are now found in the nonindustrialized countries of Asia, Latin America, and Africa. Approximately two thirds of the world population reside in these countries.

In considering whether a population problem exists in the United States, one might be influenced by examining how rates of reproduction can jeopardize existing goals of our nation. We ought to ask ourselves whether we want not only to keep what we have, but also to move ahead and reduce the number of underprivileged, lessen the amount of poverty and the numbers of unemployed, give each child the best education of which he is capable, provide for the millions of aged, and make modern medicine available to all. The higher fertility rate of the underprivileged means that a large portion of the next generation is being raised under conditions of economic and cultural deprivation. Education and income continue to influence the number of children born; that is, the higher the education or income, the fewer the children. Differences in family size on the basis of income alone also show a marked inverse relationship. High fertility among high-income groups is presumed to be a matter of choice, whereas among low-income groups it is presumed to be the result of apathy, ignorance, and inaccessibility of family planning guidance.

Charles F. Westoff of Princeton University's Office of Population Research and co-director of a national fertility study of 5,000 women of childbearing age reports that on an estimate made between 1960 and 1968, unwanted children made up 35 to 45 percent of the U.S. population increase. Some 42 percent of all poor children were unwanted, as opposed to 17 percent of children born to the near affluent and well-off. These children were conceived in spite of contraceptive measures, or because contraception was inadvertently omitted or not available.[21]

The United Nations has calculated that a continuation of current trends will give us a world population of 6.5 billion in the year 2000. An awareness of the problem of rapid population growth, coupled with newly developed methods of family limitation has lowered a previous projection of 7.4 billion at the turn of the century to the new projection of 6.5 billion.

Today the governments of half of the developing regions officially favor family planning. The advanced countries are also becoming more alert to the crises in world population. The subject of birth control has become a topic of open debate in legislative bodies and in the mass media of world news and opinion.

The problems of motivation, communication, religious acceptance, and suitable family-planning techniques are such that a rapid decline in fertility is not likely to occur. A world population of at least 6 billion in the year 2000 seems highly probable. Hope lies in the fact that as public opinion polls in various parts of the world indicate, many people would like to limit the number of children in their families to those they can adequately care for and raise.

In July, 1969, in a message on population, President Nixon recommended that

1. A Commission on Population Growth and the American Future be established.

2. Research for developing new birth control methods be increased.

3. A family planning office be opened in the Department of Health, Education, and Welfare to provide leadership and funding for United States family planning programs.

4. High priority be given to attention, personnel, research and funding of population assistance in the Foreign Assistance Program.

5. United Nations leadership, with full United States cooperation, be encouraged to meet the world challenge of too rapid population growth.[22]

Although previous presidents had shown concern about population growth, this was the first presidential message dealing with the threat posed by overwhelming numbers.

Federal expenditure programs to support family-planning projects increased the number of persons served from 863,000 in fiscal year 1968 to more than 3.4 million in fiscal year 1974. These include family-planning programs offered in hospitals, health departments, by Planned Parenthood, and other voluntary projects. Through these funded projects, continued effort is being made to promote the inclusion of family-planning services in general health delivery systems. In addition to and in collaboration with the gynecologist-obstetrician, registered nurses are assuming increased responsibility in insuring that each pregnancy is a result of an informed individual decision. Current family-planning methods which include acceptable methods of birth control, abortion, and sterilization permit each individual or couple to make a decision regarding reproduction. Every pregnancy, therefore, should be the result of an informed personal decision and the outcome a wanted child.

Women's liberation—the feminist movement—which has developed and progressed in recent years has proved to be a stimulus to the limitation of family size. Cultural and social attitudes have altered the role of women in today's society. Women are becoming more aware of the inadequate gynecological and maternal health care available to them and are currently more vocal in their demands for improving this care. The everchanging female role in our society may prove to be a dramatic force for lowering the birthrate in this country.

Control of Fertility—Female

ORAL PROGESTINS

HISTORY. After extensive investigation and experimentation, field trials of oral contraceptives began in 1956.[23] In 1960, the first oral contraceptive, "the pill," was approved for general distribution by the Food and Drug Administration. The pill is considered to be one of the major developments in medicine during the last decade. Since the approval of the pill for U.S. prescription, its use has spread rapidly throughout the world.

BIOLOGICAL ACTION. Oral contraceptives are synthetic compounds, some of which are similar in structure to the natural hormones associated with the menstrual cycle and with pregnancy in the human female. In the dosages currently used, these compounds (estrogen and progestin) inhibit ovulation. Therefore, the mechanism of action of hormonal contraception is through pituitary depression with failure of production of follicle-stimulating hormone (FSH) and luteinizing hormone (LH), thereby suppressing ovulation. The normal ovulatory cycle is controlled by the interplay of the pituitary gonadotropins secreted by the anterior pituitary gland and the estrogen and progesterone secreted from the ovary. The pituitary gonadotropins stimulate the ovary to secrete estrogen and progesterone, and these hormones act in turn to inhibit the secretion of pituitary gonadotropins. In addition to inhibiting ovulation, the various oral contraceptives are believed to interfere with the normal transport of the zygote and to create an endometrial lining unfavorable for implantation as well as a change in the cervical mucus which becomes resistant to penetration by spermatozoa.

The oral contraceptives now available are the combined, sequential and low-dose progestin preparations. Low-dose combination preparations have a small amount of the progestin combined with a much larger amount of estrogen. The sequential preparations have fairly high levels of estrogen since the estrogen acting alone is responsible for their contraceptive effectiveness.

With the combined pill, it appears that the primary effect is produced by the balance of estrogen and progesterone during the last half of a menstrual cycle, when further ovulation is inhibited by the body's own processes. The action of the pill is initiated very early in the cycle for the prevention of the release of the ovum. Without ovulation, fertilization is impossible and conception cannot occur. Under this regimen, twenty (or twenty-one) tablets, containing one of several synthetic progestins as well as estrogen, are taken from the fifth to the twenty-fourth (or twenty-fifth) day of the cycle.

The low-dose progestin preparation has the advantage of eliminating any of the side effects which may be due to the estrogenic component of other oral contraceptives. A distinct disadvantage of this preparation is that the pregnancy rate is several times greater than that for the combination preparations. In addition, with the low-dose progestin regime the menstrual pattern is often very irregular. This preparation is of value to women who may wish to take an oral contraceptive but are unable to tolerate a preparation containing estrogen. The low-dose progestin without estrogen is taken daily without interruption.

The sequential pill relies on estrogen to suppress production of FSH sufficient to prevent egg cells from maturing. With this regimen, fifteen (or sixteen) tablets, containing estrogen only, are followed by five (or six) tablets containing progestin and estrogen. The added progestin for the last four, five, or six days of the cycle is given to produce bleeding on discontinuance of use. Because estrogen alone does not eliminate the midcycle peak of secretion, there is some possibility of ovulation if a mature egg happens to be present when the LH reaches its peak. For this reason, the sequential method may not inhibit ovulation with the same degree of certainty as the balanced combination method.

Oral contraceptives not only inhibit ovulation, but stimulate growth of the endometrium as well. Menstruation occurs a few days after the pill cycle has been completed.

EFFECTIVENESS. If the pill is taken as prescribed, the effectiveness of the combination of tablets containing a progestin and an estrogen is rated as almost 100 percent. Oral contraceptive tablets are the most effective means known for the control of fertility. The sequential administration of estrogen for 15 or 16 days, followed by an estrogen and a progestin for 5 or 6 days, is also highly effective for family-planning purposes, but, as stated previously, is somewhat less effective than a progestin and an estrogen given in combination. A disadvantage of the low-dose progestin preparation is that the pregnancy rate is several times greater than that for the combination preparation. A distinct advantage of oral contraceptives is that their use is not immediately related to sexual activity.

ADVERSE REACTIONS. Most side effects reported during the use of oral hormonal contraceptives have generally been mild and have consisted of spotting and breakthrough bleeding,

nausea and vomiting, breast tenderness, weight gain, occasional emesis, and gastrointestinal symptoms. These effects are related to the estrogen present in oral contraceptives. Some progestogen-estrogen combinations are claimed to be associated with a lower incidence of breakthrough bleeding than others, but there is evidence to suggest that these compounds are also associated with a higher incidence of amenorrhea or failure of withdrawal flow. With several products available to choose from, the dosage and product can be shifted until the one best suited to the patient's physiological makeup is found. Most symptoms are relieved during the first few months of therapy; however, some women become discouraged and resort to other methods, or even abandon their efforts at family planning.

One serious condition for which an association with the use of the pill has been established is thromboembolic disease, including pulmonary embolism. In 1967, a cause-and-effect relationship of birth control pills to thromboembolism was reported in the studies of Inman and Vessey[24] and Vessey and Doll.[25] Although the validity of these studies is still being challenged, the findings have been corroborated by later investigation. The U.S. Food and Drug Administration, however, considered the results of sufficient importance to require that labeling and advertising policies for all oral contraceptives reflect possible side effects of these preparations. In a subsequent report in 1970, Inman and Vessey were able to demonstrate a positive correlation between the dose of estrogen and the risk of pulmonary embolism, deep vein thrombosis, cerebral thrombosis, and coronary thrombosis in the United Kingdom.[26] From information now available, one can conclude that there is a greater risk of thromboembolic complications from the use of oral contraceptive preparations and that low-estrogen compounds are considered more safe or less likely to cause undesirable side effects.

To allow for the possible occurrence of thromboembolism episodes, it has been recommended that women with previous vascular problems, varicose veins, or other factors which may predispose to thrombophlebitis should be watched closely for any signs of this complication, or be given another method of contraception.

In September, 1969, after an exhaustive three-year study, the U.S. Food and Drug Administration announced that the pill was safe for the vast majority of women. The FDA's advisory committee on obstetrics and gynecology, which conducted the study, did not, however, overlook the possible harmful side effects of the pill. The increased risk of blood-clotting disorders in the estimated 8,500,000 women who take the pill, it noted, was 4.4 times the normal risk of women who do not. These disorders proved fatal to three out of every 100,000 women using the pill. Physicians on this committee warned that the pill should be taken only under a physician's careful supervision and never by women with circulatory ailments or a history of persistent headaches.[27] It is recommended that the medication be discontinued immediately if there is a sudden onset of migraine. Because oral contraceptives may cause some degree of fluid retention, conditions which might be influenced by this factor (i.e., migraine, epilepsy, asthma, cardiac or renal dysfunction) require that physicians and nurses be alert to early manifestations of these conditions. Migraine headaches are believed to result from dilation of small arteries near the surface of the skull; the headaches may, therefore, be related to the pill's effect on blood vessels.

Hormone components of the pill appear to accelerate the action of other hormones that regulate blood pressure. Women unusually sensitive to this hormone effect may develop high blood pressure. In addition to this danger, the estrogen component of the pill is known to increase the coagulability of blood and, therefore, the risk of clot formation. Although strokes are uncommon in women under 40 years of age, neurologists have reported as many as 16 cases in a year among women on the pill as compared to only one or two before the advent of the pill. It is believed that the increased blood pressure and the estrogen's effect on the clotting mechanism may be responsible. A few cases of severely impaired vision, even blindness, as the result of clotting in the minute retinal arteries have been authenticated in women taking the pill.[28]

Laboratory studies of carbohydrate metabolism and hepatic and thryoid function have in some instances revealed deviations from the normal in women taking oral contraceptives. For this reason, the drugs are contraindicated in women with either a history or presence of hepatic disease or dysfunction. In addition, the presence or history of breast or genital cancer is considered a contraindication to hormonal contraception.

In 1969, a survey of women attending the Planned Parenthood clinics in New York City revealed a higher prevalence of epithelial abnormalities, diagnosed as carcinoma in situ, among women taking oral contraceptives than those using the diaphragm.[29] Data obtained from this study were not conclusive enough to establish that oral contraceptives have a carcinogenic effect. In late December, 1975, medical officers of the U.S. Food and Drug Administration warned that there may be an increased risk of cancer of the uterus with the use of the sequential contraceptive pill. This warning came as a result of a recent study done at the University of Colorado School of Medicine, where 21 women under 40 who had developed endometrial cancer were studied. Eleven of the 21 women were taking sequential oral contraceptives. No definite link could be found between this disease and the use of the combination pill. Although it was recognized that the sampling in this study was small, it was thought to be important enough for FDA representatives to meet with the manufacturers of the sequential pills and to indicate that unless drug companies are able to show that the benefits of this oral contraceptive are greater than the risks, the sequential pill will be withdrawn from the market.[30] Early in 1976, this warning was widely disseminated through the various news media.

Because oral contraceptives may suppress lactation, mothers who plan to breast-feed their babies are usually advised not to take this medication until after the milk supply has been well established.

Careful and continued medical and nursing supervision is essential for women using this method of contraception. A complete medical history, breast and pelvic examination, blood pressure reading, a urinalysis, and a Papanicolaou smear are prerequisites before this medication is prescribed. In addition, patients must be taught to recognize and report any untoward symptoms related to possible complications and the necessity for periodic medical examinations.

VAGINAL DIAPHRAGM

HISTORY. About 1882 a German physician, Wilhelm P. J. Mensinga, invented the vaginal diaphragm. Before the introduction of oral contraceptives in 1960, the diaphragm was the contraceptive method most recommended by physicians in the United States and throughout the world. Following the introduction of oral contraceptives, the diaphragm was seldom the method of choice. In more recent years, however, increasing numbers of women who cannot, for medical reasons, use these contraceptives or who have a fear of taking the pill or of using the IUD are choosing the diaphragm as the best of the remaining alternatives.

Biological Action. The diaphragm, a flexible hemispherical rubber dome, is used in combination with a spermicidal cream or jelly. This device, covering the cervix, provides a barrier to sperm. The jelly or cream acts as a spermicide and as a lubricant for inserting the diaphragm. It must be left in place a minimum of six hours after coitus; douching is prohibited. If the diaphragm is inserted more than four hours prior to intercourse or if intercourse is repeated, additional spermicidal cream or jelly should be introduced with an applicator.

EFFECTIVENESS. This method of contraception is highly effective when used consistently by women who have been taught to check for correct placement after its insertion and if left in place the recommended period. The diaphragm must be fitted by a physician, refitted every two years and after each pregnancy.

ADVERSE REACTIONS. Many women use the diaphragm successfully and find it quite acceptable. Some women have difficulty inserting it correctly, are not sufficiently motivated, or feel the procedure is distasteful. The nurse can be very helpful in explaining the anatomical relationships of the vagina and cervix and in teaching how to insert and best determine the proper positioning of the diaphragm. A pelvic model might be used for teaching purposes.

Because the use of a diaphragm requires a pelvic examination by a physician, or other trained health worker, this method of contraception is not suitable in situations where such services are not available. Privacy for the insertion of the diaphragm by the user should also be a prerequisite for its use.

SPERMICIDES

HISTORY. Chemical products to be inserted into the vagina just prior to intercourse and used without a diaphragm have been developed in recent years. These spermicidal agents include vaginal jellies, creams, foams, tablets and suppositories.

BIOLOGICAL ACTION. These materials coat the vaginal surfaces and cervical opening, immobilizing sperm on contact. The agent may act as a mechanical barrier as well. Suppositories that melt in the vagina and tablets that crumble and dissolve on contact with moisture release carbon dioxide, producing a dense foam.

EFFECTIVENESS. Chemical contraceptives used alone appear to be less effective than spermicides used in combination with the diaphragm or condom. The vaginal foams, followed by the jellies and creams, appear to be more effective than other types of spermicides. Spermicides are simple to use, do not require a pelvic examination, and are inexpensive. This method of contraception is more popular in Europe than in the United States.

ADVERSE REACTIONS. Many users complain that the drainage of the chemical materials from the vagina is objectionable and that the foaming tablets cause a temporary burning sensation. Irritation and/or inflammatory changes of the mucous membrane have been reported in rare cases. Suppositories and foam tablets require a waiting period of several minutes to allow for melting or disintegration. Spermicides provide protection for only about one hour.

POSTCOITAL DOUCHE

HISTORY. Postcoital douches with water, vinegar, or various other products have long been used for contraceptive purposes. This method was widely used until World War II. In recent years a variety of commercially available "feminine hygiene products" have been used for postcoital douching as well as for aesthetic reasons.

BIOLOGICAL ACTION.   Flushing of the vagina immediately following coitus is intended to remove or destroy sperm.

EFFECTIVENESS.   The postcoital douche is considered to be a very poor method of contraception because spermatozoa have been found in the cervical canal within 90 seconds after ejaculation.[31] The douche is ineffective, inconvenient, and useful only as an emergency measure (e.g., if a condom breaks). Douching within six hours after intercourse, when other methods such as foams or creams have been utilized for contraception can interfere with their effectiveness.

ADVERSE REACTION.   Frequent douching and use of strong solutions may damage the bacterial flora of the vaginal mucosa. Inflammation of the sensitive mucosa may result in pruritus and general discomfort.

RHYTHM METHOD

HISTORY.   The belief that women are able to conceive during part of the menstrual cycle only is very old. However, early ideas of the fertile and sterile periods of the menstrual cycle were frequently the opposite of what is known today. Based on a study of the menstrual cycle, the calendar rhythm method and the basal temperature method are practiced.

The calendar rhythm method was developed in the 1920s by two men independent of one another, Ogino in Japan and Knaus in Austria.[32,33] In this method, the day of ovulation is estimated by a formula based on the individual woman's menstrual history, recorded over a number of months. Abstinence from intercourse is prescribed for a few days before and after the estimated day of ovulation.

The basal temperature method is more recent and is based on the fact that progesterone is produced near the time of ovulation and that circulating progesterone raises the basal body temperature. Daily readings of basal body temperatures are studied over a period of at least three months in an effort to determine the time of ovulation. The accuracy of the estimated date of ovulation can be increased by this method.

BIOLOGICAL ACTION.   The rhythm method is based on abstinence on the days when an ovum and motile spermatozoa might simultaneously be present. Since ova are thought to be available for fertilization for only 24 hours and spermatozoa remain viable for 48 hours, there are, theoretically, only three days in each menstrual cycle during which conception can occur.

EFFECTIVENESS.   The contraceptive effectiveness of the rhythm method has been greatly debated. Correctly taught, correctly understood, and consistently practiced, the rhythm method, and particularly the basal temperature method, may be quite effective.[34,35] Successful practice, however, requires a great deal of self-control and a strong desire to avoid pregnancy. This method is widely used among Roman Catholics, since their faith prohibits the use of other contraceptive methods.

ADVERSE REACTIONS.   There are no side effects but several disadvantages. The method depends on abstinence from intercourse during the time of month when the women is fertile; the opportunity for coitus is, therefore, greatly reduced. It is unsuitable for women with irregular menstrual cycles. Reasons for failure of the calendar method include errors in recording the menstrual history, errors in computation, the variability of the menstrual pattern, and an exceptionally long survival of sperm in the female genital tract. Reasons for failure of the temperature rhythm method include errors in reading the thermometer and errors in interpreting the temperature curve. It should be recognized that pregnancy can possibly occur at any time during a menstrual cycle.

INTRAUTERINE CONTRACEPTIVE DEVICES

HISTORY.   Intrauterine devices (IUD) are mentioned in the writings of Hippocrates. Devices made of many different materials have been used for more than 2,000 years in a variety of gynecological disorders, as well as for the control of fertility. Intrauterine, or more accurately, intracervical devices during the 19th century were used chiefly for correction of uterine displacement, but also for contraception. Early models were in the shape of collar buttons and wishbones. Many gynecologists rejected these devices because their use was associated with inflammatory conditions of the pelvic organs which at that time were difficult to treat and frequently fatal.

In 1928, Grafenberg of Berlin reported a series of more than 2,000 insertions of intrauterine devices for contraception. These were first made of silkworm gut and later of silver wire. The failure rate with the silver ring was 1.6 percent. Although the mechanism of contraceptive action was not ascertained, Grafenberg suggested that the devices increase functional activity of the endometrium. Other researchers showed that foreign bodies in the uteri of experimental animals prevented pregnancy. After a brief period of popularity, opposition to the new device developed rapidly among gynecologists, who apparently based their objections on unfortunate experiences with earlier intrauterine devices. This method fell into disrepute and no further work was reported in this area for almost 30 years. Textbooks of gynecology, if contraception was discussed at all, condemned the Grafenberg ring.

In 1959, Oppenheimer reported results of years of experience with modifications of the Grafenberg ring. His series included 1500 patients with no serious complications. The era of the modern IUDs had to await the availability of such materials as plastics and stainless steel which could remain in the uterus indefinitely. Japanese workers were the first to utilize plastic material for intrauterine contraceptive devices. In 1962, the Population Council inaugurated an intensive research program, which includes experimentation in the laboratory, as well as clinical and field trials. The results of these studies encouraged the adoption of IUDs as the method of choice in the national family-planning programs of a number of countries.[36,37]

BIOLOGICAL ACTION. Despite extensive research during the past few years into the biological effects of intrauterine devices, the precise mode of action of the IUD remains uncertain. Explanations for its effectiveness include interference with the movement of sperm through the uterus and the fallopian tubes, or with the fertilization of the ovum, or with its transportation through the tubes, or with its implantation in the uterus. There is no evidence that the antifertility effect of the IUD involves interference with the implanted embryo. Intrauterine devices have an antifertility effect in every animal tested, but differences among species have been found. Because of the anatomical and functional differences in the genital tracts of the various species investigated, it is believed unlikely that any one mode of action will be found common to all.

Evidence of transient endometrial inflammation has been found in women with IUDs. Histological studies suggest an alternation in cyclic maturation of the endometrium. Bacterial contamination occurs almost universally after insertion of an IUD. Recent reports of infection attributed to use of the IUD have involved the Dalkon shield. Although the use of this device is being questioned, intrauterine infections may occur with any IUD. Chronic infiltration of the endometrium with plasma cells and lymphocytes almost always occurs. There is tissue edema and increased vascularity in tissues directly adjacent to the device. Delayed or asynchronous endometrial maturation may be sufficient to inhibit intrauterine pregnancy.

EFFECTIVENESS. The IUD is one of the most effective methods of birth control and, while less effective than the oral contraceptives in preventing pregnancy, its use results in a pregnancy rate of only 2 to 5 percent. The IUDs currently in wide use are the Lippes loop, Saf-T-Coil, Dalkon shield and the Copper 7. Pregnancy rates for the most effective IUDs vary inversely with the size of the device and the age of the patient.

However, higher pregnancy rates can be expected under the conditions of a community health program, which does not provide for frequent checkups, since the IUD may be expelled without its being noticed by the wearer. Frequent checkups, customary in clinical studies, increase the chance of discovering an unnoticed expulsion before pregnancy occurs.

The contraceptive effectiveness of IUDs is less reliable than either the combined or sequential oral contraceptives. IUDs are probably not more effective than the diaphragm or condom if these forms of contraception are used correctly. In clinic patients, however, IUDs have proved far more reliable than traditional methods and only slightly less reliable than oral compounds.

The IUD continues to be a popular method of contraception in the United States. The IUD is widely used in several national family-planning programs, especially in Asia, with the largest numbers of insertions reported from India, Pakistan, South Korea, and Taiwan.

The incidence of expulsion and of side effects that necessitate the removal of the IUD have been determining factors affecting the continued use of IUDs. The rate of expulsion varies markedly among the various IUDs, with about 10 percent during the first year after insertion reported for the most widely used device. The expulsion rate tends to be higher among young women of low parity than among older women of higher parity, with age being the most important factor. Expulsion after the first year is uncommon.

About 80 percent of women will continue to use the device for the first year, 70 percent for the second, and from the limited data available, about 50 percent at the end of the fifth year. These figures include women who are wearing an IUD after one or more reinsertions.

ADVERSE REACTIONS. The menstrual flow usually becomes heavier with the use of the IUD. Among the minor complications of the intrauterine devices are backaches, irregular bleeding, and uterine cramps or pelvic pain. These commonly occur during the first two or three months after insertion and tend to disappear with continued use. They constitute the reasons for about 60 percent of all removals.

Perforation of the uterus is uncommon and is often unnoticed by the physician. Most perforations of the uterus are asymptomatic and are discovered at a routine checkup, or when removal is attempted, or after delivery. The incidence of perforation varies with the skill of the operator and the type of device used.

There is no evidence at the present time that IUDs cause cancer in women. It will not, however, be possible to make a definitive statement on this point until substantial numbers of women have used IUDs for prolonged periods. Each patient, nevertheless, should have a cervical smear done before the insertion of an IUD, followed by periodic cytological examinations.

One adverse experience associated with the use of IUDs is pelvic inflammatory disease. At least one study suggests that, in a population with a high rate of pelvic inflammatory disease, the incidence is even higher among women wearing IUDs. Whether the insertion of an IUD in a woman with healthy pelvic organs can produce pelvic inflammatory disease is not known.

The incidence of abortion among women who wear IUDs may be as high as 40 percent if pregnancy occurs with the IUD in situ. When the pregnancy proceeds to full term, the device is found to be outside the membranes or occasionally beneath the placenta. No increase has been noted in the prevalence of malformations among the children born to women wearing IUDs.

Ectopic gestation occurs about once in 20 pregnancies with the IUD in place. This ratio, ten times the normal rate, is attributable to the substantial reduction in the number of intrauterine pregnancies. Although there is a lack of agreement that IUDs cause ectopic pregnancies, the possibility of an ectopic pregnancy in a woman with an IUD in place must always be considered.

SURGICAL CONTRACEPTION

HISTORY.   Dr. James Blundell of London is credited with having first suggested this procedure in 1823. Surgical sterilization was originally done to protect women whose life or health was threatened by pregnancy or delivery. Effective techniques were developed in the latter half of the 19th century when aseptic surgery and anesthesia became available.

The safety of surgical sterilization led to its being used to prevent persons with hereditary disabilities from having children. In recent years, discussion has centered on the legality of voluntary sterilization as a method of family limitation and on the use of sterilization in countries where high birthrates and rapid population growth threaten to produce serious economic and social difficulties.[38]

Voluntary elective sterilization is now a medically accepted procedure which is legal in all states. Sterilization for purposes of contraception is increasing.

BIOLOGICAL ACTION.   This method consists of surgical interruption of the fallopian tubes to block the passage of sperm. The methods used include tubal ligation, partial excision of the tubes, or total salpingectomy. Until recently this usually involved an abdominal incision so that the tubes could be ligated, a portion excised, and the two ends cauterized. Female sterilization by means of culdoscopy can be performed under local anesthesia and on an outpatient basis. A new method of laparoscopic instrumentation has advantages over the classic procedures of sterilization by means of laparotomy and colpotomy. This technique requires only a brief hospitalization of a few hours to one or two days and is safe and effective. In this procedure carbon dioxide is insufflated intraperitoneally to facilitate observation and manipulation of the fallopian tubes. The laparoscope is then inserted through a 2 cm. horizontal incision 1 to 2 inches below the umbilicus. An electrical current is passed through the laparoscope and a portion of the tube coagulated and removed. Recent advances include development of instruments enabling suture and ligation of the tubes through the laparoscope.

EFFECTIVENESS.   Surgical sterilization is considered to be virtually 100 percent effective. Failure may be due to inadequate surgery and rare anatomical aberrations.

ADVERSE REACTIONS.   The risk of surgical complications does exist, as well as the possibility of untoward emotional reactions, particularly in the event of remarriage or if the death of children creates a desire for more.

THE FUTURE.   A number of new techniques for temporary sterilization are under investigation. In one technique, the ovary is enclosed in a Silastic pouch which is then buried with the ovary in the broad ligament. With fimbriotexy, a Silastic hood is placed over the fimbria and sutured in place. Temporary occlusion of the fallopian tube has been attempted by placing a fimbrial plug inside the tube. All of these techniques require a laparotomy initially and again for removal.[39]

Other Means of Fertility Regulation—Female

Other methods of hormonal contraception have undergone clinical trials and some have been approved for general use. Still other potential methods of contraception which hold promise for the future are currently under investigation.

POSTCOITAL ORAL ESTROGENS OR ANTIESTROGEN

Dubbed the "morning after" pill, this method is claimed to be effective in preventing pregnancy following isolated exposures. Because of the high-estrogen dose involved and the accompanying nausea and vomiting, this method should be the choice only in emergency situations. Presumably this method affects the rate of ovum transport. The potent estrogen pill is started within 72 hours after unprotected intercourse and continued for five days.

ONCE-A-MONTH ANTIOVULANT PILL

This pill combines estrogen and progestin. The steroids are absorbed from the gastrointestinal tract, stored in adipose tissue, and released gradually over a month. The estrogen, quinestrol, and the progestin, quingestanol acetate, are given orally every four weeks. In one study, the pregnancy rate was 4 per 100 women years of use and the menstrual cycle control was good. Side effects were similar to those encountered as a result of the use of the more conventional oral contraceptives.[40]

LONG-TERM ANTIOVULANT INJECTION

Medroxyprogesterone acetate, an estrogen-progesterone combination, administered by injection every 90 days, has recently been approved for clinical use. This method appears to be as effective as oral contraceptives in the prevention of pregnancy. Side effects are similar to those with the use of oral contraceptives. Problems such as irregular bleeding, amenorrhea, and lack of restoration of fertility have been encountered. Because of this possible delay in fertility this should not be the method of choice for women who wish to have more children.[41]

LONG-TERM ANTIOVULANT IMPLANT

With this technique, an implant of Silastic tubing containing estrogen-progestin for chronic release is placed beneath the skin. This procedure suppresses ovulation and menstruation.[42] Absorption of the steroid has been reported to be about the same three months after the insertion as it is three days afterward. Fertility can be prevented for as long as the steroid lasts and theoretically for as long as three years.[43] The effectiveness of this method is dose related and is dependent on systemic absorption of the hormonal implant. Implant methods of contraception are still under investigation.

CONTINUOUS LOW-DOSE PROGESTIN

REMOVABLE VAGINAL RING.   A vaginal ring made of silicone rubber is impregnated with medroxyprogesterone (Provera). The ring provides for continuous absorption and may act locally on cervical mucous glands or systemically to give the low-dose progestin antifertility effect. The woman inserts the ring five days after the beginning of a menstrual period, removes it after 21 days, and throws it away. She should menstruate within two days, and start the 28-day cycle again with a new ring five days later. Clinical trials on this method are still being conducted.[44]

SUBDERMAL IMPLANT.   This method is still being investigated. It provides for continuous absorption of a progestin-impregnated capsule imbedded in subcutaneous tissue.

IUD-RELEASED.   This method provides for continuous absorption and may act either locally in the uterus, or systemically to give the low-dose progestin antifertility effect.

IMMUNIZATION WITH SPERM OR WITH SEMINAL-FLUID ANTIGENS

The objective in this method would be to protect the female from pregnancy by preventing fertilization through massive agglutination of the traveling sperm.[45]

IMMUNIZATION WITH ANTIGENS SPECIFIC TO PREGNANCY

Antigens of placental tissue, fetal membranes, and the umbilical cord tissue, would theoretically prevent the nidation process.[46]

Control of Fertility—Male

CONDOM

The condom is one of the most widely used methods of conception control. It can be purchased and used without a prescription and, in addition to serving as a contraceptive, it provides protection against acquiring or spreading venereal disease.

A condom is a sheath or cover shaped to fit the erect penis and worn to prevent sperm from entering the vagina. This device is usually made of thin, strong rubber or latex. If used correctly and consistently, the condom offers a high degree of protection against pregnancy. For added protection, the wife may also use a vaginal foam, cream, or jelly. The condom rates in effectiveness with the diaphragm. Side effects are extremely rare. Occasionally an individual may be sensitive to rubber or to the powder used on the condom.

COITUS INTERRUPTUS

This method of contraception requires that the husband practice great self-control since it means that the man must withdraw from the woman's vagina before emission of semen. However, sperm may escape before sexual climax, or the climax may occur unexpectedly. "Withdrawal" has been responsible for many failures in family planning. This is one of the oldest methods of conception control and is the principal method by which the decline of the birth rate in Western Europe was achieved from the 18th century on.

This method is unacceptable to many couples because it may interfere with sexual gratification of either partner or both. It does apparently still occupy first place in many countries of Europe and the Near East. In general, its use is inversely associated with socioeconomic status.

SURGICAL CONTRACEPTION (STERILIZATION)

The bilateral vasectomy is considered to be the most effective method for controlling fertility in the human male. This procedure is quite simple and can be performed in a physician's office in 15 or 20 minutes. An incision is made on the upper part of the scrotum and the sperm-carrying tubes or spermatic ducts are tied. The testicles continue to form sperm which are absorbed in the body, and the male will still have an orgasm and ejaculate although the semen contains no sperm. Contraceptive practices should be continued until the semen is examined by the physician about eight weeks or ten ejaculations after the operation to ensure that it is free of sperm. It must be understood that vasectomy does not provide immediate sterility, since mature sperm remain in the vas deferens and accessory glands beyond the area of ligation. Work can usually be resumed a day or two following this surgical procedure.

Some countries are relying more on male methods of contraception than on female. For example, male sterilization is being used extensively in India.

In recent years, male sterilization in the United States has become more widely accepted and is now considered a popular means of permanent contraception. It has been estimated that one million vasectomies a year are being done in the United States.[47]

Other Means of Fertility Regulation—Male

Extensive research has been conducted on a number of approaches to control fertility in the male. At present, investigators have been unsuccessful in their attempts to find a new male method of contraception that would be comparable to the pill for females. Investigation of methods for male contraception include a pill for males, suppression of sperm production, alteration of the seminal fluid by the addition of a chemical which would be picked up by the semen, interference with sperm transport, and immunological techniques. Procedures are being tested for restoring fertility after occlusion of the vas deferens and for reversible vas deferens ligation.[48]

Nursing Implications

In this Space Age, with the vast technical and scientific knowledge available, it is hard to understand why knowledge of means for temporary prevention of pregnancy is not widespread. Birth control information is readily available. Yet many couples do not seek help, or do not know that such information is accessible, or perhaps are not sufficiently motivated to utilize these recommended methods.

It is the responsibility of the nurse to maintain health and prevent illness, whatever the circumstances. The nurse, therefore, may assume responsibility for teaching family planning, for it involves the total relationship between man and woman, including health, fertility, and socioeconomics. Dissemination of information in these areas is essential for the development and perpetuation of sound family relationships.

Since women tend to relate better to other women when discussing this very personal matter, the nurse is in a unique position to assume responsibility for teaching them ways of planning for the children they want. Techniques must be explained, evaluated, and chosen on an individual basis. If the nurse is to be effective in teaching family planning, she must not only be knowledgeable in the present methods for this purpose, but also informed of current research and new developments in this area and the numerous reasons for contraceptive control.

The registered nurse in the hospital, physician's office, school, community health agency, or other community agency, is frequently asked for advice on family planning. And because of the broad scope of the subject, knowledge, understanding, and active participation in discussing it is required not only of nurse and patient, but also of the physician, the social worker, and members of other related health disciplines. A multidisciplinary approach provides the greatest benefits to the patient.

It is extremely important that nurses, as well as physicians, understand the need for information which will enable women to postpone or prevent pregnancy. No patient should be denied advice, upon request, because of the individual physician's or nurse's moral or religious beliefs. If giving advice on family planning is against one's religious mores, the patient can be referred to someone who will give her or him the information requested.

The American Medical Association and the American College of Obstetricians and Gynecologists have established similar policies endorsing control of fertility. Family planning has become an integral part of medical care. Attention has been directed, therefore, to the inclusion of courses in family planning in medical school curricula. Schools of nursing, too, are incorporating the subject of child spacing into their curricula.

In September 1966 the board of directors of the American Nurses' Association adopted the following statement:

AMERICAN NURSES' ASSOCIATION
STATEMENT ON FAMILY PLANNING
During the past years, there has been noticeable public concern over implications of the expanding world population and the human and natural resources available to maintain this population. It is evident that even the minimum in health care, food, and the other necessities of life are not now available to all individuals at a subsistence level. If the world population continues to expand at the present rate, these necessities will continue to diminish for even greater segments of the population. The American Nurses' Association, the professional organization of nurses concerned with the health and welfare of individuals and families, feels that it is the responsibility of registered nurses:

1. To recognize the right of individuals and families to select and use such methods for family planning as are consistent with their own creed and mores.

2. To recognize the right of individuals and families to receive information about family planning if they wish.

3. To be responsive to the need for family planning.

4. To be knowledgeable about state laws regarding family planning and the resources available.

5. To assist in informing individuals and families of the existence of approved family planning resources.

6. To assist in directing individuals and families to sources of such aid.

Because nurses have a real and enduring interest in the well-being of people, the American Nurses' Association endorses efforts to promote understanding of family planning methods and supports positive and realistic programs designed to cope with the implications of unchecked population growth.[49]

Concern over population growth and its bearing on community health has stimulated widespread interest in family limitation as a community health and demographic problem. Positive influences of child spacing on a woman's mental and physical health have been well substantiated. Women today are subjected to many pressures—economic, spiritual, educational, social, and physical—that affect her role in raising children. She should not be expected to bear more children than the number for which she can provide quality care. In 1959 the American Public Health Association endorsed a statement that cites the threat to health, nutrition, and standards of living of unrestricted population growth; this statement concludes in part as follows:

The American Public Health Association believes therefore that:

Public health organizations at all levels of government should give increasing attention to the impact of population change on health. . . .

Public and private programs concerned with population growth and family size should be integral parts of the health program, and should include medical advice and services which are acceptable to the individuals concerned.

Full freedom should be extended to all population groups for the selection and use of such methods for the limitation of family size as are consistent with the religion and mores of the individuals concerned.[50]

Psychological and Social Factors in Family Planning

Psychological and cultural factors of human reproduction have only recently come under scientific inquiry. Therefore, in studying human behavior one must consider the particular social class in which the individual exists. Contraceptive attitudes and behaviors must be placed within a value system determined by the person's culture. A woman's values in regard to health care may be inferred from the frequency with which she seeks medical examinations and follows medical advice on such matters as diet, exercise, medication, and contraception.

The values that a woman learns in regard to sex, marriage, reproduction, children, and family life have a profound influence on her before, during, and after pregnancy. One woman may not be aware of this influence because her behavior conforms to her value system and to various expectations. Another woman, however, may be confronted with severe conflict because of discord between the values she holds and those to which she is exposed. For example, such conflicts may arise when a woman must make a decision regarding contraceptive practices, or an abortion when she has an unwanted or illegitimate pregnancy; or, if the infant has been delivered, whether to arrange for its adoption.

Values tend to change as social, economic and technological conditions change. They are also influenced by new knowledge, as, for instance, that acquired through information about child spacing. Technological and social changes and fears of overpopulation are resulting in a shift in values, from the large family to smaller families. The Planned Parenthood Association was founded in the United States for the purpose of establishing proper values and for making opportunities for family planning more widely available.

Rainwater and Weinstein have reported that social class was more closely related to family planning and behavior than any other single factor.[51] In their investigation they found that effective and constant use of contraceptives is attained only as the attitudes of people toward sex, marital relationships, concept of parental roles, beliefs about masculinity and femininity, and other issues associated with sex and male-female relations are taken into account.

Westoff, in accounting for unplanned pregnancy, calls attention to the disposition on the part of couples to "take a chance" when they have competing values for and against having another child.

> This chance-taking behavior, whether it involves not employing any contraceptive precautions at all or risking conception through the use of ineffective methods, can be interpreted as a consequence of the competition of different values. If the values opposing the conception of another child are strong, whether these values center around mobility aspiration, the desire to send children to college, or feeling of economic insecurity, presumably, chance-taking will be less.[52]

Devereux states, from an analysis of psychoanalytic cases, that

> The adequacy or inadequacy of contraceptive measures is only marginally determined by rational considerations and by proper instruction. . . . The prime motivating factors in inadequate contraception are: masochistic brinkmanship, unconscious wishes to become pregnant, and aggressive impulses toward the partner.[53]

Obstacles to family planning have been classified under four general categories:[54,55]

KNOWLEDGE AND BELIEFS. This includes concepts, accurate or inaccurate, held by an individual concerning contraception and related sexual information. One attitude found in this investigation is: "It does not make any difference what you use or how you use it. If it is going to happen it is going to happen."

SEXUAL ATTITUDES. Sexual attitudes play an important factor in couples being able to develop effective procedures for successful family planning. The subjects in this research study revealed how they related to their marital partners or how they looked upon themselves in relation to their marital partners. Feelings toward sexual behavior were revealed: such as "The men don't care! They don't have the children, and they can walk out whenever they please."

VALUES AND MOTIVATIONS WITH RESPECT TO FAMILY PLANNING. Lack of planning for the future was prevalent among the respondents in this study. Considered in this classification were statements which reflected 1) presence or absence of a concept of family-size goal; 2) marital or personal conflict regarding family-size goal; and 3) faltering motivation at the time of sexual excitement which led to "taking a chance." For example: "If I'm making love in the living room, I can't be bothered to get up and go to the bathroom to get a contraceptive."

MARITAL RELATIONSHIPS. The Rainwater study found that working-class wives felt isolated from their husbands, whom they considered to be dominant and controlling. In order not to be deserted, they felt that they had little or no power in the marital relationship. This investigator's findings indicate that ineffective contraceptive practices, commonly used in the working class, are embodied in particular personalities, world views, and ways of life which have consistency and stability, and which do not readily admit such foreign elements as conscious planning and emotion-laden contraceptive practices.[56]

In summary, through this discussion, an attempt has been made to point out various psychological and social considerations that the nurse must consider when approaching the teaching of family planning and fertility control. It is important that the nurse be aware of women's emotions during the childbearing years. The patient's reactions to temporary or permanent contraception as they affect her personality should be noted. These reactions could be expected to affect not only her relationship to her husband, but to other children and to the extended family as well. Social class values, as they directly relate to effective contraceptive behavior, must be recognized as important issues when teaching and counseling in family planning. The nurse must be able to recognize the cultural and psychological factors that contribute to the individual's motivation for planning his or her particular life situation. The freedom to choose the size and spacing of a family offers an individual a greater freedom of choice of what she can do with her life.

The facts of life do not penetrate to the sphere in which our beliefs are cherished . . .; as it was not they that engendered those beliefs, so they are powerless to destroy them; they can aim at them continual blows of contradiction and disproof without weakening them.

Marcel Proust
Remembrance of Things Past

Nursing Implications for the Woman who Chooses to have an Abortion

In recent years existing laws prohibiting abortion have been challenged in the courts. Public support for legalized abortion increased, and, as a result, in January, 1973, the U.S. Supreme Court ruled that abortions are legal during the first three months of pregnancy. This law specifies that during this period of pregnancy, the decision to have an abortion lies with the woman and her physician. This ruling further specifies that for the next three months of pregnancy a state may regulate the abortion procedure by requiring hospitalization of the woman and licensing of the persons and facilities involved. For the last ten weeks of pregnancy, any state may prohibit an abortion unless it is necessary for the preservation of the life or health of the mother.

With legal restraints removed, a woman now has the right to personally decide whether or not to end an unwanted pregnancy and to seek an abortion. Physicians are no longer restricted from performing abortions, and, because of the Supreme Court ruling, physicians are likely to be expected to perform an abortion simply because a woman requests it. This decision has become a matter of individual judgment and choice. This choice may, of course, be influenced by one's religion, philosophy of life, or morals, or by a woman's views on her right to make decisions regarding her own body.

Now that prenatal detection of fetal defects is possible through transabdominal amniocentesis and analysis of the amniotic fluid, the woman carrying a defective child may choose to have a therapeutic abortion. Intrauterine diagnoses of a chromosomal or biochemical abnormality may give prospective parents the option to terminate the pregnancy if serious or irremediable mental or physical handicaps of the fetus appear to be inevitable. Teratogenic agents such as radiation, viruses (as maternal rubella), and chemicals may also have a deleterious effect on the intrauterine environment and cause congenital malformations. Although the susceptibility of an embryo to a teratogen largely depends upon the developmental stage at which the exposure occurs, the risk to the fetus may result in a decision by the mother and on advice from her physician to have the pregnancy terminated.

In 1970, a New York State law went into effect permitting abortions up to the twenty-fourth week of pregnancy. Statistics compiled since this time indicate that early abortions performed by competent physicians result in a lower mortality rate than term deliveries.[57] Based on the large number of abortions being performed we can conclude that although abortion is not considered a method of contraception, the procedure is widely used to prevent unwanted births. These unwanted pregnancies are usually the result of lack of knowledge about contraception, failure to use any form of contraception, or the use of an unreliable method of birth control.

It is not the writer's intent to discuss the moral aspects of abortion, but rather to look at ways in which the nurse can best provide optimal care for women who have made the decision to have their pregnancies terminated.

The professional nurse caring for the abortion patient is in a unique position to utilize nursing skills to their fullest potential. Within the scope of professional nursing practice, the nurse makes decisions related to health care assessment and counsels and plans for the maintenance of health and prevention of illness. Since a large number of women seeking an abortion report having used no method of birth control at the time of conception, counseling the woman includes helping her to decide what method of preventing pregnancy will best meet her individual needs. By the full utilization of her knowledge and skills the nurse assumes increased responsibility for primary health care for individuals and their families. She makes more independent and collaborative decisions, assumes responsibility for identifying patient needs and concerns and takes appropriate action. She is able to provide care to patients on a personal continuous basis. Because of recent changes in nursing practice, nurses are using their preparation more advantageously, accepting more responsibility in the management and counseling of abortion patients and providing information on contraceptive practices. Nursing interviews as a means of assessing patients are an integral part of the plan of care for these women. As an expert practitioner the nurse is competent to plan, implement, and evaluate the nursing process. This information will enable the nurse to determine nursing care problems, needs, and concerns that fall within the scope of professional nursing practice. The nurse is accountable for independent as well as collaborative decisions which result in improved patient care.

Hospitalized abortion patients should be placed on a separate unit. Since it is not uncommon for abortion patients to encounter hostility from new mothers and from staff members on an obstetrical unit, placing abortion patients with new mothers should always be avoided.

In caring for the woman seeking an abortion, the nurse needs to talk with her before, during, and after the procedure to learn what emotional factors are involved and what may have prevented her from using adequate contraception. Women who are ambivalent in their decision to have an abortion need time to work through these feelings. In talking with the patient prior to her decision, the nurse may have the opportunity to explore all of the alternatives available, such as adoption, single parenthood, marriage, or termination of pregnancy. Following the woman's decision, the nurse is obligated to respect and support the decision which she has made.

Little is known about the psychological effect of abortion on women. A follow-up study of 41 girls in early adolescence, carried out six months after therapeutic abortion, revealed feelings of guilt, depression, and anger; however, these feelings were confined mostly to the immediate postoperative period. If parents and health care personnel show a helpful attitude rather than a critical and punitive one toward these girls, the emotional reaction to the pregnancy and subsequent abortion will be of much shorter duration.[58] Gabrielson et al found an apparent high risk of attempted or threatened suicide in 105 pregnant young women under the age of 18. These authors stress the importance of unified medical care, social services, and special educational facilities.[59] The effect of abortion on the emotional status of the woman who has had an abortion is still controversial. Those favoring the increased availability of abortion have one point of view, the opponents of liberalized abortion quite another. In administering the Minnesota Multiphasic Personality Inventory test to 65 abortion patients, Niswander et al reported an improvement in psychological state six months after the abortion.[60] The initial feeling of elation a woman feels following an abortion and the relief of having it over with may be followed by a grief reaction and a feeling of depression. The patient may become more quiet, appear withdrawn, and cry. A woman's emotional reaction to abortion depends in part on her reasons for choosing to have the abortion and on the emotional health of the patient. For women who were emotionally stable before their pregnancy was terminated, the reaction to the procedure is likely to be mild and of short duration. Nurses can help patients during this difficult period by giving them an opportunity to verbalize their feelings, and by listening and giving them needed support. Providing emotional support to the abortion patient is one of the most important functions of the nurse. In part, the physical needs of the patient are determined by the particular type of abortion procedure performed. The knowledgeable nurse will be able to screen patients for referral to medical, psychiatric, or social services.

Following the abortion procedure, patients are usually very receptive to information about how to prevent future pregnancies. If given the opportunity, the patient may feel that the nurse is the one person with whom she can communicate freely. The abortion patient needs to be encouraged to express positive or negative feelings about her decision to end her pregnancy. This is an ideal time to correct misinformation the patient may have and to help her select that method of birth control best suited to her individual needs. Utilization of this opportunity in counseling the patient will help her to avoid any future unwanted pregnancies, and, in addition, improve her general status of health.

Attitudes and concerns of nurses caring for abortion patients must also be considered. Nurses have the responsibility of providing nursing care, but, in assuming responsibility for the care of these patients, the nurses' moral, religious, and ethical beliefs and individual rights also need to be maintained. Nurses whose views are not in accord with current abortion policies and beliefs have an obligation to inform their employer of these attitudes prior to accepting employment or, if already employed, to request a change of assignment. Personnel caring for the abortion patient should include only persons who believe that a woman has the right to decide that she will have an abortion or who have been able to resolve their personal attitudes and feelings about termination of unwanted pregnancies. Opportunities need to be provided for staff members to discuss their feelings and attitudes about abortion, for only when they understand their own feelings will they be able to effectively counsel and support women who have chosen to have their unwanted pregnancies terminated.

Summary of Nursing Management

The nurse as a recognized health teacher has a vital function in assuming responsibility for counseling individuals about fertility control. The problem of the legality of giving information on methods of contraception no longer exists, since dissemination of such information is now legal in all states.

In addition to providing this information, nurses are being taught the techniques essential to the provision of conception control. The nurse, a clinical practitioner, prepared to recognize the need or desire for conception control for individuals, can determine the level of interest and understanding and offer information and encouragement for success in the chosen method. The nurse who is prepared to take health care histories and assume responsibility for some of the techniques of health assessment, including breast and pelvic examinations, is accountable for primary care of the individual seeking these services. Improved basic and continuing education for nurses and changes in nursing practice should help to make family planning more universally accessible and acceptable for all who desire to plan the number and time spacing of their children.

Functioning within the guidelines of the profession's code of ethics and the policies of the health agency in which the nurse is employed, the nurse has many opportunities to teach fertility control and to inform prospective parents of the family-planning services available to them. For many individuals, the opportunity to choose the size and spacing of one's family may be the first opportunity they have had to influence the direction of their lives. Initial encouragement and support given by the nurse to the patient first exposed to birth control methods may be a key factor in effective family planning.

The teacher of family planning must be completely knowledgeable about the methods of birth control and be able to give directly, or through other staff members, accurate information on where, when and how these services are available. Posters, pamphlets, circulars, and visual aids as well as formal and informal discussions can supplement the education of paramedical workers. The *method* of contraception to be used must be the decision of the individual. The nurse may find it advisable to refer individuals seeking advice on child spacing to their clergy for counseling and support, before proceeding with a plan.

Nurses prepared by education and experience are assuming a primary care role in family-planning services. The nurse may function in an independent role with consultative advice being available from a physician or she may work in a colleague relationship with a physician in a clinic or office. Regardless of the situation, it is the nurse's responsibility to discuss family planning and to talk about other aspects of health care as well. Patients need to be given the opportunity to request information about birth control.

Counseling about family planning is particularly appropriate for women during the prenatal period, the hospital stay itself, and the postnatal period. It should also be included in the health teaching of all hospitalized patients—male or female.

Family-planning counseling must be nondirective; values or beliefs must not be imposed upon the patient and the right of the individual to make his or her own decision must be respected.

To be effective in family-planning education the nurse needs to

1. Understand the problems that uncontrolled fertility creates for individuals, families, and societies;
2. Be accurately informed about the methods of fertility control, their usage, dosage (pills), effectiveness, adverse reactions, contraindications, warnings, and precautions;
3. Know the facts needed to dispute myths which may occur about fertility control;
4. Know how to alleviate patient's fear and anxiety and lend emotional support. (An explanation of what will be done when a patient visits a clinic or doctor's office for family planning help for the first time will lessen apprehension);
5. Be prepared to reinforce and supplement what the doctor has told the patient about the contraceptive method of choice;
6. Be familiar with the local, state, and national agencies to which a patient can be referred for information and help on family planning;
7. Consider the social, moral, and religious attitudes of the community.[61]

The nurse who is relaxed, nonjudgmental, sensitive in approach, and uses words the patient understands, can quickly gain the individual's confidence and cooperation. Patients must be helped to express their fears, doubts and concerns. The nurse can clarify information for the patient, help the patient to use correctly the method he or she chooses and deal with any problems that may arise concerning its use. Continuity of guidance and supervision for the patient throughout reproductive years can be provided by the nurse. With so much emphasis being placed on family-centered nursing, family planning and the significant role it plays in the health of individual families and communities should be considered a vital part of nursing.

References

1. Studies in Family Planning—A Publication of the Population Council. The Behavioral Sciences and Family Planning Programs: Report on a Conference, 23:2, Oct. 1967. (From a keynote address by The Honorable Wilbur J. Cohen, Under Secretary of Health, Education and Welfare.)
2. Ogg, E.: A New Chapter in Family Planning. Pub. Affairs Pamphlet 136 c:1, 1964.
3. Arnold, E.: Individualizing nursing care in family planning. Nurs. Outlook 15, 12:26, Dec. 1967.
4. Manisoff, M.: Role of the L.P.N. in family planning. Reprint. J. Practical Nurs., Sept. 1967.
5. Family Planning With the Pill—A Manual for Nurses. G. D. Searle & Co., 1967, p. 13.
6. Guttmacher, A. F.: Family planning—the needs and the methods. Am. J. Nurs. 69, 6:1229, June 1969.
7. Searle, *op. cit.,* pp. 13-14.
8. McKay, W. J. S.: The History of Ancient Gynecology. London, Bailliere, Tindall & Cox Ltd., 1901.
9. Southam, A. L.: Historical review of intrauterine devices. *In* S. J. Segal, A. L. Southam, and K. D. Shafer (eds.): Intrauterine contraception; proceedings of the second international conference, p. 3, International Congress Series, No. 86. Amsterdam, Excerpta Medica Foundation, 1965.
10. Richter, R.: Deutsch Med. Wschr., 35:1525, 1909.
11. Grafenberg, E.: An intrauterine contraceptive method. *In* M. Sanger and H. M. Stone (eds): Practice of contraception; an international symposium and survey; proceedings of the seventh international birth control conference. Zurich, Switzerland, Sept. 1930. Baltimore, Williams & Wilkins, 1932.
12. Searle, *op. cit.,* p. 14.
13. *Ibid.*
14. *Ibid.,* p. 15.
15. *Ibid.*
16. *Ibid.*
17. *Ibid.*
18. *Ibid.,* p. 16.
19. Malthusian math is right: it's crowded. New York Times, Dec. 28, 1975.
20. *Ibid.*
21. Tie line. Psychol. Today, 12, Jan. 1970.
22. Nixon, R. M.: Presidential Message on Population. Washington, D.C., Population Crises Committee, 1969.
23. Pincus, G., et al.: Fertility control with oral medication. Am. J. Ob. Gyn. 75:1333-1346, June 1958.
24. Inman, W. H. W. and Vessey, M. P.: Investigation of deaths from pulmonary, coronary, and cerebral thrombosis and embolism in women of child-bearing age. Brit. Med. J. 2:193-199, 1968.
25. Vessey, M. P. and Doll, R.: Investigation of relation between use of oral contraceptives and thromboembolic disease: A further report. Brit. Med. J. 2:651-657, 1969.
26. Inman, W. H. W. and Vessey, M. P.: Thromboembolic disease and the steroidal content of oral contraceptives. A report to the Committee on Safety of Drugs. Brit. Med. J. 2:203, 1970.
27. Medicine. Time, Sept. 1969.
28. Medicine, Time, May 2, 1969, p. 58.
29. Melamed, M. R., et al: Prevalence rates of uterine cervical carcinoma in situ for women using the diaphragm or contraceptive oral steroids. Brit. Med. J., 3:195-200, July 26, 1969.
30. Medicine. Time, Jan. 1976, p. 60.
31. Sobrero, A. J. and MacLeod, J.: The immediate post-coital test. Fertil. Steril. 13:184-189, Mar.-Apr. 1962.
32. Ogino, K.: The ovulation and conception periods in women: their application for conception control. Fifth International Conference on Planned Parenthood, International Planned Parenthood Federation, 1955, pp. 141-144.
33. Knaus, H. H.: Human Procreation and Its Natural Regulation. Obolensky, 1964.
34. Marshall, J.: A field trial of the basal-body temperature method of regulating births. Lancet 2:8-10, July 6, 1968.
35. Tietze, C. and Potter, R. G.: Statistical evaluation of the rhythm method. Am. J. Ob. Gyn. 84:692-698, Sept. 1, 1962.
36. Segal, S. J. and Tietze, C.: Contraceptive technology: current and prospective methods, reports on population. Family Planning Population Council and the International Institute for the Study of Human Reproduction, Columbia University, Oct. 1969, p. 7.

37. Food and Drug Administration, Advisory Committee on Obstetrics and Gynecology. Report on intrauterine contraceptive devices. Jan. 1968.
38. Segal, *op. cit.*, p. 9.
39. Romney, S. L., et al.: Gynecology and Obstetrics The Health Care of Women. New York, McGraw-Hill, 1975, p. 577.
40. Guiloff, E., et al.: Clinical study of a once-a-month oral contraceptive: quinestrol-quingestanol. Fertil. Steril. 21:110, 1970.
41. Schwallie, P. C. and Assenzo, J. R.: Contraceptive use—efficacy study utilizing medroxy-progesterone acetate as an intramuscular injection once every 90 days. Fertil. Steril. 24:331, 1973.
42. Segal, *op. cit.*
43. Guttmacher, *op. cit.*
44. Glass, R. H. and Morris, J. M.: Antifertility effects of an intracervical progestational device. Biol. Reprod. 7:160, 1972.
45. Laurence, K. A.: Immunological conception control: the future? *In* F. Hoffman and R. L. Kleinman (eds.): Advanced Concepts in Contraception. Professional Conference Series, Excerpta Medica Foundation, 1968, p. 102.
46. *Ibid.*
47. Hackett, R. E. and Waterhouse, K.: Vasectomy-reviewed. Am. J. Ob. Gyn. 116:438, 1973.
48. Segal, S. J.: Contraceptive research: a male chauvinist plot? Family Plann. Perspect. 4:21, 1972.
49. Professional practice—ANA adopts statement on family planning. Am. J. Nurs. 2376-78, Nov. 1966.
50. American Public Health Association: Governing council policy statement on the population problem. Am. J. Pub. Health 49:1702, 1959.
51. Rainwater, L. and Weinstein, : And the Poor Get Children. Chicago, Quadrangle Books, 1960.
52. Westoff, C. F.: Some Aspects of Decision Making in the Family Growth Process, p. 4.
53. Devereux, G.: A psychoanalytic study of contraception. (unpublished study), p. 16.
54. Hill, R., Stycos, M. M. and Back, K. W.: The Family and Population Control. Chapel Hill, N.C., University of North Carolina Press, 1959.
55. Ring, A. E.: Psychosocial Aspects of Contraception. Bull. Am. College Nurse-Midwifery XIII, 3:76-80, Aug. 1968.
56. Davis, K.: Population policy: will current program succeed? Science 158:730-739, Nov. 10, 1967.
57. Tietze, C. and Lewit, S.: Mortality with legal abortion in New York City, 1970-1972. JAMA 225:507, 1973.
58. Perez-Reyes, M. G. and Falk, R.: Follow-up after therapeutic abortion in early adolescence, Arch. of Gen. Psych. 28:120, 1973.
59. Gabrielson, I. W., et al.: Suicide attempts in a population pregnant as teenagers. Am. J. Pub. Health, 60:2289, 1970.
60. Niswander, K. R. et al.: Psychological reaction to therapeutic abortion. Am. J. Ob. Gyn. 114:29, 1972.
61. Searle, *op. cit.*, p. 43.

Bibliography

Arnold, E.: Individualizing nursing care in family planning. Nurs. Outlook 15:12, Dec. 1967.

Alvior, G. T.: Pregnancy outcome with removal of intrauterine device. Ob. Gyn. 41:894, 1973.

Andrews, W. C.: Oral contraception: a review of reported physiological and pathological effects. Ob. Gyn. Surv. 26:477, 1971.

Bauer, R. et al: Oral contraception and increased risk of cerebral ischemia or thrombosis. Collaborative group for the study of stroke in young women. N. Eng. J. Med. 288:871, 1973.

Blake, R. et al.: Beliefs and attitudes about contraceptives among the poor. Monograph 5, Carolina Population Center. Chapel Hill, N.C., University of North Carolina, 1969.

Bracken, M. B. et al.: Contraceptive practice among New York abortion patients. Am. J. Ob. Gyn. 114:967, 1972.

Council on Drugs, American Medical Association: Oral contraceptives: current status of therapy. JAMA 214:2316, 1970.

Davis, H. J. and Lesinski, J.: Observations on the mechanism of action of intrauterine contraceptive devices in women. Ob. Gyn. 36:350, 1970.

Ewing, J. A. and Rouse, B. A.: Therapeutic abortion and a prior psychiatric history. Am. J. Psych. 130:37, 1973.

Garcia, C. R.: The oral contraceptive: an appraisal and review. Am. J. Med. Sci. 253:718, 1967.

Guttmacher, A. F.: Birth Control and Love. New York, Macmillan, 1969.

Hellman, L. M.: Family planning comes of age. Am. J. Ob. Gyn. 109:214-224, 1971.

Howells, J. G. (ed.): Modern Perspectives in Psycho-Obstetrics. New York, Brunner/Mazel, 1972, pp. 175-229.

Jaffee, F. S. et al: Organized family planning programs in the United States: 1968-1972. Family Plan. Perspec. 5:73, 1973.

Leroux, R. et al.: Abortion. Am. J. Nurs. 70:1919-1925, 1970.

Manisoff, M.: Counseling for family planning. Am. J. Nurs. 66:271-276, Dec. 1966.

Peel, J. and Potts, M.: Textbook of Contraceptive Practice. Cambridge, Mass., Cambridge University Press, 1969.

Rudel, H. W. et al: Birth Control—Contraception and Abortion. New York, Macmillan, 1973.

Stampar, D.: Croatia: outcome of pregnancy in women whose requests for legal abortion have been denied. Stud. Family Plan. 4:267, 1973.

Vital Statistics Report: U.S. Department of Health, Education and Welfare. National Center for Health Statistics, Vol. 22, No. 10, 1974.

Westoff, C. F.: Modernization of U.S. contraceptive practice. Family Plan. Perspec. 4:9-12, July 1972.

Woodruff, J. D.: Fallopian Tube. Baltimore, Williams & Wilkins, 1969.

Zahourek, R.: Therapeutic abortion and cultural shock. Nurs. Forum, 10:8-17, 1971.

6

Genetics in Clinical Nursing: caring for families who have health problems with hereditary implications

Kay Kintzel, Dolores Lake Taylor, and Richard Schwarz

Heredity and Health • Human Heredity • The Biochemical Basis of Heredity • Genetic Counseling • Caring for the Unborn.

Those whose hopes are strong
see and cherish all signs of life. . .
and are ready every moment to help
that which is ready to be born.
　　　　　—Erich Fromm

Part I. Heredity and Health

Each time parents gaze at their children and find their own features mirrored there, they observe anew the pervasive influence of heredity. Every individual represents the sum of the influences of heredity and environment, and the interplay between these two forces is evident throughout his or her life, in health and in disease. The science of genetics is currently contributing unprecedented insights into the nature of this complex interaction and its implications for the well-being of present and future generations.

The genetic view of disease takes into account the possibility that many impairments can be due to variations in genetic material and little influenced by prevailing environmental conditions, while others are primarily due to prevailing environmental factors with genetic factors playing a subordinate role. Medical genetics is concerned with the role genetic factors play in disease and the study of those pathological conditions which are primarily determined by changes in genetic material.[1] Health personnel are equally concerned with manipulation of environmental factors in order to promote optimum conditions for particular genetic endowments.

Speculations on the nature of heredity are as ancient as the history of the human race. Nevertheless, genetics is a young science that has developed mostly within the present century. In 1865, Gregor Mendel, the father of modern genetics, presented the results of his famous experiments with garden peas, but the scientific world was unprepared to understand the significance of his work. It was not until 1900 that investigators "rediscovered" Mendel's work and recognized its monumental importance. What Mendel's studies had established was subsequently confirmed: there are definite hereditary units which are responsible for the transmission of genetic characteristics; two of each type of hereditary factor exist in each body cell; when these factors differ, one is expressed or dominant and the other remains latent or recessive; these two factors segregate unchanged into the gametes so that each carries only one factor of each type; and there is a random union of gametes resulting in a predictable ratio of characters in the offspring. A provocative summary of Mendel's life and work may be found in *Biology Today*.[2]

Since the turn of the century, important contributions to the body of genetic theory have been made at an astounding rate. A summary of these, with particular reference to human genetics, is included in McKusick's *Human Genetics*.[3] During the 1960s, genetics gradually became an integral part of health care. Today, a variety of modern tools facilitates the rapid and accurate diagnosis of patients and carriers, and provides the essential framework for genetic counseling. These tools also enable scientists to probe cell structure and thus establish relationships which provide clues about the origin of hereditary diseases. Investigators are finding new ways to control and treat hereditary disorders, enabling more severely affected individuals to mature, marry and reproduce. Furthermore, a number of genetic conditions may now be accurately detected and, in some cases, treated during intrauterine life.

In the United States, the number of patients with real or potential hereditary health problems who seek medical advice and counseling is steadily increasing. Worldwide events, such as ever-growing population, the advent of nuclear energy, and the growth of interest in environmental protection, have forced new awareness of genetic issues on human society. In addition, the decline of infectious diseases has brought genetic disease to the fore. As vaccines, antibiotics, and sanitation have brought about a decrease in the rates of mortality and morbidity from infectious

disease, the relative importance of congenital disorders has increased. Experts have estimated that currently "one of every eight pediatric hospital beds is occupied by a child with a condition in which genetic factors figure," even though the actual incidence of genetic disease has remained constant over the years.[4]

Further, it is thought that perhaps as much as 20 percent of the adult members of our population have genetic concerns for either their own health or that of their progeny.

As the demand for treatment grows and health facilities respond to it, the scope of the nurse's role in genetic medicine expands. To meet the challenge of growing responsibilities in the prevention, detection, and treatment of genetic disorders the nurse needs to fully utilize a knowledge of pathology, skills in observation and health-teaching, experience in collaborating with other health team members, and an ability to establish empathetic relationships. In addition, the nurse should acquire a working knowledge of genetics, biochemistry, statistics, anthropology, interviewing and counseling methods, and the psychodynamics of human behavior in health and in disease, as well as developing a keen appreciation for the influence of cultural factors in determining attitudes toward genetic disorders. (See Chapter 1 for a discussion of the nurse's counseling role as a factor in the maintenance of health, and Chapter 3 for similar material on the promotion of mental health.)

Any nurse working with families who have genetic problems can profit by recognizing his or her personal abilities and fully using them, recognizing personal abilities that are lacking and finding ways to remedy this lack, and recognizing when, how, and where to work with others to fulfill needs that are beyond this personal scope. The number of nurses working on the hereditary clinic team or exclusively with families who have genetic problems will be small in the near future. Nevertheless, nurses in all disciplines—in the hospital, in industry, in the physician's office, and in the community—will have frequent opportunities to provide direct or indirect help to families with problems concerning heredity and their health.

Human Heredity

When egg and sperm unite, the resultant fertilized cell or *zygote* becomes a "genetic factory" that is automatically programmed to duplicate itself and direct its own future development. In the process of fertilization, both parents contribute nearly equal amounts of the hereditary material, DNA, to the zygote. In humans, as well as in other organisms, this hereditary material is contained in chromosomes.

Each human somatic cell contains 46 chromosomes arranged in pairs. They are called *diploid* cells, and contain two of each type of chromosome. In the male, each body cell is composed of 22 pairs of like chromosomes (autosomes) and one dissimilar pair of sex chromosomes, X and Y. In the female, there are 22 autosomal pairs plus a pair of identical sex chromosomes, XX. When a normal somatic cell divides by mitosis, every chromosome makes a copy of itself so that the number 46 is maintained in each of the two resultant daughter cells. The egg and sperm cells, or gametes, differ from somatic cells in chromosomal complement. Each gamete is a *haploid* cell, and contains 23 chromosomes, one of each type. Gametic division takes place by meiosis, a reduction-division process which is different from somatic cell mitosis. The student may wish to review the chromosomal events of mitosis, as a knowledge of these is a necessary prerequisite for understanding the characteristics of normal and abnormal inheritance.

GAMETOGENESIS

Before considering the mechanism of gametogenesis in detail, it is well to recall that the 46 human chromosomes exist as paired entities. Two of each kind of gene is found in each body cell, each of which is found on two different chromosomes, and these two chromosomes make up an identical pair. For every chromosome of a given type, there is another chromosome homologous to it, bearing the same genes in the same sequence. (The only exception is the sex chromosome pair XY in the male.) These 23 paired chromosomes exist in all somatic cells except the sperm and egg cells, which contain only 23 single chromosomes—one of each of the different chromosomal types.

Both sperm and egg cells divide by meiosis, but there are differences in the process. Each primordial sperm cell (spermatogonium) in the male testes contains 46 chromosomes, as do the rest of the somatic cells. As certain spermatogonial cells migrate toward the center of the seminiferous tubule and enlarge, they become primary spermatocytes, destined to divide by meiosis. As these cells enter prophase, the 46 chromosomes arrange themselves in homologous pairs, with each partner of the pair consisting of chromonemata which have divided to form two chromatids connected by a single centromere. Although each chromosome divides to form two chromatid strands, the centromere does not. The chromosomes are thus arranged in tetrads, or units consisting of four chromatids and two centromeres (Fig. 6-1,B). These tetrads arrange themselves on the equatorial plate in metaphase, and the centrioles travel toward the poles, pulling the paired chromosomes apart. When cell division occurs, the two resultant cells (secondary spermatocytes) each contain 23 "double" chromosomes, or 46 chromatids (Fig. 6-1,C).

The secondary spermatocytes now undergo another meiotic division, allowing the double chromatid strands in each cell to separate. In prophase of this division, the centromere of each chromatid pair duplicates, while the chromatids do not. The resultant chromosomes are known as dyads. The dyads arrange themselves on the spindle as in ordinary mitosis in each of the two secondary spermatocytes. Cell division results in four spermatids, each containing 23 chromosomes, one of each chromosomal type (Fig. 6-1,D). In summary, during the first meiotic division there is duplication of chromosomes (and the genes carried therein), with division resulting in cells which have one half the original chromosome number but retain the diploid number of genes. In the second meiotic division, there is division of chromosomes without duplication of genes, so that four cells result, each containing one of each kind of chromosome and one of each kind of gene.[5]

In oogenesis, the meiotic events are similar to

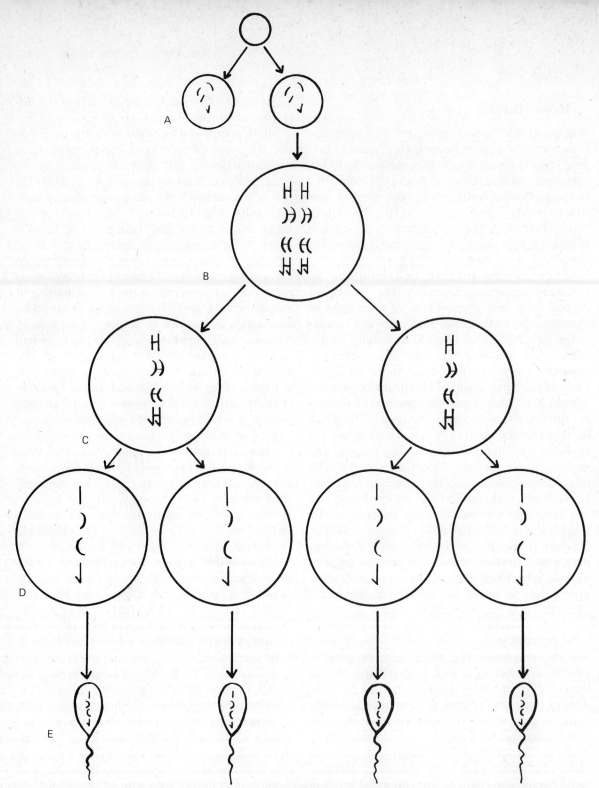

FIGURE 6-1

Spermatogenesis. *(A)* Immature gametes (spermatogonia) divide by mitosis in the testis, 46 chromosomes present in each cell in the human male. *(B)* A spermatogonium undergoes meiosis (primary spermatocyte). Homologous chromosomes pair and double, forming tetrads; 92 chromosomes present, four pairs are shown here. *(C)* Primary spermatocyte divides to form secondary spermatocytes. First meiotic division, cutting chromosome number to 46 in each cell. *(D)* Each secondary spermatocyte divides, and four spermatids are formed. Second meiotic division, cutting chromosome number to 23 in each cell. *(E)* Spermatocytes mature, developing head, neck, and tail; four mature sperm result, each carrying 23 chromosomes.

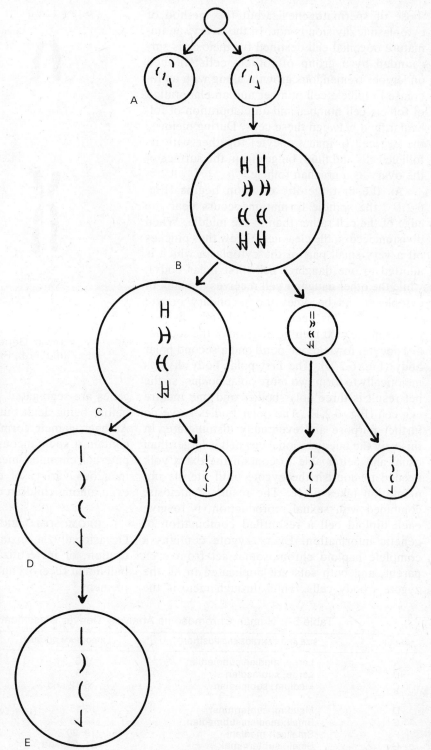

FIGURE 6-2
Oogenesis *(A)* Immature gametes (oogonia) divide by mitosis in the ovary; 46 chromosomes present in each cell in the human female. *(B)* An oogonium undergoes meiosis (primary oocyte). Homologous chromosomes pair and double, forming tetrads; 92 chromosomes present; four pairs are shown here. *(C)* Primary oocyte divides to form secondary oocyte and first polar body. First meiotic division, cutting chromosome number to 46 in each cell. *(D)* Secondary oocyte divides to form ootid and second polar body. (First polar body divides to form two other polar bodies. All polar bodies disintegrate.) Second meiotic division, cutting chromosome number to 23 in each cell. *(E)* Ootid matures into egg cell, carrying 23 chromosomes. Fertilization by mature sperm cell will restore chromosome number to 46 in zygote.

those of spermatogenesis, but the method of cytoplasmic division is not. In the ovary, an immature oogonial cell destined for meiosis is surrounded by a group of follicle cells; it then undergoes tremendous growth, along with an increase in follicle cell number and an elaboration of follicle cell number and an elaboration of follicular fluid between these cells. During meiosis, the egg cell (primary oocyte) together with its follicle cells and fluid, bulges from the surface of the ovary as a graafian follicle.[6]

As the first meiotic division begins (Fig. 6-2,B), the spindle formation occurs near the edge of the cell rather than in the middle. When division occurs, the cleavage furrow thus pinches off a very small part of the cytoplasm which is allotted to one daughter cell (first polar body), while the other daughter cell receives the bulk of cytoplasm and becomes the secondary oocyte (Fig. 6-2,C). This unequal cytoplasmic division occurs in the next meiotic division of the secondary oocyte, to yield one ootid and a second polar body (Fig. 6-2,D). The first polar body divides meiotically to form two more polar bodies, so the net result is three polar bodies and one mature egg cell (Fig. 6-2,E). The polar bodies serve no further purpose and eventually disintegrate. In this way the one functional egg cell is larger than usual and better able to contain the extra yolk needed to nourish the zygote until uterine implantation takes place. The result of meiosis, combined with sexual reproduction, is to give each diploid cell a reshuffled combination of genetic information. Every zygote contains a complete haploid chromosomal set from each parent, and both sets are duplicated in all the zygote's body cells. Thus through meiosis the

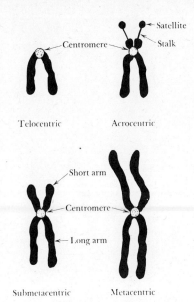

FIGURE 6-3
Types of chromosomes. Source: McKusick, V. A.: Human Genetics. Englewood Cliffs, N.J., Prentice-Hall, 1964.

genes are segregated, assorted, and recombined before being dealt out randomly at fertilization. As each gamete formed by meiosis is likely to contain a spontaneous mixture of maternal and paternal chromosomes in its haploid set, a tremendous variety of characteristics may occur even among children of the same parents.

CHROMOSOMAL ERRORS
Occasionally, a mistake occurs in gamete maturation, or in fertilization, so that a particular individual receives an abnormal chromosal complement.[7]

Table 6-1. Human Chromosome Analysis. Denver Classification System.

GROUP	SIZE AND CENTROMERE POSITION	IDEOGRAM NUMBER	NUMBER IN DIPLOID CELL
A	Large; median/submedian	1-3	6
B	Large; submedian	4,5	4
C	Medium; submedian	6-12 and X	15 (male) or 16 (female)
D	Medium; subterminal	13-15	6
E	Small; median/submedian	16-18	6
F	Smallest; median	19, 20	4
G	Small; subterminal	21, 22, and Y	5 (male) or 4 (female)

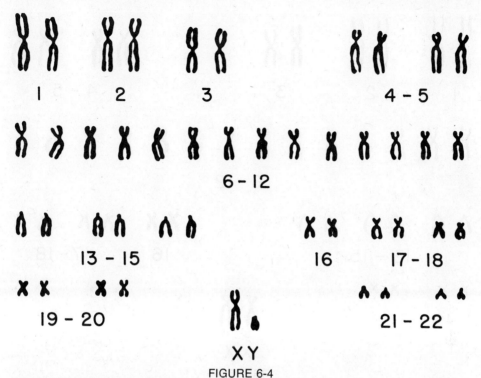

FIGURE 6-4

Normal male karyotype. Source: Reeder, et al.: Maternity Nursing, ed. 13. Philadelphia, J. B. Lippincott, 1976.

The chromosomal pattern of the individual is called his or her karyotype. A karyotype is made by examining a specimen of white blood cells (or other tissue) to find cells at metaphase. These cells are first stained to prevent further division and then photographed. After the photograph is enlarged, each chromosome is cut out, classified, and pasted in its proper place on a piece of paper to complete the karyotype. Chromosomes are classified (Denver System) by their size, shape, and the position of the centromere.[8] (See Table 6-1 and Fig. 6-3.) Figures 6-4 and 6-5 illustrate the normal male and female karyotype.

Although chromosomal problems are rare, several things can happen to one or more chromosomes so that the formation or the total number of chromosomes is abnormal.[9] A piece of chromosome may be lost (deletion), or hooked on backward (inversion), or curled around itself in a hoop (ring formation). The most frequent accident involving an entire chromosome is nondysjunction.

Usually nondysjunction is the failure of two homologous chromosomes to separate during the first meiotic cell division (i.e., failure for one to go to each dividing cell). Instead both go to one cell while the other cell fails to receive one chromosome of the pair. If the ovum with two homologous chromosomes is fertilized, the sperm adds a third like chromosome making three of a kind, or trisomy. The karyotype of the individual developing from this zygote shows 47 chromosomes, since one chromosome is present in triplicate rather than in duplicate.

Trisomies

There are several known trisomies. Since it is not possible to know exactly which member of the two or three chromosomes from a group of chromosomes is triple, the group number or letter is given (Denver System). Trisomies and other genetic defects can be detected in the nursery by the nurse's observation if she has an adequate knowledge of newborn development

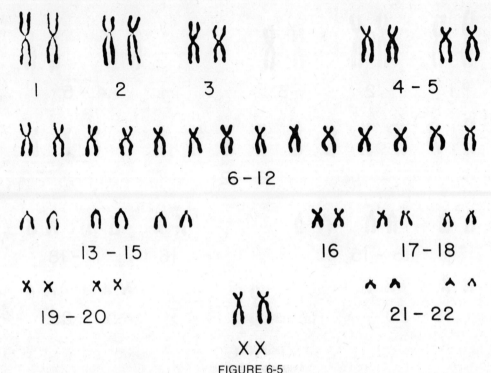

FIGURE 6-5
Normal female karyotype. Source: Reeder, et al.: Maternity Nursing, ed. 13. Philadelphia, J. B. Lippincott, 1976.

and behavior and recognizes deviations from normal.[10,11]

TRISOMY 21-22 (DOWN'S SYNDROME, TRISOMY G). The cause of Down's syndrome (mongolism) was unknown until 1959 when Lejeune discovered that individuals with this disorder have an extra chromosome. Chromosome 21 or 22 is present in triplicate. The estimated incidence of Down's syndrome is 1:600 live births. Among mothers over 40, it is approximately 1:40. The reason for this increase in the ratio of mongoloid children born to older women is still unknown. Many theories have been investigated. It is known that ova begin to develop and undergo the first meiotic division during the fetal life of each female. Further maturation of a single ovum does not occur until the onset of each monthly ovulation after puberty. During this time, the ova are thought to be in a "resting stage." In the older woman, the prolonged resting stage of the maturing ovum between the first meiotic division which occurs in her fetal life and the second meiotic division which occurs at a specific ovulation may be a factor. Other factors which have been suggested include hormonal changes, failure to abort an abnormal fetus, and the increased exposure to all forms of radiation which may result from a longer life span.

The typical newborn infant, child, or adult with Down's syndrome is quickly recognized by a round face, low-set ears, flat nasal bridge, epicanthial folds, short fat neck, short extremities, and hypotonia. A very wide space between the thumb and index finger and between the great and second toe, a single straight line across the palm of the hand (simian crease), a short and curved fifth finger, wide hands, and white speckled irides (Brushfield spots) are usually present. Cardiac and other defects occur. Recently, biochemical studies have shown that many major metabolic processes and enzyme systems are altered, since the genes governing them are present in triplicate.

All persons with Down's syndrome are mentally retarded. The degree of retardation varies among individuals. The IQ in this population ranges from below 30 to 65. Most, if not all, mongoloids have enough intellectual capacity to be trained to do simple tasks of personal care, and many can be trained to do simple jobs of a structured and repetitive nature. The degree of individual accomplishment relates directly and significantly to the person's particular environment. Where social experiences, learning opportunites, and, above all, satisfying interpersonal relationships are provided, achievement is greater.

Since parents of mongoloid children have many concerns about health, growth, behavior (particularly limit-setting), recreation, school facilities, and sometimes residential placement, they need considerable guidance and support. Nurses who are adequately prepared, especially community health nurses, are key figures in providing this necessary service. The family genetic counseling services described later in this chapter are applicable here. Several sources for further reading are included in the references and bibliography at the end of this chapter.

TRISOMY 16-18, EDWARDS' SYNDROME, OR TRISOMY E. The infant with Trisomy 16-18, Edwards' syndrome,[12,13] may have any combination of many characteristics: low-set malformed ears; receding chin; difficulty sucking and swallowing; profuse body hair; genital defects; overlapping fingers and toes; rocker-bottom feet; low birth weight; failure to thrive; kidney abnormalities, and hypotonia. Some infants have a grossly abnormal appearance while others are less obviously defective. Aspiration is a frequent problem. Feeding is always difficult. Many infants with Edwards' syndrome die in the first year of life, but some live much longer. A few children of grade school age have been reported. Others may live at home or in institutions and remain undiagnosed.

Trisomy 16-18 occurs less frequently than does trisomy 21. The estimated incidence varies considerably. The incidence has been reported as 1:1000 to 1:6000 live births. Some, but not all investigators have found more females than males with this syndrome.[14] Taylor also reports that there appears to be a particular group of

children with Edwards' syndrome for whom maternal age is a factor. Others have not reported this finding.

TRISOMY 13-15, PATAU'S SYNDROME, OR TRISOMY D. Infants with Patau's syndrome[15] show severely gross malformations including arhinencephalia, anophthalmia, skeletal, cardiac, and renal defects. Over two thirds of these children have a severe harelip and cleft palate. Almost three fourths die before six months of age. Many fetuses with this syndrome are aborted. Among live births the incidence is about 1:5000.

Corrective surgery may be done for some infants, depending upon the total extent of their problems, circumstances within the family, and many other factors. Nursing care is difficult. Often elaborate feeding techniques must be improvised. Aspiration, dehydration, infections, and many other complications frequently occur. Perhaps more difficult than trying to solve all the technical problems is being able to give emotional support to parents (and at times to staff as well).

Autosomal Deletions

Several types of autosomal deletions (missing parts of a chromosome) have been reported in current medical literature. Abortion of fetuses and death in the newborn period sometimes is attributed to chromosomal deletions. Although deletions are usually incompatible with life, this is not always so, nor do they always cause grossly apparent deformities. The cri du chat syndrome is an example.

CRI DU CHAT SYNDROME, OR THE CAT CRY SYNDROME, DELETION OF THE SHORT ARM OF THE FOURTH OR FIFTH CHROMOSOME. A peculiar and rare syndrome is found among infants of low birth weight with persistent failure to thrive: the cri du chat syndrome.[16] Usually these infants have small, delicate, elflike faces; large dark eyes; long eyelashes; low-set ears; small chins and thin extremities. A mild or moderate degree of hypotonia and epicanthic folds are sometimes present. Poor sucking and developmental retardation occur in all infants with this syndrome. Over 97 percent of the reported cases are girls. Karyotype shows a deleted short arm of the fourth or fifth chromosome. The most striking feature is a peculiar, pathetic mewing cry like that of a hungry, lost kitten. Hence the name cri du chat (French for *cry of the cat*) syndrome. Taylor reports that 100 percent of newborn infants with cri du chat have this markedly peculiar cry.[17] It may become less distinct or disappear entirely before the end of the first year. In many instances, nursery nurses are the most likely persons to first hear and report the cry.

The cry of one infant with cri du chat was so distinct that the other children on the pediatric unit insisted that the nurses had hidden a kitten somewhere. Not believing the cry was that of an infant, they continued to hunt for the kitten. Secretly, they saved food from their trays, placing it where they thought the cat might find it. Only after the nurse showed them the infant and they had personally listened to its cry, did they stop looking for a kitten on the unit.

A few older children with this syndrome have been reported. All of them are severely mentally retarded, but most walk and are toilet trained. All have a history of markedly delayed speech. None has begun to talk until five years of age. This is a most unusual finding, for in all other forms of organic or psychic developmental retardation, speech rarely, if ever, develops after the age of five. Older children with the cat cry syndrome have a strange quality about the voice that is different from that of other retarded or disturbed children. The dainty elflike features are retained so that even older children look considerably younger and usually remain quite attractive. How many older children with cri du chat might be living in institutions and other places where they have never been diagnosed is unknown.

Translocation

There are probably more disorders involving translocation than any other chromosomal accident. Translocation involves a break in one, two, or more chromosomes.[18] The broken pieces hook up with the wrong chromosomal fragments or, less often, with each other. The karyotype varies according to specific and highly individualized problems. There may be anywhere from 44 to 49 or more chromosomes, but there are usually 46 or 47.

Some individuals have a translocation and are themselves apparently normal. In these cases, two pieces of chromosome are hooked up incorrectly, but the chromosomal material is present in the correct amount (balanced translocation). Even though some individuals with a balanced translocation may have only 45 chromosomes, their genetic material is not altered in any apparent way. Yet, if they produce offspring, there is a high probability (about 1:6 if the translocation occurs in a woman) that any pregnancy may result in a fetus with an unbalanced translocation, an unbalanced translocation with a trisomy, or a deletion.

Oddly enough, approximately 5 percent of the cases with Down's syndrome occur by translocation of the twenty-first chromosome rather than by nondysjunction. Clinically, they cannot be distinguished. Only a karyotype will differentiate one from the other. Translocation mongoloids are almost always born to considerably younger mothers (in teens or very early twenties) in marked contrast to trisomy 21 mongoloids who are more likely to be born to older mothers.[19]

If either parent has a translocation, the risk of having more than one child with a chromosomal problem, and multiple abortions, is high (possibly 1:6). Whenever a karyotype shows that an infant has a translocation, the parents, especially if they are young, should be karyotyped also in order to obtain necessary information for genetic counseling. Genetic counseling involves much more than merely stating probabilities to parents or suggesting that they do or do not have more children. Each family must be considered separately and generalizations must be made with extreme care.[20] Many factors must be considered. In the final analysis, it should be the family and not the medical staff (including the nurse) who makes genetic decisions after carefully considering all available information and alternatives. Considerable skill and insight are vital in all attempts to work with parents regarding family planning and genetic counseling.

Mosaicism

Mosaicism is the coexistence of two different chromosomal patterns within the same individual. For example, some of the cells may contain 46 chromosomes while others contain 47. Mosaicism is the result of an error in mitosis, (not meiosis as in all other chromosomal problems discussed), occurring early in embryonic life. The developing embryo, then, continues to divide along two different cell lines. Mosaic mongolism and mosaic Turner's syndrome are two examples of clinical mosaicism.

PROBLEMS INVOLVING THE SEX CHROMOSOMES

Turner's Syndrome (XO)
The individual with Turner's syndrome has only 45 chromosomes. One of the female, or X, chromosomes is missing. The karyotype is therefore designated as XO. Short stature, widely spaced nipples and small, poorly developed breasts, a shieldlike chest, webbed neck, normal appearing external female genitalia, small uterus, dystrophic or fibrotic ovaries, and infertility are characteristic. Coarctation of the aorta or unexplained edema of the feet without cardiac involvement may be found in the newborn. Mental retardation is moderate. Some individuals manage to live in society, although they tend to have social and other problems. Others are institutionalized from early childhood. The incidence of Turner's syndrome is about 1:5000 female births.[21]

Klinefelter's Syndrome (XXY)
Males with Klinefelter's syndrome usually show little overt evidence of having a chromosomal problem until early puberty when their testes fail to mature, and they develop secondary female sex characteristics, particularly beginning breast development. These characteristics are associated with an extra X chromosome. The karyotype for this syndrome is XXY (47 chromosomes). Variants of more than one extra X have been found, but clinically they cannot be distinguished from the classical type of Klinefelter's syndrome.

The youth with Klinefelter's syndrome usually has long, slender extremities, poor muscular development, and wide, curving hips, accompanied by enlarged breasts. The penis may be normal to small in size, but the testes are hard, atrophied, and sometimes undescended.[22]

Klinefelter's syndrome should not be confused with homosexuality. Homosexualty is a psychodynamic problem of sexual adjustment probably having roots in very early childhood when poor emotional identification with the male prototype, role confusion, maternal overprotection, and other distortions in interpersonal relationships may occur. These and other factors may interfere with the normal psychosexual development of the male, especially with his own self-image and role concepts. However, it is possible for individuals with Klinefelter's syndrome to become homosexuals under certain environmental circumstances. Because they look "girlish" they are often treated accordingly. Also, particularly in institutional settings, they are easy targets for older homosexuals who introduce them to homosexual activities.

Nor should Klinefelter's syndrome be confused with adrenocortical hyperplasia. Females having adrenocortical hyperplasia have an enlarged clitoris (which might be mistaken for a penis) and hirsutism.[23]

Klinefelter's syndrome probably occurs in 1:500 male births, or perhaps more frequently. Although most of these individuals are mentally retarded to a mild or moderate degree, some have been accepted for military service, and manage to live within the standard deviation of normal.

Superman Syndrome (XYY)
Investigations among penal institutions in Scotland, Canada, and the United States repeatedly have indicated that a certain type of criminal (who is always tall, over 6 feet, muscular, and unusually aggressive) has an extra male (Y) chromosome: XYY.[24] Such prisoners have been involved in crime since early childhood and have committed crimes of a highly aggressive and brutal nature. The case of Richard Speck, the man accused of slaying eight student nurses in Chicago, is a well-publicized example of one whose karyotype has been reported as being XYY.[25] Efforts toward rehabilitation, sometimes including psychotherapy, have failed to change the behavior patterns of these men who, reportedly, show little or no overt evidence of remorse or guilt about the crimes they commit. Although

their IQ scores are borderline to dull, the men often are cunning and manipulative. Severe acne which persists in adulthood is usually found in the XYY male.

There is considerable controversy about the legal rights and responsibilities of the XYY criminal and society. There are those who believe that if there is a genetic predisposition toward crime in the XYY criminal, he cannot be held responsible or prosecuted for his crimes. Yet, there is certainly no clear evidence of a cause and effect relationship between having an extra Y chromosome and aggressive behavior. Some persons with an extra Y have been found among the socially normal population. These men have not had criminal records and show no evidence of abnormally aggressive behavior. Moreover, there is clinical evidence that male hormones, or hormones related to aggression, are either located on or influenced by the Y chromosome. It seems entirely possible that environmental factors may be the determining element in criminal and assaultive behavior of those having an XYY karyotype.

The incidence of the XYY syndrome is unknown. Reports vary considerably. Some suggest an approximation of 1:30 among institutionalized male criminals; 1:2000 among the general population; and even, more recently, 1:250 newborn males in the general population.[26]

The Biochemical Basis of Heredity

Chromosomes serve as vehicles, carrying as passengers the basic units of heredity. They are composed of a particular form of nucleic acid—deoxyribonucleic acid, (DNA). Genetic information per se is contained within these large molecules, and the biochemical foundation of inherited disease may be considered in terms of faulty transmission of genetic information from DNA to the organism.

Nucleic acids are made up of two organic units. One is a pentose sugar linked to an inorganic phosphate molecule. In DNA, this pentose is deoxyribose, while in the closely related molecule ribonucleic acid (RNA), the sugar is ribose. The other substance is a group of ring-

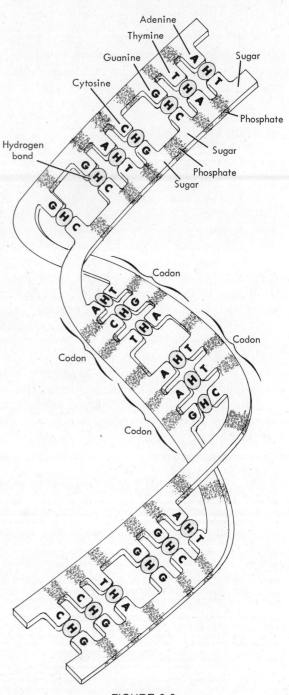

FIGURE 6-6
Structural model of DNA.

compound bases, purines and pyrimidines. The purines in DNA are adenine and guanine, and the pyrimidines are thymine and cytosine. In RNA, the bases include adenine, guanine, cytosine, and uracil.

An arrangement of the components of sugar and base that accounts for all the known properties of DNA was elucidated by James Watson and Francis Crick in 1958. According to the Crick-Watson model, DNA is a very long, double-stranded helix, with the two strands twisted about each other. Each of the strands is composed of a "backbone" chain of the phosphorylated sugars, with the bases which are attached to the sugar molecules projecting into the middle of the helix (Fig. 6-6). Bases located on opposite strands of the double helix are paired with each other via weak hydrogen bonds in a very precise fashion—each type of base is paired with only one other type of base. Adenine pairs with thymine, guanine with cytosine (Fig. 6-6). Each guanine in a DNA strand is also capable of pairing with cytosine in an RNA strand. Similarly, DNA thymine can pair with RNA adenine and DNA adenine with RNA uracil.[27] Since the sugar-phosphate chain does not vary from one molecule of DNA to another, it is in the different sequences of base pairs from molecule to molecule that genetic variation exists. The precise complementary nature of base pairing is also the foundation for DNA replication which takes place in cell division. The two helical strands separate as the hydrogen bonding breaks up, and each strand produces for itself a complementary strand like that of its lost partner. Thus, two double strands identical to the original are produced.

According to the Crick-Watson theory, a gene must be considered as being a portion of the helical DNA chain. Actually, the gene has not been specifically defined to everyone's satisfaction, but an apt operational definition is: "the smallest length of DNA that is concerned with synthesis of a single protein molecule or polypeptide chain."[28] Thus defined, a gene is responsible for specifying a certain sequence of amino acids making up a protein, and this sequence determines the overall structure and function of the protein. The set of directions, or "code," that specifies amino acid sequence in polypeptide chains is contained within the gene in terms of DNA bases in sets of three. These are known as base triplets, or codons (Fig. 6-6). Each triplet represents a coding unit which specifies the positioning of a particular amino acid within the polypeptide. Since there are four bases available to make up the "letters" in the genetic code—U, C, A, G—three-letter coding units offer 4^3 or 64 different possibilities for coding 20 amino acids.

It can be seen that some amino acids must be specified by more than one codon. Some codons act as punctuation, marking the start or completion of a protein. All 64 possible codons are used in the genetic code. The codons are universal in that they represent the same amino acids in all organisms from viruses to plants and animals, implying a common ancestor for all existing biological systems.[29]

PROTEIN SYNTHESIS

Inherited disorders are expressed through changes in the type or amount of one or a number of proteins. The method by which genetic information carried in the sequence of base pairs in a DNA molecule is converted to a functioning protein is quite complex. The gene, as defined above, may be regarded as a "structural" gene, in that it determines the primary structure of the polypeptide chain. The structural gene, composed of DNA, synthesizes a homologous RNA molecule, messenger RNA (mRNA), which carries the DNA's prescribed code for the linear assembly of amino acids in the polypeptides. This process of DNA-directed RNA synthesis is called the "transcription" of genetic information because the information contained in the DNA sequence is copied into RNA using the same alphabet (Fig. 6-7,A,B). (Uracil in RNA pairs exactly as thymine in DNA).

Cellular RNA is found in small cytoplasmic particles (ribosomes) which are closely associated with the endoplasmic reticulum. The chemistry of ribosomes is poorly understood, but their role in protein synthesis is to act as "relatively nonspecific workbenches" on which any one of a number of proteins can be made.[30] From

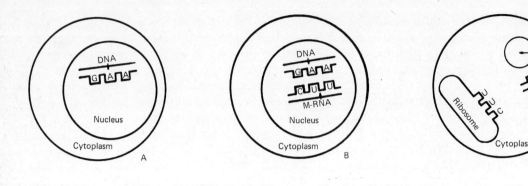

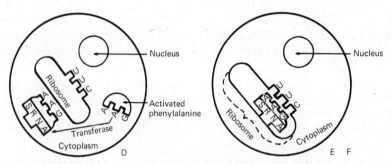

FIGURE 6-7

Diagrammatic sequence of steps in the synthesis of a protein, using the incorporation of the amino acid phenylalanine as an example. *(A)* One triplet sequence of bases for the amino acid phenylalanine is guanine, adenine, adenine, designated by the codon GAA within the DNA molecule in the cell nucleus. *(B)* The GAA codon of the DNA molecule synthesizes for itself the complementary messenger RNA codon of cytosine, uracil, uracil, or CUU. *(C)* The CUU mRNA codon leaves the nucleus and associates with a ribosome in the cytoplasm, at that site which is specific for a CUU codon. *(D)* Activated phenylalanine is attached to its specific sRNA molecule, through the action of transferase enzyme. *(E)* The sRNA-phenylalanine complex is "selected" from the cellular pool of activated amino acids by the ribosome containing the mRNA codon CUU. The complex is incorporated into the ribosome, and the three bases of the phenylalanine codon, GAA, are aligned in proper position along the CUU codon. *(F)* Within the ribosome, phenylalanine is bound to other amino acids by peptide bonds. When the prescribed amino acid chain has been completed, the finished polypeptide is released from the ribosome.

its site on the ribosome, mRNA is the template upon which proteins are built (Fig. 6-7,C). Thus, mRNA takes over the direction of protein synthesis—the process of "translation" of the genetic code specified by the nucleotide sequence into a code made up of the sequence of amino acids in a protein.

The translation process involves a number of biochemical steps, some of which remain obscure. For more detailed descriptions see Stanbury, Wyngaarden, and Fredrickson and Hartman and Susskind in the bibliography at the end of this chapter. The first step is that of amino acid activation. Amino acids are activated by a group of enzymes, each of which is specific for one of the 20 amino acids. Each activating enzyme, with the aid of another enzyme, transferase, attaches its amino acid to an RNA molecule (transfer RNA, sRNA, or tRNA) which is present in the soluble portion of the cellular cytoplasm (Fig. 6-7,D). The transfer RNA molecule is the "adaptor" between the amino acids and their coded counterparts transcribed from DNA; it "reads" the string of codons on the RNA molecule and inserts the corresponding amino acid into a growing polypeptide chain. For each amino acid there exist tRNA molecules that are specific for that amino acid.

The amino acid-tRNA complex becomes attached to a ribosome, which chemically "recognizes" appropriate tRNA molecules from the cellular pool. Thus, both the tRNA and its amino acid passenger are reversibly bound to the ribosome containing the mRNA template (Fig. 6-7,E,F). In the ribosome, the specific organization and alignment of amino acids is dictated by the mRNA base sequence, which selects the correct complementary base sequence from the pool of tRNA molecules charged with amino acids. The process may be very generally described as follows:

The first codon of the mRNA binds to the ribosome, and is then matched by the corresponding codon of the appropriate tRNA (with its attached amino acid) in such a way that the two codons become hydrogen bonded. The second codon on the mRNA directs the binding of a second "matching" tRNA amino acid. The two amino acids on the two bound tRNA's are those specified by the first two codons on the mRNA; these two amino acids are close to each other on the ribosome, allowing enzymatic action to link them together by a peptide bond. As peptide bonds are formed between succeeding amino acids, they are split from their tRNA molecules and the growing chain is moved along the ribosome as over a conveyor belt.[31]

Peptide bonds are rapidly formed with the aid of the peptide polymerase enzyme system, binding amino acids together in sequence to form the polypeptide originally prescribed in the directive mRNA molecule. Hartman and Susskind point out that observations involving the synthesis of hemoglobin show that reticulocyte cells make approximately one polypeptide hemoglobin chain per ribosome every one-and-one-half minutes; since about 150 amino acids are involved, indications are that the chain grows at the amazing rate of two amino acids per second. When a chain is completed, it folds into biologically active configuration and is released from the ribosome.

Other factors enter into the synthesis of protein. For example, regulatory phenomena have been observed and various proposals advanced to explain these. Control genes which govern the expression of structural genes are known to exist. According to one accepted proposal, one type of control gene, the operator, acts to initiate synthesis of mRNA from DNA. Operator genes are thought to be simply initial segments of the structural gene or genes which they control. One operator gene may govern the transcription process of one or more structural genes, and the whole group of genes thus functionally related is known as the operon. The activity of operator genes is in turn controlled by regulator genes. These produce a repressor substance, which when present is capable of associating reversibly with operator genes and inhibiting the initiation of transcription. This means that the extent of protein synthesis is regulated by the rate of synthesis of mRNA—the structural genes actively synthesize the messenger with the aid of the operator unless the whole process is inhibited by the repressor.[32] However, it is thought that not all protein synthesis is under the control of these regulatory phenomena. In some instances, the quantity of protein synthesis is determined only by the number of structural genes for a particular protein the individual possesses.[33]

Mutations

Mutations, or changes in the genetic material, may occur. Though these mutations might not be apparent in the individual in whom they occur, they become evident when the affected gamete is fertilized, producing offspring with the mutant genes. There are different types of mutations. For example, the replacement, insertion, or loss of a single nucleotide may occur, resulting in a "point mutation." Replacement may involve substituting one purine for another or one pyrimidine for another (transition); it may also involve changing a purine for a pyrimidine or vice versa (transversion). The changed base results in a new triplet codon which may specify the synthesis of a protein that is different from the normal pattern. The mutant protein may differ from the old with respect to one amino acid or it may be shorter or longer than the original.[34] Sickle cell anemia is an excellent example. The production of valine instead of glutamic acid in the sixth amino acid along the beta chain of the hemoglobin molecule is the only difference between the abnormal hemoglobin found on one of the beta chains in the carrier and both beta chains in the homozygote as compared to normal. When, how, and why this mutation took place is unknown. There appears to be a relationship between the presence of the abnormal hemoglobin in sickle cell anemia and greater resistance to malaria. This indicates that originally, the mutant provided an improved fitness in persons living in the tropics where malaria was a major cause of death. (That is, the carriers of sickle cell anemia and sickle cell trait lived to produce offspring, while others without the mutation died from malaria.) As far as can be determined, the sickle cell mutation was probably a natural spontaneous one.

Deletions or additions of bases in DNA molecules may produce changes in the number or sequence of amino acids in the resultant protein. In a "frame-shift" mutation, the codons may still be read three at a time, but not in the proper phase, resulting in a mutant polypeptide sequence. The mutant protein functions differently—usually either poorly or not at all. A large number of mutant hemoglobin molecules have been recognized because they incorporate a changed amino acid which causes them to move differently in an electrophoretic field. In other cases, mutations are discovered because the changed proteins impair normal metabolic pathways. The disease phenylketonuria is a classic example. In affected individuals the enzyme that normally converts phenylalanine to tyrosine is inactive. Multiple effects ensue as the phenylalanine accumulates in abnormal amounts and alternate metabolic pathways are utilized for its disposal, creating still more abnormal phenylalanine derivatives. (This series of events is illustrated in the case of Wayne and Debbie, phenylketonuric siblings who are discussed later.)

Mutations may affect an entire chromosome or a major part of a chromosome. Usually because such a large amount of genetic material is involved, chromosomal mutations occurring in gametes frequently lead to fetal death or infants born with poor chance of survival and low rate of reproduction.

Chromosomal change in somatic cells, both in utero and throughout life, is quite another matter. Many substances produce wide disruption of the genetic material, leading to either gross change or death of the involved cell. Drugs are common initiators of genetic change, especially through chromosomal breakage. Any drug may be a possible offender depending upon the precise stage of cell division which happens to be occurring at the time the drug enters the cell. Aspirin, caffeine, and LSD are reported to cause increased chromosomal breakage.[35] Since DNA has the ability to repair itself, chromosomal breakage as a cause of cell damage and possible widespread pathology remains a controversial issue. The specific time, or phase, of cell division is a major factor in whether or not cells can repair themselves. During the resting stage, mistakes in DNA can be corrected prior to replication. Once replication begins, it will go to completion. If mistakes occur during that time, or if chromosomal material is lost or altered, mutation will result. Sometimes, the chance of such a cell surviving for very long in the body is poor because of the role the immune system plays in defense.

Vinyl chloride, copper, lead, and zinc are a few of the common industrial substances which are known to produce mutation. Men working in plants where these substances are present in large quantities run the risk of severe chromosomal damage, illness, and, too often, death. Industrial substances, such as vinyl chloride and many rubber and plastic ingredients, are carcinogenic and highly toxic as well as mutenogenic.[36]

Ionizing radiation, such as x-rays, atomic fall-out, ultraviolet and cosmic rays, and cobalt, gamma rays or any other irradiated element causes mutation.[37] At what point the dosage becomes toxic is largely unknown. Many factors, including type of radiation, time of exposure, and type of tissue, are variables in the complex process of cellular change by ionization. X-ray treatment should be avoided during pregnancy, especially early in pregnancy. Sunlight, in too large an amount, can be dangerous. Light-skinned beach boys frequently develop cancer of the skin years later due to exposure to excessive sunlight. Ultraviolet rays are a potent hazard and should be treated with great respect.

Viruses are capable of producing genetic alteration in human cells. The growing fetus is especially sensitive to viral insult. Rubella, cytomegalovirus, and herpes virus are the leading offenders which produce gross fetal damage through mutation leading to widespread pathology and to death.

In extrauterine life viruses are still a problem because of their great ability to produce cellular mutation. Such mutations are likely to be carcinogenic. Mice, chickens, cats, snakes, monkeys, and many other animals can and do develop various forms of malignancy induced by viral mutation. Such problems are thought to occur in humans, but to date there is no conclusive proof, although it is highly likely that some forms of leukemia, lymphoma, and perhaps other types of cancer can be induced by viruses.

There is considerable evidence that many forms of cancer arise from mutations, perhaps from a single cell, that survive by some malfunction of the immune system. (See Chapter 22 regarding the surveillance operation of the immune system.) It is just as likely that favorable mutations may be taking place within us as individuals and as a species. However, it seems that only the pathological ones come to our attention.

Gene Action

Knowledge of the chemical nature of genes and of protein synthesis allows us to consider the ways in which genes operate to bring about the characteristics apparent in the organism. From the previous discussion, we are aware that in humans, a hereditary trait that is apparent (phenotype) is the correlate of the existence of a particular protein. This trait becomes noticeable when one of the two alternate forms of the same trait shows up. Only two forms of the same characteristic are found in any one individual, because pairs of homologous genes or alleles af-

fect the same polypeptide chain in the same way. Individuals who carry two identical alleles for a certain trait (homozygotes) are able to produce only one type of the polypeptide chain governed by that allelic pair. On the other hand, if the individual is heterozygotic (possessing a pair of differing alleles) for a particular trait, he or she will produce two types of the polypeptides controlled by the directive allelic pair. It may be recalled that each gamete possesses only one member of every gene pair, so the heterozygote has two populations of gametes, and any one allele of either population may be transmitted when random fertilization occurs. If the phenotype in a heterozygote reflects only one member of a given allelic pair, that allele is said to be dominant and the partner allele recessive. It follows that recessive genes only become recognized in the individual who is homozygous with respect to them.

The situation is complicated by the fact that various traits represent the expression of cumulative small effects of many collaborating genes interacting with intrauterine and extrauterine environmental influences. Different genetic and nongenetic factors may be operative in different cases. These are termed multifactorial or polygenic factors. Many of the basic parameters of human beings are polygenic, including intelligence, height, basal metabolism, and blood pressure. These traits show a continuous variation across a wide spectrum, with most of the population concentrated in the midrange and only a few individuals at the extremes. If this were not so, an individual would be, for instance, either tall or short but not in between. Such common diseases as diabetes mellitus and schizophrenia, in addition to congenital disorders like clubfoot and spina bifida, are examples of multifactorial inheritance. The actual basis of inheritance of these diseases is still poorly understood, though progress is being made. (See C. O. Carter in the bibliography.)

The study of genetic traits in humans is carried out chiefly by the observation of their distribution in families. Pedigrees provide information by which both traits determined by a single factor (such as polydactyly, the possession of

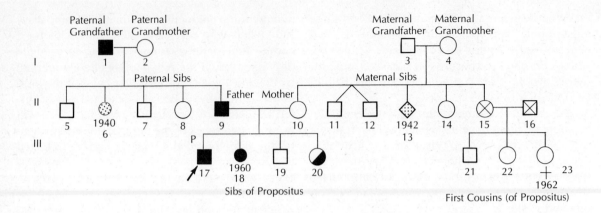

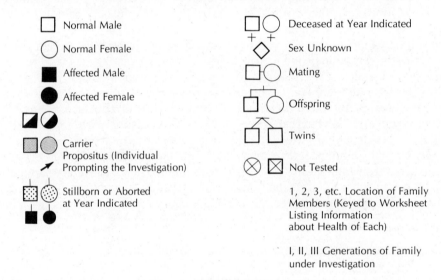

FIGURE 6-8
Standard construction of pedigree chart.

extra digits) and those due to multifactorial causes (such as stature and intelligence) may be effectively studied. Figure 6-8 depicts a representative pedigree. Such "pictorial histories" are one of the basic tools used in genetic counseling.

Given known parental genotypes for a certain trait, predictions can be made about the appearance of the trait in the progeny, in line with the principles of random segregation of alleles. The types of possible genotypes and phenotypes, along with the ratio and frequency of each, may be determined. Figure 6-9 demonstrates this in two different parental matings with respect to the hypothetical gene A. One of the illustrated matings crosses heterozygote Aa with homozygote aa, the other crosses two heterozygotes, Aa. No illustration is given for the situation in which both parents are homozygotic for either the dominant or recessive form of the same allele, as in this case all the progeny will be like their respective parents.

Dominance and recessiveness are terms frequently encountered in the study of particular traits or diseases occurring in families. However,

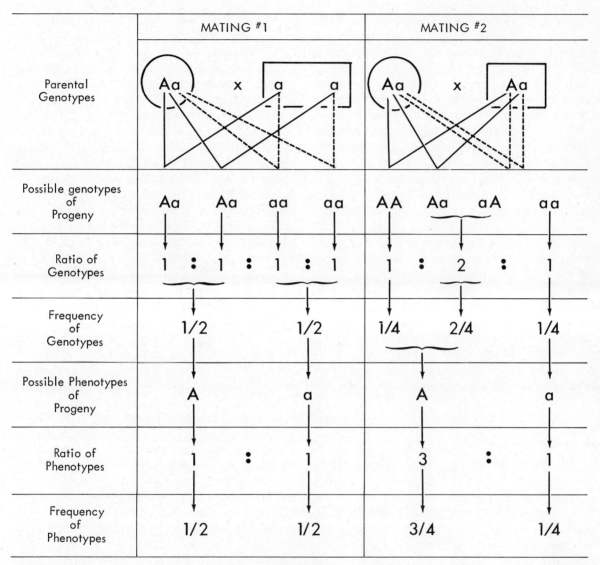

FIGURE 6-9

Gene segregation for a single allelic pair Aa in two different types of matings. A designates the dominant gene partner, a the recessive partner.

if the alleles under study are located on the sex chromosomes rather than on the autosomes, a variation of the dominance-recessiveness pattern emerges. The mature ovum carries 22 autosomes and one X chromosome, while the sperm cell carries 22 autosomes and either an X or a Y chromosome. When a Y-carrying sperm fertilizes an ovum, the zygote is male; when an X-carrier is the fertilizing sperm a female results. Although the two X chromosomes are homologous, as are the rest of the autosomal pairs, the Y chromosome probably has none or very few of the alleles found on the X chromosome. As a result, males carry only one of each of those genes located on the X chromosome, and the allelic form of each gene that is present is expressed regardless of its inherent dominance or recessiveness. Genes carried on the X chromosome are X-linked and the males hemizygous with respect to them. There are a number of disorders that are inherited as X-linked traits, but the classic example is that of some types of hemophilia. The gene for hemophilia is X-linked recessive and appears almost exclusively in males. It is transmitted by female carriers who possess the gene on one of their X chromosomes but do not show the clinical illness because they also have a normal dominant allele on the other X chromosome. (If a female carrier mates with a normal male, half of her daughters will be carriers and half of her sons will be hemophiliacs.) In addition to such sex-linked inheritance, there are a number of traits that are sex influenced or sex limited. For example, baldness behaves as an autosomal dominant in the male and an autosomal recessive in the female, who must have the gene in homozygous state in order to become bald. Its expression is therefore sex influenced. An inherited testicular disorder would express itself only in males and would thus be strictly sex limited.[38]

As described above, dominance and recessiveness do not fully apply in situations in which the more immediate products of the genes, the polypeptides, can be detected. Here the apparent phenotype of the heterozygote will be that associated with the dominant gene, but at the molecular level both alleles may be detected by chemical analysis of the differing polypeptide chains.[39] For example, individuals who are heterozygotic for hemoglobin S, which in its homozygotic form, SS, results in sickle cell anemia, can be detected by subjecting samples of their hemoglobin to electrophoresis. When this is done, these heterozygotes are shown to have both hemoglobin S and normal hemoglobin A in approximately equal amounts.[40]

There is great variability in the phenotypical expression of inherited metabolic disorders in different individuals. For example, a small number of those with untreated phenylketonuria are free of the severe mental retardation usually associated with the disease.[41] The trait is not completely penetrant; that is, not all the individuals who possess the genotype for the character actually exhibit it phenotypically. Further, although a particular trait may be completely penetrant, in some cases there is great variability in the degree of expression. Various environmental factors enter the picture and often alter the expression of a particular genotype. Clinical phenylketonuria would never occur if there were no phenylalanine in the diet of the individual with the affected genotype. Diabetes mellitus has been shown to be a complex syndrome that is definitely influenced by both hereditary and environmental factors. The most prevalent current opinion is that the disorder is probably inherited as a simple autosomal recessive trait.[42] However, studies of identical twins have demonstrated that diabetes is both incompletely penetrant and of variable expressivity. A number of environmental factors, including pregnancy, diet, and weight, are important in determining the onset, nature, and course of the disease. (Further discussion of the vagaries of diabetes mellitus may be found in Chapter 15.)

INBORN ERRORS OF METABOLISM

Inborn errors of metabolism, or disorders of molecular origin, constitute an ever-growing list of genetic disorders, which result in defective metabolism. In each inborn error, a particular block, or alteration, in biochemistry (which is itself caused by a missing or aberrant gene resulting in a missing or aberrant enzyme) is specific to that particular disorder, but responsible for elaborate metabolic disruption of a complex and far-reaching nature. Several hundred inborn errors are known, most of which have been discovered quite recently. We do not yet know how many more there are. There could be thousands.

Most inborn errors are autosomal recessive. Pathology occurs only in the homozygote who has inherited the aberrant (or missing) gene pair. The parents, both of whom must be heterozygotes, show no clinical evidence of the disorder. For each child they produce there is a 1:4 probability that the child will be normal; a 2:4 probability that he or she will be a carrier (like themselves) of that particular disorder; and a 1:4 probability that he or she will have the disorder. (See Fig. 6-9, second mating.)

Cystic fibrosis, sickle cell anemia, phenylketonuria, galactosemia, familial dysautonomia

Table 6-2. Classification of Some Inborn Errors of Metabolism
Disorders of Molecular Origin

I. Inborn Errors of Carbohydrate Metabolism
  A. Diabetes
  B. Glycogen storage disorders:
    1. von Gierke's disease
    2. Glucose-6-phosphate dehydrogenase deficiency
    3. Pompe's disease
    4. Fabry's disease
    5. Others
  C. Galactosemia
II. Inborn Errors of Protein Metabolism
  A. Single amino acid disorders:
    1. Phenylketonuria
    2. Histidinemia
    3. Tyrosinosis
    4. Hypervalinemia
    5. Homocystinuria
    6. Cystinuria
    7. Tryptophanuria
    8. Hartnup disease
    9. Hyperprolinemia
    10. Sickle-cell anemia
  B. Multiple amino acid disorders:
    1. Maple-syrup urine disease
    2. Cystinosis
    3. Fanconi's syndrome
  C. Adrenal cortical hyperplasia
  D. Porphyria
  E. Muscular dystrophy
  F. Cystic fibrosis
  G. Hemophilia
  H. Familial dysautonomia (Riley-Day syndrome)
  I. Thalassemia
  J. Agammaglobulinemia

III. Inborn Errors of Lipid Metabolism
  A. Hyperlipidemia
  B. Tay-Sachs disease
  C. Niemann-Pick disease
  D. Gaucher's disease
  E. Metachromatic leukodystrophy
  F. Refsum's syndrome
  G. Krabbe's disease

IV. Inborn Errors of Vitamin Metabolism
  A. Pyridoxine (B_6) deficiency anemia
  B. Pyridoxine (B_6) deficiency seizures
  C. Pernicious anemia (B_{12}) deficiency
  D. Celiac disease
  E. Night blindness
  F. Hyperketonemia

V. Inborn Errors of Mineral Metabolism
  A. Wilson's disease
  B. Hypophosphatemia
  C. Hypocalcemia
  D. Hypomagnesemia
  E. Hypothyroidism
  F. Hypoparathyroidism

VI. Mixed or Miscellaneous Types
  A. Mucopolysaccharidosis
    1. Hurler's syndrome (gargoylism)
    2. Hunter-Hurler's syndrome
    3. San Filippo syndrome
  B. Gout
  C. Lesch-Nyhan syndrome
  D. Disorders of lactic acid metabolism
  E. Leucine induced hypoglycemia

---

or Riley-Day syndrome, and several types of hemoglobin problems are among the many inborn errors of metabolism that are inherited as autosomal recessive traits. These and others are listed in Table 6-2. (For clinical information about these conditions, please see the bibliography at the end of this chapter and current medical journals.)

There are also inborn errors which are X linked. As previously mentioned, these disorders are transmitted to male offspring by female carriers. There is a 1:2 probability that the son of a female carrier will be affected with the disorder she carries depending upon whether or not he happens to inherit the aberrant X. One half of the daughters of the female carrier can also expect to be carriers, but they themselves will appear normal. Duchenne type muscular dystrophy,

Lesch-Nyhan syndrome, color blindness, certain types of hemophilia and gammaglobulin deficiency, and one form of glucose-6-phosphate dehydrogenase deficiency are a few examples of X-linked errors.

Inborn errors of metabolism may involve carbohydrate, protein, fat (lipid), vitamins, or minerals. They may manifest themselves in red blood cell disorders, anemia, hemorrhaging, or skin, kidney, liver, muscular, or central nervous system defects. Many cause mental retardation. Others are directly associated with blindness, deafness, muscular weakness, paralysis, sensory disturbances, or respiratory problems. When metabolic equilibrium is upset, accumulation of a specific metabolite is usually found in the blood or stored in some organ, and perhaps excreted in the urine.

Inborn errors such as phenylketonuria, galactosemia, and Wilson's disease can be treated with a special diet low in the particular substance which cannot be metabolized. Then, development is likely to be normal, or more nearly normal, depending upon how early the treatment was begun, how well it is controlled, and many other factors. Nurses, in particular, can play an important part in the detection of inborn metabolic errors in nursery and infant care centers by recognizing when and how an infant deviates from the normal pattern of eating, elimination, or other expected behavior. Nurses may also make a significant contribution in teaching parents about dietary control, child care, and genetic counseling.[43,44] To see more clearly specific activities in the role of the nurse working with children who have inborn errors, let us look at two examples—Debbie and Wayne, siblings with phenylketonuria (PKU), and Teddy, who will eventually die with a rare type of central nervous system degenerative disease, metachromatic leukodystrophy.

Wayne and Debbie, Siblings with Phenylketonuria (PKU)

A routine Guthrie test taken in the newborn nursery led to the discovery that, even though she looked and acted like a normal infant, Debbie had PKU. (PKU is an autosomal recessive inborn error of phenylalanine metabolism. The essential amino acid, phenylalanine, cannot be converted to tyrosine because the necessary enzyme, phenylalanine hydroxylase, is missing or defective. If untreated in infancy, severe mental retardation almost always results.[45,46,47]) A phenylalanine loading test on both of Debbie's parents was compatible with the expected results found in heterozygotes. Immediately, Debbie was placed on a Lofenalac diet.[48] The diagnosis was given to her parents and they were asked to take her to the state PKU Center.

The Millers were stunned and could not believe the diagnosis. Their initial denial was soon mixed with feelings of shock, dismay, fear, and guilt. Anxiety and guilt were especially poignant, since they also had a 4-year-old retarded son, Wayne, whose behavior was exceptionally bizarre.

Although the parents had consulted several pediatricians and other professionals, they had never been given a clear diagnosis about Wayne. Some said he was profoundly retarded; others that he was slow, or emotionally disturbed, or deaf. No one had given concrete suggestions or comprehensive counseling about the child's management or care. A few vague comments were made suggesting institutionalization. Still, the family had no real understanding of the nature of Wayne's problem.

At the PKU Center, Wayne was examined along with Debbie. Both had PKU. For Debbie the prognosis was good, under proper treatment, since her diagnosis was made early in infancy.[49] For Wayne, the diagnosis was made too late. Brain damage had already occurred and he would never recover from severe mental retardation. However, because behavior sometimes improves in older PKU children placed on dietary restrictions, Wayne was given a modified low phenylalanine diet.[50]

Miss Haines, the nurse in the PKU clinic, had been adequately prepared in genetics and psychodynamics so that she could relate to parents of these children in a therapeutic manner. She met the Millers upon their arrival at the clinic and, recognizing their apprehension, she explained that she would discuss with them any of their fears or problems. She remained with them while the physician examined the children and talked with the parents. As she observed and listened she detected clues to their distress and later offered appropriate clarification and reassurance.

The first few interviews were oriented toward the factual presentation of the transmission, treatment, and prognosis of PKU. Opportunity was given for the parents to express their feelings, but the deeper psychodynamics of the family and the exploration of the parents' unconscious conflicts were strictly avoided. They needed their strength to cope with the difficulties of having two genetically handicapped children. Later, if the need was indicated, psychotherapy or another form of intensive counseling could be offered.

Specific ways were explored for managing the children and coping with their diet. The importance of following the diet was stressed but it was pointed out that otherwise Debbie was to be cared for as a normal infant.

Since the PKU Center could not provide all necessary guidance and since the Millers needed particular services, it was suggested they consult various other community resources. The community health nurse assisted them in monitoring the diet and with other aspects of child care. She coordinated activities between the home and the health center. Her observations of the home, rapport with the family, and knowledge of community facilities were valuable in comprehensive treatment and planning.

After Mrs. Betz, the community health nurse, had made several visits to the Millers, she reported to Miss Haines that there was tension in the Miller home. Mrs. Miller prepared Debbie's formula precisely but was rigid and tense as she fed her. She kept both children on a strict meal schedule. In an attempt to control Wayne's diet, she rearranged the family's meal pattern. She fed Wayne first and tried to eat at the same time. She bought only enough protein food for her husband, and while he ate, she took Wayne for a walk so the child would not see and want the foods he could not have. For a few days this worked, as Wayne had never been aware of or interested in his environment, so he did not immediately notice the change. Then, apparently through smelling, he discovered the cooking meat and tried to take it. When it was denied him he screamed and fought going outside. His behavior upset his father who, as a result, would not eat. Mr. Miller grew increasingly ambivalent about the rigidity and value of the diet. As a solution, without consulting his wife, he decided to buy his meals at the diner. In turn, Mrs. Miller became angry, saying that he was beginning to spend too much time away from home and not being helpful to her when she needed him most.

The hostility and ambivalence reached a peak one afternoon when Mrs. Miller was hanging diapers on the clothesline. Wayne raided the refrigerator, spilled juice, and dumped dishes of leftovers on the floor. He opened a large jar of peanut butter, ate a considerable amount of it, and smeared even more on the table and wall. Debbie awoke from her nap and began to cry as Mr. Miller walked in from work. An argument followed. Both parents were upset and frustrated with Wayne and angry with each other. When they calmed down enough to discuss the situation, each recognized that he or she was contributing to the difficulty. However, neither knew what to do about it.

Mrs. Betz suggested that they call the PKU Center for an earlier appointment and ask for a conference. She talked with Miss Haines and sent the diet records, along with a summary of the Millers' visits, to the Center.

An analysis of the diet records revealed that Mrs. Miller was indeed rigid in the way she governed Wayne's diet. She lacked flexibility in varying the foods that Wayne ate, selecting foods that were easiest to measure. She calculated the food equivalents with compulsive preciseness. Seldom did she give Wayne snacks that were phenylalanine free and apparently Wayne was hungry.

Upon his return to the Center, Wayne's phenylalanine level had dropped considerably, but was still above normal. Although he was hyperactive and seemed hungry, his behavior was less bizarre. His previous tendencies to rock, slap himself, scream, and cry for long periods without apparent cause had lessened. His increased hyperactivity seemed related to his increased if fleeting, awareness of things around him. He started to watch TV commercials and showed definite preferences. He discovered his baby sister and frequently looked into her crib and touched her.

Debbie's phenylalanine level was well within normal limits. She took her formula well and was developing normally. She liked being held, listened to the human voice, looked attentively at toys dangled in front of her and smiled socially.

The parents were pleased with Debbie's Guthrie results and the progress she was making. Though they saw a slight change in Wayne they were distressed by what they considered their ineffectiveness in coping with him and were certain that he would have to "end up in an institution." As Miss Haines discussed this problem with them, it became apparent that they expected too much of Wayne and of themselves. With Miss Haines' guidance they set specific goals that could realistically be reached. Mrs. Miller agreed to select a wider variety of food for Wayne (for the same phenylalanine content). Mr. Miller, agreed with these diet changes and was able to look at his former behavior as being a hindrance. He had badly wanted a son and had been disappointed when Wayne could not meet his expectations. Knowing Wayne was retarded made his father feel helpless as well as hopeless. However, once he began to realize that small gains could be made through consistency, patience, and realistic firmness, he was able to more openly express feelings for Wayne through short periods of playful interaction.

As a result of improved parent-child relationships and decreased metabolic toxicity, positive changes in Wayne's behavior can continue to develop. Yet, he will always remain severely retarded, even though he has learned to feed and dress himself and has become toilet trained. A day nursery school program, or some other special community education program can be helpful to Wayne and his family. Because Wayne does not have the ability to function semi-independently in society, he will always need constant supervision in a protective and structured environment, and eventually will probably need a special residential setting.

On the other hand, Debbie's future is much brighter. Because she received adequate early treatment and lives in a basically wholesome family environment, she could continue to do well. Although islands within the major seas of developmental tasks may be difficult for her to reach at times, her overall development should be within the normal range. One of the major hindrances to such development (especially personal-social development) could be imposed upon her by Mrs. Miller's rigidity and compulsiveness.

Initially, the nurse did not attempt to change Mrs. Miller's behavior because it served as a means of coping with the extreme anxiety and guilt which she felt so strongly. Eventually, through the listening, supportive attitude of the nurse, Mrs. Miller's insecurity and lack of confidence in preparing Debbie's meals decreased as she became familiar with the mechanics of using dietary exchanges. Also, she began to recognize that she was rationalizing many of her negative feelings so that the diet became the scapegoat for deeper insecurities. In time, she was able to develop insight into her much deeper feelings of inadequacy as a mother. Her fears and worries not only involved the present, but extended into the future. She feared that her children would never be normal and that there would be no hope for having normal grandchildren. She was painfully aware that Wayne would always be too retarded to marry and carry on his father's family line. What would Debbie's future be? What were her chances of ever marrying and having normal children? As time passed, Mrs. Miller worried about this more and more. Here, genetic counseling became of great value. As she explored her concerns with the genetics nurse, she began to understand her own needs and behavior more clearly. Major changes in her outlook and attitude about the future began to take place when she became aware that there was hope for the future. She learned that females who have PKU can grow up, marry, and have normal children. Their chances are especially good when dietary treatment had been started in their infancy. Even though they may not have had to adhere to the diet as adolescents and young adults, the low phenylalanine diet is recommended during pregnancy for expectant mothers who are known to have PKU. If during pregnancy the diet is properly maintained, the mother who has been a lifetime victim of PKU can have a normal child. The child will, of course, be a carrier of PKU (assuming the father is normal), but should not suffer brain damage prenatally if the pregnancy is well monitored. Usually the infant born to a PKU mother is of low birth weight, perhaps because of protein restriction. Otherwise these infants are usually reported to be normal at birth and to maintain normal patterns of development as infants and toddlers.[51] If the mother had not been diagnosed prior to pregnancy, or had not had the benefits of a well-controlled diet early in life, it is extremely difficult and dangerous to restrict phenylalanine intake during gestation. The added stress in such cases often leads to abortion. Given proper health care, including pre-prenatal care, Debbie presumedly has good opportunity for becoming a happy mother of a normal infant when she herself becomes ready for this. Meanwhile, it is of great importance that her current health care as a child be adequate.

How long the diet must be controlled during the years of childhood remains controversial. Some clinicians begin to take children off the PKU diet when they are about five or six years old.[52] It is certain that older children have more difficulty with the diet, not only because of their own increased metabolic needs which come with growth, but also because of increased awareness of restrictions placed upon them and not on other children. Most older children attempt to get forbidden food by trading toys for it or by "snitching" food from pets. Sometimes, in a misguided attempt to avoid such incidents, parents restrict the child's play and other social experiences. Parents must learn to cope with these problems and many others yet still give their children everything needed for normal development, including opportunities for learning independence, and responsibility.

It takes the comprehensive efforts of many professionals who communicate freely with each other to work effectively with a family like the Millers, or any family with a genetic problem. Because of the kind of interaction and rapport she promotes, the skillful nurse who is adequately prepared is undoubtedly a key figure in that team of professionals. Through her professional use of self, she conveys that concern essential for a therapeutic relationship which is based upon trust and is open to communication of thoughts and feelings. Only in coming to recognize their thoughts and feelings can parents begin to solve old conflicts, face new problems, and feel secure in acting as partners in the kind of parent-child relationship that brings satisfaction and promotes healthy development.[53]

Teddy, a Boy with Metachromatic Leukodystrophy

Teddy White, 7-years-old, was admitted to the pediatric research unit after his first grand mal seizure. He was given anticonvulsants and placed under careful nursing observation while his medical evaluation was being completed.

Teddy was thin, awkward, irritable, and walked with a jerky, poorly coordinated gait. Though he appeared oriented in all spheres, his behavior was marked by many peculiar mannerisms and inappropriate responses. He often seemed indifferent to the presence of others, was preoccupied with thoughts of fire and snakes, and sometimes said he could not see. It was learned that around home Teddy frequently played with gasoline.

The Whites had other small children at home and lived a long way from the hospital. But they were concerned about Teddy and anxious that the physicians "find out what's wrong with him and correct it." They reported that he was a "loner" and slow in school, having to repeat first grade. They were unable to give precise developmental landmarks but considered his early development normal. During her pregnancy, Mrs. White had experienced some spotting during the first trimester, but the remainder of it and Teddy's delivery were normal. About two months before Teddy's seizure he had suffered a "mild virus" infection accompanied by fever and headache.

Each time the Whites visited Teddy, the genetic nurse, Mrs. Scott, (whose role here was of consultant), talked with them about their concerns and what was being done for their son. Helping the family to bear the burden of fear and uncertainty by giving the support of a professional relationship founded on trust and empathy is a difficult but essential nursing responsibility. The nurse must try to promote trust without giving false reassurance or false hope. All factors must be considered in a family-centered approach to genetic counseling.[54]

Teddy's laboratory studies, including skull x-ray series, arteriogram, and brain scan, were negative. His EEG was abnormal. He had brisk deep tendon reflexes, and a bilateral Babinski was present. After his seizures had been controlled with medication, which was continued at home, his parents were consulted and Ted was discharged with plans to return for appropriate follow-up as an outpatient. His diagnosis still remained uncertain. Postencephalitis, early cerebral macular degenerative disease (type of lipid storage disease uncertain), or organic and behavioral changes from the ingestion of toxic agents could not be ruled out. More information about Teddy's history and family was needed. Consequently, Mrs. Scott arranged to visit the Whites at home.

Before the visit, Teddy was readmitted in the throes of another grand mal seizure. When his convulsive movements ceased, he awoke disoriented, hyperactive, aggressive, and obviously hallucinating. He saw snakes on the wall and an alligator on the bed. The child psychiatrist visited with him to comfort him. Tranquilizers were administered, and a few days later Teddy seemed improved. One afternoon, however, he told the nurse, "Mickey Mouse and Donald Duck were here. I saw them through the window." No one was certain what this apparent return of hallucinatory behavior meant.

During Teddy's hospitalization, Mrs. Scott made careful observations of him. With her consistent and reassuring approach, he became more trusting and less fearful. By talking with the other nurses who cared for him, she was able to guide them in maintaining continuity of nursing care.

While Ted was still in the hospital, Mrs. Scott drove out to visit his family. The Whites lived in a shabby house at the end of a dirt road in the pines. Periodically, Mr. White worked in the nearby sawmill. He had frequent vague episodes of headache and fatigue, stayed home from work often, and had difficulty sticking to any task for long. Usually he remained very quiet and passive, but occasionally became very agitated and aggressive. He and his brother were known to have had convulsive disorders (of unknown etiology) since childhood. Mrs. White, the more verbal and responsible parent, had left home at 17 to marry (she may have been pregnant). There had always been instability in Mrs. White's family, a fact which contributed greatly to her anxiety. From time to time her parents and siblings moved in with her and stayed for extended periods of time. While they were there, there was always confusion, but when they left, she became sullen and depressed.

The following picture came into focus as Mrs. Scott delved further into the family structure. The Whites have four living children, the oldest of whom is Teddy. Donald, age 5, is healthy and active, with a vivid imagination which gains him considerable attention at home and in kindergarten. By friends and family he is teasingly called "Donald Duck." Michael, age 3, is small, thin, and appears slow. He is not toilet trained and is just beginning to talk. His articulation is poor and he is rather clumsy. His family nicknamed him "Mickey Mouse." Sally, 18 months, is a robust toddler. She feeds herself, is toilet trained and talks well for her age. Another child, Alvin, one year older than Teddy, died three years before in a house fire.

Mrs. Scott asked if the children missed Teddy or seemed worried about him. Mrs. White answered that they did, and added, "So on our last visit we took Mickey Mouse and Donald Duck with us to see Teddy. They were not allowed inside the hospital, so Teddy could only see them through the window." It is through such skillful communication and observation that the child-oriented nurse finds information pertinent to distinguishing fantasy, or hallucinatory behavior, from behavior which is reality based!

During the home visit, Mrs. White reported that Teddy had seemed to be all right after his "virus," but was irritable and played less. He had started school at the beginning of the term, but would not participate in classroom activities. He became more and more withdrawn as his behavior became more regressed. Finally, the Whites were asked to keep him home from school (there were no special education facilities in the area) and to see a physician. They were, in fact, considering taking Teddy to a "city doctor" just before he had his first seizure. The Whites were unable to understand what was happening to their son. They were very worried about him and anxious to have anything done to help him. They knew he was "going downhill" (i.e., his condition was degenerating) and just could not understand why "the doctors could not find the answer."

Unless it is possible to have the benefits of enzyme studies to detect carriers and affected individuals, it is seldom easy to make an early diagnosis in childhood degenerative disorders of the central nervous system, especially if psychiatric and social issues complicate the picture while organic evidence is still very scant. Herein lies the value of skillful interviewing by the psychodynamically orientated genetic nurse. Valuable information about the family, environment, medical and social history help significantly in making a differential diagnosis. Often this includes the tracing of a family pedigree, or "tree," wherein all pertinent information is recorded about each member of the family for several generations. Data obtained by the genetic nurse (assuming they are valid and reliable) can suggest either the presence or absence of specific hereditary disorders in the family.

By carefully interviewing the family, Mrs. Scott obtained a helpful social history, but was unable to find anything suggesting a familial disorder, except possibly seizures. In several weeks, additional laboratory studies were completed, making it possible to diagnose a specific lipid storage degenerative disease, metachromatic leukodystrophy. This is an autosomal recessive disorder affecting sulfatide metabolism, the exact nature of which is unknown.[55] Sulfatide is one of the many types of lipid products normally found in the white and gray matter of the central nervous system. In metachromatic leukodystrophy, the sulfatide level is significantly elevated, and enzyme sulfatase levels are low. The heterozygote's levels lie between the normal and disease states.[56]

Metachromatic granules are found in the adrenals, kidneys, and urine. As the disorder progresses, peripheral nerves, the midbrain, the cortex, and gray matter become involved. Sural nerve biopsy (preferred to brain biopsy because it is safer and more likely to show degenerative pathology earlier in this disorder) was performed on the calf of Teddy's leg. It showed abnormalities compatible with metachromatic leukodystrophy. Metachromatic granules were found in his urine. In time, total macular and optic tract degeneration, blindness, deafness, inability to swallow, and increased involuntary movements will occur. How this extensive

pathology occurs is still unknown, but it may be associated with electrolyte imbalance induced by the sulfatide. In addition, secondary metabolic disruption in catecholamines can produce psychoticlike symptoms. The progression of the disease varies in each individual. Eventually, all cortical and midbrain functions are lost. Decerebrate posture and death occur in six months to ten years. There is a 25 percent chance, or 1:4 probability, that each sibling of an affected child could inherit the disorder. No treatment is yet available except supportive care to the child and his family. (Interesting work by Jergen Clausen and Johennes Melchoir in Denmark [see bibliography], suggests that vitamin A is necessary in the first step of the synthesis of the sulfatides that accumulate in the central nervous system. Therefore a vitamin-A-restricted diet may prove helpful in preventing symptoms.)

Thorough supportive nursing care, frequent turning, skin care, positioning, and feeding not only help prevent complications such as pneumonia and decubitus ulcers in the latter stages of the disorder, but also convey the attitude that someone cares about the comfort and dignity of a dying child. Parents can be somewhat comforted in knowing that their child receives conscientious care. Often, having the parents actively assist in administering body care gives them some tangible way in which to help their child. The activity and the energy it consumes temporarily serve to reduce some of their anxiety. Since the child probably will not remain in the hospital for the duration of his long illness, but will go home for periods of time, parents must be taught more difficult procedures such as tube feeding and suctioning in addition to general basic nursing care.

There is no simple way to alleviate the impact that the diagnosis of a hereditary disorder leading to early death has upon the family. The far-reaching effects of guilt and sorrow disrupt individual and family life, sometimes to catastrophic proportions. This is especially true when other problems and strained relationships already exist. Some parents find strength and comfort in each other, in friends, and in God. If, during their child's illness, they have had a supportive and trusting relationship with a nurse like Mrs. Scott, this relationship can be of comfort to them. No nurse can take away parents' agony and grief as they wait hopelessly by their dying child, but her empathy for them and her compassion for their child will let them know that they do not await death alone.

Genetic Counseling

The March of Dimes Foundation urges parents to "be good to your baby before it is born." In the fullest sense, this means that, whenever possible, parents should be encouraged to begin caring for their baby before it is even conceived. There are distinct advantages in seeking pre-prenatal care. Primary among these is the opportunity for genetic counseling, if needed, in order that the stresses attending hereditary illness might be circumvented at the outset.

In a recent review, Danes reflected that, although twenty years ago genetic counseling was such an esoteric specialty that only ten professional counselors were counted in the United States, today it is available in most major medical centers.[57] She points out that early counselors usually could only estimate the risk of a given couple bearing an affected child in broad generalities, and that virtually the only possible therapeutic measure they could recommend for the couple at risk was to avoid pregnancy. Currently, however, a number of genetic diseases may be detected in utero early enough to permit selective, therapeutic abortion, and in more and more cases, counselors are able to inform parents whether or not they carry the abnormal gene for a specific condition so that future pregnancies may be monitored.[58] Our understanding of genetic illness has grown immeasurably in recent years. However, though the list of treatable conditions continues to grow, successful reversal or alleviation of the manifestations of genetic disease remains limited. Thus, if we are to reduce the amount of ill health caused by hereditary disorders, we must still focus on preventing the transmission of injurious genes.[59] This kind of preventive health care is the province of genetic counseling.

Genetic counseling is more than simply giving parents numerical risk figures concerning the probability that hereditary disease will occur in their offspring. Careful consideration of the numerous medical, psychological, religious, and social factors pertinent to the problem and its impact on the family is required. Hence, counseling embodies the total dynamic process of exchange of information relative to genetic prognosis and its attendant problems. Empathy, of course, is a necessary, but not sufficient ingredient of genetic counseling. The full range of counseling services requires an impressive array of specialized knowledge, for misguided, incomplete, or inaccurate information is often worse than no counseling.[60] Nevertheless, most professional genetic counselors agree that successful counseling depends as much on an understanding of the emotional matrix of the family as on a knowledge of genetics. The specially prepared nurse may function as a member of the hereditary counseling team and personally counsel families who seek this health service. In addition, the nurse may facilitate the efforts of the professional counselor and ensure that the patient, the patient's family, and the community derive maximum benefit from the latter's recommendations.

We have referred to the advisability of genetic counseling before pregnancy is initiated. However, the most common counseling situation is the investigation initiated by a couple who has one child affected with a disorder that is not obviously environmental in origin.[61] According to Fraser, such couples are primarily seeking an answer to the question, "Should we have another baby?", although they also want to know the cause of their present problem.[62] It is worth noting that this situation is most often first encountered by the family physician, so that, by reason of accessibility, the nurse who practices in a physician's office has frequent opportunities to aid the counseling process in some way. Patients with genetic problems may also come to the attention of the counseling center via the general hospital, a consultation, personal referral, or community health screening programs.[63] Hence, nursing personnel may be directly or indirectly involved in referral at any step in the process. Since no one center will have all possible resources or facilities available for performing tests, a complementary continental treatment and referral network has been established. The National Foundation—March of Dimes (P.O. Box 2000, White Plains, N.Y. 10602) publishes a directory of genetic counseling centers, listing the various services available at each referral center. Any individual living anywhere in North America may obtain counseling assistance through this directory. Physicians may also refer patients with rare and complex hereditary disorders to the network of counseling centers coordinated by the National Genetics Foundation, or seek assistance in genetic diagnosis from the Syndrome Identification and Consultation Service founded by the March of Dimes.[64]

When a family is referred to the professional counseling team, the first problem is to determine whether the person causing the investigation (the propositus or proband) actually has a transmissible hereditary disorder. To this end, appropriate diagnostic laboratory and clinical studies are obtained, and a family pedigree is constructed (see Fig. 6-9, p. 126). A primary source of confusion in completing this study involves misunderstanding of the terms congenital, familial, and genetic. Congenital conditions are present at birth; they may result from genetic or environmental causes or a combination of both. A familial disorder is one which "runs in families." It, too, may be produced by genes or by environmental agents present in the family, like pinworms or syphilis. The terms genetic and hereditary may be considered to be synonymous, and refer to any condition involving genes or chromosomes. These may or may not be congenital, familial, or transmissible.

Hereditary problems fall within one of three general categories. First, there are point mutations, which are transferred in accordance with the Mendelian patterns of autosomal dominant, autosomal recessive, or sex-linked inheritance. Many of these can be diagnosed by symptomatic and physiological criteria. Second, there are chromosomal aberrations. These can usually be studied and defined by cytogenetic investigation of the propositus and, if necessary, his or her parents. Finally, multifactorial or polygenic inheritance may be the source of the problem. This involves changes in groups of genes on one or more chromosomes in which environmental factors play a large part in clinical expression. (Disorders such as diabetes mellitus, schizophrenia, atherosclerosis, rheumatoid arthritis, clubfoot, congenital heart disease, and various central nervous system anomalies are examples of this inheritance pattern.)[65]

In this situation, each of a number of genes contributes a small amount to the individual's phenotype, but the intrauterine and extrauterine factors which contribute to the expression of these may be unpredictable or undetected. Thus, only an empirical risk of recurrence may be calculated, "based on statistical studies of recurrence in the population at large and on the prevalence of the disease in the family history."[66] For example, it has been estimated that the risk of coronary thrombosis for first-degree relatives of a victim is two-and-one-half times that of the general population, and six times that of the general population for first-degree relatives of victims of thrombosis before age 55 in men and age 60 in women.[67]

It can be appreciated that a careful family history related to all three categories of inheritance is imperative in genetic counseling. Every member of a hereditary counseling team may contribute to the process of uncovering information. Queries are made about each family member. It must be determined if any female in the family has had a miscarriage or stillbirth, and the age, sex, and state of health of each person are recorded in standard pedigree pattern.[68] (The family physician is an invaluable source of much of this information when recall is vague or medical facts are not completely known by the family members themselves.) A minimum of three generations is shown in the family's pedigree, including the siblings, parents, grandparents, first cousins, aunts, and uncles of the propositus. When a significant fact is uncovered, follow-up by personal conversation, telephone call, or letter is made to the appropriate individual or agency.

Following the establishment of an accurate diagnosis, the genetic workup may be focused on pinning down recurrence risks more specifically. In addition to information learned from the family's pedigree, karyotyping (see p. 115), amniocentesis, and carrier state tests may be considered. It has been noted that as a genetic investigation becomes more and more specific, family resistance may occur. This may be because desire for the truth is accompanied by the thought that a hereditary "taint" is a moral offense, because of a wish to keep genetic facts secret to avoid compromise of marriage prospects of children, or because of numerous other intrafamily stresses and tensions.[69] Offering information that is not wished for will frequently reap only hostility if the situation is not handled with understanding and diplomacy.

Counseling the family after a genetic investigation is completed ceases to be merely the sum of factual information gathered from charts and studies. The counseling content may proceed along several avenues: when relatives of an affected person are found to be at no greater risk for the given condition than the population at large, strong reassurance may be given; when a condition is both genetically and environmentally produced, the importance of environmental control may be stressed; when the disorder is largely due to genetic factors, the family may be informed of the risks as clearly as possible. The parents must understand the meaning of probability figures as they apply to their particular situation. Not only the risk of transmission, but the amount of distress the disease in question is likely to cause the patient and family must be considered. This should be assessed in terms of both the degree and the duration of distress. For example, some disorders are lifelong but produce very little impairment (color blindness), while others are so severe as to cause spontaneous abortion of affected fetuses (incontinentia pigmenti).[70] Other problems are characterized by fairly early impairment that may last for years before death (Duchenne type muscular dystrophy), while some extremely severe disorders allow an affected individual to enjoy many years of life before impairment supervenes (Huntington's chorea).[71]

Noninterference in an informed parental decision is the wisest course, even in cases in which parents choose not to have children for what may be regarded as a trivial reason. (In these instances, parents may be using the genetic problem to avoid the responsibilities of parenthood.) In any situation, particularly careful explanations must be given and repeated after the parents have had time to discuss and digest their meaning. Frequently, "the arithmetic is understood but the reality is comprehended only dimly." Visual aids may be a necessary adjunct to comprehension.

Counseling is frequently the difference between partial and complete success in any therapy . . . "if it is not provided when indicated it is as much a therapeutic omission as failing to provide digitalis in congestive heart failure."[72] One of the most difficult jobs in genetic prognosis is dealing with the reaction generated by the information the genetic workup provides. No one wants to hear they carry less than superior traits. Sometimes one parent will "blame" another, with the hostility spreading to involve other relatives and resulting in a family feud. Most often, however, there are intense guilt feelings involved. The parents may feel that they are being "punished" for past transgressions of their own or of their forebears, or that they have unwittingly done something to cause the situation, such as engaging in sexual intercourse or taking unprescribed medicines during pregnancy.[73]

Parents are frequently stunned after learning the mechanics of the hereditary problem, so that further counseling will have to await their readiness to hear what is being said. Whatever the reaction, follow-up of the counseling process is necessary to reinforce the parents' understanding, correct misapprehensions, reveal attitudes about the problem and the previous counsel given, and provide support. This family might be regarded as a family in a crisis situation, and the problems involved are multifactorial. (See Chapter 3 for a discussion of crisis intervention and the multiproblem family.)

When a genetic problem is one that requires long-term management, effective counseling appears to be directly proportional to the amount of contact maintained with the family.[74] According to Clow et al., "constant monitoring of therapy and support given in the home to patients can close the gap between theory and practice for many potentially treatable genetic diseases.[75] A supportive care system must meet continuing counseling needs as well as the more technical demands of genetic disease control, and it must be flexible enough to undergo changes necessary to deal with many different kinds of problems as they arise. Nurses and other nonphysician personnel may be particularly effective in performing the health supervision needed by the family requiring continuous long-term treatment and counseling.

In one highly effective program for in-home care of patients with ten different types of genetic disease, two nonphysician personnel perform most of the health care, utilizing a variety of institutional resources for back-up needs.[76] One of these personnel, a nurse, performed all the home visits. An analysis of the tasks performed by the nurse during these home visits showed that she was most frequently called upon to give support-ive care, including listening, explaining, and examining health care status; she also rendered health and genetic counseling, gave dietary advice, delivered medications, and transmitted instructions for their use, interpreted disease and laboratory results, and collected samples (such as venous blood) for testing.[77] Job analysis of tactics for the delivery of health care also showed that the nurse associate spent 30 percent of her time talking to and meeting patients and 21 percent of her working day traveling to meet patients in their homes. The technician associate spent 18 percent of her time talking to patients on the telephone or in person and 23 percent of her time on care-oriented laboratory work. Both spent 20 percent of their time recording data and keeping notes and charts on their patients' progress.

Such a program illustrates how a realistic health service may be provided along the lifetime continuum so often desperately needed by the family with problems attributable to hereditary disease.

PART II. Caring for the Unborn: Current Status and Future Challenge

In the author's opinion, one of the greatest inconsistencies of modern medicine is that we are frequently willing to spend thousands of dollars, not to mention the time and efforts of many skilled professionals, to prolong the lives of the aged and incurable, while often the unborn patient with a life expectancy of several decades is treated so casually that the hospital setting and the attention of health professionals might as well be dispensed with. In caring for the unborn, we are dealing not only with the absolutes of life and death, but, perhaps even more important, with the quality of life. As couples have come to desire fewer children, they have also heightened their concern about the quality of these children. It is becoming less and less acceptable to assume that the majority of babies will be healthy. There must be a continuing attack on both the perinatal mortality and morbidity rates. Expanded efforts are also called for in the recognition of major congenital malformations, their prevention and correction. Finally, the effort must be a continuation of the birth process which follows through into intensive care of the neonate. Although many critically ill newborns have been saved by transporting them to regional centers, it should be obvious that far better results might be achieved had the high-risk mother, her fetus and subsequent newborn all been cared for in such a center. Thus, the charge of fetal medicine is to do everything possible to assure the quality of the new life, from prepregnancy counseling, to early pregnancy screening and care, through the parturition process and the care of the newborn. This is quite obviously a team effort with major nursing roles at many levels.

Prepregnancy Counseling and Population Screening

All too often the high-risk patient does not seek advice about the feasibility of a pregnancy until she is already pregnant, commonly at an advanced point. Given appropriate counseling prior to pregnancy, such patients might make a variety of decisions, including not to undertake a pregnancy at that time or ever, to undergo further study prior to conception, to reproduce selectively utilizing antenatal diagnosis, as in the case of Tay-Sachs carriers, or to go ahead with pregnancy, reassured that the risk is indeed low. It is not sufficient for the patient to know that she falls into a high-risk category; she must understand the nature of the risks. A good example is the juvenile diabetic. She is at risk in numerous ways, including progressive, albeit temporary, worsening of her diabetes, increased perinatal mortality, increased incidence of congenital malformations in the offspring, and probably increased incidence of diabetes in the children. In addition to these medical risks, there is the added cost of care during her pregnancy because she is diabetic, and the strong possibility that she might have to spend extended periods in the hospital away from her family. There is also an emotional "cost"—the uncertainty about the outcome, fear for her own health and life, and a realistic concern about whether she will live to see the child grow up. Some of these risks can be easily described and will be handled comfortably by the patient. Others, such as her own longevity, are generally not confronted directly in these sessions, since often the patient handles such a threat by denial. However, it may be well to take the opportunity to see that the husband is aware of the situation.

Inherent in the concept of prepregnancy counseling is the identification of the patient at risk. Obviously there are many factors which can be identified only after conception, permitting counseling only at that time or prior to a subsequent pregnancy. These situations are more common in primigravidas and would include such factors as age (at either extreme), toxemias, premature labor, and the like. However, other patients can be identified on the basis of prior performance or of known preexistent problems. A third group includes patients identified by population screening studies. This is a rapidly expanding area which, unfortunately, is not necessarily accompanied by sound planning and adequate education of the public. Screening programs deal almost exclusively with disorders following autosomal recessive inheritance patterns,

for the obvious reason that the carrier is phenotypically normal and unaware of the disorder unless he or she is mated with another carrier, in which case there is a 25 percent chance of an affected child. To make such screening an effective and meaningful program, certain prerequisites must be met.

1. The screening test must be reliable, practical, and inexpensive.
2. The carrier frequency must be reasonably high.
3. There must be preferably an identifiable population at higher risk (e.g., Ashkenazi Jews for Tay-Sachs disease).
4. Antenatal diagnosis must be available.
5. Pregnancy termination must be an option, or some form of fetal therapy is available as an alternative.
6. The information obtained in screening must be appropriately handled to protect the civil rights of the individual.

Point 6 is emphasized in the recent interest in sickle cell screening. Individuals with sickle cell trait have been denied jobs, insurance, and a variety of other rights even though they are healthy. Some have suggested that all newborns should be karyotyped even though normal phenotypically. How will this information be used?

To illustrate the way population screening can work and the magnitude of a project, let us assume a theoretical disease of autosomal recessive inheritance with a carrier frequency in the population of 5 percent. If we begin by screening 12,000 women premaritally or at least preconceptionally, we will find the following:

Women screened	12,000
Female heterozygotes (carriers)	600
Men requiring screening	600
Male heterozygotes (carriers)	30
Couples at risk	30

Assuming each couple desired two normal children:

Pregnancies required	80
Amniocentesis for antenatal diagnosis	80
Affected fetuses aborted	20
Normal pregnancies	60

It must be understood that, although population screening is an effective means of identifying carriers and helping mated carriers to selectively reproduce, it is not an efficient means of wiping out the recessive gene. To do this would necessitate the identification and abortion of all carrier fetuses, which would be economically, if not otherwise, unacceptable. This would certainly be true in the case of diseases with high-carrier frequency, such as sickle cell anemia. In the case of diseases with low-carrier frequency, it would be possible to eliminate the recessive gene (i.e., the number of abortions required would be small); however, there would be no practical reason to do so since heterozygote matings are rare and could be monitored by antenatal diagnosis. In addition to the impracticality of eliminating recessive genes, many geneticists feel that the possessors of these genes are in other ways privileged and that their elimination might jeopardize the population. Thus, at present, population screening cannot be considered a eugenic tool, but rather a method for the identification of a specific population at risk which can then be offered the opportunity for selective reproduction.

Postconceptional Identification of Patients at Risk

When presented with a pregnant patient, although the situation is less desirable, one can still accomplish a considerable improvement in perinatal statistics by identifying the high-risk patient. This is particularly true if the identification is made early in pregnancy. In general, the factors which categorize the patient as high risk are either antepartal or intrapartal. The latter are acute, generally requiring prompt action and not permitting preventive measures.

Antepartal factors include:

1. Prior obstetric problems such as stillborns, repeated abortions, premature labor, difficult deliveries, cesarean sections, babies with birth trauma, toxemias, and Rh sensitization.
2. Maternal problems such as diabetes, hypertension, heart disease, renal disease, hyperthyroidism, anemia, and obesity.
3. Sociomedical factors, including extremes of maternal age, poor nutrition, out-of-wedlock pregnancies, low income, distance from medical facilities, low educational levels, drug usage, and language barriers.
4. Genetic factors, including prior children with birth defects, known carrier states, exposure to known teratogens in early pregnancy, drug ingestion, and suspicious family pedigrees.
5. Prelabor pregnancy complications, including toxemias, anemias of pregnancy, bleeding, pyelonephritis, and hyperemesis.

Intrapartal factors include:

1. Premature labor.
2. Premature rupture of the membranes.
3. Prolonged labor.
4. Malpositions.
5. Operative delivery.
6. Intrapartal bleeding.
7. Alterations in the fetal heart rate.
8. Meconium in the amniotic fluid.
9. Multiple pregnancy.
10. Relative fetopelvic disproportion.
11. Excessive sedation, analgesia, or anesthesia.

Although these lists are far from complete, it is obvious that a great variety of factors can place the patient in a high-risk category and that some of the factors must present more concern than others. Many centers are now utilizing computer programs to evaluate and weigh the various factors, and it has become apparent that several categories of patients exist when evaluated in light of the outcome. Patients with the poorest perinatal outcome comprise that small group who have both antepartal and intrapartal problems. However, the next poorest results are from patients who have no antenatal problems, and are regarded as low risk but suddenly develop major intrapartal complications. With careful supervision high-risk antepartal patients can often avoid further complications and, in fact, can have better perinatal statistics than those with isolated intrapartal problems.

Fetal Evaluation and Diagnosis

What can be done to evaluate the high-risk fetus vis-à-vis its particular problem or suspected problem? The diagnostic aspects of the practice of fetal medicine are currently focused in three major areas: 1) the prenatal diagnosis of congenital disorders; 2) the determination of fetal age; and 3) the evaluation of fetal well-being, both antepartal and intrapartal.

PRENATAL DIAGNOSIS OF CONGENITAL DISORDERS

This relatively new concept began in the mid-1950s when Fuchs demonstrated that sex chromatin could be determined in amniotic cells, and was elaborated in 1967 when Steele and Jacobsen successfully cultured and karyotyped amniotic cells. Since then, the list of diseases that may be diagnosed antenatally has grown exponentially, and there has been a rapidly expanding methodology as well. The following are the current methods of diagnosis:

ULTRASONOGRAPHY. With the use of the B mode scan, the fetus can be outlined relatively early, allowing the elimination of certain major malformations, such as anencephaly. Multiple pregnancy can also be diagnosed, and some clinicians feel they can differentiate the normal from the abnormal conceptus in the case of a threatened abortion. As an adjunct, this technique can also be used to localize the placenta preliminary to amniocentesis. Low-energy ultrasound has been felt to be entirely innocuous to the fetus, although reports have indicated that amniotic cells did not grow as well in tissue culture after exposure to diagnostic ultrasound. There is no doubt that there will be advances in ultrasonography as more sophisticated equipment and uses are developed. In fact, studies are being done in such areas as the development of the cerebral ventricles and even the cardiac chambers and valves in the fetus. These studies show promise for the future.

AMNIOGRAPHY is a technique in which a water-base radiopaque medium is placed in the amniotic fluid to provide more detailed visualization of the fetus. With this approach, the fetal skull can be outlined, ruling out anencephaly and, hopefully, less obvious neural defects, such as meningomyelocele. This can be done prior to visualization of the fetal skeleton with x-ray studies. The dye is swallowed by the fetus, and, when the water is reabsorbed, it is concentrated in the gastrointestinal tract, thus providing a means for determining obstruction of the upper tract. The major risks in amniography are the amniocentesis, radiation, and the effect of the hypertonicity of the opaque medium. The risks of amniocentesis will be discussed below. Using appropriate filters and fast film and taking only one exposure, can markedly limit the radiation risk. The hypertonic contrast medium can initiate uterine contractions by the same mechanism as hypertonic saline. This can be avoided by using small amounts and, perhaps, by premedicating the patient with ethyl alcohol. The future of this approach may lie in the development of contrast material which will better outline the fetal soft tissues. Work has already been done with the technique of fetography using lipid soluble material which will be picked up by the vernix. If such a material can be found which is nontoxic, the method will become more valuable.

AMNIOSCOPY. The technique of amnioscopy is currently receiving wide attention. The goal of the experimentation is to develop an endoscope which can be introduced transabdominally under local anesthesia, provide clear visualization of the fetus, and be small enough to avoid the risk of consequent abortion. Numerous instruments are currently being studied, but as yet, none has resolved all the problems. When the instrument becomes available (and it should be soon), it will provide not only the opportunity to visually inspect the fetus for defects, but also to biopsy fetal skin (a more efficient means of doing karyotypes) and even to collect fetal blood samples. The latter could provide the key to a variety of problems, including the diagnosis of sickle cell anemia, monitoring RH disease, and allowing intrauterine transfusion without x-ray studies or fluoroscopy.

AMNIOCENTESIS. For the present, amniocentesis and the study of amniotic fluid are the main tools of antenatal diagnosis. Although direct studies on fresh cells and supernatant fluid can be done, such determinations are not generally regarded as definitive. For example, sex chromatin determinations leave too great a margin of error to be used as a final criterion for fetal sex, especially if pregnancy termination hangs in the balance, as in the case of sex-linked diseases.

Biochemical studies on fresh cells are not valid because this mixed population of cells from normal amniotic fluid contains a great many desquamated nonviable cells which would have little or no biochemical activity. This problem can only be overcome by doing the studies on living cells growing in tissue culture. Viral studies, as in the case of Rubella exposure, are of less value because of the length of time required to perform viral cultures in relation to the acceptable period of gestation for therapeutic abortion. Amniotic cells include desquamated squamous epithelium as well as cells from the urinary tract, gastrointestinal tract, and the amnion. These cells were first successfully cultured and karyotyped in 1967 and are more difficult to grow than skin fibroblasts or lymphocytes. Culture conditions are extremely fastidious and the average time from planting the culture to karyotyping is two to three weeks. When biochemical studies, which necessitate larger volumes of cells, are required, the time averages four weeks or more. The rapidly growing list of disorders amenable to antenatal diagnosis can be split into three categories: chromosomal disorders, sex-linked diseases, and metabolic defects. Despite the fact that these disorders comprise a growing group, it is important to recognize that they represent only 80 to 85 percent of all congenital disorders, the vast majority of malformations being multifactorial or polygenic in origin and not amenable to antenatal diagnosis.

Chromosomal disorders include trisomies, translocations, deletions, and sex chromosome abnormalities. Of these the trisomy, specifically trisomy 21, represents the most common indication for amniocentesis for prenatal diagnosis. The association of trisomic mongolism with advanced maternal age is well recognized, reaching 1:100 at age 40 and 1:40 by age 45. (See discussion of mongolism earlier in this chapter.) The question of the lower limit of age for this procedure is a debatable one, with most authorities agreeing to accept age 40 and some age 35, although the risk of mongolism may be less than the risk of the procedure producing an abortion. The second most common indication for antenatal diagnosis is previous trisomic mongolism.

In the past, a trisomic mongol child born to a young woman was not thought to increase the risk of recurrence in subsequent pregnancy; however, more recent data indicate the recurrence risk is 1 to 2 percent. Although these two groups, advanced maternal age and previous trisomy 21, constitute the bulk of cases for prenatal diagnosis, they are in the relatively low-risk category.

Sex-linked diseases have higher risks of recurrence. Of the sex-linked diseases, Lesch-Nyhan and Hunter's syndromes can be specifically diagnosed prenatally. However, in Duchenne type muscular dystrophy and hemophilia, this cannot be done. In the former, sex determination can shorten the time to decision, since it would be unnecessary to proceed with biochemical testing if the fetus were female. In the case of diseases not specifically diagnosable biochemically, the determination of sex will either eliminate or clarify the risk for the couple, that is, if female, no risk, if male 50 percent risk, in which case abortion may be elected. If the sex determination is to be utilized for abortion decisions, sex chromatin cannot be considered adequate because of the margin of error. Therefore a full karyotype must be done.

Metabolic disorders encompass a large group of relatively rare diseases, most of which are autosomal recessives. Table 6-2 lists those which are amenable to antenatal diagnosis. In most cases, attention is drawn to the problem by the birth of an affected child, although in some cases, such as Tay-Sachs disease, population screening provides the impetus for study. Although studies can be performed on fresh amniotic cells and on the supernatant fluid, such studies are generally not regarded as accurate. The reason is that the cells in amniotic fluid are a mixed population most of which are nonviable desquamated cells. If nonliving cells are included in a study of specific enzyme activity, obviously the activity will be low. To avoid this problem, only living cells in cultures are used for the studies, and, because relatively large numbers of cells may be required, a longer time (three to four weeks) may be necessary to obtain the results. It is also especially important that there be advance notice to the laboratory when these biochemical studies are contemplated; time is needed to set up the assay and to provide adequate controls. Without such attention to details, it may not be possible to separate the heterozygote (phenotypically normal carrier) from the affected fetus. Using this approach a couple, both partners of which are known carriers, can selectively reproduce unaffected children if they can accept the idea of aborting affected fetuses (theoretically one in four will be affected). Being phenotypically normal, the heterozygote is not aborted and poses no great risk for future reproduction, since the carrier state is rare, and, therefore carrier matings are even more rare. For example, the carrier frequency is 1:30, the carrier matings will be 1/30 x 1/30 or 1:900.

When one considers using amniocentesis to make a prenatal diagnosis, one must consider not only the risk of occurrence or recurrence of the disease, but also the risks, if any, of the procedure. Until recently, the magnitude of the latter risks was unknown, glibly regarded as negligible or interpolated from data on late pregnancy amniocentesis. However, recent collaborative studies have quantified these risks as suggested below. The risks can be classified as maternal, fetal, or technical. Maternal risks include sepsis, hemorrhage, syncope, and uterine contractions. Transient leakage of amniotic fluid through the vagina occurs occasionally, probably as the result of fluid escaping at the puncture site into the extravascular space. This is almost always transient with the pregnancy continuing uneventfully. A more serious consequence for a few patients is fetomaternal bleeding, the frequency of which is not known, but which does occur with greater frequency in the case of bloody taps and which could be a sensitizing event in an Rh-negative patient. It is well to look for this occurrence in the Rh-negative patient by a technique such as the Kleihauer Betke smear. If a significant number of fetal cells are present after the procedure, one must seriously consider the use of human anti-D globulin (Rhogam), despite the stated contraindication to antenatal use. In such a situation, a well-calculated dose would be largely tied up in clearing the transfused cells,

leaving little to cross the placenta and cause fetal red cell hemolysis.

Of the fetal risks, the most important is the danger of abortion. There are two mechanisms by which amniocentesis can lead to abortion. Disruption of the placenta would likely result in rather prompt abortion, whereas fetal hemorrhage and death would more likely cause a delayed loss. It seems apparent from data now available that the risk of abortion is less than 1 percent. This information must be presented to the patient in order that a reasonable decision can be reached. An unsettled issue at present is whether preliminary placental localization is indicated in an effort to avoid this problem. Enthusiasts for ultrasonography favor it as an innocuous approach while others say it does not help and may, in fact, not be completely innocuous. This question should soon be answered. In general, risks are minimized by having an experienced person do the procedure and by desisting if the first attempt is unsuccessful.

Finally there are the technical risks. Despite successful performance of the procedure, there are still pitfalls to the technique. Occasionally cells fail to grow, a problem which can be minimized by obtaining an adequate volume of fluid, handling it efficiently (transported specimens fail to grow more often than do non-transported ones), and even dividing the initial specimen for two primary cultures. Another mishap occurs if maternal cells contaminate the specimen and grow out, giving erroneous results. This is a particular concern in the case of a bloody tap. Potential difficulties in biochemical tests include failure to have adequate controls, inability to discriminate the affected fetus from a heterozygous carrier, and the time required to get an adequate volume of cells to do the study.

To apply the techniques of prenatal diagnosis effectively certain prerequisites should be met:

1. The gestational period of 14 to 16 menstrual weeks is as early as it may be considered both practical and safe to obtain amniotic fluid. Because of time pressures regarding the termination of pregnancy and the time required for the studies, it must be done as early as possible.

2. Required study available pertains particularly to

the biochemical disorders. It is too late to set up an assay when the sample has already been obtained.

3. The information obtained must be essential to the patient's plan of action. In most instances, it would seem foolish for a patient to take the risk, if, in fact, she could not morally accept abortion if the fetus were affected.

4. The technique is applied as a part of a total counseling service and not as an isolated laboratory procedure. The indications, risks, and information obtainable from the procedure must be thoroughly explained, generally at a preliminary interview. In most centers many more patients are referred and counseled than ever actually resort to the tests.

Such is the state of prenatal diagnosis at this point; permitting the identification for purposes of abortion of certain pregnancies. Undoubtedly, in the future effective forms of fetal medical and surgical therapy will be developed for some of these disorders.

STUDIES OF FETAL AGE AND MATURITY

This group of studies constitutes the most commonly used diagnostic approach to the fetus. All too frequently the patient in the higher risk category is uncertain about the date of her last menstrual period and often reports late for care, so that uterine size is less reliable. Another obvious pitfall in determining fetal age is irregularity in the menstrual cycle. A common example of this is the patient who conceives after discontinuing oral contraceptives, a time when ovulation is notoriously delayed. What then are the circumstances under which the determination of fetal age is needed?

1. Unreliable or unavailable menstrual history—a common occurrence even in the intelligent patient (perhaps a sign of a healthy attitude).

2. Indicated induction of labor for complications requiring early delivery.

3. Postdate pregnancy.

4. Repeat cesarean section.

5. Elective induction of labor.

Obviously for some of these indications, one would wish to do all available studies to determine maturity, while in other cases, for example,

elective induction of labor, one could justify only clinical determination, and, if these findings were inconclusive, one would be better off deferring the induction. A basic assumption made in all studies of fetal maturity, and even in the postnatal pediatric assessment of gestational age, is that although growth may be retarded, maturation continues. If this were not so, a growth-retarded (and maturity-retarded) baby would be indistinguishable from a premature infant of the same size. A second assumption is that organ systems mature at the same rate. This assumption is probably not completely valid but, nonetheless, forms the basis for a number of studies using skin maturity as an indicator. Clinical means for assessing fetal age and maturity include:

1. Last menstrual period.
2. Onset of pregnancy symptoms.
3. Uterine size (especially in early pregnancy).
4. Quickening.
5. Auscultation of fetal heart sounds.
6. Cervical changes.
7. Fetal size.
8. Lightening.

All of these clinical parameters are fraught with a degree of unreliability, some more than others. They do, however, suffice for the majority of cases in which more sophisticated methodology is not indicated. When a greater degree of accuracy is necessary, the following laboratory methods can be used:

1. Radiology.
2. Ultrasonography.
3. Amniotic fluid studies.
4. Maternal endocrine assays.
5. Maternal enzyme assays.

RADIOLOGIC METHODS are among the oldest but, unfortunately, the most variable methods. The use of x-ray studies to establish the age of a second trimester pregnancy is too variable and probably imposes more risks than it provides information. The calcification of certain crucial ossification centers in the last month of pregnancy provides useful information when these sites can be visualized. They are the distal femoral epiphysis (usually appears at 36 weeks), the proximal tibial epiphysis (38 to 40 weeks), and the femoral head (40 weeks). Unfortunately, there is variation according to the age, sex, and weight of the fetus, so that the study is valuable only if positive (epiphyses definitely seen); a negative study is difficult to interpret. One must also be aware of technical problems: occasionally an x-ray study is reported as not showing the epiphyses but the reason is technical, the fetal knee perhaps overlying the maternal spine.

UTRASONOGRAPHY offers assistance in two ways. It can, using the B mode scan, identify the gestational sac early in pregnancy and thereby fix the point of conception. Later in pregnancy, using the A mode linear scan, one can measure the biparietal diameter of the fetal head and from that interpolate fetal weight with reasonable accuracy. In addition, using serial measurement of the fetal head, it is possible to determine whether or not growth rates are normal. Since the brain is often spared to some extent in fetal growth retardation, some clinicians now suggest that other measurements, such as those of the thorax will produce even more reliable evidence in these cases.

AMNIOTIC FLUID STUDIES for fetal maturity have found increasing favor in recent years. Since the risk of amniocentesis has been discussed in a previous section, it goes without saying that these studies should be undertaken only for good indications and that once fluid is obtained it should be screened by all available methods.

Cytology. The cells in amniotic fluid come from the fetus and the membranes. The majority of fetal cells are desquamated squamous epithelium although one also finds cells from the respiratory, gastrointestinal, and urinary tract. If one stains the cells using the Papanicolaou technique, one notes that the more mature the fetus, the more anucleated superficial type cells one sees, whereas in the immature fetus one sees intermediate, or para-basal cells. This is analogous to a maturation index for determining estrogen effect in the vaginal smear. A simpler technique involves the use of a stain for fat, (Nile blue sulfate). Increasing numbers of cells which take the stain are seen as the fetus matures. At term, one sees 50 percent fat (orange) cells and

even free-fat globules. Any percentage exceeding 15 to 20 indicates maturity. The source of these fat-containing cells was thought to be the developing sebaceous glands of mature skin, but this is in doubt, and the changes may simply be degenerative ones. In any case, the correlation with gestational age is good, the test simple, and the break point (cutoff between immature and mature) is at a good practical point, approximately 36 to 37 weeks. Although one is studying skin maturation, the correlations with overall maturity are good.

Creatinine. In early pregnancy, most solutes in amniotic fluid reflect the concentration of solutes in maternal plasma. As pregnancy progresses creatinine increases in concentration absolutely and in relation to the maternal plasma level. This is a reflection of two factors: increased fetal muscle mass (creatine-creatinine metabolism) and the maturation of the fetal kidneys and their ability to excrete creatinine into the amniotic fluid (the near-term fetus has a urinary output of 400 to 500 ml per 24 hours). Amniotic fluid creatinines of 2 mg per 100 ml or greater indicate fetal maturity and correlate reasonably well with important parameters such as pulmonary maturity. The ready availability of the determination is a great advantage.

Bilirubin. In the absence of Rh sensitization, the level of bilirubin (as measured by the ΔOD_{450}) falls in late pregnancy. This is presumed to be the result of the increased efficiency of the placenta in clearing the bilirubin and the maturation of the fetal liver permitting bilirubin conjugation. The ΔOD_{450} falls to 0.010 by 36 weeks and disappears at 37 to 38 weeks. As with a number of studies, the critical gestational age of 35 to 36 weeks may be a little short of the time required for pulmonary maturation or the disappearance of the risk of respiratory distress.

Osmolality. Amniotic fluid in early pregnancy is isotonic to plasma but becomes progressively more hypotonic as the pregnancy progresses. However, this change is gradual, without a sharp cutoff; thus its diagnostic value is diminished.

Phospholipids. The most useful of all the studies of maturity is the measurement of lecithin, the major constitutent of pulmonary surfactant. (See Chapter 13 for further discussion.) Largely through the work of Gluck, it became clear that, with maturation of the lung, there appears in the pulmonary fluid a surface active material, surfactant, which acts to permit permanent expansion of the alveoli. Lack of this material is associated with risk for the respiratory distress syndrome. The fetus develops a pathway for the synthesis of surfactant at about 35 to 36 weeks of gestation, and at the same time there is an abrupt increase in the concentration of lecithin in amniotic fluid. Techniques for measuring this material have been developed using thin layer chromotography. Since the concentration of another constituent of amniotic fluid, sphingomyelin, remains relatively constant, it is used as the standard and the results are expressed as the lecithin sphingomyelin (L/S) ratio. Ratios of greater than 2:1 are indicative of pulmonary maturity, and generally appear at 35 to 36 weeks. Recent reports indicate that, in some pregnancy complications, surfactant production may be induced early and that the administration of large doses of corticosteroids to the mother may have the same effect. Because the L/S ratio is a relatively complex study to perform, an alternative study called the Shake test has been developed. This test is based on the ability of surfactant to maintain a stable form on the surface of an amniotic fluid alcohol mixture. Serial dilutions of amniotic fluid are shaken with equal volumes of 95 percent ethanol for 15 seconds. The tubes are inspected after 15 minutes for the presence of surface bubbles. Results are expressed in terms of the last dilution in which the foam remains. A positive result at the 1:2 dilution is equivalent to a 2:1 L/S ratio and indicates lung maturity.

MATERNAL ENDOCRINE ASSAYS. Because of their progressively rising levels during the course of pregnancy, estrogens, progesterone, and human placental lactogen (human chorionic somatotropin) have all been used to establish fetal age, although for the reasons defined below they constitute a group of studies which are more applicable to the study of placental function or fetal well-being.

Estrogens. Of the three natural estrogens (estradiol, estrone, and estriol), estriol predominates in pregnancy, constituting 90 to 95 percent of the total. However, estrone and estradiol follow the same progressively rising sigmoid curve; consequently, one can obtain the same information from the assay of total estrogens as from the measurement of estriol. Determinations have been made for the most part on 24-hour urine collections, but can be done on serum samples as well, bearing in mind that there is a diurnal variation and one cannot compare samples obtained at different times of the day. The difficulty encountered in using this assay for estimating fetal age lies with the wide range of normal in late pregnancy. A given value may be within that range at both 35 to 40 weeks, providing there is no age discrimination.

Progesterone. Urinary pregnanediol, the major metabolite of progesterone, and serum progesterone also follow a rising pattern quite similar to that of estrogens and have similar disadvantages. There is the additional disadvantage that progesterone is a reflection of placental function alone, while estrogens require fetal precursors.

Human placental lactogen (human chorionic somatotropin) also follows a flat curve and presents the same difficulties as those encountered when estimating gestational age.

MATERNAL ENZYME ASSAYS. A group of enzymes which increase in concentration in maternal serum have been studied in relation to fetal age and well-being. The group includes diamine oxidase (DOA), the heat stabile fraction of alkaline phosphatase, and oxytocinase (cystine amnio peptidase). Like endocrine assays, these studies are more useful in determining fetal well-being than age because of their wide range of normal.

Of all the methods presently available, the L/S ratio probably is the most valid estimate of fetal age, at least in circumstances when delivery is being considered. This study assesses that aspect of maturity, the pulmonary, which is most critical to extrauterine survival. While amniotic fluid creatinine and fat-cell levels correlate well, they are, in fact, measuring less pertinent aspects of maturity. Earlier in pregnancy (second and third trimester), ultrasound measurements would seem to provide the most help. In some situations, only clinical judgment will be required to make the estimate, while with the most difficult problems, a battery of studies may be necessary. Some have suggested complex scoring systems which utilize the results of several studies. In the last analysis, there is still considerable lack of scientific precision, for even after the newborn is available for direct determination, the estimate must be based upon such vagaries as neurological development and cutaneous manifestations, for example, foot creases, breast bud development, and the like. Nonetheless, when faced with a perplexing pregnancy complication and confusion regarding gestational age, the modern clinician has many tools available for obtaining that information.

STUDIES OF FETAL WELL-BEING

Until recently, studies to determine the well-being of the fetus were applied only when it had been determined that the fetus was at increased risk. However, as the reliability, availability, and the practicality of these methods increases they will be applied to the screening of apparently normal uncomplicated pregnancies. To a significant extent, this is already being done.

Intrapartal fetal monitoring is now being used in a number of institutions for normal as well as abnormal pregnancies. This is especially important since poor outcome is common in patients who are considered low-risk antepartum but develop intrapartal complications: One can also envision a time when the routine prenatal visit will include not only routines now performed, but also the screening of a urine and/or blood sample for a variety of enzymes, hormones, and so on to detect the occasional unsuspected problem.

Of the studies currently available for determining fetal well-being, most are applicable to the antepartal period, although heart rate monitoring and fetal scalp sampling are specifically applied to the intrapartal period. The following are the currently available antepartal studies:

1. Clinical methods
2. Radiographic
3. Ultrasound
4. Maternal hormone assays
5. Maternal enzyme assays
6. Oxytocin challenge test
7. Amniotic fluid studies
8. Amnioscopy

Intrapartal techniques include:

1. Fetal heart rate monitoring
2. Fetal scalp blood sampling
3. Amniotic fluid evaluation

Antepartal Evaluation

CLINICAL ASSESSMENT of fetal well-being is the theoretical justification for much of what is done in the course of routine prenatal care. If critically analyzed, however, we see that these maneuvers provide no more information than the presence or absence of fetal life, and even that is sometimes difficult to ascertain. Subjectively, the patient may judge the health of her fetus by the pattern and the amount of fetal movement she experiences. This is not totally without justification, since increased fetal movements are a common consequence of acute fetal distress, albeit such an increase is often an agonal event. Diminished fetal movement is also difficult to interpret, although many clinicians do pay it heed, especially in the presence of an etiology for a problem such as maternal diabetes. The elements of the physical examination are somewhat more objective. If done consistently and carefully, observation of uterine and fetal growth can provide early evidence of fetal growth retardation or (if growth is increasing rapidly) suggest hydramnios commonly associated with significant fetal problems. Auscultation of the fetal heart, however, is usually perfunctory in the routine prenatal examination, providing little more than assurance that the fetus is alive. To provide additional information, one can evaluate the response in the fetal heart rate to such stimuli as compression of the fetal head or atropine administered to the mother. Even with these referents, the ability of the obstetrician to evaluate the well-being of the fetus clinically is quite limited and is perhaps best done by singling out patients with the potential for problems and applying the appropriate studies.

RADIOGRAPHIC STUDIES are of little value in determining the status of the fetus. There are definitive signs of fetal death, including collapse of the skull, marked flexion of the spine, gas in the heart, and the like, which appear late after the demise, but there are no signs which antedate them. Amniography is a technique in which water soluble contrast material is injected into the amniotic fluid. The healthy fetus constantly swallows fluid (<450 ml per day at term) and absorbs the water leaving concentrated dye in the gastrointestinal (GI) tract. Although this serves as a good indicator of fetal viability if present, absence of a "GI series" may indicate either a sick or a nonviable fetus and cannot be quantitated. Some clinicians have done retrograde femoral arteriography to evaluate the adequacy of the uteroplacental circulation; however, the information obtained can scarcely justify the radiation exposure.

ULTRASOUND is being used more and more to evaluate the fetus. In the first trimester when symptoms of a threatened abortion appear, a B mode scan can be used to define the presence or absence of a fetal sac. In its absence, one can assume a nonsalvagable pregnancy and proceed with evacuation of the uterus. Beginning in the second trimester, ultrasound measurements of the biparietal diameter of the fetal head, done serially, can be used to detect growth retardation, a sign of fetal jeopardy. Since the brain and, consequently, the head are spared to an extent in growth retardation, some clinicians are now concentrating on other measurements, for example, the thoracic diameters. Measurements of the biparietal diameter can also be used to estimate fetal weight with reasonable accuracy and, as a result, are a good adjunct in making decisions regarding the feasibility of premature delivery and about suspected cephalopelvic disproportion.

MATERNAL ENDOCRINE ASSAYS, particularly for estriol or total estrogens, have been the backbone of fetal evaluation for the past several years. Although all estrogens rise progressively throughout pregnancy, estriol predominates, constituting the major portion, approximately 90 to 95 percent of the total (see p. 147). The major advantages of estriol over other endocrine assays is that fetal precursors are essential. For example, 16 hydroxydehydroepiandroosterone is produced by the unique fetal or x zone in the fetal adrenals, modified by the fetal liver, converted to estriol by the placenta, and cleared by the maternal kidneys. Thus, the recovery of a normal amount of estriol in the urine of a pregnant woman indicates that the entire three-compartment system is intact and functions normally. An abnormal value may indicate a problem in any of the three areas. In contrast, progesterone and human chorionic somatotropin are of placental origin and can theoretically be in the normal range with a nonviable fetus as long as the placenta continues to function. The collection of a 24-hour urine specimen presents certain disadvantages, including the delay of the collection, the possibility of an incomplete collection, and the role of maternal renal function which may have an actual bearing on the well-being of the fetus. These factors can be circumvented by measuring serum estriol, although this technique is more difficult and there is a diurnal variation in serum levels so that comparisons of serial studies are valid only when taken at the same time of the day. Despite the disadvantages, 24-hour urinary estriol determination remains the most practical study for evaluating fetal well-being in the face of such maternal problems as hypertension and diabetes. Most important is the negative value of the study, that is, the ability of the obstetrician to delay intervention in the presence of a normal value.

MATERNAL ENZYME ASSAYS have the great advantage of being technically easy to perform and very reproducible as opposed to endocrine assays which are much more difficult and variable, making it impossible to compare results from one laboratory to another. The enzymes commonly determined are of placental origin making these studies less specific for fetal well-being than estriol assays. Diamine oxidase (DOA) has proved disappointing in evaluating late pregnancy, but it is valuable in early pregnancy with threatened abortion. The heat stabile fraction of alkaline phosphatase rises progressively in normal pregnancy. In complications such as diabetes, values are all below the normal range while in toxemia, particularly, values are higher than normal; according to some clinicians, this rise may antedate the overt signs of preeclampsia. An oxytocinase, cystine aminopeptidase (CAP), also has a progressively rising pattern with lower than normal values indicating fetal jeopardy. Because of their simplicity, these assays provide a reasonable backup for estriol studies and perhaps will make up part of a battery of studies of fetoplacental function similar to those done for liver function.

THE OXYTOCIN CHALLENGE TEST (OCT) offers one of the few simple and practical tests of fetoplacental function and requires no complicated equipment or extended periods of time. The principle involved is that the forces of uterine contractions are applied to the uteroplacental circulation, and, if it is compromised to begin with, fetal hypoxia will result and be signaled by alterations in the fetal heart rate. During the first stage of labor, normal contractions peak at 40 to 50 mm of mercury with a resting tone of 10 to 15 mm Hg. Although much higher pressures are achieved in the second stage, the normal first-stage contraction will interfere with uteroplacental venous outflow at its peak. With normal circulation, there is compensation and no alteration in the fetal heart rate. When the circulation is impaired, as in diabetes or hypertension, a later deceleration (Type II dip) pattern appears. This involves a baseline tachycardia with deceleration, which begins at the peak of a contraction and does not recover until the contraction has ended. Such a positive test confirms other evidence of fetal distress and is generally accepted as an indication for prompt delivery. To consider a test negative, good contraction (30 mm Hg) must be maintained for at least 30 minutes without decelerations. Although the use of an external fetal heart rate monitor makes the evaluation simple and provides a permanent record, it can be done with a hand-held Doppler probe or an ordinary fetal stethoscope by counting 15-second intervals. The advantages of the method are obvious, enabling the obstetrician to quickly evaluate fetal well-being at any time in an hour or less. Large studies are now in progress to correlate the OCT with other studies of fetal well-being as well as with pregnancy outcome. These studies indicate, tentatively at least, that as long as no acute problem supervenes, a negative test provides reassurance regarding fetal status for the ensuing week. Other forms of the stress test have also been tried. These include maternal exercise (as in the Masters 2 step ECG test) which causes some problems in the recording of the fetal heart and a maternal hypoxia test in which the mother breathes less than 20 percent oxygen. The latter offers some concern regarding potential fetal damage but can probably be standardized at an oxygen concentration which is safe but yet provides a critical test. The disadvantage of all of those tests is that they are cumbersome if serial studies are needed, tying up labor room personnel and equipment. At this point it would not seem advisable to attempt such studies in other than a hospital (labor room) setting.

AMNIOTIC FLUID STUDIES. Although more useful in estimating fetal age, amniotic fluid studies also are of value in assessing fetal well-being.

1. The presence or absence of meconium in the fluid is helpful information in certain clinical syndromes, especially in the postdate pregnancy. Meconium is passed by the fetus as the result of hyperperistalsis in response to a variety of stresses including hypoxia. Although clear fluid is reassuring in certain situations, especially the postdate fetus, it is not universally so and thereby lacks reliability. On the other hand, the meconium may have been passed in response to a single transient stress and be insignificant at the time of the observation. Quantitation is also a problem and quite imprecise terms, such as light staining, heavy, "pea soup," and so on, have been applied. Generally the more meconium present, the more severe and proximate the stress; however, this is only a very general correlation. Nevertheless, large quantities of meconium do provide a hazard in that aspiration by the baby at birth causes serious respiratory problems for the newborn. The ubiquitous problem in evaluating amniotic fluid is that it must be obtained, meaning that in the antepartal patient,

amniocentesis with its inherent risks must be used (see p. 144). Alternatively, transcervical amnioscopy (see below), or, if the patient is in labor, amniotomy can be used.

2. Bilirubin is normally present in small and decreasing amounts in amniotic fluid except in the case of Rh sensitization. The quantities are so small that they are not measurable by standard colometric methods. To determine these quantities, fluid samples are filtered, centrifuged, and examined in a spectrophotometer to determine the optical density deflection at a specific wavelength (450 mu). This number, the ΔOD_{450} is a reflection of the quantity of bilirubin in that fluid sample, and in the case of Rh disease, correlates far better with the outcome (cord blood hemoglobin, for example) than any other information available, including maternal antibody titers and past performance which are rather nonspecific. Ideally, of course, one would like to know the hemoglobin or hematocrit of the fetus to determine the degree of hemolytic anemia and the course of action to be taken. Since this study is not obtainable, the ΔOD_{450} is the next best, showing a good inverse correlation. A lower zone value indicates a fetus that is either Rh negative, unaffected or, at most, mildly affected without need for intervention. A midzone result indicates that the fetus is affected, but not in imminent jeopardy and that the test should be repeated at regular (weekly) intervals. When values reach the upper zone, the indication is that the fetus is severely anemic and will not likely survive two weeks unless there is intervention (delivery or intrauterine transfusion) depending upon the age of the fetus). The zones which leave a downward slope toward term make a given value more ominous later than earlier, probably because the placenta becomes increasingly efficient in clearing fetal bilirubin. Amniocentesis is indicated in all Rh-sensitized patients but is generally not indicated before 20 to 24 weeks since no therapy is available to the fetus before that time. Pitfalls include a bloody tap in which case the oxyhemoglobin peak (415) may obscure the ΔOD_{450} and the possibility that the development of polyhydramnios may falsely lower the value by dilution. The latter can be obviated by

doing protein determinates each time, since they remain relatively constant. (If the protein decrease is equivalent to the ΔOD_{450} decrease, it is due to dilution and not a real fall.) Despite pitfalls, amniotic fluid bilirubin determination has provided a solid scientific basis for the management of the Rh-sensitized patient.

3. Other amniotic fluid studies for fetal wellbeing have proved of less value. The pH, Po_2, and Pco_2 have been measured but seem to be slow to reflect the true status of the fetus. Estriol in amniotic fluid has been studied and is of some predictive value but is not as helpful as urine or serum determinations. Alpha-l-fetoprotein has also been used as an indicator of fetal distress, being increased in both amniotic fluid and maternal serum, but confirmation must come from further studies.

AMNIOSCOPY via the cervix is a technique advocated by Saling as a means of evaluating amniotic fluid without rupturing the membranes or performing amniocentesis. A conical metal endoscope, or preferably one of light-conducting plastic can be inserted through the cervix with as little as 1 to 2 cm of dilation. Through the cervical portion of the membrane, one can visualize the amniotic fluid and make gross determinations, for example, of the presence or absence of meconium and vernix. Use is obviously limited to near-term pregnancies when cervical dilation has begun and rupture of the membranes is a hazard especially to the inexperienced observer. Another obvious flaw is the inability to obtain a sample of amniotic fluid for analysis. Nonetheless in certain situations, especially the postdate pregnancy, it is a simple, safe office procedure which can be used to check for the presence of meconium.

Intrapartal Techniques

These methods are utilized to evaluate the fetus during the course of labor and delivery, a time when the fetus is subjected to a variety of stresses. Two categories of patients must be considered: patients whose fetuses are known to be at increased risk and those who are normal in all ways but have the ever-present small chance of developing unexpected intrapartal problems. In the first case, one can justify significant steps, even those which might involve small risk, for example, fetal scalp blood sampling. However, in the normal uncomplicated patient, such steps cannot be justified. To be acceptable for routine use, a technique must be essentially free of risks, reliable, relatively inexpensive, uncomplicated to use (could be applied and interpreted by nurse specialist) and productive of minimal anxiety in the patient.

FETAL HEART RATE MONITORING. At present, fetal heart rate monitoring is the one technique for intrapartal evaluation of the fetus which comes closest to the above ideals. It seems natural that the most objectively definable parameter of fetal well-being, a physical examination, is the focus for the development of continuous monitoring techniques. Three basic approaches have been used in the systems developed to date. Simple amplification of the heart sounds has proved to be the least efficient because it is so directionally sensitive (minimal movement may cause loss of the sound) and because other sounds (muscle contractions, maternal pulses) are amplified as well. The Doppler probe operates by transmitting a low-energy ultrasound wave which is reflected back to a receiver in the same probe, the angle of reflection being related to the difference in tissue density at a given interface. Maternal as well as fetal pulses can be detected, and, although this instrument is somewhat directionally sensitive, it is less so than the amplifier and picks up less noise. This is the most reliable of the commercially available systems and can be used in the normal patient. It can be applied by the nurse. The fetal electrocardiogram is the most obvious source of a signal for heart rate monitoring, but this method also has its problems. The electrical activity of the fetal heart produces only a fraction of the voltage produced by the maternal heart. Thus, when recorded with leads placed on the maternal abdomen, the maternal ECG is superimposed on the fetal, obscuring many of the fetal complexes and making interpretation extremely difficult. The one obvious way to avoid this is to place an electrode directly in contact with the fetus. This can be done via the cervix, if there is cervical dilation and the membranes are ruptured. A variety of clips and, more recently, a corkscrew type electrode have been developed to accomplish this. This equipment provides the cleanest possible tracing but has the obvious disadvantages of being invasive (requiring a physician to apply) and having some perinatal complications (for example, scalp lacerations and abscesses). These factors would seem to indicate that the use of the scalp electrode should be limited to known high-risk patients, patients with intrapartal complications, and patients in whom monitoring is desirable, but noninvasive methods fail for technical reasons. Another approach to the ECG involves the use of an analog computer to "subtract" the maternal tracing. This approach may prove to offer a superior noninvasive recording.

Regardless of the type, the signal is fed into a cardiotachometer (heart rate recorder) and then to a paper recorder or oscilloscope as a line tracing of fetal heart rate. (Attempts to interpret changes in the fetal QRS complexes have been unsuccessful to date; thus, only rate is used.) Simultaneously with the heart rate, a recording is then made tracing uterine contractions. This is done noninvasively by a tocograph attached by a belt, or invasively by a catheter inserted through the cervix and attached to a pressure transducer. The former gives only an estimate of the intensity of contractions while the latter is calibrated to give precise information.

How, Caldeyno, Barcia and other pioneers in fetal monitoring have described a number of abnormal heart rate patterns but there are three classic patterns which should be recognized by anyone dealing with the patient in labor:

The *early deceleration, or Type I dip* is a slowing of the fetal heart rate which is the mirror image of the contraction wave. It begins and ends with the contraction. This pattern is caused by compression of the fetal head and represents a compensatory mechanism for maintaining cerebral blood flow in the face of increased intracranial pressure (the same mechanism, that is, hypertension or bradycardia occurs in the adult). Type I dips are most commonly seen in advanced labor when the head is deeply engaged in the pelvis and are *not* associated with poor neonatal status.

Late decelerations, or Type II dips begin at

the peak of a contraction. This pattern is commonly associated with a baseline tachycardia (more than 160) which indicates the first response to hypoxic stress, catecholamine release. The bradycardia is thought to be a later, vagal response. Type II dips can occur at any point in labor or in the oxytocin challenge test and indicate uteroplacental insufficiency and true fetal jeopardy. The occurrence of Type II dips is an indicator for prompt delivery.

Variable decelerations are dips in heart rate which bear no constant relationship to the uterine contraction pattern. This pattern is caused by compression of the umbilical cord. Such compression is often transient and can commonly be relieved by changes in maternal position. If the pattern persists despite positional changes and the administration of oxygen to the mother, prompt delivery is indicated to avoid a depressed neonate.

A variety of other patterns may be encountered. *Persistent tachycardia* is especially common with maternal fever, and, if this is present, is not an indication for intervention but rather for treating the cause of the fever. Occasionally a uterine abnormality in the fetal heart such as a 2:1 heart block may occur, in which the rate may jump from 140 to 70 and back. However, such situations are rare and bradycardias are almost always ominous. Recently, more attention is being paid to the beat to beat variations in the fetal heart rate. The normal heart rate tracing is not a straight line; there is normally beat to beat variation. The absence of this variation is ominous. Other parameters may lend themselves to monitoring as the technology develops. Continuous recording of pH, Po_2 or fetal temperature are all potentially feasible. For the time being, heart rate monitoring is the most practical of the intrapartal techniques, and there are a number of most satisfactory systems commercially available and constantly being improved. Most units have both invasive and noninvasive sensors and many can be set up with a central display as well as the bedside unit. Although fashionable, central monitoring is not a substitute for bedside observation, and in many hospitals in which central units have been installed, usage does not justify the cost. The future of monitoring undoubtedly involves more sophisticated, smaller wireless noninvasive sensors which will give tracings comparable to those now obtained only by direct fetal application of electrodes. Much of this technology has already been developed, for example, in the biomedical aspects of the space program. It is quite clear that within the next decade, fetal monitoring will be a routine part of intrapartal care.

FETAL SCALP BLOOD SAMPLING was popularized by the same physician (Eric Saling) who promoted transcervical amnioscopy. Unfortunately, fetal blood is not readily and safely obtainable until cervical dilation, rupture of the membranes, and descent of the fetal head have occurred. These limitations constrict the usefulness of the technique; nonetheless, it is very helpful in specific situations. One major concern expressed by many at the initiation of the approach was that the blood sample obtained from the fetal scalp was not pure blood but a mixture of blood, edema, and tissue fluid resulting from the pressure on the head and caput formation. However, extensive clinical correlations have established that at least for pH (Po_2 and Pco_2 are less reliable) the scalp sample is representative of the fetal status. The approach has also proved useful in the study of other substances, including fetal concentration of local anesthetics and glucose. These latter studies are of more research than clinical interest.

The technique involves the use of the conical amnioscope, as described previously, placed through the cervix and firmly against the fetal scalp. The exposed area of the scalp is wiped clean with cotton balls and silicone grease is applied so that the blood will form a drop. Using a special blade with limited exposure, a nick is made and the sample is collected in a long heparinized capillary tube. A pH determination can be done very quickly, and the results available in 5 to 10 minutes. Hemeostasis is accomplished by holding pressure against the site with a cotton ball.

The pH determinations are particularly useful since the fetus, when subjected to hypoxia, promptly initiates anerobic glycolysis with the accumulation of lactate and pyruvate, producing a metabolic acidosis. The magnitude of the acidosis is an accurate reflection of fetal status. One can be reassured by a pH of 7.25 or higher. A pH of 7.20 or below indicates significant hypoxia and, in general, warrants prompt delivery. Values between 7.20 and 7.25 are inconclusive and must be followed with repeat determinations. Scalp sampling is most often used and is most helpful as an adjunct to heart rate monitoring. With heart rate changes which are not conclusive or persistent, the pH will often provide the basis for a management decision. A good pH will permit further expectant management, whereas a low one would dictate intervention. If the heart rate pattern is obvious, as in the case of persistent Type II dips, a scalp sample would be superfluous.

One pitfall in the technique is that the fetal pH rate could be a reflection of maternal changes. If for any reason there is a suspicion of maternal acidosis, simultaneous maternal and fetal samples will clarify the situation. Complications of the procedure include bleeding from the puncture site, scalp hematoma, and scalp abscess. If good judgment is used in selecting patients and careful technique applied, these can be minimized. Presentations other than vertex are generally considered a contraindication.

AMNIOTIC FLUID EVALUATION. For the most part, intrapartal amniotic fluid evaluation consists of observation for the presence of meconium. If conditions permit early rupture of the membranes, this will permit this observation in the high-risk patient. Occasionally when the presenting part is deeply wedged the forewaters are clear while the fluid behind may be meconium stained. That problem can be avoided by periodic sampling of fluid through the catheter used for intrauterine pressure recording or by amniocentesis. The latter is probably too strenuous a procedure to do repeatedly during labor. In early labor prior to rupture of the membranes, amnioscopy can be used to check for the presence of meconium. Specific clinical measurements such as pH and Po_2 have not proved to be of value.

At present, noninvasive heart rate monitoring and observation of amniotic fluid are the only means justified in the normal patient, while invasive monitoring and scalp sampling can be used in the fetus already determined to be at risk.

Fetal Therapy

Techniques for fetal treatment have been slower in developing than has the diagnostic methodology. A considerable amount of what can be accomplished is very nonspecific and indirect, involving the treatment of maternal disease, good maternal nutrition, prenatal care, and the like. One can certainly be assured that careful diabetic management in the mother is, in fact, treating the fetus, albeit indirectly. One must also include in this general category, pregnancy termination in the case of genetic studies indicating an affected fetus. This is admittedly a negative approach but is the only one available at this time. There are examples of specific fetal treatment which are now available and undoubtedly the number will be greater in the near future.

INDUCTION OF CHEMICAL PATHWAYS IN THE FETUS

BILIRUBIN CONJUGATION. Being immature, the fetal and early neonatal liver has inadequate glucuronyl transferase, an enzyme necessary for the conjugation of bilirubin. The synthesis of this enzyme occurs spontaneously in the early neonatal period with adequate levels being available in a few days in the full-term infant and somewhat later in the premature. The fetus does not require the enzyme before birth, since it is the unconjugated form of bilirubin which is cleared via the placenta to the maternal circulation. The administration of certain agents to the mother can induce the synthesis of the enzyme before it would occur maternally, thus affording protection to the newborn if problems with jaundice are anticipated, as in the case of Rh disease. It is only the unconjugated fraction which is a threat to cause kernicterus; consequently, the neonate can safely tolerate a higher total bilirubin once the enzyme system is activated. Although this approach is helpful, it is not a substitute for the other accepted approaches to Rh disease. At best it can probably reduce the number of exchange transfusions required in a marginal case.

SURFACTANT. One of the most critical biochemical pathways in the fetus and newborn is that for lecithin, the major constituent of pulmonary surfactant. Without this, the newborn is subject to respiratory distress syndrome. Under normal circumstances, this occurs at about 35 weeks gestation and perhaps earlier in some pathological conditions. Recent evidence suggests that lecithin synthesis may be induced early by the administration of corticosteroids. When betamethasone is administered to patients in threatened premature labor or to those who require premature delivery for pregnancy complications, there is a significant reduction in respiratory distress, provided at least 48 hours elapse between administration of the drug and delivery. Although reasonably large, the dose of steroid required carries no particular risk and on that basis alone, is probably indicated in the face of imminent premature delivery. Further studies will be required before the value of this approach is finally clear.

MATERNAL DIET THERAPY

In some of the metabolic disorders, a heterozygous fetus being carried by a heterozygous mother may be subject to some in utero damage, albeit much less extensive than that encountered in the homozygous state. Such damage can be obviated by placing the mother on the appropriate diet, for example, galactose free if the concern is galactosemia. Since it is possible in many of these diseases to detect and abort the affected fetus, this approach permits the protection of the heterozygotic fetus from metabolic damage.

INTRAUTERINE TRANSFUSION

This technique, developed by Dr. William Liley approximately ten years ago, is undoubtedly the most striking example of fetal therapy currently in use. There are a small number of fetuses of Rh-sensitized mothers that are so severely affected so early in pregnancy that premature delivery cannot salvage them; that is, they die of prematurity or if delivery is delayed, they are stillborn as a result of hemolytic disease. These fetuses are identified by the amniotic fluid OD_{450} with upper zone values prior to the 32 to 34 week of gestation (see p. 151). Since bilirubin is effectively released via the placenta, jaundice and kernicterus are not the risk, but rather anemia so severe as to cause high output cardiac failure. Hydropsfetalis is the descriptive term used for

such a stillborn, which connotes the massive edema with hepatosplenomegaly and pleural, pericardial, and peritoneal effusion. Generally this stage of the process occurs only after several progressively more severely affected pregnancies. Unfortunately, in other cases, especially when sensitization has resulted from incompatible transfusion, this disastrous result may come in a first pregnancy.

The problem then, which Liley was the first to solve, was how to correct the severe fetal anemia (hydropic fetuses often have hemoglobins in the range of 2 to 4 per 100 ml) sufficiently to avoid heart failure until the fetus is mature enough to deliver. In solving the problem, he utilized the approach of intraperitoneal transfusion which had been applied for some time in newborns and young children. Red cells are absorbed intact from the peritoneum quite efficiently in young children and do not cause sequelae as the result of peritoneal infection. To help localize the peritoneal cavity of the fetus, an amniogram is performed, the dye being injected 12 to 24 hours prior to the transfusion. Dye concentrated in the fetal gastrointestinal tract then provides a target for the needle, with a combination of preliminary x-ray studies and fluoroscopy during the procedure. Premedication with narcotics and/or barbiturates not only helps to reduce maternal anxiety, but also decreases fetal movement, making needle placement simpler. Under fluoroscopic control, an amniocentesis is performed with a long, large bore needle (7 inch 17 gauge) and the needle is then thrust into the abdomen of the fetus, preferably in the lower quadrants away from the large liver and spleen. However, the ability to be that accurate in needle placement is a function of fetal size and with very small fetuses the operator is satisfied to find the cavity regardless of the quadrant. Position is checked by injecting a small quantity of contrast material which produces a rather typical picture as it coats the loops of the bowel. Blood may then be injected either directly through the needle or through a polyethylene catheter placed through the needle. The former is much faster while the latter lessens the risk of injury should the fetus move during the procedure. The quantity of blood used has been determined empirically, the limiting factors being the size of the fetus, abdominal muscle tone, and pressure increases within the peritoneal cavity which could effect blood flow through the intraperitoneal portions of the umbilical veins. The latter has been postulated as a cause of sudden fetal death during the procedure. The milliliters used are generally 6 to 8 percent of the fetal weight in grams. Thus in a 1000 gm. fetus, one would administer 60 to 80 ml. Packed cells are used since fetal needs are for hemoglobin not volume and the cells are O negative and crossmatched to the mother's serum to be sure they will not be attacked by circulating maternal antibodies. The procedure is repeated at 10 to 14-day intervals until the fetus reaches a size and maturity compatible with good survival chances (generally delivery at 34 to 36 weeks.)

Although the plan as described appears straightforward, the problems are many. Each transfusion has an operative fetal mortality of 5 to 10 percent and the more required (the earlier they must be started), the poorer the outcome. Direct injury to the fetus by the needle and fetal hemorrhage secondary to placental puncture are common causes of fetal death. Overall, one can expect to salvage 40 to 50 percent of the fetuses in whom intrauterine transfusion must be undertaken. Although this represents a sizable mortality, the theoretic mortality is 100 percent for fetuses without the procedure. Even for babies born alive, there are concerns. What are the long-term effects of the radiation? Theoretically there may be concerns as a result of infusing immunologically competent lymphocytes which in animals causes the graft vs. host reaction and runt disease. Since the first intrauterine transfusion was done only ten years ago, many long-term follow-up questions remain unanswered. One interesting, less serious complication which is seen in these babies is a higher incidence of inguinal hernia due to the distention of the abdominal cavity by the blood.

To avoid some of the serious complications of this rather crude technique, some clinicians have tried to use "open" techniques in which a uterine incision is made, an extremity brought out, and a fetal vessel cannulated. Although this is successful in the experimental animal, in humans labor normally ensues and until this can be controlled the method is not useful. Another possible modification of the technique involves the use of an amnioscope to help with needle placement. This awaits only the development of a more efficient instrument. Fortunately, because of the development of Rhogam, the procedure will likely be obsolete within the next two decades.

The future of fetal treatment is bounded only by the limits of imagination. Operating amnioscopes should provide an access to the fetal circulation as well as a means to perform "closed" surgical procedures. Temporary exteriorization of the fetus would provide the ability to do more extensive surgery and replace the fetus. An artificial placenta might provide salvage of a fetus when there is a placental insufficiency. In utero nutritional supplements might be placed into the amnion. These are but a few rather obvious examples in a mushrooming technology.

The Goldbergs—A Family Requiring Genetic Counseling and Prenatal Diagnostic Services

It is evident that caring for the unborn is a task that requires a wide variety of professional skills. To point out some of the nursing challenges inherent in working with families who have hereditary health problems, we will describe the situation of a particular family, the Goldbergs. Although this family is fictitious, the services required by the family members illustrate the actual operation of the professional genetic counseling—antenatal diagnosis team at the Hospital of the University of Pennsylvania. Ms. Eileen Rawnsley, the nurse member of this health team, recounts the story of the Goldbergs.*

Amniocentesis is a very specific diagnostic tool requiring medical expertise. Although the procedure takes only 10 to 15 minutes, the actual laboratory work takes 3 to 4 weeks to complete. A significant amount of preparation and counseling is involved prior to the tap. The follow-up is not completed until after the baby is born or even

*The authors are indebted to Ms. Eileen Rawnsley, R.N., who expertly prepared the case material concerning the Goldberg family and assisted in reviewing the manuscript.

longer. For the family members, the decision to have an amniocentesis is not an easy one. They must face the possibility of spontaneous abortion as a consequence of the tap. Even more difficult is serious consideration of the possibility of a therapeutic abortion, should the fetus be affected (see the discussion of abortion in Chapter 5). For the family who has elected prenatal diagnosis, the baby is usually very much wanted. The anxiety of waiting 4 weeks until diagnosis is completed intensifies the ambivalent feelings that are normally present in pregnancy. The value and desirability of the child increase. In addition, there is the viability of the 20-week fetus: the mother may have felt fetal movement before the diagnosis was made. During this period, the family needs a great deal of support. The amount of interaction with the nurse counselor will depend on the severity of the problem and the family's capability of coping with stress. The nurse's ability to assess the family situation and plan the specific support that may be necessary can alleviate the crisis situation. After the diagnosis, which most of the time will be reassuring, the family initially experiences great relief, and continues the pregnancy with more confidence and less fear. However, the family does not really relax until the child is born or even until he or she is 6 to 12 months of age and healthy.

To provide the best possible service to the family, the genetic counseling-antenatal diagnosis team meets to share information. This team is composed of an obstetrician, pediatrician, geneticist, laboratory technologist, and nurse. When necessary, other consultations are made. The nurse functions as coordinator. She is usually the first person with whom the patient has contact and the one continuing individual who will follow the family over a period of time. She also screens incoming requests, handling some counseling herself and involving the appropriate physician in others.

The Goldbergs were discussed repeatedly at these staff conferences. This is a couple heterozygous for Tay-Sachs disease who illustrates some of the elements involved in prenatal diagnosis.

Tay-Sachs disease (an accumulation of ganglioside GM_2) is an autosomal recessive disease which occurs in all ethnic groups, but is most common in Ashkenazi Jews of Northern and Middle European origin. It probably first appeared about 1000 A.D. for some unknown reason. In this select group, the carrier rate is about 1:25 to 1:30, which means that statistically about 1:900 Jewish couples are at risk. This leads to a projected occurrence of one child with Tay-Sachs disease in every 3,000 births to Jewish couples.

In 1970 probably no more than 40 cases of Tay-Sachs disease were diagnosed in the country.[78] With a total of 19,142,000 live births that year, this seems like an insignificant number, but the disease is catastrophic to the family both emotionally and financially. It is estimated that the care of an affected child would cost over $35,000.[79]

The cause of GM_2 gangliosidosis is the complete absence of an enzyme, hexosaminidase A, which is necessary for the terminal cleavage of gangliosides. Without this enzyme, gangliosides are stored in the central nervous system, specifically the brain, eventually causing complete destruction of the neurons. There is no treatment for the condition and it is invariably fatal by age three or four.[80]

The disease was first described clinically in the 1880s. In 1964, the specific enzyme deficiency was discovered.[81] This opened the avenue for identification of carriers. In 1970, after the successful development of cell culture techniques, prenatal diagnosis by the use of amniocentesis became feasible.[82] With the development of an inexpensive, reliable screening method, adequate public education, available counseling for carriers, and expertise in prenatal diagnosis, it is now possible to prevent this fatal disease.[83]

Mrs. Goldberg is a 40-year-old woman, now in the twelfth week of her third pregnancy. Her first child died ten years ago. The medical records confirmed the diagnosis of Tay-Sachs disease on the basis of clinical symptoms and pathological examination at autopsy. The second child is now five-years-old and was conceived with artificial insemination. The third pregnancy

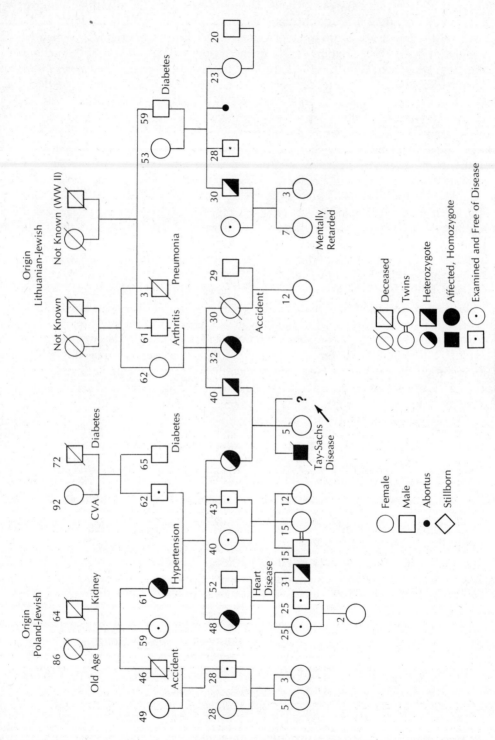

FIGURE 6-10
Pedigree of the Goldberg family.

was unplanned, as both Mr. and Mrs. Goldberg felt they were "too old to reproduce." Mrs. Goldberg is extremely anxious, has considered abortion, but was advised to seek genetic counseling before making a decision. The geneticist felt that if the Goldbergs decided to continue the pregnancy, they should first be screened for Tay-Sachs disease. Although the diagnosis seemed conclusive, we now have the technical means to substantiate this and should do so. The level of hexosaminidase A in the heterozygote is approximately half of the normal value.

The obstetrician agreed and suggested they also be counseled concerning the risk of chromosomal aberration on the basis of maternal age. About 1 percent of mothers at the age of 40 produce a child with Down's syndrome.[84] We would also discuss with them the 2 to 3 percent general population risk that any couple faces of having a child with defects.

When the couple arrived, they were interviewed by the nurse, who obtained a family history (Fig. 6-10). At times other syndromes of a hereditary nature become evident when not previously mentioned. In this pedigree, no other significant hereditary diseases were elicited that were amenable to prenatal diagnosis. As the nurse talked with the family, the reasons for their anxiety became evident as they discussed their experience with their son vividly.

"I just cannot face the thought of watching another baby die."

Jay, the Goldberg's Tay-Sachs son, was a beautiful baby until about six-months of age, when he did not want to eat and did not seem interested in anything. Worry increased when he had trouble sitting up. The doctor agreed something was wrong, but it was about four months and six doctors later that the diagnosis of Tay-Sachs disease was made. No one else in either family had had this experience. He was kept at home as long as possible. His deterioration was progressive, with convulsions preceded by spastic motions and explosive laughter; he became hypotonic and eventually blind. Feeding became an ordeal and when it was necessary to feed him by tube, he was placed in a nursing home. He then developed pneumonia and died. "Truth-

fully," they said, "it was a relief." Mrs. Goldberg admitted that her current pregnancy was a mixed blessing. Her husband had agreed to have a vasectomy, but never went through with it. Now, at her age, she said she did not know if she had the strength to care for a baby.

Mr. Goldberg expressed no regrets about the pregnancy; he wanted a son. He felt some guilt about bringing a sick baby into the world and did not want to have another sick child. He was relieved that both he and his wife were equally responsible for the disease and that neither was at fault.

"Our little girl is beautiful. I'm glad we decided to have her, but artificial insemination was a difficult decision. We had also considered adoption, but found it difficult, with a waiting period of two to three years. Now that it is possible to have a healthy child of our own, I want to take the chance."

The obstetrician presented the possibilities of prenatal diagnosis, discussed the general population and age-related risks (pp. 157-159). Problems related to her own health could be treated if any arose. The limitations and risks of the procedure were explained. It would be known whether the cells did not grow well within seven to ten days; and the Goldbergs would be asked to come back for a repeat tap. The obstetrician also explained that there was no way of knowing if Mrs. Goldberg was carrying twins. If they were identical twins, the fluid sample would represent both of them. If fraternal twins, only one sac would be penetrated, and the status of the other twin would not be known. This could lead to abortion of a healthy twin plus an affected child, or conversely, the delivery of an affected and a healthy child. The amniocentesis could be done at 15 to 16 weeks gestation. When the diagnosis was made at 19 to 20 weeks gestation, should termination be necessary, the procedure of choice would be saline abortion, and Mrs. Goldberg would be admitted to the hospital for a few days.

At the end of four weeks, they would be told if the child was affected with Tay-Sachs disease. However, it would not be possible to absolutely distinguish between the carrier and the normal. When the Tay-Sachs assay was completed, a karyotype would be done and they would be told if the chromosomes were normal, and also, if desired, the baby's sex. The Goldbergs were further advised that they could not be assured of a healthy normal child as there was still the possibility of defects that could not be diagnosed.

The Goldbergs were to think and talk about their options and make a final decision later. Blood was drawn from both of them for Tay-Sachs screening. Mrs. Goldberg's blood was specifically labeled that she was pregnant because this affects the enzyme level in the red cells, and the assay would have to be done on the white cells. (The usual screening procedure is done on red cells.)

The nurse would call in a week with the results of the screen and was available for any further discussion. Later that week the nurse spoke with the Goldbergs and reviewed the counseling session. They had a good understanding of the situation.

As expected, both were identified as carriers of Tay-Sachs disease. In the next conversation, Mrs. Goldberg expressed great anxiety about having an abortion at 20-weeks gestation. She had told her parents about the plans, and they had cited the Jewish religious ban against abortion. In discussing this, it appeared that the Goldbergs needed support in their own philosophy, that this was a decision that they would have to make themselves. They were advised to discuss the situation with their Rabbi, who supported them in their decision to attempt prenatal diagnosis.

When it appeared that the Goldbergs had worked through their ambivalent feelings about abortion, an appointment for amniocentesis was made. The laboratory was notified, as preparation time was needed. It is necessary to obtain control fluids from women undergoing therapeutic abortion at 16-weeks gestation to assay independently of the patient and to run as a comparison control with the patient.

On the day of the tap, Mrs. Goldberg was extremely apprehensive, her fears centering on the damage that could possibly occur to the baby. Mr. Goldberg, however, was calm, and matter-of-factly stated that they were prepared to take the risk of spontaneous abortion, that the risk of misdiagnosis seemed very small; and that they were confident this would not be in error. He also stated that, realistically, he felt they really had no choice, as this fetus had a 25 percent chance of having Tay-Sachs disease, 25 percent chance of being normal, and 50 percent chance of being a carrier.

In preparation for the tap, the nurse again explained the procedure. After the bladder was emptied, the abdomen was prepared with tincture of iodine: 2 cc of 1 percent procaine (Novocain) was used for local anesthesia. A number-18 spinal needle with stylet was inserted through the abdominal wall and the uterine muscle. As the pressure in the cavity is greater than air pressure, as soon as the stylet was removed, clear, straw-colored fluid was immediately obtained. Two cc were discarded, as a precaution against contamination by maternal cells which may have entered the needle. Twenty cc of fluid were obtained in two separate 10 cc syringes. Each specimen was taken to a different laboratory to be prepared for culture. The fluid was spun down, the liquid, or supernatant, set aside, and the cells placed in one or two bottles containing culture media and placed in an incubator where they remain undisturbed for about one week, during which time, they should begin to grow.

During the procedure, Mrs. Goldberg was kept advised of exactly what was happening step by step. After the needle was withdrawn and an adhesive bandage applied, Mrs. Goldberg burst into tears, saying "I hope the baby is alright, but it really wasn't as bad as I thought it would be. All I felt was pressure."

After resting for ten minutes Mrs. Goldberg got up and dressed.

"If I lose the baby, how soon will it happen?"

The obstetrician replied that it was a very clean, uncomplicated tap, and no problems were expected. However, if persistent cramping, vaginal spotting or leakage of amniotic fluid was observed, Mrs. Goldberg should call immediately.

One week later, Mrs. Goldberg was contacted. She had no complications of any kind following the tap. She was informed that the cells seemed to be growing satisfactorily. She stated that she had heard there was a quick method of diagnosing Tay-Sachs disease in several hours. It was explained that there was a fluorescent method of determining the activity of hexosaminidase A in the amniotic fluid.[85,86] However, at this time it has not been demonstrated to be as reliable as cell culture. The fluid is apt to contain some maternal cells and many dead cells which make the results indefinite: we could not use this alone as a criterion to advise abortion or continuation of pregnancy.

It became apparent that Mrs. Goldberg needed frequent information about the progress of the culture, and was in contact with the nurse once or twice a week. The assay for hexosaminidase A was completed and found to be normal. The family was informed. They were greatly relieved. One week later, a karyotype was completed, a normal male chromosome analysis.

Two weeks later the Goldbergs were again contacted by the nurse and the possibility of screening other family members was discussed. Mrs. Goldberg said that it had been discussed with them and they were very interested in doing this. A meeting was arranged for the nurse counselor and the geneticist to meet with five members of the family to discuss the value of screening. The problems in screening were also explored. There seems to be no ideal time in the life span to screen for a recessive disease. It is useful to screen couples at risk when they are contemplating pregnancy or are in early pregnancy because something can be done at this time to prevent the birth of a defective child. Many of the questions concerning screening are not yet answered. How will the grandparents of an affected child react when they learn one of them passed this trait on to the next generation? If a young adult is found to be a carrier, will this effect mate selection? If newly wed couples are found to be carriers, how will this influence their decision to produce offspring? It has been known that young children identified as carriers are treated as sick or different even though they are normal and healthy. We are prepared to screen anyone interested, but generally our policy is to advise it only for couples at risk who are of childbearing age.

Continuing contact through the next five months completed the screening of many individuals in the Rubin-Goldberg family. Of the ten members screened, six were found to be heterozygotes (see Fig. 6-10). No other couples were found to be at risk of producing a child with Tay-Sachs disease. This is quite common with autosomal recessive syndromes. It is unlikely to find more than one affected couple in a family group unless there had been some intermarriage which would increase the probability of expressing a recessive gene.

Mrs. Goldberg delivered a healthy male infant, who when tested was found to be a normal individual. The family expressed great pleasure in their healthy son: Mrs. Goldberg was euphoric, but definitely decided not to attempt another pregnancy, primarily because of her age. Mr. Goldberg was extremely proud of his son.

At our staff conference, we discussed this happy ending and made loose plans for follow-up to include these elements:

1. Health of the baby at age one.
2. Parental attitude toward both children.
3. Provide screening for Tay-Sachs disease for other family members when this becomes useful to them.

Although far from being an ideal solution, prenatal diagnosis is one option open to couples who are at significant risk of bearing defective children.

Summary

The care of the unborn has for too long been passive and fatalistic, based on the assumption that the healthy mother would have a healthy baby and that complications, if they arose, could be handled as they came. The technology described in this chapter represents most of that which is practical today but obviously only a minute fraction of that which will be available in the future. Fetal medicine is an exciting field in health care delivery, with opportunities for participation by a variety of workers at the professional as well as the nonprofessional level.

References

1. Bartolos, M. (ed): Genetics in Medical Practice. Philadelphia, J. B. Lippincott, 1968.
2. Mendelian genetics. *In* Biology Today. DelMar, Calif., CRM Books, 1972, Chapter 12.
3. McKusick, V. A.: Human Genetics. Englewood Cliffs, N.J., Prentice-Hall, 1964.
4. Davis, B. S.: Genetic counseling. Med. World News, Nov. 6, 1970.
5. Cell division. *In* Biology Today, Chapter 13.
6. *Ibid.*
7. Genetics and your health. World Health, Aug.-Sept. 1966.
8. *Ibid.*
9. Sergovich, F. et al: Chromosomal aberrations in 2159 consecutive babies. New Eng. J. Med. 851-855, April 17, 1969.
10. Genetics and your health, *op cit.*
11. Hillsman, G. M.: Genetics and the nurse. Nurs. Outlook 14:34-39, Jan. 1966.
12. German, J. L. et al: Autosomal trisomy of a group 16-18 chromosome. J. Pediatrics 60:503.
13. Taylor, A.: Patau's, Edwards' and cri du chat syndromes: a tabulated summary of current findings. Develop. Med. Child Neurol. 78-87, Feb. 1967.
14. *Ibid.*
15. Patau, K. et al: Multiple congenital anomalies caused by an extra chromosome. Lancet I. 790, 1960.
16. Taylor, *op cit.*
17. *Ibid.*
18. McKusick, *op cit.*
19. Sergovich, *op cit.*
20. Tips, R. L.: The whole family concept in clinical genetics. Am. J. Diseases Child. 107:67-76, Jan. 1964.
21. McKusick, *op cit.*
22. *Ibid.*
23. Williams, R. H. (ed.): Textbook of Endocrinology, ed. 4. Philadelphia, W. B. Saunders, 1968.
24. Price, W. H. et al: Criminal patients with XYY sex chromosome complement. Lancet I:565, 1966.
25. Stock, R.: The XYY and the criminal. The New York Times Magazine, Oct. 20, 1968.
26. Sergovich, *op cit.*
27. Hartman, P. E. and Susskind, S.: Gene Action. Englewood Cliffs, N.J., Prentice-Hall, 1965.
28. Epstein, C. J.: Biochemical aspects of human inheritance and hereditary disease. Human Genetics, Birth Defect Original Article Series, IV:6, Nov. 1968.
29. Molecular genetics. *In* Biology Today, Chapter 15.
30. Stanbury, J. B., Wyngaarden, J. B. and Fredrickson, D. F. (eds): The Metabolic Basis of Inherited Disease, ed. 3. New York, Blakiston-McGraw, 1972.
31. Biology Today, Chapter 15, *op. cit.*
32. Stanbury, *op cit.*
33. *Ibid.*
34. Epstein, *op cit.*
35. Taussig. H.: The thalidomide syndrome. Sci. Am. 207, 2:29-35, 1962.
36. Schwanitz, G. et al: Chromosomal injury due to occupational lead poisoning. German Med. Month. 15, 12:738-746, 1970.
37. Udalov, G.: Bone marrow transplants in irradiated monkeys. Nature 266, 5249:956-958, 1970.
   Bloom, A.: Chromosomal aberrations and malignant diseases among A-bomb survivors. Am. J. Pub. Health 60, 4:641-644, 1970.
38. Cann, H. M.: Principles of human inheritance. Human Genetics, Birth Defect Original Article Series, IV:6, Nov. 1968.
39. *Ibid.*
40. *Ibid.*
41. Mabry, C. C.: Maternal Phenylketonuria. New Eng. J. Med. 269:1404-1408, Dec. 26, 1963.
42. Stanbury, *op cit.*
43. Hsia: Inborn errors of metabolism. Clinical Aspects, ed. 2. Medical Yearbook, 1966, Part I.
44. McKusick, V. A.: Mendelian Inheritance in Man: Catalogs of Autosomal Dominants, Autosomal Recessives and X-linked Phenotypes. Baltimore, Johns Hopkins Press, 1966.
45. Stanbury, *op cit.*
46. Forbes, N.: The nurse and genetic counseling. Nurs. Clin. N. Am. I:4, 679, Dec. 1966.
47. Hillsman, *op cit.*
48. Anderson, J. A. and Swaiman, K. F.: Phenylketonuria and allied metabolic diseases. Washington, D. C., U.S. Department of Health, Education and Welfare, 1967.
49. Lake, D.: Nursing implications from an investigation of mothering, diet and development in two groups of children with phenylketonuria. ANA

Clin. Sess. 1968. New York, Appleton-Century Crofts, 1968.

50. Ragsdale, N. and Koch R.: Phenylketonuria: detection and therapy. Am. J. Nurs. 64:90, Jan. 1964.

51. Arthur, L.: Intelligent, small for date baby born to ologophrenic phenylketonuric mother after low phenylalanine diet during pregnancy. Pediatrics 46, 2:235-239, 1970.

52. Anderson, *op cit.*

53. Lake, *op cit.*

54. Tips, *op cit.*

55. Stanbury, *op cit.*

56. Hackett, T. et al: chemical detection of metachromatic leukodystrophy in disease and carrier states. Am. J. Diseases of Child. 122, 3:223-225, 1971.

57. Danes, *op cit.*

58. *Ibid.*

59. Fraser, F. C.: Genetic counseling. *In* V. A. McKusick and R. Claiborne (eds): Medical Genetics. New York, H. P. Publishing Co., 1973.

60. Hillsman, G. M.: Genetics and the nurse. Nurs. Outlook Jan. 1966.

61. Fraser, *op. cit.*

62. *Ibid.*

63. Clow, C. L. et al: On the application of knowledge to the patient with genetic disease. *In* A. Steinberg and A. Bearn (eds): Progress in Medical Genetics, Vol. IX. New York, Grune and Stratton, 1973.

64. Genetic counseling. Patient Care May 15, 1972, p. 135.

65. Genetic counseling. Patient Care, April 30, 1972, p. 18.

66. *Ibid.* p. 25.

67. *Ibid.* p. 32.

68. *Ibid.*

69. Patient Care, *op. cit.*

70. *Ibid.*

71. *Ibid.*

72. Korneesk, E. J.: They're ready to listen—are you talking to your patients? Med. Dimensions Feb. 1973, p. 10.

73. Patient Care, May 15, 1972, *op cit.*

74. Clow, et al, *op cit.*

75. *Ibid.*

76. Clow, C. L., Reade, T. M. and Scriver, C. R.: Management of hereditary metabolic disease: role of allied health personnel. New Eng. J. Med. June 10, 1971, p. 1292.

77. *Ibid.*

78. Harris, M. (ed): Early diagnosis of human genetic defects. H.E.W. Publications, 1970, p. 62.

79. *Ibid.*

80. Stanbury, *op cit.*

81. Kolodny: Biochemistry, Biophysics, p. 37, 1969.

82. Schneck C., Valenti, C., Amsterdam, D., Friedland, J., Adachi, M. and Volk, B. W.: Prenatal diagnosis of Tay-Sachs disease. Lancet I:582, 1970.

83. Kaback, M.: Time, Sept. 18, 1971, p. 54.

84. Milunsky, A., et al: Prenatal genetic diagnosis. New Eng. J. Med.

85. Brady, R.: Hereditary fat metabolism diseases. Sci. Am. 88, Aug. 1973.

86. Hultberg, B.: N-acetylhexosaminidase activities in Tay-Sachs disease. Lancet II:1195, 1969.

Bibliography

Anderson, R. E.: From peas to people. Nurs. Sci. 1:2, 94-104, June-July 1963.

Aronson, S., Aronson, B. and Vold, B.: A genetic profile of infantile amaurolic family idiocy. Am. J. Diseases of Child. 98:50, 1959.

Brady, Roscoe: Hereditary fat metabolism diseases. Sci. Am. 88-98, Aug. 1973.

Carter, C. O.: Multifactorial genetic disease. *In* V. A. McKusick and R. Claiborne (eds): Medical Genetics. New York, H. P. Publishing Co., 1973.

Chase, G. and McKusick, V. A.: Founder effect in Tay-Sachs disease. Am. J. Human Genetics 24:339-340, 1972.

Clausen, J. and Melchoir, J.: Lancet I. 7520:834, 1967.

Crick, F.: Of molecules and men. Seattle, University of Washington Press, 1966.

Davis, B. D.: Prospects for genetic intervention in man. Sci. 170: 1279, 1970.

DiFerrante, N., Nichols, B. L., Donnelly, P. V., Neri, G., Hrgovcic, R. and Berglund, R. K.: Induced degradation of glycosaminoglycans in Hurler's and Hunter's syndromes by plasma infusion. Proc. Natl. Acad. Sci. 68:303, 1971.

Hermann, R. E. and Mercer, R. D.: Portcaval shunt in

the treatment of glycogen storage disease: report of a case. Surg. 65:499, 1969.

Hitchcock, J. M.: Crisis Intervention. Am. J. Nurs. 73, 8:1388, Aug. 1973.

Holtzman, N.: Prevention of retardation of genetic origin. Pediatric Clin. N. Am. 151, Feb. 1973.

Jampel, R. and Quaglio, N.: Eye movements in Tay-Sachs disease. Neurol. 14:1013, 1964.

Journals: Am. J. Human Genetics and Ann. Human Genetics.

Kanoff, A., Aronson, S. and Vold, B.: Clinical progression of amaurotic family idiocy. Am. J. Diseases of Child. 97:656, 1959.

Knudson, A. G. Jr., DiFerrante, N. and Curtis, J. E.: Effect of leukocyte transfusion in a child with type II mucopolysaccharidosis. Proc. Natl. Acad. Sci. 68:1738, 1971.

Mahoney, C. P., Striker, G. E., Hickman, R. O., Manning, G. B. and Marchioro, T. L.: Renal transplantation for childhood cystinosis. New Eng. J. Med. 283:397, 1970.

Merril, C. R., Geier, M. R. and Petricciani, J. C.: Bacterial virus gene expression in human cells. Nature 233, Oct. 8, 1971.

Montagu, M.F.A. (ed): Genetic Mechanisms in Human Disease: Chromosomal Aberrations. Springfield, Ill., Charles C Thomas, 1961.

Moore, M. L.: The Newborn and the Nurse. Philadelphia, W. B. Saunders, 1972.

Myrianthopaulos, N., Naylor, A. and Aronson, S.: Founder effect in Tay-Sachs disease unlikely. Am. J. Human Genetics 24:341-342, 1972.

Nurs. Outlook 14, Jan. 1966.

Peters, J. A. (ed): Classic Papers in Genetics. Englewood Cliffs, N.J., Prentice-Hall, 1959.

Roberts, J. A. F.: An Introduction to Medical Genetics, ed. 4. London, Oxford University Press, 1967.

Roslansky, J. D. (ed): Genetics and the Future of Man. The Nobel Conference, Gustavus Adolphus College. New York, Appleton-Century Crofts, 1966.

Stahl, E. W.: The mechanics of inheritance. Englewood Cliffs, N.J., Prentice-Hall, 1964.

Starzl, T. E., Brown, B. L., Blanchard, H. and Brettschneider, L.: Portal diversion in glycogen storage disease. Surg. 65:504, 1970.

Stevenson, R. E. and Howell, R. R.: Some medical and social aspects of the treatment for genetic-metabolic disease. Annals Am. Acad. Pol. and Soc. Sci. 399:30, 1972.

Sutterly, D. C. and Donnelly, G.: Perspectives in Human Development. Philadelphia, J. B. Lippincott, 1973.

Thomal, G. and Scott, C.: Genetics disorders associated with mental retardation: clinical aspects. Pediatric Clin. N. Am. 151, Feb. 1973.

Thomas, G. and Scott, C.: Laboratory diagnosis of genetic disorders. Pediatric Clin. N. Am. 105, Feb. 1973.

U.S. Department of Health, Education and Welfare, Social and Rehabilitation Services, Children's Bureau, International Seminar in Medical Genetics, 1966.

Watson, J. D.: The Double Helix. New York, Atheneum, 1968.

7

Providing Primary Health Care for the Growing Child

DONNA NATIVIO

Fundamental Skills Required • *Specific Services Provided* • *Case Examples*

For many years, millions of people around the world have received all or most of their professional health care from nurses. These nurses, usually employed by religious, social, or governmental agencies, often have to work quite independently. The kinds of services that they are able to provide are largely governed by common sense and the highly individualized limits of their own knowledge. One does not have to look far into the literature to find evidence that the basic concept of the nurse as a provider of primary care has historical precedent.[1] Moreover, in recent years the terms "expanded role," "extended role," and "primary care giver" have occurred with increasing frequency in health care journals that discuss the role of the nurse.[2]

The move to legitimize the expanded/extended role through education and practice began full swing in the mid-1960s. The earliest efforts were in child health.[3,4] Programs to teach nurses to deliver primary care to the pediatric population sprang up under the auspices of universities, health departments, the armed forces, and individual physicians.[5] Most programs received at least part of their financial support directly or indirectly from the federal government. Entrance requirements, length of programs, units of study, and awards at completion varied greatly from program to program.

To encourage some standardization, in 1971, a joint committee of the American Nurses Association and the American Academy of Pediatrics issued "Guidelines on Short-term Continuing Education Programs for Pediatric Nurse Associates."[6] These guidelines outlined the functions and responsibilities of the pediatric nurse practitioner and provided some reassurance for those who recognized the need for the role to develop in an organized manner. Based on a review of existing programs, the guidelines set up ground rules for the establishment of future programs. They represented a recognition by both professions that the nurse is a logical individual to collaborate with the physician in the management of care for the patient. Perhaps most significantly, these guidelines are tangible evidence of an effort by both professions to work together toward the common goal of providing an improved level of health care for the children of our nation.

Fundamental Skills Required

Nursing is a profession whose tenet is one of service to people. The pediatric nurse practitioner specializes in providing health care to children directly and through their parents. It was once said that 90 percent of the health care in the United States is provided by mothers of families. To a great extent, the role and goal of the pediatric nurse practitioner is to help that mother, (or father), do the job in the best possible way. The following sections discuss the basic skills necessary for the nurse if that goal is to be attained.

INTERPERSONAL AND INTERVIEWING SKILLS (HISTORY TAKING)

Establishing rapport is a term used so commonly in nursing that it has become a cliché. Nevertheless, the process is far too often given only lip service rather than the serious consideration it really deserves. Setting up a mutually comfortable and trusting relationship is a sine qua non when working with children and adolescents.

Most educational programs for nurses teach the principles and techniques of interviewing. However, there is great variety in the degree to which the student has an opportunity to practice these skills in a clinical situation. Real skill in interviewing and establishing rapport comes only with experience and considerable effort on the part of the learner. The nurse who works with children has a dual task, for the parent/child dyad, most often the mother/child dyad, is inseparable. Both must trust and respect the nurse.

The interviewer must be so comfortable in her role that she is able to focus all of her powers of observation on the person being interviewed. She must be skillful enough to obtain the information she needs while allowing the client to freely express his or her feelings and concerns.

When possible within the employment setting, it is helpful to have one or both parents come in for a "Comprehensive Health History." This includes all of the traditional medical information such as family history of inheritable conditions, a review of development and previous illness, and a discussion of current concerns.

However, it is much more than a simple medical history. It is an opportunity to learn about the family members: how they function, how they fit into their social setting, their relationships to each other, and how these parents view their parental role. The skilled interviewer can put together a picture of the environmental and social setting in whch they live. For instance, how does the sports-enthusiast father of a little girl sublimate his desire to rear an All-American? Does the mother who was abandoned by her own parents as a child show signs of being overprotective toward her child? Does the father's job require him to travel and thus be absent from home frequently? This can place the burden of child rearing and discipline on the mother. Does she accept this responsibility and manage it easily or is there smoldering anger and resentment of her solitary burden? Perhaps both parents work. If so, responsibility for the children may be shared by yet another—a relative, a paid sitter, or a day care center. Does this situation allow for the security of consistent support and discipline? It is often helpful to know why both parents work. The reason may be financial need or a desire to have interests and commitments outside of the home. Such situations affect family relationships which, in turn, affect child-rearing practices.

Circumstances surrounding the pregnancy greatly influence parental feelings and response to the child. Perhaps this is the last birth for a woman who enjoys having a small baby to cuddle. How will this influence her response to this last child's striving for independence? Were conception and birth anxiously awaited by a couple desiring children or was it unplanned, unwanted, and disruptive to a comfortable way of life? Was infertility a problem? Special anxieties accompany the birth and rearing of a child conceived via fertility drugs or artificial insemination.

Adoptive children predictably are viewed and treated differently by their parents, albeit in subtle and hard-to-define ways. These parents may always harbor concern about the unknown heredity and its effects on the growth and development of their child. They may use this unknown to explain problems that are really produced primarily by the environment.[7] They may be reluctant to talk about some of these situations unless specific opportunity is given.

The environment varies for each child, even in the same family. Birth order, age and education of parents, health of other family members, financial status, availability and influence of grandparents and siblings are all factors that alter the child's life style.

Such broad-based information provides a background for looking at each child's total health picture as he or she grows and develops within the social/environmental setting. The extent to which environmental stress influences physical illness still eludes scientific measurement, but few would dispute its effect. Awareness of the total situation helps us and the colleagues with whom we consult to be more exact in our application of therapeutic techniques.

In addition to obtaining information and establishing a relationship, the history-taking session can provide an opportunity to begin counseling. Through this the parent learns another dimension of the pediatric nurse practitioner role. The nurse should not try to do too much in one session, especially if the material being discussed is highly emotional. Generally, neither parent nor interviewer absorbs much if the session is prolonged beyond 45 to 50 minutes. It is important for the nurse to assure the parent of her willingness to continue the discussion at another time.

After a "good" interview session, clients will often spontaneously remark that they feel better or relieved. They may express surprise at their ability to talk about their concerns. Occasionally they may regret having revealed so much of themselves. It is important that they be reminded of the confidential nature of the interview. Even parents who have no specific family concerns will enjoy pondering and putting their feelings about their families into words. This opportunity for guided reflection often seems to enhance their views of themselves as parents. A good initial contact can set the tone for a successful working relationship between parents and nurse. Conversely, if the initial contact is poor, there is often no opportunity for a second try.

Establishing rapport with the child will be discussed under physical examination, since this is where many of the techniques can be most appropriately illustrated.

INDEPTH KNOWLEDGE OF DEVELOPMENT

Nurses wishing to work as pediatric nurse practitioners must review and expand their knowledge of child development. Indepth knowledge of physical, mental, emotional, and social growth and a succinct family and personal history enable them to formulate a composite picture of the individual child. This dynamic composite forms a foundation on which nurses can base their decisions on how best to assist a specific child and his or her family. Nurses must be comfortable and secure in the appropriate knowledge and versatile in the use of written and spoken language so that they can explain their concerns and plans for therapy with clarity to families and professional colleagues alike.

Developmental rate varies greatly from child to child. Physical, mental, emotional, and social development frequently do not progress at the same rate in the same child. Children whose physical growth outruns the rest of their development may be made to feel inadequate and insecure because they cannot perform to the level their appearance leads one to expect. The intellectually precocious youngster of small physical stature may be rejected by intellectual equals who are older and more developed physically. Likewise, the late maturing adolescent may develop an inadequate sex image while his or her early maturing peers may find themselves in social and emotional situations with which they are not yet able to cope.[8]

What is viewed as adequate social adjustment in one setting may be interpreted as deficient in a different milieu. In our increasingly mobile society, this is frequently demonstrated. It is faced by the child whose family moves from a small rural community into the center of a bustling city or into a highly sophisticated suburban neighborhood. Modes of social interaction, dress, and even language may seem disturbingly foreign to the newcomer. The impact of such cultural shock may manifest itself as depression, somatic complaints, school refusal, or delinquent behavior. A patient and understanding approach to counseling in such situations can speed up resolution and make the process of adjustment less painful.

A clash between social and environmental situations and developmental phases is often manifested in physical symptoms that are interpreted as illness. One example is the 14-month-old boy who is toilet trained in a crash course because his mother wants to finish the job before the new baby arrives. This puts great pressure on a child who is probably not yet able to conform to her wishes. The mother, who is also under stress, may punish him for his accidents, producing guilt for herself and greater anxiety for the child. Sometimes the child does manage to conform, only to find that, in spite of his great effort, his mother has turned her interest to the new baby. He may attempt to attract her attention either by stool holding or regressing to his earlier habits. Either way, the mother expresses concern about a physical defect that is causing the problem.

Similarly many parents grow anxious when their one-year-olds refuse to eat or show considerable appetite decline. Many can be comforted by an explanation of the normal slowdown in growth and appetite at this age and the transfer of the children's interest from food to the job of mastering mobility and exploring their expanded world.

If the nurse has ongoing contact with a family, it is often possible to anticipate such situations. Prevention of concerns and problems is, of course, highly desirable and often easier to deal with than the complicated situations that can develop when anticipatory guidance is not possible.

Other illustrations of the interplay of development, environment, and health can be found in the case examples which are presented later in this chapter.

PHYSICAL EXAMINATION

The examination must be organized and thorough. Each examiner should establish a repetitive routine which enables him or her to remember to cover all areas. This routine must vary according to the purpose of the examination and the person being examined. When reasonable, the initial examination should be complete.

When the same child returns with a specific complaint, the examiner may choose to perform a partial examination depending upon the presenting history (see Chapter 4, The Assessment of Physical Health).

The approach to the child must be as varied as children themselves. One important variable is the age of the child. If the examiner observes well and has a healthy background in child development, the child will provide clues to guide his or her actions.

The sleeping infant can be examined easily if approached quietly and slowly. If handled gently, he will usually awaken slowly allowing sufficient time to evaluate his heart, lungs, and abdomen without interference from crying and tense muscles. The screaming infant can often be quieted with a familiar bottle or pacifier or by having his mother nearby.

The six-month-old who pulls at the stethoscope can be distracted by placing some toy in his hand or dangling a bright object in his line of vision. The eight-month-old exhibiting stranger anxiety may best be examined on his mother's lap. Unless specifically indicated, intrusive examination of ears, nose, mouth, and rectum might wisely be deferred. The child with only mild anxiety will often submit to examination if allowed time to become familiar with the examiner and the surroundings. While staying a comfortable distance away, the examiner can observe the activities of the child, including his interaction with his mother. This warm-up time can also be used to talk with the mother about her concerns.

As soon as the child has learned to identify body parts, the examiner can enlist his cooperation by asking him to point to his eyes, ears, and nose. His anxieties are forgotten as his energies are used in playing the game. He should be allowed to examine the otoscope, stethoscope, and tongue blade before they are used to examine him. If he refuses to accept them from the examiner, he may feel safer accepting them from his mother since security comes to him through her. Sometimes curiosity will overcome anxiety if the examination equipment is simply left within his reach. Of course, all of this is time consuming, but the rewards are great. A cooperative child allows the examiner to be more secure in the findings since the examination can be carried out more carefully and completely.

At the same time, parent and child are also learning. They learn that a visit for health care need not be terrifying and upsetting to the child or guilt producing and embarrassing for the parent.

The previous experience of the child and parent with health care workers is another important variable. A child who has undergone a frightening or painful experience in one setting will frequently generalize his anxiety to all health care settings. Fears are often built up as a result of separation for hospitalization, surgical procedures, or stories related by adults or other children. It is wise to ask parents beforehand how their child feels about coming in for an appointment and how he has reacted in the past. The frightened child requires a slow and cautious but persistent approach. If an older child can verbalize his fears, the examiner is sometimes able to allay the fright through careful explanation.

The budding adolescent may wish to avoid undressing for a physical examination. For some, the situation can be made more comfortable if the examiner is of the same sex. The examination should be carried out without delay and in a matter-of-fact manner while care is taken to avoid any unnecessary exposure.

The physical examination provides a good opportunity to talk with adolescents about sexual development. Though the examiner may get little verbal response from them, it is reassuring if he or she at least points out that they are healthy and developing normally. If the approach is interested and matter-of-fact, the examiner can often provide answers to questions that they have not had an opportunity to ask before (see Chapter 8, Health Problems During the Adolescent Years).

The preceding paragraphs have been largely a discussion of how to approach the child. The actual step-by-step direction of how to complete a physical examination is the subject of several well written textbooks and can be reviewed in detail there,[9] as well as in Chapter 4 in this text.

Real skill in perfecting organization, examination techniques, and ability to detect deviation increases with experience and personal effort to learn. It is wise for the examiner to take advantage of every opportunity to consult with more knowledgeable and experienced colleagues to verify his or her findings and for continued learning opportunity. Most of us retain best the knowledge we have gained through experience.

DIAGNOSIS OR ASSESSMENT

The use of the term diagnosis in relation to nursing practice has been the subject of much discussion and of some verbal acrobatics in the writing of nurse practice acts. In fact, the dictionary definition of diagnosis generally points out the relationship of the word to disease, that is, the act or process of identifying or determining the nature of a disease through examination,[10] the art of distinguishing one disease from another,[11] and the determination of the nature of a case of disease.[12] On the other hand, assessment has not yet found its way into medical dictionaries. Its first three definitions in the *American Heritage Dictionary of the English Language* relate to the setting of fees for tax, fine, or other payment.[13] However, the fourth definition, to evaluate or appraise, more clearly relates to nursing's increasingly popular use of the word. The term "diagnosis" with its disease orientation is much too narrow to describe all that is included in the examination of a child. For that reason, the broader term, assessment, seems preferable. The pediatric nurse practitioner looks at all aspects of the child in an effort to identify wellness and to rule out illness rather than vice versa. When one sets out to make a medical diagnosis the approach is largely the reverse.

Findings on physical examination must be coupled with information gained through history taking and, often, laboratory tests. If wellness cannot be ascertained, the deviations are enumerated and a list of problems or symptoms compiled. In some instances, the pediatric nurse practitioner may indeed add up a list of symptoms and identify a problem in a manner consistent with that followed by a medical colleague.

Once a list of deviations, symptoms, or problems has been enumerated, the next step is to formulate a plan for action. A decision here is based upon the knowledge, skills, and experience of the individual practitioner. She will be influenced by the policies of the employer, the availability of other professional disciplines and her relationship with them, and the wishes of the client and the client's family.

The nurse practitioner may decide that she is able to handle the situation independently and prepare to do so. She may need a verifying opinion and seek consultation from a peer or medical colleague. Or, the situation may clearly be beyond her capabilities, and she will make an appropriate referral.

The skills of the pediatric nurse practitioner can blend into and complement the services of other professionals in a health care facility. How well this is accomplished will depend largely on the practitioner's ability to make her role acceptable to coworkers and clients.

Specific Services Provided

PARENT/CHILD EDUCATION FOR HEALTH

The pediatric nurse practitioner can play an impressive role in the education of parents and children. Each parent brings his or her own collection of ideas about health and illness to the situation. Superstition and myth abound. Treatment is handed down from generation to generation. Almost anyone who is asked (and some who aren't) have advice to give about child rearing and illness care. The nurse practitioner must be aware of the conflict that develops for a parent when professional advice differs from that of grandparents and friends. It is also important to note that opinion among professionals varies, which often adds to the confusion. The nurse practitioner should discuss this conflict situation with the parent when it seems advisable. When a family member is part of the problem, it is helpful to invite that person to sit in on the discussion.

It is worth noting here that grandparents are very special people. They can be immensely supportive to parents and important to the child's development of trust and security. It behooves the pediatric nurse practitioner to view them as allies and to capitalize on their potential value.

One of the most common conflict situations that develops in illness care is related to the use of medications. Although there has been progress, we live in a culture where many feel that all discomforts can and should be quickly relieved by medication. This low tolerance for discomfort that we teach our children may be one of the reasons for the problems of addiction and drug abuse that we face today.

Illness produces anxiety which adds to the discomfort for most children. Much of this can be relieved by sympathetic and gentle handling by parents. Before parents can act in a therapeutic way, they must be convinced that the care they have been advised to give is appropriate. This is more readily accomplished if there is a good and trusting relationship between practitioner and parents.

Nurses are aware of techniques for bringing comfort that do not require specific medical direction. The pediatric nurse practitioner can advise the parent to employ some of these same measures at home. Fever alone usually does not call for antibiotic therapy and can be relieved by antipyretics, fluids, and tepid baths. Vomiting and/or diarrhea often responds to diet alteration, nasal congestion to humidity control, and mild cough to increased fluid intake and a soothing hypertonic solution such as honey and lemon. Pruritic rashes can be relieved by baking soda baths, local applications of lotions, and avoidance of drying and overheating. I do not mean to discount the importance and efficacy of medications. It is, however, important to be sure that their use is appropriate and clearly necessary.

Another area of teaching that is often overlooked is the need to help a parent decide if an ailment is minor or serious. Advising parents before the fact that all children will sooner or later develop fever, cough, vomiting, and diarrhea and providing them with some methods of coping can be extremely helpful and reassuring.

Health care crises are defined in different ways depending on the knowledge and emotional state of the person doing the observing. Many concerns that parents view as critical may seem minor to the professional who can be unemotional and objective in viewing the situation. It is important to remember that if the situation is anxiety producing for the parent, it is necessary for the nurse practitioner to take the time to ease those concerns. Knowing that they have quick access to advice is reassuring to most parents. This access is often via the telephone.

Telephone consultation is an important service that the pediatric nurse practitioner can provide for clients. The most effective method of doing this will depend upon the individual work setting. Many practitioners like to set aside time in the early morning exclusively for answering calls. Parents can be encouraged to call at this time to have their questions answered. An effort should be made to assure them that the nurse practitioner views this consultation time as an important part of her job, that she expects them to call and that their call will not be viewed as an unnecessary interruption to her regular work routine.

For the pediatric nurse practitioner, the telephone as an instrument of communication may be a mixed blessing. It is certainly more convenient than a trip to the office and usually more economical from the patient's point of view since most practices or agencies do not bill the patient for this service.

An interesting finding in my experience is that some people seem to find telephone conversation more comfortable than face-to-face discussion. They are better able to ask questions that may make them feel embarrassed or a little foolish. On the minus side, the nurse practitioner's ability to assess the situation depends upon the caller's skill as an observer and the ability to verbalize concerns in a manner that helps the practitioner to make the right decision. It is helpful if she knows the parents and has some feeling for their ability to observe and report reliably. Remember that no parent can be unemotional when concerned about his or her own child.

A variety of questions can be appropriately fielded over the phone if both nurse and parent are comfortable with the situation. Questions related to feeding, elimination, minor illness, and development can often be answered without actually seeing the patient. When advice is given over the phone, all conversations should end with a request that parents call back to report on progress. They should be told to call back at once if the child's condition seems to worsen or if their concern increases for any reason. In general, a visit should be planned for the child with ear pain, dyspnea, significant blood loss, vomiting or diarrhea severe enough to raise the concern of dehydration, or when suturing or x-ray examination seems indicated. In addition, a visit should be the option of all parents who feel they are not comfortable with phone advice or the condition of their children necessitates examination.

A third area of teaching involves development, anticipatory guidance, and safety. Although each of these subjects could be discussed separately, they are often so dependent on one another that it seems appropriate to look at them together. Most parents delight in every skill that their children demonstrate. In their rejoicing they may be oblivious to the need to protect the child from the hazards of learning while continuing to encourage him to master skills. The infant who learns to roll over is in immediate danger of rolling off something. When he learns to pick up objects and bring them to the mouth for investigation, it becomes important to see that he does not pick up objects that can be swallowed or cause external injury. Walking and climbing skills greatly increase the size of the child's world. Electric cords, wall sockets, hot stoves, fire places, and stairs pose particular hazards. Exploration often leads to cupboards full of medicines, cleaning fluids, and other poisons. Some might feel that appropriate discipline could take care of the situation, but the young child is impulsive, curious, unaware of danger, and simply unable to control his desire for mobility and investigation. No amount of verbal warnings and no type of punishment will insure protection. The most dependable method is to simply remove the temptation. Even the child who is old enough to understand danger may need to frequently test the limits set by parents and injure himself in the process.

Many of the situations mentioned above can be avoided if parents are given advance warning. They can learn about and prepare for developmental stages. They can better understand their child's actions and reactions if they have an opportunity to anticipate rather than be taken by surprise. Avoidance of accidents can spare a parent the pain of guilt.

Nutrition and feeding is another area in which there is ongoing need for education of parents. The expectant parent faces the dilemma of choosing between breast- and formula-feeding. Breast milk is of course good for babies, but more important than the nutritional aspects is the relationship that develops between mother and baby as part of the feeding process. If the mother breast-feeds because she feels that she must rather than because she wants to, the whole experience may be unpleasant and disrupting for both.

The mother who truly enjoys breast-feeding and whose baby is content and thriving should be encouraged to continue until either she or the baby loses interest. When possible, weaning should be a planned and gradual process allowing time for the baby to adapt to a new mode of taking in food and for the comfort of the mother whose milk supply will usually decrease in proportion to the decrease in the amount of stimulation provided by sucking. Experienced mothers will say that the eruption of teeth does not mean that weaning must take place immediately. Abrupt weaning is disruptive and confusing to the baby and uncomfortable for the mother. Many mothers choose to continue a single breast-feeding (usually at bedtime) long after the baby has mastered taking fluids from a cup.

Conversely, the mother who finds breast-feeding distasteful or unpleasant should not be made to feel inadequate or guilty about "depriving" her baby. Babies thrive very well on cow's milk and feeding can still be a time of mutually satisfying closeness. An advantage to bottle-feeding is that the father can participate more actively in sharing the experience. Fathers of breast-fed babies may truly feel left out and unnecessary unless special effort is made to include them.

There is often much concern about the appropriate time for the introduction of solids into the infant diet. There is no magic time or mysterious sequence for the introduction of foods. In general, the role of the pediatric nurse prac-

titioner is to encourage parental self-confidence and self-sufficiency. If the mother prefers vegetables rather than cereal or fruit as a first solid, it will not damage the baby, and the mother will gain confidence in her ability to make decisions about the care of her child. Rough guidelines that I like to share with parents are as follows:

1. In the early months of life, milk will provide all of the essential nutrients with the possible exception of vitamin C and iron (many prepared formulas have these added).
2. The bottle-fed baby who takes 8 ounces at a feeding or more than 32 ounces in a 24-hour period is generally ready for solids.
3. The breast-fed baby who requires feeding at less than two-hour intervals is generally ready for solids.
4. New foods should be introduced one at a time.
5. Mixtures should be avoided until each food in the mixture has been given separately.
6. Citrus and eggs should be withheld until the child is four-to-six-months old, especially if there is a family history of allergy.
7. Any food that seems to cause distress, that is, diarrhea, vomiting, cramping, or rash, should be discontinued and tried again in a week or so.

A few parents will be unable to accept a permissive approach to feeding and will continue to seek specific directions. Most of them will master the feeding process in a few months.

Concern again arises during the second year when the apparently healthy toddler loses interest in food. A classic article, "Johnny won't Eat," by Dr. Platou aptly describes the anxiety of parents and the frustration of the physician who is unable to convince them that tonics, vitamins, and extreme diagnostic measures are not necessary.[14] In fact, this period of minimal weight gain is physiological. The child at this age is so busy developing skill at locomotion that he is simply too busy to eat. Growthwise he is trading baby fat for muscle, tissue for tissue, rather than adding to his total mass. If this expected decline in growth rate and food intake is anticipated, parents are better able to take it in stride. They can avoid providing the child with the opportunity to use their concern about eating as the perfect attention-getting mechanism.

Some basic guidelines for feeding the pre-school and school-age child are helpful, but should not be rigidly enforced. Children should be offered a variety of foods at mealtime and required to try a little of each. Dessert may be granted as a reward and need not be part of every meal. Meals should be on some fairly regular schedule, and the child should be required to come to the table at mealtime. Between meal snacks, especially of high-carbohydrate foods, have no virtue. The child's need for frequent intake of snack food may be an indication that his diet is generally lacking in foods of high-nutritional value.

Finally, it is advisable for parents to practice what they preach. Children learn their mealtime habits and food choice, including size of portion, from others in the family. They also learn the social significance of food and that it pleases some parents if the children eat often and eat a lot. The tendency for exogenous obesity develops from early eating habits. Overweight without question is a problem which is easier to avoid than to solve. The battle to lose pounds and keep them off is never ending and far too often unsuccessful. The psychological factors in obesity have been well analyzed and are much too broad to cover here. However, the bibliography includes several references that should be helpful to those who want to pursue that aspect of the problem.

During adolescence, the appetite is usually greatly increased. This is due largely to an increased metabolic rate, accelerated growth, and the deposition of body fat that is a normal secondary sex characteristic. Like the two-year-old, the adolescent is too busy to eat. Unfortunately, this is also the age of food faddism and dieting. The teenager who sets a goal of either gaining or losing a certain number of pounds will not be influenced by tears, pleas, or threats of parents. Acceptance by his or her peer group is a dominant drive and his or her will to conform to their values is all consuming.

Part of the developmental work of adolescents is to decrease their dependence on their parents. For this reason, dietary or other counseling is often better received and has a greater chance of being successful if it comes from adults that they respect but with whom they have no emotional ties. Adolescents generally want to be responsible for decisions about themselves. Thus they are more apt to respond to advice if one "treats them like adults" while still being aware of the tenuous nature of their independent decision making.

An emotion-laden area in which there is much parent and child concern is sex education. Most of the concern focuses on the adolescent years when mature sexual function occurs. However, children begin to learn about sex very early in life. Given the opportunity, they will observe the difference between the anatomy of their parents and be comfortable in comparing their own bodies to those of mom and dad. They learn that daddy is a man and mommy a woman. They clarify their own sex identity by practicing both roles, largely through imitation of their parents.

The three- or four-year-old asks many questions and displays much interest in a pregnant lady and how she got that way, the new baby and where it came from and why only mommies have babies. In general, it is wise to give information when it is sought and to avoid confusing the child by providing him with more detail than he is asking for. Answers should be straightforward and in a language that the child will understand.

Ideally, information about sex should be available from the school, church, and home. However, there continues to be much disagreement about who should do the teaching and how old the child should be when information is presented. Some parents prefer to personally control all teaching of sex information while others want no part of the responsibility and prefer that school or church do the job. In fact, the sexual education of a child has progressed to a considerable degree prior to adolescence with or without the participation of home, church, and school.

No matter who does the teaching, adolescents must be provided with more than anatomical facts and a list of secondary sex characteristics. They need help in understanding that hormonal changes will produce new emotional response. With advance knowledge, the experience of nocturnal emissions and menstruation and the accompanying feelings and urges will be less confusing and better understood. Anxiety and guilt can be minimized if adolescents know that they are free to discuss homosexual feelings and masturbation and are assured that these are normal components of sexual development.

Adolescents who wish to be sexually active are not dissuaded by threats of venereal disease or unwanted pregnancy. Teaching them the symptoms of venereal disease and methods of preventing spread is likely to be a far more effective deterrent than the use of scare tactics. Further, it is less than honest to ply the adolescent with information on the joys of love, marriage, and parenthood unless this is realistically coupled with the responsibility to others that each entails. Contraceptive information is being requested with increasing frequency by young people and the request is often suggested or supported by their parents. The pediatric nurse practitioner who feels she is unable to discuss birth control because of personal religious or moral beliefs should at least be prepared to refer a client desiring such information to an appropriate source (see Chapter 5 for further discussion of birth control and related family health services).

PREVENTIVE SERVICES

Many references have been made to prevention of problems in the previous sections of this chapter. All of these could be appropriately reiterated here.

Most parents are quick to seek care if they feel their child is ill or failing to grow and develop normally. Most see a need to have an infant seen at periodic intervals but are less convinced that the same care is appropriate for their healthy-appearing older child. Largely this is because our traditional approach to teaching health care personnel has been to focus on medical care (illness care) and not the broader concept of health care which encompasses prevention and early case finding, as well as treatment and rehabilitation. In addition, our actions support this traditional teaching stance. It is much easier to get an appointment for care if one presents symptoms of illness than if one asks for a routine checkup. Many hospital ambulatory care centers maintain a variety of specialty clinics for treating illness but provide almost no service for well children.

Proponents of the current system are quick to point to the well baby clinics operated in many areas by community health agencies as sources of preventive care. Many of us know, however, that services offered in these clinics run the gamut from very good to deplorable and often are little more than "shot clinics." Further, access to these clinics is often restricted by age, income, and geographical limits. In some areas, neighborhood health centers offering comprehensive care present a glimmer of hope, but they are few and far between.

The expressed reason for this lack of preventive service is that of too many people and too few prepared personnel. Whether this is a fact or an excuse, the pediatric nurse practitioner can begin to provide a solution to the problem. She can focus on the element of prevention as an important part of primary health care whether her employment setting is a hospital, health center, private office, school, or well baby clinic. Her greatest task is to convince parents and others that children of all ages should be seen for periodic evaluation. The purposes of these visits are to keep the healthy child healthy, to detect impending problems, and to detect and treat minor problems before they become major. Periodic visits for preventive services should include interim history, physical examination, developmental assessment, and other screening procedures such as vision and hearing. A laboratory screening of blood and urine as well as immunizations should be provided when appropriate.

Perhaps the most tangible and best known preventive service is the provision of immunizations against common childhood illnesses. The most up-to-date recommendations for scheduling are published periodically by the American Academy of Pediatrics[15] (see Chapter 22 for material on immunization and the immune process).

For the nurse practitioner, the provision of immunizations provides an opportunity to help the child and parent learn to tolerate a painful procedure without producing permanent trauma. Honesty is important. The young child should know that an injection is painful, but with cooperation it will not hurt very much and will be over very quickly. When the child must be restrained, he should know that the nurse practitioner understands that it is sometimes hard to hold still and for that reason his mother is going to help him. This allows for safety in giving the injection while providing the child with security and preserving his self-esteem.

Developmental screening also warrants a brief comment here. Each contact with the child should include some evaluation of his development—social, emotional, and physical. It is often helpful for the nurse to share with the parents those things that she observes that point to normal developmental attainment. For instance, the three-month-old who smiles in response to a smiling face, the ten-month-old who is nearly impossible to diaper because of his desire to practice standing up, and the six-year-old who rejects the adults in the family when there is opportunity to spend time with his peers.

Standard developmental tests, such as the Denver Developmental Screening Test, are often helpful in showing parents that their child is functioning within the range that is expected for his age. They can also be used to verify suspicions that a developmental delay is present and serial testings can help keep track of the child's progress. However, screening tests have little predictive value and should not be used to project ultimate developmental outcome.

Family planning can also be viewed as preventive pediatrics. For some professionals, the use of birth control measures is more acceptable when viewed from this perspective (see Chapter 5 concerning Family Planning).

Frequent pregnancies can produce both physical and emotional stress on the mother, thus increasing the threat of poor pregnancy outcome. Generally, she will have more time and energy to devote to giving each baby a good start if there are at least two years between the birth of one child and the conception of another.

ADVOCACY

One of the most helpful roles that the pediatric nurse practitioner can assume is that of client advocate. She may need to represent the child's point of view to the parent or vice versa in an effort to help each understand the other a little better.

She can help the physician to be more precise in his understanding of a family's concern by sharing her knowledge of background information that contributes to the anxiety. Some parents find it difficult to sort through the confusion and impersonal attitudes of a large busy medical center and turn away without getting the help that they need. The pediatric nurse practitioner can smooth the path considerably by alerting someone inside the institution of the need to intercede.

Finally, the nurse must act as an advocate for child health in the community. She has responsibility to evaluate factors which influence the health of the child and act with others to remove health hazards. She can contribute to the development of new and improved community resources and patterns of health care delivery and participate in establishing standards for child health care.[16]

CARE FOR THE ILL CHILD

As mentioned earlier, the skills and knowledge of the pediatric nurse practitioner are more geared to health maintenance than to illness control. However, the treatment of common illness is certainly part of primary health care. The experienced nurse practitioner generally spends part of her time advising parents on the management of minor illness and discomforts. Examples of these are fever, gastroenteritis, colds, sore throats, childhood communicable diseases, rashes, and minor injury.

Some nurse practitioners pursue the policy of recommending the use of mild nonprescription drugs when indicated, while others, by prior agreement with their physician consultant, may recommend the use of prescription drugs. In the case of chronic illness, the pediatric nurse practitioner may help the parent to decide when it is appropriate to alter dosage or switch from one prn medication to another.

It is the responsibility of the pediatric nurse practitioner to determine the extent of illness and arrange for medical intervention if necessary. The treatment of acute illness and complicated disease remains the province of the physician. In these instances the nurse practitioner may work with the physician but not in his stead. In all aspects of illness, the nurse still has responsibility to provide teaching, support, and guidance for the patient and his family.

Summary

The pediatric nurse practitioner is a registered professional nurse who has chosen to work with children. She has completed a special program of education in which she expands her knowledge and extends her skills in the area of child and adolescent health care. She assesses the health status of her clients by obtaining a comprehensive history, performing a physical examination, and utilizing appropriate screening and laboratory data. She helps parents and children to manage illness and to understand and cope with the problems arising from their own particular environmental, social, and developmental milieu. She cooperates and collaborates with other professionals in providing health care and in establishing standards for that care. Finally, she constantly seeks to increase and improve her own professional knowledge and skills.

Case Examples

The following examples are taken from the caseload of practicing pediatric nurse practitioners. They represent typical situations and are presented here in an effort to illustrate, by clinical example, the role of the pediatric nurse practitioner in providing health services to children and their parents. I hope that they point out strong components of education and support as well as physical assessment and treatment.

AUDREY

Audrey was adopted at five days of age. She was eight-days-old when she was brought in for routine care by her adoptive mother and father. Mr. Watts is a 37-year-old chemist. His wife is 35 and has recently resigned from a secretarial job. They have been married nearly five years. Both seemed tense and they were unable to quiet their crying infant. She was passed back and forth be-

tween them several times during our conversation. She fell asleep only after I suggested that they lay her on the exam table and cover her with a blanket.

Mrs. Watts did most of the talking but frequently looked to her husband for reinforcement. He responded by nodding in agreement. They admittedly were concerned about their lack of experience with infants. They were quite anxious to have me answer their questions about infant supplies and physical care and wanted to be assured that their infant was well and normal.

On the second visit, when Audrey was one-month-old, Mr. Watts did not accompany his wife. She and I had had many phone conversations since the first visit, so we had gotten to feeling quite comfortable with each other. I believe that Mr. Watt's single visit had been to satisfy himself that we (PNP and MD) would be able to provide the kind of help and support that his wife and baby needed.

Mrs. Watts again had many questions but was also ready to discuss her feelings and concerns about the adoption. She told me that during the early years of their marriage, she and her husband had not wanted children. "We had always thought that we could have a child when we wanted to and were very upset when we were unsuccessful." Mrs. Watts described their experiences as they went through fertility testing as "degrading, embarrassing and hard to talk about." Mr. Watts had a particularly hard time because the doctor kept telling him that he simply, "wasn't trying hard enough." The studies were finally reported as negative for both of them. Mrs. Watts began taking a fertility drug but this was ineffective also. "My husband buried himself in his work and we actually saw less of each other. I found a part-time job and tried to keep myself busy."

They learned that friends of theirs planned to adopt a child and began to think of adoption as a solution for their problem. One day the friend called to say that she was pregnant and didn't want the baby that they had planned to adopt. She asked if the Watts wanted to take the baby, who had been born the day before. Mrs. Watts said yes immediately but Mr. Watts wasn't sure.

He said that it "didn't seem right to get a baby that way." They didn't know that it was a girl until they got to the hospital. They were told that the mother was an unwed college student. Mrs. Watts saw a young girl there and asked if that was the baby's mother. She was told that it was not but, "they didn't convince me."

Mrs. Watts talked of her curiosity about the "other parents." She said that it worried her not to know more but added that she did not expect to ever learn any of the details. On two occasions Audrey had sounded congested and Mrs. Watts wondered if she could have inherited some allergies.

Mrs. Watts asked me if it was "normal" for an adoptive mother to "feel as if she is caring for someone else's child." We talked about experiences during the nine months of pregnancy that help a man and woman to prepare for parenthood; experiences that she and her husband had not had opportunity for. Accepting the newborn as quickly as they had allowed little time for either mental or physical preparation. We also talked of the delay in the development of maternal feelings experienced by many women who do carry their babies through a normal pregnancy.

Mrs. Watts said that her husband helped with infant care when asked but usually just stood looking at the baby. She admitted to being angry with him when he got the baby "all fussed up." I encouraged her to talk with him about his feelings on becoming a father and suggested that he also be allowed a chance to get to know the baby in his own way and in his own time.

At the third visit when the baby was nearly three-months-old, Mrs. Watts seemed relaxed and handled the baby easily. She proudly announced that Audrey smiled and talked to her. She had a small pink ribbon scotch taped to the baby's scant hair. Without being asked, she related that her father fed her dinner almost every night. Previous concerns seemed to be under control but Mrs. Watts was distressed by a neighbor who had asked, "Whose little girl is she?" When told, "She's my little girl," the neighbor persisted and said, "I mean who's little girl is she really?" Mrs. Watts was hurt and angry, as was her husband. We talked of the real possibility of this situation being repeated and agreed that she and her husband needed to discuss ways of handling the question comfortably.

Mrs. Watts relationship with her baby is warm and comfortable. She has continued to share her plans for the baby with me and is quick to seek advice when she is concerned. These parents will continue to have a need to share some of their concerns that are common to many adoptive as well as natural parents.

To a certain extent, couples who adopt children feel that they have settled for second best. They have often tried for a number of years to produce a child. This desire usually leads them to see one or more physicians who may put them through a series of physical and psychiatric tests. The process of the fertility studies intrudes upon an area that is usually viewed as a very personal matter between husband and wife. A spontaneous act of expressing love may be reduced to following a prescription.

Choosing to adopt often means admitting to your family and friends that you are sterile. This implies loss of masculinity/femininity; it implies deficiency. I must assume that some people would never be able to make this admission and because of this remain childless.

Adoptive parents need to be reminded that they can be loving and competent parents without physically producing the child themselves. They should not feel guilty about taking someone else's baby. I think it helps to remind them of the importance of environment and that adoptive parents can do much to shape the character and personality of the child. Some children do begin to look like their adoptive parents as they learn to imitate facial expressions and gestures.

I think the potential is good for this child and the parents are sincere in their desire to be good parents. I am sure that they will have doubts from time to time and will need to seek continued support from their own peer group and from professionals.

SARA AND MARY

Sara, age five, and Mary, age three, are sisters. Sara is blond and shy and stays close to her mother initially. She is anxious to help discipline her younger sister. Mary is dark and devilish. She approaches quickly and is eager to explore. She accepts discipline only if it is firm, and she continually tests limits.

Mrs. Lane, their mother, is blond and pretty. I liked her immediately and was impressed by her commonsense approach to child rearing. She is patient, kind, and firm with the children. She did not ignore their questions, but asked them to wait until she was free to answer them.

During our history session, Mrs. Lane told me that she had been divorced a year ago. Mr. Lane lives nearby and has frequent contact with the children, seeing them at least once a week and phoning almost daily.

On one occasion, both parents brought the girls into the office. The children climbed all over their father and seemed to be competing for his attention. He demanded strict obedience and kept reminding them to, "act like ladies."

Sara has had much difficulty with ear infections since infancy and recently had tubes inserted in hopes of preventing further problems. Mary is troubled mostly by frequent colds.

On one visit Mrs. Lane brought Mary for a routine examination. Initially the girls were the same, coaxing to be first and wanting to tell me about their latest adventure. Mrs. Lane asked me to check to see if Sara's ear tubes were still in place. A chunk of cerumen occluded my vision. I reached for an ear curette, as I was explaining to Sara what I planned to do. She immediately became very fearful, held her ears and clung to her mother. Both Mrs. Lane and I were surprised by this reaction, since Sara had tolerated this intrusive procedure well on several occasions in the past. Because of her extreme anxiety, I told her that I would look at her ears on another day. When asked why she was afraid, she tearfully acknowledged that she didn't know.

I asked Mrs. Lane to see if she could think of any experience in the past few months that might have caused a change in Sara. She related the following incident. Three weeks ago, when they had gone out of town for a weekend, Sara had complained of abdominal pain and had a fever. She was seen in a hospital emergency room and admitted for observation. Mrs. Lane was told

that all tests were normal and Sara had not complained again. I was ready to believe that the hospital experience was the reason for the change in Sara, when at that point Sara walked in and announced, "I vomited last Sunday when Daddy was there." I looked at Mrs. Lane who looked as if she had suddenly thought of something. Sara returned to the play area and Mrs. Lane and I continued our conversation.

She told me that she had been dating her former husband for the past few months. Along with this he had fallen into a pattern of having dinner with them and helping to put the children to bed. About a month ago they had decided to remarry and had set a date. Mr. Lane had asked the children if he could, "move back into the house, be a real Daddy and make them a family again." Mrs. Lane remarked that she had not wanted him to discuss the plans with the children but he had insisted upon doing so. What Mrs. Lane had just remembered was that on the day of Sara's episode of abdominal pain, Mr. Lane had called to tell her that he was not ready to remarry and felt they must change their plans. "I got very upset and cried in front of the children, I couldn't help myself." Sara was very upset at her mother's crying and pleaded to know what was wrong. Mrs. Lane told her that, "Daddy has changed his mind again."

Although they were not currently dating, Mrs. Lane had asked her former husband to keep in touch with the children. She now wonders if it was a good idea since they are always upset when he leaves. On his last visit, Mr. Lane became very angry at Sara for putting her shoes on the wrong feet. He left soon after and Sara told her mother, "I won't make him mad next time."

After talking with Mrs. Lane, I asked Sara to tell me about the hospital. She told me in several ways that she was all alone there. "No Mommy, no Daddy, and no Mary;" a poignant expression of abandonment. She also said that she liked the nurses, but they did not like her.

It seems that these children would very much like to have their parents together again. They had reason to think that this wish was coming true. Mr. Lane's indecision has disappointed and confused them. The separation conflict has been recreated. One might think that the parents need to be advised to make a decision and stick with it for the sake of the children. Mrs. Lane is aware of the impact on the children, but she, too, is torn. She would like to be reconciled with her husband and is not able to pressure him in fear of driving him further away.

Sara, who is very oedipal, feels rejected by her father and may fantasize that her mother and sister will also leave and she will be truly alone. The hospital experience could only add to this fear. She knows that her father gives her special attention when she is ill. The abdominal pain and vomiting episode could represent an unconscious effort to hold onto him.

When dealing with this increasingly common situation in a family, it is important to remember that divorce is a process and not a solitary event. It is a disruptive, stressful experience for the children involved and most certainly will either alter or end their relationship with their parents. The child's reaction depends on his age, sex, extent and nature of the disharmony prior to divorce, the relationship of each parent to the child prior to and after divorce, and the parents' basic personalities. Children may manifest their concern through depression, neurosis, sleep disturbances, developmental regression, or physical illness. They may feel that they are the cause of the trouble between their parents, and may attempt to make things right by working to get them back together again.

The pediatric nurse practitioner can be most helpful in these situations by being available to listen, support, and interpret. Mrs. Lane seemed to need to be reassured that she was doing a good job with the children. Obviously, this is a problem that this family must handle for themselves. Perhaps in time they will find a workable solution. Until then, their uncertainty and unhappiness will continue to produce stress for them all.

KIMBERLY

Kimberly Max is six-months-old and the youngest of five children. She has four brothers ranging in age from six to two years. During a well child visit, Mrs. Max expressed concern that Kim seemed slower than the boys. When asked to be more specific, she pointed out that Kimberly was still on the breast, did not seem interested in sitting, made a mess when trying to drink from a cup, and preferred her mother to all others. On physical and developmental examination, Kim was found to be a normal healthy infant whose development was within normal limits for her age. It would have seemed reasonable to convey this to the mother, reassure her, and plan to follow this infant at regular intervals. However, I decided to further explore this mother's concerns.

This interview/observation and a review of the initial history brought out the following significant details. Mr. and Mrs. Max had decided that they were unable to provide for more than five children, so he had had a vasectomy. Mrs. Max expressed great affection for Kim and repeatedly said that she loved cuddly little babies. Her nickname for Kim was "Princess." In spite of her husband's protests, Mrs. Max seldom left Kim with a sitter because, "she cries so for me and doesn't want anyone else to hold her." While talking, Mrs. Max held Kim to her for a breast-feeding. I observed that the baby was easily distracted by sounds and objects in the room. Mrs. Max seemed to be unaware that she was actively forcing Kim to stay in the cradled-feeding position. When I remarked that the baby seemed a little restless, her mother replied that she was always like that but, "If I don't make her stay she will be hungry again in an hour or so." After the feeding, Mrs. Max encircled Kim with her arms and rocked her on her lap. When I indicated that it would be all right to put her on the floor, Mrs. Max responded that it was easier to keep her there because once down she would only get into everything.

In summary, (Princess) Kimberly is the last child and only girl of a mother who loves small cuddly babies. She had breast-fed and weaned four boys each by six months of age. She continued to keep Kim at the breast despite the infant's obvious efforts to push away. She interpreted her messiness with a cup as a lack of readiness to learn. She rarely separated herself from the child even for an evening out. Kim's normal striving for independence is being unconsciously thwarted by her mother. Mrs. Max feels that something is wrong but is unable to identify the cause.

The pediatric nurse practitioner had a close and comfortable relationship with the mother and was able to discuss the situation with her. Even with good rapport, the approach to such a sensitive situation must be cautious and words must be carefully chosen.

A few weeks after our discussion, Mrs. Max called to tell me that she and her husband wanted some advice on how to remedy the situation. It was necessary to meet with her several times to support her effort to slowly allow some separation. It was a difficult process for her, but she was able to slowly turn her attention to the other children instead of concentrating on the youngest as had been her pattern over the past several years. She found that she and her husband were sharing more and she admitted to being amazed at how each child had developed his own personality and interests. It was as if she was meeting each of her children all over again. In fact, she remembered each of them only as an infant and, although she had not neglected their physical needs, she had lost track of them as individuals.

She continues to need support. Her intellectual understanding of the situation is good, but emotionally she feels a great loss as her child separates from her. She must replace that loss by learning to enjoy the children as they are now rather than as they used to be.

MICHAEL

The mother of five-year-old Michael is very distressed that he has begun to urinate whenever and wherever he pleases. He had been toilet trained since age two with only occasional accidents, usually during illness. One week ago, he was seen by a physician who has assured the mother that no infection or physical defect was responsible for the change. However, the symptoms continued and the mother's distress increased. She had recently begun to punish Michael for urinating in the yard and in his sandbox. A careful history of recent events failed to identify any stress-producing events. We did

learn that Michael, his brothers, and his father spent a week together at a father-son campout. I asked the mother to question her husband about Michael's reaction to camping.

The precipating cause became obvious when the father told us that all of them had urinated in the woods around the campsite. Further, they had all been amused by Michael's delight with the new game.

This is an example of poor sharing within a family. The father's job required him to travel and he discouraged his wife from talking of problems during the brief time that he was home with the children. Because of this, the mother felt that she must solve this problem alone. She became quite distressed when she was unable to do so. The pediatric nurse practitioner was able to help with the solution and also to point out the need for greater sharing of concerns within the family. This case also again points out the need to look closely at the history before undertaking a series of diagnostic tests.

MARION

Marion and her husband were heroin addicts. Bouts of nausea sent Marion to the hospital where she learned of her pregnancy. Her immediate plans were for abortion. However, two weeks later, her husband died of an overdose. She then wanted desperately to have his baby. In her third month she enrolled in a Methadone maintenance program and discontinued her use of heroin. An amniocentesis in her fourth month revealed normal genetic studies, and she was encouraged to continue the pregnancy. As often happens with addicts, her baby was born early and there was no opportunity to withhold her regular Methadone dose. Because of this, narcotic withdrawal occurred. Marion saw her tiny baby in great distress. She was twitching, irritable, unable to suck properly, and unable to sleep. Marion's thoughts as she expressed them were, "All I could think as I watched her cry and fuss was she's so sick and its all my fault." Although at four months, the baby is doing quite well, Marion is unable to erase her concern that her addiction and early thoughts of abortion have in some way caused permanent damage to her baby. Every small rash, spitting episode, even hiccups are interpreted as impending crises.

The pediatric nurse practitioner's most important role here is to help Marion develop confidence in her ability to mother and to decrease her feelings of guilt and inadequacy. It has also been important to examine the baby frequently and assure the mother that she is growing and developing normally. This is a very vulnerable child and Marion will continue to need much support throughout the early years if she is to avoid becoming an overprotective mother. An ongoing relationship with the same nurse practitioner and doctor could be very important here since Marion does not have a close relationship with her own family, and her friends, thus far, are mostly addicts and generally undependable. She has recently been willing to allow us to involve some community agencies and is currently showing some interest in job training and day care.

BRETT

Brett Hartman was seen initially for a six-week checkup. His weight gain was inadequate and he was irritable and pale. His mother expressed concern about a "cold" that he had had for three weeks. He had been seen twice in a local emergency room and she had been advised to use a vaporizer and was given some medicine which did not seem to help. Further physical assessment revealed bilateral bulging immobile tympanic membranes, white plaques in his mouth that left a bleeding surface when removed, and a maculo-papular rash in the diaper area with peeling of the skin.

He was seen by the physician and treated for acute bilateral otitis media and oral and cutaneous moniliasis. In further discussing the feeding process, I learned that Mrs. Hartman was attempting to feed him a great variety of baby foods since, "he sucks a lot and doesn't drink much milk so he must not like it." I found that the nipple had only a tiny opening. I pointed out to her that Brett was drinking poorly because he was getting tired from sucking so hard.

She also needed specific directions and demonstration in other aspects of child care including the administration of medications. She was able to accept and follow directions well but required frequent reinforcement and did not seem to be able to transfer learning from one situation to another.

Brett was seen frequently over the next two months, usually in consultation with the physician. His condition did not improve significantly and he ultimately needed to be hospitalized for a myringotomy with tube insertion. Mrs. Hartman was fearful of hospitalization and tearfully asked if I thought he was going to die. I accompanied her through the admission process and was able to inform the inpatient personnel of her extreme anxiety and need for careful interpretation of what was happening to her baby.

Brett is now home again and beginning to show improvement in his growth and physical development. He and his mother will continue to be seen frequently for monitoring of care and support.

SEAN

Mrs. Mickell called our office to say that she was expecting her first baby and was looking for a convenient pediatric service. As is our practice, the receptionist invited her to come to the office to meet us and to provide us with a family history prior to delivery. Both she and her husband came.

I learned from them that the pregnancy was planned and eagerly awaited. They had recently moved here and had some concern that they had no close-by family or friends to depend upon. Neither had had any child care experience.

The Mickells were attending prenatal classes and hoped to deliver without anesthesia. They also had many questions about the pros and cons of breast-feeding. They were pleased to learn that we would support them in their plans. I invited them to call me if there was anything else that they wished to discuss.

The delivery went well and Mrs. Mickell was able to breast-feed successfully. She brought Sean in for periodic visits and immunizations and was always anxious to talk about his progress and what she could expect him to do next.

That was two years ago and Sean has grown and developed normally. His relationship with his parents and with the world is secure. His parents enjoy him and are proud of his accomplishments. Together they have weathered several bouts of gastroenteritis and one ear infection. The parents have learned to handle minor illness and accidents and are quick to consult me if the situation seems to be getting out of hand. The Mickells are now looking forward to the birth of their second child. Mrs. Mickell recently called to discuss her plans for preparing Sean for the new baby.

NOTE: This abstract is typical of many families in my caseload. They need support and guidance in coping with the day-to-day concerns of child rearing but are not deeply troubled by serious social or emotional problems.

KAREN AND KENT

The Luke family was introduced to our practice when Kent had a hypoglycemic reaction in the newborn nursery at two days of age. The physician asked me to see them because, "We need a good history, this is an extremely anxious mother and I don't know why."

On the first visit I was able to do little more than confirm the physician's feeling that this was indeed a very anxious mother. She and her husband both came, but Mrs. Luke was so concerned about having left the children with her mother that she was unable to participate in the history. Mr. Luke appeared much calmer and somewhat embarrassed by his wife's behavior, but was unable to reassure her. He felt certain that the children were fine, but thought it would be better if he took his wife home. I invited them to bring the children with them on the next visit.

Mrs. Luke called me the next day expressing concern that Kent was unable to move his bowels properly. I advised her on some dietary changes and offered reassurance. However, she called me each morning with the same concern until finally on the third day, I asked her to bring the baby in. His physical assessment was normal and, in addition, the rectal examination stimu-

lated a soft normal bowel movement. Mrs. Luke promptly dissolved in tears of relief. She thanked me profusely and apologized for bothering me so much. Her relief was short-lived however, for she called for the next three days to describe each bowel movement in detail and also was concerned that Kent was irritable and not eating or sleeping properly. I arranged a visit with myself and the physician. Kent was tense and crying and difficult to comfort but showed no other symptoms of physical illness. The physician prescribed a mild sedative for the mother, and Mr. Luke arranged for the grandmother to stay with them that night and care for the children.

They came the next day for the history and Kent slept in his mother's arms for most of the session. I learned that they had moved here from another state about a year ago. Mrs. Luke had grown up in this area and her mother still lives nearby. Mr. Luke is a history teacher at the local junior high. Both parents seemed to have a great need to discuss their feelings and concerns about their children. They were both intelligent and well-informed young people. They were quick to "look things up," and had read many child care books. They had initially decided upon a permissive approach to child rearing but that had gotten out of hand with Karen who is now five. They told me of the "terrible things" they had done to Karen and expressed concern about how this would affect her in later life. From the start she had been permitted to set her own routine for sleep, play, and mealtimes. There were no guidelines and no attempts at any sort of scheduling or discipline. By age three she was a terror who wouldn't eat, screamed until she got her way, and aroused great anger in her parents. When they became "angry enough to kill her," she would be sent to stay with her grandmother for awhile. They had sought help through a child psychologist and felt that he had been helpful. He had also advised that they have another child so that Karen could learn to share and perhaps learn to live by rules along with her sibling. Mrs. Luke had discontinued her birth control pills and became pregnant just prior to moving here. Now they both had doubts as to the wisdom of that decision but realized that it was too late to change anything. Both expressed continued guilt feelings about the mistakes they had made with Karen and fluctuated between determination to do better and doubting that they would be able to. They agreed that for a time Karen had seemed to do better, but had recently begun to refuse to go to school and to disrupt all conversations with constant demands for attention. They felt this was out of proportion to the expected reaction to the birth of a new sibling.

During her pregnancy, Mrs. Luke had feared that God might punish them for their bad parenting by giving them a baby with some congenital defect. An episode in the hospital had confirmed this fear in her own mind. Kent was not brought to her for two feedings. When she asked why, she was told that she could go to the nursery to see him. "I almost died when I saw him with tubes in his head. Now I always think of him as sick instead of well."

I also learned of a long history of bowel problems in the maternal family. Some of these conditions had required surgical intervention.

Both parents seemed more relaxed after they had told their story. Mr. Luke felt that his wife worried too much and that the experience with Karen had only made it worse. I encouraged Mrs. Luke to call me anytime and she took full advantage of this offer. Her husband and mother later told me that they both encouraged her to call since life was more pleasant for all when Mrs. Luke was able to relax.

Unfortunately, Kent suffered from ear infections and this was predictably upsetting to Mrs. Luke. Finally he had to be hospitalized for the insertion of myringotomy tubes. Although I spent considerable time with Mrs. Luke explaining the reason for the surgery and the expected outcome, she was certain that, "something would go wrong."

At one point, Mrs. Luke's fanatical concern about the children threatened their marriage. The Lukes had left the children with their grandmother and had gone out to dinner to celebrate their anniversary. Mrs. Luke telephoned home every half hour and insisted upon going home early because she was sure that something was wrong. Mr. Luke angrily informed her that he was fed up with her paranoia. I saw Mrs. Luke a few days later and she expressed concern about ruining her marriage as well as her children. Also, after that episode, Mrs. Luke's mother felt that she was contributing to their problem and refused to do any further baby-sitting.

Both Mr. and Mrs. Luke had serious doubts about their ability to be effective parents. Mrs. Luke expressed many guilt feelings and expected (needed) to be punished for the "terrible" handling of Karen. She expected that punishment to be in the form of some sort of damage to Kent. For that reason, she felt responsible for his every discomfort. She felt a great need to protect him and consequently refused to allow anyone else to become involved in his care. Her obsessive concern for Kent nearly shut out her husband, mother, and other child.

Mr. Luke also felt guilt and fluctuated between sympathizing with his wife and being angry with her. The grandmother was willing to be helpful, but was confused by her daughter's actions and began to back away. Kent's development was being stifled by extreme overprotectiveness and Karen responded to the tension and confusion in the family with regressive and disruptive behavior.

I offered these parents a relationship with a consistent professional who knew their story and their concerns. I think I was successful in decreasing Mrs. Luke's anxiety by being available, by explaining each situation, and by helping her to anticipate and to understand what was happening to her children. I tried to focus on their wellness and normal development rather than dwelling on their problems. They needed help in recognizing the fact that all parents have some problems with the rearing of normal children and that having made some mistakes does not mean that the product (i.e., the child) is a lost cause.

Although I felt that psychiatric intervention could have been helpful, such a referral was unacceptable to these parents. With their approval, I did discuss their case with a psychiatrist and was able to utilize some of his suggestions in working with them. I was also able to help other health workers (both in the hospital and in our office) to work with these parents by explaining the reasons for their excessive anxiety and their need for adequate explanation and frequent reassurance.

Problems such as those described here are not easily resolved, but the current situation is better. These parents seem to have a greater respect for their own parenting ability and their relationship with each other is not as strained. Mrs. Luke has been able to renew contacts with her friends and to share the children with their grandmother and others. She still needs to call for consultation but proudly reminded me recently that it had been more than three weeks since she has needed my help.

References

1. For example, see Schutt, B.: Frontier's family nurse. *Am. J. Nurs.* 903-909, May 1972; Cipolla, J.: Nurse clinicians in industry. *Am. J. Nurs.* 1530-34, Aug. 1971; and Employment opportunities for nurses with the foreign service. Washington D.C., Employment Division, Department of State, Sept. 1974.
2. Primary care is that health care that most people need most of the time. It involves both the entry contact to the health care system and the continuum of management including referral and evaluation of care for diagnosed problems. It includes the basic determination of wellness-unwellness, institution of measures for the maintenance of health, treatment of some conditions, and proper referral of indicated cases to other health practitioners.

    An expanded role is a spreading out or a process of diffusion in which the nurse role is not only expanded, but the very nature or composition is changed. The range of cues utilized in decision making is broad.

    An extended role is a unilateral lengthening process in which the nurse takes on new functions essentially designed to help in the cure function of medicine. The range of cues utilized is restricted.
3. Ford, L. and Silver, H.: The expanded role of the nurse in child care. *Nurs. Outlook* 43-45, Sept. 1967.
4. ———: Directory of current programs for the training of pediatric nurse associates, pediatric assistants and pediatric aides. Evanston, Illinois, *Am. Acad. Pediatrics,* Apr. 1971.
5. *Ibid.*
6. ———: Guidelines on short term continuing education programs for pediatric nurse associates: a joint statement of the American Nurses Association and the American Academy of Pediatrics *Am. J. Nurs.* 509, Mar. 1971.
7. LeShan, E.: You and Your Adopted Child. Pub. Affairs Pamphlet #274, New York, Pub. Affairs Comm. Inc., June 1959.
8. Group for the Advancement of Psychiatry, Committee on Adolescence: Normal Adolescence. New York, Charles Scribner's Sons, 1968.
9. Alexander, M. and Brown, M.: Pediatric Physical Diagnosis for Nurses. New York, McGraw-Hill, 1974.
10. Morris, W. (ed.): The American Heritage Dictionary of the English Language. New York, Houghton Mifflin, 1969.
11. ———: Dorland's Illustrated Medical Dictionary, ed. 25. Philadelphia, W. B. Saunders, 1974.
12. ———: Stedman's Medical Dictionary, ed. 22. Baltimore, Williams & Wilkins, 1972.
13. American Heritage Dictionary, *op. cit.*
14. Platou, R. V.: Johnny won't eat. The New Physician 62-64, July 1962.
15. ———: Report of the Committee on Infectious Diseases. Evanston, Illinois, Am. Acad. Pediatrics, 1974.
16. ANA Council of Nurse Practitioners in the Nursing of Children: Scope of Practice for Pediatric Nurse Practitioners. Kansas City, Missouri, American Nurses Association, Apr. 1974.

Bibliography

Andrews, P.: The pediatric nurse practitioner, the concept, her role and responsibilities, Parts I and II. Pub. Health Currents, Columbus, Ohio, Ross Laboratories, 1971.
———: A Summary Statement on Manpower. Evanston, Illinois, Department of Community Services, Am. Acad. Pediatrics, May 1973.
Bruch, H.: Physiologic and psychologic aspects of the food intake of obese children. Am. J. Diseases of Child. 59:739, 1940.

Brunetto, E.: The primary care nurse—the generalist in a structured health care team. Am. J. Pub. Health 785-93, June 1972.

Cominos, H.: Teaching infant care to adopting parents. Nurs. Outlook 19:421, June 1971.

Day, L. and Egli, R.: Acceptance of the pediatric nurse practitioner. Am. J. Diseases of Child. Mar. 1970.

Driscoll, V.: Liberating nursing practice. Nurs. Outlook 20:24-27, Jan. 1972.

Eyres, P.: The role of the nurse in family centered nursing care. Nurs. Clin. N. Am. 7, 1; Mar. 1972.

————: Fact About Nursing 72-73. Kansas City, Missouri, American Nurses Association, 1974.

Fagin, C. and Goodwin, B.: Baccalaureate preparation for primary care. Nurs. Outlook, 240-44, Apr. 1972.

Hershey, N.: Expanded roles for professional nurses. Nurs. Digest, 18-29, Jan. 1974.

Lambertsen, E.: Perspectives on the physician's assistant. Nurs. Outlook 20:1, Jan. 1972.

Leininger, M. et al.: Primex. Am. J. Nurs. 1274-77, July 1972.

Levin, P. and Berne, E.: Games nurses play. J. Nurs. 483-87, Mar. 1972.

Mayer, J.: Correlation between metabolism and feeding behavior and multiple etiology of obesity. Bull. N. Y. Acad. Med. 33:747, 1957.

McDermott, J. F.: Divorce and the psychiatric sequelae in children. Pediatrics 46:588-95, Oct. 1970.

Nightingale, F.: Notes on Nursing, What It Is and What It Is Not. London, Harrison and Son, 1859.

Rogers, M.: Nursing: to be or not to be? Nurs. Outlook 42-46, Jan. 1972.

Robertson, A. and Lowery, G.: Overweight children. Mich. Med. 63:629, 1964.

Schafer, M.: The political and economic scene in the future of nursing. Am. J. Pub. Health 73:10, 887-89.

Schlotfeldt, R.: Nursing is health care. Nurs. Outlook 245-46, Apr. 1972.

Sugar, M.: Children of divorce. Pediatrics 46:588-95, Oct. 1970.

Yankauer, A. and Connelly, J.: Assessment of pediatric nurse practitioners. Bull. Pediatric Prac. Am. Acad. Pediatrics, Dec. 1971.

Yankauer, A. et. al.: The cost of training and the income generation potential of pediatric nurse practitioners. Pediatrics, June 1972.

Young: Physicians' assistants and the law. Nurs. Outlook 36-41, Jan. 1972.

8

Health Problems During the Adolescent Years

MARY EVANS MELICK

Health-related Problems of Adolescence • General Considerations

He was tall and awkward. Acne marked his unsmiling face. He wore no shoes and both feet were badly blistered. His body smelled strongly of urine. He had just been admitted to a residential treatment center for emotionally disturbed adolescents when the director brought him to me. "Here, Nurse, do something with him."

One of the challenges of nursing adolescent patients, such as this young man, is helping them to deal with the multitude of changes taking place within and around them. Adolescence is a period of life characterized by change. Changes occur in physical growth and development causing the child to acquire the stature, strength and reproductive potential of an adult. Adolescents gain the ability to engage in deductive reasoning. Their general outlook becomes future-oriented. There is an increased sensitivity to the contrasts between idealism and the official goals of their culture and realism and the ways in which they see adults behaving. Adolescents are in the process of acquiring stable sex roles and identities. Because of all of these changes, persons associated with adolescents treat them differently than younger children. They, as well as the adolescent, vacillate between fostering dependence and independence.

Partly as a result of these changes, and especially because of the hormonal changes and physical sexual maturation, many persons have labeled adolescence a period of storm and stress. However, much of this stress may be culturally induced. The distinction has been made between puberty, a physiological occurrence, and adolescence, a cultural and psychosocial phenomenon. Some writers believe that adolescence is an American invention.[1] Until the last two decades of the 19th century, one was either a child or an adult. Children under the ages of five to seven were not employed. Older children were employed either on farms or in factories and were, for many purposes, considered adult. Compulsory schooling and child labor laws helped to create periods of childhood and adolescence. The emphasis on higher education has prolonged the period of adolescence.

At present, there are no firm limits to the period of adolescence. Pediatricians may consider as adolescent children age 13 through 18. Depending on the commonwealth or state, adolescence may last until full adult privileges are obtained, up to age 21. With the emphasis on higher education, the period of adolescence may be undergoing a prolongation, or a period of young adulthood, characterized by financial dependence, may be emerging. The term youth appears with increasing frequency in the literature. This term is generally used to refer to a segment of the population, some of whom are adolescent while others are beyond adolescence, but have not yet attained full adult status.

Adolescents are viewed by adults as being neither children nor adults. They are denied the dependency of childhood and admonished to, "Grow up" or "Stop behaving as children." At the same time, many adult privileges and responsibilities, such as full-time employment and access to alcoholic beverages, are denied them either by law or by parental fiat. For these reasons, adolescents are considered as marginal persons in American society. Many adults consider adolescents irresponsible,[2] and this cult of irresponsibility is reinforced by adults failing to give adolescents responsibility. Adults often see adolescents as a group with much leisure time and little or no social value. This may be the reason that many adults direct angry feelings at adolescents as a group. In American society, groups seen as nonproductive, such as adolescents and the elderly, are low-status groups. Bettelheim believes that young people feel that they have no future because technology has made them obsolete, socially irrelevant, and insignificant. He postulates that activism, such as student protest, makes young people feel active and gives them a sense of community with other youths.[3]

Despite their low social value, adolescents have important developmental tasks to accomplish which will vitally affect their participation in society as adults. The overall goals of adolescence could be considered to be the development of selfhood and a stable identity and the achievement of intimacy. The latter, especially, may extend into the period of young adulthood. Developmental tasks include physical growth and maturation, achievement of independence from parents, development of a sense of responsibility, self-discipline, and worthwhile goals, acquisition of a stable set of values,[4] adjustment to sexual maturation, learning to handle dating and heterosexual relations, planning of an educational and vocational future,[5] refinement of peer relationships, acceptance of one's physique

and use of one's body effectively, and achievement of a sense of economic independence.[6] Not all of these tasks, for example, financial independence, can be accomplished in their entirety during the period of adolescence.

Many of these tasks involve choice, which emphasizes the fact that adolescents need reliable information and consistent support from others to allow them to make appropriate choices. The turmoils experienced by adolescents result from factors characteristic of adolescence, such as physical development, and from the culture in which they live. Cultural stressors include the decreasing importance of religion and the continued necessity of a search for a relevant value system, living in a drug-oriented culture, affluence with leisure time often devoid of meaningful activities, and adult idolization of the concept of being young.

Despite intra- and interpersonal stress and cultural stress, most adolescents make what is considered to be a healthy adjustment to the period of adolescence. Important socializing agents at this time include family, peer group, school, religious institutions, and employers. The family and peer group are of primary importance.

The family continues to be a source of affection and values for the adolescent. However, as the adolescent moves through adolescence, the importance of the parents as socializers decreases. This is true because the adolescent is trying to gain independence, especially psychological independence, from them and also because the parents are members of another generation and may be perceived as being less relevant than peers. A direct relationship probably exists between the rapidity of social change and the size of the generation gap. Studies have attempted to demonstrate which is the more important influence on adolescents—peers or parents. Results are inconclusive, with some studies noting the supremacy of the peer group in affecting values and behavior and others showing that parents are a more important source of values.[7,8,9,10,11] Conger believes that the peer-oriented child is more a product of parental disregard than of the attractiveness of the peer group.[12]

If any conclusion can be drawn, it is that the peer group, always present in life as a socializing influence, becomes more dominant during adolescence and, to an extent, replaces the family as an important primary group. However, because of affectional ties and the durable nature of childhood socialization, and because peer group membership consists of persons holding at least some similar values (acquired from parents and the larger society), parents continue to be an important socializing influence on their adolescent children.

The primary purpose of the adolescent peer group is to aid in shaping the adolescent's identity—to answer the question, "Who am I?" The norms of the group are enforced by applying or withholding group approval and social interaction. Dunphy studied the urban adolescent peer group and divided adolescent groups into cliques composed of 8 to 9 members, and crowds of 15 to 30 members. The major function of the clique was to provide information, for example, about dating and sex, while the function of the crowd was recreational. Cliques began as unisexual in early adolescence, progressing to heterosexual and eventually dissolving as couples became engaged or married.[13] Functions of the peer group include shaping identity, providing information, and influencing attitudes and values.

On a larger scale, the youth culture, with its distinctive style of dress, music, and behavior patterns, provides the identity that peer groups provide locally. This may be a positive factor for the adolescent seeking identity in a complex, pluralistic culture, but it also permits adults to stereotype adolescents. Young people can be labeled as hippies, drug-taking drop-outs, and so on. On the other hand, adults may be labeled by adolescents as "straights," "unhip," or whatever jargon is in vogue. This tends to polarize adolescent-adult interactions and may tend to widen the generation gap between the two groups.

An understanding of the social and cultural factors influencing adolescents is important for all health professionals. Even though close in age to adolescents, health professionals may be viewed as a part of the establishment adolescents are learning to distrust because it labels them, treats them as roles instead of persons, and denies them first-class citizenship. For contacts with health professionals to be productive, adolescents and adults need to be able to see each other as persons as well as group members.

Health-related Problems of Adolescence

In general, the adolescent period is characterized by little morbidity or mortality. For this reason, nurses may see few adolescents as patients unless they specifically work with this age group. However, there are a number of health-related problems which occur primarily in adolescence or which cause particular psychosocial problems when they do occur.

Leading causes of death in adolescence include suicide, homicide, and accidents. It is difficult to obtain precise statistics on adolescent suicides, homicides, and accidents; however, federal statistics on the death rate per 100,000 population show that, for youths 15 to 24 years of age, the death rate from suicide is 9.7, from homicides it is 12.4, and from accidents it is 67.2[14] Adolescent females make the highest number of per capita suicide attempts of any group, although two thirds of all suicides committed in this age group are by males. Girls prefer to use drugs while boys more frequently use shooting or hanging in their suicide attempts.[15] Investigating the relationship between physical illness and suicide, Weinberg found that physical illness seemed to influence suicidal preoccupation in males when illness was seen as an insurmountable barrier to the achievement of masculine identity. Females tolerated illness to the extent that it induced the care and support of significant others. All 13 adolescents in Weinberg's study had notified someone of their suicide intent.[16]

Males are more frequently involved in accidents; for example, three times as many adolescent males as females die in motor vehicle accidents. This ratio approaches five to one in college students.[17] Suchman also noted the importance of the sex variable; in addition, his data supported the hypothesis that the more deviant a person is, the more likely he or she is to have an accident. This may be because the person rejects society with its protective measures.[18]

Mike is an example of an adolescent who rejected the protective measures of society. Fourteen-year-old Mike and some friends were swimming in a quarry posted No Trespassing. The boys were taking turns showing their skill in swimming and diving. One of the boys dared Mike to dive off a particular rock. Mike accepted the challenge and dove into the water. The water was more shallow than he had expected and he struck bottom. The impact caused a fracture of the sixth cervical vertebra, producing sufficient damage to the spinal cord to leave Mike a quadraplegic.

The majority of physical illnesses occurring in adolescence are acute, and most of these illnesses are accounted for by respiratory and infectious diseases. These illnesses place only temporary restrictions on the adolescent. More important in the development of the adolescent are chronic diseases or problems requiring a lengthy period of treatment. Examples of such problems are muscular dystrophy, asthma, and scoliosis. Many of these conditions limit the mobility of the adolescent which has special meaning for them. Since adolescence is a period of developing the potential of the body for strength and energy, adolescents, especially males, may be very angry about their handicapping condition. This anger may be expressed by such failures to cooperate with the treatment regimen as refusing to wear a brace (scoliosis) or smoking (asthma). Also, limited mobility means one cannot easily get away from home to be with one's peer group. In addition, chronic conditions often affect the development of heterosexual relationships, which has important implications for the development of self-esteem and identity.

It is important to note that adolescents and adults may perceive health problems differently. What appears to be a minor, acute illness to an adult may be perceived as being more serious to an adolescent. For this reason, it is important to assess what an illness means to an adolescent. One study of adolescent health in Harlem pro-

vided for input from adolescents about major health problems. They saw drug abuse, smoking, drinking and unsanitary living conditions as being most important. They tended to report health problems such as trouble seeing, frequent colds, and repeated headaches. Health examinations found more dental problems than any other health problem. Visual, upper respiratory tract, heart and blood pressure, and nutritional problems were also frequently identified.[19]

Failure of adolescents and adults to communicate their perceptions of health problems results in less than optimal care. If they do not understand the nature and importance of a health problem, adolescents are not likely to seek treatment or to follow suggested health practices. If health personnel fail to understand the adolescent's perspective, they may lose an opportunity to provide information and explanation or may provide information the adolescent sees as irrelevant and, therefore, is likely to disregard.

The establishment of trust is a necessary component of all helping relationships. By nature, adolescents are not inclined to trust health personnel; such trust must be earned. Adolescents with chronic problems have more frequent contact with health personnel; thus demonstrating concern, treating the adolescent as a person, and respecting confidences are basic behaviors which may promote the establishment of a trusting relationship between the adolescent with a chronic health problem and the personnel who will be providing care over a period of time. Once established, this type of relationship is valuable for obtaining information essential for care and for ensuring that the adolescent will perceive information and suggestions coming from health personnel as being related to his or her welfare.

Sometimes adolescents with chronic diseases become interested in pursuing health professions so that they can help others like themselves. Often they will discuss these goals with health personnel. It is important to provide information about these careers and about their health problems in order to differentiate between idealism and realism. In some cases, their goals may be appropriate and specific information about the chosen career may be offered. In others, the goal may be inappropriate and other life goals should be explored.

Sally was an example of the latter situation. At age 18 she decided, during the course of a hospitalization, to enter the school of nursing sponsored by the hospital. Her goal seemed inappropriate because of polycystic kidney disease. Her physicians and nurses discussed with her the problems of long hours, irregular schedules, hard physical work, and exposure to infectious agents and what these might mean in terms of her prognosis. Other occupations, such as medical secretary, were explored with her.

A trusting relationship with parents is of equal importance. Parents need information about the medical condition, medications, treatments and prognosis for their child. They need support in coping with their child's illness. They need someone to talk to about the child's behavior and someone who can interpret this behavior for them. Many times they will need assistance in securing services for their child, such as appliances or school programs. Health personnel should also discuss growth and development with parents so that they understand why the child behaves as he or she does. Such discussions provide an opportunity to suggest, for example, that parents of an adolescent with limited mobility could provide opportunities for peer group gatherings at their home.

Adolescents are very concerned about their changing bodies and may seek validation that they are developing normally. In a school or camp situation, the nurse soon learns the attraction of a well-placed scale and height and weight charts. Adolescents compare themselves with their previous weight, with the norm, and often with their peers. Such opportunities can be used for instruction in nutrition and other aspects of health.

The relationship between developmental parameters and self-esteem is striking in the case of the obese adolescent. Becoming obese during adolescence is more likely to be associated with body image disturbances than becoming obese during other periods of life.[20] Obese adolescents receive continual negative feedback from peers, health personnel, and sometimes from family.

They may become social isolates, sharing in few of the activities of their peer groups, especially athletics and dating. Introducing them to a new peer group of obese adolescents who want to decrease their weight may be an effective means of treatment. Parents should also be involved because there may be a faulty dietary pattern or interpersonal conflicts. The latter is important because parents assuming control over the adolescent's dietary habits may be just another source of family conflict and serve to increase food intake as a means of rebellion. Obese adolescents need information about diet and exercise and consistent, long-term support. They should be encouraged to take responsibility for their own food intake and exercise schedule.

Another group of health-related problems centers on sexual maturation. Dramatic changes in sexual behavior occur in adolescence as the child moves from a person incapable of reproduction to one capable of both reproduction and formation of mature interpersonal relationships. Probably no other area of adolescent development evokes more parental anxiety and has such long-term implications for society than that of sexual adjustment.

Girls in this country are experiencing menarche at an earlier age, and a teenager is frequently as fully developed physically as an adult.[21] However, there is a time lag between the onset of physical maturity and the official granting of adult sexual prerogatives. It is this period which is of concern to parents, adolescents, and society.

A debate is raging in the literature about whether or not a sexual revolution is or has been taking place. Morgenthau and Sokoloff, for example, believe that the major change in sexual behavior took place in the 1920s. They see no evidence that a revolution is taking place now. Although behavior has not changed, attitudes have finally caught up with behavior.[22] Osofsky also believes that attitudes may have caught up with existent behavior, but that adolescent sexual behavior is or may soon be changing.[23] In 1968, Bell and Chaskes replicated a 1958 study of premarital sexual experience among coeds and found that the commitment of engagement has become a less important condition for many couples engaging in coitus. In 1968, women were more likely to have their first experience while dating or going steady. Also, the percentage of women feeling guilty about their coital activity decreased by approximately one half. There is some evidence that young women who are having premarital coitus, whose numbers have remained stable at about 50 percent, are having it with more partners.[24] Zelnick and Kanter's more recent study on a national probability sample of women 15 to 19 years showed that for those currently aged 19, 97 percent were virgins when they reached age 15 while only 91 percent of those now 15 years reached it as virgins. It is their provisional conclusion that there has been a real and rather dramatic shift in the sexual behavior of females who are coming of age in this country.[25] Other changes include the fact that on the average, adolescents have more permissive views about premarital sex than their parents; there is more willingness to talk about sex; college-educated women are having coitus at an earlier age; and there are more couples living together before marriage. Evidence has also shown that although adolescents approve of premarital sex for themselves and their peers, they may not approve of it for their hypothetical daughters 20 years from now.[26] Whether or not these changes imply revolution is not clear, but they do have implications for health personnel.

Nurses in particular need to be more involved in the establishment and ongoing maintenance of sexuality education programs. Sexuality involves more than sex education. Education for sexuality involves assisting persons to develop a sexual identity in conformity with their anatomical sex, to learn to understand themselves and others as sexual beings, and to learn to live with and manage their genitality and reproductivity.[27] The primary place to begin such education on a planned basis is the home. Many parents are not comfortable with this aspect of their child's education because of lack of information or inability to provide information without guilt or anxiety. One way of educating children for sexuality involves educating parents. Parents need information about sex, a nonthreatening environment in which to share and analyze feelings about sex, and information about the growth and development of their children and their ability to understand information about sex. Nurses are ideal persons to provide such parental information because they have access to the homes of the community, they are seen as legitimate sources of information about sex, and they are often viewed in the wise sister role. A wise sister is a person who comes to one's aid and to whom one turns in time of trouble. She acts as a troubleshooter and comes whenever she is informed about trouble or the need for care.[28] There is much informality in this role allowing the transcendence of social distance so that advice may be offered to those in need.

The other means of promoting education for sexuality is the establishment of programs for children and adolescents. Again, nurses are in a good position to establish such programs or to facilitate their establishment in schools, clubs, or religious organizations. Programs need to be appropriate for age, and dividing adolescents into coed groups of early (age 11 to 15) and later (above age 15) adolescents may be appropriate.[29] Early adolescents are concerned with the changes occurring in their bodies while later adolescents focus on interpersonal relationships. All will want to know if they are normal, how the other sex develops, and what is "normal" sexual behavior. Later adolescents should be given information about birth control. Such information has not been found to increase the incidence of premarital coitus—values determine this—but it does provide security for those who choose to engage in coitus. Information about venereal disease—its cause, treatment, and prevention—should be discussed. Adolescents should know their rights as persons seeking treatment for venereal disease. At least 48 states permit the physician to diagnose and treat venereal disease in minors without parental consent. However, only 16 states have statutes which explicitly allow an adolescent to seek care for pregnancy on his or her own consent and only 19 states and the District of Columbia have laws specifically permitting minors to consent to contraceptive services.[30]

Pregnancy in adolescents has important implications for the couples involved, their families, and for society. Even when pregnancy occurs within marriage or culminates in marriage, teenage marriages frequently end in divorce.

Pregnancy is a sociomedical problem. Social aspects of the problem include dropping out of school with consequences for the mother's educational and occupation career and unwanted children. The younger a woman is when she begins having babies, the more babies she is likely to have.[31] In addition, children of young mothers are at greater risk of being reared by persons other than their biological parents and they are likely to live in households with more people.[32] In comparison with older women, medical problems include increased incidence of hypertension, toxemia five times as frequent, more fetal loss, more premature deliveries, more low weight placentas, shorter and longer labors, more frequent uterine inertia, contracted pelvis, and more frequent stillbirths and deformed infants. Operative deliveries are needed twice as frequently.[33] A recent study of 471 women under 15 who delivered babies between 1968 and 1972 compared their pregnancies and deliveries with the same number of control patients between 19 and 25 years, matched on race and socioeconomic status. The younger patients differed significantly from the control group in having had an earlier menarche and a greater number of recurring pregnancies within 18 months of the initial pregnancy. Younger women experienced pregnancy-induced hypertension and pelvic inlet contraction more frequently. In contrast to other studies, the incidence of toxemia was no more frequent in the younger than in the older group.[34]

For all of these reasons, prevention of unwanted pregnancy in adolescence should be a priority for health professionals. Birth control information plays a primary part, but understanding the motivations for coitus is also important. Examples of motivation are: release of anxiety and tension, expression of intimacy, proof of identity, proof of self-worth and value, pleasurable experience, escape from loneliness, and a means of expressing anger.[35] For middle-class girls pregnancy may serve as a means of rebellion while lower-class girls may desire affection, acceptance by peers or to have something to call their own.[36] Ignoring the reason for the pregnancy fails to deal with the problem in its entirety and may result in a subsequent pregnancy under similar circumstances.

Once pregnant, the adolescent has several choices: abortion, placing the child for adoption, or keeping the child. At this time, she needs both information and support. Significant others should be included in the decision-making process.

Since the advent of legal abortion, the proportion of adolescents seeking and receiving abortions exceeds other age groups. For example, in California in 1969, 31.6 percent of all legal abortions performed were for adolescents while the proportion of adolescent live births was 17 percent of all live births.[37] In 1972, 10 percent of all women having legal abortions in New York State were 17 years or younger while in 1974, 31.4 percent of all legal abortions in California were performed on women less than 20 years.[38] However, statistics in no way express the magnitude of the problem. Adolescents seeking abortions tend to be further along in their pregnancies than are older women. This may necessitate the use of saline to produce abortion which is associated with the risk of complications not seen with the suction dilatation and curettage method used prior to the fourteenth week of gestation.

Nurses need to be aware of how adolescents view abortion in order to provide supportive care. One study investigated attitudes of three groups of adolescents: those seeking contraceptive measures, candidates for abortion, and residents of a maternity home. Those favorably disposed toward abortion tended to be higher in socioeconomic status, without current religious affiliation and older. Guilt was apparent from their answers to a hypothetical situation and 37 percent of the maternity home group felt that a pregnant adolescent is at fault and should not be permitted to get an abortion.[39]

To minimize the psychic trauma of abortion,

the nurse needs to know how the patient feels about the pregnancy and the abortion procedure. Providing information and personalized supportive care are the two most important functions of the nurse. A nonjudgmental attitude is crucial. (See Chapter 5 for further discussion of abortion.)

Adolescents who choose to retain the pregnancy also need information and support. The nurse should provide information about nutrition or make referral to a dietitian, if one is available, because the nutritional patterns of many adolescents are poor. Information needs to be provided on the minor discomforts of pregnancy, physiology of pregnancy, progress of labor and delivery, general health measures, and care of the infant or procedure for placing it for adoption. Support again must be individualized, and the adolescent should be given opportunity to discuss her feelings about this pregnancy, sex, and interpersonal relationships. The use of group sessions for providing information and support seems to be an effective technique.

The teenage father should also receive attention. Health personnel usually assume he is uninterested. He should be involved in exploring alternative ways of dealing with the pregnancy. He needs to know his legal responsibilities and rights.[40] He may benefit from a discussion of his feelings about sex and knowledge of contraceptives. With guidance from mature adults, pregnancy, like other crisis situations, can be a maturing experience for both male and female adolescents.

All adolescents known to be sexually active should be given birth control information. Ideally, this should be given before they become sexually active, but this is not always possible in our society. Many adolescents are not knowledgeable about contraception, and many myths passed on by the peer group are accepted as fact. Hausknecht reports that well over 95 percent of those seeking abortion have never used any method of contraception.[41] Data from the Pregnancy Counseling Service, operated by Planned Parenthood of Alameda, California, show that only 50 percent of all clients had ever used an effective contraceptive method; 30 percent had no knowledge about contraceptives available without prescription and 30 percent had had previous pregnancies.[42]

It is to prevent repeated unwanted pregnancies that many contraceptive programs have been established.[43] Some programs have been initiated for providing services to adolescents who have not been pregnant or programs directed primarily at adolescent males.[44] Successful programs have been reported using condoms, birth control pills, and intrauterine devices. An important ingredient of success is the nurse who advises and counsels adolescents about reproduction, interpersonal relationships, and the use of the contraceptive of choice.

There seems to be a developing trend to provide contraceptive services to sexually active adolescents. The American Medical Association House of Delegates at its 1971 Convention and the American Academy of Family Physicians at its April 1971 Board Meeting endorsed the recommendations made by the American College of Obstetrics and Gynecology and the American Academy of Pediatrics that the teenage female whose sexual behavior exposes her to possible conception should have access to medical consultation and the most effective contraceptive advice and methods consistent with her physical and emotional needs. The physician so consulted should be free to prescribe or withhold contraceptive advice in accordance with his medical judgment in the best interests of his patient.[45]

In the community, the nurse has frequent contacts with sexually active adolescents and other adolescents seeking information about birth control. The nurse should utilize all opportunities to provide information and/or appropriate referral. (See Chapter 5 for further discussion of contraception and the nurse's role in providing information concerning family planning.)

Another concern of adolescents and society is drug use. In general, American society seems to be drug-oriented and drugs are available for many social and individual uses. Some drugs have not been legalized and the use of others has not been legitimized. When these drugs are used, people talk about drug abuse, although such drugs as aspirin, alcohol, caffeine, and tobacco may also be abused.

When drug abuse was considered a problem of the ghetto, it was of little concern to the average citizen, and law enforcement authorities were empowered to deal with the problem. However, when use of illegal drugs moved into middle-class neighborhoods other groups, such as teachers and health personnel, were called on to stem the rising tide of drug use. Many surveys were commissioned and drug education programs were established.

For purposes of analysis, drug users can be divided into such groups as oblivion seekers and experience seekers.[46] The former come primarily from the lower socioeconomic strata and use drugs to escape from the painful realities of their lives. Experience seekers come from middle and upper socioeconomic strata and use drugs to produce novel experiences and feelings of liberation denied them by their culture. It is the latter group's rebellion, not their addiction, which is viewed with alarm.[47] To these groups Blaine adds personality change seekers who have underlying personality problems.[48]

Oblivion seekers tend to be associated with heroin use. Adolescent narcotic addicts constitute 24 percent of the total addict population. Of these, 93 percent are addicted primarily to heroin, although the adolescent addict is much more likely to be a poly-drug addict than are other addicts.[49] Adolescents who are making satisfactory progress in their development toward maturity rarely become addicted.[50] In general, if they seek help, treatment is the same as that given adult addicts. The exception is that, in some cases, groups of adolescent addicts, such as gangs, undergo treatment together.[51]

A larger group of adolescent drug abusers are the experience seekers. A survey in middle-class public schools in Milwaukee found that 6 percent of the students smoked more than five cigarettes a day, 62.5 percent used alcohol at least occasionally, and 21.5 percent admitted to having used illegal drugs other than alcohol.[52] A cross-sectional study of high schools in Oregon showed that drug use varied with grade—lowest users

being 3.4 percent of freshman females and the highest 24.9 percent of senior males. The incidence of tobacco, alcohol, and pot use was found to increase with grade.[53] Recent longitudinal surveys in New York support this finding. The mean self-reported age for onset of smoking was 12 years, for alcohol 12.6 years, and for pot 14.4 years.[54]

A Children's Bureau study found that at least one half of the respondents knew something about drugs. The same percentage accepted the use of marijuana while nearly two fifths expressed disapproval of all types of drugs. These adolescents gave the following reasons for using drugs: impulse to escape, rebellion, inner psychological problems and having nothing better to do, curiosity, need for status or conformity, excitement, or to expand the mind. Reasons for nonuse were avoiding the harm that drugs do and having inner strength and worthwhile things to do.[55] There may be different reasons for students initially trying drugs or continuing to use them. For example, one study found 47.7 percent first tried drugs out of curiosity, while the most frequent reason for maintaining drug use was escape (40.3 percent).[56] The peer group appears to have a socializing influence. Adolescents having a good friend who smokes have been found to be nine times as likely to smoke as adolescents without smoking friends.[57]

Adolescents use a wide variety of drugs, the type used varying with age. For example, glue sniffing occurs in early adolescence while smoking tobacco and using alcohol and pot tend to increase as the adolescent grows older.

Implications for health personnel can be divided into three areas. The first concerns education. There is a lack of agreement on who knows more about drugs—adolescents or adults. Nurses should familiarize themselves with drugs commonly used by adolescents so they are prepared to discuss both the actions of these drugs and the psychological, social, and cultural implications of taking drugs. It is important to stress the facts and avoid moralizing. Literature from state health departments and other reputable sources may be used effectively in groups and on a one-to-one basis. In discussing tobacco use, it may be most beneficial to focus on the relationship between smoking and diseases other than lung cancer and on immediate concerns of the adolescent, such as impairment of athletic performance.[58] The approach should be geared to the development of the adolescent with younger adolescents being present-oriented and becoming more future-oriented as they approach adulthood.

The second concern is drug users who become patients. If the person is an addict or known abuser of a particular drug, it is relatively easy to watch for specific signs of drug use or withdrawal. However, some patients are not known drug users and nurses should be aware of withdrawal symptoms, flashbacks, needle tracks, and equipment used for drug administration. If the adolescent is brought to the emergency room following drug ingestion, it is important to find out how much was taken of what drug at what time. Friends may be the best source of such information. Assessment of the physical and psychological status of the patient is important since dilatation or constriction of pupils, lethargy or excitement, and hallucination may give clues as to the type of drug used.

Steve is an example of a young adolescent who took an overdose of several drugs. He wandered into an ambulatory care clinic looking dazed and reported to the nurse that he had taken a "lot of drugs," but could not remember what they were. Vital signs were stable and within normal limits, but Steve was becoming increasingly drowsy. The nurse noted that Steve's breath smelled like alcohol. There were no needle marks on his body, no evidence of marijuana seeds or leaves and no cigarette papers or drug paraphernalia. Steve's wallet contained his home phone number, and, after providing for his immediate safety, the nurse contacted Steve's mother. She was able to tell the nurse that she found a number of empty bottles of cough syrup and an empty decongestant bottle in Steve's room. Steve was given central nervous system stimulants and admitted to the hospital for observation.

The similarities of agent-host-environment interactions in communicable disease and drug dependence have been pointed out by Cameron. He notes that a significant difference exists in that drug dependent hosts seek the agent while hosts do not seek infectious agents.[59] Therefore, for treatment to be effective, the supply of drugs must be decreased at the same time the patient is treated; that is, the demand for the drug is decreased.

This type of approach was used with John, an adolescent who was a heavy user of combinations of hallucinogens and pot. He had been caught selling drugs to peers, and was arrested and assigned by the judge to a residential treatment center for emotionally disturbed adolescents. At the center John continued to use drugs which he easily acquired in a nearby town. He made poor progress in school and rarely interacted with fellow students or staff. As part of the school program, all students were sent to an isolated summer camp. All John's mail was carefully monitored and all trips away from camp were closely supervised. John was unable to acquire any drugs. An intensive educational program and group and individual therapy sessions were initiated. At the end of three months John had completed his grade level and was more at ease in interactions with staff and students. At present, the effects on John of re-entry into an urban environment where drugs are easily acquired are unknown.

The final area of health concerns is emotional health. Some aspects of this have already been discussed in relation to suicide and drug use; however, emotional health in adolescence is a broader area than this. It depends on feelings of adequacy and self-esteem. Whatever disrupts development of self-identity and self-esteem has important implications for emotional health. Examples of such deleterious factors are rejection by peers because of physical appearance, continued failure experiences in school, and statements by parents implying worthlessness. To cope with these experiences, adolescents may develop patterns of acting out behavior or withdrawal that are troublesome to them, to their parents, or to society. It is at this time that the individual is referred for treatment. The outcome of therapy often depends on the way in which the adolescent sees the therapist.[60] For example, if the therapist is seen as another authoritarian adult, like the parents, therapy may not be as successful in effecting behavior change.

The goal of nursing should be the prevention of emotional problems by promoting health through positive relationships with adolescents. (See Chapter 3 concerning the establishment and maintenance of mental health.) When working with emotionally disturbed adolescents, three general guidelines are establishing and maintaining consistent limits on behavior, pointing out the reality of the situation, and providing success experiences in skills and interpersonal relationships.

Gregg was a 17-year-old referred to a residential treatment center following discharge from a state mental hospital. He was the younger of two sons and believed his parents greatly favored the older son. He always tried to be like his brother, but his parents continued to favor the older son. A number of asocial acts resulted in Gregg's hospitalization with the diagnosis of schizophrenia. At the treatment center Gregg would go from person to person telling them he was sick and that he felt worthless ("I feel like shit.") His failure to make progress in school, despite exceptional ability, led to his presentation at staff meeting. The staff decided to focus on changing his perception of himself as sick and providing success experiences. One therapist and one male staff member were assigned to Gregg for special care. The nurse played an important part because Gregg came to her for validation of physical and emotional problems. She stressed that perhaps he had been ill, but he was ill no longer. Physical complaints were carefully evaluated, but, if believed to be psychophysiological their importance was minimized. The nurse was able to provide success experiences in the areas of biology and histology, favorite areas of Gregg's. They both enjoyed afternoons preparing and examining slides. Gregg eventually came to the nurse just for rap sessions or to present her with his latest creative work—a poem, a picture, or a slide. Eventally Gregg was able to teach another student how to scuba dive, and the other students praised him for this.

Slowly he is learning to view himself as a person with unique talents capable of relating effectively with others.

General Considerations

Some general principles of interaction could apply to adolescent-nurse interactions, regardless of the setting. One is the importance of eliciting the adolescent's perception of his or her present problem and usual health-related problems. This often proves revealing and serves as a basis for counseling and teaching. The small cut on the adolescent's face that one cleans and dresses so easily may cause him or her uneasiness because it may leave a scar and if it does so, what implications might this have on dating relationships? This opens the door to a discussion of these relationships.

To communicate effectively, one must understand the idiom of young people. They use some of their distinctive language in communicating with adults, and it is important to understand it. This prevents the continued interruption to ask for meanings and ensures that one understands what is being said. A favorite informer may keep one posted on new language developments or songs and discussion on radio programs aimed at adolescents may keep one current. However, there is no necessity to use their distinctive language in communicating with adolescents. If they do not come naturally, such attempts can be very awkward and disrupt communication.

Several aspects of relationships with adolescents can be uncomfortable for the nurse. One of these is the keeping of confidences. Adolescents may approach the nurse with the bargain of revealing information to her if she promises not to tell anyone. Sometimes such secrets are relatively trivial, such as a practical joke they are planning to play, but sometimes they have serious implications, such as the possibility of pregnancy. In all cases, it is best for the nurse to tell the adolescent that she will keep the confidence if it does not prove harmful to do so. This shifts responsibility back to the adolescent. By the time the adolescent comes to the nurse with such a bargain, he or she may have already decided that he or she wants the nurse to know and is willing to take the risks involved.

Another problem in relationships with adolescents is termination of relationships. Adolescents frequently form strong attachments to people and are uneasy about changes. If they know that they may be in contact, either by mail or return visit, this usually gives them enough security to tolerate the termination and to form new relationships. Of course, the nurse must be mature enough to permit dependency when it is therapeutic and to encourage independence when this becomes a therapeutic goal.

Assumption of responsibility is another area in which conflict may arise between patient and nurse. Because of the cult of irresponsibility associated with adolescence, the nurse may not be inclined to give adolescents responsibility for their own care. In general, if adolescents can perform a task, such as leg exercises, they should be instructed, supervised, and left to perform such exercises on whatever schedule is appropriate. Asking them about the exercise or dropping by when they are performing them lets them know you are still interested in them, but trust them enough to perform the tasks satisfactorily. Parents should be instructed as to what adolescents are expected to carry through at home, but they should also know that they can perform these activities with minimal supervision.

Related to both dependency and responsibility is the tendency to use relationships with adolescents to get them to perform an activity. If they are learning to give themselves insulin and are hesitant to inject themselves, the approach should not be, "Do it for me." Adolescents need to understand why this self-injection is important so that the emphasis is shifted from the nurse to the patients who do the procedure for themselves.

The environment in which care is given frequently affects its outcome. For this reason, adolescent in-patient units and youth clinics, either independent or associated with hospitals, have been established. In attempting to assess the effectiveness of separate adolescent units, a survey was conducted of a sample of institutions with separate adolescent in-patient units and those

with separate clinics, but not in-patient units. Both adolescents and nurses were interviewed. The patients liked the separate units because they enjoyed the peer support. The nurses liked separate units because of continuity of care and teaching, good support from other disciplines, and because the units met the needs of patients. Problems identified were difficulty with discipline, the need for special background in growth and development, and the social and emotional factors affecting this group. Despite its problems, the overwhelming concensus was that adolescent units were worthwhile.[61]

Discipline is frequently a source of frustration for nurses working with groups of adolescents either within or outside of the hospital. If at all possible, adolescents should be involved in establishing the rules governing their conduct and in decisions regarding infractions. Therapeutic communities provide for this. For example, if the rules are already established by hospital or unit policy, adolescents must understand why such rules exist and what consequences result from disregarding them. Consistency in enforcement is important in discipline, although flexibility is not excluded if all members of the group understand the rationale for altering the rules.

Discipline often becomes a less important concern if adolescents have something to do in the hospital. Recreational therapists, school programs, and planned unit activities may be useful. Also, providing adolescents with familiar sources of entertainment, favorite reading material, radios, and phonographs helps to pass time. The activity which occupies most of the adolescent's time is talking, and a gathering area should be provided for patients where they can meet to share meals and entertain friends. Access to a telephone is also an important means of keeping in touch with one's peers.

More recently, youth clinics are being established. Some are associated with hospitals and function to follow up previously hospitalized patients, to provide services for adolescents with chronic health problems, and, sometimes, to provide care for acute problems. Examples of the type of patients seen are those with obesity, acne, allergies, and respiratory diseases. Some institutions are establishing separate clinics for adolescents with obstetrical and gynecological problems.

Another type of youth clinic, operated by health departments or voluntary groups, tends to see patients with problems related to drug use, pregnancy, or venereal disease.[62] Some of these clinics use indigenous community workers. Hallmarks of such clinics seem to be availability (evening hours, central location), low cost for service, and few hassles about ability to pay, style of living, and other personal information. In some ways the establishment of free clinics and alternative health services points out inadequacies in the present health care system. These clinics are meeting needs of the youth community and professional nurses should be there to counsel and teach. (See Chapter 2 for more detailed discussion of methods of health care delivery.)

Medicine is evolving the speciality of ephebiatrics, adolescent medicine. Nursing should take a broad view of American youth, recognizing that wherever they are, they want information about health, they need health care, and they need mature role models of adult behavior. Nurses can provide these services and ought to take opportunities to do so, both at their place of employment and in the community.

Some further aspects of working with adolescents can be illustrated by reviewing the interactions between a young man and health team members. Ken, a 15-year-old, had been enrolled in a residential treatment school for two years. He had been doing poorly in school and was difficult to get along with at home. He had been diagnosed as having diabetes mellitus at age nine, and he used this disease to control his parents. He threatened to eat excessive amounts of carbohydrates in order to obtain whatever he wanted. In turn, they allowed him little independence, and his mother continued to test his urine, administer insulin, and admonish him about his diet.

In the residential school setting he formed few friendships and continued to use manipulative behavior. A staff nurse administered his in-

sulin each morning and whenever he needed coverage. One of the male staff members tested his urine twice a day. A recreation staff member, of whom he was fond, convinced Ken to go out for football. Training took place in a camp setting. Ken showed up for the first two days of practice; after this he became increasingly angry and seclusive, refusing to talk with either students or staff. On the fourth day of training, Ken came for his morning insulin as usual; however, after the insulin administration, he went back to his cabin to lie down. About 11:30 A.M., a staff member found him in hypoglycemic shock. Fruit juice followed by lunch was all that was necessary to correct the hypoglycemia. However, staff members concerned about his behavior, viewing it as a request for help, scheduled a special meeting to discuss Ken. A variety of disciplines were represented: education, nursing, psychology, and recreation therapy. In addition, Ken's cabin counselor attended. Following a general discussion, the major objective established was to collect information about Ken's current behavior. The psychologist and cabin counselor were designated to gain information from Ken.

A second meeting was held two days later to discuss the findings and modify the plan of care. The nurse had been gathering information about Ken's feelings concerning diabetes and its treatment. She learned of his resentment concerning dependence in diabetic care. The psychologist and cabin counselor had both learned that Ken really did not want to play football; he had been doing it to please the recreation staff member. The educator noted Ken's increasingly poor academic performance and the need to successfully complete two courses before entering the next grade in September. The following objectives and methods of implementation were established:

1. *Self-care of diabetes:* Ken already knew how to test his urine. He would be instructed in keeping a record and reporting results. He would also be instructed in the administration of mixed insulins. Diet would be reviewed and Ken would be encouraged to join several students, who were using an exchange list diet for weight loss, in their

daily weight checks. In addition, a special serving area was to be added to the dining room to include a selection of fruits, vegetables, hardboiled eggs and other foods requested by weight watchers.

2. *Improvement of academic performance:* In addition to class periods, special tutoring sessions were to be held two days each week.

3. *Participation in activities program:* Football would no longer be a required activity. Ken had expressed an interest in gymnastics, and a recreational therapist would work with him in this activity.

4. *Learning more effective coping behavior:* The number of individual therapy sessions would be increased to provide a better opportunity to form a relationship with Ken and to explore alternative coping behaviors.

The therapeutic plan was evaluated weekly at staff meetings and modified as necessary. When Ken was hospitalized a short time for minor surgery, the camp nurse communicated pertinent aspects of the treatment plan to the charge nurse.

At the end of the summer, Ken was scheduled to spend two weeks at home with his parents before school started. The family was going to spend a few days sightseeing in the area of the camp before the trip home. Staff members took advantage of this time to meet with Ken and his parents to discuss the treatment plan, Ken's progress, and the family involvement in carrying out the plan at home.

A final evaluation of Ken's behavior prior to vacation revealed that all staff members had noted more cooperative behavior, independence in self-care, completion of the required courses, and the beginnings of friendships with other students in the gymnastics group.

Summary

If any summary statement can be made about nursing adolescent patients, it must be that such nursing is challenging. Nurses can work effectively with adolescents by including them, and important others, in all steps of the nursing process. When nurses listen to and observe adolescents, they learn what the adolescent can contribute in terms of perceptions of illness, likes and dislikes and identified goals. Very often adolescents will express priorities in health goals or suggest preferred means of implementation. The nurse uses this information in formulating a plan of care. The plan is evaluated jointly by adolescent and nurse based on criteria designed to assess the attainment of mutually formed goals.

The word process is an important one in nursing adolescents because of the use of the nursing process as a tool and because of the importance of the process of forming relationships with adolescents. Nursing adolescents is a relational process with possibilities for growth and change.

References

1. Demos, J. and Demos, V.: Adolescence in historical perspective. J. Marriage and the Fam. 31:623-638, Nov. 1969.
2. Poveda, T. G.: A perspective on adolescent social relations. Psychiatry 35:32-47, Feb. 1972.
3. Bettelheim, B.: Obsolete youth: towards a psychograph of adolescent rebellion. Encounter 33:29-42, Sept. 1969.
4. Schneiders, A. A. (ed.): Counseling the Adolescent. San Francisco, Chandler, 1967, pp. 10-12.
5. Weiner, I. B.: Perspectives on the modern adolescent. Psychiatry 35:20-31, Feb. 1972.
6. Barber, J. M., Stokes, L. G. and Billings, D. M.: Adult and Child Care. St. Louis, C. V. Mosby, 1973.
7. Kandel, D. B. and Lesser, G. S.: Parental and peer influence on educational plans of adolescents. Am. Soc. Review 34:213-223, Apr. 1969.
8. Floyd, H. H., Jr. and South, D. R.: Dilemma of youth: the choice of parents or peers as a frame of reference for behavior. J. Marriage and the Fam. 34:627-634, Nov. 1972.
9. Larson, L. E.: The influence of parents and peers during adolescence: the situation hypothesis revisited. J. Marriage and the Fam. 34:67-74, Feb. 1972.
10. Smith, T. E.: Foundations of parental influence upon adolescents: an application of social power theory. Am. Soc. Review 35:860-873, Oct. 1970.

11. Larson, L. E.: An examination of the salience hierarchy during adolescence: the influence of the family. Adolescence 9:317-332, Fall 1974.

12. Conger, J. J.: A world they never knew: the family and social change. Daedalus 100:1105-1138, Fall 1971.

13. Dunphy, Dexter C.: The structure of urban adolescent peer groups. *In* R. E. Grinder (ed.): Studies in Adolescence. London, Macmillan, 1969, pp. 188-202.

14. U.S. Bureau of the Census: Statistical abstract of the United States, ed. 93. Washington, D.C., U.S. Government Printing Office, 1972.

15. Weinberg, S.: Suicidal intent in adolescence: a hypothesis about the role of physical illness. J. Pediatrics 77:579-586, Oct. 1970.

16. Weinberg, *op cit.,* pp. 579-586.

17. Adolescents and Summer Accidents. Clin. Pediatrics 6:323, June 1967.

18. Suchman, E. A.: Accidents and social deviance. J. Health and Soc. Behav. 11:4-15, Mar. 1970.

19. Brunswich, A. F. and Josephson, E.: Adolescent health in Harlem. Am. J. Pub. Health, Supplement, 62, Oct. 1972.

20. Craft, C. A.: Body image and obesity. Nurs. Clin. N. Am. 7:677-685, Dec. 1972.

21. Lamers, W. M., Jr.: Problems of teen-agers presented to obstetricians and gynecologists. Clin. Ob. and Gyn. 13:727-733, Sept. 1970.

22. Morgenthau, J. E. and Sokoloff, N. J.: The sexual revolution: myth or fact? Pediatric Clin. N. Am. 19:779-789, Aug. 1972.

23. Osofsky, H. F.: Adolescent sexual behavior: current status and anticipated trends for the future. Clin. Ob. and Gyn. 14:393-408, June 1971.

24. Bell, R. R. and Chaskes, J. B.: Premarital sexual experience among coeds, 1958 and 1968. J. Marriage and the Fam. 32:81-84, Feb. 1970.

25. Zelnick, Melvin and Kanter, John F.: The probability of premarital intercourse. Soc. Sci. Research 1:335-341, Sept. 1972.

26. Morgenthau and Sokoloff, *op. cit.,* pp. 779-789.

27. Woody, J. D.: Contemporary sex education: attitudes and implications for childbearing. J. School Health 43:241-246, Apr. 1973.

28. Taylor, C.: In Horizontal Orbit: Hospitals and the Cult of Efficiency. New York, Holt, Rinehart and Winston, 1970.

29. For example, see Pion, R. J.: Family planning education. Clin. Ob. and Gyn. 14:409-419, June 1971.

30. Hoffman, Adele D. and Pilpel, Harriet F.: The legal rights of minors. Pediatric Clin. N. Am. 20:989-1004, Nov. 1973. For further information see also Irwin, T.: The rights of teenagers as patients. New York, Pub. Affairs Pamphlets, 1975 (35¢) or contact a regional affiliate of Planned Parenthood-World Population or write to Planned Parenthood-World Population, 810 Seventh Avenue, N.Y., N.Y. 10019.

31. Brunswich, A. F.: Adolescent health, sex and fertility. Am. J. Pub. Health 61:711-729, Apr. 1971.

32. Oppel, W. C. and Royston, A. B.: Teen-age births: some social, psychological and physical sequelae. Am. J. Pub. Health 61:751-756, Apr. 1971.

33. Faigel, H. C.: Unwed pregnant adolescents. Clin. Pediatrics 6:281-285, May 1967.

34. Duenhoelter, Johann H., Jimenez, Juan M. and Baumann, G.: Pregnancy performance of patients under 15 years of age. Ob. and Gyn. 46:49-52, July 1975.

35. Friedrerich, M. A.: Motivations for coitus. Clin. Ob. and Gyn. 13:691-700, Sept. 1970.

36. Daly, M. J.: The unwanted pregnancy. Clin. Ob. and Gyn. 13:713-726, Sept. 1970.

37. Ballard, W. M. and Gold, E. M.: Medical and health aspects of reproduction in the adolescent. Clin. Ob. and Gyn. 14:338-366, June 1971.

38. Hausknecht, R. V.: The termination of pregnancy in adolescent women. Pediatric Clin. N. Am. 19:803-810, Aug. 1972. See also *Abortion*-Part I. Hearings before the subcommittee on constitutional amendments of the committee on the judiciary of the United States Senate, 93rd Congress. Washington, D.C., U.S. Government Printing Office, 1974, p. 442.

39. Gabrielson, I. W., et al.: Adolescent attitudes toward abortion: effects on contraceptive practice. Am. J. Pub. Health 61:730-738, Apr. 1971.

40. Pannor, R.: The teen-age unwed father. Clin. Ob. and Gyn. 14:466-472, June 1971.

41. Hausknecht, R. V., *op. cit.*

42. Ballard and Gold, *op cit.,* p. 350.

43. For example, see Finkelstein, R.: Program for the

sexually active teenager. Pediatric Clin. N. Am. 19:791-794, Aug. 1972, and Marinoff, S. C.: Contraception in Adolescents. Pediatric Clin. N. Am. 19:811-819, Aug. 1972.

44. For example, see Arnold, C. B. and Cogswell, B. E.: A condom distribution program for adolescents: the findings of a feasibility study. Am. J. Pub. Health 61:739-750, Apr. 1971, and Gordis, L., et al.: Adolescent pregnancy: a hospital based program for primary prevention. *In* J.Kestenbergled (ed.): The Adolescent: Physical Development, Sexuality and Pregnancy. New York, MSS Information Corp., 1972, pp. 184-193. See also Hambridge, William R.: Teen clinics. Ob. and Gyn. 43:458-460, Mar. 1974.

45. Pilpel, Harriet F. and Wechsler, N. F.: Birth control, teenagers and the law: a new look. Fam. Plan. Perspec. 3:37-45, July 1971.

46. Zinberg, N. E.: Facts and fancies about drug addiction. *In* R. E. Grinder (ed.): Studies in Adolescence. London, Macmillan, 1969, pp. 309-323.

47. *Ibid.*

48. Blaine, C. B., Jr.: Are Parents Bad for Children? New York, Coward, McCann and Geoghegan, 1973, p. 72.

49. Boyd, P.: Heroin addiction in adolescents. J. Psychosom. Research 14:295-301, Sept. 1970.

50. *Ibid.*, p. 299.

51. For example, see Levitt, L.: Rehabilitation of narcotics addicts among lower-class teenagers. Am. J. Orthopsych. 38:56-62, Jan. 1968.

52. Jackson, B., Lange, R. and Lehmann, R. P.: Teenage drug abuse in middle class Milwaukee. Wis. Med. J. 71:210-212, Sept. 1971.

53. Johnson, K. G., et al.: Survey of adolescent drug use. I—Sex and grade distribution. Am. J. Pub. Health 61:2418-2432, Dec. 1971.

54. Kandel, Denise and Faust, Richard: Sequence and stages in patterns of adolescent drug use. Archives Gen. Psych. 32:923-932, July 1975.

55. Herzog, E., Sudia, C. E. and Harwood, J.: Drug use among the young—as teenagers see it. Child. 17:206-212, Nov.-Dec. 1970.

56. Jackson, Lange and Lehmann, *op cit.*, pp. 210-212.

57. Lanese, R. R., Banks, F. R. and Keller, M. D.: Smoking behavior in a teenage population: a multivariate conceptual approach. Am. J. Pub. Health 62:807-813, June 1972.

58. Boyle, C. M.: Some factors affecting the smoking habits of a group of teenagers. Lancet 2:1287-1289, Dec. 14, 1968.

59. Cameron, D. C.: Youth and drugs: a world view. JAMA 206:1267-1271, Nov. 4, 1968.

60. Rouslin, S.: The adolescent in psychotherapy. Perspec. Psych. Care 7:263-266, Nov.-Dec. 1969.

61. Rigg, C. A. and Fischer, R. C.: Is a separate adolescent ward worthwhile? Am. J. Diseases of Child. 122:489-493, Dec. 1971.

62. For example, see Krain, L. S. and Heidbreder, G. A.: Health department youth clinic facilities: a nationwide survey. Inquiry 9:73-76, June 1972, and Minkowski, W. L., Weiss, R. C. and Heidbreder, G. A.: The county of Los Angeles health department youth clinics. Am. J. Pub. Health 61:757-762, Apr. 1971.

Bibliography

Adolescence. An international quarterly journal devoted to the physiological, psychological, psychiatric, sociological and educational aspects of the second decade of human life. Libra Publishers, Inc.

Bakwin, R. M.: Self abuse with drugs (drug abuse in adolescents). J. Am. Med. Women's Assoc. 24:482-487, June 1969.

Berman, S.: Alienation: an essential process of the psychology of adolescence. J. Am. Acad. Child Psych. 9:233-250, Apr. 1970.

Brown, F.: Sexual behavior of the adolescent girl. Pediatric Clin. N. Am. 19:759-764, Aug. 1972.

Clancy, B.: The nurse and the abortion patient. Nurs. Clin. N. Am. 8:469-478, Sept. 1973.

Cobliner, W. Godfrey, Schulman, Harold and Romney, Seymour L.: The termination of adolescent out-of-wedlock pregnancies and the prospects for their primary prevention. Am. J. Ob. and Gyn. 115:432-444, Feb. 1973.

Coleman, Janes S., et al.: Youth—Transition to Adulthood. Chicago, The University of Chicago Press, 1974.

Dambacher, B. and Hellwig, K.: Nursing strategies for

young drug users. Perspec. Psych. Care 9:200-205, Sept.-Oct. 1971.

Daniel, W. A., Jr. (ed.) The Adolescent Patient. St. Louis, C. V. Mosby, 1970.

Daniels, A. M.: Reaching unwed adolescent mothers. Am. J. Nurs. 69:332-335. Feb. 1969.

Daniels, A. M. and Krim, A.: Helping adolescents explore emotional issues. Am. J. Nurs. 69:1482-1485. July 1969.

Deisher, R. W. et al.: Drug abuse in adolescence—the use of harmful drugs—a pediatric concern. Pediatrics 44:131-141, July 1969.

Dempsey, M. O.: The development of body image in the adolescent. Nurs. Clin. N. Am. 7:609-615, Dec. 1972.

Fleshman, R. P.: (ed.): Symposium on the young adult in today's world. Nurs. Clin. N. Am. 8:1-104, Mar. 1973.

Forsythe, M. J.: Youth and drugs—use and abuse: educational and sociological aspects. Ohio State Med. J. 65:17-23, Jan. 1969.

Furstenberg, F., Jr., Gordis, L. and Markowitz, M.: Birth control knowledge and attitudes among unmarried pregnant adolescents: a preliminary report. J. Marriage and the Fam. 31:34-42, Feb. 1969.

Gordon, C.: Social characteristics of early adolescence. Daedalus, 100:931-960, Fall 1971.

Gordon, S.: What adolescents want to know. Am. J. Nurs. 71:534-535, Mar. 1971.

Grinder, R. E.: Studies in Adolescence. London, Macmillan, 1969

Hammar, S. L.: The obese adolescent. *In* J. Kestenberg (ed.): The Adolescent: Physical Development, Sexuality and Pregnancy. New York, MSS Information Corp., 1972, pp. 41-44.

Harmer, S. L. and Eddy, J. A.: Nursing Care of the Adolescent. New York, Springer, 1966.

Heald, F. P.: Growth and development. Clin. Ob. and Gyn. 14:327-337, June 1971.

Hoffman, A. D. and Shenker, I. R.: Medical care of adolescents and the law. N.Y. State J. Med. 70:2603-2611, Oct. 15, 1970.

Johnson, K. G. et al.: Survey of adolescent drug use. II—Social and environmental factors. Am. J. Pub. Health 62:164-166, Feb. 1972.

Johnson, K. G. et al.: Survey of adolescent drug use. III—Correlations among use of drugs. Am. J. Pub. Health 62:166-170, Feb. 1972.

Kestenberg, J. et al.: The Adolescent: Physical Development, Sexuality and Pregnancy. New York, MSS Information Corp., 1972.

Kramer, J. P.: The adolescent addict. Clin. Pediatrics 11:382-385, July 1972.

LeShan, Eda J.: Mates and roommates: new styles in young marriages. New York, Pub. Affairs Pamphlet, 1973.

Levy, N.: The Use of Drugs Among Teenagers. Canad. Psych. Assoc. J., Supplement 2, 17:31-36, 1972.

Litt, I. F. and Cohen, M. I.: The drug-using adolescent as a pediatric patient. J. Pediatrics 77:195-202, Aug. 1970.

Lordi, W. M.: Drug use and abuse in adolescence: a twenty year perspective. Va. Med. Monthly 99:632-636, June 1972.

Luckey, E. B. and Nass, G. D.: A comparison of sexual attitudes and behavior in an international sample. J. Marriage and the Fam. 31:364-378, May 1969.

Marinoff, S. C. and Schonholz, D. H.: Adolescent pregnancy. Pediatric Clin. N. Am. 19:795-802, Aug. 1972.

Miller, John P.: Suicide and adolescence. Adolescence 10:11-24, Spring 1975.

Nosphitz, J. D.: Certain cultural and familial factors contributing to adolescent alienation. J. Am. Acad. Child Psych. 9:216-223, Apr. 1970.

Osofsky, H. F. and Osofsky, J. D.: Let's be sensible about sex education. Am. J. Nurs. 71:532-535, Mar. 1971.

Rigg, C. A.: Approaching the adolescent in the office. Pediatric Clin. N. Am. 19:727-733, Aug. 1972.

Rogerson, K. E.: Psychiatric emergencies. Nurs. Clin. N. Am. 8:457-466, Sept. 1973.

Russell, Lynette K.: Sexual counseling: an approach to the integration of sexual counseling into the antepartal management of teenagers. J. Nurse Midwifery 20:24-30, Spring 1975.

Saltman, Jules: Drug-abuse—what can be done? New York, Pub. Affairs Pamphlet, 1975.

Schonfeld, W. A.: Adolescent turmoil and the search for identity. Am. J. Psychoanal. 31:19-34, 1971.

Schorr, B. C. Sanjur, D. and Erickson, E. C.: Teenage

food habits. J. Am. Dietetic Assoc. 61:414-420, Oct. 1972.

Schowalter, John E. and Anyan, Walter R.: Experience on an adolescent inpatient division. Am. J. Diseases of Child. 125:212-215, Feb. 1973.

Shamon, P. D.: The adolescent experience. Am. J. Occupational Therapy 26:284-287, Sept. 1972.

Smith, D. M.: Adolescence: a study of stereotyping. Soc. Review 18:197-211, July 1970.

Symposium on Adolescent Medicine: Pediatric Clin. N. Am. 20, Nov. 1973.

Tanner, J. M.: Sequence, tempo and individual variation in the growth and development of boys and girls aged twelve to sixteen. Daedalus 100:907-930, Fall 1971.

Thomas, D. L. and Weigert, A. J.: Socialization and adolescent conformity to significant others: a cross-national analysis. Am. Soc. Review 36:835-847, Oct. 1971.

Wein, B.: The Runaway Generation. New York, McKay, 1970.

Youth and society, a quarterly journal. Sage Publications.

9

Health Horizons of the Aged: influences and myths

NANCY PERPALL KELLY and LAWRENCE J. HOURANY

Attitudes Regarding Aging • Who are the Elderly? • Physiological Factors in Aging • Life Expectancy • Illness • Genetics and the Elderly • Mortality • Sexual Vistas • Sociological Factors • Stereotypes • The Impact of Attitudes Toward the Elderly • A Positive Approach

In a world in which change is the rule, ours is a time when the rate of change seems to be accelerating. The knowledge we use to guide our existence seems to be part of a cultural fund that increases at an exponential rate. Very possibly we are living in a time when a greater than ever percentage of human energy is devoted to the expansion of that knowledge. And we have become painfully aware that opposing and sometimes even erroneous information may be current at any given moment. Moreover, there is frequently a lag between scientifically verified "truth" and common practice. So it is with our attitudes regarding old age. In this chapter we will explore some psychological, sociological, and biophysical aspects of the aging process, particularly as these parameters influence health and nursing needs of the elderly.

Attitudes Regarding Aging

In other cultures and in other times, old people are and have been accorded more respect than they receive in contemporary Western society. Now, in an affluent youth-oriented society in which there is a greater percentage of people living to old age than ever before, we have no time for those who cannot "keep up." When they slow down they cannot produce efficiently—and this is a very product-oriented society. Hence, the elderly join other marginal, minority groups and frequently face a forced reduction in economic pursuits, social activities, and responsibilities. This is called societal disengagement and it may have beneficial aspects. However, through whatever process it occurs and for whatever reasons, it constitutes an unwanted and disturbing reality for the old.[1] For their part, younger members of society often contribute to this disengagement. The old person may no longer be sought out for leadership in organizations or in the community. In terms of jobs, he may be acknowledged as competent, but the younger

TABLE 9-1
Life Span Outline

YEARS	PERIOD	MAIN CHARACTERISTICS
Birth to about 20	Childhood Adolescence	
21 - 30	Early adulthood	Acquisition of adult roles, economic responsibility, marriage, employment, children; full engagement in activities; peak years for athletic achievement (to about 35).
30 - 45+	Middle adulthood	Consolidation of social and occupational roles; peak years for most kinds of intellectual achievement; slight decline of some physical and mental functions apparent in tests of maximum performance; accumulation of material possessions and establishment of lifetime social relations.
45+ - 55+	Late adulthood	Continuation of established social and occupational roles; departure of children; diminution of sexual and reproductive functions; re-entry of some women into jobs; broadening disuse of physical and mental functions.
55+ - 65	Preretirement	More obvious declines, but peak years for some kinds of social achievement of authority, or partial disengagement from occupational roles and community affairs; especially notable divergence between those who show further diminution and those who show continued sexual function and interests.
65+	Retirement	May be disengagement from occupational role; reassessment and reorientation of life goals; possible withdrawal from community affairs, or continuation of some kinds of social authority; greater prominence of kinship and primary group relationships; in most cases an increased susceptibility to physical disorders.
Men - 71 Women - 74	Average life expectancy U.S.A.	Changes in biological and psychological condition largely dependent upon continued involvement; reduction in elasticity, a function of previous life styles *and* current efforts to maintain self; mental, physical, sexual, and emotional behavior reflect enduring dispositions more than inherent limitations; some people will show *improvement* in some abilities.
75+	Old age	Certain inadequacies may begin to develop, but, while incapacitation may characterize more people, many people show continued maintenance of general functional levels.
To a maximum of 113	Terminal illness and death	Gradual breakdown of critical biological functions; in some instances senile dementia is present but most people show only slight memory loss and disorientation; impairments accumulate and may lead to incapacitation, but many people show little loss until shortly before or even up to death.

Modeled on an outline developed by D. B. Bromley: The Psychology of Human Aging. Baltimore, Penguin Books, 1966.

worker will be preferred, both for hiring and promotion. Even in the home he is not expected to participate in financial decisions, and he may not be included in social activities. His progress through life seems to be marked by an accumulation of negative characteristics and experiences (see Table 9-1).

There is, of course, a profound difference in voluntary and involuntary changes in one's life style. While many of our social institutions *seem* to thrive on infusions of "young blood," there is by no means a clear-cut point at which the skill that the young person brings to a position outweighs the contributions of the older adult. Certainly few older persons agree with the social demarcation that indicates that they have exceeded their period of usefulness. This is true whether the person is a manual laborer, a typist, a dentist, a nurse, or a teacher. And while there are differences in interest and job satisfaction related to occupational level and to age, even if provided with economic independence and even though the percentage goes down with age, the majority of employed people would prefer to continue working and maintaining their established life style.[2]

Actually job satisfaction may be the key variable in determining work longevity. If a job is viewed as an avocation rather than as work, the person can be expected to be more accepting of and dedicated to his or her role. Thus the role developed by the values, talents, and conflicts encountered during years of productive work will be maintained. On the other hand, if the job has not been internally satisfying, the worst aspects of job performance might be expected to come to the fore: lack of attention to detail, failure to be competitive (concerned?), loss of efficiency, exaggeration of physical disabilities, and so on. In fact, this process may become as evident in a 35-year-old as in a 70-year-old.*

The bulk of evidence indicates that, in most instances, most people at all ages would prefer to select their own life styles, but it is *society* which often dictates role selection.[3] With regard to age designations, it would appear that an arbitrary delineation at age 65 transforms individuals from middle age to old age as though some alchemy were performed at that time. The effect is exceptionally strong, despite the fact that during their 40s and 50s these people recognized that their age group had the most power and control in setting standards and making decisions.[4] Of course, the dislocation experienced during these transition years may be due precisely to that removal of power. That is, children certainly experience long periods of powerlessness, but, as part of their increasing engagement with their environment, their expectations and roles are preparatory for assuming greater control. Instead, the

*This possibility was pointed out by Roger Moss (personal communication).

older person is *deprived* of power he or she once had. Hence, for any role or capacity the sense of loss is greatest for those who have enoyed it most.

Therefore, it seems that the psychological and sociological conditions occurring at approximately age 65 for most Westerners bring a peculiar blend of conditions which almost force a transition.[5] But the elderly are not a uniform, unvarying group, and any effort to delimit even the term will necessarily produce arbitrary and only partially satisfying guidelines.

Who Are the Elderly?

Is there a specific age at which one clearly becomes part of a new subgroup, or is age a totally abstract variable? Do lay people and professionals agree when they refer to a specific age group? These questions are crucial because the definitions people use affect their attitudes toward themselves and their behavior toward others.[6] Also, if the findings of researchers are to have any generality, the parameters they use should resemble to a degree conventional usage. Fortunately there seems to be agreement on this. Cameron asked 571 people ranging in age from 11 to 80 and from all walks of life what they thought of when they heard or used such terms as "young adults" The age categories were established as: young adult—18 to 25; middle age—40 to 55; old—65 to 80; and aged—80 and older.[7]

There is general conformity to these parameters in the professional literature. However, some experimenters might include 50-year-olds with their "old," group[8] and some may select an arbitrary age, such as 40, at which to divide their overall sample.[9] Selection of sample age limits can serve to either sharpen or attenuate the results of experiments. For example, a sample including 50-year-olds will not yield the same results as a sample restricted to people 70 years and older. These age divisions are especially important because recent research is supporting the contention that many mental abilities remain essentially undiminished until at least age 75 if the person is in good health.[10]

Is good health the answer to the "who" and "when" questions of ability loss? There is no simple answer. Of course, physical disability is not coordinate with mental disability, but general mental decline does seem to accompany loss of physical vigor. This may occur at fairly young ages for some people who show marked loss during their 50s. On the other hand, there have been many remarkable achievements by people in their 70s and 80s.

The picture is clarified when old age is viewed as

> a period of rapid, profound and multiple changes of varying intensities, physiological and social, which influence subjective experience, behavior and adaptation. Characteristics possessed prior to old age modify the extent and the nature of these influences but do not fully account for the changes themselves.[11]

This description could apply to any age, but it clearly underscores the progressive and cumulative nature of the changes characteristic of the later stages of the aging process. Thus, it is not chronological age but the interaction of a number of influences which affects behavior and produces the condition known as old age.

Physiological Factors in Aging

Each older person is a member of a subpopulation consisting of other older individuals that actually has more in common with the general adult population, particularly in the physiological process of aging, than it has differences. Indeed, following the common tendency to treat this subpopulation as different may, in fact, be creating the differences we have been assuming exist, that is, that the elderly person is an isolated patchwork of malfunctioning organs and shriveled skin; that the aged have little value as participating, contributing members of society.

Gerontological nursing does not deny that the alteration of organ systems and functional body parts occurs as a result of the aging process; however, death remains a consequence of disease, not of age.[12] It is the nurse's responsibility to care for the gerontological patient with the same intensity as she would the pediatric patient.

In fact, the study of pediatrics and gerontology may be considered as mirror images on opposite ends of the life cycle spectrum. The recognition that age is directly related to health and disease, via the inception of pediatrics as a specialty, clarified the misconception that a child was merely a "little man." Including functional, chemical, nutritional, metabolic, structural, and psychosocial differences, the stages of the life cycle, from infancy to old age, are classified by age and growth continuance. The elderly are not just "old people"; they are individuals who toward the end of the life cycle continue to change physiologically and psychosocially, thus continuing the developmental process.[13]

PHYSICAL CHANGES

Although there are individual differences, anatomical changes and changes in physiological functioning inevitably occur with age. The main anatomical changes consist of two types—the first is evidenced by a decrease in functional (parenchymal) cells of organ systems and an increase in supporting connective tissue (stroma). This results in the tendency for the total weight of an organ to decrease with age thus decreasing the functional weight as well. Second, as age progresses, pigments, fat, calcium, and amyloid may begin to appear and tend to accumulate in excess quantities.[14]

Loss of cells and accumulation of inert materials cause certain functional changes and body disturbances. The most obvious characteristic of the aging process is a decline in the ability of body organs to do work.[15] Although the rate at which each organ is subject to the effects of age varies, physiological function of all organs tends to decrease with increasing age, leaving the older person with less "reserve capacity" (Figs. 9-1 and 9-2). That is, organs operate well under conditions of rest but not under an increased workload or in situations of stress to which the younger person may more easily adapt. For example, muscles used in exercise require increased amounts of oxygen and other nutrients and produce increased amounts of waste which need to be carried away; increased heart action is needed to move blood through the body during

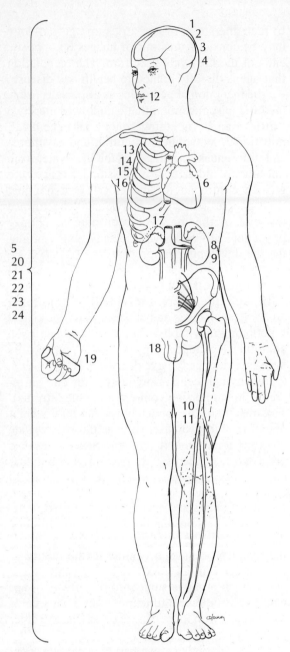

exercise. However, with advanced age, the heart is less able to do this, pumping only 65 percent of the blood at age 75 that was provided at age 30. At rest the aging individual's heart rate may be within normal limits (44 to 108 beats per minute). During periods of exercise, the heart rate increases as it pumps more blood at higher pressure, the duration of systole being slightly increased. However, the heart of the elderly person cannot achieve as great an increase in rate as the young individual. Thus, during exercise, the increase in the older person's heart rate is more than that of the younger individual performing the same exercise.[16]

Perhaps the most notable event in recent times which might best exemplify these data was the tennis match between Billie Jean King and Bobby Riggs. Pregame publicity billed this as a contest of male chauvinistic standards versus the woman's movement for equality. However, as the match progressed and it became evident that the 58-year-old Riggs was having trouble "keeping up" with someone 30 years his junior, sports commentators and observers alike spoke of the disparity in years that separated the players, ultimately attributing age rather then sex as the cause of Rigg's defeat.

There are many theoretical answers to the question of what causes biological aging and resultant physiological change. Two of the more popular theories follow.[17] The "accumulation of copying errors" is a theory that assumes correct replication of cells may only occur a limited number of times. As the organism ages, "copying errors" occur in cellular replication (DNA transfer to RNA messenger) and cellular muta-

FIGURE 9-1.

Physiologic decline accompanying age appears in many measurements throughout the body. Changes are great in some cases, small in others. Figures in brackets are approximate percentages of functions or tissues remaining to the average 75-year-old male, taking the value found for the average 30-year-old as 100 percent. 1 brain weight [56]; 2 memory loss; 3 slower speed of response; 4 blood flow to brain [80]; 5 speed of return to equilibrium of blood acidity [17]; 6 cardiac output (at rest) [70]; 7 number of glomeruli in kidney [56]; 8 glomerular filtration rate [69]; 9 kidney plasma flow [50]; 10 number of nerve trunk fibers [63]; 11 nerve conduction velocity [90]; 12 number of taste buds [36]; 13 maximum oxygen uptake (during exercise) [40]; 14 maximum ventilation volume (during exercise) [53]; 15 maximum breathing capacity (voluntary) [43]; 16 vital capacity [56]; 17 less adrenal activity; 18 less gonadal activity; 19 hand grip [55]; 20 maximum work rate [70]; 21 maximum work rate for short burst [40]; 22 basal metabolic rate [84]; 23 body water content [82]; 24 body weight for males [88].

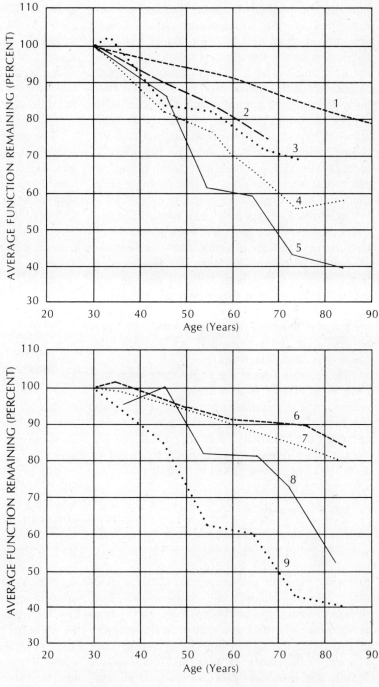

FIGURE 9-2.
Percentage changes with age for nine different physiological functions. The average value for each function at age 30 is 100 percent. small drop in basal metabolism is probably due simply to loss of cells. Source: Shock, N. W.: The physiology of aging. Sci. Am. 206:100 (January 1972).

1 Basal Metabolic Rate
2 Work Rate
3 Cardiac Output (At Rest)
4 Vital Capacity of Lungs
5 Maximum Breathing Capacity
(Voluntary)

6 Nerve Conduction Velocity
7 Body Water Content
8 Filtration Rate of Kidney
9 Kidney Plasma Flow

tion results. Inefficient cellular metabolism follows and further deleterious effects cause generalized organ decline. This theory has been the spring board for the "mean time to failure theory" which is basic to engineering principles. Supporters of this theory espouse that the human body has a limited potential longevity because its organs and organ systems are finite matter being affected by various traumas throughout the life cycle. Although the body may be repaired via medical/surgical intervention, total organ replacement is not possible, so that at some point failure of each organ system will occur.

In addition, it has long been recognized that "repeated exposure to small doses of radiation" may increase the rate of aging. The precise cause of cellular alteration is unknown. However, it has been noted that both radiated animals and aging animals show a rise in somatic cell mutations. Not accumulation of radiation per se but the "accumulation of deleterious material," such as lipofuscin (fatty pigments), in the cell may cause loss of cellular vitality.

These are a few of the many theories which have been offered in an attempt to explain the reasons for the inevitable physiological decline of the human body. It will be through answering correctly the questions about aging that our life expectancy (or years we may anticipate based on a statistical probability) will be lengthened.

Life Expectancy

Medical breakthroughs in drug therapy, such as, vaccines and antibiotics, and improved diagnostic ability of acute infectious diseases have primarily been an aid to increasing life expectancy of young children and young adults. Two thousand years ago a Roman baby had a projected longevity of 22 years. It took 19 centuries of slowly increasing life expectancy to raise the average to 40 years in 1850 in the New England States. This rose to 49 years for the total population of the United States in 1900. Dramatic increase has occurred since the turn of the century with a life of 60 years expected in 1930, and 63 years in 1940. In 1959 life expectancy in the United States was 66.5 years for males and 73

years for females. The average length of life in 1966 was 70 years, with the female outliving the male by 7 years (74 years, 67 years). However, since 1900 less than 3 years (2.3) have been added for men over age 40 and 6 years for women over age 40. That is, if a person survives to his fortieth year, his life expectancy is little improved over that of 70 years ago.[18]

The most important factor in reviewing data on projected longevity is that for individuals over 40 the percentage reaching old age has doubled, approaching a ratio of 1 in 10. Every 20 seconds someone turns 65. Although 3,000 persons age 65 and older die each day, by the end of the century, there will be 32 million citizens age 65 or over.[19] Substantial additional research must be done to discover the secrets of physiological aging and in treating its effects—those of chronic degenerative diseases that attack organ systems, particularly the cardiovascular.

Illness—Acute and Chronic

Due to the impact of age-linked functional disturbances on organs and organ systems, those who survive to age 65 or over most often suffer from chronic rather than the more easily cured acute diseases. When acute illness occurs, it may be due to influenzal illness, upper respiratory infection and/or other respiratory diseases, which taken together are the primary category of acute illness in the elderly. Accidental injury is the second most frequent cause of acute incapacitation in the aged, with approximately 3,500,000 cases reported. Injury is most often attributed to decreased visual acuity, hearing loss, and decreased speed of movement. The most common type of trauma sustained is contusion, followed by fractures, sprains, and dislocations. Digestive distress ranks as the third most common cause of acute illness among the aged.[20] However, Bromley suggests that rather than being due to atropic changes caused by the aging process, acute discomfort from heartburn, gas, indigestion, and constipation is usually caused by poor dietary habits. Constipation, an acute complaint, is usually due to observance of rigid bowel habits established in childhood rather than organic dysfunction.[21]

Chronic disease is usually marked by insidious onset. It is diagnostically difficult to delineate the effects of the physiological aging process from those of disease entity. Therefore, chronic illness may, in part, be attributed to the effect each has on the other. Compounding factors are a lessened level of immunity to pathogens, reduced awareness of disease symptoms, and possibly even a diminished concern over bodily health.[22] An example of the insidiousness of chronic ailment may be taken from prehistoric man who suffered from arthritis, the world's oldest known chronic disease. He did not wake up one morning with a sudden inability to grasp his spear. Rather, changes in bone and supporting tissue began to occur early in childhood and progressed throughout the life cycle. Today approximately 13 million Americans suffer from arthritis, which ranks second to heart disease as a cause of activity limitation in the elderly. The main types are osteoarthritis and rheumatoid arthritis. While the ratio in women is 3 to 1, 15 percent of the total population age 65 or over are affected by arthritis.[23] Other commonly diagnosed chronic diseases of old age are obesity, cataracts, varicose veins, abdominal cavity lesions, neurological disorders (dementia and parkinsonism) hypertension without heart disease, hemorrhoids, and among men, prostate disease. There are 400 chronic diseases per 1,000 of the population under age 15. At age 65 or over, 4,000 chronic diseases appear per 1,000 of the population.[24] Albeit some aged individuals may exhibit numerous disease entities while others will only manifest one or two.

A limited environment resulting from decreased mobility is perhaps the most debilitating effect of chronic disease. The rise in prevalence of chronic disease with age is reflected by the increased number of days spent in restricted activity. This increase is true for both sexes after age 25. The number of days of restricted activity is also influenced by family income, with lower income families having more ill days resulting from chronic disease than those at higher income levels. However, Kimmel suggests that low income may be a reflection of the effect of chronic conditions on the earning power of family members.[25] It is obvious that the older people become, the more effort they should give to keeping themselves in a state of good health. Illness in old age, whether acute or chronic, not only affects the diseased organ, but may also cause the failure of other organ systems which have undergone physiological aging or the attack of unrecognized disease.

Genetics and the Elderly

The role hereditary influences play in the old person's susceptibility to acute or chronic illness is certain only to the extent that genetic factors are known to operate throughout the life cycle. Specific gene mutations may introduce disease or disability that may modify the normal aging process. Chronic disability and even minor anomaly of long duration may considerably influence the elderly individual's psychosocial and physiological adjustment to the latter part of the life cycle. Although manifested in childhood, early adulthood, or middle age, genetic disease may assume greater consequence with advancing age.[26] For example, Mr. T., who has had diabetes mellitus in control since onset at age 32, may indeed find its control more difficult in advanced years. Age has brought on a forced retirement and retirement has meant a reduced income. Now unable to buy the same quality and types of food he was accustomed to, Mr. T. eats food high in starch and carbohydrate.

Multiple genetic factors also operate on each individual, young or old, in terms of longevity. Some families produce a high proportion of individuals who survive to advanced ages; others do not. Investigators in gerontological longevity find that individuals who survive to old age usually had parents and/or grandparents who also did. Kallman et al., studied 2,536 sets of twins, both monozygotic (twins identical in genetic constitution), and dizygotic (twins genetically as similar as any other siblings)—of which at least one member had passed age 60. Of 180 sets of twins, both having died after age 60, the average intrapair difference in life span was 36 months for monozygotic pairs, and 74.6 months for dizygotic pairs of the same sex. The average difference in life years for dizygotic twins of opposite sex was 106 months. These findings include the tendency for greater longevity among females. A direct relationship between parental age at time of death and the life span of the offspring has been established. Children of parents age 70 or over had average life spans of 62 years. Kallman concludes that genetic factors are significant determinants of potential longevity and health factors among the aged.[27] (See Chapter 6 for further discussion of genetics and health).

However, there is the problem, intrinsic to longevity, of being able to live through the latter years of the life cycle, well or ill, in an environment that encourages the creative expression of genetic abilities. An example might be Mrs. O'L., a 72-year-old widow, who was returned to her hospital room after successful surgery for a fractured right hip sustained by a fall at home. Several days postop, Mrs. O'L. continued to ring her call bell with minor requests for attention and had constant tasks for any nurse who ventured into her room. Mrs. O'L.'s roommate, Mrs. H., was disturbed at these events since she felt she was being overlooked by the nurses, who in an attempt to avoid Mrs. O'L.'s commands, did not come into the room. Mrs. H., a 41-year-old art teacher, was empathetic about Mrs. O'L.'s lack of visitors and attention. Mrs. H. questioned her roommate as to possible hobbies she had pursued prior to her fall. Inquiry revealed Mrs. O'L. to be an accomplished painter who subsequently spent much time talking to Mrs. H. about techniques in oil painting which she had developed. The constant demands made on the nursing staff by Mrs. O'L. ceased as she was encouraged to renew her identity as a talented painter.

Mortality

Death as the final stage of the life cycle may occur in "old age" but does not occur *because* of "old age." As previously stated, death is a consequence of a specific disease entity. The chief cause of mortality at all age levels, and of approximately 80 percent of deaths after age 65, is cardiovascular disease (including coronary heart disease and stroke). Cancer and accidental injury rank second and third respectively. For 1968, the eight leading causes of death for the general population of the United States was 1) heart disease; 2) cancer: The American Cancer Society reported that over half of all diagnosed carcinomas were among those over 65; 3) stroke: 1.6 million Americans are stroke victims each year and it accounts for 12 percent of deaths in the elderly; 4) influenza and pneumonia; 5) arteriosclerosis; 6) accidents; 7) diabetes mellitus: each year 2 million new cases are reported and an additional 2 million undiagnosed are estimated, with 40 percent of these occurring in those over 65 years; and 8) respiratory disease (bronchitis, emphysema, and asthma) in which there has been an 800 percent increase in incidence in the past ten years. Men died more often than women from 1) bronchitis; 2) emphysema and asthma; 3) vehicular accidents; 4) cancer; 5) influenza and pneumonia; and 6) heart disease. Blacks and other races age 65 to 74 died twice as often as whites of the same age from 1) cardiovascular disease; 2) diabetes mellitus; 3) influenza and pneumonia; and 4) arteriosclerosis.[28]

The impaired function of organs and organ systems with age obviously increases the probability of disease and death. In 1825, Benjamin Gompertz, an English insurance actuary, realizing that the mortality rate (excluding premature and accident-related deaths) increases exponentially with age, published a mathematical equation with which projected longevity could be calculated. Gompertz' equation is $R = R_0e^{at}$ the letter R represents the chance of dying at any age, R_0 represents a mathematical constant related to the predicted chance of dying at age 0, and a is a constant that describes the rate of increase of mortality as a function of age; e is the base of natural logarithms, and t is age in years.[29] The application of this equation demonstrates the increased occurrence of death among those members of the population who have undergone the physiological aging process (Fig. 9-3).

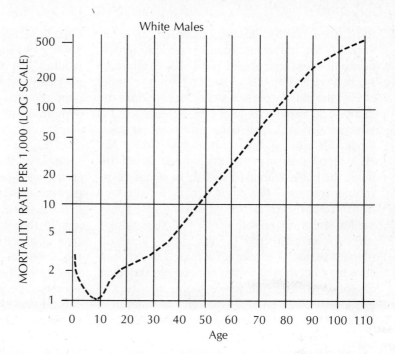

FIGURE 9-3.
Gompertz plot. Mortality rate as a function of age, United States, 1938-41. Between age 30 and 90 the data obey the equation $R = R_0 e^{at}$. R_0 (the initial mortality rate at time 0) and a (the increase in the mortality rate over time) are constants which depend on the population; e is the base of natural logarithms and ^{t} is the age in years. Source: Busse, E. and Pfeifer, E.: Behavior and Adaptation in Late Life. Boston, Little, Brown, 1969, p. 15.

Cardiovascular Decompensation

One author projects that if an individual's organs and organ systems were always in the same state of resistance to disease, stress, and/or injury as was present at age 12, it would be possible for that person to live another 700 years.[30] Currently in America, it is not possible to live much beyond 20 years without being affected by cardiovascular disease.[31] Beginning early in life and progressing throughout the life cycle, arteriosclerosis is the major contributing factor to cardiovascular decline. (See Chapter 12 concerning the heart, in health and in disease.)

HEART

Except for the collection of lipofuscin within the cardiac muscle cells, the generalized effect of the physiological aging process on the myocardium is negligible when compared to the effects of hemodynamic stress. Contrary to most body tissues, the amount of connective tissue in the myocardium does not increase concurrently with age. Hypertrophy is not a result of age, but rather a response to increased demands on the heart muscle. Fragmentation of elastic fibers, lipid de-

posit, accumulation of collagenous tissue and smooth muscle changes occur, but are for the most part specific to the endocardium.[32]

Reduced cardiac output occurs with age and is contributed to by the effects of arteriosclerosis on coronary vessels. Preferential areas of lipid deposit in coronary vessels occur at the first portion of the anterior descending branch of the left coronary artery, the first part of the descending branch of the right coronary artery, and the bend of the acute margin in the right coronary artery. Although how much of arteriosclerosis is due to aging and how much to disease is not known, there is increased prevalence of arteriosclerosis with advancing age. Generally, incidence is lower in females than males during early adult life, a sex difference which has been attributed to protective properties of estrogen.[33]

Correct evaluation of the aging patient occurs when the nurse is cognizant of the effects that ensue from a compromised cardiovascular system. For example, Mr. H., an 83-year-old retired sheet metal worker, was brought to the emergency room for removal of a foreign body from the right eye. The ER nurse recorded initial vital signs as Bp 200/108 p 90 r 16. After making the patient comfortable and offering verbal assurance, the nurse rechecked the vital signs to determine the effect the patient's excitement might have had on the admission findings. Under stress, the elderly person's cardiac rate does not increase as rapidly as might be expected in the young individual, and once increased, it takes longer for vital signs to return to normal.[34] Mr. H.'s blood pressure was unchanged at 200/108 while the pulse decreased slightly to 86 and respirations remained 16. Blood pressure rises with age in response to increased arterial resistance. Under stress, increased stroke volume compensates for an ineffective cardiac rate to raise the blood pressure. Therefore, increased blood pressure may be viewed as the normal physiological response to insure adequate blood flow to kidneys, heart, and brain. However, the amount of increase in systolic and diastolic pressures, resulting from the compensating mechanism is not yet agreed upon.

The rule of thumb for determining the appropriate level of increased blood pressure is 100 mm Hg plus the age of the patient. Perhaps this formula seems too simplistic for some researchers who believe the "normal" limits for the elderly should be higher than those allowed by this means of evaluation. According to W. Ferguson Anderson, who considers a systolic pressure between 215 and 230 mm Hg and a diastolic pressure of 110 to 120 mm Hg within normal limits, a blood pressure reading of 200/108 mm Hg would be an essentially normal finding. He espouses that exuberance in artificially lowering the blood pressure in the elderly patient may cause hypotension and resultant inadequate blood flow to heart, brain, and kidneys.[35]

Other researchers of hypertension such as Edward Freis, Herbert Benson, and John Laragh, would disagree. Rather than causing hypotension in the elderly, their treatment is aimed at averting stroke, heart disease, and kidney ischemia by decreasing dangerously demanding levels of pressure on physiologically aged arteries. Since there seems to be a correlation between levels of blood pressure and projected longevity (see Fig. 9-2), and in view of the current hypertensive research, it would be the

nurse's responsibility not only to advise the attending physician of the increased blood pressure reading, but also to encourage the patient to report any dizziness, blurred vision, precardial pain, reduced urinary output, or other associated symptoms of ischemic responses to hypertension.

BRAIN

In the aged population the cumulative effects of cardiovascular changes are evident not only as heart disease, but also as cerebral ischemia (at age 75 the brain receives 20 percent less blood than at age 30), and infarction. More than being the result of brain hemorrhage, stroke is now seen to be the result of thrombosed intracranial vessels superimposed on already arteriosclerotic carotid and extracranial arteries.[36]

Stroke may be diagnosed as 1) transient ischemic attack (TIA, neurological deficit occurs abruptly and lasts a few minutes to 24 hours then disappears completely); 2) reversible ischemic neurological deficit (RIND, in which neurological deficit lasts from several hours to two or three days before complete recovery is observed; 3) stroke, in-evolution (begins initially as small neurological deficit but over several hours or days evolves into full insult); 4) completed stroke, or abrupt neurological deficit without remission for several days to years, and in which there is no complete recovery.[37]

Neurological deficit resulting from the physiological aging process manifests itself within the central nervous system (CNS), where complex connections are made (See Chapter 20). There is relatively little deficit at the level where nerve fibers connect directly with muscle cells. The physical changes exhibited by the CNS are the result of loss of nonreplicating neural cells, and the accumulation of lipofuscin in the remaining neurons throughout the brain (which results in disturbance of liposomal function). Reduced numbers of basic functioning neurons increase progressively with age. Increased amounts of connective tissue take the place of nerve fibers, thus reducing the capacity for impulse transmission to and from the brain. Although Shock reports that speed of nerve impulses along single fibers is not seriously affected, with only a 10 percent to 15 percent loss in elderly people when compared to the young, clinically the old individual presents a slowed reaction time (time between a signal and the subject's response) and increased time needed for decision making and task completion.[38] The "old man" who takes "all morning" to fill out the day's menu is a classic example.

Difficulty in remembering recent events or recently learned facts is the clinical manifestation of neurochemical changes, albeit long-term memory such as vocabulary skills, personal history, past experience, and knowledge appears unaffected by such changes.[39] The elderly patient recovering from cataract surgery who must learn how to wear and care for contact lenses need not be a teaching problem. Given sufficient time in an unpressured atmosphere, the aged learn. When learning, they focus their attention on detail and specifics, rather than on ideas or concepts. Therefore, it would be helpful to employ teaching aids which would physically demonstrate the material given in verbal instruction. For example, visual demonstration of proper insertion and cleansing of contact lenses repeated at frequent intervals will reinforce what has been communicated verbally.

ORGANIC BRAIN SYNDROME. Most often associated with symptoms of memory loss and impairment of intellectual functioning and judgment is organic brain syndrome, a diagnosis most commonly given the aged who present psychiatric symptoms. This may be the result of the broad definition given by the Diagnostic and Statistical Manual of Mental Disorder published by the American Psychiatric Association. It describes organic brain syndrome as a "basic mental condition characteristically resulting from diffuse impairment of brain tissue function from whatever cause." As a result, 2.3 percent of the elderly are considered to have organic brain syndrome. Depending upon the level of reversibility, the syndrome may be acute, as in TIA, or chronic, with permanent brain dysfunction.[40]

Included as a division of organic brain syndrome are degenerative dementias (Alzheimer's disease, arteriosclerotic disease, Pick's lobar atrophy, subacute spongiform encephalopathy, parkinsonism-dementia complex, and a few rarities), in which the elderly person presents gradual loss of memory, impaired judgment, general decrease in intelligence (as measured by tests of comprehension), loss of general knowledge, and lessened learning ability. Early clinically observed signs of loss of sociability, mobility and impaired affect, and depression give way to symptoms of advanced dementia in which delusion, hallucination, and disorientation appear.[41] Postmortem examinations of elderly persons diagnosed as having organic brain syndrome show senile brains as atrophic, changed in convolution, and having thickened cerebral arteries and reduced numbers of neurons, with those remaining being discolored and shrunken.[42]

Perhaps one of the most difficult encounters in nursing assessment and care of the elderly is that which occurs when a patient presents the pattern of faulty perception, slowed reaction, and difficulty making an appropriate response (see Chapter 20). Often the elderly patient labeled uncooperative, confused, or senile may have difficulty perceiving verbal and environmental cues, thus giving inappropriate responses to them. Speaking slowly in a normal tone of voice (unless the patient has an obvious auditory deficit) and waiting until the initial question or statement is responded to before initiating further communication often aids the patient in making an appropriate response.

COMMUNICATION SYSTEMS. Stone suggests that the intercommunication system used in hospitals or other institutions may distort the nurse's voice so that the elderly patient may not understand what is being said. "If the older person presses the button and a disembodied voice replies, 'yes, can I help you?' he can become so confused that in attempting to reply he forgets his reason for ringing the bell and fails to make his need known."[43] A test conducted by the nurse to evaluate the patient's ability to understand what is being said over the call system may avoid many anxious moments for both the patient and the nursing staff. Another call system, such as providing a dinner bell to be rung for attention, may need to be instituted.

KIDNEY

Renal disease among the aged is rarely diagnosed as an acute condition. Usually years of gradual degeneration of renal tissue occur before kidney reserves become exhausted and renal disease becomes evident. White reports that autopsy findings of old people show cardiovascular change to manifest itself in the form of nephrosclerosis.[44] A serious complication of the aged, ischemia, atrophy of parenchyma, and fibrosis of the kidney results from the nephrosclerotic process.

Physiological decline of kidney function occurs with age as the kidney becomes smaller in size, and there is a decreased number of functioning glomeruli (see Fig. 9-1), some having been worn out or destroyed by disease and replaced with scar tissue (see Chapter 17, the Insulted Kidney). Glomerular filtration rate decreases, and at age 75 is 69 percent of what it was at age 30.[45] Because of decreased glomerular filtration rate (GFR), the level of blood urea nitrogen accepted as normal increases with advancing age, rising from 12.9 mg per 100 ml at age 40 to 21.2 mg per 100 ml at age 70. Further, due to the combined effects of decreased GFR and the kidney's reduced ability to concentrate urine, prompt replacement of any lost body fluids or gastrointestinal contents is essential. Thus, Papper suggests the parenteral hydration of aged patients during preparatory enemas, catharsis, and restriction of oral intake involved in gastrointestinal X-ray studies.[46] Second only to the brain, which requires 15 to 20 percent, the kidney at rest requires 9 percent of the total body consumption of oxygen. At age 75, blood flow to the kidneys is reduced to 42 percent of the amount it received at age 30. Shock suggests that this is an adaptive mechanism to allow greater blood flow to the brain.[47] However, it leaves the kidneys susceptible to any bodily insult, such as infection, anemia, surgical trauma, or the like, which might further decrease blood flow to an already compensated renal system.

Since the length of time a drug is capable of acting on the body is contingent upon the amount of time it stays in the body in active form, reduced renal blood flow and decreased numbers of functioning nephrons may result in inadequate elimination of administered drugs.[48] The nurse should be acutely aware of signs and symptoms of drug toxicity and should discourage the use of self-administered "over the counter" drugs.

Sexual Vistas and the Elderly

It is frequently thought that there is no sexual activity over age 60. Certain physiological changes occur in both male and female; however, neither sex loses sexual needs or function concomitant with age. Most researchers feel that sexual patterns established in the earlier years of the life cycle are reflected in later life. Masters and Johnson's studies of human sexual behavior in the elderly conclude that males who have experienced high sexual "output," in their earlier years will be more likely to continue those sexual habits in old age. Females who have engaged in regular sexual relations throughout the life cycle will also desire its continuance.[49] Comfort states that: "The things that stop you having sex with age are exactly the same as those that stop you riding a bicycle (bad health, thinking it looks silly, no bicycle). The difference is that they happen later for sex than for bicycles."[50]

Frustration and anxiety about meeting such needs may well underlie or contribute to ill health or exacerbation of already present disease. Freeman reports a case in which a 72-year-old widow contacted a physician for complaint of periodic abdominal pain. Routine studies and hospital evaluation were negative for organic cause. The patient, who was accompanied at each office visit by her spinster daughter, was unable to offer any clues. One day in the absence of her daughter, the patient began to cry and related that she had been troubled for months by a recurring dream in which her deceased husband returned and made love to her, leaving her sexually satisfied. The patient felt guilty and ashamed about these experiences, fearing that her daughter might find out. When it was explained that this was a normal response, the patient became irritated and refused further treatment. It was later learned that her abdominal pain disappeared.[51]

In the male, testicular changes occur in terms of reduced size and firmness of the organ, as well as a thickening of membranes within the tubules of the testicles, which are responsible for the production of sperm. Although there is reduced sperm production with age, the male's capability to produce progeny never ceases. Seymour and associates report a case history of a man born in 1840 who had had 16 children by his first wife who had died in 1924. In 1932, he remarried a 27-year-old woman, and at the age of 95 fathered another child. That man died at the age of 103. Postmortem examination of his sperm showed the spermatozoa to be of average size and 65 percent normal in number.[52]

The organic changes in the genitourinary system specifically resultant from an increase in the size of the prostrate may cause sexual dysfunction. However, barring disease, the only significant change in the male over the first seven decades of the life cycle is that spontaneous erection occurs less frequently, ejaculation takes longer, and there is more concern over performance of the sexual act.[53]

Women differ from men in their sexual aging in that there is clear delineation of the end of reproductivity via cessation of menstruation. For most women, climacteric occurs in the late 40s or 50s with women who begin menstruating early in life ending menstruation later in life. The progressive decline of gonadal endocrine stimulation to reproductive organs which occurs at this time causes physiological aging of genital tissue and reproductive organs. As the pituitary-gonadal-uterine mechanism reaches a nonfunctionary activity level, specific physical changes in both internal and external reproductive organs occur. For example, vulvar hair becomes sparse and gray; the vulva becomes pallid and the labia shrunken; thinning and atrophy of the vaginal wall occur; the vaginal canal shortens and loses elasticity and moisture; and there is regression of mammary tissue.[54] However, there is little if any physical change related to sex function (except in frequency, which may be attributed to the death of a partner) to age 75 and beyond. Contrary to the belief that diminished sexual function, when it occurs, is a result of impotence or frigidity, the causes of sexual decline are those imposed by diseases such as arthritis, arteriosclerotic heart disease, genitourinary dysfunction, and the like and not by the aging process per se. Comfort states that up to one half of the couples of the age group 75 and above have sex on a regular basis.[55]

In search of an attractive, attentive partner, increasing numbers of individuals are looking for ways to make themselves more attractive. Many find the answer in plastic surgery. In fact, it has been the rhytidectomy (face-lift) that has given the pseudonym "applied geriatrics" to plastic surgery.[56] For the most part, it is the increased amount of collagen fiber in the connective tissue which surrounds the cells that causes facial change with age. Although the rhytidectomy is the procedure most commonly employed, brow-lift, blepharoplasty, rhinoplasty, and surgical abrasion (to eradicate fine wrinkles) are performed as well.

At this juncture, it may be assumed that a review of the data presented on the physiological effects of the aging process will show positive proof of the negative factors involved in reaching the latter years of the life cycle. However, the factors of disability attributed to physiological aging severely limit only a small number of elderly people. The belief that most "old people" are relegated to "old age homes" simply is not true. In 1970, only 5 percent of persons over 65 recorded permanent residence as a nursing home or other institution. The remaining 95 percent resided in the community. Of these, 81 percent reported no physical impairment that limited ability to move about and 14 percent reported no chronic impairment.[57]

Whether as members of the majority living in the community or of the small number residing in a nursing home or other institution, the elderly continue the developmental process. How they perform the developmental tasks at each stage will be reflected by their performances in meeting the developmental tasks involved in aging, that is, retirement, widowhood, loss of life long friends, and so on. Sutterly and Donnelly describe the individual as an open system (see Chapter 1). The physiological process of aging may constrict that system, but does not stop the flow of the developmental process which continues throughout the life cycle. The chronological age of 65 or older does not surreptitiously leave an individual insensitive, unperceptive, or asexual.

Sociological Factors in Aging

Although no one group of factors constitutes the single means by which old age is determined, social factors have particular and sometimes unexpected potency. However, these factors seldom act in concert to produce distinct, readily observable results. For example, group identity is a means by which individuals adopt standards that provide legitimacy and security for their behavior. Thus, it is permissible for someone who is 75 to be crotchety, but not to be a "cry-baby." In the first instance he is merely "acting his age," while in the second supposedly he is not (even though both behaviors may be essentially equivalent as short-tempered, ill-humored responses). Consequently there is a "sorting-out" process whereby both the individual and his observers learn to catagorize behavior, and there appears to be a tendency for stricter observance of behavioral standards as age increases.[58]

Certainly most people behave in accordance with prevailing group standards. But group standards and norms are not all that clear, nor will everyone adopt them, at least not all of the time. Even among the standards that people adopt there will be many they do not share. In addition, each person will not be identically perceived by other people. For example, a 50-year-old may be perceived as old by a 20-year-old and as young by someone who is 70, each of whom would expect certain behavior. This is especially true if the 50-year-old is relatively feeble or relatively robust. Hence, group identity can strongly influence behavior, but at the same time it is not irresistible or unchanging.

Of course, there are a number of extrinsic factors which have worked to shape the elderly into a minority group. Certainly in terms of number they are a minority group. Even though the number of people age 65 and older increased from 3 million to over 20 million between 1900

and 1970—nearly double the rate of increase for the overall population—they still represent only 9.6 percent of the population.[59] But more than statistical infrequency or visual cues are necessary before the aged can be considered a minority group. Various influences and conditions have to produce stable differences within the group to establish characteristics which not only distinguish them from the general population, but are also somewhat self-perpetuating.[60]

Even though the necessary conditions might not prevail which would technically qualify those over 65 as belonging to a minority group, the conditions that do exist seem to be changing. For example, factors such as the sheer increase in numbers, employment, compulsory retirement, social activities, living conditions, and the structure of the family are all creating new problems for the aged. Consequently, more attention than ever before is being directed toward solution of these problems.[61] In addition, a subculture is being produced by the increased interaction of the elderly with each other.[62] Group consciousness is heightened by such events as enforced retirement, the availability of pensions, and even by admission into retirement communities. Changes in the family structure contribute indirectly to the formation of Golden Age or Senior Citizen clubs in which many elderly engage in the majority of their socializing.

The combination of increased problems and heightened awareness has led to the development of organizations such as the Gray Panthers, which are devoted to the alleviation of problems specific to old people. The old are being courted by politicians who are becoming aware of their special interests and emerging cohesiveness. And the old are becoming increasingly and vocally dissatisfied with the image that has developed of their inadequacies.[63]

Stereotypes

Among the more damaging influences shaping the environment and thinking of the elderly are the prevailing social stereotypes. One of the most widespread beliefs in Western society is that old people don't have "it." Even within the scientific and health communities, it was and is believed that by the time someone is 70 he has lost most of his abilities, a process of loss which is felt to start in the 30s or 40s. It was maintained that the average 80-year-old functioned at the intellectual level of a 12-year-old. This accorded with "common sense"—which translates as a willingness to think in terms of averages. Of course, one of the unfortunate aspects of living is that, if people live long enough, they will become less able—a "fact" which has received considerable scientific verification.[64] But these findings are interpreted in the light of assumptions which are currently receiving critical re-examination.

When stereotypes deteriorate into subtle forms of prejudice, they become particularly harmful. Stereotypes result from efforts to give coherence to a set of facts. Prejudice is the formation of opinion in the absence of facts. It is this distinction which is commonly lost. One of the distinguishing features and more devastating consequences of prejudices is that the holder typically imputes negative attributes to outgroups.[65] And possibly at no time in history have the elderly been more of an outgroup. The exercise of authority, responsibility for finances, caretaking of tradition, being sought for counseling, and so on have all passed from the hands of the elderly. Present social institutions and even the very pace of modern living tend to deny the elderly their previous roles. They no longer have traditional rites of passage to ease their transition into new roles. Butler and Lewis suggest that this can be "disconcerting and disorienting, particularly if the older person feels or is some way personally victimized by change."[66] Often the burden of "ageism", is added to the prejudices the elderly have been dealing with all of their lives. This is especially true for women and blacks.[67]

Ageism is a prejudice founded on a number of myths, four of which are related to aspects of aging which are especially susceptible to distortion: chronological age, senility, tranquility, and unproductivity.[68] The particularly strong impressions surrounding the myth of chronological age are partly responsible for the efforts to establish retirement at age 65. Yet the evidence is clear that the rates of psychological, social, and physiological aging vary widely among individuals.[69] With advancing years, differences among people in the relative effects of "age" tend to *increase*.

Most stereotypes concerning chronological age can more accurately be applied to the young, for example, running speed. If any "stereotype" were to be valid, it would be that almost all healthy 30-year-olds can run quite well. On the other hand, at 70 years of age some people can run nearly as fast as they could at 30, most would be slower, and some could only manage a fast walk. With regard to verbal abilities, the same kind of distribution would exist, but some people in their 70s would actually show improvement relative to age 30. For those showing loss, the degree would be less than it would be for running. Yet regardless of this retention and even improvement in verbal skills, there is no shift in social expectancies. For example, a brick layer may experience a reduction in work proficiency and an improvement in other skills. But society has made no provision for his making a shift to a new job. There are new efforts to educate both the individual and the public, but they have not been adequate. Many people are forced to continue in jobs for which they are becoming less suited while being excluded from jobs they could easily handle. Perhaps the efforts at re-education need especially to deal with sex role stereotypes—other stereotypes would indirectly but necessarily be modified. Then it may be that the future will see a merging of work and social expectancies that would capitalize on shifting individual proficiencies.

Our social stereotypes and programs also need to consider the unlimited examples of people who maintained their overall vigor when they were in their 80s and 90s. Despite evidence that undiminished activity is a possibility *and* an attraction for many older people, they are still admonished, by health professionals and others, to "slow down" and to "act your age." In contrast, it is not only a more positive attitude, it is more accurate to acknowledge that "you're as old as you feel." A 1975 television program on aging presented interviews with people who had changed occupations after "retirement." Some had earned their first million when in their 70s and *after* starting new careers. All reported that the chance to remain active or to reinvest their energies was like "a new lease on life." They became what they saw themselves as becoming.

Senility is a frightening spectre associated with old age and it, too, is largely a myth. It is assumed by most laypeople, and many in the health professions, to be inevitable—it will happen to all of us and much too soon. The evidence indicates that this is not the case. First, senility is not a medical term. It is an overused and misused term referring to a wide variety of unrelated disorders, chief among them being the functional— as opposed to organic—disorders, such as depression, apathy, and so on. Second a small positive correlation exists between intellectual deterioration and the degree of brain impairment for persons exhibiting signs of disorder. This is called senile dementia, and "is characterized neuroanatomically by cerebral atrophy, senile plaque formation, neurofibrillary tangles, and lipid accumulation."[70] The relationship between the senile psychosis observed as part of this condition and the mild memory loss and confusion occurring among nonpsychotic older persons is not known. However, for people residing in the community and in relatively good health the incidence of senile dementia is rare.[71]

Related to the above is the misconception that a large percentage of the over 65 live in various institutions. As stated previously, actually only 5 percent of people past 65 live in institutions.[72] The vast majority are self-sufficient and although there is a trend toward separate households for the elderly, the extended family is still the rule.[73]

A third myth is that of old age as a period of tranquility. It is considered to be a time of peace and ease, a time when the old can reap the fruits of their labors. Yet the news media are replete with stories of the hardships experienced by the elderly, including poor housing, inadequate medical care, and meager recreation. A trend noted by newspapers and newsmagazines is the increase in sales of canned dog food to the elderly and other minority groups as food prices escalate. The phrase "their savings were wiped out" is particularly applicable to the old. Even retirees who have some savings, income from social security, and possibly a part-time job find that one medical problem can become a financial disaster. Medicare is only partial protection—inflation reaches everywhere. Thus, the emotional tranquility that might be anticipated is frequently destroyed by unexpected events and by a sense of loss and betrayal. Rather than tranquility, old age may be a period of frustration for many.

Another unsubstantiated belief is that the late years are necessarily or voluntarily a period of unproductivity. It is assumed that old people do not want to work and are no longer capable of high level performance. Actually many people past 65 are still employed and given a chance many more would be.[74] The forces operating to remove the older person from the work force are almost entirely independent of personal choice. For example, there is constant updating of job skills which leaves a growing proportion of older workers untrained, even if not unfit. There is a negative attitude toward hiring older workers. There is also a host of factors, not substantial by themselves, which contribute to unemployment for the elderly: more jobs once held by older males are being filled by younger females; there is less self-employment retirement benefits are often contingent upon reduced earnings; increased mechanization is simply eliminating some jobs (e.g., train conductors and switchmen); and there are simply more people in general competing for fewer jobs.[75]

THE PERPETUATION OF MYTHS

Part of the reason certain stereotypes and myths regarding the elderly have achieved such potency is because of the apparent support from developments in the field of mental measurement. Toward the end of the last century, the primary concern of psychology was how the "mind" worked, how people did their thinking. Then, in the 1890s, a major bifurcation took place. Freud began his studies of personality and Binet began his work on the measurement of mental abilities. Until Binet's time, mental functioning had been measured by such things as the size and shape of one's head, visual acuity, and physical reactions.

Binet was asked to provide a stable means of differentiating those who would benefit from schooling and those who would not be able to deal successfully with school work.

Thus, the impetus for the construction of tests of intelligence was directly related to the prediction of success in school. Previous measures had not been able to do this. Binet's scales did because they were designed to include aspects of behavior integral to school performance. He used test items which were appropriate to each of the grade levels. This was the key to his success. His intuition was that for his purposes, the most crucial feature of intelligence was its developmental nature. It seems obvious now, but it was a major breakthrough to think of intelligence as age related. He was the first to use the age-level approach in which items are included in the test which have been correctly answered by a majority of children at each age level. For example, a child earned a mental age rating of seven if he passed the test items which had been included because the *average* child of seven had successfully answered them. Binet's working assumption was that an item was appropriate to a given age level if approximately 70 percent of children at that age could "pass" it while a lower percentage of younger children would not pass it and a higher percentage of older children would.

Of course, these items were relevant to the school environment and were drawn from the experience of a child growing up in turn of the century Paris. A straight translation of the Binet items into other languages for use in their respective countries proved fruitless—the scales did not predict school success. So the items were modified or replaced. But somehow the use of the scales grew to include adult performance. Assumptions were made regarding the construct of intelligence which were not intended by the early test constructors and which have developed into the "myth of intelligence."

Intelligence became not only a description of behavior, but a permanent and unquestioned *cause* for certain behavior.[76] Intelligence was something one inherited, like height or an endocrine system. It was a biological entity and, as such, was subject to the same laws and influences as all biological structures or processes.[77] But intelligence remains a description of behavior, not an explanation for behavior. It is a *way* of responding to events; it is not something we have. The difficulty in making a clear distinction here may be because it may be impossible to separate what we can do from what we have learned or "know." Yet these tests which do so well in predicting scholastic aptitude seem not to do at all well in predicting success in later life endeavors including learning and assimilating regimens to maintain or restore health.[78] This simple but critical fact is disregarded by those who insist on using intelligence measures in ways inappropriate to the important changes in what a person knows or can do.[79]

A RECONCEPTUALIZATION OF ABILITY

The same considerations apply to the concept of creativity. It, too, is assumed by some to be an entity, a special ability that only a few favored mortals possess and which is only poorly or fleetingly available to the rest of us. Instead, creativity, like intelligence, seems to be a functional modality—a way of responding.[80] It is the resultant operation of all of the acquired skills, preferences, and momentary urges a person can bring to bear. It is directly franchised by the personal history, immediate circumstances, and special concerns that exist for a person at any point in time. It is the particular combination of acquired abilities relevant to the achievement of a desired goal (See Chapter 1 regarding the creative process, systems theory and human development). In other words, one uses those abilities one has learned to use.

The abilities a person uses will include skills in which he or she has achieved special proficiency, skills he or she has developed a preference for, and those his or her perception of the situation indicate may be appropriate. This process is the result of experience and conscious decision. The importance of personal choice should not be underestimated, for there is growing reason to believe that performance styles are primarily determined by personal choice, often in interaction with situational variables.[81] The manner in which this process might be enacted is

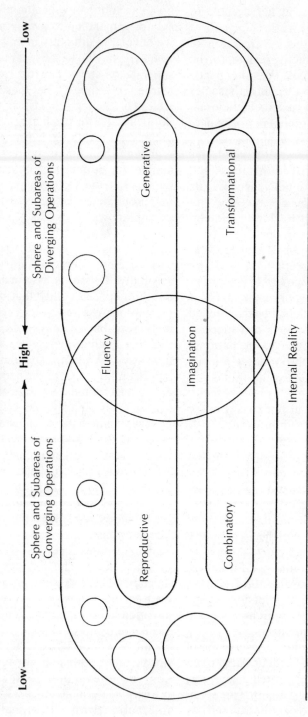

Performance Effectiveness

FIGURE 9-4.

Model representing the acquired skills and functional modalities through which the individual interacts with his environment. Contact with the environment can occur at any point and to any extent.

at that point which, according to the person's perception, his or her skills match the demands of the environment (Fig. 9-4).

Performance efficiency will be determined by factors not specified in this model, but the particular approach to dealing with a situation or a problem will be governed by factors represented here. Broadly conceived, the intellective and creative "spheres" are seen as two general modalities or ways of responding to a problem. Then there are two general skills which operate as messengers linking the more specific skills together: fluency, which ranges from the reproduction of acquired knowledge to the generation of new items;[82] and imagination, which ranges from the combination to the transformation of elements in the acquired repertoire.[83]

Importantly, this conceptualization of performance provides a broad outline for understanding the operation of various skills in relation to age. First, it can deal with the evidence that is accumulating that personality factors govern the selection and even the application of cognitive skills.[84] A performance style may interfere with, rather than facilitate performance; yet the person will insist on employing that combination of skills. This is interpreted as rigidity, and, although it has traditionally been considered as a cause of lowered performance in the elderly, new evidence indicates that it may be due to learning inadequacies and that it is not a permanent condition inevitable with age.[85] (This certainly has implications for nurses working with and teaching elderly patients in a variety of settings.)

Second, it can deal with the strong experimental evidence that concerns the loss of memory with age.[86] Here the memory loss may be shown to be due as much to personality factors as to permanent (organic) debility. Thus, fear and uncertainty result in interference in the retrieval mechanism essential to facile access to the memory store. Once this process begins, it is compounded by a reluctance to experiment or take chances and the person begins to rely increasingly on his best-learned skills—even when they are less appropriate to the task demands. These well-learned skills are part of the ensemble of skills subsumed under the term intelligence.[87]

The Impact of Attitudes Toward the Elderly

One of the ironies of stereotypes is that they are most devastating to those who are weakest to defend themselves: the socially disenfranchised, the young, the old, and the sick. Being old *and* sick leaves one especially vulnerable to intrusions from a world structured around the young and the healthy. The old not only occupy a peripheral role in Western societies, they also come to feel they are held in diminished perspective by others.[88] What was once theirs by request must now be shouted for—and even then they may be ignored. They feel rejected and may interpret this as a form of contempt. This leads to a subtle and irresistible erosion of their self-concept. They feel they are no longer masters of their own fates. They begin to become passive, to withdraw, to "give up." When the perceived violations of their sanctity become too great, they may "strike out." This may manifest itself in irascibility, petulance, or noncooperation. They may want to be pleasant, but physical discomfort and/or mental distress and uncertainty may lead to contradictory behavior. They may demand attention, then, when they get it, behave as though they wish to be left alone. Their "timing" is affected. Their participation may have been spurned so often that they may no longer know when or how to cooperate. Well-meaning relatives, friends, nurses or other caretakers may compound their plight by being overly-solicitous or protective. In these instances, the tendency is to strive for *maintenance* or restoration of the old person's capacities. On the other hand, the old person sees his existence in terms of a continuing process, however interrupted. He is, in large measure, growth-oriented and adapted to *change*.[89] Accordingly, he will resist importunities to "relax and get some rest." He accepts confinement to bed and dependence on others not so much because of physical need, as because of learned tolerance and emotional resignation. When first confronted with illness, he may hold his personal goals in abeyance. Then, because he is related to as though he has no goals, he begins to yield his image of himself and to abandon his tendency toward self-actualization. If told what to do often enough, his self-determination and willingness to make decisions become impaired.

Of course, not all people wish to be self-determining nor do all people have the energy or resources with which to accomplish their goals. They are more reactive than active.[90] They prefer to acquiesce to the demands and pressures of their environment. The prognosis for their physical and mental health is poor. Yet this need not be so. The nurse should consider that even withdrawn, retiring people are goal directed and have special preferences—it may not seem so because these preferences are so readily abandoned. But this is precisely the point. They, as well as the strong person, will benefit from support, encouragement, and the freedom to exercise personal choice when healthy or when ill. Such choice may entail little more than the wish to be kindly remembered or to have one's pets taken care of, but it can provide a core around which a positive outlook can be built. In this situation, even an "outsider" can make a substantial contribution to help ward off discontent and uncertainty. Fear, lack of cooperation, and even mental instability may be caused less by specific problems than by lack of direction and purpose.

Both the forward-moving and the stagnating aspects of psychological development are part of an essentially unconscious process and may, therefore, be difficult to influence. However, the person subjects this process to a self-evaluation that is largely conscious. The strength of this conscious awareness can overwhelm the unconscious infrastructure that generally governs behavior. This tendency toward self-evaluation is typically ignored, but it could form the basis of true communication. For example, through sensitive intervention, a nurse could disrupt a patient's developing pattern of self-pity by working with the patient's relatives. Each could inform the other of the way the patient is responding to various experiences. They could cooperate to contribute to his strengths and to avoid feeding his weaknesses. Improvement in a patient's behavior and even in his medical condition can result from the simple communication of en-

thusiasm and liking. Thus, even long-standing behavior patterns can be altered.

A Positive Approach

Opportunities to help the aged patient are often lost because of negative attitudes of health team members—attitudes which lead one to think "there's so little here to work with, it's not worth the effort." These attitudes are the product of years of thinking in stereotypes, stereotypes based on inadequate or incomplete data and on "common sense." Of course when pressed, each of us is able to see that what passes for "common sense" is neither all that common nor all that sensible. These "off course" attitudes with regard to the capabilities of the elderly have prevailed for so long that it will take conscious effort by everyone who comes in contact with older persons to divest themselves of such beliefs. It is time to deemphasize the infirmities and to pay attention to the considerable residual capacities of the elderly.[91] As we shift from a child-based orientation in our thinking about abilities, particularly about intelligence, we become aware of the remarkable potential that often remains untapped within many older people.[92]

The suppression of effort that typifies so many elderly people and that obscures their true potential is caused by a wide variety of factors. Two deserve special attention in the immediate context.

The first relates to the unique problems of sick older people. In their weakened conditions they need the support and protection of family, friends, and the health team. But each of these must be aware of the magnitude of the gains and losses in the daily turn of events *as perceived by each older person*. What may seem trivial or even pass unnoticed by a younger, healthy person may assume crucial importance to an older, infirm individual. Perceived losses become especially important for those who have little to bargain with.[93] For example, a bedridden individual may see himself as mistreated or ignored, and may feel as though he must barter for his wants, perhaps even for his needs. He may feel he has to be nice to someone he would like to "tell off."

He may feel frustrated at not being able to express to the nurse or the physician his negative feelings about them—just as they may not feel free to express their negative feelings about dealing with an aged patient. There is a—sometimes pathetic—drama that takes place "when a spirited old man or woman gives of whatever is left in order to get whatever is wanted."[94] On the other hand, this may be the only challenge that is left to them and signs hastily interpreted as irascibility may in fact be evidence of a spark of courage and independence.

The importance of some form of challenge being present should not be underestimated. In fact, perhaps one flaw in patient care may be the removal of most or all "demands."[95] A consequence of no demands is to lose skills, for example, the rapidity with which the skill of walking deteriorates as the musculature of a bedridden patient atrophies. This is true of almost all skills. And the effects proliferate, as the bedridden patient's "cardiovascular control also becomes impaired."[96] How quickly this extends to social skills can readily be seen with regard to interpersonal or social expectations. If the members of one's social environment expect a certain kind of behavior, and if the individual accepts this, his or her behavior will probably come close to matching such a standard. The converse is also readily apparent in institutionalized settings where few demands are made and the individual shows rapid withdrawal and deterioration.

Also, almost everyone connected with medical care has seen or heard of recovery rates that seem attributable to the ebullience of the practitioner rather than to his or her expertise. Good spirits should be accompanied by genuine concern, but even when this is not the case, the patient will often translate the pleasantness of the practitioner into positive social reinforcement—and anything positive can be beneficial. Of course, if the medical treatment and "demands" are routinized and required, the "involvement" becomes onerous for all concerned, and something to be avoided.

The second factor relates to specific nursing care. Remarkable advances have been made in improving nursing care.[97] One way to ensure that this trend continues is to utilize advances and contributions from other areas, for example, the emerging picture of retained abilities of the elderly.[98] For instance, as we move away from broadly based achievement (i.e., intelligence) tests we become aware of the special abilities of the older person.[99] This refocuses our attention on the underlying competence that is still present for many elderly.[100] Once we become aware of this, we can break out of the "vicious circle" of fake beliefs that produce their own predictions.

In addition to being aware of the contributions coming from other areas, in order to maximize effectiveness, the nursing profession needs to *contribute to* social trends.[101] That is, nurses need to be aware of and to incorporate current advances, and to predict and promote future trends. Active participation in the course of one's profession is the best guarantee that we won't be engaged in yesterday's practices when tomorrow arrives.

References

1. Atchley, R. C.: The Social Forces in Later Life: An Introduction to Social Gerontology. Belmont, California, Wadsworth, 1972, p. 220.
2. *Ibid*. See also Maddox, G. L.: Persistance of life style among the elderly: a longitudinal study of patterns of social activity in relation to life satisfaction (1966). *In* B. L. Neugarten (ed.): Middle Age and Aging. Chicago, University of Chicago Press, 1968.
3. Nardi, A. H.: Person-perception research and the perception of life-span development. *In* P. B. Baltes and K. W. Schaie (eds.): Life-span Developmental Psychology. New York, Academic Press, 1973, pp. 285-300. See also Smith, E. L.: Handbook of Aging. New York, Barnes and Noble, 1972.
4. Neugarten, B. L.: The awareness of middle age (1967). *In* Neugarten, *op. cit.*, p. 93.
5. Rose, A. M.: A current theoretical issue in social gerontology (1964). *In* Neugarten, *op. cit.*, p. 187; and Tournier, P.: Learn to Grow Old. New York, Harper & Row, 1972.
6. Ahammer, I. M. and Baltes, P. B.: Objective versus perceived age differences in personality:

how do adolescents, adults, and older people view themselves and each other? J. Gerontol. 27:46-51, 1972; Anderson, N. N.: Effects of institutionalization on self-esteem. J. Gerontol. 22:313-317, 1967; and Carp, F. M.: Senility or garden/variety maladjustment? J. Gerontol. 24:203-208, 1969.

7. Cameron, P.: Age parameters of young adult, middle-aged, old, and aged. J. Gerontol. 24:201-202, 1969.

8. Gilberstadt, H.: Relationships among scores of tests suitable for the assessment of adjustment and intellectual functioning. J. Gerontol. 23:483-487; 1968; Riegel, K. F.: Speed of performance as a function of age and set: a review of issues and data. In A. T. Welford and J . E. Birren (eds.): Behavior, Aging, and the Nervous System. Springfield, Illinois, Charles C Thomas, 1965.

9. Jamieson, G. H.: Prior learning and response flexibility in two age groups. J. Gerontol. 24:179-184, 1969.

10. Baltes, P. B. and Schaie, K. W.: The myth of the twilight years. Psych. Today 7:35-40, March 1974; Birren, J. E.: Toward an experimental psychology of aging. Am. Psych. 25:124-135, 1970, Botwinick, J.: Aging and Behavior. New York, Springer, 1973; and Hourany, L. J.: Differences in Verbal Abilities in Relation to Age. Unpublished doctoral thesis. London, Ontario, Canada, University of Western Ontario, 1974.

11. Butler, R. N.: The facade of chronological age (1963). In Neugarten, op. cit., pp. 235-242.

12. White, P. D.: Cardiovascular disorder. In E. V. Cowdry and F. V. Steinberg (eds.): The Care of the Geriatric Patient. Saint Louis, Missouri, C. V. Mosby, 1971, p. 53; and Bierman, E. L. and Hazzard, W. R.: Biology of Aging. In D. W. Smith and E. L. Bierman (eds.): The Biologic Ages of Man. Philadelphia, W. B. Saunders, 1973, p. 17.

13. Stieglity, C. J.: Foundations of geriatric medicine. In E. J. Steiglity: Geriatric Medicine: Medical Care of Later Maturity. Philadelphia, J. B. Lippincott, 1954, p. 9.

14. Moore, M. E.: Physical changes. In M. W. Riley and A. Foner (eds.): Aging and Society. New York, Russell Sage Foundation, 1968.

15. Shock, N. W.: The physiology of aging. Sci. Am. 206:100, Jan. 1962.

16. Ibid., pp. 100-103.

17. The following material draws heavily from Busse, E. W.: Theories of aging. In E. W. Busse and E. Pfeiffer (eds.): Behavior and Adaptation in Late Life. Boston, Little, Brown, 1969, pp. 18-22.

18. Estes, E. H., Jr.:Health experience in the elderly. In Busse, op. cit., p. 119; and Newton, K. and Anderson H. C.: Geriatric Nursing. Saint Louis, Missouri, C. V. Mosby, 1966.

19. Jaeger, D. and Simmons, L. W.: The Aged Ill. New York, Appleton-Century Crofts (Educational Division/Meredith Corporation), 1970, p. 3.

20. Estes, op. cit., pp. 116-117 and Newton and Anderson, op. cit., p. 63.

21. Kimmel, D. C.: Adulthood and Aging. New York, John Wiley & Sons, 1974, p. 36.

22. Estes, op. cit., p. 116.

23. Birchenall, J. and Streight, M. E.: Care of the Older Adult. Philadelphia, J. B. Lippincott, 1973, p. 106.

24. Estes, op. cit., p. 118.

25. Kimmel, op. cit., p. 359.

26. Herndon, C. N.: Medical genetics. In Cowdry and Steinberg, op. cit., pp. 126-127.

27. Ibid.

28. Kimmel, op. cit.; Birchenall and Streight, op. cit.; and Newton and Anderson, op. cit.

29. Busse and Pfeiffer, op. cit., p. 15.

30. Smith and Bierman, op. cit., p. 15.

31. White, op. cit., p. 52.

32. Bourne, G. H.: Structural changes in aging. In N. W. Shock: Aging . . . Some Social and Biological Aspects: Publication No. 65, Washington, D. C., Am. Assoc. Advance. Sci., 1960, pp. 133-134, and Moore, op. cit., pp. 225-226.

33. Bourne, op. cit. pp. 133-134; Riley and Foner, op. cit., pp. 226-228; and Estes, op. cit., p. 121.

34. Shivak, M.: Caring for the aged. page 2049-2053. In Browning, M.: Nursing and the Aging Patient. New York, Am. J. Nurs. Company, 1974, pp. 2049-2053.

35. Ibid.

36. White, op. cit.,p. 52; and Shock, Sci. Am., op. cit., p. 102.

37. Hardin, W. B. and O'Leary, J. L.: Neurologic aspects. *In* Cowdry and Steinberg, *op. cit.*, p. 311.

38. Stone, V.: Give the older person time. *In* Browning, *op. cit.*, pp. 20-21; Shock, Sci. Am., *op. cit.*, pp. 102-103; and Riley and Foner, *op. cit.*, p. 224.

39. Shock, Sci. Am., *op. cit.*, pp. 102-103.

40. Wang, H. S.: Organic brain syndrome. *In* Busse and Pfeiffer, *op. cit.*, p. 263; and Kimmel, *op. cit.*, p. 226.

41. Hardin and O'Leary, *op. cit.*, p. 316.

42. Kimmel, *op. cit.*, p. 226.

43. Stone, *op. cit.*, p. 21.

44. White, *op. cit.*, p. 33.

45. Shock, Sci. Am., *op. cit.*, pp. 104-105.

46. Papper, S.: The effects of age in reducing renal function. Geriatrics 83-87; May 1973.

47. Shock, Sci. Am., *op. cit.*, pp. 101-102.

48. Schwab. *In* Neugarten, *op. cit.*, pp. 11-12.

49. Pfeiffer, E.: Sexual behaviour in old age. *In* Busse and Pfeiffer, *op. cit.*, p. 156.

50. Comfort, A. (ed.): The Joy of Sex. New York, Simon & Schuster, 1972, p. 224.

51. Freeman, J. T.: Sexual aspects of aging. *In* Cowdry and Steinberg, *op. cit.*, p. 175.

52. *Ibid.* p. 185.

53. Comfort, *op. cit.*, p. 224.

54. Soule, S. A.: Gynecologic disorders. *In* Cowdry and Steinberg, *op. cit.*, pp. 105-106.

55. Comfort, *op. cit.*, p. 224.

56. McDowell, F.: Plastic surgery. *In* Cowdry and Steinberg, *op. cit.*, p. 236.

57. Kimmel, *op. cit.*, p. 365.

58. Nardi, *op. cit.*, p. 294.

59. Atchley, *op. cit.*

60. Streib, G. F.: Are the aged a minority group? (1965). *In* Neugarten *op. cit.*, p. 35.

61. Eisdorfer, C. and Lawton, M. P. (eds.): The Psychology of Adult Development and Aging. Washington, D. C., Am. Psych. Assoc., 1973.

62. Rose, A. M.: The subculture of the aging. (1962). *In* Neugarten *op. cit.*, p. 29.

63. Offir, C.: Old people's revolt. Psych. Today, 40, March, 1974; and Pressey, S. L. and Pressey, A. P.: Genius at 80 and other oldsters. Gerontologist 7:183-7; 1967.

64. See, for example: Botwinick *op. cit.*, Eisdorfer and Lawton, *op. cit.*

65. Brown, R. Social Psychology. New York, Free Press, 1965.

66. Butler, R. N. and Lewis, M. I.: Aging and Mental Health. Saint Louis, C. V. Mosby, 1973; p. 126.

67. *Ibid.*, p. 84

68. *Ibid.*, pp. 21-3.

69. Eisdorfer and Lawton, *op. cit.* Welford, A. T. and Birren, J. E. (eds.): Behavior, Aging, and the Nervous System. Springfield, Illinois, Charles C Thomas, 1965.

70. Jarvik, L. F. and Cohen, D.: A biobehavioral approach to intellectual changes with aging. *In* Eisdorfer and Lawton, *op. cit.*, p. 250.

71. Wang, H. S.: Cerebral correlates of intellectual function in senescence. *In* L. F. Jarvik, C. Eisdorfer, and J. E. Blum: Intellectual Functioning in Adults. New York, Springer, 1973.

72. The Aging, Trends, Problems, Prospects. Toronto, Ontario, Social Planning Council of Metropolitan Toronto, Mar. 1973.

73. Atchley, *op. cit.*, p. 12.

74. Butler and Lewis, *op. cit.*, p. 22.

75. Gordon, M. S.: Work and patterns of retirement. *In* R. W. Kleemeier: Aging and Leisure. New York, Oxford University Press, 1961, pp. 25-27.

76. Ebel, R. L.: And still the dryads linger. p. 486. Am. Psych. 29, 7:486, July 1974.

77. Jensen, A. R.: How much can we boost IQ and scholastic achievement? Harvard Ed. Review 39:100-123, 1969; and Wechsler, D.: The Measurement and Appraisal of Adult Intelligence. Baltimore, Williams & Wilkins, 1958.

78. McClelland, D. C.: Testing for competence rather than for "intelligence." Am. Psych. 28, 1:3, Jan. 1973.

79. *Ibid.*, p. 8.

80. Ebel, *op. cit.*, p. 489.

81. Guilford, J. P.: The Nature of Human Intelligence. New York, McGraw-Hill, 1967; and Shouksmith, G.: Intelligence, Creativity, and Cognitive Style. London, Batsford, Ltd., 1970, p. 153.

82. Cattell, R. B.: Abilities. New York, Houghton Mifflin, 1971; and Clark, D. M. and Mirels, H. L.: Fluency as a pervasive element in the meas-

urement of creativity. J. Ed. Measurement 7:83-86, 1970.

83. Hoepfner, R., Guilford, J. P. and Bradley, P. A.: Information transformation abilities. Ed. Psych. Measurement 30:785-802, 1970. Shouksmith, *op. cit.*

84. Cattell, *op. cit.;* Fredricksen, C. H.: Abilities, transfer, and information retrieval in verbal learning. Multivariate Behavioral Research Monographs, No. 69-2, 1969; and Renner, V.: Effects of cognitive style on creative behavior. J. Personal. and Soc. Psych. 14, 3:257-262, 1970.

85. Jamieson, *op. cit.;* and Monge, R. H.: Learning in the adult years—set or rigidity. Human Develop. 12:131-140, 1969.

86. Botwinick, *op. cit.*

87. Cattell, *op. cit.*

88. Tournier, *op. cit.*

89. Buhler, C.: Meaningful living in the mature years. *In* Kleemier, *op. cit.,* pp. 345-387.

90. *Ibid.*

91. Butler and Lewis, *loc. cit.;* and Granick, S. and Friedman, A. S.: Educational experience and maintenance of intellectual functioning in the aged—an overview. *In* L. F. Jarvik, C. Eisdorfer and J. E. Blum (eds.): Intellectual Functioning in Adults. New York, Springer, 1973, Chapter 7.

92. Baer, *op. cit.;* and Honzik, M. P. and Macfarlane, J. W.: Personality development and intellectual functioning from 21 months to 40 years. *In* Jarvik, Eisdorfer, and Lawton, *op. cit.,* p. 56-7.

93. Jaeger and Simmons, *op. cit.,* p. 7.

94. Brown, E. L.: Nursing Reconsidered—A study of change. Philadelphia, J. B. Lippincott, 1970.

95. Jaeger and Simmons, *op. cit.,* p. 22.

96. *Ibid.*

97. *Ibid.*

98. Baltes and Schaie, *op. cit.*

99. Kuhlen, R. G.: Age and intelligence. *In* Neugarten, *op. cit.,* p. 552.

100. Baer, *op. cit.;* and Cole, M. and Bruner, J. S.: Cultural Differences and Inference About Psychological Processes. p. 872.

101. Brown, *op. cit.*

Bibliography

Anderson, H. C.: Newton's Geriatric Nursing, ed. 5. Saint Louis, Missouri, C. V. Mosby, 1971.

Andrew, W.: Structural alterations with aging in the nervous system. J. Chronic Diseases 3:575-596, 1956.

Barrows, C. H., Jr.: The challenge—mechanisms of biological aging. Gerontol. 115:5-11, 1971.

Bender, A. D.: Effects of age on intestinal absorption in the elderly. J. Am. Geriatric Soc. 16:1331-1339, 1968.

Birren, J. E. (ed.): Handbook of Aging and the Individual. Chicago, University of Chicago Press, 1959.

Blumenthal, W. T. (ed.): Medical and Clinical Aspects of Aging. New York, Columbia University Press, 1962.

Boyd, D. R. R. and Oakes, C. G.: Foundations of Practical Gerontology. Columbia, University of South Carolina Press, 1973.

Cowdry, E. V. and Steinberg, F. U.: The Care of the Geriatric Patient. St. Louis, Missouri, C. V. Mosby, 1971.

Field, M.: Depth and Extent of the Geriatric Problem. Springfield, Illinois, Charles C Thomas, 1970.

Franks, L. M.: Cellular aspects of aging. Experimental Gerontol. 4:281-290, 1970.

George, J. A.: Teaching the young adult about the old. Nurs. Outlook 20, 6:405, June 1972.

Gotto, A. M., Scott, L. and Manis, E.: Prudent eating after 40—relationship of diet to blood lipids and coronary heart disease. Geriatrics 29, 5:109-118, May 1974.

Hamburger, F. and Bonner, C.: Medical Care and Rehabilitation of the Aged and Chronically Ill. Boston, Little, Brown, 1964.

Harris, R.: The Management of Geriatric Cardiovascular Disease. Philadelphia, J. B. Lippincott, 1970.

Johnson, W.: The Older Patient. New York, Paul B. Hoeber, 1960.

Knowles, L. (ed.): Putting geriatric nursing standards into practice. Nurs. Clin. N. Am. 7, 2, June 1972.

Krehl, W. A.: The influence of nutritional environment on aging. Geriatrics 29, 5:65-76, May 1974.

Long, J. M.: Caring for and Caring About Elderly People. Philadelphia, J. B. Lippincott, 1974.

Mayer, J.: Aging and nutrition. Geriatrics 29, 5:57-59, May 1974.

Myers, J.: An Orientation to Chronic Disease and Disability. New York, Macmillan, 1965.

Palmore, E. (ed.): Normal Aging, Vol. II. Durham, Duke University Press, 1974.

Rossman, I. (ed.): Clinical Geriatrics. Philadelphia, J. B. Lippincott, 1971.

Stevens, C. B.: Special Needs of Long Term Patients. Philadelphia, J. B. Lippincott, 1974.

Townsend, C.: The Nader Report. Old Age: The Last Segregation. New York, Grossman Publishers, 1971.

U. S. Veterans Administration, Department of Medicine and Surgery: Nursing Care of the Long-Term Patient (G-8, M-2, Part 5). Washington, D.C., U.S. Government Printing Office, 1963.

Recommended Sources
Psychosocial Aging

Atchley, R. C.: The Social Forces in Later Life. Belmont, California, Wadsworth, 1972.

A much needed text in an area that is little cultivated. The author covers many topics and, while a number of topics receive only brief treatment, he does succeed in giving both sides of many important issues.

Baltes, P. B. and Schaie, K. W.: The myth of the twilight years. Psych. Today, Mar. 1974.

An up-to-date, sock-um article which should go a long way toward displacing the shibboleths that abound. This article gathers together the crucial issues regarding age and mental ability and clearly examines each, presenting strong evidence for the maintenance of ability well into old age. This is must reading for laypeople and professionals alike.

Butler, R. N. and Lewis, M. I.: Aging and Mental Health. Saint Louis, Missouri, C. V. Mosby, 1973.

This book discusses the medical and psychosocial influences that contribute to the dispropor-

tionate distress encountered by older people. It works to dispel the spectre of ageism and is a unique attempt to counter it with positive interpretations and recommendations.

Eisdorfer, C. and Lawton, M. P. (eds.): The Psychology of Adult Development and Aging. Washington, D.C., The Am. Psych. Assoc., 1973.

This volume represents the combined efforts of experts organized into a Task Force on Aging by the American Psychological Association. It attempts to bring up-to-date what is known regarding aging and to give special attention to areas of neglect and misperception. Thus, it constitutes an authoritative statement of the current scientific findings and speculations. It attacks myths and outdated assumptions directly as in its very first subheading: Alleged Loss of Intellectual Functioning.

Hunt, J. McV.: Intelligence and Experience. New York, Ronald Press, 1961.

A book that, if not already, will probably become a classic. Hunt presents a careful analysis of evidence and theories regarding the development of abilities and concludes that experience leads to the formation of abilities; they are not innate, fixed entities. Essentially his position is that you are what you do, the more you do, the more you *want* to do; the more you *can* do, the more you'll *try* to do.

Kimmel, D. C.: Adulthood and Aging. New York, John Wiley & Sons, 1974.

This book treats the aging process within a developmental framework. There are three guiding assumptions. (1) People grow, change, develop *throughout* their lives. (2) There is a sequential, orderly progression to aging, and it has both quantitative and qualitative milestones. (3) Development is not a simple extension of occurrences in childhood. This is a highly competent treatment of the psychology of aging by a person under 30 who had a need to know but did not have the burden of historical commitment and misperception.

Neugarten, B. L. (ed.): Middle Age and Aging. Chicago, The University Press, 1968.

Possibly the most comprehensive review available of the social and psychological aspects of aging. Articles range from analyses of the aged as a group, to their family and social relationships, and to the technical issues involved in understanding the aging process.

Smith, E. D.: Handbook of Aging: For Those Growing Old and Those Concerned With Them. New York, Barnes and Noble, 1972.

A brief book (105 pages) written expressly for the nontechnically prepared person. It is beautifully written—clearly and sensitively—by a person who is both professionally trained and retired. It deals with the conditions of aging, major problems encountered, and with social relations—all with a view toward applying the knowledge we have to the problems of today.

Tournier, P.: Learn to Grow Old. New York, Harper & Row, 1972.

This book provides a rather complete overview of the life experiences of the older person—his work, leisure, retirement, the contempt he faces, his health, new careers, and his confrontation with death. It is written with a spiritual orientation but has a message for everyone.

10

Intensive Care Nursing

MARY RIESER, ELIZABETH MOIR CARMELITE and MARTHA TAYLOR

Evolution of the ICU • Purpose and Objectives • Pathophysiological Needs and Prevention of Further Complications • Immediate Psychosocial Needs • The Physical Environment • Environmental Stress • Nursing Intervention • Opportunities for Research

A rapidly growing part of the hospital setting today is the intensive care unit (ICU). An accelerating number of such special units have been established and are organized in several ways: 1) traditionally as medical and surgical ICUs; 2) by organ systems or clinical syndromes (coronary, respiratory, burn, shock and trauma); 3) by special patient population such as the pediatric or obstetrical ICU.[1] Some health care experts predict that increased technology, cost, and demand for specialized units will greatly influence the design of hospitals of the future.[2] Patients in such units share in common the admission criterion: an illness or injury which is presently or imminently serious, and which, hopefully, can be reversed through constant surveillance and concentrated care.

Evolution of the ICU

The genesis of the ICU may be traced to the front line hospitals in World War II. These postoperative shock and trauma victims were cared for in units staffed by personnel specifically trained for this purpose and supplied with the necessary medical and surgical equipment. Physicians, nurses, and hospital administrators returning to civilian hospitals incorporated this concept in the postanesthesia or recovery rooms of hospitals. The surgical ICU followed as a logical extension for patients who required continued vigilance after recovery from anesthesia. Recognizing the need for such units in its hospitals, the Veterans Administration appointed a subcommittee, comprised of administrators and surgical chiefs, to study the problem of intensive care. The inclusion of a surgical intensive care unit for patients "whose therapeutic requirements cannot be met adequately in a ward or postanesthetic recovery room"[3] was recommended for all VA hospitals.

To help hospital administrators with the dilemmas brought on by rising hospital costs, shortage of qualified personnel, and advancing medical technology, a federally sponsored project was undertaken to classify patients according to their care needs and to determine the type of nursing unit to which they should be assigned. This concept, known as progressive patient care, included:

Intensive care: For critically and serious ill patients who are unable to communicate their needs or who require extensive nursing care and observation.

Intermediate care: For patients requiring a moderate amount of nursing care.

Self-care: For ambulatory and physically self-sufficient patients requiring therapeutic or diagnostic services, or who may be convalescing.

Long-term care: For patients requiring skilled prolonged medical and nursing care.

Home care: For patients who can be adequately cared for in the home through the extension of certain hospital services.

Outpatient care: For ambulatory patients requiring diagnostic, curative, preventive, and rehabilitative services.[4]

At Bethany Hospital, Kansas City, Kansas, in 1962, Dr. Hughes W. Day opened the first coronary care unit in the United States. With a grant from the John A. Hartford Foundation, Day and associates set out to lower the mortality rate of coronary patients and to achieve a higher incidence of successful cardiac resuscitation. Shortly thereafter, the Heart Disease Control Program of the U.S. Public Health Service awarded Presbyterian Hospital in Philadelphia a one year contract to establish a coronary care unit. Thereafter the Division of Nursing of the Service supported a pilot study of nursing patterns within this coronary care unit.[5] Out of this project came the first nursing text on intensive coronary care.[6] Between 1962 and 1966, 250 hospitals established coronary care units, using local funds to do so. Another 250 hospitals established medical intensive care units in the same period. The Public Health Service provided guidelines in a booklet, "Coronary Care Units," which stressed the importance of this concept in the delivery of health care to the nation.[7]

The success of coronary care units and the acceptance of the recovery room as a part of routine hospital care, along with the lack of skilled private duty nurses to care for the critically ill, have been responsible for mounting interest in other intensive care units. The newborn infant, or the child or adult in respiratory distress, the stroke victim, the burned patient, the patient with renal failure, or combinations of the above patients are found in the ICU. The coronary care unit is a prime example of the successful ICU where recognition and treatment of serious arrhythmias, the original and primary objective of the unit, have now been replaced by prevention of serious arrhythmias.

As the concept of the ICU continues to evolve, a number of small, isolated units are being centralized to form an intensive care service in both large and small hospitals which cares for all seriously ill patients, not just a specific class of patients.[8] Several hospitals within a community can provide excellent intensive care by utilizing a cadre of community physicians and specially trained nurses to staff the community ICU, while permitting the patient's physician to maintain primary control.[9] As nursing has prepared the acute care nursing generalist to staff ICUs, medicine is currently developing the intensive care physician.[10] Both provide expertise in the care of the seriously ill, regardless of age, medical diagnosis, or specific therapy.

The development of ICUs has brought to the hospital many problems in terms of manpower and costs. The health care industry must continue to address itself to the problems of finding the best ways of supplying ICUs with personnel who require time-consuming and expensive, continuing education; of demanding meaningful directives which spell out responsibilities of those personnel; and of meeting the need for personalizing the care of patients surrounded by increasing numbers of machines and technicians. In reality, costs of ICUs will continue to rise geometrically in relation to the increase in highly technological medical care.[11]

Purpose and Objectives

A 1961 Kellogg Foundation Report defined the purpose of the ICU as the provision of "high level nursing care for patients who require continuous and detailed intensive care in an atmosphere of compassion and understanding."[12] Intensive medical care, of course, is crucial to the ICU patient, but the nurse remains the vital link for providing continuous patient observation and care, despite sophisticated, electronic monitoring equipment.[13]

Nursing objectives, which flow logically from the purpose of the unit, are: 1) the detection of and participation in treatment of life-threatening crises; 2) the preservation of the patient's physiological defenses and the prevention of further bodily complications; 3) the provision of comfort which does not conflict with the second objective and serves as a beginning implementation of the next objective, and 4) the establishment and maintenance of meaningful communication with the patient, reflecting an attitude of respect for the person and his or her emotional reactions and concerns. The critical nature of the patient dictates setting a hierarchy of objectives without relegating his or her psychosocial needs to the realm of unimportance. The patient is a whole being, a complex entity, whose needs are often in reciprocal relationship, each capable of intensifying or diminishing the other. For example:

Lucy is a 15-year-old girl with a diagnosis of schizophrenia (of seven months' duration), compounded more recently by anorexia nervosa, whose therapy, in the psychiatric unit of the hospital, included reward-punishment conditioning and finally feeding by large vein parenteral hyperalimentation.[14] This method provides an adequate amount of nitrogen, calories, and other nutrients, thereby achieving tissue synthesis and anabolism.

Lucy's condition deteriorated to the point where she developed progressive neuropathy (because of her poor nutritional state) and respiratory distress. She was immediately transferred to the medical intensive care unit. A synopsis of her history, her medical treatment and nursing care, her response to it, and her present status were communicated to members of the medical and nursing staff before Lucy's arrival in the unit.

On admission Lucy was 5 feet 8 inches tall, weighed 62 pounds, and had 2+ bilateral, pitting, pedal edema. She could not or would not speak, was withdrawn, and severely debilitated. Immediate ECG monitoring showed a sinus tachycardia of 150 to 170 beats per minute, and congestive heart failure was ruled out. Lucy's respiratory distress was obvious despite use of oral airway and administration of oxygen through a mask. She had developed all the signs and symptoms of Landry's ascending paralysis and her respiratory involvement necessitated tracheostomy and the support of a volume-cycled ventilator. (She subsequently developed Friedländer's pneumonia.) Loss of bladder function required the use of an indwelling catheter.

Although her psychosocial needs were significant, immediate priority was demanded by her pathophysiological problems. Assessment of her needs resulted in these priorities in her nursing care:

Pathophysiological Needs and Prevention of Further Complications

MAINTENANCE OF CIRCULATION AND VENTILATION. Details of the specific nursing care required to meet these needs are part of the written standards of nursing practice established for the ICU. These include such procedures as aseptic tracheostomy care with hyperinflation and aspiration as needed, and hourly repositioning to reduce physiological shunting; manual chest physical therapy techniques of percussion and vibration; continuous monitoring of ECG; monitoring of arterial and /or central venous pressure, and so on. Nursing observation centered on the detection of arrhythmias, and signs and symptoms of hypoxia and hypercapnia, with attention to blood gas values and their significance. All stools were hematested because of the association of stress ulcers and hemorrhage with patients on ventilators.

METABOLIC NEEDS. Parenteral hyperalimentation was discontinued by the medical staff so it would not "cloud" Lucy's medical evaluation. She was maintained with routine IV solutions with electrolyte additives prn. She remained NPO and parenteral hyperalimentation therapy was restarted after several days. Her urinary output was measured hourly and checked for specific gravity and glucose.

PHYSICAL THERAPY. To prevent further musculoskeletal deterioration, passive range of motion exercises were carried out twice a day.

SKIN CARE. Lucy's skin over all bony prominences, particularly the spinal column and sacral area, was prone to breakdown. An alternating pressure mattress was employed. Lubricating lotion was used with her bath water and frequent skin care with germicidal solution and thorough rinsing was given. Lucy was massaged frequently—gently but firmly over all bony prominences—and a padded bedpan was used.

Immediate Psychosocial Needs

COMMUNICATION. The two methods Lucy used to attempt to control her environment were refusal to eat and speak. These methods were no longer under her control. She was NPO and because of the tracheostomy could not speak even if she wished to. Moreover, she was too weak to move, so that writing was impossible. Therefore, communication was established by Lucy's nodding her head. The nursing staff explained to Lucy (prior to the emergency tracheostomy and after) that nodding would be a satisfactory, temporary method of communication. (Fortunately, she did not withdraw completely.) Questions were phrased so that she could answer with a *yes* or *no* nod. Chatter of interest to a typical teenager was conducted by the nursing staff in an effort to kindle interest. However, because of Lucy's flat affect and lack of ability to communicate except by nods and facial grimaces, it was difficult and occasionally impossible to determine her interest. When silence was felt to be therapeutic, it was employed.

IMPACT OF THE ACUTE ILLNESS AND TRANSFER TO ICU. A conference (the first of many) with Lucy's psychiatrist and the nursing staff of the ICU was held concerning the impact the acute medical illness and transfer to the ICU had made on Lucy, and the best approach to helping her. The importance of misinterpretation of tactile communication by the schizophrenic was discussed and the consensus was to use no more physical contact than was necessary. The basic approach of the nurse remained friendly, encouraging, and as natural as possible. Every effort was made to prevent Lucy's further withdrawal. Praise was used when warranted and disapproval was not verbalized. However, even in her debilitated state, after being weaned from the ventilator, Lucy had the ability to manipulate others; therefore, the nurses could not be totally permissive. The same nurse on each tour of duty was assigned to Lucy in an attempt to help her form a therapeutic relationship. However, other nurses on the unit were encouraged to "pop in" and, in general, to display an interest in her as a person.

NEED FOR COMMUNICATION WITH HER PARENTS AND SIBLINGS. Lucy expressed a desire to see her parents, but their visits seemed to upset her. Therefore, the restrictive visiting hours on the ICU were strictly enforced. Visits by the five younger siblings were postponed over concern that the children would become extremely upset by Lucy's physical condition and would be unable to prevent Lucy from realizing the cause of their distress.

NEED TO MAINTAIN CONTACT WITH THE OUTSIDE WORLD. Lucy displayed interest only in TV and radio. Because TV shows are often depressing, the TV was not left on indiscriminately. Because Lucy also liked rock music, it was played on her radio a great deal of the time (to the delight of some staff members and to the dismay of others.)

NEED FOR PATIENT TO MAKE CHOICES.
Physical appearance. Every effort was made to make Lucy feel as attractive as possible, and to allow her a choice—the style of her hair, with or without ribbon, shade of lipstick, and the like.

Food preferences. Although Lucy was NPO for awhile after admission, it was decided to determine in advance her favorite foods (from her family and her nursing care plan from the psychiatric floor). The dietitian also was contacted in preparation for Lucy's eating again and choosing her favorite foods.

Prior to the development of the ICU and sophisticated respiratory care, Lucy might not have been saved. After five weeks in the ICU, Lucy has made much physical and some mental progress. She now weighs 72 pounds. Her affect is not as flat; she smiles and talks now that her tracheostomy has been occluded. She is eating fairly well and thoroughly enjoys hamburgers and milkshakes. In anticipation of her transfer, one of the ICU nurses took Lucy in a wheelchair to the hospital snack bar where she ordered from the menu. Hopefully, this may make the necessary adjustment upon transfer less abrupt and traumatic. Lucy is being encouraged to view her transfer as a sign of progress. The priorities of Lucy's nursing care have shifted frequently and her grave psychiatric problem now assumes top priority.

The Physical Environment

The design of the ICU has been influenced recently by the concept of the critical care service or center. The problems of operation, replacement, and equipment repair of monitoring facilities can be simplified when a number of ICUs are centrally located.[15] A center may consist of two or more special care units in which a total of 30 to 60 patients are housed. For example, these may be: a 5-bed coronary care unit, and 8-bed surgical ICU, a 5-bed respiratory unit, and a 20-bed intermediate care unit. The center is designed to more patients progressively from the specific ICU to intermediate care and back again, if necessary, under optimal physical conditions and with staff in close communication with each other. For any one ICU nursing unit, no more than 12 to 15 patients or less than 5 or 6 have been recommended.[16,17] To provide continuous surveillance, a U-shape or half circle design has proved to be quite effective. Although more costly, it is preferable that single rooms (or cubicles) have solid partitions rather than curtains to separate one patient from another. Cross-infection is thereby cut down and privacy is provided. The goals of surveillance and privacy need not be mutually exclusive. A glass wall of the patient's room (or cubicle) facing the nurses' station permits surveillance; curtains may be drawn across the glass wall when privacy is desired. An alternative design consists of a half-glass, half-solid partition or no partition at all on the side of the room next to the nurses' station. The room (or cubicle) itself should contain supplies to make it as autonomous as possible, color-corrected fluorescent lighting,[18] and a variety of lighting for examination and treatment purposes.

A well-controlled study indicates that patients in rooms with windows are less prone to develop delirium or depression than patients in windowless rooms.[19] Lavatory facilities (and toilets for coronary units) are essential. Noise control is aided by carpeting made of low-static-resistance materials. Medication rooms should be separate from the nurses' station, which is basically an observation post.

Patients' families prefer to wait out their vigils in close proximity to their loved ones. A waiting room adjacent to the ICU, preferably with its own partitions (if only floral arrangement), provides comfort and some privacy. Ideally, the waiting area includes separate rooms for the counseling of family members by clergy, social services, and ICU personnel. In the larger hospital, several units may share these more elaborate facilities.

Beside the obvious need for multiple-wall outlets for suction and oxygen, it is the presence of electronic monitoring equipment in the ICU which sets it apart from other patient units. Electronic equipment provides a link between the patient and the highly trained ICU personnel. Characteristics of the ICU monitoring system include:

1. A signal generator—the patient.
2. Data acquisition systems (e.g., the cardiac monitor).
3. Data displays to facilitate decision making (e.g., the tachometer).
4. The personnel.[20]

Decisions are made and actions taken not through or to the electronic system, but directly on the patient. Continuous monitoring equipment serves as an ancillary tool, assisting the physician and nurse in their observations, decision making, and actions.

Systems are available for the continuous monitoring of the electrocardiogram, arterial and venous pressures, including intracardiac pressures, and intracranial pressures. Digital displays can indicate numerical values for blood pressure, heart rate, body temperature, blood and fluid infusions, and fluid outputs. The computer stores an increasing variety of data which is easily retrieved for the study of the natural history of the disease process. The computer is programmed not only to log data, but to reduce and compute complex information and even to suggest necessary intervention. Presently, computer systems which analyze and make patient care decisions are being studied in relation to the extent to which automation can free highly trained persons for those interventions that absolutely demand human skills.[21]

The advance of electronic monitoring has been rapid and the ICU nurse must be alert to this fact, watching for achievements and limitations. Because the human factor still needs more consideration, with respect to the equipment, the nurse is ideally suited to criticize and to suggest changes in monitoring equipment— alarms which are too soft or too loud; poor location of on-off alarm switches; display devices which are difficult to see under varying conditions; complex alarm resetting procedures.[22] At all times, the nurse must have convenient access to the patient, and the electronic equipment must not be allowed to restrict the patient's movements. Understanding of the limitations of electronic equipment is essential. The nurse who fully comprehends electronic limitations and who has confidence in her own observational and decision-making abilities does not place much confidence in the alarm system which cannot pick up early arrhythmia changes.

Environmental Stress

EFFECT ON THE PATIENT

Superimposed on the physiological stress experienced by every ICU patient, as well as his or her individual psychic reaction to bodily injury, is the potential stress imposed by the very environment of the ICU. It is the conclusion of systematic investigations made over the past 20 years[23] that marked subjective states and behavioral disturbances are often associated with extremes in environmental stimulation. For example, Kornfeld et al have implicated the isolation of the open-heart recovery room in the behavioral disturbances of postcardiotomy patients.[24] A psychoticlike state associated with environmental extremes includes symptoms of

pathological anxiety, delusions, and hallucinations—visual and sometimes auditory and somesthetic.[25] This clinical state, of course, closely resembles toxic delirium, which is often found in the patient with infection, neoplasm, hypoxia, drug ingestion, dehydration, or another metabolic disturbance. In particular, postcardiotomy patients are subject to delirium which appears to be associated with the severity of preoperative disease, extent of surgical stress, and increased age. The relationship of time on cardiopulmonary bypass and delirium has been given considerable attention in the literature.[26]

Disturbances in environmental stimulation or sensory input may be classified into three operational processes: 1) sensory deprivation, in which the amount or variability of stimulation is markedly reduced; 2) sensory overload, in which multiple stimuli are in action simultaneously at levels of intensity above normal; and 3) sensory distortion, in which an auditory stimulus, for example, is presented out of proper time sequence with tactile or visual stimuli.[27] (See Chapter 19.)

Evidence of these processes can be found in the ICU[28] and should be identified if the nurse is going to manipulate the patient's environment therapeutically. How much of the ICU environment acts to deprive the patient of sensory input? Immobility and estrangement from a familiar environment, heightened by the severity and longevity of the illness, promote sensory deprivation. Immobility, particularly as exemplified by the tank respirator and the narrow "coffinlike" Stryker frame, confines the patient mentally and emotionally to a monotonous environment. Davis et al showed that, rather than quantity or variation in sensation, volunteers placed in tank respirators required continuous, meaningful input to prevent disordered thinking.[29] Patients with bandages over the eyes and ears are known to develop aberrant behavior, even delirium.

Sensory overload occurs in the ICU, particularly when continuous surveillance of patients takes priority over privacy. Thus, the patient, often in pain or discomfort, is exposed to the stimulus of staff members interacting with each other and with other patients, the strange sounds of electronic equipment with visual and auditory alarm systems, and the continuous noise of ventilators. The monotonous, rhythmic sounds of ventilators and audible ECG monitoring induce in some patients auditory hallucinations of musical content. Under experimental conditions, normal subjects have responded with hallucinations when subjected to regular, intermittent, auditory stimulation.[30] Compounding these sensations are the more highly personalized and frequent physical examinations, irrigations, aspirations, and injections. Lack of privacy for very modest patients in an ICU is a source of considerable distress. ICU patients readily become upset with the staff discussion which they cannot quite overhear, but can see, noting with distress the solemn-faced discussants gesturing in their direction. Sensory overload induced by intensive medical and nursing attention to the patient or to his or her fellow patients can result in sleep deprivation, implicated by some investigators as a causative agent in psychological disturbances.[31,32,33,34]

Katz et al describe a simple mental status test which can be helpful in detecting the type of cognitive impairment operating in the patient.[35] These authors distinguish between global cognitive impairment which they found in patients with organic abnormality and selective cognitive impairment in patients with delirium more likely secondary to environmental factors. The implication is that the type of impairment detected by testing may become an important indicator of the underlying cause, thus expediting effective intervention.

Delirium in a coronary care unit (CCU) occurs less frequently than in a surgical ICU, and it appears that the tranquil periods which counteract periods of crisis and hectic activity help to keep psychological trauma down.[36] Hackett and his fellow psychiatrists, studying a one-room, multibed coronary unit, found patients contented with the physical setting and reassured by the cardiac monitor.[37] Although there were violent fluctuations in sensory input ranging from monotony to the sudden terror of witnessing an emergency or experiencing incapacitating chest

pain, psychological disturbances such as delirium occurred in only 10 percent of the patients. Denial was the dominant defense mechanism used in coping with anxiety, a mood admitted to by 80 percent. Patients who witnessed a cardiac emergency grasped the most comforting aspect (i.e., the astonishing efficiency of the staff) while denying the obviously more threatening aspects. In this case 33 out of 45 patients said that they were reassured by news of their transfer from the ICU. With the exception of a very few areas of stress, Cassem and Hackett concluded that the medical and nursing CCU staff should be able to manage the emotional stresses of most of their patients without psychiatric consultation.[38] After experience with 145 CCU patients, they identified the most frequent psychological problems as anxiety, depression, and management of inappropriate behavior and set guidelines for their management. The data suggest that emotions in normal people not only respond predictably, but usually follow a foreseeable course.

Another opportunity for stress may occur on transfer. Some patients become anxious about lack of surveillance or staff expertise in the new patient area. In a study of coronary patients, Klein et al found adverse emotional reactions and cardiovascular complications in some patients following transfer from the ICU.[39] Marked differences in the two environments and the attitude of the medical and nursing staffs in the new unit were associated with the stress experienced by the patients: sudden transition from dependency to an environment interpreted to be fraught with neglect and rejection.

EFFECT ON THE NURSE

Hay and Oken perceive the ICU as a setting in which the psychological threat of object-loss to the nurse is pervasive.[40] She is bombarded by anxiety, grief, and overstimulation. Work pressures are often intense, at least qualitatively, and threaten to overcommit her; guilt and anger are inevitable.

To protect herself, the nurse may respond to these stresses with a variety of defense mechanisms. Sometimes, the ICU nurse is criticized for being "too technically oriented."

Technical competency, an essential quality in ICU nurses, may act as a psychological defense against the high mortality of the ICU. Denial is a major defense mechanism, as evidenced by the joking and light chatter often heard among ICU personnel. We have found most experienced ICU nurses, particularly charge nurses, quite aware of the delicate balance between considerate interaction with frightened patients and grieving relatives and protection of their own morale. As one nurse put it: "We can't walk around looking morbid all the time, who would want to work up here? Our patients don't want that either." A respiratory ICU is nicknamed "Mucus Manor" by a nursing and medical staff.[41] The descriptive name, "Mucus Manor," although used only in jest, indicates another release valve for the emotional stress of staff continuously responsible for keeping ventilator patients out of difficulty. A room or lounge adjacent to the ICU, sufficiently private to permit staff to really "let off steam" is a priority item in planning an ICU. As identified by Vreeland and Ellis, stresses on the ICU nurse may include those of feeling insecure about the knowledge and skill needed to meet life-threatening, complex situations; of maintaining an appropriate balance between sympathy for the patient's comfort and carrying out pain-producing but essential procedures; of communicating with patients who cannot speak; of making emergency decisions in the absence of a physician; and of the frustration arising from lack of quiet periods of time to talk with anxious patients or to reflect on one's own ministrations.[42]

Continuing education for the ICU staff is essential to meet the demands for emergency decision making and minute-to-minute assessment of critical patients. Indeed, inadequate or lack of available training is cited as a source of stress by ICU nurses. That critical care courses must be made available is no longer challenged. It is the quality of program which is the variable today. Regionalization of staff development programs and the pooling of resources and faculty offer the best hope for solution of this problem.

In caring for a number of unconscious patients, the ICU nurse suffers from sensory deprivation; despite the skill and all-out efforts of the ICU team, she must live with a number of unfavorable outcomes for patients. It is important that the ICU nurse understand that temporary reassignment to another part of the hospital is available, and is considered desirable. In our experience, it often restores perspective and permits the nurse to sharpen her communication skills in an intermediate unit where many of the ICU patients are located pre-and post-ICU. The realities of staffing a nursing department usually demand the nurse's replacement on the ICU. Where more than one ICU exists, we believe these nurses are the most interchangeable. Intermediate unit nurses may serve in the ICU in a secondary role for that rotation. They have received some training in arrhythmia detection, ventilator care, and the like, but are not expected to perform with the degree of sophistication of the ICU nurse in her own environment, nor as charge nurses or even as primary decision makers for ICU patients.

When staff morale is low, a group conference on the stresses being experienced may be all that is needed to "break the tension." The choice of a leader for such a conference must depend on its purpose. For example, a mental health nursing specialist may be required to work through suppressed intragroup hostilities;[43] the head nurse or unit instructor may promote, especially with new staff, the conviction that anxiety, guilt, and uncertainty are acceptable feelings that need to be shared; the supervisor takes the opportunity to encourage staff to offer solutions to administrative problems.

To combat the frustration of too little time to talk to patients and families, the ICU nurse must remember that, although only short periods of time may be available for quiet communication, the nurse-patient relationship still can be a strong one. Persons under considerable stress, both patients and their families, seek support in reducing emotional pressure. They often respond, even in the short time available with the rapid turnover of patients on the surgical ICU.[44] Newman illustrates how the nurse can identify the hospitalized patient's psychological needs and initiate appropriate nursing action by spending relatively short periods of time with him or her.[45] As identified by Newman, the three major psychological needs of the medical-surgical patient are: 1) need arising from fear, anxiety, pain, and loneliness, 2) need to exercise control over him- or herself, and 3) need to have his or her identity recognized and maintained in the face of disability. The most frequent need is the first of these three. However, the ICU nurse must not ignore the other two.

What are the rewards of intensive care nursing? Being a member of an expert team of observers and decision makers in critical situations is a highly satisfying and ego-rewarding experience. This is enhanced by physician-nurse communication and collaboration in the ICU which, in the writers' opinion, are very favorable. The lifesaving nature of the care has demanded that both disciplines sit down together, assess their strengths and limitations, and establish their protocols for patient care. The mutual respect and camaraderie which prevails is a recruitment plus for ICU nursing.

Nursing Intervention

The process of nursing intervention in an ICU is identical to that of any other unit; assessment, planning, implementation, and evaluation. The whole process must be ongoing and repeatedly revised as the patient's condition changes. This is particularly true in the care of the high-risk ICU patient whose condition is subject to rapid and frequent variation. However, one major difference between nursing in an ICU and in another unit is in establishing and maintaining priorities. Unlike the nurse in other units, the ICU nurse usually cannot fully involve the patient in setting priorities for his or her care. Patients in the ICU are in either a potential or immediate life-threatening crisis. Their pathophysiological needs must be met first. Life-threatening arrhythmias, respiratory and cardiac arrest, shock and hemorrhage can and do occur so quickly and so often that nursing action centers on maintenance and support of respiration, circulation, and metabolism, particularly fluid and electrolyte balance, and relief of pain. The

nursing care and skills involved in meeting these needs are described in other chapters in this text.

The psychosocial needs of the ICU patient are important, and, under most circumstances, the nurse begins to meet these needs while caring for the pathophysiological needs. The antediluvian attitude of concentrating solely on present physical problems, if it ever really existed, is certainly not in evidence at present. Behavior problems, including psychosis, are often precipitated in the ICU. Although the typical patient remains oriented and rational, he or she demonstrates verbally or nonverbally the nerve-racking effect of pain, anxiety about the future or death itself, and loss of positive body and/or self-image. The feeling of impotence which the busy ICU nurse sometimes experiences when she attempts to help the patient with these problems is understandable. However, there are a number of concrete suggestions which the ICU nurse can use in coping with these problems and even in preventing or minimizing the behavioral problems.

THE PATIENT FACTOR

PIECE TOGETHER A "PORTRAIT" OF THE PATIENT AS AN INDIVIDUAL AND AS A MEMBER OF A FAMILY. Include in the assessment, whenever possible, information about the patient's family and social life, previous reaction to illness, and other life crises. Family and other visitors on the ICU may exert desirable or disastrous influences which must be evaluated by the staff. Our experience indicates that a significant and stable family member or friend may need to be available beyond the usual five-to-ten minutes visiting intervals typical of ICUs. For some patients, the significant visitor serves as the vital bridge to reality. Whenever there is opportunity, use a few, simple clues to assess role determination within the patient's family. This information should make the nurse more helpful in assisting family members to cope as their stress continues or increases in severity.

When the patient is transferred to the ICU from another area within the hospital, insist upon a nursing care plan which provides such data. Ideally, a nurse who has been caring for the patient accompanies him to the ICU, introduces him to the staff, and communicates his nursing care needs directly, both verbally and through the written care plan. It is advantageous for some patients to visit an ICU preoperatively, providing the visit is carefully cleared beforehand with ICU staff. For most patients, it is often more satisfactory to plan for the surgical ICU head nurse or one of her staff to visit the patient in the preoperative unit. Large photographs of the ICU serve to orient the patient to its emphasis on constant surveillance. Upon transfer from an ICU, include the patient, when possible, in the discussion of some carefully chosen aspect of care with the nurse in the intermediate unit, thereby reinforcing concern for continuity of his therapy and rehabilitation. For example, visiting by the ICU

staff to patients before admission to surgical ICU and after transfer from an ICU is most helpful when specific problems, possible solutions, and objectives are formulated with the intermediate unit nursing staff. The following care plan illustrates the above points (Figs. 10-1 and 10-2).

On ICU, Miss J. experienced a fairly uneventful postoperative recovery. The ICU nursing staff identified the following as some specific ways in which they used the preoperative care plan in caring for Miss J. for several days postoperatively.

1. Communicated with mother, most significant family member to patient, as link between hospital staff and family.

2. Encouraged patient to ask for analgesics; could

Nursing Care Plan

Goal of Nursing Care: 11/15/75 To prepare Miss J for surgery (mitral valve replacement) on or about 11/8

Date	Patient's Needs/Problem	Nursing Approach
11/15	A 22 year old former nursing student (completed 1 year of diploma program — voluntarily withdrew). Apparently satisfied in present vocation - zoo technician. Lives with parents, 18 year old brother. Athletically oriented and increasing SoB and fatigue convince her that "surgery is now although I'm more apprehensive than I should be."	Support her right to be apprehensive "more than I should be." Appears to be tied to Nursing School experience. Encourage her to express her specific concerns. Approach: "Sometimes our nursing knowledge may make us fearful. Can we talk about how we can use it in a positive way?"
11/16	Uses medical terminology she does not fully understand, appears to have need to present herself as a knowledgeable professional	Don't permit Miss J to "lose face," e.g. confused terms stenosis and regurgitation. Given booklet which defines terms, without any reference made to her use of terms.

FIGURE 10-1.
Nursing care plan.

TEACHING PLAN

Type of Teaching Needed	Date Taught	Instructions Given and Reactions	Specific Reinforcement Needed
Valve replacement technique	11/15/75 A.M.	Simple illustration by Dr Jackson of artificial valve and cardeopulmonary by-pass. (Mother and patient hesitant to ask for clarification)	Use heart model to emphasize points made by M.D. RN praised patient for her learning—
Preoperative Prep	11/15 P.m.	Explained skin prep, medications, Foley. Called SICU head nurse to visit.	began to ask more questions
Respiratory Care	11/16 Am	Began diaphragmatic and lateral costal exercises after assessing breathing patterns. Discussed endotracheal tube and use of ventilator postoperatively.	Needs little reminder to practice breathing exercises. Coughs well.
Respiratory Care cont'd.	11/16 Pm.	Chest tubes, chest films discussed. Percussion & vibration techniques demonstrated.	Reluctant to discuss discomfort and pain with procedure. "I can take pain."
Other Postop Care	11/17 A.m.	Monitoring of vital signs, leg exercises, fluid restriction, diet progression, ↑ activities	
Visit from SICU head nurse	11/17 P.m.	SICU head nurse discussed ICU layout; again gave simple briefing on ventilator	Reassured by this visit of HN and information he ventilators.
Review	11/18 Am	Questions by Miss J. are realistic ones, seems to value our help. Still guarded in discussion of pain.	Mother attended this session and is able to interpret to other family members

FIGURE 10-2.
Teaching plan.

carry over her facade of the "brave professional."

3. Anticipated postoperative events in which she could have "lost face," such as removal of chest tubes. Provided as much privacy as possible.
4. Reassured about pacemaker even though she might not ask specifically about it.

In transferring the patient to 3 East, the ICU nurse communicated pertinent information concerning her postoperative course, identified an emerging problem and discussed it with Miss Smith, the nurse who would care for Miss J. Although Miss J. had been well taught and understood generally what progress to expect, she was becoming increasingly anxious about setting a performance record beyond her physical capacity. In pushing herself, Miss J. was becoming irritated and demanding. The staff of 3 East soon found evidence of the problem for themselves. Shortly after transfer, on her third postoperative day, Miss J. became exasperated when asked by Miss Smith to wait a few minutes for nursing attention. "You're holding me back! No wonder patients take so long to get well in hospitals." After praising Miss J. for her fine efforts as a patient, which she obviously needed to hear, Miss Smith reflected on her accusatory words. There began to unravel a deeper reason for Miss J.'s "professional facade." Part of her dissatisfaction in nursing school had arisen from her feelings of "hypocrisy" about patients who demanded much but did not seem to try hard enough on their own to get better. Preoperatively, Miss J. could not admit this, nor had she realized that she would live through even a brief experience where she would begin to feel alienated from the hospital staff. With Miss Smith's acceptance of the patient's ambivalent and somewhat guilty feelings about her nursing school experiences, Miss J. developed insight into her own behavior as a patient. She began to relax and her need to be a "superior patient" was significantly reduced. Discharge teaching proceeded smoothly.

A criticism of progressive patient care has been the fragmentation of the care and the additional numbers of personnel to whom the patient must become adjusted. This becomes a valid criticism when transfer of patients to and from the ICU is not considered an important nursing responsibility.

ANTICIPATE THE PROBLEM OF PAIN, ESPECIALLY ACUTE PAIN. In the surgical ICU, pain is predictable as to site, intensity, and usually duration. A written assessment by the nurse on the preoperative floor indicates the patient's attitude toward the surgery and his or her instruction about pain and its alleviation. By pointing out to the patient in advance the characteristics of the postoperative pain and assessing his or her psychological response to the surgery and pain, the program to minimize pain is well established.

When the ICU nurse initiates the assessment, both the patient's verbal and nonverbal behavior should indicate how he or she copes with pain and discomfort. Family members can be helpful here. Nursing comfort measures, distraction, suggestion, even the knowledge that the patient will not be rejected if he or she cries out in pain, all can help the patient to deal with moderate to severe pain. Nevertheless, analgesics, sedatives, and tranquilizers are often vital for patient comfort. Children below age ten rarely require narcotics and are most amenable to suggestion;[46] the elderly require analgesics or sedation to assure adequate rest, although sensitivity to these drugs necessitates smaller doses.

DESCRIBE CAREFULLY AND DOCUMENT THE BEHAVIOR OF PATIENTS AS THEY COPE WITH THEIR ANXIETIES. This is where deliberate planning to meet specific psychological needs begins. Share observations about the patient's behavior with the physician and other team members, thereby avoiding actions and statements which enhance feelings of tension and discouragement in the patient. Such an evaluation may demonstrate the need for expertise beyond that of the ICU staff.

Permit patients to discuss their fears of death, or find someone qualified and willing to talk with them if you cannot bring yourself to listen. "If the patient wishes to discuss his death, he should not be cajoled into changing the subject. This way comforts the listener, but it does not change the character of the patient's preoccupation."[47] If the patient has suffered a loss of positive body image, the nurse's reaction of acceptance is crucial and therapeutic. The family often requires counseling about the importance of acceptance, too.

PLAN ESPECIALLY FOR REGULARLY SCHEDULED COMMUNICATION WITH PATIENTS WHO ARE SEVERELY IMMOBILIZED, ELDERLY, OR WHOSE FAMILY AND OUTSIDE-WORLD CONTACTS ARE RESTRICTED OR INEFFECTUAL. Show your interest in the patient as a person by listening and talking with him or her when you are not doing something to, with, or for him or her. The ICU nurse has an important "cure" role as a valuable ally of the physician, but her "care" role in an ICU is more vital, if the patient is to be sustained through the crucial period of life. TV, radio, travel slides, and records often provide relief from monotony or loneliness. Calendars and clocks are helpful in preventing or correcting loss of the sense of time.

TREATMENT FACTORS

MINIMIZE TREATMENT-PRECIPITATED FACTORS BY EXPLAINING MONITORING AND TREATMENT EQUIPMENT TO THE PATIENT IN TERMS HE OR SHE CAN APPRECIATE. Repeat and restate the explanation until his or her apprehension is sufficiently allayed to permit comprehension and retention. This habit of meaningful explanation should be practiced even when there is real doubt that the patient can comprehend. The cardiac monitor is looked upon by most patients as tangible evidence that surveillance is continuous. False alarms, at best, are a nuisance, but the "mechanical guardian angel"[48] is well received by patients.

RECOGNIZE THAT THE DEGREE OF ARTIFICIAL ASSISTANCE REQUIRED TO SUSTAIN THE PATIENT IS RELATED TO THE FREQUENCY OF BEHAVIORAL DISTURBANCES. Check monitoring and lifesaving equipment periodically. Avoid speaking about the "Bird" or the "Bennett," instead of "Mrs. N. on the Bird or the Bennett ventilator." Do not assume that the obtunded patient is oblivious to staff comments concerning equipment. Several postcardiotomy patients, following a period of delirium, commented on their belief that personnel were more concerned with the equipment than with them. Their feelings of hostility and paranoia were very real to the patients, no matter how silly these feelings appeared to them when the delirium passed. Several years ago, one woman who developed paranoid delusions and visual hallucinations had been attached to a Bird ventilator for three days. Upon weaning from the machine, she imagined that she was a "bird" or was imprisoned like a "bird in a cage." When patients experience such delusions, support them by showing you are there to keep them from harm, but do not reinforce the delusion by referring specifically to it.

PLAN THE CARE OF THE PATIENT TO PERMIT AS MUCH UNINTERRUPTED SLEEP AS POSSIBLE. Sleep deprivation, or at least sleep that is not satisfactory, is a common patient complaint. Remember also, that the patient whose sleep is interrupted is more likely to develop an increased sensitivity to pain.[49] There is room for improvement in the coordination of the care given by the total health team, and it falls to the nurse who observes the patient over eight hours to bring this to the attention of the physician. It is not unlikely that the nurse may be the first to suggest that some monitoring equipment or treatment may no longer be needed as frequently, thereby facilitating more or better rest.

ENVIRONMENTAL FACTORS

RECOGNIZE THE UNFAVORABLE PHYSICAL ASPECTS OF THE UNIT WHICH AFFECT SENSORY INPUT. The one-room, multibed unit demands more frequent assessment of noise levels and that portion of the emergency protocol which calls for screening of other patients. It is necessary to consider that some patients are "deprived" when physical structure prevents their view of the nurse on whom they feel so dependent. Simply seeing the nurse can act as a comfortable, familiar bulwark for the patient in a stressful environment.

Examine periodically the noise levels and the character of the noise in the ICU (with tape recorder, if necessary). Minckley's findings in a study of noise in the recovery room environment supported the hypothesis that the postoperative patient is made more uncomfortable as noise in the environment increases.[50] Reactions to noises appeared to depend upon the patient's interpretation of the noises. The most pronounced reaction was one of resentment of the laughter and jovial verbal behavior of recovery room staff. Patients' subjective sensations of pain were increased at times when noise levels were high. These findings are readily applied to the ICU, particularly in the unit which may have no area apart from the patients for personnel to discuss care or converse together in normal tones.

Karen—SICU Nursing Intervention

As you read the highlights of this patient's clinical course, think of the nursing intervention you would attempt if you were the patient's nurse.

Karen, an 18-year-old girl, was in an auto accident and struck her head, neck, and chest on the dashboard. She was taken to a nearby hospital. She never lost consciousness, but developed increasing respiratory distress and suffered a respiratory arrest, necessitating an emergency tracheostomy. (The site of the tracheostomy was lower than usual due to the trauma site and edema.) Her airway was then adequate, her respirations spontaneous, and there was no apparent deleterious effect from her brief respiratory arrest (spinal and chest films were negative). However, Karen was immediately transferred to the SICU of a University Medical Center for continuous observation and further evaluation, because of possible pneumothorax and/or cardiac tamponade.

Upon arrival in the SICU, Karen was placed on the ECG monitor, tracheostomy care with cautious aspirations only prn, hourly I and O, vital signs every 15 minutes, including complete CNS evaluation. She was kept NPO and on IV therapy.

The nursing staff gave Karen calm, matter-of-fact explanations for all the procedures that were being done to, for, and with her, and emphasized that these were precautionary measures. A clipboard and pencil were quickly provided, and Karen was reassured that she could communicate in this manner. The almost constant presence of her nurse, plus the fact the the SICU is an "open" unit where other nurses are always visible, was also comforting to her. A "clapper" bell was taped to the siderail of her bed for added reassurance.

Karen began to complain of tenderness in her upper sternum and chest wall. Subsequently, subcutaneous emphysema in her neck and upper chest wall was noted. She then developed a pneumomediastinum and her trachea was deviated to the right. A tomogram of the larynx revealed an interruption of the normal air column just underneath the left vocal cord, with escape of air into the surrounding tissues.

Early the next morning, a bronchoscopy and revision of the tracheostomy was performed. But an ominous sign had developed; the tracheostomy tube began to visibly pulsate, indicating its

Right   Left

proximity to the innominate artery. "Massive hemorrhage from erosion of the innominate artery is the most common delayed fatal complication of tracheostomy."[51]

For the next few days, Karen tolerated liquids well, and her pulmonary status improved. The size of the tracheostomy tube was decreased and the pulsations ceased. After six days in the SICU, she was transferred to the Oto unit. The day prior to transfer, a nurse from the Oto unit came to the SICU, reviewed the care plan and chart, and was introduced to Karen so she would have a familiar face to identify with on the other unit, and to reassure Karen that the staff of the Oto unit would be familiar with her care. A full report on the nursing care was given by the nurse from the SICU to the nurse from the Oto unit, and the transfer was accomplished smoothly. Karen appeared "out of the woods," but was extremely disappointed because her sister was being married the next day, and Karen very much wanted to participate in the wedding. Because of her steady physical progress, but mental depression, Karen was issued a pass to attend the wedding. Unfortunately, only a few hours after her return to the hospital, Karen suddenly spurted blood from her trachea 6 to 8 inches in the air due to erosion of the tracheostomy tube into the innominate artery. She was whisked to the OR where a thoracotomy was performed to ligate the innominate artery. It was necessary to place Karen on the ventilator on 70 percent oxygen. She was transferred back to the SICU postop.

Over the next nine-and-one-half months, Karen alternated between making progress and suffering relapses. She required 18 stat surgical procedures for massive hemorrhages (blood loss ranging from 3,000 ml to 9,000 ml). She bled from the innominate artery, and later from the aorta itself. After the third thoracotomy, Karen's sternum and chest were left open and her mediastinum packed, because of infection. Twice daily, thereafter, her physician and nurse removed the packing, irrigated her chest with 1,000 ml sterile saline, retrieved the solution with suction, and repacked the wound. (Because Karen's chest was open, it was possible upon subsequent hemorrhages, for her nurse to apply direct pressure on the bleeding site in order to gain the precious seconds necessary to rush her back to the OR.)

Karen's infections were caused by a variety of organisms, and the numerous antibiotics, hypothermia, and antipyretics could not control her temperature which frequently remained between 103° and 105°. She had bilateral lung infections as well as a resistant pseudomonas mediastinitis.

Two months after admission, Karen passed a 12-week-old fetus, which was not anticipated. According to her normal cycle, she had missed only one menstrual period, and this was assumed to be due to the severity of her illness. Following the abortion, Karen bled moderately, but an IV pitocin drip controlled this. She later passed the placenta with very little blood loss. Because of Karen's depression, she was not told of the abortion—she thought she had irregular bleeding and clots because of her illness.

In addition to all of Karen's physical complications, her mental status was also of prime concern. Although her depression was realistic considering her complications and length of stay on the SICU, it had to be dealt with. We held many conferences on Karen's care with representatives of all services involved: otorhinolaryngology, cardiothoracic surgery, neurology, anesthesiology, gynecology, psychiatry, cardiology, ophthalmology, infectious disease, hematology, occupational therapy, inhalation therapy, and dietary, as well as nursing. A concerted effort was made by all to approach Karen in a consistent and positive manner and to gently, but firmly, reinforce that the behavior she had regressed to was not going to manipulate us or be an attention-gaining mechanism. For example, Karen had begun to refuse her bath, would not cooperate with her chest irrigations, would not

remain still for her portable chest films, threatened to pull out her tubes (but never attempted to do so), and so on. The psychiatrist felt these were manipulative measures to keep as many people at her bedside for as long as possible because of intense fear. By continuing to assign the same nurses that Karen was fond of to her care as much as possible, and using a firm but understanding approach, we managed to change the above behavior. The nursing staff had suggested that hypnosis might help, but Karen was too depressed for attempts at hypnosis to be successful. But we did gain Karen's confidence to the point when, during one of her hemorrhages, she calmly pointed to her chest and said, "I've done it again."

Over two months postadmission, during repair of one of Karen's hemorrhages, it was noted that the tear in her trachea had increased considerably: there was only a small piece of tissue holding the trachea together 1 to 2 cm above the

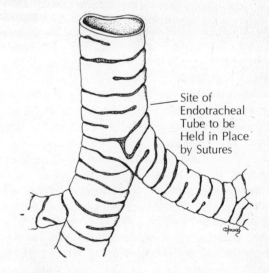

— Site of Endotracheal Tube to be Held in Place by Sutures

carina. For the next few days Karen's condition was stable. A tracheal prosthesis was attempted and an anode tube placed in the trachea.

Karen continued her up and down course, and nearly ten months postadmission, she bled for the eighteenth time. The attempt to repair the hole in the aorta was not successful and she died from circulatory collapse secondary to uncontrolled hemorrhage. Clinically, on the OR table that day, a 19-year-old girl died from complications following an automobile accident. Almost ten months of effort, anguish, sweat, apprehension, concern, heroic performance, and conscientious care for Karen also died that day. Our grief was deep and profound.

The nursing care Karen required, even for an ICU patient, was great. Attempting to meet the four objectives of ICU nursing was challenging and frustrating for this chronically, critically ill patient.

The first objective was detection of and participation in life-threatening crises. Obviously, maintenance of Karen's circulation was a repeated crisis. Each hemorrhage required immediate detection and nursing intervention. The phychological impact on the patient and the nursing staff was traumatic. It may seem obvious that massive hemorrhage would be easily detected immediately, but Karen's chest dressings were usually pink to bright red in color, and her chest could not be left exposed. Frequent observation was necessary, but we did not want to increase Karen's apprehension, nor did we wish to deprive her of sleep. So we were as gentle and as casual as possible.

Maintenance of adequate ventilation for Karen was a problem from the moment she was admitted. A whole chapter could be written about her respiratory care: the frequent blood gas values, the number and various types and sizes of tracheostomy tubes, the irritation of numerous anesthetics, the laryngeal stents and revisions, the attempted tracheal repair, pulmonary infection, and the like. Of utmost importance was repetitive sterile, meticulous, yet gentle aspiration by the nursing staff. The IPPB, chest physiotherapy, and hyperinflation were coordinated with aspiration. Frequent "stripping" of chest tubes to assure patency and to observe the character and amount of drainage, and amount of "bubbling" to indicate the presence and amount of air leak were also of high priority. The nursing observations each time Karen was weaned from the ventilator were also important.

The second goal of Karen's care was preservation of her physiological defenses and prevention of further complications. Despite "isolation technique" and all the antibiotic agents employed, the complication of infection could not be prevented, and the severity of Karen's infections was a major factor in preventing healing, and, therefore, contributed greatly to her fatality.

The nursing observations and treatments recorded during Karen's hospitalization including vital signs (TPR, CVP, neuro check, I and O, ECG, and so on), medications, respiratory care, comments not only on her care, but her reaction to it, her mental status, reaction to visitors, and the like were so numerous that the nursing record portion of her chart was over 8 inches thick. Obviously, her care plan was changed frequently and rapidly.

Karen's metabolic needs were also a challenge. When she was NPO, "regular" IVs could not supply the calories and nutrients she needed for healing. Nasogastric tube feedings at times were tolerated, but when Karen developed diarrhea or regurgitated the feedings, parenteral hyperalimentation was necessary, although this method of meeting nutritional requirements was used only when necessary because of the hazard of the subclavian line becoming another source of infection.

Passive range-of-motion exercises were successful in preventing contractures. Skin care might seem of low priority considering Karen's multitudinous problems, but it was not. Frequent turning and good back care prevented decubitus ulcers and another focus for infection. It was previously stated that during Karen's depressed, negative state, she refused her bath. In some instances, this might not be important. But Karen was a teenager with excessively oily skin and acne—a further source of infection. So a daily bath was important. Karen also had very long hair which became dirty and greasy quickly (particularly with her temperature elevations and perspiration). The nurses, with difficulty, managed to wash her hair about once a week. But due to her illness, Karen's hair began to fall out and became much thinner. This did not help her appearance or self-image. Karen expressed a desire to have her hair cut, so the nurses arranged for the hospital beautician to cut Karen's hair in a cute "pixie." Karen loved the style; it improved her appearance, and made it easier to keep her hair clean.

The third goal of Karen's care was to provide comfort which did not interfere with the second goal, and would serve as implementation of the fourth goal which was to establish and maintain meaningful communication with the patient and her family.

It was necessary to administer morphine prior to Karen's chest care. She also had pain as a result of her multiple surgical procedures. It was necessary to relieve her pain, and this was accomplished with judicious use of narcotics. Smaller doses were administered more frequently which relieved her pain, but gave her less of a "high." Because Karen had "experimented" with drugs prior to admission, a concerted attempt was made not to create an iatrogenic addict.

Because Karen required so much care involving so many medical services, it was difficult to coordinate her care to allow as much rest as possible, but her nurses planned her care toward this aim.

To allow Karen to participate in her care, she was allowed to sleep late, and her treatments and procedures planned accordingly, since sleeping late was her normal habit. Although Karen had a choice of foods from the menu (when she was on oral feedings), she did not like many of the foods offered, and the dietitian could not please her. Therefore, to encourage her to eat, the nursing staff made and/or bought some of her favorite dishes. They also managed to obtain a portable TV for her. Karen's sister brought in a portable radio, and between the TV and the radio, Karen's spirits improved.

Upon admission, Karen's relationship with her parents was not good: they did not approve of her friends; they had forbidden her to "keep company" with the individual driving when the accident occurred, and in general considered her a rebel. Fortunately, Karen and her sister were close. By using her sister as the significant family member, we were able to build a meaningful

bridge between Karen and her parents. Eventually they visited Karen regularly and this was helpful, even though some of their visits were not therapeutic because they began to harp on Karen's choice of friends. The nurses at this point would intercede with some excuse or reason, such as it was time for a treatment. As time passed, with the nurses' repeated explanations of Karen's need for demonstration of her parents' love and understanding, they began to develop a positive attitude and more patience with Karen and this was therapeutic for all three of them.

Karen's nineteenth birthday occurred during her stay on the SICU and at a time when she was NPO. But the nursing staff had a party, and made a cake. The physicians allowed Karen to partake of some cake and they supplied the ice cream. Even though Karen could not swallow the "goodies," she could at least taste—she expectorated them. Although this was not the greatest party in the world, Karen enjoyed it and appreciated the presents from her family and the nursing staff.

The nurses identified closely with Karen. Grief accompanies the loss of any patient, but Karen's age and her length of stay on the SICU made her loss even greater. The staff, in spite of her recalcitrant behavior, had come to know and love her. They also had become involved with Karen's family. They were aware of why Karen's parents had originally felt as they did, and were sympathetic. The stress on the nursing staff was extremely great, and this was further increased when Karen's family invited the nursing staff to the funeral services. They felt the nurses had done and cared so much for Karen, that they considered the staff "part of the family." As difficult as it was, those members of the staff who were not on duty, did attend the services.

Opportunities for Research

The ICU nurse is committed to action—quick, sure, and safe—in her objective of patient care. But if nursing is to advance, it is necessary to analyze such actions and formulate nursing theory from them.[52] What patient information is important for ICU nurses to receive from nurses on the preoperative or intermediate unit? In what form can this information be meaningfully communicated? A one-page, easy-to-complete but comprehensive, assessment tool developed by Winslow and Fuhs, the result of their research study, provides baseline physiological and psychological data which the ICU nurse uses to evaluate postoperative responses.[53] To promote a sense of security and relaxation in the seriously ill patient, communication skill, especially nonverbal interaction, is very important. The skillful ICU nurse observes for nonverbal clues, interprets the patient's communication, and responds accordingly. What system of communication develops between nurse and patient? How can she teach this skill to others? It is necessary to describe and analyze what this nurse does, to conceptualize the interaction, if possible, and to test, practice, and teach it. Similarly, the so-called intuition of the highly experienced ICU nurse that the patient is "going sour" (and he or she does), needs study. The prodromal signs and symptoms of the psychoticlike state seen postoperatively need further verification, both qualitatively and quantitatively. We have observed, for example, very short periods of staring or eye movements which seem to indicate suspicious feelings in patients who later demonstrate bizarre behavior.

Administering the simple mental status test developed by Katz, et al, to patients with cognitive impairment and documenting the results would be most worthwhile in attempting to assess the underlying cause, and thus, the more appropriate intervention.[54] The study on training cardiac surgical patients in relaxation methods preoperatively is encouraging in illustrating a more specific, tangible method of psychological intervention to reduce postoperative emotional stress. Further study should be done on the effect of telling the patient in advance that hallucinations and sensory distortions can occur. Our experience has been limited; but we are encouraged by the response of selected patients who are informed of these events, presented as normal and self-limiting which should be reported to the staff if they occur.

ICU nursing is often in the forefront of medical and technological advance. The nurse's clinical experiences need to be documented so that these data may be incorporated into nursing school curricula and continuing education programs for practitioners. One early study attempted to identify nursing actions during the first four postoperative hours for the cardiac surgical patient.[55] Methods for analyzing such actions were developed as a basis for relating practice to scientific content. The study by Schmitt, et al, illustrates the ICU nurse's colleague relationship with the physician in examining the effects of armchair treatment of myocardial infarction.[56] Nursing members of the health team were responsible for data collection, hypothesis formation, and analysis of study findings. Nursing must continue to be intimately involved in research dealing with the extent to which computer skills can replace human skills.[57] Because of the nurse's proximity to the patient, she is in an excellent position to assess any possible "dehumanizing" aspects and to determine how the nurse may better serve the patient when machinery relieves her of some time-consuming tasks.

The electronic equipment of the ICU is an excellent research tool, for data describing the patients's clinical course can be stored in it and retrieved for analysis. These data can be studied in relation to a time-related activity or situation. Work done by faculty and graduate students at the University of Washington examined the usefulness of electronic monitoring in identifying stressful situations for the patient.[58] In three separate studies, nursing researchers identified electrocardiographic changes in both patients and healthy volunteers during such nursing activities as feeding and bathing. More prolonged rather than shorter periods of nursing activity were associated with ischemic ECG changes, a concept which needs to be validated if nursing practices are to become more explicit.

A word of warning is required when surveying the subjective responses of the patient to the ICU experiences. Extreme dependency on and feelings of gratitude toward ICU personnel appear to affect the patient's objectivity in reporting his or her reactions. It is helpful to validate such responses with biochemical and polygraphic data.[59]

Finally, the ICU nurse needs to become involved in the study of nursing the chronically ill and in multidisciplinary research of systems of health care for the chronically ill. Because the ICU cares for many chronically ill patients during the acute phase, the ICU nurse needs to become more familiar with the preventive and rehabilitative aspects of chronic illness. Then, in turn, she can contribute to the study of the patient during exacerbation.

References

1. Special care units.: Mod. Hosp. 118:81, Jan. 1972.
2. Benner, P. and Kramer, M.: Role conceptions and integrative role behavior of nurses in special care and regular hospital nursing units. Nurs. Research 21:30, Jan.-Feb. 1972.
3. Gerwig, W. H., Jr.: The surgical intensive care unit. Surg. Clin. N. Am. 48:955, Aug. 1968.
4. U.S. Public Health Service, Division Hospital Medical Facilities. Elements of Progressive Patient Care. U.S. Public Health Service Publication, No. 930-C-1. Washington D.C., U.S. Government Printing Office, Sept. 1962, p. 2.
5. Coswell, J. E.: A brief history of coronary care units. Pub. Health Reports 82:1105-1107, Dec. 1967.
6. Meltzer, L. E., Pinneo, R. and Kitchell, J. R.: Intensive coronary care. A manual for nurses. Presbyt. Hosp. Philadelphia, Coronary Care Unit Fund, 1970.
7. Coswell, *op. cit.*
8. Dammann, F. J., Jr.: Intensive care service contributions and costs. JAMA 206:2319, Dec. 2, 1968.
9. Maddox, D.: Community hospital gears up to provide intensive care. Mod. Hosp. 118:100-102, Jan. 1972.
10. New organization seeks to set guidelines for special care. Mod. Hosp. 118:86-87, Jan. 1972.
11. Martin, L. E.: Cost and management: problems of intensive care units. Mod. Hosp. 118:99, Jan. 1972.
12. W. V. Kellogg Foundation: The Planning and Operation of an Intensive Care Unit. Battle Creek, Michigan, Sept. 1961.
13. Hochberg, H., et al: Coronary care unit ECG monitoring by digital computer. Biomed. Sci. Instrum. 5:11-15, 1969.
14. Grant, J. A., Moir, E. and Fago, M.: Parenteral hyperalimentation. Am. J. Nurs. 69:2392-2395, Nov. 1969.
15. Automation helps treat patients in center for the critically ill. Mod. Hosp. 118:95, Jan. 1972.
16. Features to consider in designing an ICU. Hosp. 43:18, 36, June 1, 1968.
17. Kinney, J. M.: Design of ICU, common problems in operation. Hosp. Top. 47:87-88, Feb. 1969.
18. Morgan-Hughes, J. O.: Lighting and cyanosis. Brit. J. Anaesth. 40:503-507, July, 1968.
19. Wilson, L. M.: Intensive care delirium. Arch. Intern. Med. 130:225-226, Aug. 1972.
20. Hanish, H. M.: Telemetry in the intensive care ward. Biomed. Sci. Instrum. 5:30, 1969.
21. Sheppard, L. C., et al: Surgical intensive care automation. J. Assoc. Adu. Med. Instrum. 6:74-78, Jan.-Feb. 1972.
22. Cohen, G. S.: State of the art: intensive care equipment. Biomed. Sci. Instrum. 5:15, 1969.
23. Solomon, P., et al: Sensory Deprivation. Cambridge, Mass., Harvard University Press, 1965, p. 1.
24. Kornfeld, D. S., Zimberg, S. and Maln, J. R.: Psychiatric complications of open-heart surgery. New Eng. J. Med. 273:287-292, Aug. 5, 1965.
25. Leiderman, H., et al: Sensory deprivation. Clinical aspects. Arch. Intern. Med. 101:393, Feb. 1958.
26. Elsberry, N.: Psychological responses to open heart surgery. Nurs. Research 21:226-227, May-June 1972.
27. Lindsley, D. B.: Common factors in sensory deprivation, sensory distortion and sensory overload. *In* P. Solomon, et al: Sensory Deprivation. Cambridge, Mass., Harvard University Press, 1965, p. 193.
28. Abram, H. S.: Adaptation to open-heart surgery: a psychiatric study of response to the threat of death. Am. J. Psychiat. 122:659-667, Dec. 1965.

29. Davis, J. M., McCourt, W. F. and Solomon, P.: The effect of visual stimulation on hallucinations and other mental experiences during sensory deprivation. Am. J. Psychiat. 116:892, 1960.

30. Egerton, N. and Kay, J. H.: Psychological disturbances associated with open-heart surgery. Brit. J. Psychiat. 110:436, 1964.

31. *Ibid.,* p. 435.

32. Kornfeld, *op. cit.,* p. 290.

33. Blachly, P. H. and Starr, A.: Post-cardiotomy delirium. Am. J. Psychiat. 121:373, 1964.

34. McFadden, E. and Giblin, E.: Sleep deprivation in patients having open-heart surgery. Nurs. Research 20:249-254, May-June 1971.

35. Katz, N. M., et al: Delirium in surgical patients under intensive care. Arch. Surg. 104:310-313, Mar. 1972.

36. Parker, D. L. and Hodge, J. R.: Delirium in a coronary-care unit. JAMA 201:132-133, Aug. 28, 1967.

37. Hackett, T. P., Cassem, N. H. and Wishnie, H. A.: The coronary-care unit. An appraisal of its psychological hazards. New Eng. J. Med. 279:1365-1370, Dec. 19, 1963.

38. Cassem, N. and Hackett, T.: Psychiatric consultation in a coronary care unit. Annals Intern. Med. 75:9-14, July 1971.

39. Klein, R. F., et al: Transfer from a CCU. Some adverse responses. Arch. Intern. Med., 122:104-108, Aug. 1968.

40. Hay, D. and Oken, D.: The psychological stresses of ICU nursing. Psychosoma. Med. 34:114, Mar.-Apr. 1972.

41. Fuhs, M., Rieser, M. and Brisbon. D.: Nursing in a respiratory intensive care unit. Chest 62:18S, Aug. 1972, Supplement.

42. Vreeland, R. and Ellis, G. L.: Stresses on the nurse in an intensive-care unit. JAMA 208:332-334, Apr. 14, 1969.

43. Reres, M.: Coping with stress in the ICU and CCU. Supervis. Nurs. 3:32, Jan. 1972.

44. Egbert, L. I.: Psychological support for surgical patients. *In* H. S. Abram: Psychological Aspects of Surgery. Boston, Little, Brown, 1967, p. 49.

45. Newman, M. A.: Identifying and meeting patients' needs in short-span nurse-patient relationships. Nurs. Forum 5:76-86, 1966.

46. Swafford, L. I. and Allan, D.: Pain relief in the pediatric patient. Med. Clin. N. Am. 52:135, Jan. 1968.

47. Robinson, L.: Psychological Aspects of the Care of Hospitalized Patients. Philadelphia, F. A. Davis, 1968, p. 60.

48. Hackett, *op. cit.,* p. 1370.

49. Long, B.: Sleep. Am. J. Nurs., 69:1898, Sept., 1969.

50. Minckley, B.: A study of noise and its relationship to patient discomfort in the recovery room. Nurs. Research 17:247-250, May-June, 1968.

51. Utley, R. J., et al.: Definitive management of innominate artery hemorrhage complicating tracheostomy. JAMA 220:577, Apr. 24, 1972.

52. Ellis, R.: The practitioner as theorist. Am. J. Nurs., 69:1436, July, 1969.

53. Winslow, E. and Fuhs, M.: Pre-operative Assessment for Post-operative Evaluation. Am. J. Nurs., 73:1372-1374, Aug., 1973.

54. Katz, et al: *op. cit.*

55. Chow, R.: Postoperative cardiac nursing research: a method for identifying and categorizing nursing action. Nurs. Research 18:4-13, Jan.-Feb., 1969.

56. Schmitt, Y., Hood, W. B., Jr. and Lown, B.: Armchair treatment in the coronary care unit: effect on blood pressure and pulse. Nurs. Research 18:114-118, Mar.-Apr., 1969.

57. Sheppard, L. C., et al, *op. cit.*

58. Mansfield, L. W.: The use of electrocardiographic monitoring in nursing research. In Second Nursing Research Conference. Phoenix, Ariz., American Nurses Association, 1966, pp. 100-137.

59. Hackett, *op. cit.*

Bibliography

Andreoli, K. G., et al: Comprehensive Cardiac Care. St. Louis, C. V. Mosby, 1975.

Ayres, S. M. and Giannelli, S., Jr.: Care of the Critically Ill. New York, Appleton-Century Crofts, 1967.

Bendixen, H. H., et al: Respiratory Care. St. Louis, C. V. Mosby, 1965.

Burrell, Z. L., Jr. and Burrell, L. O.: Intensive Nursing Care. St. Louis, C. V. Mosby, 1973.

Bushnell, S. S., et al: Respiratory Intensive Care Nursing. Boston, Little, Brown, 1973.

Druss, R. G. and Kornfeld, D. S.: The survivors of cardiac arrest. JAMA 201:291-296, July 31, 1967.

Hamilton, W. P. and Lavin, M. A.: Decision-Making in the Coronary Care Unit; A Manual and Workbooks for Nurses. St. Louis, C. V. Mosby, 1972.

Meltzer, L. E., Abdellah, F. G. and Kitchell, J. R.: Concepts and Practices of Intensive Care. Philadelphia, Charles Press, 1976.

Little, D. E. and Carnevoli, D. L.: Nursing Care Planning. Philadelphia, J. B. Lippincott, 1969.

Wade, J.: Respiratory Nursing Care; Physiology and Technique. St. Louis, C. V. Mosby, 1973.

11

The Burned Patient: current concepts of medical and nursing management

CURTIS P. ARTZ, PAULETTE MILLER and ELIZABETH W. BAYLEY

Causes of Burns • Prevention of Burns • Incidence of Burns • First Aid • Assessment of the Injury • Small Burns • Hospital Management • Care of the Burn Wound • Psychological Factors • Narcotics • Nutrition • Infection • Chemical Burns • Electrical Injuries • Burns About the Head • Curling's Ulcer

Because of the complexity of the illness, the burned patient presents a challenging problem to the medical-nursing team. It is essential that the team concept be utilized.

The nurse who cares for the burned patient should have an understanding of the physiological problems involved, and thus be better able to cope with the minute-to-minute bedside problems that this patient presents.

Unlike wounds that can be closed immediately, the deep burn requires time for removal of the dead eschar before closure. The persistence of this dead tissue furthers the injury and additional systemic derangements occur. This makes the extensive deep burn one of the most severe injuries to which the human body is liable. On the other hand, there are many first- and second-degree burns that heal in a few days if kept free from infection. It is this wide range of injury that makes it difficult to understand the burn problem. In addition, for the past half century, a number of recommendations for treatment have been in vogue, so that no best single treatment for all burns exists. However, since no two burned patients are alike, it is gratifying to know that there are a number of acceptable ways to attack the problem. It is in this complex challenge of the burned patient, and the further complex maze of treatment regimens, that the nurse must try to gain an understanding of each particular burned patient.

Causes of Burns

In children under age three, scald burns are most common—usually the result of an overturned container of hot liquid or of a bathtub accident; from ages three to fourteen, flame burns due to ignited clothing predominate—from the misuse of matches and fire, as well as from open fires and space heaters. Because of the flammability of their attire, girls are more prone to clothing burns. A common burn occurs in the little girl who, clothed only in a flammable housecoat, backs up against an open fire. The coat catches fire, the girl runs, fans the flames, and becomes the victim of a severe burn. In adults, burns are generally caused by home, auto, or industrial accidents. Major burn injuries in adults usually result from ignition of clothing—frequently from the misuse of combustible liquids in starting fires and, especially among the elderly, from smoking in bed.

Burns are common among military personnel and frequently are quite extensive—often caused by aircraft accidents, flame throwers, explosions, white phosphorous, and accidents involving aviation fuel. Chemical and electrical injuries are more frequent in industrial accidents than in home injuries.

Prevention of Burns

A better educational program would undoubtedly prevent a large number of burns. Most of the injuries that occur in and around the home are preventable. A broad educational program against the practices that lead to burning insults might be very beneficial. Two major factors should be considered in prevention: 1) the type of heating appliance used in the home; and 2) the type of clothing. Household heating units should be adequately protected so that children's clothes cannot catch fire. Parents should not use heating appliances that are dangerous to their children. Safer clothing could be made. The most critical garments are the nightclothes of children and the elderly, and particularly girls' dresses, certain fabrics being highly combustible. It is now practical to treat various flammable fabrics with chemicals which make them sufficiently flame retardant.

Education through community health nurses, school nurses, and teachers concerning the hazards accompanying fire in and around the home could significantly reduce the number of victims of fire.

Incidence of Burns

Annually, between 7 and 10 thousand persons die in the United States from burns. Each year about 7.5 persons per 1,000 population in the United States are injured by contact with hot objects or open flames. Accidents in the home are responsible for more than three-fourths of all the deaths from fire and explosions.

In the 1958 Report of the Oklahoma Crippled Children's Commission, Foerster found that the burn is the leading single diagnosis of these children when ranked by the number of cases, the number of days hospitalized, or Commission dollars expended. In the survey, burns seemed to be the number one problem of crippled children.

It is obvious that burns are a major problem in the United States, although the number of deaths is small in comparison with the number caused by the leading killers—heart disease, cancer, and stroke. The number of working years lost is appreciable because of the younger age group in which burns take their toll.

First Aid

The person whose clothes are burning should never run, since this only fans the flames, nor remain standing, since this position may cause him or her to inhale flames or cause his or her hair to be ignited. The person should lie in a horizontal position and roll him- or herself in some type of coat or rug to choke out the flames.

The objectives of first aid are to prevent further wound contamination, to alleviate pain, and to transport the patient safely to a location where professional care is available. Initially, the wound should be covered, since this minimizes contamination and inhibits pain by preventing the air from coming in contact with the injured surface. The most useful emergency dressing is a clean sheet. Probably the greatest advance in first aid in burns in the past decade has been the utilization of cold applications. Towels soaked in ice water bring almost immediate relief from pain and also stop the burning insult, thus limiting the injury. If possible, time should be taken at the scene of the accident to apply bath towels soaked in ice water to the burned areas. This may be done while arrangements are being made to move the victim to a physician's office or a hospital. Any burn involving more than 10 percent of the body surface should be seen by a physician.

Medication or home remedies should not be applied, nor should the patient with an extensive burn be given water because of the danger of vomiting. Stimulants, of course, are contraindicated. If the patient is suffering from a respiratory arrest due to smoke inhalation, he or she should receive artificial respiration by the mouth-to-mouth technique.

Chemical burns caused by acid or alkali should be washed immediately with large quantities of water to remove the injurious agent. One should not waste time looking for a specific antidote. All clothing should be removed, and, if a large quantity of the chemical burning agent remains in contact with the skin, the patient should get into a shower immediately.

Burned patients usually tolerate transportation well during the immediate postburn period. Although many times it is felt that burned patients are too sick to travel and that one should wait for a few days before transferring them over long distances to specialized centers, it is not true. Burned patients can be moved best in the first few hours after injury, if they have good airways and fluids are administered. Burn shock is insidious in its onset. If one predicts from the size of the injury that burn shock may occur, it can usually be prevented by adequate infusion of fluids. If the transportation is expected to require a prolonged period, lactated Ringer's solution should be started. Frequently, a nurse is asked to accompany a patient with critical burns in transit.

The nurses' role at this point is two-fold. First, she must insure adequate and proper delivery of medical services (a good airway with or without administration of oxygen and suctioning if needed), assure the intravenous fluid infusion rate, observe the amount and character of urine output, promote body temperature, relieve pain, and maintain position of comfort along with first aid treatment for other related injuries if present.

Second, and equally important, she must provide emotional support and comfort during this period of great fear. The patient is usually alert and able to communicate. The nurse can gather assessment data pertinent to the circumstances of the injury, the patient's social status, and prior medical history. She needs to be alert to the patient's concerns for his or her own life as well as questions regarding others who may have been involved in the same accident. Frequently a parent or spouse will want to accompany the patient during transport. The nurse then has the responsibility for explaining procedures and providing reassurance to both the victim and the anxious family member. A straightforward, calm approach will help to establish trust between the medical personnel and the patient who is being taken to a strange place.

Adequate preparation of the patient for transport is essential. The referring physician must assure not only the airway, but also an intravenous lifeline so that fluids can be administered. Because peripheral intravenous lines are more prone to dislodgement during transport, a central route may be more reliable. A Foley catheter should be inserted and connected to a drainage bag.

If inhalation injury has occurred, the airway may be maintained with a cuffed endotracheal tube or tracheostomy prior to moving the patient. Suction equipment, an oxygen cylinder, and an Ambu-bag should be available.

A patient is always transported more comfortable if the wound is covered by a dressing. Many patients treated by the exposure method, or one of its modifications, with the use of local antibacterial agents, may have dressings applied for the period of transportation, mainly because of comfort. If wet dressings are used, additional care must be taken to prevent chilling and to keep the patient comfortably warm during transport.

Assessment of the Injury

Although it is difficult to appraise the relative magnitude of different types of mechanical injuries, the severity of a burn injury can be satisfactorily assessed by taking into consideration the percentage of body surface burned and the depth of the burn. However, there are other factors that determine the seriousness of the injury, such as its location, the cause of the burn, the age and physical condition of the patient, any preexisting disease, and the presence of concomitant injury.

The extent of a burn is usually expressed as the percentage of the total area of body surface injured. A rapid method of estimating percentage of body surface burned is the Rule of Nines, a simplified rule that is sufficiently accurate for immediate appraisal. According to the Rule of Nines, the body surface is divided into areas representing 9 or multiples of 9 percent: the head and neck, 9 percent; the anterior trunk, 9 × 2 or 18 percent; the posterior trunk, 18 percent; each lower extremity, 18 percent; each upper extremity, 9 percent, and the perineum, 1 percent. An area equivalent to one side of the hand is approximately 1 percent of the body surface (Fig. 11-1).

A much more accurate method is the use of a Lund and Browder chart (Fig. 11-2). This chart takes into consideration the changes in percentage of various parts of the body surface that occur during stages of development from infancy through childhood. These charts are used in al-

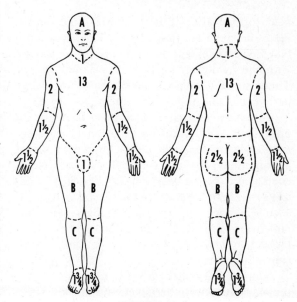

FIGURE 11-2.
A Lund and Browder chart is used for more accurate estimation of extent of injury.

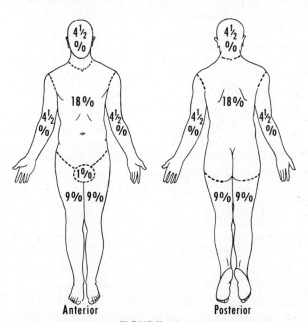

FIGURE 11-1.
The Rule of Nines provides a rapid method of estimating percentage of body surface burned. Source: Artz, C. P. and Moncrief, J. A.: The Treatment of Burns. Philadelphia, W. B. Saunders, 1969.

most every hospital to map out the areas of injury; usually a blue pen is used for marking second-degree injury and a red pen for indicating areas of third-degree burn. This determination is done best immediately after the burn wound has been cleansed and is usually an integral part of all burned patients' hospital charts.

The seriousness of the injury usually is determined by the volume of tissue destroyed. Of course, the deeper the burn, the more serious it is. Although several classifications have been used to differentiate various depths of burns, in this country they are commonly divided into three categories: first degree, second degree, and third degree. First- and second-degree burns are partial-thickness burns. Third-degree burns are full-thickness burns.

The first-degree burn involves only the epidermis. It is characterized by erythema that appears a few hours after exposure. The first-degree burn may follow injury from bright sunlight or instantaneous exposure to a more intense heat. Since tissue destruction is superficial, minimal systemic derangements occur; pain and a slight amount of edema are the chief problems. Usually the uncomfortable burning sensation and pain subside after 48 hours, unless the burn is really deeper than first degree. Healing usually takes place uneventfully within five to ten days, with the epidermis peeling off in small scales. There may be some residual redness for a short period, but scarring is very rare.

A second-degree burn involves all the epidermis and much of the corium. Most second-degree burns are characterized by blister, accompanied by considerable subcutaneous edema. All second-degree burns heal in 16 to 21 days, unless complicated by infection. A second-degree burn is usually moist and rather pink in appearance. It is quite painful because the protective covering of the nerve endings of the skin has been removed.

Third-degree burns involve all the layers of the skin. The entire dermis including skin structures such as hair follicles, sweat glands, nerves, and sebaceous glands down to the subcutaneous fat is destroyed by coagulation necrosis. Thrombosis occurs in the small vessels of the underlying tissues. Increased capillary permeability and edema are greater than in second-degree burns. In two or three weeks, liquefaction of the dead skin occurs which is usually accompanied by suppuration. Capillary tufts and fibroblasts organized into the granulating tissue are found beneath the eschar. Most third-degree burns are caused by flame or contact with hot objects. Most electrical burns are third degree. The third-degree burn is dry, nonviable, and may be white, waxy-yellow, mottled red, or charred in appearance. The skin feels leathery in contrast to the moist, soft surface of a partial-thickness burn. Third-degree burns are not very painful; in fact, the area is almost insensible to pain, because the terminal nerve endings are inactivated by the deep-burn injury. This impairment in sensation has been used clinically as a test for depth of skin loss. One of the best ways of differentiating between second- and third-degree burned areas is by pulling on a hair. If the hair pulls out easily and painlessly the burn is third degree; if the hair seems attached and causes pain, the burn is probably a partial-thickness injury.

The age of the patient is important in estimating severity of injury. Although a 20 percent third-degree burn in a 60-year-old individual usually results in death, a younger person with the same lesion may be expected to recover without unusual complications. In burns of 30 percent of the body surface in patients under 50, the mortality rate is quite low. In elderly individuals, even small third-degree burns carry a high mortality rate. Infants also tolerate burn poorly, and the mortality rate for those younger than one year is much higher than for older children. In general in a healthy individual under the age of 40, a 50 percent second- or third-degree burn carries about a 50-50 chance for survival. In some specialized centers, the chance for survival may be a little better.

Small Burns

Minor burns include partial-thickness burns of less than 10 percent of the body surface and full-thickness burns of less than 2 percent of the body surface. They do not usually require fluid replacement and can be treated with local cleansing and the appropriate type of wound care. Usually, patients with such injuries are treated on an outpatient basis. Minor burns also should be cared for as aseptically as possible by attendants wearing masks. Debris and loose devitalized tissue should be gently removed and the wound cleansed with warm water and soap.

The patient with a minor burn should be made as comfortable as possible. Initially, the burn should be treated by cold application followed by cleansing and then covered with a dressing. The method may be a semi-open or closed technique depending on the patient's ability to care for the wound.

The patient who has difficulty managing wound care at home or whose environment may increase the likelihood of infection, should have sterile, nonadherent, fine-mesh gauze placed over the wound and fixed in place with a bulky dressing. Such patients should report to their physicians or outpatient clinics every two to five days or, if the dressing becomes grossly wet or soiled, for observation of the wound and redressing.

Some patients can be taught to utilize a light,

sterile, dry dressing which they or a family member can change once or twice a day. The patient is instructed to wash the burn with soap and water, observe for any redness or purulence, and redress the area with sterile gauze. Any signs of infection should be reported to the physician.

If the burn is very minor, some type of anesthetic ointment can be applied without dressing. This usually alleviates pain and does not complicate healing.

Hospital Management

EMERGENCY MEASURES

In the emergency department, speed is not necessary in the case of a patient with a major burn. There should be an orderly execution of all the various established routine procedures.

As soon as the patient arrives, the responsible physician should be contacted with someone on the spot making arrangements for adequate assistance. Several nurses and technicians, medical students, and house officers may be profitably utilized in the expeditious emergency department care. All attendants should wear caps and masks. The patient's clothing or initial dressing must be removed and all burned areas exposed for evaluation. If reasonably good dressings have been applied for transportation, these should be removed so that someone can estimate the size and severity of the injury.

A brief history should be obtained including how and when the injury occurred, the age of the patient, any allergies or chronic illnesses he or she may have, medications currently taken, the status of tetanus immunizations, and any associated injuries.

Burns of more than 20 percent of the body surface (15 percent in children) usually require intravenous fluid therapy. A large bore needle should be inserted into any available vein and blood obtained for baseline determinations of hemoglobin, hematocrit, BUN, blood sugar, and electrolytes. Through the same needle, replacement therapy may be started and a narcotic (also an excellent analgesic) may be given to allay apprehension. Such medication should be given intravenously in acutely burned patients, because

subcutaneous medications are not readily absorbed due to the circulatory derangements occurring in the burned area.

The life of the burned patient frequently depends upon intravenous replacement therapy. Some type of intravenous cannula should be inserted in all adult patients with burns of more than 20 percent of the body surface and in children with burns of more than 10 percent. Usually an intracath is used. This should be inserted in an unburned area when possible; the antecubital veins are the sites most frequently used. Occasionally a cutdown is necessary. If the burn is extensive, the jugular or subclavian veins are used so that central venous pressure monitoring can be accomplished. Indwelling cannulas are usually changed every four or five days. The site of insertion is usually dressed with some type of antibacterial ointment and a sterile occlusive dressing. This dressing is changed each day in an attempt to keep the site as free of bacteria as possible and thus prevent infection in the vein.

On all patients with major burns, the hourly measurement of urinary output by means of an indwelling catheter in the bladder is the most reliable method for determining adequacy of replacement therapy. The catheter is usually inserted while the patient is in the emergency department, and fluids are infused until there is a reasonable urinary output. As soon as replacement therapy is assured, the local burn wound is examined and treated. All devitalized and loose tissue should be removed along with dirt and debris. The burned surface, irrespective of the method of local care, is treated by washing with warm water and bland soap.

In many hospitals, entire local care may be accomplished in the emergency department. In others, the patient is taken to a dressing room, a treatment room, or to one of the operating rooms for initial local care.

Tracheostomy is indicated in all patients with respiratory tract injury from the inhalation of noxious gases and in some patients with very deep burns of the face and neck. In such patients, an endotracheal tube is passed through the nose and allowed to remain in place for one or two days. These patients' arterial blood gases are monitored frequently. It may be necessary to do a tracheotomy later. The tracheotomy should not be performed through burned tissue because purulent drainage from the wound carries organisms into the lower respiratory tree with resultant fatal pulmonary infection.

The initial effect of inhalation of flames, smoke, and noxious irritants associated with flame burns of the face and upper chest is laryngeal edema. The edema may appear early, but in most cases symptoms of respiratory distress are delayed for hours. It is most often the bedside nurse who first notices a change in the patient's respiratory condition. A cough, labored breathing, progressive hoarseness, increased rate with shallow chest movements, or sometimes stridor may develop quickly. The patient may become extremely restless because he or she is fighting for air. The nurse must be careful to distinguish restlessness due to pain from that caused by hypoxia. Any significant change which the nursing team observes should be passed on to the physician immediately.

Anticipation of the patient's and the physician's needs should be every nurse's goal. An intubation tray or tracheostomy tray should be present at the bedside of all patients suspected of having inhalation injury. A suctioning apparatus and oxygen delivery system should also be available. Laryngeal edema and inhalation injury are treated with endotracheal intubation or tracheotomy.

The nurse attempts to keep the pulmonary tree as free from secretions as possible with frequent suctioning. Every precaution is taken to minimize the introduction of infection into the tracheobronchial tree. Sterile, single-use suction catheters and sterile gloves should be used. Before and after suctioning, the nurse listens for breath sounds and records the findings. The character of the secretions is observed for the presence of soot or sloughed tissue. A chest x-ray study should be done on admission and may be required periodically to check endotracheal tube placement, subclavian catheter placement, and to document changes in the lungs noted on auscultation.

All patients with severe burns should receive prophylaxis against tetanus. If the patient has maintained appropriate basic immunization, prophylaxis consists of a booster dose of 0.5 ml of alum-precipitated toxoid administered subcutaneously. In patients who have had basic immunizations but have not had a booster dose within five years, passive immunization may be provided by the use of human immune globulin, given in one arm and a booster dose of alum-precipitated toxoid in the other.

A nasogastric tube for low-volume intermittent suctioning may be necessary. The patient can be put on a clamping schedule and antacids given as ordered through the nasogastric tube as prophylaxis against Curling's ulcer.

FLUID REPLACEMENT THERAPY

A patient with a major burn should be given nothing by mouth for the first day or two, because paralytic ileus is often a complication of severe burn injury, and gastric dilatation may occur. Adequate fluid replacement can be given by the intravenous route. All well-treated burned patients in the first 48 hours are thirsty so that the nurse should explain to them why they cannot have water. Many times cold water put on a piece of gauze and placed in the patient's mouth alleviates some of the discomfort, and is better than giving the patient quantities of ice chips which could cause nausea and vomiting.

Good mouth care is essential not only for comfort, but also to prevent introduction of candidiasis infections via the oral passage way. Small electric toothbrush can gently clean the teeth and massage the gums. The use of ointments applied to the lips helps prevent drying and cracking. Frequency of care is the key to good oral hygiene. A solution of equal parts of 3 percent hydrogen peroxide and normal saline is a useful adjunct for cleaning crusts in the mouth or on the lips. A bland lubricant to keep lips moist also promotes comfort. Cleaning the mouth should be done at least every four hours with facial burn victims, and routinely after meals and at bedtime for other burned patients.

The burned patient requires considerable fluid resuscitation, due to the obligatory accumulation of fluids in the burn wound and adjacent areas. This is secondary to the increased capillary permeability and to vasodilatation. There is a significant loss of fluid from the burned surface as insensible water loss.

During the first 48 hours, calculation of fluid replacement can be aided by the use of a burn fluid formula. Because of the complexity of the burn wound and its associated variables, it is impossible to state the required fluids exactly. It is important that the formula be used only as a general guide to the amount and type of therapy but that the exact amount administered be according to the clinical response of the patient. It is usually the nurse who measures the urinary output and adjusts the speed of infusion (Fig. 11-3). (See Chapter 16 for discussion of nursing measures for patients with fluid-electrolyte imbalances.)

It is essential that an accurate record of hourly intake and output be maintained, especially during the first 72 hours of resuscitation. Realizing the frequent changes made in the in-

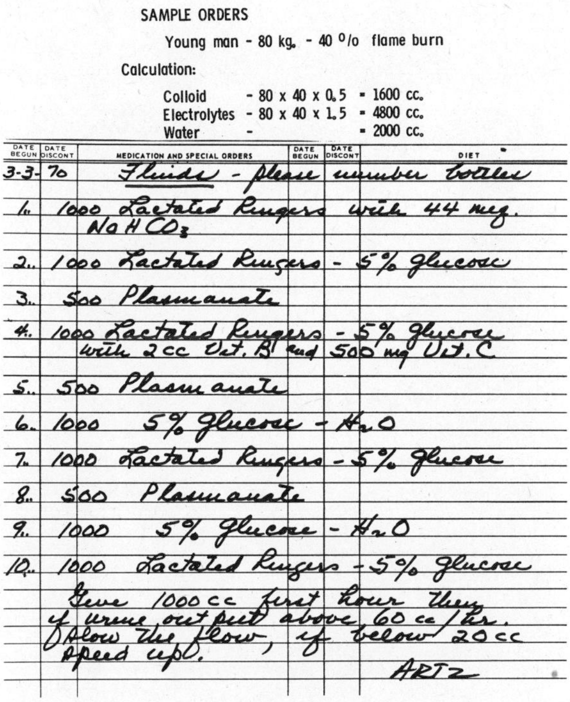

SAMPLE ORDERS

Young man - 80 kg. - 40 % flame burn

Calculation:

Colloid — 80 x 40 x 0.5 = 1600 cc.
Electrolytes — 80 x 40 x 1.5 = 4800 cc.
Water — = 2000 cc.

DATE BEGUN	DATE DISCONT	MEDICATION AND SPECIAL ORDERS	DATE BEGUN	DATE DISCONT	DIET
3-3-70		Fluids - please number bottles			
1.		1000 Lactated Ringers with 44 meq. NaHCO₃			
2.		1000 Lactated Ringers - 5% glucose			
3.		500 Plasmanate			
4.		1000 Lactated Ringers - 5% glucose with 2 cc Vit. B and 500 mg Vit. C			
5.		500 Plasmanate			
6.		1000 5% glucose - H₂O			
7.		1000 Lactated Ringers - 5% glucose			
8.		500 Plasmanate			
9.		1000 5% glucose - H₂O			
10.		1000 Lactated Ringers - 5% glucose			
		Give 1000cc first hour then if urine output above 60 cc/hr. slow the flow, if below 20 cc speed up.			
		ARTZ			

FIGURE 11-3.
Initial fluid orders are written with adjustments noted according to clinical response of the patient. The nurse has a major role in fluid administration.

travenous solutions administered and their rates, it becomes the nurse's responsibility to keep a record of what fluids the patient actually received. The use of metrisets to help record fluid intake are invaluable. Likewise it is important to be able to record the urine output per hour and its specific gravity. A low-specific gravity (1.000 to 1.005) may indicate an overload of fluid and a high-specific gravity (1.020 to 1.030) may indicate a need for more fluid. This value and all vital signs should again be reported to the physician quickly if a change occurs. Labstix may also be used to determine the presence of blood glucose, ketones, and protein in the urine as well as the pH.

Numerous burn fluid formulas have been proposed. The Brooke formula, a modification of the Evans formula, has proved adequate and is popular with American surgeons. The Brooke formula estimates the following fluid requirements for the first 24 hours after injury:

Colloids (plasma, Plasmanate, or dextran): 0.5 ml per kg per percent body surface burned
Lactated Ringer's solution: 1.5 ml per kg per percent body surface burned
Water requirement: 2,000 ml dextrose in water for adults; children correspondingly less.

According to the Brooke formula, one half of the first 24-hour fluid requirement should be given in the first eight hours postburn and the remaining one half over the following sixteen hours. The second 24-hour requirement for colloid and lactated Ringer's solution is about one half that for the first 24 hours.

Many years ago at the Parkland Hospital in Dallas, Moyer initiated a regimen for initial fluid replacement for burns. This regimen consisted entirely of lactated Ringer's solution. Since that time, Shires and Baxter have continued the enthusiasm for this regimen and now use the following formula: During the first 24 hours postburn, lactated Ringer's solution is given in the amount of 4 ml per kg per percent of body surface burned.

Obviously, there are many ways of calculating fluid requirement in burns. Usually, the physician uses the one with which he is most familiar.

It is generally understood today that very little colloid can be retained within the vascular system during the first 24 hours after injury. Therefore, many physicians modify the above two formulas to give about 3 ml of lactated Ringer's per kg. of body weight per percent of body surface burned in the first 24 hours. In the second 24 hours, they add colloid and glucose in water to maintain an adequate urinary output.

Undoubtedly the most valuable single index for fluid replacement for the first 48 hours is the urinary output. In adults fluids should be given so that the output is maintained in the range of 30 to 50 ml per hour. A decreasing blood pressure and decreasing urinary output mean that more colloid should be given. A decrease in urinary output with normal blood pressure indicates that additional electrolyte solution or water is required. When one fears that too much fluid is being given but the urinary output is low, central venous pressure helps to determine further therapy. Diminution of the urinary output usually calls for an increase in fluid replacement, but if the venous pressure is rising, fluids must be restricted. In such instances, it may be necessary to give isoproterenol (Isuprel), digitalis, or a diuretic.

Central venous pressure measurements are very valuable in the care of the severely burned patient during initial replacement therapy. The tip of the intravenous catheter is usually in the superior vena cava. When measuring the central venous pressure, the position of the patient and bed must be flat. The slightest alteration in body alignment will affect the reading because of the gravitational effect on the manometer. The lower part of the manometer must be level with the heart each time a reading is taken. A normal central venous pressure reading is usually about 5 to 15 cm of water pressure. In burned patients during the early phases after injury, the central venous pressure measurement may be zero. This usually increases as fluid resuscitation improves. The main value of central venous pressure observations is to prevent overloading. This is indicated by a rapid rise in the central venous pressure or a central venous pressure significantly above normal. Usually the physician leaves instructions with the nurse concerning frequency

of central venous pressure measurements and the changes that should be reported to him.

Usually the physician writes orders to increase fluids if the urinary output falls below 20 ml per hour and to decrease them if it goes above 60 ml per hour (See Fig. 11-3). If fluids are given at a rate so that the urinary output is above 100 ml per hour, the patient may become overloaded with fluids and go into pulmonary edema. After the first 48 hours, the urinary output is not a good method of determining adequacy of fluid therapy. At this time serum sodium should be watched carefully. Lesser quantities of fluid are required and usually electrolyte-free water is given. If sodium-containing solutions are given, the serum

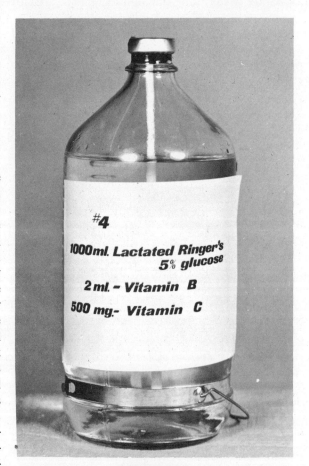

FIGURE 11-4.
Bottles should be numbered for accuracy in following fluid orders and for rapid assessment of fluid intake.

sodium has a tendency to rise and may become too high. Generally the serum sodium should be kept a little less than normal, about 135 mEq per L. If it is higher than this, additional quantities of sodium-free water should be given. At this time, the patient can usually take food and fluid by mouth and will not need additional quantities of potassium. However, if the patient is not eating, it may be necessary to give 60 to 80 mEq of potassium each day in his intravenous fluids, along with 1,000 to 1,500 mg of ascorbic acid and an ampule of vitamin B complex (Fig. 11-4).

Signs of hyperkalemia (increased potassium levels in the blood) are sometimes seen early in the postburn period due to the release of potassium from injured cells. The nurse should be aware of laboratory results and report abnormalities in these and patient symptoms to the physician immediately.

Blood transfusions are required throughout the entire burn period but are rarely used before the fifth to seventh days. Hematocrit and hemoglobin are usually high or normal in the initial postburn days. The anemia seen later in the burned patient is due to a number of factors:

1. Many cells are actually destroyed by heat at the time of burning.
2. In burned patients the life of red cells is considerably shortened, because they are rendered abnormally fragile.
3. Red blood cells are trapped in dilated capillaries and sludging occurs.
4. Infection may occur and depress the function of the hematopoietic tissue.
5. Considerable quantities of blood are lost from the granulating wound at each dressing change.

A good rule to remember is that transfusions are necessary in amounts sufficient to maintain a hematocrit of 38 in a well-hydrated patient. The hemoglobin and hematocrit should be determined twice weekly during the patient's hospitalization.

Care of the Burn Wound

Local management of the burn wound continues to be a controversial subject, but major advances in this field have been made in the past several years. The burn wound serves as a massive open portal of entry for invasive sepsis and every effort should be directed toward preventing this. However, until the burn wound is closed, invasive sepsis is a constant threat. The primary aims in management are: 1) control of infection; 2) early removal of eschar; 3) wound closure by skin grafting in full-thickness burns, and 4) minimization of scarring. There are a number of ways to treat partial-thickness burns; all seem to be effective as long as the area is kept free from infection. A common technique in the hospital is the exposure method with an antibacterial agent, such as silver sulfadiazine (Silvadene) or mafenide (Sulfamylon), applied once or twice each day. This is particularly effective in deep second-degree burns. In third-degree burns the techniques of wound care are initial excision, dressings, exposure, topical antibacterial therapy, or any combination of the above methods. Each of these techniques is useful in certain circumstances. Topical chemotherapeutic agents are commonly used at present for deep burns.

EXCISION

Initial excision with grafting has one great advantage in that all the burned area can be excised soon after injury and a graft applied two days later, permitting the patient to be discharged from the hospital much earlier than by other methods of management. The technique is particularly indicated in small full-thickness burns with clearly defined edges, and in some types of electrical injuries. Excision is usually accomplished in the first 48 hours under general anesthesia. The burned skin and underlying subcutaneous tissue down to the fascia are completely excised in the operating room and a large, bulky dressing applied. Skin grafting is performed two to four days later. For patients with burns not exceeding 15 percent of the body surface, and when there is definite evidence that the injury is third degree, initial excision followed by grafting is desirable.

ELEVATION AND ESCHAROTOMY

In addition to prescribed topical wound therapy in the early postburn period, the nurse performs several independent activities. Extremities should be elevated for the first few days to decrease edema and prevent interstitial tissue pressure from decreasing distal circulation. This can be accomplished by placing some type of tubular elastic netting or stockinette over the length of each arm and suspending arms from ceiling-mounted IV poles or an overhead frame. Pillows under the upper arms offer support. The arms can be let out of suspension for a short period each hour or two and range-of-motion exercises implemented to enhance circulation and absorption of edematous fluid.

The legs can best be elevated by putting them in sling suspension using an overhead frame. The patient can then exercise the legs as well.

Whatever dressing method is used, the fingers and toes should be left exposed so that hourly checks of circulation can be made. Peripheral pulses should be checked using a Doppler flow meter or similar method if edema prevents accurate palpation.

If circumferential, full-thickness burns are present on the extremities or trunk, the nurse must anticipate the need for escharotomy to relieve difficulties resulting from edema and constricting eschar. Any signs of decreasing distal circulation or decreasing tidal volume should be reported to the physician at once. An electrocautery unit, sterile gauze sponges, and suture supplies should be ready. Escharotomy, which involves linear incisions through dead tissue to the subcutaneous fat can be done without anesthesia. Dramatic relief of compromised circulation and greatly improved chest expansion may be seen immediately following this procedure.

OCCLUSIVE (PRESSURE) DRESSING

Occlusive dressings may be used when exposure is not applicable (Fig. 11-5). The method should be used for almost all patients treated on an outpatient basis. The aim of good dressing is to cover the open wound to protect it from infection. The material placed next to the wound may be dry, fine-meshed gauze, lightly impregnated petrolatum gauze, Carbowax gauze, commercially prepared nylon fabric or antibacterial ointment-impregnated gauze. The dressing must

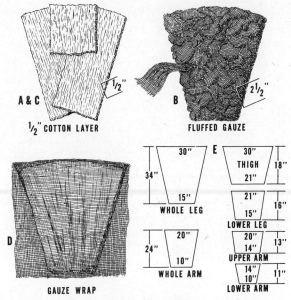

FIGURE 11-5.
Diagram for making Brooke burn dressings. This is an inexpensive one-piece dressing made of standard materials of various sizes for different parts of the body. Usually these standard dressings are made in the central supply area and put up sterilely for use. Source: Artz, C. P. and Moncrief, J. A.: The Treatment of Burns. Philadelphia, W. B. Saunders, 1969.

be occlusive, to prevent the invasion of bacteria; absorptive, to keep the wound surface dry and thereby inhibit the growth of bacteria; bulky and applied with even compression, to eliminate dead space, give vascular support, and produce a splinting effect (Fig.11-6). Burn dressings should be changed every two to five days. For children they are very comfortable and make the children easy to handle, but for adults the dressings are bulky, hurt each time they are changed, and cause the patient to feel hot. Dressings can be soaked with sterile saline to decrease the pain of removal.

SEMI-OPEN METHOD

A semi-open method of wound care incorporates a topical agent with a gauze dressing which is generally changed once or twice daily. This method is combined with hydrotherapy or another means of wound cleansing. It allows for

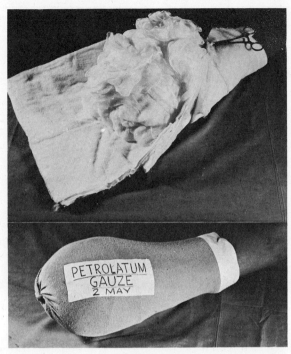

FIGURE 11-6.
Typical occlusive dressing for the hand. The fingers are separated, the hand is put in a position of function and a large bulky dressing is applied with some type of nonstick gauze next to the wound. In this instance even, resilient compression is made by using stockinette. Source: Artz, C. P. and Moncrief, J. A.: The Treatment of Burns. Philadelphia, W. B. Saunders, 1969.

frequent observation of the wound. The topical agent helps to control bacterial growth on the wound, thus decreasing the possibility of invasive sepsis. The frequent removal of the fine-mesh gauze assists in wound debridement, as necrotic tissue and products of infection are removed with each dressing change. This method helps keep the patient warm and allows for range of motion during and between dressing changes. Narcotic analgesics may be required prior to this procedure which is particularly useful for patients with extensive burns.

EXPOSURE METHOD

The exposure method is preferred for most burns. Its chief advantage is that it can be used with the application of one of the local antibacte-

rial agents. It is particularly well suited to burns of the head, neck, and perineum where dressings are difficult to apply. In many second-degree burns, simple exposure is adequate. In deeper burns, exposure with the use of a chemotherapeutic ointment is best.

TOPICAL AGENTS

In recent years, a number of topical agents to prevent or control infection have been tested. One widely used agent has been 0.5 percent silver nitrate solution applied as continuous wet dressings. The chief disadvantage of this form of treatment is severe electrolyte disturbances. The hypotonicity of the silver nitrate solution, as well as the ion-binding potential of the silver ion, results in serious sodium chloride and potassium deficiencies. These changes seem to be particularly noticeable in children. The staining qualities of the silver nitrate solution also proved objectionable to patients, to physicians, and, most of all, to nurses. Silver nitrate dressings must be rewet every two to four hours so that the concentration provides effective antibacterial action without allowing damage to re-epithelizing tissue. A dry top sheet or bath blanket will help to decrease evaporative water loss and promote patient warmth and comfort.

Currently the most popular topic antibacterial therapy is the use of either Silvadene or Sulfamylon ointment. Sulfamylon is supplied in the form of Sulfamylon acetate in a water-soluble cream base. Likewise Silvadene is in a cream base. Silvadene is frequently preferred especially in deep burns of less than 40 percent of the body surface because it is easily applied and gives a soft pliable eschar. Silvadene does not cause pain. On the other hand, Sulfamylon, causes pain in some patients and produces a firm eschar that remains in place for a long time. Many surgeons feel, however, that Sulfamylon penetrates the burned tissue better than Silvadene and, therefore, is more effective in minimizing the growth of bacteria under the eschar. Most burn centers use both creams and the specific indications are usually determined by the attending surgeon. Both agents are used in a similar fashion. As soon as the burn wound has been cleansed and all loose

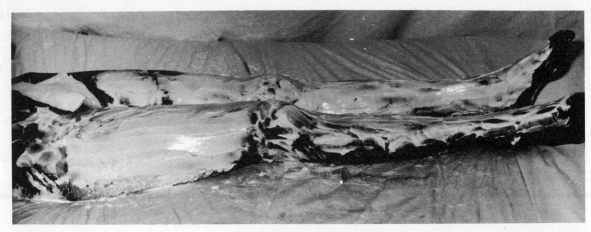

FIGURE 11-7.
Sulfamylon ointment on second- and third-degree burns of the legs. The ointment is placed on the burned surface once each day. It is usually applied by the nurse who wears a pair of sterile gloves. Each morning the Sulfamylon ointment is washed off either in a tub, a shower, or a Hubbard tank.

devitalized tissue is removed, the area is covered with the cream (Fig. 11-7). It is usually applied with sterile gloved hands and reapplied every 12 to 24 hours. Before each reapplication the cream is removed either by washing or by placing the patient in a tank of warm water, such as the Hubbard tank. This not only makes the patient feel better, but allows some exercise and is a simple method of removing the cream and cleansing the surface in preparation for the next application. Sulfamylon frequently causes a burning sensation for 45 minutes to an hour after application which may be relieved by the use of narcotics. Sulfamylon does not give pain on full-thickness burns, but it is frequently painful on partial-thickness injury.

HYDROTHERAPY

There are many varieties of tanks or tubs. The Hubbard tank is a large stainless steel tub with extensions of the sides for the arms. Newer materials, such as fiber glass, are being used for modified versions of the tank and are less expensive.

The objective of the tanking procedure is to clean and debride the wound, and to exercise the burned patient as comfortably as possible. At each cleansing procedure the patient is allowed to stay in the water 20 to 30 minutes. All loose tissue is pulled or cut away using forceps and scissors. There are two methods of performing this tanking procedure. The first requires immersing the patient into the water so that the body is actually covered from the neck down, much like a relaxing bath. The water level is approximately 18 inches from the top of the tank to provide for displacement. The addition of a mild detergent agent to tap water has been found helpful both for cleansing the wound and to meet the basic hygienic needs of the human body. Electrolytes such as sodium chloride and potassium chloride, and a disinfectant agent such as calcium hypochlorite may also be added to the water. Normal body perspiration and odor can cause any person to feel self-conscious and withdrawn, especially the person who has already experienced a great injury to his or her image. The temperature of the water varies according to each patient but should be within the range of 95 to 100° F.

The second method of tanking is simply to secure the stretcher on which the patient is placed over the tank and rinse the body with tap water. An ordinary hose can be adapted for this purpose with or without autoclavable nozzle heads for each patient. However, most centers use the immersion method.

Regardless of the method used, certain

equipment is essential and certain guidelines should be followed.

Equipment:

1. Hubbard tank or similar structure; plastic disposable protective liners are optional.
2. Gauze or foam rubber surgical sponges, washclothes or large burn dressings, as desired, for gently but thoroughly washing the burn wound.
3. Debridement instruments; a small tray can be set up including curved scissors and forceps.
4. Gloves for staff's protection against transfer of infection; long plastic disposable gloves, extending up to the shoulder are available commercially.
5. Warm blankets and towels; this comfort measure is especially appreciated by patients following the tanking because of the chills experienced. An inexpensive roaster oven can be used to warm the blankets to about 130° F. rather than investing in high-cost warming cabinets.
6. Ceiling-mounted heat lamps or shields assist in maintaining optimal environmental temperature.

Procedure:

1. Explain the procedure to the patient if this to be his or her first tanking. Never forget to try and alleviate a patient's fear.
2. If necessary, premedicate the patient according to the physician's orders.
3. Fill the tank with tap water or insure proper functioning of the hosing apparatus. Note temperature of the water. A simple thermometer mounted in a wooden holder works well and can be left in the water while the tank is being filled. Add detergent agent if requested.
4. Transfer the patient to the tank on a stretcher; if ambulatory, a patient may walk to the tank, step in and assume a sitting position rather than a reclining one.
5. The stretcher can be raised and moved over the tank by means of a hoist and then lowered to desired level.
6. Remove all topical agents and as much necrotic tissue as possible by gently washing. At this time the nursing staff can give special care to the patient's basic hygienic needs, such as washing the hair, shaving the faces of males and hair in proximity to wound, perineal care, and nail care.
7. Put patient through active and passive range-of-motion exercises depending on his or her capabilities. A physiotherapist may come and work with the patient at this time.
8. Remove the patient from the water; dry and warm patient; either proceed with dressings in the tank or dressing room or return to the patient's room.
9. Drain the tank and clean according to designated procedure. Frequent culturing of tanks and all objects which can lead to cross-contamination as well as close supervision of staff responsible for cleaning tanks is essential.

REMOVAL OF ESCHAR

During the first two weeks of management of a full-thickness burn, the primary aim is to keep the burn wound clean and free from infection. After approximately 21 to 30 days, it becomes important that preparation be made to remove the dead eschar and apply a skin graft.

There are several acceptable techniques for the removal of the eschar and their desirability depends upon the type of local care, location and extent of the burns, general condition of the patient and the facilities available. These methods include repeated changes of dry dressings, daily soaking in the Hubbard tank, wet soaks, and surgical excision under anesthesia. The surgeon usually selects the methods best suited to the patient and the institution. Sometimes two or three methods are used for the same patient.

Frequently a patient with injuries on the posterior surface who is treated by exposure has a tendency to stick to the bedsheet. A special type of nonstick sheeting is available and may be used underneath the parts with posterior injury (Fig. 11-8, p. 266).

Repeated change of dry dressings is an acceptable technique, especially in burns of limited extent treated initially by the occlusive dressing method. Usually the dead skin softens under the dressing, and the bacterial activity beneath the eschar causes it to loosen. If this method is used, the dressings must be changed every two days; sometimes this is done under light general anesthesia. With this technique all the loose tissue should be removed. A good rule of thumb is to

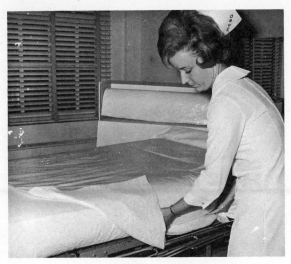

FIGURE 11-8.
Nonstick sheeting made by 3M Company. Whenever burns are exposed and an antibacterial ointment is used there is frequently sticking of certain portions of the body to the bed. As shown in the photograph, this sheeting comes in a large roll and can be placed over the patient's bed and changed each day.

use a pair of scissors to cut the collagenous strands that hold the eschar but not to cut deeply enough to cause bleeding.

A daily bath in the Hubbard tank is another excellent method of removing eschar (Fig. 11-9). It provides drainage for the wound, keeps the area clean, and softens the eschar, thus hastening its removal.

Wet soaks are also a good method of preparing the recipient site for grafting (Fig. 11-10). The wet dressings keep the eschar soft, and, when they are changed, any loose areas of dead tissue are removed. When the wound is severely infected, the wet soak method is particularly desirable, since it provides good drainage, accomplishes some debridement, and permits frequent inspection of the area. The best technique is the application every four hours of comfortable wet saline soaks with coarse-mesh gauze. Frequent removal of the wet gauze pads pulls away dead tissue. The dressings are more comfortable when kept warm. Although this is difficult, an Aqua-K pad over the wet dressings provides heat and comfort. At least once a day, forceps should

be used to clean the wound as thoroughly as possible. As soon as the eschar loosens, scissors may be used to cut the collagenous bands that hold the eschar. Extensive nursing care is required to apply wet dressings properly and on schedule, but they are effective in cleaning a dirty burn wound, removing the eschar, and getting the area ready for grafting.

Gridding, a method which employs escharotomy in a gridiron pattern creating 1-inch squares, is also useful in assisting eschar removal. By exposing more wound edges, it becomes easier for the nurse or physician to get scissors under the eschar and lift off the eschar. It also allows drainage of purulent material and prevents wound abscess formation.

In addition to natural and sharp debridement, enzymatic debridement is useful in some patients. Daily or twice daily application of commercially prepared concentrated enzymes to small areas of the burn can produce dissolution of the eschar in a few days. This application should be covered with an antibacterial ointment such as Silvadene to prevent wound infection,

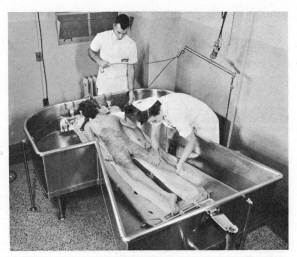

FIGURE 11-9.
A Hubbard tank. It is excellent for physical therapy for burned patients. When local ointments are used the patient can be bathed each day in the tank for removal of the ointment. This also provides a good means of exercise. Source: Artz, C. P. and Moncrief, J. A.: The Treatment of Burns. Philadelphia, W. B. Saunders, 1969.

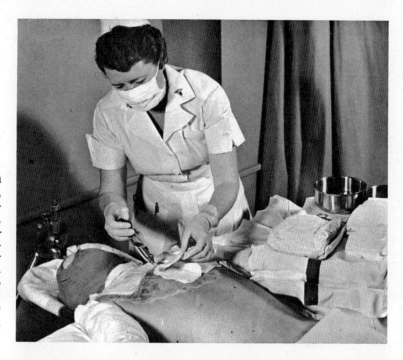

FIGURE 11-10.
Wet dressings are used for a number of reasons in burns. First, they are excellent for the treatment of infection and, second, they provide a good means for aiding the débridement of the third-degree eschar in preparation for grafting. Wet dressings are usually removed and reapplied every four hours. Source: Artz, C. P. and Moncrief, J. A.: The Treatment of Burns. Philadelphia, W. B. Saunders, 1969.

and it must be kept moist continuously with a saline dressing. Sometimes it is wise, if the patient is in good condition, to take him or her to the operating room, anesthetize him or her, and pull away all the dead, devitalized tissue, cutting collagenous bands with scissors.

BIOLOGICAL SKIN DRESSING

In recent years the use of biological skin dressings as temporary grafts has been very advantageous. These dressings can be obtained from another human being (homografts) or from another species (porcine heterografts). The skin is put on for one or two days then removed and another dressing applied. Homografts are excellent and can be left on up to three weeks, but they are not readily available. Fresh or frozen porcine heterografts are available at all times. Some institutions prefer to obtain pigskin in their own laboratories, whereas others obtain it from one of the reputable commercial skin banks that provide excellent service.

Both heterografts and homografts protect the burn wound from invasive infection and diminish the losses of protein and other nutrients from the wound. As dead tissue is removed from the wound biological dressings may be used until the area is cleaned and ready to accept a graft from the patient's own body (autograft). The usual technique is that the patient is placed in a Hubbard tank, all loose devitalized tissue removed and the strips of skin applied immediately after the patient is removed from the water. These dressings are very comfortable. One or two days later, when the patient is put in the tank, pigskin dressings are easily removed in the water with no bleeding. Homograft usually sloughs off within a few weeks. Sometimes it may begin to "take" and cause a sensitization reaction. To avoid systemic effects it should be removed before this occurs.

In many recent reports biological skin dressings have been suggested in the treatment of second-degree burns. Large, partial-thickness burn wounds are very comfortable and seem to heal more rapidly when treated with pigskin dressings that are applied every two or three days (Fig. 11-11, p. 268).

GRAFTING

The earlier a graft can be applied the more rapidly the wound is closed. Therefore, every ef-

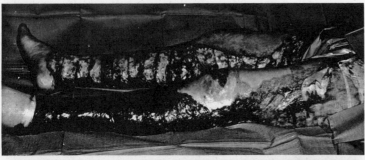
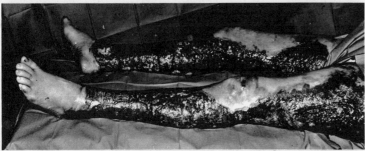
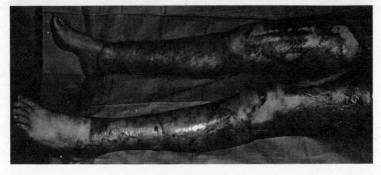

FIGURE 11-11.
Series of three photographs depicting the use of heterografts and homografts as biological skin dressings. (Top) The legs of this patient were not ready for grafting because the surface was not totally free of dead tissue. Homografts were placed on the left leg and heterografts from a pig on the right leg. After three days they were removed and another crop applied. (Middle) The areas are ready for grafting. The heterografts from the pig were as effective as the postmortem homografts. (Bottom) Good results were obtained on both legs.

fort is made to prepare the recipient site for grafting as early as possible.

Grafting should be planned carefully on extensively burned patients. Sometimes when there is a circumferential burn of the trunk, it is wise to graft one side from donor sites on the same side, and then turn the patient over two weeks later grafting the other side with donor sites from that side.

A CircOlectric bed may be used to facilitate tilting and turning and to help in changing the patient's position. This is important to prevent decubitus ulcers, pneumonia, and orthostatic hypotention during long periods of immobilization. One should keep in mind the priority of certain areas for skin coverage as well as the availability of donor sites. Usually as much of the burn wound is covered at the first grafting procedure as is reasonable. Sometimes autografts are used to cover most of the burn wound; but if they are not available for total coverage, homografts or heterografts are applied to close the rest of the wound. These homografts or heterografts come off after a short period of time and autografts are then applied. The patient should be kept in as good condition as possible for operation. The hematocrit should be maintained at 38 or above.

Certain areas of the body should be given consideration for coverage before others. Areas around joints should be grafted before large flat surfaces. Priority for skin coverage is as follows: hands and face first, with special priority to the hands; then areas of motion, especially those about the elbow. When skin coverage of the arms and hands is achieved early, it permits patients to do things for themselves, such as feeding, thus improving their morale and nutrition. When a leg is burned, the area around the knee is usually covered first, then the lower legs are given priority over the thigh.

Selection of a donor area is usually determined by the distribution of the surfaces to be grafted. The donor areas are usually taken from convenient places and areas that afford the most comfortable position for the patient. If there is a choice between using the chest and abdomen, the selection probably depends upon the type of dermatome used (see below). With a Brown air-driven dermatome, it is much easier to take skin from the chest than from the abdomen. However, the abdomen and the buttocks are excellent areas from which to take skin because scars will not show. When there is a choice, it is best to select a donor site on the anterior surface of the body rather than on the posterior, because the patient is more comfortable on his or her back during the convalescent period. Though it is easy to obtain skin from the arms, it is best not to incapacitate the arms if skin is available from other surfaces.

Several crops of skin may be taken from the same area if the patient has extensive burns. Depending upon the thickness of the skin, it may be possible to take a second crop approximately three to four weeks after the first graft has been removed.

Skin grafts may be taken with a variety of instruments and are usually about 0.008 to 0.012 of an inch in thickness (about half the thickness of the skin). The donor site usually heals in about two weeks providing that infection is prevented.

The Brown air-driven dermatome is one of the most useful instruments in cutting skin for grafting, because many sheets of skin can be removed rapidly (Fig. 11-12). It takes a piece of skin about 3 inches wide. Its construction is simple and little experience is required for the successful removal of a large amount of skin.

There are two drum-type dermatomes in common use, the Padgett and Reese. The Padgett dermatome is particularly useful in obtaining grafts from uneven surfaces. It furnishes the best method of cutting skin when a thicker piece is desired. A wider piece of skin can be removed than with the Brown air-driven dermatome, but the piece is not as long, since the standard Padgett instrument cuts an area 10×20 cm. The Reese dermatome is essentially a modification of the Padgett. The instruments are identical in basic design, but the Reese is much heavier and more solidly built. The method of regulating the depth of cut has been modified on the Reese dermatome and for a beginner, the Reese is much easier to use than the Padgett. The Reese dermatome uses dermatape as a backing for the skin. This green rubberized material fits over the

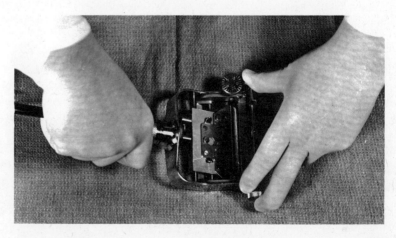

FIGURE 11-12.
Air-driven dermatome. This is the best dermatome for cutting skin for burns. It is rapid, easy to operate and provides long strips of thin skin for coverage of large granulating wounds. Source: Artz, C. P. and Moncrief, J. A.: The Treatment of Burns. Philadelphia, W. B. Saunders, 1969.

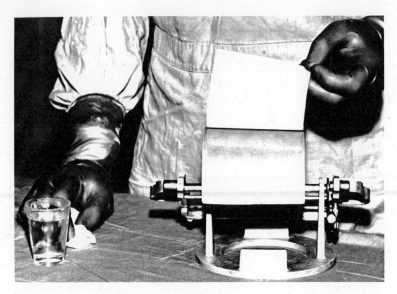

FIGURE 11-13.
Reese dermatome. There are two types of drum dermatomes, the Reese and the Padgett. The Reese instrument is a highly precisioned instrument and uses a dermatape. It is more cumbersome to use than the air-driven dermatome. It takes a wider strip of skin and is more effective on difficult donor areas. Source: Artz, C. P. and Moncrief, J. A.: The Treatment of Burns. Philadelphia, W. B. Saunders, 1969.

back of the drum, is attached to one end, than placed over the drum and tightened by means of a worm gear spool at the other end. Dermatome cement is painted on the skin allowing the adhesive layer of the green backing dermatape to adhere to the skin (Fig. 11-13).

The above instruments are almost always used in the operating room. When small pieces of skin are needed to fill in open areas, the Davol dermatome or a Weck skin knife may be used on the ward for cutting small strips of skin. These instruments are highly advantageous because many small areas can be covered by taking skin at the bedside under local anesthesia. Sometimes, when it is inadvisable to take seriously ill patients to the operating room for a major procedure, small strips of skin may be taken under local anesthesia every other day and applied to the burn wound.

The aim in the management of the burn wound is to cover it as rapidly as possible. Skin must be obtained by the method that best fits the situation.

In recent years mesh grafting has become very popular. When mesh grafting was first introduced by Tanner, it was for the primary purpose of stretching the available donor skin to fit a large area. Currently mesh grafting has been used in a variety of ways. It stretches well to fit an uneven area and does not contract as much as unmeshed skin. It allows drainage and, therefore, can be put on wounds that are not perfectly clean. Scars following grafting using skin meshed in a 1½ to 1 ratio are very little different from scars after sheets of thin split thickness skin.

When there are large areas to be covered and only a limited amount of skin, grafting using skin meshed in a 3 to 1 or even a 9 to 1 ratio makes the amount of available skin cover a larger area. While this type of grafting leads to increased scarring, it is not excessive. After mesh grafts are applied, a dressing is used for a period of at least 72 hours.

Care of Donor Sites

Donor sites are treated in a variety of ways. All of the methods are good as long as they keep the area free from infection. Methods such as large bulky dressings, coverage with nylon, or the use of scarlet red ointment have been suggested. The simplest, easiest, and probably the best way to handle a donor site and expect it to heal without infection is by exposure. Immediately after the graft has been removed, the donor area is covered with dry fine-mesh gauze. A wet gauze pack is placed over this to achieve hemostasis. At the end of the operation, the gauze pad is removed and the blood-soaked fine-mesh gauze is allowed to remain as the only covering of the wound. A firm coagulum soon forms by the blood that is caught in the interlacing fibers of the gauze. When this dries and hardens, in about 24 hours, it makes a protective covering for the wound. There may be a moderate amount of pain until the coagulum dries and hardens, but this is not severe. Epithelization proceeds beneath the coagulum and the area is usually healed in 14 days. After about 2 to 6 days, the patient may be put in a bathtub without any deleterious effects to the exposed donor areas. The area is then left open to air and any loose edges of gauze may be trimmed.

After Care of Grafts

Grafts may be applied in lay-on fashion to most burned surfaces. Sometimes it is necessary to put in a few sutures on such areas as the hands, face, and around joints. A graft takes best when it is exposed and the nurse or physician rolls it out each day—that is, after the graft is placed over the area and as serum or air collects beneath it, a cotton-tipped applicator is used to roll it out, thereby preventing the collection of fluid in any area. Meshing helps to prevent the accumulation of fluid bubbles under the graft. Exposure is advantageous in allowing frequent observation of the graft. Nursing measures and patient cooperation to provide immobilization for several days postgrafting are important.

Excellent takes of grafts can also be expected when a large, bulky dressing is applied. The dressing must be firm and put on with even compression. Such dressings are usually removed after three to five days.

The Hubbard tank is an effective method for stimulating motion and keeping the grafted areas clean. As soon as the dressings have been removed, or after the fourth postgrafting day in an exposed graft, the patient may be placed in the Hubbard tank at least once each day. Early motion and early ambulation are desirable.

When a patient with burns of the lower legs becomes ambulatory, he or she should wear elastic rubberized bandages. If the legs are wrapped with gauze such as Kerlix prior to the application of Ace bandages, the patient may be more comfortable and irritation of the grafts is decreased. Such a bandage should be worn over the grafts or donor sites on the lower extremities for a period of two or three months. This support for freshly grafted areas and donor sites is necessary to prevent breakdown of epithelium and subsequent small ulcerations. Elevation of the grafted legs or other dependent parts when the patient is not walking also helps to prevent the formation of blisters. The patient usually has a burning or stinging sensation when he or she stands if the circulation of the lower extremities is unsupported.

Physiotherapy is an essential part of the team approach to caring for the burned patient. The physiotherapist formulates the plan of exercise for each patient to maintain full range of motion and to prevent contractures. The therapist or nurse actively and passively exercises the patient daily, sometimes several times a day. Many units employ a therapist solely for the care of the patients in the burn unit, but this is not always possible. If the physiotherapy department of a hospital provides the service, a rotation of one month intervals for the therapist is found to be very satisfactory. This guarantees a patient the same person working with him or her for four weeks and also enables the therapist to know the patient and his or her limitations better.

The best time for exercising is when the patient is in the tank or immediately after any type of cleansing. Proper movement can not be achieved if bulky dressings are intact. It is the nurse's role to plan the day's care so that the therapist can visit when the patient is free of dressings and ointments. It is also the nursing staff's duty to continue the exercising program throughout the shifts when the therapist is not present. Active and passive exercises should be done with each dressing change.

Proper positioning is also an important nursing activity to prevent formation of deformities. The patient with burns of the ears should not be allowed to have a pillow, as this will cause pressure on this difficult-to-heal area. The use of a pediatric crib mattress on top of a regular mattress on the bed of an adult with anterior neck burns will allow hyperextension of the neck and prevent neck contracture.

Patients with axillary burns need to be positioned with their arms in abduction. Pulleys and slings or traction may be added to a basic overhead frame with side bars to meet individual needs. Footboards and long leg splints help to prevent footdrop while the patient is in bed. Dorsal hand splints will prevent wrist drop and maintain hands in a functional position when they are not involved in exercise activities or self-care such as feeding.

Occupational therapy stimulates patients' desires to rehabilitate themselves and also improves their morale. As soon as the granulating wounds are covered, a complete change usually occurs in the patient's general condition. There is less pain, the appetite improves, there is weight gain, and the patient feels much better in general. The occupational therapist can channel the patient's energy into activities which promote physical and social functioning.

Care of Specific Wound Sites and Equipment

CARE OF EYES

In the treatment of burns about the eyelid, keeping the cornea moist to prevent ulceration and infection is important. The eyes should be irrigated with normal saline with a bulb syringe at least every six hours and sometimes more often. After irrigation, an ophthalmic ointment should be instilled. Special care should be given to prevent cross-contamination from one eye to the other. Steroid ointments used as topical therapy for the face should be kept away from the eyes so that their normal inflammatory response to infection is not masked.

If the lids are not in apposition, a moist pad must be kept over the eye to prevent drying of the cornea; this is especially important at night. While eye care is being given, the nurse must be careful to reassure patients that they will be able to see. Sometimes it is wise to pull the eyelids apart to convince patients of their sight, especially if they have visitors. If some corrective measure on the eyelids is necessary it is important to inform patients before the operation about the type of procedure involved; and it is essential to tell them that they will be unable to see for several days because their eyes will be bandaged. When patients' eyes are closed because of edema or a bandage, it is advisable to speak to them

before touching them for any nursing procedure. Many patients have real psychological difficulties when their eyes are bandaged and they cannot see for more than three days (see Chapter 19).

CARE OF TRACHEOSTOMY

A tracheostomy is required in many severely burned patients, especially those with respiratory tract irritation. Careful nursing measures are extremely important following a tracheostomy. A clean dressing should be kept around the tracheostomy tube to cover the wound until healing is complete and to help absorb secretions from around the stoma. This dressing must be changed as often as indicated to prevent infection of the trachea. Cleansing around the tube may be done with peroxide, saline, or any mild cleansing agent. Humidification of the inspired air is required for all patients who have a tracheostomy to prevent drying of the mucous membrane which favors infection and the formation of obstructing mucopurulent plugs. An ultrasonic nebulizer either with or without oxygen attached provides a good humidity source (Fig. 11-14). Respirators are all equipped with humidity at-

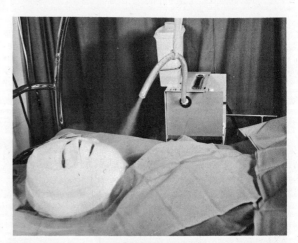

FIGURE 11-14.
This type of nebulizer provides humidified air or oxygen in very fine particles. It is always advisable to keep moist air going into a tracheostomy tube, otherwise the secretions may dry and form plugs in the bronchi. Source: Artz, C. P. and Moncrief, J. A.: The Treatment of Burns. Philadelphia, W. B. Saunders, 1969.

tachments but should be checked to insure proper functioning. If other methods are not available, a damp sponge may be placed over the tracheostomy opening to provide moisture. The better technique of course is the use of the humidifying apparatus mentioned above, since this provides much more efficient moistening of the airway. It should be used in cases with significant pulmonary problems. Simple bubbling of oxygen through water does not provide adequate moisture. The rapid expansion of the compressed oxygen cools the gas so much that its vapor-carrying capacity is lowered below that of ambient air and actual drying occurs.

The tracheostomy tube may be metal (or Shiley) with an inner cannula or portex with or without an inflatable cuff. If a double cannula tube is used, the inner cannula should be removed and cleansed at least every eight hours. The procedure is simple and quick but certain points must be emphasized: suction the patient well before removing the inner cannula using sterile technique; remove the cannula; clean with peroxide and saline; check for and remove mucoid obstruction within the inner cannula; before reinserting, suction the outer cannula.

The obturator should be kept strapped to the bed to facilitate reinsertion of the tube should it come out. It is extremely important to make sure the tracheostomy is functioning well both before and after a patient is turned onto his or her abdomen. Sometimes the curved tracheostomy tube abuts against the front of the trachea or slips out, causing respiratory obstruction. A plastic or portex tracheostomy tube has no inner removable part; if an obstruction develops that cannot be removed by suctioning, the entire tube must be replaced.

Suctioning techniques vary at different institutions; however, certain principles never change. Suctioning must be executed properly or the tracheal epithelium may be damaged (Fig. 11-15). Excessively vigorous tracheal suction is the most frequent error in the management of the tracheostomy. Absolute sterile technique should be followed and broken only in cases of extreme emergency. Many types of commercially packaged suction catheters are available which are

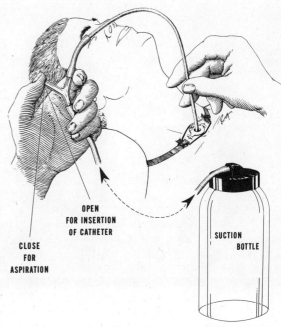

OPEN
FOR INSERTION
OF CATHETER

CLOSE
FOR
ASPIRATION

SUCTION
BOTTLE

FIGURE 11-15.
Technique of suctioning trachea. The clean catheter is placed in the tracheostomy tube with the Y adapter open. As soon as the catheter is well into the trachea, the Y tube opening is closed permitting suction on the catheter as it is withdrawn. When there is suction on the catheter as it goes into the trachea it may damage the lining. Source: Artz, C. P. and Moncrief, J. A.: The Treatment of Burns. Philadelphia, W. B. Saunders, 1969.

often prepackaged with a glove. A box containing 20 to 25 sets can be kept at the patient's bedside. The principle of placing a patient on 100 percent oxygen several minutes before suctioning to prevent hypoxia during the procedure is followed by many hospitals. Instillation of saline and bagging the patient periodically may also be part of the procedure. Generally, it is the nurse who will be suctioning the patient and her words of reassurance can be most comforting during this apprehensive period. After suctioning a patient, the nurse should not leave the bedside until she is certain the patient has no respiratory distress and is exchanging well. If the patient cannot make him or herself heard by covering the tracheostomy opening, an alternate means of communication should be provided.

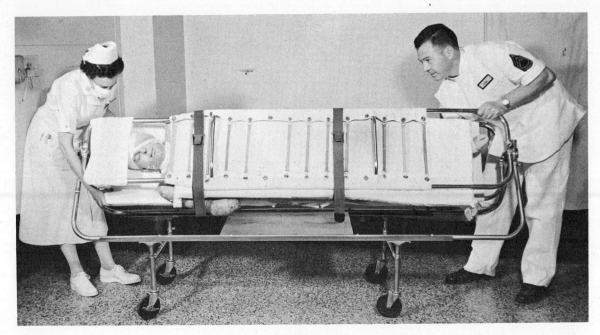

FIGURE 11-16.
A Stryker frame is convenient for turning burned patients. Unfortunately, this is a very narrow frame and is rather uncomfortable. Source: Artz, C. P. and Moncrief, J. A.: The Treatment of Burns. Philadelphia, W. B. Saunders, 1969.

TURNING BEDS

Several types of turning frames, or beds, have been used for the treatment of patients with circumferential burns. The Stryker and Foster frames have been popular for a number of years (Fig. 11-16).The electrically operated CircOlectric bed is much more useful. A patient is less afraid of and more comfortable on the CircOlectric bed than on the narrower turning frames (Fig. 11-17). The CircOlectric bed is a device consisting of two separate stretchers which electrically allow a patient to be rotated 360° from a supine to a prone position or to any degree of variation. The patient need not move at all to undergo this position change, making it extremely beneficial in cases of extensive burns. The head may be raised or lowered, allowing for better respiratory movement. The head may be lowered for better drainage from the lungs by means of gravity. Complete exposure of the anterior and the posterior surface by planned turn-

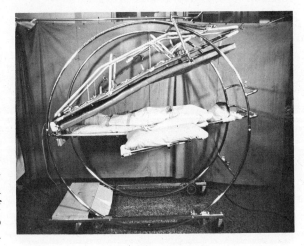

FIGURE 11-17.
CircOlectric bed. This is a wide frame and the patient can be turned from side to side without a great deal of difficulty. It is a very good turning frame for burned patients. Source: Artz, C. P. and Moncrief, J. A.: The Treatment of Burns. Philadelphia, W. B. Saunders, 1969.

ing enables better wound care in circumferential injury. Certain precautions must be taken when the bed is in use. Before the patient is turned, it should be explained to him or her how the bed operates and what movement is going to be accomplished. The anterior frame foam mattress pad should be placed on top of the patient with the headrest in the proper position. Before the patient is turned, the anterior frame should be fastened to the bed frame very securely, using the two turn screws provided. Before the patient is turned, the nurse should check the intravenous tubing and catheters to make sure they will not be pulled out during the turning procedures. Safety straps around the two stretchers at strategic areas should always be used when turning to prevent injury to the patient should the turn screws loosen or other malfunctions occur.

Turning on a CircOlectric bed should be done on a scheduled basis. This not only helps the patient's circulatory system, but also prevents pressure sores. Whenever the patient is kept face down for a long period of time there is increased edema of the eyes and face. If the patient shows any respiratory distress, he or she should be carefully observed when placed in this position. The amount of time that the patient is placed on one side or the other depends upon the need of the burned surface and the patient's ability to withstand the prone position.

THE AIR-FLUIDIZED BED

In the care of the burned patient, the air-fluidized bed can be one of the nurse's most valuable instruments (Fig. 11-18). Experience has proved its application for immediate postburn care, for grafting, and for patient comfort. Properly utilized it can effectively reduce the nursing effort required in the most difficult cases and still provide for the patient an environment not obtainable in any other system. It is extremely comfortable and very beneficial in burns of the back.

Essentially the bed consists of a large metal tank filled with approximately 2,000 pounds of glass beads ranging in size from 73 to 105 microns. The beads are covered with a monofilament, polyester sheet with a controlled pore space of 32 microns. A regular sheet is placed over the filter sheet before the patient is put in the bed. A blower provides the air which fluidizes the mass. Controls provide for the degree of hardness of the bead mass and regulation of temperature up to 103°F (39.5°C).

Proper installation requires an air-conditioning system that will maintain the room at 72°F (22°C), when the bed is circulating 50

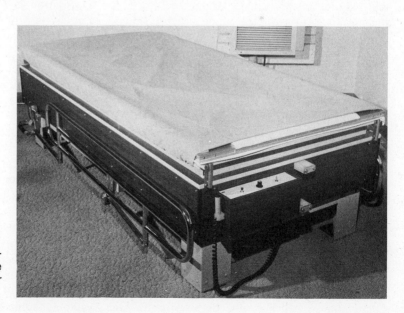

FIGURE 11-18.
The air-fluidized bed floats a patient. There are no pressure points. It is very comfortable for some burned patients.

cubic feet per minute of 95°F (35°C) air around the patient. At times this requires a window air-conditioner in addition to the air available from the hospital air-conditioning system.

The air issuing from the bed is free of bacterial contaminants; its temperature is controlled to within one degree of that found to be most desirable by the patient. When necessary the bed can be used for hyper- or hypothermia.

There is an increase in evaporative water loss in the bed and additional water is always given. The degree of loss is usually monitored by frequent measurement of the patient's serum sodium. The conscious patient usually will protect him- or herself against excessive water loss if permitted to drink ad lib; the unconscious patient must be carefully watched.

Routine care of the patient is more easily accomplished in the air-fluidized bed than in most other types of support. Patients, regardless of size, can be easily turned for any treatment. Bedpans are easily inserted and withdrawn, and, since they are displaced into the bed, patients can remain on them for extended periods without problems.

Should cardiac resuscitation be required, it is done by simply turning the bed off and climbing upon it in order to pump the chest. Since the bed will become instantly hard when the blower is turned off, this procedure is not difficult.

Care of the filter sheet, which is the most expensive item associated with the bed, is quite important, for it is this which separates the patient from the beads. Nothing is ever pinned to the sheet. Pin-sized holes will permit beads to come through. While the beads are innocuous as far as the patient's safety or well-being are concerned, they can be a nuisance if they get on the surface of the sheet and into the eyes or mouth. The glass from which the beads are produced contains no free silica and, therefore, cannot under any circumstances cause silicosis.

Nurses will find the air-fluidized bed most useful during the reconstructive phase of burn care. Skin grafts can be taken from, or placed upon, the patient's back, and the patient can be safely placed in the bed in a supine position. The circulating air will keep the donor site dry and relatively comfortable while it heals. Experience suggests that there is no need to turn patients who spend an extended period of time in an air bed. Stasis pneumonia has not been a problem with burned patients convalescing on these beds.

Filter sheet changes are recommended weekly; minor soilage can easily be handled without removing the filter sheet by washing the soiled spot with a very moist, soapy cloth and then wiping away the excess with a clean, damp cloth. The moist spot which remains will be dry in a matter of minutes. Generally speaking, if the room is maintained at the required temperature and the patient is well supervised, the air bed will make his or her care considerably easier for the staff and provide a more comfortable environment in which to recover.

THE INSERT MATTRESS

The insert mattress is a new design of mattress for the prevention and treatment of decubitus ulcers (Fig. 11-19). The unique waffle design of the insert causes a much larger area of the patient's back to be in contact with the mattress. This increase in surface contact substantially reduces the pressure in the areas normally associated with skin breakdown and ulcer development. Maceration is of little concern because of the ventilation provided in this design.

The mattress is similar in appearance to all others except that it is 7 inches thick and has a cavity provided on one side to accept the insert. The insert is 30 inches long, 20 inches wide, and 5 inches thick. It will provide a supporting surface from the neck to mid-thigh on the majority of patients. A loose sheet covers the mattress when it is in use. Although the insert is disposable, considerable care is taken to prevent soilage. Patients are either continent or catheterized.

Experience indicates that patients can rest on these mattresses for extended periods without developing pressure points or skin breakdown.

With an insert in place, waffle side in, the mattress can be turned over and used as a standard bed mattress; thus, it is unnecessary to store these units until needed since they can always be made available by simply reversing them.

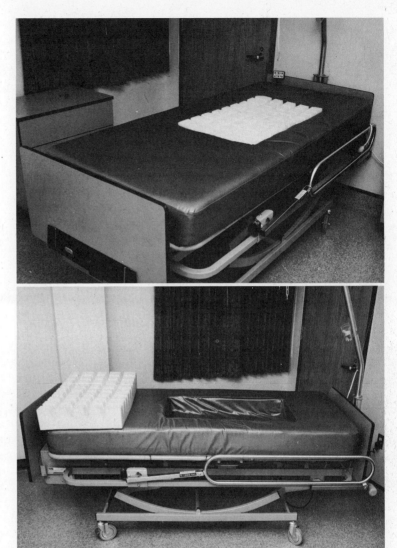

FIGURE 11-19.
The upper photograph shows a bed with the new insert mattress in place. As seen in the lower photograph, the cavity in the mattress holds an insert of foam rubber cut with a waffle design. The insert is changed with each patient. If the insert is not necessary, the mattress is turned over and it serves as the usual mattress for a hospital bed. Nursing services have found the insert to be very beneficial in the prevention of sacral decubitus ulcers.

Psychological Factors

There is no aspect in the therapy of burns in which a nurse can be more decisively helpful than in the promotion of a patient's emotional well-being. Attitudes of callousness as well as oversolicitude must be avoided. If a nurse is somewhat unstable emotionally, she may tend to react to a patient's complaining with one or the other of these extreme modes of behavior. Callous treatment reinforces the patient's fear of rejection. Oversolicitude may promote regression to childlike behavior. The effective nurse must be kind but firm. Burned patients must be disciplined to maintain a well-planned schedule.

When a severely burned patient is admitted to the hospital, he or she is not only in a state of severe physical pain, but also undergoing serious emotional disturbances. Many burned patients are difficult to manage because they are unable to adjust to their physical incapacity and to their surroundings. Emotional instability is reflected in abnormal behavior. Some patients are noisy, loud, and demanding; others are markedly depressed, often refusing to cooperate. It is important for the nurse responsible for the care of these patients to have some understanding of the adaptive problems and of the adaptive mechanisms they use.

The primary problems to which recently burned patients must adapt are threat to survival, fear of disfigurement, prolonged physical discomfort, frequent anesthesia and surgical procedures, and a long tedious convalescence. In addition to these primary adaptive problems, others appear in varying combinations as secondary problems, including separation from family and friends, feelings of inadequacy and rejection, emotional overtones associated with the accident, possible effect of the injury on future plans, and conflict engendered by a state of utter dependency.

Sometimes a patient believes that the burn was caused by his or her own negligence or through the fault of a close friend. Patients may have strong feelings of guilt, especially if a loved one was burned in the same accident. Separation of the patient from family and friends deprives him or her of a main source of emotional gratification. Sometimes a feeling of loneliness leads to depression and self-pity. Many patients, particularly women, interpret their injury as a threat to their capacity to be loved. Such patients are often hypersensitive to the slightest indication of personal rejection and need to be constantly reassured. Patients who have been active in athletics are particularly disturbed by burns of the lower extremities, and patients with extremity burns frequently fear the possibility of amputation.

Previously healthy, independent patients suddenly become dependent upon others for aid after a burn. The victim is totally incapacitated. He or she must be fed and even helped in voiding and defecating. All this may be a very difficult adjustment.

The multiple severe psychological threats involved in the near fatal injury cause patients to be placed in the dangerous situation of becoming overwhelmed by physically and emotionally painful stimuli. The major initial responses are repression and suppression of unpleasant thoughts, feelings, and sensations. Patients' attitudes are that they will not think about these unpleasant things and above all they will not allow themselves to have any feeling.

At times the patient may so completely shun the reality of the problems as to present a peculiar clinical picture. Badly burned patients may indicate in their conversation that they consider their injuries trivial and expect to go home in a few days. At other times, verbalization of fear of dying and dreams in which they relive the accident may be noted. Euphoria may occur followed by a long period of disorientation that may be psychogenic in origin. Sometimes disorientation is a toxic manifestation of extensive sepsis and should be so considered unless proved otherwise.

Friendly, personal contacts provide elements of hope that may aid the patient in giving up emergency repressive and constrictive techniques and in substituting mechanisms of constructive appraisal and planning, as well as direct action. Visitors and friendly patients diminish the feeling of separation and fear of not being loved. If patients are encouraged to attempt some constructive activity early in their treatment, the conflict over their dependency may be removed and they may feel that they are contributing some direct action toward their future recovery. The nurse must encourage patients to think constructively about their future plans. It is always wise to inform them when they may do something for themselves, such as eating and getting out of bed.

It is essential that the nurse understand the general nature of the patient's adaptive problems and assist him or her in his or her psychological adjustments. The nurse should attempt to learn about the patient's preburn personality. Family and friends may be helpful in giving information regarding the patient's usual coping mechanisms and behavior patterns. Effective burn therapy involves not only the management of the physical injury, but also a constant effort to make the situation less difficult for the patient and more bearable emotionally. It is essential for a patient to have confidence in the competence of the staff. Many burned patients are deeply discouraged and see little prospect of recovery, but they do exhibit a form of primitive childlike faith in the ability of a physician. This faith of the patient needs to be stimulated by an attitude of genuine interest on the part of all attendants and a truthful but hopeful approach.

Families of burn patients may go through the same stages of reaction to the burn as the victim. They deserve an opportunity to ask questions, to ventilate feelings, and to share concerns with the nurses for at least a brief time each day. Group meetings of families led by a staff nurse, clinical specialist in psychiatric nursing, or social worker may help them to share and profit from common feelings. Nurses need to help define a definite role for close family members such as parent, spouse, son, or daughter so that this person can actively participate in care and express his or her desire to do something for the loved one.

Severely burned patients are sometimes better off on a ward than in a private room. Isolation reinforces their impressions that they are alone and suffering whereas exposure to the plight of others lessens the significance of their wounds. (See Chapter 19.) While one cannot disregard obvious disability, the fact that others may be suffering more has a peculiarly comforting effect. If several patients have been involved in the same accident, placing them in the same cubicle is particularly beneficial to group morale.

Visual evidence of the likelihood of uneventful recovery is especially encouraging in the early phase of hospitalization. Contact with patients who have had similar burns and are almost recovered is an excellent source of encouragement. Some patients are reassured by seeing photographs of other severely burned patients showing burned areas at the time of injury and after recovery.

Unfortunately, patients who have recovered from severe burns are often quite reluctant to help those who are acutely ill. Evidently, they are striving to forget the physical and emotional suffering they have endured. Any contact with others who are suffering from thermal injury reminds them of their own painful experience. In the experience of others, burn patients who are returning for clinic appointments may be happy to visit inpatients and give them encouragement.

Some metroplitan areas have seen the formation of groups of burn victims and families who meet regularly for discussion, mutual support, social activity, and community-aimed burn prevention programs. Staff morale is also boosted by the opportunity to see ex-patients return to a productive life.

Isolation of patients should be avoided as much as possible. Early in the course of treatment diversional measures such as reading, music, and television are helpful. During the first two weeks some patients may be too frightened and bewildered to ask about their condition. After the acute effects of the injury have diminished, however, they begin to ask questions. It is most helpful at this time to explain what can be expected in the ensuing months. It frequently is a great source of help if someone can state that the hands and face will not be scarred. This is always a great fear of most patients, and if they are not badly burned, this fear can frequently be alleviated early in the course of therapy.

The patient with a face burn that causes closing of the eyes due to edema of the lids, impairment of hearing due to fluid collection in the ears, and edematous interference with smell and taste has had his or her sensory contact with the environment severely limited. Such patients tolerate this for a short period but soon begin to lose contact with reality and eventually become completely detached. Under such circumstances it is mandatory that frequent contact be made with the patient by touch, loud talking, feeding or radio. These patients characteristically are totally disoriented unless brought back to reality by vocal and tactile stimuli. (For further discussion, see Chapter 19).

Lack of sleep due to the frequent nursing activities and pain on movement required for a critical patient also are detrimental to a patient's mental status. It is necessary to group nursing activities and coordinate the interventions of other burn team members so that periods of solid sleep are available. A balance between sensory overstimulation which causes "ICU psychosis" and sensory deprivation resulting from the effects of the burn, must be effected by the nurse as she organizes her plan of care.

Narcotics

Treatment of a severe burn is accompanied by some pain, and minor physical discomfort persists over a long period of time. However, physical pain is considerably less severe than is generally supposed. In contrast, emotionally induced pain is a much more serious problem. Frequently, patients do not distinguish between physical pain and emotional tension and report all discomfort as pain. In patients whose emotional needs are neglected, regressive behavior sometimes occurs as manifested by moaning, complaining, and demanding.

Physical pain should be treated with narcotics, initially given intravenously. As soon as possible, however, narcotic administration should be limited. Narcotics, tranquilizers, and sedatives should be used to make the patient as comfortable as is reasonable, but he or she should not depend upon these drugs. Some type of narcotic can be given immediately before such painful episodes as washing the wound, getting the patient out of bed, and putting him or her in the bathtub. If patients learn that they will be given something for pain when they actually experience it, they will call for medication only when they have physical pain. Narcotics have a tendency to cause constipation and lack of appetite. They should be used when needed, but every effort should be made to relieve emotional anxiety by methods other than narcotic administration.

Nutrition

The survival of a severely burned patient frequently depends upon nutritional replacement. Studies in energy metabolism show that severely burned patients develop marked metabolic deficits and when they die they have essentially "run out of gas." The needs of proteins and calories are two to three times normal during the first three weeks after injury. Every effort should be made to encourage the greatest possible intake of proteins and calories to maintain the patient in as good a nutritional status as possible. It is unwise to institute immediate forced-feeding

programs to offset all nitrogen losses. The patient should receive increasing quantities of nutriment, when his of her gastrointestinal tract is capable of accepting them and when reasonably efficient utilization can be expected.

A high-protein, high-calorie intake should be prescribed as soon as peristalsis has returned after the injury. In a patient without complications, a good intake should be obtainable in ten days. The aim is to achieve a daily protein intake of 2 to 3 Gm per kg of body weight along with an intake of 50 to 70 cal per kg. A healthy individual lying quietly in bed requires 1 Gm of protein and 30 cal per kg of body weight per day to maintain protein equilibrium. Obviously considerably more is required to meet the needs of the hypermetabolic burn patient. The routine serving of three standard hospital meals is totally inadequate for severely burned patients. To achieve an acceptable protein intake, the patient should be put on a selective, high-protein, high-calorie diet and given supplemental high-protein liquid nourishment between meals (Fig. 11-20). The nurse should take great care to explain to the patient the importance of an adequate nutritional intake. Since standard menus rarely suffice for the patient's protein and caloric needs, various supplements are used. Almost every hospital dietary department has a standard high-protein supplemental feeding formula. Several excellent commercial preparations are available. It is extremely important that the supplemental feeding

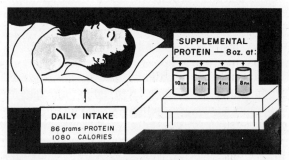

FIGURE 11-20.
Schematic diagram of sample high-protein supplementary feedings. The use of additional proteins and calories, as between meal feedings, keeps up the energy reserve of the burned patient.

be a palatable liquid. Changes in the flavor may be necessary from time to time. Nutritious snacks available 24 hours a day and favorite foods from home should be utilized to increase total dietary intake. The nurse must be ever mindful of the needs of burned patients for a high-nutritional intake and use her ingenuity in aiding the dietitian to provide the most palatable of high-protein, high-calorie support for the patient.

It is difficult to give positive indications for the institution of tube feedings. An indwelling nasogastric tube is uncomfortable and its use may be followed by complications, such as aspiration, respiratory infection, and gastric dilatation. One of the common causes of deaths in burned children is the aspiration of tube feedings. Sometimes this occurs because the nurse administering the tube feeding does not notice that there is gastric atony with dilatation, and, after the tube feeding is instilled, the patient regurgitates, aspirates, develops a pneumonia, and dies. Before tube feeding is initiated and during the first few hours thereafter, the abdomen should be examined for the presence of bowel sounds and to make sure that the gastrointestinal tract is not atonic. The endotracheal or tracheostomy tube should have the cuff inflated, and the patient should be positioned to prevent aspiration of vomitus. An adequate amount of water must always be given when tube feedings are used. It is usually wise to flush out the tube with water after the tube feeding has been given.

Tube feeding can be used as an adjunct to the patient's regular meals. Feedings are scheduled between breakfast and lunch, lunch and dinner, and every three hours during the night. Once the patient meets his or her calorie goal by the oral intake, the nasogastric tube can be removed.

All burn patients should be weighed without dressings daily. This weight can be graphed to give a visual record of fluid and nutritional balance. The dietitian sets a calorie goal for each patient based on age, preburn weight, and extent of injury. By sharing the goal with the patient and keeping him or her informed of his or her progress, the nurse can often get patient support in meeting the required calorie intake. Food in-

gested at mealtime is recorded on the patient's menu which is saved. This and a daily record of between-meal nourishment intake will allow the dietitian to maintain an accurate calorie count.

Since it is so important that an adequate intake of proteins and calories be maintained, intravenous hyperalimentation is used in some extensively burned patients. It would seem that this would be an excellent method of maintaining a good protein and calorie intake which is so essential in the burned patient, but because infection is such a problem in these patients, prolonged hyperalimentation is used cautiously. The problem of infection in and around the tip of the catheter which may eventually lead to an overwhelming systemic infection is very common in extensively burned patients. The decision to start hyperalimentation is often difficult. The patient really needs the increased calories and proteins, but the fear of a fatal infection is ever present. Usually the physician selects hyperalimentation for a short period of time when it is felt that there is no other method of maintaining a reasonable intake. Frequently hyperalimentation is used for seven days and then every effort is made to get the patient to take food by mouth or tube feeding. If hyperalimentation is used, the catheter site is rotated approximately every seven days. In extensively burned patients, hyperalimentation has saved many lives but it must be used judiciously because of the ever present threat of overwhelming sepsis.

It should be emphasized that total enteral support of nutrition is possible in most cases unless the patient has a nonfunctioning gastrointestinal tract. However, a great deal of nursing time and effort and ingenuity is essential.

Infection

Infection is one of the common problems in burns. Most second-degree burns, if kept free from infection, heal in a very short time. All third-degree burns become infected. The degree of infection is important and if the infection is kept at a minimum, the surface can be grafted, and healing with little scarring can be expected. On the other hand, if large open wounds become severely infected, many systemic problems follow. Infection is the cause of pain, nutritional disturbances, conversion of second-degree burns to third-degree injury, failure of skin grafts to take, and may be the cause of death. Obviously, the aim in the treatment of a third-degree burn where the barrier against infection, namely, the skin, is totally destroyed, is to treat the wound in such a way that infection is minimized.

Since infection is such a common problem, burned patients in many hospitals are isolated in the belief that harmful organisms can be kept away from them. Unfortunately, this is impossible, for even in strictest isolation extensively burned patients develop infection from their own organisms. At one time it was believed that cross-infection could be minimized by strict isolation. In recent years, with the advent of local antibacterial agents such as Sulfamylon, cross-contamination has been minimized and isolation is unnecessary. In fact, isolation of a burned patient probably means that he of she will not receive the careful attention that is necessary; therefore, it is strongly contraindicated. If there is a local antibacterial agent covering the wound, it is doubtful that any organisms that fall on the wound will multiply. Thus, patients treated with local antibacterial agents are essentially isolated from their own environment.

Local infection is limited to the burned area and is manifested by cellulitis, lymphangitis, and enlargement of the regional lymph nodes. There is usually fever and an increase in white blood cell count. The common causes of this type of infection are the beta hemolytic streptococcus and the staphylococcus. Local infection may complicate both second- and third-degree burns. In the period prior to the use of antibiotics, local infection was common in many burns, but in more recent years it has been rather well controlled by the use of appropriate antibiotics given systemically. When local antibacterial agents are used, local infection is rare.

When partial-thickness burns and some full-thickness burns and donor sites become locally infected, a culture should be taken and a systemic antibiotic given, according to the sensitivity of the organism. In addition, the wound should be made as clean as possible. Local antibacterial ointments may be applied or continuous wet dressings used, this being one of the best techniques for managing local infections in any burn wound. The dressings should be kept moist and warm, and changed every four hours. Because this technique increases nursing time, it is not always used. The use of a local antibacterial ointment applied daily may be satisfactory and is certainly less time consuming than the wet dressing method.

Burn wound sepsis is a recent term used to describe the massive invasive bacterial involvement of the burn wound and the adjacent tissue. Quantitative bacteriology routinely reveals 10^7 to 10^9 organisms in each gram of involved tissue. Wound sepsis is predominantly due to a mixed flora of gram-negative organisms. About half the cases have positive blood cultures. This unusual serious complication occurs most frequently in patients who sustain extensive full-thickness burns but is rare in partial-thickness burns, or in full-thickness burns of relatively small extent. The primary manifestations of burn wound sepsis are the topical appearance of the degenerating wound and the clinical appearance of the patient. The onset of sepsis may be insidious or acute—a gradual rise or drop in temperature being the earliest manifestation. The complete burn wound sepsis syndrome then develops gradually within two or three days.

Observation of early signs of systemic sepsis is an important nursing responsibility. Decreased appetite, flushing of the face, and a brief period of increased urine output may be warnings of impending sepsis. When output drops, the nurse can act quickly to increase IV fluid rate to fill the temporarily enlarged vascular compartment. She may give antipyretics and apply cold packs or a hypothermia blanket to decrease the high fevers often seen with gram-negative sepsis. Oral intake should be held until the episode is over. Continued close observation of the patient's vital signs and response to treatment are necessary. Frequent consultation with the physician is essential to bring the patient through this life-threatening situation.

Sepsis due to gram-negative organisms more

characteristically is associated with a leukopenia relative hypothermia and rapid wound deterioration. There may be a bleeding tendency manifested by petechiae, ecchymoses, and oozing from the wound. When sepsis is due to gram-positive organisms the temperature usually rises to 102° F (39°C), and there is a marked increase in respiratory rate. In all types of burn wound sepsis, disorientation usually occurs. Paralytic ileus is common and one of the most distressing findings, preventing gastrointestinal feeding and thus contributing substantially to debilitation. In the final stages, hypotension and oliguria occur. If the offending organism is a staphylococcus, the prognosis is a little better than if it is a gram-negative organism. Few patients with gram-negative burn wound sepsis survive. (See Chapter 13 for a discussion of shock secondary to sepsis.)

Treatment consists of supportive therapy such as fluids and blood transfusions, systemic antibiotics in large doses, and the best possible local wound care. Subeschar antibiotic therapy may be of benefit if the causative organism and its antibiotic sensitivity are known. The selected antibiotic is injected beneath the eschar. The common technique is to dissolve the daily dose in a reasonable quantity of saline and inject this through multiple portals beneath the eschar every 24 hours. This allows for a diffusion of the antibiotic into the subcutaneous tissue where bacteria are proliferating.

In recent years with the use of local antibacterial agents, it has been possible in many instances to prevent burn wound sepsis in the extensively burned patient. This is one of the major advances in the past decade in the treatment of burns.

Chemical Burns

Most chemical burns are either acid or alkali burns. In some instances, mustard gas or tear gas has caused burns. The mechanism of injury is usually a combination of chemical and thermal alteration of tissue. The depth of cellular damage depends upon the duration of exposure and concentration.

Acid burns are usually the result of some type of industrial or home accident. The wound is extremely painful, often for long periods because of the continued chemical reaction. The appearance of the wound varies according to the depth of burn from erythema in the more superficial to a gray, yellowish brown or black in the deeper wound. The treatment of acid burns is most effectively accomplished immediately after onset and, thus, becomes both a first aid and a definitive action. The most readily available substance for effective treatment of chemical burns is water. Copious rinsing with water as soon as possible is a most effective therapy. In some instances, neutralization may be beneficial. Specific management of acid burns is outlined in Table 11-1, page 284. General support and fluid resuscitation are the same as for a flame burn. After initial care the local treatment of acid burns is the same as that for thermal burns.

Alkali burns should be treated in essentially the same way as acid burns. Copious rinsing with water is most important.

Phosphorus burns are extremely painful, penetrating deeply into the tissue, and may emit smoke if the phosphorus is exposed to air. The phosphorus should be removed as soon as possible. Sometimes the wound is soaked in copper sulfate which makes the phosphorus a little more evident. This is not a common civilian injury, but is more often seen in time of war.

In any chemical burn of the eyes, extreme care must be exercised. It is much better to rinse with large quantities of water than attempt to use any type of neutralizing agent.

Electrical Injuries

Electrical injury is frequently referred to as an electrical burn. Electrical burn is a poor term because the effect of electricity passing through the tissues makes a deeper injury than the usual partial- or full-thickness burn. In many instances, a flame burn is associated with electrical injuries.

Because of the different types of burns associated with electrical accidents, there is a wide variation in electrical injuries. Most skin burns occur at the entrance and exit of the current,

TABLE 11-1
Management of Chemical Burns

Agent	Cleansing	Neutralization	Débridement
Acid Burns			
Sulfuric	Water	Sodium bicarbonate solution	Débride loose,
Nitric			nonviable tissue
Hydrochloric			
Trichloracetic			
Phenol	Ethyl alcohol	Sodium bicarbonate solution	Débride loose,
			nonviable tissue
Hydrofluoric	Water	Same as other acids plus magnesium oxide, glycerin paste, local injection, calcium gluconate	Débride loose, nonviable tissue
Alkali Burns			
Potassium hydroxide	Water	0.5-5.0% acetic acid or	Débride loose,
Sodium hydroxide		5.0% ammonium chloride	nonviable tissue
Ammonia			
Lime	Brush off powder	0.5-5.0% acetic acid or 5.0% ammonium chloride	Débride loose, nonviable tissue
Phosphorus	Water	Copper sulfate soaks	Débride and remove particles of phosphorus
Mustard gas	Water	M-5 ointment	Aspirate; then excise blebs during flushing with water
Tear gas	Water	Sodium bicarbonate solution	Débride loose tissue

damage at the entrance of the current being generally more severe than at the exit. The burns may vary from small circular spots to large areas of destruction, and the depth and extent of injury is usually underestimated when first seen. There is usually an extension of the necrosis because of arterial thrombi common after electrical injury. Necrosis deep to the lesion and the subcutaneous tissue is common. A limb may appear viable soon after an electrical injury, but, in a few days, it becomes ischemic and finally gangrenous (Fig. 11-21).

Burns associated with electricity may be divided into three categories: 1) true electrical injury caused by the electrical current passing through the skin after the contact with the conductor; 2) electrothermal burns that result from electrical generation of heat outside the skin, such as flash or arc burn; and 3) flame burns that result from ignition of clothing by electrical sparks and arcing. Many times the extensive area of flame burns is much greater than that of other burn lesions. The type of injury varies according to the type of the accident; often all three types may be present.

One of the immediate effects of electrical injury is tetanic contraction of the muscle. It may be so severe that fractures and dislocations occur. A delayed effect of electrical injury, especially about the head, is the development of cataracts which usually become evident four to six months after the accident.

The victim of an electrical shock should be freed from the electric current as quickly as possible. The rescuer must make sure that the current is off before touching the victim so that he or she is not injured by the current. If the patient is not breathing, artificial respiration must be

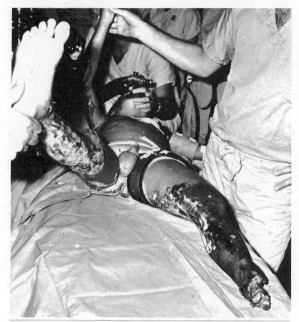

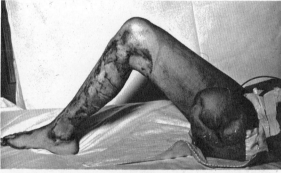

FIGURE 11-21.

(Top) Photograph of a 10-year-old boy who came in contact with a high-tension wire. There was a marked amount of necrosis of the left leg with dead muscle. The right leg had thermal injury caused by his clothing's igniting. (Bottom) An amputation of the left leg plus reamputation was required to eliminate all the dead muscle. The right leg was grafted about three weeks after injury. The patient recovered. Source: Artz, C. P. and Moncrief, J. A.: The Treatment of Burns. Philadelphia, W. B. Saunders, 1969.

started immediately. Mouth-to-mouth resuscitation has saved many lives. If the heart is not beating, there is probably ventricular fibrillation and cardiac massage should be instituted.

The amount and type of replacement therapy after electrical injury depends upon the type and extent of the injury. Electrical injury has been likened to crush injury. The usual formulas for thermal burns do not apply. The volume of tissue destroyed, because of the deeper injury from electricity, means that more fluids are required than are generally used with thermal burns of the same extent. One of the great problems in electrical injury is the high frequency of renal failure, which is usually out of proportion to the total extent of skin involvement and probably caused by the precipitation of myoglobin in the renal tubules following muscle death. Sometimes alkaline solutions are given in an attempt to prevent renal complications. Resuscitative fluids are usually administered in a rate sufficient to maintain a urinary output of approximately 30 ml per hour. When urine flow is not adequate, mannitol may be used. (See Chapter 17 for further discussion of renal failure.)

Local wound management is similar to that for thermal injury except when there is evidence of tissue damage beneath the skin and subcutaneous tissue. Frequently the physician incises one or two areas and looks at the underlying muscle. If it is normal, the area is treated as a thermal burn; if the muscle is dead the patient is usually taken to the operating room, as soon as his or her general condition permits, and the dead tissue excised (Fig. 11-22). After excision, the wound is dressed and inspected in two or three days. The nurse should observe the electrical injury sites carefully for signs of vascular collapse. This may occur gradually over a period of several days and lead to gangrene. Initial excision or amputation may be conservative requiring close attention to signs of additional tissue death following the first operative procedure. If there is no further evidence of dead tissue, the wound is then closed by a graft.

Burns About the Head

Management of burns about the head is particularly difficult because of the many important functional organs involved. A more marked systemic derangement appears to be associated with deep burns about the face and neck than with

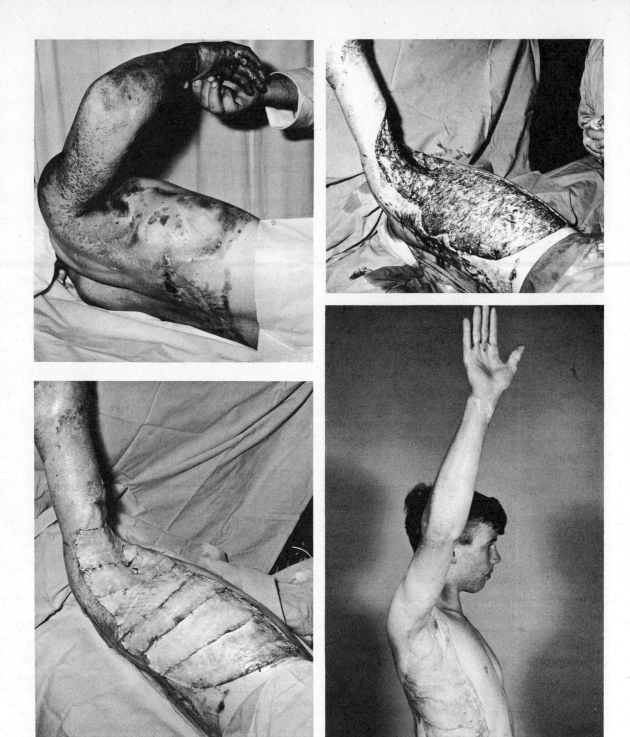

FIGURE 11-22.
(Top left) Photograph of electrical injury and thermal burn incurred when a 17-year-old boy came in contact with a high-tension wire. (Top right) There was a question of dead muscle around the anterior aspect of the axilla. This was incised. The dead muscle was removed and the remaining full-thickness burn on the right chest was excised. (Bottom left) Grafts placed in lay-on fashion on the third postexcision day. These grafts were treated by exposure. (Bottom right) Final result showing excellent mobility of shoulder. Source: Artz, C. P. and Moncrief, J. A.: The Treatment of Burns. Philadelphia, W. B. Saunders, 1969.

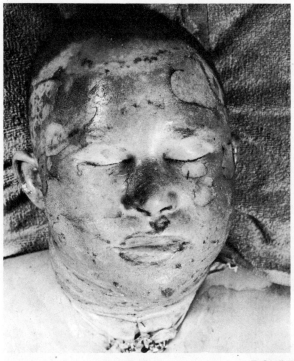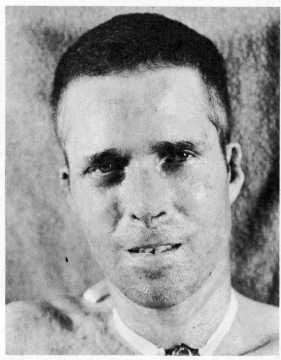

FIGURE 11-23.
(Left) This photograph shows marked edema of the face 48 hours after a second-degree burn which occurred in a racing accident. The eyes are closed by edema which subsided two days later. (Right) Only two months after the injury the face had completely healed. Source: Artz, C. P. and Moncrief, J. A.: The Treatment of Burns. Philadelphia, W. B. Saunders, 1969.

burns of comparable extent in other areas. Extensive edema occurs because the loose areolar tissues around the face and neck offer little tissue pressure to resist extravasation of edematous fluids. Convulsions occurring in children with head burns are frequent. Cerebral edema has been demonstrated by special autopsy techniques in such instances.

In burns of the face, the eyelids become edematous and are usually closed tightly within six to eight hours after injury. Most of the edema occurs in the first 24 hours, although it does not reach its maximum until about 48 hours (Fig.11-23). The edema of the eyelids usually begins to disappear on the third day, and the patient can frequently see by the fourth day.

It is difficult to determine accurately the initial depth of a burn on the face. Occasionally the burn appears to be third degree initially, but, with proper care, epithelial growth occurs in

many areas from the lining of the hair follicles. One of the primary problems in nursing care of burns about the face is to keep the area as clean as possible. The patient is most uncomfortable unless the nares, eyes, ears, and mouth are kept clean.

Burns of the eyelids are common in face burns; however, burns of the sclera and cornea are rare. In burns of the eyelids, it is important to irrigate with saline and instill an antibiotic ophthalmic ointment to prevent infection. In full-thickness burns of the eyelids, the chief danger is rapid contracture and ectropion formation (Fig. 11-24). The resulting incomplete closure of the lids causes drying of the cornea and ulcer formation. If infection supervenes, a panophthalmitis may develop. Therefore, the important aim in treating burns of the eyelids is protection of the cornea. Sometimes it is necessary to suture the eyelids together to protect the

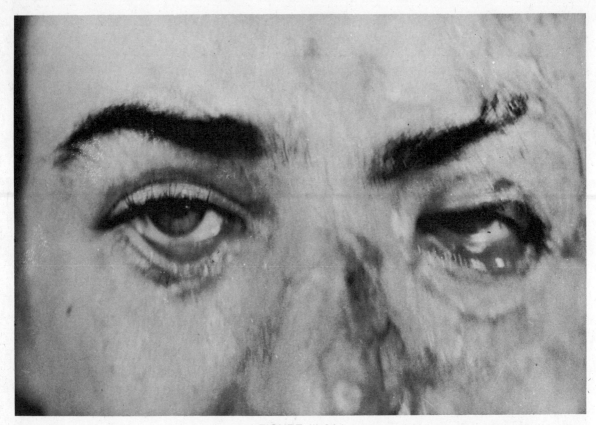

FIGURE 11-24.
Close-up photograph showing scarring with ectropion of the left eye. There is also minimal extropion on the right. Unless these are repaired the eyelids cannot be closed and a corneal ulcer may develop. Source: Artz, C. P. and Moncrief, J. A.: The Treatment of Burns. Philadelphia, W. B. Saunders, 1969.

cornea, but the best procedure is the tarsor-rhaphy.

In rather deep burns of the face, the best way to prepare the area for grafting is by wet soaks. Priority for grafting is usually given to the face, since the eschar of the full-thickness burn on the face seems to come off a little earlier than it does in other areas of the body. The nurse must use every effort to keep the face as clean as possible and to assist in the removal of the dead tissue so that a graft can be applied early.

Thermal injury to the skin of the external ear may result in direct destruction of the cartilage or necrosis subsequent to infection. Early inflammatory necrosis is not usually associated with demonstrable bacterial involvement, and as the process progresses, more cartilage is liquefied

and an abscess of the auricle is formed. Every effort should be made to minimize bacterial infection in burns of the auricle and it is vital that a local antibacterial agent be used in such burns.

Once chondritis has developed, the aim is to minimize infection and prevent further destruction of the cartilage. The best method of treatment is wet soaks and, if necessary, early and wide excision of the necrotic cartilage. Because burns of the auricle are frequently very painful, warm compresses may be used.

Respiratory damage is most frequently associated with burns about the face and neck, especially in individuals burned in a closed space. Respiratory irritation results from inhalation of noxious fumes and gases and should be termed inhalation injury, not respiratory burn.

Inhalation injury is recognized clinically by redness and edema in the posterior pharynx, coughing, and hoarseness. Singeing of the nasal hairs may be present and bronchospasm with prolonged wheezing may be a prominent finding. If there is appreciable injury to the lower respiratory tract, treatment is very difficult.

Use of a fiberoptic bronchoscope to determine the extent of respiratory injury shortly after admission has been a recent aid to respiratory care. Aggressive chest physiotherapy, postural drainage, and frequent auscultation of the lungs are nursing activities of much therapeutic and diagnostic value.

The management of respiratory tract injury includes tracheostomy followed by diligent, gentle aspiration of tracheobronchial secretions, administration of moist oxygen, antibiotics, and corticosteroids. In all patients with clinical evidence of respiratory tract damage, tracheostomy is indicated. These patients are in danger of asphyxia both from swelling of the air passages and from accumulated excessive secretions. The danger is lessened if early tracheotomy is performed and efficient tracheobronchial toilet is maintained. The tracheobronchial tree must be kept free of excessive secretions by gentle suctioning. Great care must be taken to prevent infection of the trachea. Mucolytic agents are of great assistance in loosening secretions, while intermittent positive pressure breathing can be effective in maintaining or reinstituting expansion of the parenchyma of the lung. A tracheostomy is frequently lifesaving in pulmonary injury; unfortunately, it may be a source of serious complications, the most dramatic being those associated with improper care. All too often the stoma is made so low that the tracheostomy tube either rides on the carina or slips down one main stem bronchus, thereby occluding the other. Poor ventilation, coughing, and bronchospasm may result. Failure to provide adequate moisture to the inspired air is a common fault. Because of the frequent suctioning and constant abutment of the tube on the anterior tracheal wall, erosion of the area with invasive infection is not uncommon. Sometimes actual perforations occur. (See Chapter 14 regarding acute respiratory insufficiency

and the use of intermittent positive pressure breathing machines.)

Shock lung, associated with a variety of conditions in which trauma and sepsis are present may also develop in burn victims. The nurse caring for the patient with shock lung should be cognizant of blood gas results and must be familiar with the goals and associated nursing care of the patient who requires mechanical ventilation, including positive end expiratory pressure (PEEP). She may be responsible for maintaining arterial monitoring equipment when the physician inserts a Swan-Ganz catheter to enable measurement of pulmonary artery pressures. A sound understanding of the cardiovascular and cardiopulmonary dynamics involved will make the nurse a most valuable participant in the frequent decisions which the physician must make regarding therapy.

Curling's Ulcer

Acute gastroduodenal ulceration associated with thermal burns is commonly referred to as Curling's ulcer. Curling reported 12 such cases in 1842. It is generally believed that these ulcers are associated with the acute stress common in extensively burned patients. Such ulcers have been seen in burns of as little as 10 percent of the body surface, but they are most commonly found in the patient who has more than 30 percent full-thickness injury.

It is difficult to diagnose the lesion unless some type of catastrophe, such as massive bleeding or perforation, occurs. Frequently there are no signs or symptoms of ulcer formation. The patient may complain of abdominal discomfort and, if a gastric tube is in place, small amounts of blood may be seen. The first sign is usually an acute hemorrhage. Ulcers may develop as early as the first or second postburn day, but the usual time for manifestation of hemorrhage is near the end of the first week.

Bleeding Curling's ulcers are usually treated the same as are other bleeding ulcers. If initial attempts at conservative management fail (such as irrigation of the stomach with ice water), some type of surgical procedure with the arrest of hemorrhage from the ulcer is mandatory. Since Curling's ulcers occur primarily in extensively burned patients, the mortality associated with bleeding requiring operation is quite high. It may be possible to manage the bleeding ulcer by surgical means, but other complications of the severe burns may cost the patient's life. The use of antacids (given in amounts to maintain the gastric pH at 7.0) has been helpful in preventing stress ulcer.

Bibliography

Achauer, B. M., et al: Pulmonary complications of burns: the major threat to the burn patient. Annals Surg. 177:311-319.

Andreason, N. J. C., et al: Management of emotional reactions in seriously burned adults. New Eng. J. Med. 286, 2:65-69, Jan. 1, 1972.

Arney, G. K., Pearson, E. and Sutherland, A. B.: Burn stress pseudodiabetes. Annals Surg. 152:77, 1960.

Artz, C. P.: Understanding thermal burns and principles of management. *In* J. H. Davis (ed.): Current Concepts in Surgery. New York, McGraw-Hill, 1965, p. 247.

———Electrical injury simulates crush injury. Surg. Gyn. Ob. 125:1316, 1967.

———Improving oral protein nutrition. Postgrad. Med., 43:223, 1968.

Artz, C. P., Bronwell, A. W. and Sako, Y.: The exposure treatment of donor sites. Annals Surg., 142:248, 1955.

Artz, C. P. and Moncrief, J. A.: The Treatment of Burns. Philadelphia, W. B. Saunders, 1969.

Baxter, C. R., Curreri, W. P. and Marvin, J. A.: The control of burn wound sepsis by the use of quantitative bacteriologic studies and subeschar clysis with antibiotics. Nurs. Clin. N. Am. 53:1509-1518, 1973.

Bayley, E. W., et al: Breaking the anger-despair cycle. Nurs. '75 May 1975.

Bowden, Marjorie: Helping the burn patient return home. Am. Operat. Room Nurses J. 69-72, Jan. 1971.

Bowden, Marjorie and Feller, Irving: Family reaction to a severe burn. Am. J. Nurs. 73, 2.

Bull, J. P. and Squire, J. R.: A study of mortality in a burns unit: standards for the evaluation of alternative methods of treatment. Annals Surg. 130:160, 1949.

The Burn Patient, Management and Operating Room Support. Ethicon, Inc., 1969.

Caring for the critically burned in your hospital. Nurs. Update 3, 2:3-11, Feb. 1972.

Colyer, B. L., Cox, J. J. and Vogel, E. H.: Principles of nursing care in the management of burns. U.S. Armed Forces M. J. 10:1428, 1959.

Crikelair, G. F.: Solution to the burn problem: prevention. *In* J. B. Lynch and S. R. Lewis: Symposium on the Treatment of Burns. St. Louis, C. V. Mosby, 1973, p. 243.

Davidson, Shirley P.: Nursing management of emotional reactions of severely burned patients during the acute phase. Heart Lung 2, 3:370-375, May-June 1973.

Fagerhaugh, Shizuko Y.: Pain expression and control on a burn care unit. Nurs. Outlook 22, 10:645-650, Oct. 1974.

Feller, I. and Archambeault, C.: Nursing the Burned Patient. Ann Arbor, Institute for Burn Med., 1973.

Feller, I., Koepke, G., Richards, K. E. and Withey, L.: Rehabilitation of the burned patient. *In* J. B. Lynch and S. R. Lewis: Symposium on the Treatment of Burns. St. Louis, C. V. Mosby, 1973, p. 241.

Hamburg, D. A., Artz, C. P., Reiss, E., Amspacher, W. H. and Chambers, R. E.: Clinical importance of emotional problems in the care of patients with burns. New Eng. J. Med. 248:355, 1953.

Hartford, C. E.: The early treatment of burns. Nurs. Clin. N. Am. 8:447-455, Sept. 1973.

Haynes, B. W.: Outpatient burns. *In* Symposium on Burns. Clin. Plastic Surg. 1, 4:645, Oct. 1974.

Haynes, B. W., Jr.: Patient isolation systems in burn care. *In* J. B. Lynch and S. R. Lewis: Symposium on the Treatment of Burns. St. Louis, C. V. Mosby, 1973, p. 135.

Jacoby, Florence Greenhouse: Nursing Care of the Patient with Burns. St. Louis: C. V. Mosby, 1972.

Knorr, J. N. and Sheehan, J.: Burn unit; patient team interaction. *In* J. B. Lynch and S. R. Lewis: Symposium on the Treatment of Burns. St. Louis, C. V. Mosby, 1973.

Larson, D. L., Abstan, S., Willis, B., Linares, H., Dobrkovsky, M., Evans, E. B. and Lewis, S. R.: Contracture and scar formation in the burn patient. *In* Symposium on Burns. Clin. Plastic Surg., 1, 4:653, Oct. 1974.

MacMillan, B. G.: Burns in children. *In* Symposium on Burns. Clin. Plastic Surg. 1, 4:633, Oct. 1974.

Margolius, Francine: Burned children, infection and nursing care. Nurs. Clin. N. Am. 5, 1:131-142, Mar. 1970.

Monafo, W. W. and Moyer, C. A.: Effectiveness of dilute aqueous silver nitrate in the treatment of major burns. AMA Arch. Surg. 91:200, 1965.

Moncrief, J. A.: Topical antibacterial therapy of the burn wound. Clin. Plastic Surg. 1:653, Oct. 1974.

Moncrief, J. A., Switzer, W. E. and Teplitz, C.: Curling's ulcer. J. Trauma 4:481, 1964.

Moylan, J. A., et al: Post-burn shock: a critical evaluation of resuscitation. J. Trauma 13:354-358, Apr. 1973.

Muir, J. F. K. and Barclay, T. L.: Burns and Their Treatment. Chicago, Yearbook Publishers, 1974.

Order, S. E. and Moncrief, J. A.: The Burn Wound. Springfield, Illinois, Charles C Thomas, 1965.

Polk, Hiram C., Jr. and Stone, H. Harlan (eds.): Contemporary Burn Management. Boston: Little, Brown, 1971.

Pruitt, B. A.: Complications of burn wound injury. *In* Symposium on Burns. Clin. Plastic Surg. 1, 4:667, Oct. 1974.

Rappaport, F. T., et al: Mechanisms of pulmonary damage in severe burns. Annals Surg. 177:472-477, Apr. 1973.

Reiss, E., Pearson, E. and Artz, C. P.: The metabolic response in burns. J. Clin. Invest. 35:62, 1956.

Soroff, H. S., Pearson, E. and Artz, C. P.: An estimation of the nitrogen requirements for equilibrium in burned patients. Surg. Gyn. Ob. 112:159, 1961.

Soroff, H. S., Pearson, E., Reiss, E. and Artz, C. P.: The relationship between plasma sodium concentration and the state of hydration of burned patients. Surg. Gyn. Ob. 102:472, 1956.

Sutherland, A. B. and Batchelor, A. D. R.: Nitrogen balance in burned children. *In* A. B. Wallace and A. W. Wilkinson (eds.): Research in Burns. Edinburgh, E. & S. Livingstone, Ltd., 1966, p. 147.

Teplitz, C., Epstein, B. S., Rose, L. R. and Moncrief, J. A.: Necrotizing tracheitis induced by tracheostomy tube. AMA Arch. Path. 77:14, 1964.

Wood, M., et al: The use of pigskin in the treatment of thermal burns. Am. J. Surg. 125:720-723, Dec. 1972.

Zaroff, L. I., Mills, W., Jr. Duckett, J. W., Jr., Switzer, W. E. and Moncrief, J. A.: Multiple uses of viable cutaneous homografts in the burned patient. Surg. 59:368, 1966.

Zschoche, Donna A.: The burned patient, a symposium in critical care. Heart and Lung 2, 5:686-719, Sept.-Oct. 1973.

12

The Heart: principles of function, pathophysiology, and goals of cardiac nursing care

WEALTHA COLLINS MCGURN

Principles Relating to the Function of the Heart • Principles of General Nursing Care • Focus on Prevention • Principles of Nursing under Special Conditions: Rheumatic Heart Disease, Arrhythmias, Hypertension, Electrolyte Disturbances, Coronary Artery Disease, Myocardial Infarction, Cardiac Surgery, Cardiogenic Shock

The heart is a common subject of literature whether is is described in physical or metaphysical terms. The ancients supposed it to be the seat of emotions and the essence of life. It is often thought to be the reservoir of the soul. Our language reflects the importance we ascribe to the heart in such familiar phrases as, "Let's get to the heart of the matter," or, "His heart wasn't in it," or, "He died of a broken heart." Semantics aside, we cannot overestimate the importance of normal heart function in relation to health maintenance. The U.S. Public Health Service reports that approximately 1,000,000 deaths a year are attributed to diseases of the cardiovascular system.[1]

During the past few years, several trends have been noted:

1. The number of coronary care units has increased rapidly across the country. Such units have effected a significant reduction in deaths from arrhythmias following myocardial infarctions. Problems which remain include a better system of delivery of health care. Since people must often travel long distances or through heavy, slowly moving traffic to reach a hospital, many arrive dead. The federal subsidized program for the development of the Emergency Medical Technician (EMT) represents an attempt to deliver life-sustaining measures on the scene and, hence, to reduce this cause of mortality.[2]

   Little progress has been made in dealing with "power failure" and acute circulatory collapse which are frequent complications of infarction and which result in very high mortality rates. "Shock" accounts for many of the deaths after myocardial infarction and for a number of deaths from congestive heart failure. We have found little systematic study of the relative merits of home versus hospital care for patients following myocardial infarction, nor have we found any study providing criteria for a selection process.

2. The findings of the Framingham study have diffused into both lay and medical literature and into medical therapy. The American Heart Association provides a pamphlet for the development of a coronary risk profile.[3] Data from the patient's health history is utilized to determine which risk factors are relevant for that patient. This information is then used as a basis for determining the probability of infarction. Low cholesterol and polyunsaturated fat are household words and advertising gimmicks. Unfortunately, the ability of the body to synthesize cholesterol from triglycerides, including the sucrose so prevalent in the American diet, is not so well known. No proof exists as to the efficacy of low-cholesterol diets.

3. Increasing attention has been given to the deleterious effects of stress in "causing" myocardial infarction and hypertension. Attempts to reduce stress range from the sublime to the ridiculous: from ascetic religious practices (which may include yoga in its pure form to personal isolation from the "rat race." Somewhere in between lie alpha wave control, relaxation techniques, and advocation of moderation in life style.

4. Medical research has advanced rapidly, despite federal cutbacks in subsidies. Notable discoveries have been made in pharmacology in terms of developing new agents and contesting the efficacy of several traditional remedies. Similarly, surgical technology has also advanced. Of particular note are coronary artery bypass—still in full bloom despite a gathering cloud of doubt; heart transplantation—on which a virtual moratorium has been declared due to abominably poor results; and mechanical circulatory augmentation—which still appears to hold promise. Surgical correction of congential anamalies, of vessel thrombi or emboli, and of damaged heart valves has proceeded with a steady decline in operative mortality rates.

5. Concern with quality of life, what constitutes death, and the responsibility of health care personnel with respect to each, appears to be nationwide.

These and other concerns will be discussed in this chapter.

Principles Relating to the Function of the Heart

THE RELATIONSHIP OF STRUCTURE AND FUNCTION

Any changes in the normal structure and position of the heart usually compromise the organ to the extent that cardiac output is diminished. While it is assumed that the reader is familiar with the gross anatomy of the heart, several details relevant to cardiac function bear reiteration.

Differences in functional requirements are reflected in structural differences between the right and left ventricles. The pulmonary circulation has a low resistance which requires only a pressure of from 15 to 20 mm of mercury for optimal blood flow. Therefore, the right ventricle can be regarded primarily as a volume pump, returning the deoxygenated blood to the lungs. In contrast, the left ventricle must develop enough energy to eject its contents against a high peripheral vascular resistance. It functions as a pressure pump. The "normal" systolic pressure is 120 mm of mercury, but, under various stressfull stimuli, the heart can generate pressure as high as 300 mm of mercury, due to its thick muscular wall.

Structural integrity of the cardiac valves is essential to cardiac efficiency. Stenotic or incompetent valves increase the workload of the cardiac muscle which may result in dilatation and failure. For example, a stenotic mitral valve retards the flow of blood from the left atrium. It results in dilatation of the atrium, subsequent engorgement of the pulmonary vessels, and respiratory distress.

A stenotic valve may not impair circulatory dynamics enough to produce symptoms at a normal resting cardiac rate. However, when exercise places increased demands on the circulation, the reduced functional reserve will result in markedly impaired cardiac output at the more rapid cardiac rate. When incompetency or insufficiency (incomplete closing) of the mitral valve develops, a fraction of the left ventricular output is ejected back into the left atrium. Consequently, the ventricle must work harder to maintain a normal cardiac output through the aortic valve. Dilatation of the left atrium and hypertrophy, dilatation, then failure of the left ventricle often develop.

The position of the heart in the thoracic cage renders it susceptible to several forces. For example, the bellowslike action of the lungs contributes to atrial filling and blood propulsion in the following manner. Upon inspiration, lung tissue compresses the great veins, retarding the flow of blood. On the other hand, expiration advances the flow of blood and, by increasing the amount of intrathoracic *negative* pressure, it actually helps pull blood upward through the great veins. In addition, the emptying of the right ventricular chamber creates a vacuum. The venous blood rushes in to fill the void. Because of their less muscular construction, the veins are much more influenced by the pumping action of the lungs than are the arteries. Systemically, skeletal muscles perform a similar function by "massaging" the veins, alternately compressing and releasing them. In the latter case, venous valves preclude the backward flow of blood which would otherwise be caused by gravity.

Differences in general body configuration and concomitant differences in the shape of the thoracic cage also affect the heart. The tall, angular individual has a narrower, longer thoracic cavity in which the heart literally hangs down in a more vertical position. This position accounts for a greater degree of rotation of the left ventricle and a difference in the electrical axis. The thin person also tends to present electrocardiographic configurations of greater amplitude because he has less fatty tissue to interfere with the conduction of electrical potentials. In an endormorphic or frankly obese person, impingement of the abdominal viscera on the diaphragm compresses the thoracic space and forces the heart into a more horizontal position which presents a more nearly horizontal electrical axis. Consequently, the configuration of the complexes is quite different. A reduction in the amplitude of heart sounds and graphic recordings also results from obesity.

THE WORK OF THE HEART

In any tissue in the body only part of the energy released by metabolism is delivered as work. The remaining (and often far greater) proportion of energy is dissipated as heat. It is desirable, of course, that the maximum amount of work be produced in relation to the amount of oxygen and nutrients consumed. Rushmer states that only 23 percent of the energy generated in the heart is delivered as work.[4] Work is defined as the energy delivered by systole to the propulsion of blood. *Cardiac output* is the index of cardiovascular efficacy. It is governed by the combination of heart rate and stroke volume. In turn, stroke volume is governed by the degree of ventricular filling and the force of contraction.

Many internal conditions change the requirement for heart work. They include the amount of muscular activity, emotional or physical stress, digestive requirements and internal organ system functioning. In general, the more active the system is, the more work it requires of the heart. The heart itself often creates a need for a substantial increase in heart work, as pointed out above.

Maximal exercise requires an increase in cardiac output of approximately 250 percent. The body modifies the degree to which the heart needs to work under conditions of increased cellular demands by increasing the amount of oxygen extracted by the tissue around the capillary beds. The resting, recumbent subject extracts about 3 volumes percent, while during exercise the extraction may be as high as 16 volumes percent. It is clear then that not all of the difference in body needs is accounted for by the approximately 10 percent increase in stroke volume and the two-and-one-half fold increase in the rate of the heartbeat that are attained by normal individuals during maximal exercise.

External environmental conditions also affect the amount of heart work that must be performed. Variation of the oxygen content in air brings about dramatic fluctuations in heart rate, even in a resting individual. In rarified air, such as that found at high altitudes, the individual must allow time for adjustment of the hemopoietic system before undertaking vigorous exercise. Until the body has compensated, the necessary oxygen delivery is accomplished mainly by an increase in heart rate. Increasing the oxygen level above that usually present in air brings about a decrease in heart rate. (This is the major rationale for the use of oxygen therapy.) When an increased amount of oxygen is delivered under increased pressure (such as in experimental hyperbaric units) the result is an increase in both the oxygen tension and the oxygen saturation of the blood. The increased amount of oxygen then delivered to the tissues creates a condition allowing drastically decreased heart work.

Temperature and humidity both affect the heart. As the temperature rises, more blood is circulated to the skin and lungs in an attempt to dissipate internal heat. Increasing humidity intensifies the work of heat dissipation by decreasing the rate of evaporation of sweat. Lowered external temperature reduces heart work by decreasing the metabolic demands of the cells. This principle is typified in the current use of hypothermia units, although it occurs as a natural phenomenon also.

The position of the body alters the manner in which gravity acts on the circulatory system. The volume of blood in the heart, the cardiac output, and the central venous pressure diminish as a person stands quietly. The effect of gravity is most demonstrable in the veins. The veins derive little benefit from the contraction of the heart. Because of their thinner walls, they react to gravitational force by distending with blood. If the veins distend, their valves become incompetent and cannot prevent the backward flow of blood. A vicious cycle of decompensation may occur, an early symptom of which is pretibial edema. Normally, the pumping action of the muscles corrects the condition. But, should muscular action be impaired, the individual faints as a result of decreased cerebral circulation. When the person is in the horizontal position, venous pressure rises, cardiac output increases, and the cerebrum receives a richer supply of blood.

THE CORONARY CIRCULATION
The heart musculature receives its blood supply from the coronary arteries. These two arteries arise from the sinuses of Valsalva behind the aortic valve cusps. The right and left coronary arteries branch off under the right and left valve leaflets respectively.

The left coronary artery divides into anterior descending and circumflex branches. The musculature supplied by these arteries is variable. Schlesinger studied the distribution of each main branch and found that in nearly 50 percent of his cases the right coronary artery and its tributaries supplied a preponderance of myocardium.[5] About one third of his subjects had balanced circulation; the remainder demonstrated left coronary artery preponderance. Theoretically, having a very large amount of tissue supplied by one arterial trunk may increase the risk of myocardial infarction.

Collateral circulation develops in the normal heart according to its needs for blood. Relative muscle ischemia is the strongest stimulus for new vessel formation. Wiggins proposes that three elements are necessary for the formation of collateral circulation: adequate nutrition, time, and a difference in pressure between two arterial branches.[6] When the need for a richer blood supply increases over time and there is an adequate supply in at least two tributaries adjoining the area, fingerlike projections of vessels grow out and interweave to form a vascular network across the deprived myocardium. When there is no difference in pressure between the tributaries or when myocardial deprivation is sudden (or relatively so), no new network can be formed.

The terminal ends of coronary arteries are buried in myocardium at varying depths. During systole, the contracting musculature squeezes the coronary arterioles and capillaries, hastening flow into the coronary veins. Blood flows into the main trunks of the coronary arteries during diastole. Diastole permits the re-expansion of the circulation. The coronary arteries then fill with the aid of the hydrostatic pressure lent by the heart.

The coronary veins empty into the coronary sinus, which in turn drains into the right atrium. When the heart rate is accelerated beyond normal limits, a dual threat to the heart occurs. Because the period of diastole is shortened, coronary artery filling may be inadequate. Second, the metabolic requirements of the myocardium increase. Myocardial ischemia is the logical result of prolonged tachycardia.

CARDIAC REGULATION

Intrinsic Regulation

Cardiac muscle has characteristics of both skeletal and smooth muscle. Like skeletal muscle, it can generate a forceful contraction at a rapid rate, but it does not fatigue as readily. Like smooth muscle it is innervated by the autonomic nervous system. Unlike either, it has its own intrinsic rhythmicity.

The usual progression of electrical impulses is from the sinoatrial (S-A) node to the atrioventricular (A-V) node to the bundle of His and Purkinje fibers. The S-A node retains its pacemaker function by virtue of the speed with which it generates electrical potential. The A-V node contains specialized tissue that takes a much longer time to generate potential. It has an intrinsic rate of about 40 to 60 beats per minute as opposed to the S-A node's ability to "fire" at 60 to 180 beats per minute. In general, as the focus of myocardial stimulation descends in the heart, the intrinsic speed with which impulses are generated decreases. However, conduction speeds vary (Table 12-1).

The S-A node seems to retain its function as the pacemaker only as long as it remains more irritable (more amenable to the dynamic exchange of sodium and potassium ions and, hence, more able to generate an impulse) than any other site within the heart. When other cells become more irritable and an impulse is conducted from an ectopic focus, the heart may beat prematurely or fibrillation may ensue. Occasionally the ectopic site is within the normal conduction system and, if conduction proceeds in the normal pattern, a compensatory pause may

TABLE 12-1
Cardiac Conduction Rates and Velocities

ANATOMIC SITE	INTRINSIC RATE	VELOCITY MM./SEC.
S-A node	60-110	1000
Atrial tissue		800-1000
A-V node and bundle of His	40-60	200
Purkinje fibers	30-40	4000
Ventricular tissue	30-40	400

From C. H. Best and N. B. Taylor: The Physiological Basis of Medical Practice, ed. 9. Baltimore, Williams & Wilkins, 1974. Reprinted by permission of the author and publishers.

follow the premature beat. Fibrillatory activity results only when impulse conduction is chaotic, causing repolarization of adjacent tissues at differing times. Then there is no unity of action so no effective contraction can take place.

Neurohumoral Influences

The autonomic division of the nervous system provides a means for adaptation of the heart rate. When the need for a greater cardiac output arises, the sympathetic nervous system fibers release norepinephrine to effect an increased heart rate and increased force. The sympathetic fibers descend through the intermediolateral columns of the spinal cord to the level of T_1, T_4, or T_5. They then form the stellate ganglion from which the postganglionic fibers help form the cardiac plexus. Sympathetic fibers also extend from the cervical ganglia 6, 7, and 8. They are named the superior, middle, and inferior cardiac nerves. The cardiac nerves form the other component of the cardiac plexus. Together they supply the S-A node and the myocardial tissue itself with sympathetic innervation.

The vagus nerve (cranial nerve X) also distributes branches to the heart. Efferent fibers of the vagi supply the S-A node and A-V nodes, while afferent fibers transmit impulses primarily from the aortic arch, right heart, and carotid sinus. Afferent fibers of cranial nerve IX (the glosso pharyngeal nerve) also arise from the carotid sinus. The two cranial nerves comprise a cardiac decelerator system. Acetylcholine is the neurohumoral transmitter for the parasympathetic system. It is activated in response to vagal stimulation. Its net effect is to slow the heart rate and permit a reduction of the force of contraction.

The exact means by which the autonomic nervous system and the neurohumoral transmitters affect the heart on the cellular level is still under investigation. Norepinephrine is believed to increase permeability of the cells of the S-A node to sodium. The application of norepinephrine to the cardiac muscle results in a shortened refractory period and faster depolarization. It seems possible that such an effect is related to an increase in the movement of sodium and calcium into the cell. Calcium increases the force of contraction, and sodium is thought to be the major ion determining the degree of irritability. Potassium moves in opposition to sodium and calcium to create membrane potentials.

The combination of a faster rate with a more forceful and complete ejection of blood raises the mean arterial pressure. It is believed that the sympathetic nerves are always in a state of some tonic activity which can be increased by stimulation of an area just under the floor of the left ventricle.

Acetylcholine liberated under the influence of parasympathetic stimulation also alters the ionic flux. It is thought that increased cell membrane permeability brings about depolarization. The higher the concentration of intracellular potassium, the slower the repolarization of the heart because potassium must be made to move out of the cell in order for sodium to move back in and recreate the action potential.

A SYSTEMS APPROACH TO CARDIAC ADAPTATIONS

The diffusion of an adequate amount of oxygen and nutrients into the cells depends on the maintenance of an adequate volume of blood within the vascular compartment. In other words, osmotic and hydrostatic gradients must be high enough between blood and cell to permit the blood to exchange raw materials for waste products. To understand cardiac physiology and pathophysiology, one must understand the meaning of the word "adequate." What is adequate in one situation is not in another (e.g., an adequate amount of oxygen for the resting person would not be adequate for the working person). Whether or not the blood supply is adequate depends partly on its pressure and composition. Pressure depends on the relationship of blood volume to the size of the vascular compartment as well as on the osmolality of the various components. The concept of adequacy must be expanded to include the fact that differences exist among the various body tissues in their need for nutrients. Differences also exist in the degree of adaptability (the reserve factor) of the various tissues.

The most consistent aids to the heart in maintaining adequate blood pressure are the vascular network and the kidneys. The vascular compartment (or portions of it) adapts to changing tissue needs in two ways: 1) dilatation to increase the flow to needy cells, and 2) constriction in some areas to shunt more blood to others. The contraction or expansion usually acts to maintain perfusion to the tissues vital to life.

The kidneys also effect cardiac efficacy by monitoring and adjusting the amount of electrolytes which remain in the body, particularly sodium, hydrogen, and potassium. Current research implies a vital role for the kidneys in the pathophysiology and treatment of congestive heart disease and shock.[7]

There is a series of systems for assessing and regulating blood volume and vessel caliber in relation to body needs (Table 12-2, pp. 298 and 299). These systems will be discussed below.

Mechanisms Altering Cardiac Rate

Stretch receptors in the carotid sinus regularly discharge impulses to the cardioregulatory center by means of the glossopharyngeal nerve and the medulla. As arterial pressure rises, many more impulses are initiated. The vagal system is stimulated and the heart rate decreases. A similar mechanism of action occurs by means of pressure receptors in the aortic arch. When a rise in pressure occurs, afferent fibers of the vagus are stimulated. The resulting impulses travel to the vagal motor nucleus whose efferent nerves cause deceleration of the heart. In both cases, a decrease in peripheral resistance is effected. The process is self-limiting. When the stretch receptors are no longer stimulated by high pressure, the barrage of impulses along the afferent nerves decreases and parasympathetic stimulation is reduced.

The opposite effect is achieved through stimulation of the stretch receptors in the right atrium by increased pressure there. Some researchers state that increased blood pressure in the viscera or in the systemic arteries in general can also activate the stretch receptors within them and bring about an increase in heart rate. The mechanism has not been demonstrated.[8]

TABLE 12-2
Stimuli Affecting Blood Volume, Cardiac Output, and Blood Vessel Caliber

STIMULI	MODE OF ACTION	EFFECTS
Adrenal Cortex	Mineral corticoids secreted under the influence of antidiuretic hormone (ADH) cause retention of sodium (water retention then occurs).	Increased blood volume
Medulla	Epinephrine: mixed dilatation (voluntary muscle) and constriction (skin and splanchnic areas).	Increased heart rate and output
	Increased heart rate and force.	Increased blood flow to dilated beds
	Norepinephrine: vasoconstriction. Cardiac output not increased generally.	Increased blood pressure; little or no increase in cardiac output
Thyroid Hyper-	Thyroxine: increased metabolic rate and increased resistance.	Increased heart rate
Hypo-	Atherosclerotic plaques causing increased peripheral resistance.	Decreased blood vessel caliber
Kidney Juxtaglomerular cells	In response to decreased renal perfusion, they secrete renin-angiotensin-angiotensin II-aldosterone production.	Vasoconstriction and increased vascular volume; sodium reabsorption is increased
Nephrons and collecting ducts	Volume regulation, sodium balance.	Adjustment in blood volumes
Spleen	Contracts under sympathetic stimulation, releasing blood cells.	Increased blood volume
Gastrointestinal	Requires approximately 30 percent more heart work for digestion.	Increased heart rate
Lungs	When decreased ventilation occurs, it is partially compensated by the cardiovascular system rate. Increased hematocrit occurs in chronic conditions.	Increased heart rate Increased blood volume

The area of the carotid sinus (at the bifurcation of the common carotid artery into the internal and external carotid arteries) also includes the carotid body. The carotid body is a specialized mass of tissue richly supplied with blood vessels and nerves. It is highly sensitive to an increase in the partial pressure of carbon dioxide Pco_2, to decreased partial pressure of oxygen (Po_2), and to pH. When a phenomenon such as cardiopulmonary incapacitation or inability to adapt to changing bodily requirements occurs, there is a need for an accelerated cardiac rate. Stimulation of the carotid body brings about the increase.

Mechanisms Affecting Blood Volume and Osmolarity

Hyperosmolality is also monitored by cells in the carotid body. It has been shown that osmoreceptors also exist in the diencephalon.[9] Normally, changes in antidiuretic hormone production (ADH) and the resultant renal conservation of water act to maintain equilibrium of blood volume and osmolarity. However, it serum osmolality rises, there is a need to conserve water. Then ADH is secreted by the cells of the supraoptic nuclei. The collecting duct of the kidney becomes less permeable to water in response.

Extracelluar fluid volume regulation is in part

TABLE 12-2
Stimuli Affecting Blood Volume, Cardiac Output, and Blood Vessel Caliber (Continued)

STIMULI	MODE OF ACTION	EFFECTS
Arterial pressure	Sensors in aortic arch and carotid sinus cause vagal stimulation when walls are distended.	Decreased heart rate
Venous pressure	Sensors in right atrium cause sympathetic response.	Increased heart rate
Environment Heat Cold	Peripheral vasodilatation. Perspiration may cause decreased volume. Peripheral vasoconstriction. Increased heart rate for heat production.	Increased heart rate and increased vessel caliber Increased blood pressure primarily from decreased vessel caliber
Oxygen rarification	Less oxygen concentration in blood until more cells are produced.	Increased heart rate
Stress	Acute sympathetic mobilization. Decreased blood vessel caliber and increased cardiac output.	Increased heart rate, stroke volume, and increased blood pressure
Neurohormonal Cholinergic	Vagal effects	Decreased heart rate and increased blood vessel caliber resulting in reduced cardiac output and lower blood pressure
Sympathetic	Catecholamine effects depend on receptor areas particularly in smooth muscle.	
	1. Alpha adrenergic effects stimulated by epinephrine and norepinephrine.	Vasoconstriction, increased blood pressure and heartbeat but with little or no gain in output
	2. Beta adrenergic effects may result from epinephrine or norepinephrine if alpha receptors are blocked.	Increased force of cardiac contraction and relaxation of nonvascular smooth muscle
	Exclusive beta adrenergic effects are stimulated by isoproterenol.	Vasodilatation and smooth muscle relaxation
Central nervous system	Catecholamine production after perception of threat or at stress.	Same effects as under sympathetic stimulation

maintained by the same factors which control sodium balance. During extracellular fluid expansion, tubular sodium reabsorption is decreased, resulting in a natriuresis (sodium diuresis). This depends not only upon the glomerular filtration rate of the kidney, but also upon a hormone, "Factor III," which specifically inhibits sodium reabsorption in the proximal tubule.

Substances Affecting Blood Vessel Size

The adrenal medulla secretes both epinephrine and norepinephrine in the approximate proportion of 4:1 respectively. The action of these catecholamines formerly confused investigators, since catecholamines seem to act differently depending on where they are produced and with what tissue they react. Now, the presence of two different kinds of receptors in skeletal, smooth, and cardiac muscle has been demonstrated.

Alpha receptors are present in smooth muscle (such as that in the intestine and the walls of its blood vessels). Under the influence of both catecholamines, they cause smooth muscle excitation (contraction). In the case of the blood vessels, constriction occurs. Beta receptors are present in the smooth muscle of the blood vessels of skeletal muscle and myocardium. They

TABLE 12-3

Comparison of the Effects of Various Chemical Substances on the Heart and Blood Vessels

DRUG	HEART					BLOOD VESSELS					
	RATE	FORCE	OUTPUT	ECTOPIC BEATS	MODE OF ACTION	INTES-TINES	KIDNEY	MUSCLE	SKIN	BLOOD PRESSURE	MODE OF ACTION
Norepinephrine	+,—*	++	0,+	+	Direct beta	C	C	C,D	C	Rise	C, direct alpha; D, direct beta
Epinephrine	++,—*	++	++	+	Direct beta	C	C	D,C	C	Fall or rise	C, direct alpha; D, direct beta
Isoproterenol	+++	+++	+++	(+)	Direct beta	D	D	D	D	Fall	D, direct beta
Methoxamine	—*	0	0,—	0	None	C	C	C	C	Rise	D, direct alpha
Tyramine	+,—*	+	0,+	+	Indirect beta	C	C	C,D	C	Rise	C, indirect alpha; D, indirect beta
Dopamine	+,—*	+	+	+	Direct beta	D	D	C	C	Rise or no change	C, direct alpha; D, unknown
Phenoxybenzamine	+	+	+	0	Indirect; reflex, beta	D	D	D	D	Fall	D, alpha adrenergic blockade
Phentolamine	+	+	+	0	Indirect; reflex, beta	D	D	D	D	Fall	D, alpha adrenergic blockade and histamine-like
Propranolol	—	—	—	0	Beta adrenergic blockade	0	0	C?	0	No acute effect	C, beta adrenergic blockade?
Angiotensin II	—*	+?	+?	0	Unknown	C	C	C	C	Rise	Unknown
Aminophylline	+	+	+	0	Unknown	D	D	D	D	Fall	Unknown
Glucocorticoids	0	+?	+?	0	Unknown	D?	D?	D?	D?	?	Unknown

C = constriction; D = dilatation; + = increase; — = decrease; 0 = no change; ? = uncertain; * = reflex bradycardia; ( ) = masked by sinus tachycardia.

From: N. C. Moran: Evaluation of the pharmacologic basis of the therapy of circulatory shock. Am. J. Cardiol., 26:250-258, Dec. 1970.

may respond to epinephrine with vasodilatation, if the alpha receptors should be blocked. Both agents have a role in increasing cardiac output but epinephrine increases both the strength and rate of contraction to a greater degree. Table 12-3 summarizes the effect of several inherent and applied chemical substances on the heart and blood vessels. See Chapter 13 for an elaboration of the interactions of the heart and vessels in response to these substances.

Several other substances affect blood vessel caliber under some conditions. Unfortunately, the means by which they do so and the conditions under which the substances are usually produced are not completely known.

1. Angiotensin II. Its production is related to the release of renin by the kidney when blood pressure in the renal arteries is decreased. It acts as a vasoconstrictor.
2. Serotonin has a vasodilatory effect on peripheral capillaries and the coronary vessels. Normally it is not liberated in sufficient amounts to be physiologically active. However, when massive destruction of platelets and mast cells occurs, it is liberated and it will produce vasodilatation.
3. Histamine produces a localized vasoconstriction surrounded by an area of vasodilatation. Its role under normal conditions has not been completely demonstrated.
4. Vasopressin secreted by the neurohypophysis may produce splanchnic vasoconstriction. The mechanism affecting its release is that of volume receptors in the left atrium which react to decreased blood pressure.
5. Plasma kinins. The plasma kinins, kallidin and bradykinin, have precursors omnipresent in the blood as well as other secretions. Activation of the kinins results in profound vasodilatation, pain, and an inflammatory response.

Throughout this section we have stated principles of cardiac adaptation to physiologic need. In a later section, aberrations in physiology, cardiac compensatory mechanisms, and their consequences will be discussed (see pp. 328 to 330). The most important concept the reader should have attained is that no part of the body is independent of another and that changing conditions within one organ system must necessarily influence others.

Principles of General Nursing Care

ASSESSING THE CARDIAC PATIENT: COMPONENTS AND A MODEL

The condition of the cardiac patient must be assessed in detail; that is, every pertinent aspect of the patient's physical and psychological status must be systematically reviewed (Fig. 12-1). Such an assessment is a prerequisite for effective, meaningful, and efficient nursing care. As the physical or emotional state of the patient changes, so should nursing care.

The following factors determine the usefulness of an assessment of normality versus pathophysiology, and of the manifestations and the interpretation of pathophysiology:

1. Knowledge.
2. Skilled observation and communication of data.
3. Efficiency. A system that minimizes the time spent by the observer and that provides a maximum of accurate, pertinent information.
4. Comprehensiveness. All pertinent sources of information should be reviewed and compiled in a manner that reveals overall patterns and their effect on the damaged part.
5. Usefulness. Data should be frequently recorded and made available to all personnel caring for the patient, in order to provide continuity in the therapeutic regimen, a minimum of disturbances to the patient, and optimal utilization of staff members.

THE PARAMETERS OF ASSESSMENT

Emotional Stress

There are three general sources of emotional stress relevant to all patients: 1) concern for their welfare, 2) the everyday concerns from which they have been suddenly removed, and 3) their environment. Cardiac patients often suffer greater emotional stress than do most other patients. Their being is often at stake. Their hospitalization is usually relatively long; often their way of life must change during and after hospitalization. They are frequently admitted not only to a hospital (fear provoking in itself to many) but also to a specialized unit where they are confronted with a variety of frightening equipment and other very ill people.

There are two general principles for alleviating emotional stress in any patient: 1) find out

Emotional status:

Calm_____ Restless_____ Agitated_____ Depressed_____

Defensive behavior? Describe

Orientation: Self_____ Interest in surroundings_____

Withdrawn_____ Influenced by sensory stimuli_____

Pain:

Description   Duration

Location   Intensity

Cardiac status: *How relieved*

*ECG: Usual pattern

Arrhythmias, describe

Vital signs: Changes of pattern

Heart sound: Describe abnormalities

B/P: Patient's norm_____   *CVP: Patient's norm_____

Reading_____   Reading_____

Changes_____   Changes_____

Pulses: radial   apical   neck vein

Respiratory status:

Rate_____ Quality_____ Therapy_____ Problems_____

Skin color and turgor_____ Lung sounds_____

Fluid balance:

In   Route(s)   Out   Route(s)

Cerebral perfusion:

Pupil reflexes

Mental alertness

GI status:

Diet_____ How taken_____ How tolerated_____

Sensory perception:

Sight   Hearing   Smell   Temperature

Sleep/activity:

Resting hours

Recreation

Patient educational status:

Level of learning

Plans for next experience

Complications or problems:

Iatrogenic potentials:

General information:

FIGURE 12-1.

Areas for assessment of the cardiac patient. An assessment guide such as this could be completed in a minimum of time by coordinated staff efforts and be a reference point for reporting changes at the end of a shift. "Repeat time can then be utilized for discussion of problems and methods of nursing intervention."

*Parameters which may or may not be monitored. Nurses should assess all others with or without directions to do so.

what the stressor is, and 2) find a way to deal with it. The first principle requires that an informed and skilled person interview the patient in a manner that conveys calm and concern. It is not enough to encourage ventilation of feelings; those feelings must be dealt with. In addition, the nurse must develop sensitivity as to when the patient should stop. Some patients say more than they intend and then withdraw or exercise some other form of defense. They often have to protect themselves from dealing with the threat imposed by their surroundings, of which the nurse may be one part.

"Finding a way to deal with the stressor" means that the nurse may, and often should, look beyond the immediate health care team to help the patient deal with his problems. This can mean something as simple as calling a clergyman or as unusual as providing for tutoring. In any case, there is a protocol to be observed and the intelligent nurse practitioner considers it his or her role to observe the protocol and to deal with any facet of the patient's existence which requires attention or intervention.

The nurse performs an ego-supportive function. Ego support may include the support of primary defenses until the patient can muster his coping abilities. Wholesale intervention with denial is unwise. Ego support also includes presenting reality in "tolerable" doses. In general, the nurse is the person best equipped to assess the patient's problems and facilitate adjustment to his environment and illness. Whether or not the nurse can accomplish these things depends on the problems presented by the patient. Often the nursing role requires bringing problems to the attention of someone better equipped than the nurse to deal with them.

Fear plays a major role in cardiac illness. The illness itself generates fear and fear constitutes a stressor to the patient. In a study of patients hospitalized for cardiac surgery, Janis devised criteria for the assessment of fear levels.[10] Patients after surgery were found to react with relatively high predictability on the basis of their preoperative fear levels. Janis's categories are paraphrased here as an important dimension of the assessment of cardiac patients:

Low Anticipatory Fear. Patients display practically no signs of fear or emotional disturbance. No sleeping disturbances are present. Little or no effort is made to seek information. These patients make use of denial and isolation mechanisms most frequently. They often develop strongly negative attitudes during the stressful recovery period, which can persist long after convalescence.

Moderate Anticipatory Fear. Patients may display symptoms of emotional tension. Usually they are relatively calm and well controlled with only infrequent signs of inner agitation. At night they may suffer from insomnia, but will respond to mild sedation. They usually ask for and pay attention to information. They utilize the information to reassure themselves, but they include objective data regarding real dangers and deprivations. They can utilize information regarding: 1) realistic dangers, 2) how the dangers can be surmounted, and 3) the mitigating or protective features of the environment.

High Anticipatory Fear. Patients display overt symptoms of sustained emotional tension with occasional spells of trembling, flushing, and/or agitated weeping. They are usually markedly restless and may have difficulty concentrating. At night they may require heavy sedation to sleep. They may maintain a relatively high level of fear during convalescence and lack confidence about fully recovering. They will probably make strong efforts to be in frequent contact with members of the staff and to obtain attention. They try to be cooperative. They attempt to distract themselves, to think about personal gains, or to adopt a fatalistic attitude. They need reassurance in order to reduce their fear level and help to develop defenses. Corrective communications may be of help. Attempts should be made to reduce fear-provoking stimuli.[11]

Although Janis's study utilized surgical patients, his modalities and commonsense comments about effective intervention with patients categorized in each one could be generalized to relate to many patients. The implications for teaching are clear with regard to diagnostic tests, the illness experience, and adjustment after hospitalization. It has been estimated that fear, apprehension, and excitement increase the cardiac output by 50 to 100 percent.[12]

Pain

Pain is a physical and emotional stressor. It cannot be reiterated too frequently that pain is a complex phenomenon which has both physical and emotional components. The nurse who deals with only one component may have left more than half the job undone.

Assessing pain in order to intervene is frequently a nursing problem. Patients may present chest pain which has arisen from the lungs, pericardium, digestive system, or the heart in a manner that suggests myocardial damage. There are many excellent guides on this subject which can be consulted.[13]

Perceptual Disturbances

Perceptual disturbances often occur in cardiac patients. They are subject to several circumstances which may promote sensory distortions or misperceptions: 1) They are frequently on bedrest. Their view of the world is different because of their position in space. 2) They are under stress. 3) They may be subject to sensory deprivation resulting from the lack of usual orienting stimuli such as diurnal variations, clocks, or calendars (to say nothing of familiar people). 4) They may be subject to sensory bombardment from machinery and traffic, as well as from visual, auditory, or tactile stimuli.

If mild sensory disturbances are manifest, the nurse may be able to prevent gross distortion by simple methods of orientation and explanation of the phenomena. If patients manifest poor reality orientation and/or hallucinations, they may require medical intervention. The nurse may augment the work of the physician by spending extra time with these patients and by presenting "normalizing" information.

Cardiac Status

A recent study found that severe trauma, particularly that which resulted in unconsciousness, resulted in definitive psychological aberrations. Although the study was done with patients who experienced accidental truama, it is likely that those undergoing therapuetic trauma may behave similarly.[14]

ELECTROCARDIOGRAPHY. Electronic monitoring of the electrical activity of the heart has been practiced for several decades. Every cardiac patient will have an electrocardiogram (ECG). Oscilloscopes presenting serial recordings are now standard equipment in most hospitals. The monitors visually display the electrical activity of the heart on an oscilloscope and most monitors have additional sound devices. More sophisticated monitors sound an alarm when the heart rate goes above or below predetermined levels, initiate a permanent recording ("write-out" of the ECG), trigger memory loops which record events preceding the alarm, record the number of abnormal beats during a given period of time, and even activate pacemaking apparatus under appropriate circumstances.

It was not electronic equipment, but human knowledge that led to the widespread use of constant monitoring of the ECG: the knowledge that 1) arrhythmias were a common cause of death, 2) certain apparently inconsequential arrhythmias indicated a predilection to more ominous and life-threatening arrhythmias, and 3) one can successfully interrupt the progression of events toward death. Treatment based upon information processed and recorded by electronic instruments (in some respects more sensitive than the human ear and eye), has significantly reduced cardiac mortalities.

When the critically ill cardiac patient is monitored electronically, the nurse trained in cardiac techniques is responsible for screening the constant flow of ECG information. The nurse must understand the information appearing on the oscilloscope. *Minimal requirements are that any nurse be able to distinguish major arrhythmias from normal variants and proceed according to the policies of the institution.* At that point another person may be called to administer treatment, or the nurse may do it according to hospital policy and her proficiency.

The following definitions are related to the electrical activity of the heart:

Action potential. Loss of the electrical gradient across the cell membrane accompanied by ionic shifts, resulting in conduction and causing contraction of the muscle.

Resting potential. The electrical gradient across the cell membrane, negatively charged on the inside and positively charged on the outside, resulting from repolarization and maintained during the period of electrical diastole.

Polarization. The period of electrical diastole between repolarization and depolarization and accounting for the resting potential.

Depolarization. Reversal of the electrical gradient across the cell membrane accompanied by an increased permeability to sodium and resulting in conduction of the impulse.

Repolarization. The buildup of the electrical gradient across the cell membrane accompanied by sodium and calcium moving into the cell and potassium moving out.

Vector. A force symbolized by an arrow representing intensity by its length, sense by its orientation and direction by the head of the arrow.[15]

The flow of current accompanied by ionic shifts during depolarization and repolarization of the heart is monitored on the body surface; then it is transduced, amplified, and visually displayed on the oscilloscope or recorded on the ECG paper. There are 12 standard ways to place the recording electrodes (leads) on the body. They monitor the electrical phenomena in different areas and highlight different aspects of the electrical phenomena. The placement of the electrodes in relation to the heart determines the pattern which is recorded. The recorded pattern should always be compared to a previous recording because there is a wide range of normal variation. The normal ECG pattern and its major aberrations should be learned by every nurse.

Depolarization and *repolarization* result in a flow of electrical current, the intensity, source, and direction of which correspond to the cardiac *vector*. Lead II displays the vector which most nearly corresponds to the mean electrical axis of the heart—the hypothetical line representing the greatest magnitude of electrical activity because it represents the largest mass of cardiac muscle. This line passes diagonally from the right atrium across and through the left ventricle. The apex of the heart is considered positive in relation to the

base of the heart because impulses proceed from top to bottom. Externally, this phenomenon is recorded as the positive deflection in Lead II.

To monitor Lead II, the electrodes are placed on the right arm or under the right clavicle and on the left leg or over the eighth or ninth left interspace slightly lateral to the nipple line. The right arm electrode is negative and the left leg is positive. Impulses flow from negative to positive so the flow of current is represented as a positive (or upward) deflection on either the oscilloscope or ECG (See Figs. 12-2 to 12-4).

When they are made by a skilled technician, ECG recordings of the electrical patterns are more accurate and have the advantage of permanency. The ECG recording paper is divided into squares measuring 1 mm by 1 mm. The paper usually runs at a speed of 25 mm per second so the 0.04 second elapses between one vertical line and the next. To facilitate reading, every fifth line is heavier (darker), and the interval between two such heavy vertical lines is 0.2 second. The horizontal lines of the ECG quantify the amplitude (voltage) of the cardiac activity. The recorded amplitude, in camparison to the voltage generated by the heart, may be modified by increased air space in the chest (such as em-

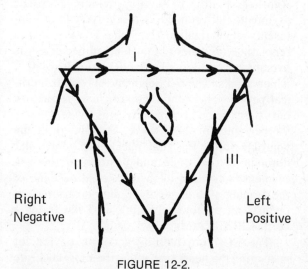

FIGURE 12-2.
Einthoven's triangle. The vectors in the three bipolar leads and the electrical axis of the heart are schematically presented.

physema), a fatty chest wall, or the presence of pericardial fluid. If none of these conditions exists, the amplitude should correspond to the voltage generated by the heart after standardization. The recording or oscilloscopic monitor is usually standardized in such a way that 1 cm between horizontal lines (ten light lines or two heavy lines in the vertical plane) represents one millivolt (mv).

In the normal electrocardiographic sequence the atria depolarize almost synchronously in a wavelike manner, spreading from the S-A node, to produce a shallow, rounded, and nearly symmetrical positive (upward) deflection. The Q wave marks the beginning of ventricular depolarization and the R wave the peak of ventricular activity. The amplitude of the R wave is usually from 2 to 20 mm. The interval from the beginning of the P wave to the point of the R wave corresponds to the conduction time from the atria to the Purkinje fibers of the ventricle. The normal value is 0.12 to 0.2 second. The interval from the beginning of the Q wave to the end of the S wave corresponds to the time of ventricular depolarization; it should occur within 0.12 second. The completion of the S wave represents the end of ventricualr depolarization and the onset of the refractory period of the heart. Another shallow deflection, which is broad, asymmetrical, rounded, and relatively long, represents repolarization. It is the T wave. Atrial repolarization cannot be visualized because it is overshadowed by the large QRS complex within which it falls. The S-T segment represents a critical period. The ventricles are, first, refractory but, then, begin to repolarize, as evidenced by the beginning of the T wave. Stimulation of the ventricle during this time may cause ventricular fibrillation. The slope and position of the S-T segment in relation to the electrical baseline of the tracing is indicative of many varieties of myocardial pathology. Figure 12-3 illustrates a normal ECG pattern.

The ECG provides an accurate device for measuring the heart rate and is the most accurate available measure of the regularity of ventricular contractions. Since the paper runs through the machine at a speed of 25 mm per second, one can

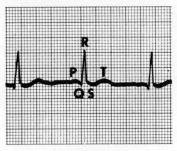

FIGURE 12-3.
A normal ECG tracing.

assess the heart rate simply by counting the number of R waves that occurred in one minute. However, the usual practice is to count the number of R waves in 3 seconds and then to multiply by 20 to obtain the rate of ventricular contractions each minute. This procedure lends an accurate assessment only as long as the beat is regular. Unless it is, the "shorthand" technique may obscure important data. For convenience, the paper usually has dots or slashes every 75 mm which represents a time interval of 3 seconds.

If the tracing demonstrates a normally functioning heart, the rate will be between 60 and 120 beats per minute, the amplitude will be between 5 and 20 mv, and the rhythm will be regular. A regular rhythm exists when the space between R deflections is identical. The measurement should be made with calipers. If a variation of more than 0.04 seconds—one space—is observed, the ventricular contractions are not considered regular. Data which the tracing reveals regarding the presence of arrhythmias, and their origin and nature, constitute the importance of ECG monitoring to patient care. The tracing should be systematically reviewed on several points.

The dominant rhythm. In the normal heart, a P wave precedes each QRS-T complex. The P wave should be rounded in contour and deflected in the same direction as the QRS complex. No more than 0.2 seconds (five spaces) should elapse between the P and the R waves. If the preceding qualifications are met, the heart is said to be in normal sinus rhythm, whatever its rate may be. The outer limits of the normal rate are defined by bradycardia or tachycardia. Rhythms other than normal sinus rhythm are usually described in terms of the point of origin of the impulse. They will be described below.

Figure 12-4 will help the reader to coordinate the physiological events of cardiac action with the electrographic and auscultatory findings.

One can see that high heart rates and arrhythmias reduce the time of diastole, which necessarily compromises both the filling and the repolarization of the heart muscle. Not only is there increased heart work, but there is less efficiency. Sustained high demands on the heart jeopardize the myocardial perfusion as a result of a shortened diastolic period for coronary artery filling. If the cardiac output drops, the heart rate increases and a vicious cycle of decreasing cardiac efficacy is set in motion. The underperfused heart is vulnerable to life-threatening arrhythmias and ischemic damage.

Occasionally, even in the normal heart, slight irregularities occur. When the P-QRS-T sequence is preserved, but one or more beats occur before the normal interval, the phenomenon is called a premature atrial contraction (PAC). (Fig. 12-5.)

Fortunately, the heart has built-in protection against the usurpation of the SA node as the pacemaker and the occurrence of too rapid rates.

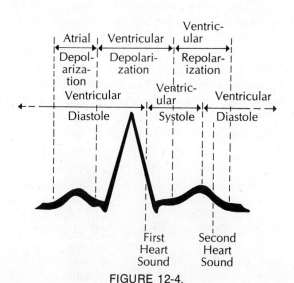

FIGURE 12-4.
Schematic representation of the electrical and mechanical events of the cardiac cycle.

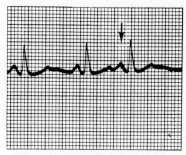

FIGURE 12-5.
Premature atrial contraction.

By virtue of the physiological limits of impulse conduction in the various components of its innervation system ectopic impulse propagation is quite unlikely. The speed at which the A-V node can conduct an impulse is far less than any atrial site. (Table 12-1 on p. 296 shows the potential impulse velocities of various components of the cardiac nerve tissue.) Because of the barrier to impulse bombardment of the ventricles that is formed by the AV node, the atria may beat very rapidly or even fibrillate without causing a hemodynamic state that is incompatible with life. Atrial flutter and atrial fibrillation may occur coincidentally with a ventricular rate within normal limits.

In *atrial flutter,* the rate of atrial contraction is so rapid that the atria seem to be in constant motion rather than, "contracting-resting-contracting." Usually, not all of the impulses can be conducted to the ventricles due to the A-V node. If the ventricular rhythm is regular and the atrioventricular blocking action is predictable, the ratio of atrial to ventricular beats is described. For instance, a patient may be described as having atrial flutter with 2:1 block. Some patients demonstrate a ratio of 4:1. The ventricles sometimes fail to respond to atrial impulses and contract in a totally unpredictable manner. The resulting condition is *atrioventricular disassociation.*

Atrial fibrillation is utterly chaotic atrial activity. Although several theories have been advanced to explain exactly what occurs and why, none has been proven. Both atrial flutter and atrial fibrillation predispose the patient to intramural thrombus formation because they allow a relative stasis of blood in some portions of the atria. In addition, while either condition persists, there is an increased risk of deleteriously affecting the ventricles. Cardiac output is at least minimally compromised when atrial flutter or fibrillation exists. For these reasons, an attempt is usually made to convert the heart to a normal sinus rhythm by means of medications or electrocardioversion. Figure 12-6 shows atrial flutter with two degrees of block and atrial fibrillation. (Treatment of atrial fibrillation will be discussed in a later section.

Ectopic focus. If the P wave is bizarre in shape or position or not discernable at all, the impulse was not generated by the S-A node and an ectopic focus is said to be present. The dominant rhythm is then usually named in terms of the area of the heart in which the impulse appears to be generated. It may be called atrial, A-V (upper, middle or lower) nodal, supraventricular, or ventricular rhythm.

Atrial and A-V nodal rhythms. As long as the pacemaker is in the atria, some form of P wave will be present. It may, however, be abnormal in shape or position or the P-R duration may be prolonged. The configuration depends on the site of the ectopic focus, which in turn governs the direction(s) in which the impulse will travel. If the ectopic focus is in the A-V node, the impulse will be conducted upward into the atrial *and* down through the ventricles. Under such circumstances, the P wave will be inverted (deflected in a direction opposite the normal for that lead). If the focus is in the lower portion of the A-V node, a P wave will not be discernible because the venticular depolarization will obscure it. Figure 12-7 demonstrates an A-V nodal rhythm.

As a rule of thumb, we will state that the lower in the heart an ectopic focus is, the more dangerous it is to the patient. When the impulse is low in the A-V node or below it, the QRS complex must be examined to determine the dominant rhythm and to assess the patient's condition.

Supraventricular and ventricular rhythms. If atrial impulses fail to reach the ventricles, if they are of insufficient magnitude to trigger systematic ventricular conduction and contraction, or if the ventricles are irritable and generating competing impulses, the ventricles may be said to behave as their own pacemaker. Since they do so in an erratic fashion—often too fast, too slow, or irregularly—the condition is extremely dangerous for the patient. If the rate is too slow *or* too rapid, cardiac output is impaired. If the ventri-

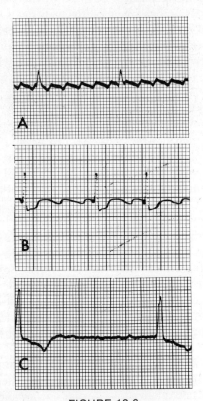

FIGURE 12-6.
Electrical cardiographic tracings. (A) Atrial flutter.
(B) Varying 2:1 block. (C) Atrial fibrillation.

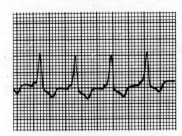

FIGURE 12-7.
A-V nodal rhythm.

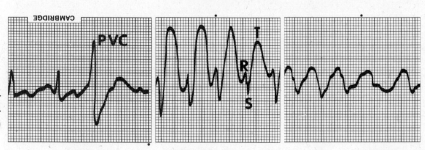

FIGURE 12-8.
(Left) Premature ventricular contraction. (Center) Ventricular tachycardia. (Right) Ventricular fibrillation.

cles become irritable, premature ventricular contractions (PVCs) usually occur. Runs of ventricular tachycardia are also a signal of decreasing cardiac control. Either condition may progress, aided by the poor cardiac perfusion that inevitably accompanies each, to ventricular fibrillation or ventricular standstill. Neither of these conditions is compatible with life. Should increasing ventricular irritability be recognized by the appearance of frequent PVCs (more than six per minute), runs of PVCs, or ventricular tachycardia, prompt intervention is necessary. Some patients show a sequential worsening of their condition (Fig. 12-8); but, it must be reiterated that more than six PVCs per minute or runs of either PVCs or ventricular tachycardia warrant immediate medical attention.

The nurse must be able to differentiate between premature atrial contractions (PACs) which do not usually warrant more than a note, and PVCs, which may require "emergency" intervention. Premature atrial contractions have the following characteristics:

1. The usual P-QRS-T sequence is preserved (The P wave may *not* be discernible in some patients due to tachycardia), but it may be difficult to distinguish the P waves from the preceding T wave.
2. Interpolation occurs. The PAC is truly an extra beat which is evident between two regular beats.
3. Compensatory pausing is rare; if it does occur, it is usually only partial.

Occasionally, a PAC is not conducted to the ventricles.

In general, PVC have four identifying features:

1. They are not preceded by a P wave.
2. The configuration and duration of the QRS complex is abnormal.

3. The QRS complex is deflected in the direction opposite to that which is normal for the patient.
4. A full compensatory pause follows the premature beat. That is, the interval after the premature beat includes the time to the next regular beat *plus* the normal R-R interval.

All of the above identifying features may not be present, but practice enables the observer to differentiate PVCs with a high degree of reliability. In this case, "When in doubt . . . do check with someone else!"

If PVCs occur in succession or at a frequency of more than six per minute, myocardial depressants are usually ordered. Table 12-4 summarizes the myocardial depressants in common use as well as antiarrhythmic agents which act in other ways.

If the depressants are ineffective or if the patient proceeds to ventricular fibrillation, electrocardioversion may be used. To become proficient with the technique, the nurse must observe several principles and must practice under supervision the following:

1. The patient needs oxygen as well as an effective cardiac output. Whether or not an electrocardioverter is immediately available, resuscitation procedures should be begun immediately with mouth-to-mouth or bag breathing and a sharp blow should be administered to the precordium followed by external cardiac massage.
2. Acidosis develops quickly and must be corrected. Until potassium is driven back into the cells, the heart rarely resumes or maintains normal rhythm. Usually, the physician injects a buffering agent by the intravenous route. However, in some locales, the nurse does this.
3. Most electrocardioverters can be synchronized to avoid the "vulnerable" period, that is, the

TABLE 12-4
Antiarrhythmic Agents

AGENT	USES	DOSAGE	REMARKS
Digitalis preparations	1. Congestive heart failure to increase force of contraction. 2. Atrial tachycardias to reduce A-V nodal conduction and prolong the refractory period.	Depends on the form.	Toxic doses increase ectopic impulse formation. Theorized as a cause of atrial conduction decrease. Effects increase in the presence of potassium.
Quinidine	1. Atrial arrhythmias and abnormal conduction circuits. a. slowed depolarization b. decreased conduction velocity c. lengthened refractory period 2. Atrial arrhythmia with fast ventricular response conjunctively with digitalis or when ventricular ectopic focus is present.	May give large first dose. Maintenance dose is 0.8-1.6 Gms daily po. Rarely used IV.	May cause increased ventricular rate if irritable foci are present. May cause asystole by depressing S-A node. People may acquire sensitivity with allergic reactions. May cause profound hypotension.
Quinaglute (quinidine gluconate)	Sustained action form of quinidine.	Tab. 1, 2-4 x daily	
Pronestyl (procainamide)		0.25-0.5 Gm, 4 x daily.	The same toxic effects as quinidine. Positive LE preps may result after prolonged usage.
Xylocaine (lidocaine)	Local anesthetic used IV for the treatment of ventricular arrhythmias, tachycardia, or frequent PVCs.	50-100 mg bolus then 1-3 mg/min IV drip.	Toxic doses may cause massive CNS stimulation. It is still under investigation. It should not be given without monitoring.
Sodium bicarbonate	Correction of acidemia.	pt. wt. x time since arrest in min. = dose in mEq.	

time after the refractory depolarized state and before complete repolarization has occurred. An electrical shock administered during the vulnerable period often causes ventricular fibrillation, since some fibers are repolarized while others are not.

4. Patients who are in ventricular fibrillation or in cardiac standstill have no vulnerable period. If the synchronizer is activated and no QRS complex is recorded, *the apparatus will not deliver an electrical impulse*.

5. Ground the machine and stand away from the patient and from any conductive material with which he is in contact.

6. The responsibilities of various categories of personnel during resuscitation varies from place to place. The nurse must take the responsibility for knowing the policies of her agency in performing her role.

It is obvious that there is a great deal more to ECG interpretation than has been reviewed here. We have covered only the most pertinent points which would allow the nurse to give responsible care, regardless of the agency in which she is working. The nurse who typically deals with patients who are prone to arrhythmias should have a thorough course of training. For the general practitioner, several self-instruction manuals are available. (See bibliography at the end of this chapter.)

THE HEART SOUNDS. Though less dramatic than electronic monitoring techniques, auscultation of the chest has been a medical diagnostic tool for centuries. More recently, nurses in specialized units have been learning the principles involved in order to give better nursing care. The criterion for evaluating the efficiency of coughing and suctioning is the absence or reduction of rales and rhonchi. These are usually best heard by listening at the bases of the lungs. Practice in listening to the chest of a patient with diagnosed rales will help the nurse learn to distinguish rales and rhonchi.

Standard procedure before giving digitalis products is to check the apical heart rate. The apical rate is much more accurate than the radial or other peripheral pulses when a patient is in shock or is severely arteriosclerotic. The nurse who is working with the cardiac patient, especially one critically ill, must learn to recognize the normal heart sounds and to detect and describe murmurs. This is particularly important in the care of fresh myocardial infarction and postoperative cardiac patients. How much the nurse improves in this skill may be a function of individual interest and job capacity, but the rudiments are necessary to all. A brief description of the procedure is given below.

First locate the cardiac valves from external landmarks. Then listen over each of the pertinent areas of the chest to detect unusual sounds. The normal sound and duration of the heart sounds are shown in Figure 12-9.

The first heart sound is caused by closure of the mitral and tricuspid valves. It is longer and louder than the second normal sound and can be heard best 1 or 2 inches from the left of the sternum at about the fourth or fifth interspace. The second sound is better heard at the base of the heart, since it is caused by closure of the semilunar valves. A fourth sound, just after the second, may be heard. It is called a ventricular gallop. Greatly distended hearts produce an atrial gallop rhythm which includes a third sound, occurring just before the first.

Having learned the normal and the commonly heard abnormal heart sounds, listen for murmurs. They are usually caused by increased turbulence of blood in the heart. To carry out nursing functions most effectively, answer the following questions regarding the heart sounds.

1. Is the rhythm regular?
2. Is the amplitude or cadence normal?
3. Are there abnormal sounds?
4. Where is the unusual sound heard best?
5. When in the cycle do unusual sounds occur?
6. Do these data represent a change for this patient?

THE PULSE. Many cardiac malfunctions can be detected by "taking" the pulse. In addition to counting the number of pulsations, the skilled nurse notes the quality of pulsations. An interesting phenomenon occurs in relation to the pulse during the respiratory cycle. During inspiration, the increased degree of negative pressure in the thorax allows an unusual amount of blood flow into the lungs; thus the amount flowing into the left ventricle is decreased. The situation reverses itself with expiration. It is essentially normal.

In conditions such as cardiac tamponade, this normal occurrence is grossly exaggerated. The radial pulse is alternately full and thready, in harmony with the respiratory cycle. This condition is called paradoxical pulse or *pulse paradoxicus*. Patients are often conscious of the rebound of pulse during expiration. It may occur in any condition causing a depressed myocardium and is a common feature of bigeminal rhythm. Bigeminy is characterized by a normal beat followed by a PVC. The phenomenon is also called *coupling*. Digitalis intoxication or an incomplete block of the Purkinje fibers often provokes bigeminy.

Counting apical beats and comparing the

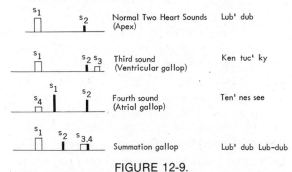

FIGURE 12-9.
Heart sounds. Source: Adapted from Andreoli, K.: Comprehensive Cardiac Care. St. Louis, C. V. Mosby, 1968. Used with permission of the author and through the courtesy of C. V. Mosby, publisher.

figure with that of the radial pulse may demonstrate a pulse deficit. Any time the ventricles do not fill adequately, a radial pulsation will not follow. If the bigeminal rhythm occurs in a weakened heart, the premature beat may take place but be so weak that a pulse is not conducted at all.

The peripheral pulses are an important index of cardiac efficacy and peripheral vessel patency. Nurses should routinely palpate for peripheral pulses on admission assessment. A change in the occurrence or character of a peripheral pulse lends useful information.

BLOOD PRESSURE. A sharp drop in blood pressure usually captures attention, but an insidious decrease, such as that occurring with internal hemorrhage, may not be observed. There are several "rules" which should be remembered:

1. A "normal" reading must be established for each patient.
2. The patient's state of activity (and mind) should be taken into account before recording an unusual reading.
3. Whether or not Korotkoff's sign is considered to be the point at which to ascertain the diastolic reading, all personnel should be consistent in the method used.
4. Diastolic reading is less influenced by other factors than the systolic and is more indicative of the degree of equilibrium between the blood supply and the arterial compartment.
5. Pulse pressure tends to decrease in mitral and aortic stenosis and to widen with aortic regurgitation. A widening pulse pressure in a patient with valvular replacement may indicate torn sutures or beginning thrombus formation.
6. The time intervals between blood pressure measurements ordered by the physician represents a *maximum* interval!

VENOUS DISTENTION. Distention of the neck veins is a simply observed index of venous distention. Neck veins should be flat when the torso is at more than a 30° to 45° angle in relation to the lower body. When distended neck veins occur in conjunction with falling blood pressure, cardiac decompensation and shock may be imminent.

CENTRAL VENOUS PRESSURE (CVP). The pressure in the right atrium reflects the dynamic equilibrium between gravity and cardiac output, as well as between vessel caliber and blood volume. A catheter threaded into the right atrium is attached at its other end to a three-way stopcock on the end of a water manometer. Intravenous solution is also attached to the stopcock. When the stopcock is at the level of the right atrium and opened, the height of the fluid in the manometer will equilibrate at a figure representing the CVP. The accuracy of measurement depends on unobstructed lines and the correct placement of the manometer in relation to the patient. The IV fluid is allowed to fill the manometer to a level above the patient's usual reading. The stopcock is then turned to allow fluid from the manometer to equilibrate. Filling the manometer above the level necessary is to be discouraged. Most patients are usually on fluid restrictions, and frequent readings contribute an unnecessary and often large increase in fluid and sodium intake.

Although IV therapy, CVP lines, and even arterial catheters are now common, they are far from innocuous. The nurse should be aware that they constitute a portal of entry of pathogens and frequently cause local inflammatory responses. Also, a patient may hemorrhage from the site—a problem most acute with arterial catheters. Puncture of the vessel with local extravasation is painful if the catheter is in an extremity. It may be lethal if this happens with a central venous catheter.

Another major nursing consideration is that of keeping the catheter clear. Some institutions use heparinized solution for the venous pressure apparatus, others instill heparin before each reading. An obstructed line usually has a thrombus at the end of it; forcing fluid through the line is a risky procedure.

The venous pressure must be evaluated in the light of 1) the arterial blood pressure; 2) the hematocrit; 3) myocardial activity; and 4) fluid intake and output. As with arterial pressures, venous pressure readings must be standardized for each individual and each reading should be assessed in the context of its predecessors.

URINE OUTPUT. Since most patients needing close urinary output monitoring have indwelling catheters, the nurse must first consider the jeopardy to the kidneys if the system is not kept sterile. Second, the nurse must determine whether urine is to be drained from the catheter at each reading. The osmotic diuretics are routinely used in many institutions. If the patient has suffered renal shutdown, these diuretics will not be excreted but will remain in the bloodstream. They pull fluid into the vascular compartment and may add to the burden of an already damaged heart under these circumstances. The patient with myocardial pathology must be closely watched. If the administration of a diuretic does not produce diuresis, another dose should not be given until the patient is reevaluated.

TEMPERATURE. Patients who are severely ill often suffer variations in temperature. The temperature usually rises in response to stress and may then fall. Patients who have been cooled during cardiac surgery are particularly prone to temperature increases. At first the rise occurs as a rebound phenomenon, while the body's thermostatic mechanism becomes reset. Any increase in temperature above the patient's norm represents increased work for the heart. For the severely ill cardiac patient, antipyretics and/or methods of reducing the temperature by external cooling are applied, in addition to treating the cause of the increase. In assessing the latter, especially after one or two days of illness, the nurse must check on the condition of the lungs and on "cutdown" sites. Urinary drainage apparatus also provides a portal of entry for infectious agents, although signs do not usually develop as quickly.

Patients subjected to hypothermic treatments are usually uncomfortable. Simple measures, such as frequent repositioning, oiling body prominences, replacing sheets with bath blankets, and reducing the amount of cooling at least one or two degrees before the desirable level to compensate for "drift," help the patient to tolerate the procedure. Shivering can double or triple the body's heat production. Sedatives such as pro-

methazine (Phenergan) are effective in blocking the sympathetic response of the hypothalamic center.

Iatrogenic Hazards

The cardiac patient is particularly vulnerable to three types of iatrogenic hazards: 1) prolonged hospitalization, usually under life-threatening circumstances, 2) long periods of at least relative inactivity and 3) drug and drug and diet interactions. With respect to the first, the hospital is an alien, stress-producing environment replete with unpleasant sights, sounds, and smells, as well as lethal microorganisms and people who through human error may administer the wrong or inadequate treatment. Some of our usual measures to aid the cardiac patient include rest, special diets, and oxygen—none of which is without accompanying hazard. Hospital personnel have at their disposal lethal poisons which they casually call "meds." With estimates of iatrogenic drug effects requiring hospitalization now ranging beyond 15 percent of those hospitalized, nurses must do their share of primary prevention. While we cannot discuss the interactions between drugs commonly prescribed for the patient with cardiac problems with the detail it deserves here, we refer the reader to an excellent article by Jan Koch-Weger for the most complete and lucid presentation we have seen.[16]

NURSING MEASURES TO PROMOTE THE HEALING OF THE HEART

REST. In the case of the patient with cardiac decompensation or acute myocardial infarction, there is always a physician's order for rest. However, a glance at the hustle and bustle around the bed of the postsurgical cardiac patient would make one think that he had not suffered a great insult to his heart. Frightening sights and sounds are kept to a minimum in coronary care units, why not in intensive care units? Temperature and humidity control are as important in one case as in another. Measures to decrease noise and noxious sensory stimuli are equally important. The difference is not in the need or assessment between the two types of patients. In fact, we do not think the difference can be *rationally* explained.

Opportunities for rest can be planned and implemented by nurses. There are four general measures to encourage rest which every nurse can practice within any physical plant:

1. Organize care in order to prevent disturbing the patient.
2. Practice self-discipline in terms of conversation and producing noise.
3. Teach all members of the therapeutic team the importance of patient rest and plan with them means of facilitating it.
4. Provide for "quiet hours," a time when lights are dimmed, visitors are asked to leave, and staff members refrain from any but absolutely necessary contacts with patients and from actions which might disturb them.

We believe that rest regimens are of vital importance to all patients and of particular importance to the person with cardiac pathology.

Oxygen. Oxygen, comfortably administered, also provides rest for the patient. The administration of oxygen increases the amount of oxygen that is present in a given volume of blood, which results in a decrease of the heart rate. There is another factor which aids in decreasing heart work—the administration of oxygen primarily decreases respiratory work: when less blood is required by the muscles of respiration; less energy is used in the work of breathing; thereby the work of the heart is decreased. For most persons who are having difficulty breathing, the administration of oxygen signals relief and their anxiety level decreases. Well-humidified oxygen also helps to loosen secretions and aids the patient in coughing effectively. Since most cardiac patients are on bed rest, at least initially, hypostatic pneumonia is a real threat. The simple measures of taking a few deep breaths every hour and coughing are as important for the medical patient as for the surgical one.

There are advantages and disadvantages to each technique of oxygen administration (Table 12-5). In addition it should be remembered that oxygen administration in any form carries two inherent dangers: 1) it is a fire hazard; 2) it is potentially toxic to the body.

TRACHEOTOMIES AND THE USE OF RESPIRATORS. There are several therapeutic goals for performing a tracheotomy: reduction of dead space; assurance of oxygen and humidity delivery; and provision of a direct route for suctioning the patient. Tracheotomies are usually utilized postsurgically for patients with increased pulmonary artery pressure and decreased compliance. These patients are more prone to lung infections and pulmonary edema. Generally, they have less ability to absorb oxygen from the lungs. Occasionally a tracheotomy may be performed when a patient's lungs do not re-expand adequately after surgery or if he cannot cough effectively. He may become severely hypoxic under such conditions.

There are several risks which can be minimized by proper care of people with tracheotomies.

1. Introduction of microorganisms. Cleaning trays should be kept sterile. The hand dipping into the solution, while cleaning the inner cannula, should be gloved. Each catheter introduced must be sterile and handled with a sterile glove.
2. Trauma to the trachea. To minimize trauma, lubricate the catheter and pinch it off prior to reaching the maximum endotracheal depth.
3. Forgetting that the patient must breathe. When the catheter is left in the trachea, vagal tone is increased. In effect, the patient is forced to perform the equivalent of the Valsalva maneuver. Proper positioning of the patient, with the head to one side, then the other, allows for quick introduction. The nurse should encourage the patient to cough. He will also cough during and after the procedure if it is done correctly. How much suctioning an individual needs will depend on how much he is secreting, how effectively he can cough, and how skilled the person suctioning him is. The only way to be assured that suctioning has been effective is to listen to the chest.

Many hospital procedures advocate instilling a few ml of sterile saline into the trachea. To gain the optimum effect from the installation, the patient must take a few breaths and cough before suctioning begins. In this manner, loosened mucus is brought within reach of the suction

TABLE 12-5
Methods of Oxygen Administration, Oxygen Concentrations Provided, Advantages and Disadvantages
Each Type

METHOD	L/MIN	CONCENTRATION PERCENTAGE	ADVANTAGES, DISADVANTAGES, GENERAL COMMENTS
Nasal catheter	6-8	30-50	Causes little restriction of movement. Mouth breathing prevents an adequate concentration. If inserted too deeply can cause gastric distention from swallowing air. Some nasal irritation usually occurs.
Nasal cannula	4-6	30-40	The general comments above pertain. Cannulas can cause severe irritation.
Mask—without bag —bag	6-8 10-12	35-55 55-65	Can be removed easily by patient. It is hard to fit. May allow CO_2 retention at lower liter flows. Some patients complain of moisture around face.
Tent	10-15	21-50	Provides cool environment and relative freedom of movement for patient who needs bed rest. Expensive. Some patients complain of coolness and moisture accumulations. Patient may feel claustrophobic.
IPPB units pressure-controlled	0-15	0-100	Depends on cooperation of conscious patient. Helps overcome pulmonary resistance. Medications may be nebulized and instilled with air.
Volume-controlled respirators	0-25	0-100	Best method in respiratory insufficiency. Size and noise of machine may bother conscious patient if used long-term. Patient is immobilized while it is in use.

catheter. Most people withdraw the saline from a sterile vial as it is needed. When this is done, the needle *must* be removed before instilling the saline into the cannula. Failure to observe this simple precaution constitutes negligence if the patient aspirates a needle.

There also seems to be a need to advocate removal of the inner cannula before beginning suctioning. The resulting opening is larger, providing a better airway; The outer cannula is cleaned as the catheter passes through it; the inner cannula can be soaking (to facilitate cleaning) while the nurse is suctioning the patient.

Not everyone knows *how* to cough. The most effective cough requires a deep inspiration, holding the breath a few seconds to build up pressure, and a two-stage expiration. It would sound something like a A-HU, A-HAAH.

The tracheotomized patient often must be taught to cough effectively. The patient who does not have a respirator, with its benefits of mucolytic agents and detergent, particularly needs to be taught. The patient must hold his finger over his stoma for a few seconds after taking a deep breath and then cough.

Patients who are on intermittent respiratory therapy should cough before and after their treatment. Coughing prior to treatment helps avoid the possibility of forcing mucous plugs more deeply into the lungs. Coughing after treatment makes the best use of the extra humidity supplied by the nebulizer and of the medications, if they have been added. Caution should be observed in the use of the bronchodilator group of medications, because many of them increase the heart rate. The pulse should be checked during and after treatment.

The nurse has a role in improving the efficacy of IPPB therapy, whether or not she administers it. She will probably ready the patient for treatment, helping him to cough by helping him, if possible, into an upright position. Patients in severe pain often will not cough. If it is possible to administer an analgesic prior to suctioning and IPPB therapy, the patient will probably respond better. Provision for splinting the incision, and any other means of making the patient physically comfortable, will usually facilitate more effective coughing. Breathing exercises without the machinery also help.

The patient having continuous mechanical respiratory assistance also needs periodic deep breathing, coughing, and suctioning. He is frequently apprehensive without his machine; therefore, the nurse will have to assess the length of time the patient can tolerate being without it. The rate and depth of respiration, the pulse, and the patient's color constitute good measures of his tolerance. At first, it may be necessary to restart the respirator before suctioning is completed. In that case, suctioning must be performed more frequently.

Endotracheal cuffs (balloons) are commonly employed for patients with continuous respirator therapy, and are usually considered necessary for patients using pressure or volume respirators. They constitute a hazard if they are not periodically deflated to allow better tracheal circulation. The time between deflations and the duration of them is usually ordered by the physician. Institutional policies vary as to who is responsible for deflating and reinflating the balloon, but it is always a nursing function to make sure that is done when the patient needs it. The nurse can also detect leakage around the balloon by being alert to an increased rate of cycling by the respirator or its failure to "trip" correctly.

PROVISION FOR THERAPEUTIC NUTRITION. In the case of the cardiac patient, discussion of nutrition can be confined to three important principles.

1. Nutrients, particularly protein and vitamins, are necessary to healing tissue.
2. Digestion takes energy.
3. Sodium in excess retains water.

The nursing role in relation to these three principles is clear-cut. Patients should be en-couraged to eat small amounts at any given time. Emphasis should be placed on eating those foods which are rich in protein and vitamins. Every attempt should be made to decrease the sodium content while retaining the palatability of food. In the case of patients on low-fat and/or low-calorie diets (especially triglyceride), the nurse must work with the dietary department in order to communicate what the patient will and will not eat, and to provide for allowable substitutes to meet his nutritional needs.

The nurse must be on the alert for iatrogenic hazards of dietary as well as pharmacological interactions. Interaction between the two therapuetic modes may occur. The problem of low potassium intake compounded by potassium wasting diuretics and the administration of digitalis preparations is a prototypical case.

FLUID CONTROL. In addition to salt restrictions, many, if not most, cardiac patients have limited fluid allowances. Most of them suffer from thirst, some to the extent that they will either sneak fluids or become very upset over the limited allowance. There are several aids which may be permitted; such as rinsing the mouth with a lemon and water solution, sucking hard candies, and pressing damp sponges to the lips. Often ice chips, supplied in small amounts, can be computed into the daily fluid allowance. If the diet tray is received holding the complete complement of fluids for the whole shift, some may be removed for later in the day. The nurse should be considerate of the patient as well as those on the following shifts with respect to the amount of fluids she allows the patient during her tour of duty.

The following distribution seems to suit most patients. It refers to the oral intake of fluids and assumes that the patient receives breakfast and lunch during the day shift.

Suggested Percentage of Oral Fluid Allotment on Each Shift

	DAY	EVENING	NIGHT
Acute phase	50-55	30-35	15-20
Convalescent phase	55-65	35-45	5-10

The acutely ill patient usually sleeps only intermittently throughout a 24-hour period and will be thirsty during that time. The evening allowance for the convalescent patient should generally be more liberal so that he can partake of the "goodies" frequently brought in to him by his family and friends. He is likely to sleep during the night, allowing a reduction in the night allotment of fluids.

A great deal of variation exists among institutions regarding what substances are considered a part of the fluid allowance. One may find that blood is included while packed cells are not, and similar discrepancies. Whatever the policy may be, the nurse has the responsibility of alerting the medical team to symptoms of overloading. Less dramatic occurrences also need to be communicated. Instances have been observed in which an order for fluids or blood (without reduction of the IV solution) has resulted in no allowance for oral fluid for the patient. Such situations are usually oversights, but they are costly in terms of patient morale and well-being and should be brought to the attention of the physician.

BLOOD ADMINISTRATION. Blood is given to virtually every postsurgical cardiac patient for replacement and to many other cardiac patients. The nurse must be constantly alert to the signals of transfusion reaction, such as chills. However, chills may also be occurring from the administration of cold blood. The need for prompt action in the case of reactions should not cause panic. Should symptoms suggestive of an incompatibility reaction occur, they will usually be present after 100 to 200 ml of blood have been administered. Usually flank pain will occur, caused by hemoglobin precipitation into the renal tubules. The following treatment is then directed toward preventing or modifying kidney damage: infusion of dilute IV solutions; administration of diuretic (usually mannitol) to prevent water reabsorption and overcome vasoconstriction; and alkalinization to reduce the amount of hemoglobin precipitating out into the renal tubles.[17]

Blood containers are frequently hung in a tandem method. When D/W is contained in the second bottle and follows blood down the tubing, small clusters of red blood cells occur. This should be brought to the physician's attention.

PROVISION FOR ELIMINATION. Most cardiac patients receive stool softeners, because constipation and resultant straining at stool are to be avoided in their case. Many patients suffer from constipation with the change in environment, food or water, or from performing this private function in close proximity to others. It is no wonder that problems arise. In addition, the patient may not be able to assume his usual position for defecation. Although the matter may seem mundane, its importance cannot be overemphasized. It can be a daily trial to patients. The nurse may intervene in some cases by finding out what the patient's usual habits are and by providing all possible privacy and comfortable positioning. Means for encouraging defecation should be instituted if the patient does not have a bowel movement *at his usual time*. However, the nurse must not try to change bowel habits and cause needless anxiety to both patient and nurse.

Focus on Prevention

The terms primary, secondary, and tertiary prevention have come into common usage. The nurse, in whatever capacity she works, is in a key position to influence the patient to adopt better health habits. Habits of living are the key to primary prevention and to individual health maintenance.

We say *influence* advisedly. The primary prevention of illness requires a healthy sociocultural milieu. Habits detrimental to health often begin in infancy. Sometimes genetic background, maternal diet, or prenatal occurrences predetermine that an individual will never be healthy as we currently conceptualize health. He may never even be free of disease. In addition, some external conditions require more generalized solutions which cannot be effected at the individual level.

Because health maintenance is a most difficult goal to achieve, we in the health professions have adopted as an operational definition of health, "optimal health for the individual in his circumstances." The phrase acknowledges the current impossibility of changing genetic endowment. It recognizes that life style—the habits of living—is deeply ingrained in the individual and difficult, if not impossible, for him to change. It also recognizes that there are many events in the social context of a person's life which are unhealthy, but which require broad and unified programs of social action (and time) to effect change.

But, change is often a question of *relative* difficulty. The effort to change must always be weighed in the perspective of human and material resources, of which motivation is a primary resource. Given enough interest and money, poverty—which is the major variable that raises our statistics on infant mortality to an embarrassingly high level—can be reversed. Obviously we have not systematically given the problem that much attention. "Optimal health," may be a pragmatic—even a necessary—definition of heath. It also can be, and sometimes is, a "cop out."

Secondary prevention is closer to the interests of nurses. In general, it may be defined as prevention of complications of an acquired (or congenital) disease. Specific measures of secondary prevention range from delineating populations at risk (and monitoring their health status more closely) to preventing what we usually think of as complications, from decubitus ulcers to shock.

Tertiary prevention deals with rehabilitation, the optimal minimization of the effects of a disease, for example, the prevention of the "cardiac invalid." Another important focus for nurses is that of crises intervention with the family whose member is ill. For the patient, such action may constitute tertiary prevention; for the family, it may well constitute secondary prevention.

The patient whom we so frequently see—the person with a myocardial infarction—is an important focus for prevention. We know now that his "disease process" began in his very early years. We recognize that a genetic background involving parents with diabetes or coronary artery disease already predisposes him to an increased risk. Superimposed on his genotypical

background is his personality structure and his life style (phenotypical considerations). What stressors does he have and, more important, how does he deal with them? *Can* he deal with them? What is his diet like? Does he smoke? Does he fail to get regular physical exercise? In general, these coronary risk factors constitute the focus for primary prevention. They should be a focus for secondary prevention for the patient with angina. They *are* usually a focus of tertiary prevention for the patient who has had a myocardial infarction.

We have made inroads into the problems of cardiovascular health. We have increasingly recognized the differential health care accorded the poor. It *is* poor—poor in terms of education and health maintenance, poor in terms of accessibility to diagnosis and treatment, and poor in terms of effecting conditions which prevent relapses or complications. To a certain extent we have devoted some time and attention to improving prenatal health for mother and child.

Research on predispositions to heart disease and efforts to disseminate the findings to the public have been nationwide. Cholesterol and polyunsaturated fats are household terms. Unfortunately, information about triglycerides, the substances which contain them, and the fact that the body can synthesize cholesterol from them is less well disseminated. Smoking is a well-known hazard which receives ongoing attention and increasing attempts at intervention. The effects of chronic emotional stress are well recognized as potentially disease-producing factors.[18]

In the area of secondary prevention, we have produced coronary care units all over the country. Less effectively, we have trained people to staff them. Still less effectively have we provided transportation—support systems to get people to them "in time." Despite the problems mentioned, we have reduced the mortality from myocardial infarction *for those who arrive in time for treatment* by approximately 15 percent. However, literature from other countries suggests that the reduction in mortality rates is not as closely associated with the improved detection of arrhythmias and treatment (especially in coronary care units) as it is purported to be in the United States.[19]

The procedures of myocardial revascularization have been widely advocated as treatment for coronary atherosclerosis and prevention of myocardial infarction.[20] They have even been advocated as emergency treatment for the patient who has myocardial ischemia and/or cardiogenic shock.[21] The general value of the procedures in effecting long-term benefits is under heated debate.[22] (For further discussion of these procedures, see pp. 343 to 346.) Even these procedures may constitute attempts at primary, secondary, or tertiary prevention, depending on the condition of the patient involved. The point at which the risk of such procedures does not outweigh the expected advantages is also the subject of heated debate.[23]

For most nurses, the key to prevention lies with the individual rather than with the broad social context. However, we have shared with other health care providers a focus on the dramatic and immediately threatening event rather than on the formulation of a relationship within which we may help the patient to make decisions about his life, formulate *his* goals of optimal health, and decide how to effect them. Here we are combined educators and supporters. It is most difficult work; the burdens of other people's dependency are heavy.

Knowing how to foster independence and when may be even more difficult. It is also very important. Perhaps we have been guilty of seeing support in too narrow a perspective in one sense and in too broad a perspective in another. Support may mean supporting defenses as well as supporting reality. We have narrowly focused on the latter. (Cardiac invalidism may be associated with attempts to deal with denial until other less fragile ego defenses can be mobilized.)

We have been too broad in our "supportiveness" when we assume that another must and wants to depend on us, on our value orientations, and on our concept of how he should conduct his life. It is as difficult for nurses as it is for others to recognize and honor the patient's decision that the changes in life style required by *the* treatment

and *his* treatment of an illness do *not* permit a quality of life as he sees it. When this is true, he may not accept treatment. When all is said and done, he has that right.

REHABILITATION OF THE CARDIAC PATIENT: A COMPONENT OF PREVENTION

THE ROLE OF TEACHING. Patients need to be taught about many aspects of hospitalization that the nurse takes for granted. In effect, he may have to learn *how* to be ill. Whether he is a medical or a surgical patient, he will have some diagnostic procedures. Woytowich interviewed patients who had undergone cardiac catheterization to determine what information they wanted.[24] In general, her findings may be applied to any patient. She stated that patients should know what the procedure is for, what it is like, and what will be expected of them. The same guidelines may be applied to any patient—his feelings must be, "worked through," before real adjustment to illness can take place. Teaching concerning his regimen upon discharge is not enough.[25]

Effective teaching is a complex process to analyze. However, several principles are particularly applicable to patients.

1. The patient is ill; he has many concerns; his attention will be restricted to information that is meaningful to him.
2. Physical and emotional stimuli which cause anxiety reduce a person's capacity to learn and his attention span.*
3. Inappropriate information, in terms of the learner's physical or emotional condition or his readiness to learn, may be either disregarded or become an obstacle to progress.
4. Learning is an active process. It implies, and sometimes necessitates, change. The learner must become involved in order to learn.
5. Learning is a prerequisite to healthy adjustment.

SPECIAL PROBLEMS IN THE REHABILITATION OF THE CARDIAC PATIENT. The severely ill cardiac patient has suffered an overwhelming

---

*Except in the case of the patient whose denial jeopardizes his life. In this case, the presentation of stimuli that may produce anxiety may be necessary so that they patient can "deal with" the situation more constructively. The decision requires a team approach.

threat. The beginning of rehabilitation is the beginning of assessment. What does the patient think and feel; how is he coping with his experience; what is his anxiety level? The patient must then be helped to integrate his experience and to plan how he will deal with it. He must learn to walk the middle road between imposing severe unnecessary restriction on himself (the cardiac cripple), and refusing to believe that anything with permanent implications has happened to him. During this difficult period of adjustment and readjustment, the nurse also has several things to learn. She must ask herself:

Who is this patient?
What does he need?
How can he be helped?

Principles of Nursing Under Special Conditions

RHEUMATIC HEART DISEASE

One of the greatest problems in medicine today is still the control of rheumatic fever. Its disabling effect, whether on the heart or the musculoskeletal system is costly not only in terms of public health, but also in terms of the immediate home environment of the afflicted individual. While pharmacological means of combating rheumatic fever have been widely used, their efficacy has been questioned. Rushmer states that active lesions are often discovered upon operation and so he poses a very pertinent question, "Is the disease active subclinically for many years despite the use of antibiotic therapy and a strict regimen of rest?"[26] If this is so, current methods of treatment and prophylaxis are ineffective for at least a proportion of patients. Grossman represents the opinions of what seems to be the majority of physicians.[27] By presenting several impressive studies regarding the effective use of prolonged prophylactic antistreptococcal chemotherapy, he makes a strong case for its continued use. Most patients receive some form of antistreptococcal chemotherapy for a prolonged period of time *if they are diagnosed,* but rarely for the five years recommended by Grossman.

One of the obvious problems in controlling rheumatic fever is diagnosing it. The disease is so insidious in its origin that it may be obscured among the miscellany of "colds," sore throats, and "growing pains," of active children and young adults. While medical technology is at an all time high, there are still people admitted to hospitals with severe valvular disease who do not remember having had rheumatic fever or a severe infection of any kind. Unfortunately, the population most prone to the development of streptococcal infections is that which is poorly housed and poorly nourished. This is the same population who is less likely to see a physician for treatment of a bad cold or a sore throat.

The pathogenic mechanism of rheumatic fever is still the subject of controversy. There are two major avenues of investigation which are clearly summarized by Brown and Epstein.[28] *Infectious agents* have been implicated in the rheumatic diseases (particularly streptococci). If they exist they do not seem to be transmitted in the usual manner. They seem to belong either to the virus class or to one composed of other filterable agents. *Immunologic mechanisms* may play a role in pathogenesis by causing the production of an antibody in response to the presence of an antigen, such as the antigen contained in group A beta-hemolytic streptococci. The antigen is purported to cross-react with the host's own tissue —heart, glomerulus, and the like. A second possible immune-type mechanism cited is that of the occurrence of an antigen-antibody reaction in vivo, with the antigen-antibody complex then becoming trapped in the glomerulus (and perhaps in other organs), causing extensive tissue damage.

According to Brown and Epstein, rheumatic diseases include those in which " . . . the eventual outcome of the acute inflammatory onslaught is widespread tissue injury involving some or all of the connective structures and at times including synovium, serous membranes and glomerulus.[29] This would logically include rheumatoid arthritis, rheumatic heart disease, systemic lupus erythematosus, scleroderma, and some forms of nephritis.

However the process is initiated, its effects

on the heart are: 1) edema and inflammation of the connective tissue stroma, 2) appearance of a modified collagenous material, 3) appearance of Aschoff bodies or diffuse and scattered accumulations of cells; and 4) healing with scar formation. The scar formations shrink and cause shortening. Affected valvular cusps no longer meet and their supporting chordae tendineae are shortened. The cusps are often thickened around their edges and fused with their neighbor near the valvular ring. The preceding events lead to the combination of valvular stenosis and insufficiency typical of rheumatic heart disease.

Medical therapy is presently aimed at preventing further cardiac damage. Steroids are usually given during the acute phase, along with penicillin (or a substitute for it for the sensitive patient, or for the patient with penicillin-resistant organisms). Strict bed rest is ordered to reduce heart work. Good nutrition and limited salt intake are emphasized. These therapeutic goals can be extended to include patients with bacterial endocarditis, myocarditis, and pericarditis.

The major adjustments in medical treatment are based on the differences in chemotherapeutic agents which are employed and the amount of time that bed rest is necessary (which varies according to the disease process). The sedimentation rate and body temperature are commonly used indices of the progression of the disease. Antistreptolysin titers above 500 Todd units, the presence of pain, the continued presence of C-reactive proteins, and leucocytosis are usually considered indications for prolonged bed rest and for continuing bacteriocidal doses of drugs. The major adjustments in nursing care depend on the patient's ability to cope with his illness, and more broadly, with his life afterward.

A prolonged course of chemoprophylactic therapy (such as oral penicillin) is frequently recommended to prevent subsequent beta-hemolytic streptococcal infections. For this purpose, penicillin V or penicillin G may be used. The former is more expensive, but is not inactivated by gastric acid as is the latter form of the drug. Intramuscular benzathine penicillin G (Bicillin) may also be given, on a schedule of one injection per month. However, some authors contest the regimen as being either dangerous or ineffective.[30]

Once sequelae of rheumatic heart disease have occurred, care is directed toward maintaining optimal function of the heart by moderation of activity and prevention of further cardiac damage. Table 12-6 summarizes the intracardiac and systemic effects of valvular disease and illustrates the concept of the heart as a closed system. Discussion of pulmonary valvular insufficiency was not included because, except in strenuous exercise, it is rarely incapacitating. It is the least dangerous of the valvular lesions. The pulmonary valve is frequently left incompetent after widening of the pulmonary infundibulum and correction of pulmonary valvular stenosis. The latter is often necessitated in the repair of Tetralogy of Fallot. With its improved results, cardiac surgery is now being performed for people with valvular lesions long before cardiac decompensation occurs.[31]

Nursing intervention in the progression of the disease is most important. First, prevention: school, industrial, and community health nurses, alert to the factors predisposing to the development of rheumatic fever and to exacerbation of acute processes, can with knowledge, insight, and persistence, teach families and individuals better health habits. These habits must be workable within the person's socioeconomic framework and his value system.

Teaching should include instruction in good nutrition, principles of medical asepsis, and, when necessary, how and where to contact social agencies to improve general housing facilities.

Imparting general awareness of what kinds of conditions warrant the physician's consideration is also a necessary part of health teaching. People who have been in close proximity to the patient with rheumatic disease should also receive a medical checkup. Anyone with a sore throat or any other condition suspected of being caused by streptococcal infection should be evaluated immediately.

The nurse is also responsible for aiding the physician in preventing any of the iatrogenic hazards of antimicrobial therapy. She may also

TABLE 12-6
Physiological Effects of Valvular Lesions

LESION	PRIMARY CARDIAC EFFECTS	PRIMARY SYSTEMIC EFFECTS
Mitral stenosis	L. atrial hypertrophy → dilatation and de-compensation.	Pulmonary hypertension → R. heart compensation → decompensation.
Mitral insufficiency	L. atrial hypertrophy or massive enlargement → L. ventricular hypertrophy—decompensation. Decreased coronary perfusion.	Low cardiac output → increasing pulmonary artery pressures in advanced stages.
Aortic stenosis	L. ventricular compensation by hypertrophy →decompensation. Poor coronary perfusion from decreased cardiac output. Angina occlusion of coronary ostia.	Low cardiac output. Brain particularly vulnerable to lowered systolic pressure. Signs of systemic hypoxia. Eventual symptoms of pulmonary hypertension as with L. heart decompensates.
Aortic insufficiency	Leakage back into ventricle causes eventual ventricular decompensation; coronary perfusion poor. Extreme dilatation may lead to ventricular fibrillation.	Dyspnea related to left ventricular failure. Eventual pulmonary hypertension.
Tricuspid stenosis	Blood pressure in atrium increases.	Systemic venous engorgement and edema.
Tricuspid insufficiency	Blood leaks back into R. atrium. Decreased amount propelled to pulmonary artery.	In severe cases heart failure occurs.
Pulmonary stenosis	R. heart hypertrophy → compensation. R. heart dilatation → decompensation.	In severe cases heart failure occurs.

be involved in the care of a patient with a valvular repair or a prosthetic valve.

ARRHYTHMIAS, HEART-BLOCK AND THE USE OF PACEMAKERS

Heart block occurs when conduction through the A-V node is inhibited. It is classified according to the degree of block.

First-degree heart block is a prolonged P-R interval (over 0.20 second). The rhythm is usually regular and the QRS complex is usually normal. This delay in conduction is rarely serious, but it may be progressive. The administration of digitalis or quinidine may provoke higher degrees of A-V block in susceptible patients. Isoproterenol (Isuprel) or atropine may be administered to reduce the degree of block. Usually, cardiac output is not significantly altered, but if the heart rate is slow or the myocardium is impaired and a more rapid rate is desired, a temporary cardiac pacemaker may be utilized.

Second-degree heart block frequently leads to reduced cardiac output. The atrial impulses are conducted at a ratio of 2:1, 3:1, or 4:1 and two or more atrial impulses precede each QRS complex. The precipitating factors and the treatment are essentially the same as for first-degree heart block. However, there is controversy as to whether or not a permanent cardiac pacemaker should be utilized for all patients in second-degree heart block who do not respond to medication. The most reasonable index would seem to be the extent of the heart's ability to supply the body needs. A variation of second-degree heart block, Wenckebach syndrome, occurs when the P-R intervals become progressively prolonged until, finally, one QRS complex does not occur.

In third-degree heart block, none of the atrial impulses are conducted to the ventricles. The conducting tissue or ventricles may then initiate the ventricular impulse. The rhythm may be slightly irregular and is usually slow. In this case, a permanent cardiac pacemaker is frequently necessary.

Impulses may also be blocked in either or

both of the bundle branches of the conducting system of the ventricles. A 12-lead ECG is usually necessary to determine which branch or branches are blocked. Again, permanent cardiac pacemakers may be necessary if the rate is slow and/or if the patient seems to be predisposed to ventricular irritability (ventricular ectopic beats, paroxysmal ventricular tachycardia, and ventricular fibrillation). Occasionally they are used as emergency therapy.

Cardiac pacemakers are now available for temporary and permanent pacing. Table 12-7 lists the major types available.

The care of the patient with a temporary cardiac pacemaker depends upon whether the pacemaker is completely external (i.e., current applied to the skin), or has an electrode passed transvenously into the right atrium or right ventricle. External cardiac pacemakers tend to produce pain and burns and can be used only for short periods of time. An alternative emergency method for temporary cardiac pacemaking is to thread a pacemaker wire through a spinal needle which has been inserted through the chest wall into the heart. This method is a "blind" technique and the risks are obvious. Most patients requiring a temporary cardiac pacemaker have the transvenous type.

Good nursing care requires information regarding the function of the pacemaker and the surgical procedure for inserting it. The nurse should be aware that this type of cardiac pacemaker is subject to interference from other electrical sources. Any time the power unit is attached to the patient externally, both the patient and the nurse must be aware of hazards from other electrical machinery and substances affecting conduction such as oil and water. Although the treatment may be of short duration, the patient may react negatively to his "dependence upon the machine." Despite the fact that the pacemaker is a lifesaving device, the patient may show apprehension of death. Such emotional reactions must be dealt with on an individual basis.

The power sources of permanent cardiac pacemakers are usually implanted in subcutaneous pockets in the axilla-subclavicular space or in a space over the upper abdomen. The electrodes may be passed transvenously or directly applied to the heart through a thoracotomy. The latter is a major surgical procedure and must be treated as such in preparing the patient. Because of the permanency of the cardiac pacemaker, major adjustments in the patient's life are necessary. One of these is frequent medical checkups to check the rate of the pacemaker. A failure at the power source may cause either an increase or decrease in rate. If the wires become dislodged or broken, the pacemaker will fail. Despite the

TABLE 12-7
Types of Pacemakers; Their Advantages and Disadvantages

TYPE	METHOD OF OPERATION	ADVANTAGES AND DISADVANTAGES
Fixed rate	Impulses generated at a predetermined (fixed) rate.	Can be used transvenously. Not altered by physiological demands. It may compete with the intrinsic rhythm. Cardiac output may be reduced because of the lack of the atrial systolic contribution to ventricular filling.
Synchronous	A sensing device in the atrium triggers an impulse to the ventricles after a predetermined appropriate interval.	Many of the disadvantages of a fixed rate pacemaker are overcome. Implantation requires a thoracotomy because a sensing electrode must be attached to the atrium and a stimulating electrode to the ventricle.
Demand	A ventricular impulse is triggered when a predetermined interval has elapsed since the last spontaneously occurring ventricular impulse. It will discharge at a fixed rate if ventricular standstill occurs.	Can be applied transvenously. Will not compete with the intrinsic rhythm and, consequently, is useful for slow rates. Not affected by physiological demands

problems cardiac pacemakers have caused, they are being used more frequently and have allowed patients to lead more productive lives.

HYPERTENSION AND OTHER CONDITIONS REQUIRING INCREASED CARDIAC WORK

Hypertension

A description of the nursing care of the hypertensive patient requires a chapter in itself. Here we can only summarize the controversies of etiology and delineate the main principles of care. (For further information see bibliography at the end of the chapter.)

Hypertension is perhaps the most commonly found chronic medical condition in the community. Figure 12-10 demonstrates its prevalence on the basis of a community sample. The community studied was a section of a large city. Ninety-five percent of the community was black.

It has been found that urban living, poverty, and belonging to an ethnic minority group all contribute to a higher incidence of hypertension; purportedly because they all add to the "stress of life."[32] It is estimated that any *unselected* group of the population will yield an incidence of 15 percent of hypertensive people.[33] When the researchers in the study reviewed here combined the categories "borderline" and "hypertensive" from their selected sample, the prevalence was 40.2 percent.[34] The role of the nurse in effecting community health screening—especially in communities at high risk—is clear! A recent study of a program of screening, treatment and follow up at a work site illustrates an innovation worth pursuing. Nurses were integrally involved.[35]

There are several postulated mechanisms of "essential" hypertension as well as several other

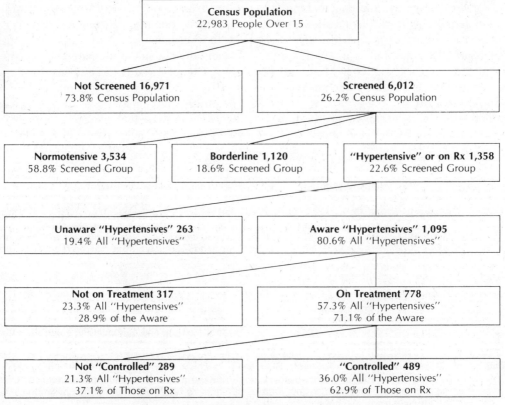

FIGURE 12-10.
Status of the screened population at time of initial interview.

forms of hypertension. We will focus here on the care of the person with essential hypertension. Care of the patient who suffers hypertension secondary to renal artery incompetency or endocrine disturbances centers on treatment of the primary conditions (although antihypertensive therapy may also be instituted). Essential hypertension has no known cause; however, although it cannot be cured, it may be modified and, hopefully controlled.

Treatment of essential hypertension involves two major forms of therapy: 1) medication and 2) modification of life style. Once the patient is diagnosed and has become stabilized on medication, the nurse in the hospital, clinic, or home must assume responsibility for helping him to maintain himself. Nursing responsibilities include listening, interviewing, teaching, and assessing the patients' progress.

The nurse *must* listen to the patient describe his illness, the conditions he feels are associated with it, and how he expects to deal with it before she can expect to assess his needs for information or support. Historically, the "drop-out rate" for patient teaching and even for treatment has been extremely high.[36] It has been found that patients often feel angry that they are burdened with such a troublesome condition; it may seem unfair. In addition, the knowledge that there may be exacerbations and the problems in initially stabilizing the disease process often provoke fear. Under these conditions, the often observed long waits of patients and the bureaucratic runarounds in some agencies are extra aggravations to the patient's problems of dealing with stress. They are stressors in themselves—as are perfunctory treatment, chiding, and all forms of depersonalization which are so readily documented in every type of health care facility. Trying to understand the patient's view is a good antidote to depersonalization.

Much of the teaching of hypertensive patients in most settings revolves around medications. Figure 12-11 and Table 12-8 may help the nurse

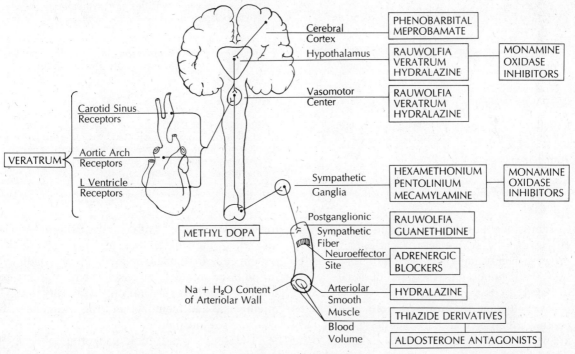

FIGURE 12-11.
Anatomical sites of action of various drugs that decrease blood pressure. Several of these exert hypotensive effects through action at more than one site.

TABLE 12-8
Drugs Frequently Used in the Treatment of Hypertension

DRUG	UPPER LIMITS OF DOSE	CLASS	ACTION, ANTIDOTES, OTHER INFORMATION
Phentolamine (Regitine) Phenoxybenzamine HCl (Dibenzyline)	varies with purpose 60 mg	Alpha adrenergic blockade	Drugs are competitive with adrenergic catechol-amines. Effects may be counteracted by using them. Levarterenol is the antidote of choice.
Hexamethonium Pentolinium (Ansolysen) Mecamylamine (Inversine) Trimethaphan (Arfonad)	60 mg 20 mg variable	Ganglionic blockage Used with reser-pine 50 mg in 500 ml IV	Venous dilatation—peripheral pooling—decreased cardiac output—hypotension. Transmission across both sympathetic and parasympathetic ganglia occurs. Therefore, decreased GI motility, loss of pupillary accommodation, urinary retention and impotence may occur. Latter may be ameliorated with neostigmine, etc.
Thiazides		Diuretics	Often used as conjunctive therapy for hypertension.
Reserpine Crude root (Raudixin, etc.) Alseroxylon (Rauwiloid, etc.)	.25-50 mg 100 mg 2 mg	Sympatholytic (Allows para-sympathetic dominance)	Tranquilizer. Depletes body of norepinephrine and serotonin. Used with ganglionic blocker and diuretic.
Guanethidine sulfate (Ismelin) Methyldopa (Aldomet) Hydralazine (Apresoline)	50 mg 2000 mg 200 mg	Adrenergic neuron blockade (also an MAO-inhibitor)	Acts as the ganglionic blocking agents without parasympathetic blockage. The latter system pre-dominates. Interrupts norepinephrine and sero-tonin synthesis. Intensifies beta sympathomimetic effects. Used with other hypotensives.
Veratrum Alkaloids (Veriloid) Protoveratrines A & B (Veralba)	4 mg IV 0.5 mg IV	Sympathetic inhibition	Inhibition of sympathetic tone and vagal augmenta-tion by baroreceptor sensitivity. Prevent resultant bradycardia with atropine.
Caffeine Theophylline (Quibron) Aminophylline	20 Gm 0.5 Gm 1.5 Gm	Xanthines	Stimulation of CNS. Relax smooth muscle, espe-cially bronchiolar. Act on the kidney to produce diuresis. Stimulates cardiac muscle, increases blood pressure and intensifies effect of narcotic analgesics and anesthetics.

Adapted from Meyers, F. H., Jawetz, E. and Goldfein, A.: Review of Medical Pharmacology. Los Altos, Medical Publications, 1969.

to remember the agents used and their effects. However, the responses of patients to these drugs is highly individualized. For this reason, we have included only the maximum safe levels of the drugs as a guideline.

We suggest that nurses help patients to routinize their medication schedules so that daily events help them to remember what is to be taken when. A second important point of teaching is the effect of undermedication or overmedi-cation so that the patient knows when to report

for additional care. Third, and frequently over-looked, is the nurse's role in making sure the patient can administer the medications. Included in the later area are the assessment of ability to obtain the drugs—financial and physical—intelligence and memory, and the willingness to take the responsibility.

The support the nurse can offer may be of crucial importance to the patient with hyperten-sion. We feel that nurses are often more in-terested in the supportive role with chronic patients than are other members of the health care team and *are able* to undertake it by virtue of their education. If nurses continue their trend of seeking employment in facilities which make more use of these skills (and less use of their feet) they are likely to be rewarded with a greater sense of personal accomplishment.

High Output Syndrome

Any condition which causes the heart to work harder to supply blood may be categorized as a "high output syndrome." In this sense, physical and emotional stress can cause high output syndrome because they increase the metabolic needs of the body. However, one must evaluate stress as a pathogenic agent in terms of several factors. The degree of stress, its frequency and duration, and the subjective reactions of the person stressed all act to determine individual reactions to stress. Moderate degrees of stress, applied intermittently and followed by effective physical responses to reduce it, serve to exercise the heart and other muscles and to preserve the body's adaptive mechanisms. Prolonged and severe stresses may give rise to high output syndrome and to resultant cardiac pathology. Stress increases the vasomotor tone, a condition which may lead to the irreversible arteriosclerotic changes which accompany hypertension.

HYPERVOLEMIA may also result in high output syndrome. Usually the condition is transitory; the administration of IV fluids too rapidly or too generously causes a volume overload of the vascular compartment that is transient in the relatively healthy patient. When the condition of a fluid overload becomes permanent—as it does with some kidney diseases and "congestive" heart failure—it often leads to cardiac damage. The patient with underlying kidney or cardiac pathology has a reduced ability to deal with transient increases in vascular volume. Patients who suffer from aldosteronism or renal insufficiency retain sodium and, therefore, water. The chronic fluid overload places an increased workload on the heart, despite the capacity of the extravascular compartments to store a large proportion of the excess.

BERIBERI results in massive vascular dilatation as a result of its effects on the nervous system. At first, the heart rate increases in an attempt at compensation. But, as the disease progresses, the nerves supplying the heart also lose their capacity to conduct the impulses necessary for increased rate and tone.

THYROTOXICOSIS jeopardizes myocardial health in two ways. First, the increase in the amount of circulating thyroxine causes an increased metabolic rate in the tissues. Heart work is subsequently increased for the transport of vital oxygen and nutrients to meet tissue demands. Second, the increment of internal heat generated by the increased metabolic rate results in massive peripheral vessel dilatation as the body attempts to dissipate it. As a consequence of the lowered peripheral resistance, the heart is stimulated to increase its rate and force of contractions to maintain adequate pressure for perfusion.

Several conditions necessitate a relatively high cardiac output to compensate for decreased pulmonary ventilation or oxygenation of the blood. Most prevalent among these are chronic obstructive pulmonary disease (which is coincident with both hypoventilation and hypooxygenation through atelectasis and arteriovenous shunting in the capillary beds). Fistulae, congenital anomalies such as septal defects of overriding aorta, and Paget's disease of the bones illustrate the wide range of conditions which may result in the poor oxygenation of blood and a subsequently increased cardiac workload. Anemia is another prevalent stimulus to cardiac compensation for tissue underperfusion with oxygen.

Parodoxically, the result of chronically high output states is an insufficient supply of blood to the tissues. The overworked heart eventually decompensates. The net result of the reduced cardiac efficacy adds a poor blood supply to the problems already manifested. Often the end of the cardiac compensatory period is signalled by the occurrence of a myocardial infarction because the cellular demands of the heart itself have been compromised. We will discuss these two mechanisms of cardiac disease below.

CARDIAC COMPENSATION AND DECOMPENSATION

There are various terms purported to describe the pathology of cardiac decompensation. We will discuss each nomenclature briefly since texts vary in their use of these terms. Each system of classification also reveals a theory about the causes of cardiac decompensation. The controversy regarding the best nomenclature underlies some basic differences of opinion as to the primary etiologies of cardiac decompensation. It may be useful first to discuss compensation and to review the mechanisms by which it is made possible.

People move back and forth between the states of cardiac compensation and decompensation, depending on their general health, environmental demands, and cardiac assistance through rest and medication. Therefore, nurses should bear in mind that decompensation is a relative term, applied at the appearance of certain symptoms but occurring with various degrees of severity. Conceptualizing congestive heart failure (CHF) in this way, makes it clear that the nurse must be alert to methods of preventing episodes of decompensation for patients who are prone to them.

The process of compensation implies greater work on the part of the heart. The capacity for more effective pumping is called the cardiac reserve. It is made possible not only by short term increases in the rate and force of contractions, but also by hypertrophy of the heart muscle; the walls then exert more pressure on the blood to eject it. The extracardiac mechanisms mentioned previously are particularly valuable adjuncts to the heart in meeting tissue needs for oxygen. Under the condition of increased tissue demands for nutrients, the cells extract more oxygen from the blood, thereby increasing the oxygen utilized from a given volume of blood. A consequent decrease in the arteriovenous oxygen saturation ratio occurs. Given adequate supplies of nutrients and oxygen, the myocardium itself is able to transfer more energy to useful work and less to the production of heat. In some conditions, the body's needs for oxygen are met not only by an increase in respirations, but by the mobilization of the erythropoietic system.

In view of the existence of the cardiac reserve and the adjunctive means of adaption by other organ systems, it can be readily seen that cardiac decompensation usually occurs after a long period of time. The point at which a patient presents the classic symptoms are often preceded by a period of general malaise and easy fatigability which may not have been defined by the patient as a condition warranting medical attention. By the time the cardiac reserve is compromised, cardiac dilatation is present. The patient is usually edematous and short of breath, and precordial pain on exertion also is often reported.

Figure 12-12 illustrates the continuum of cardiac compensation-decompensation and shows the roles of other organs in the process.

The reader can readily see the potential for any one of a number of conditions to act as the "triggering mechanism" of cardiac decompensation. Let us return now to the nomenclature controversy over decompensation and the opinions it reveals regarding the primary pathology of the decompensated state.

BACKWARD FAILURE AND FOWARD FAILURE. A conceptualization of a decompensated state as *backward failure* assumes that the blood becomes "dammed up" behind the chambers of the heart. This process would lead to congestion of the systemic veins and generalized edema formation. Consequently, the tissues are deprived of an effective volume of blood. Mechanical cardiac obstructions can be readily appreciated as primary etiologies of backward failure. The term *forward failure* is applied to a situation in which the primary pathology is diminished cardiac output. Logically there must be some reason for that! Subsequent to reduced output, the hypoxic tissues become more permeable and compound the problems of diminished renal perfusion, causing massive electrolyte shifts and the movement of sodium and water into the extravascular spaces. As a theory of etiology, the foregoing conceptualization belies the nature of the cardiovascular system as a closed system. The designations of backward or forward failure as primary to the process of decompensation seem arbitrary and artificial in this light.

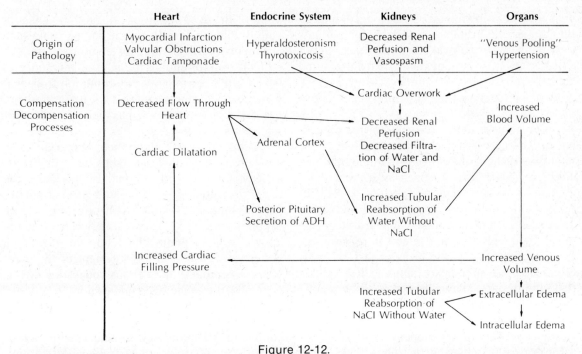

Figure 12-12.
The continuum of cardiac compensation-decompensation with the effects of other organ systems on the process.

RIGHT-SIDED FAILURE AND LEFT-SIDED FAILURE. Advocates of this nomenclature purport that it isolates the site of decompensation and allows the therapist to deduce the effects the patient will suffer as a result. The term failure is a short way of stating that some part of the heart has failed to act effectively as a pump. It is often called simply "congestive failure" and the designation right or left is not applied. Since decompensation of only one side rarely exists for any length of time, it can be seen that the conceptualization shares the same faults as that of backward and forward failure although it is somewhat more descriptive. The idea of congestive heart failure also obscures the fact that there are *degrees* of decompensation and that the pathology may be a result of several processes which affect the heart only secondarily. Treatment directed to the heart without correction of the underlying cause may fail.

HIGH AND LOW OUTPUT SYNDROMES. High output syndrome was discussed previously (see page 327). Low output syndrome appears in response to such factors as arterial hyperten-sion and hypovolemia. Arterial hypertension may precipitate decompensation because, although the heart is initially healthy, the resistance against the flow of blood is so great that a deficit in tissue perfusion occurs. Secondarily, the heart may decompensate from its increased workload. Mechanical obstructions to the flow of blood act in the same manner to produce low output. Low output is also the obvious result of hypovolemia. This nomenclature reveals two factors relevant to the treatment of people with cardiac decompensation. First, by using the word syndrome, it is made clear that decompensation represents a reaction rather than a primary pathology. Second, the fact that the body is a system is incorporated into this concept. As a result, the reader is led to appreciate the roles of other system components in the process of decompensation and the therapy directed to restoring compensation or removing the need for it; one example is the cure of thyrotoxicosis. However, the isolation of initiating mechanisms is often a most puzzling process: we do not mean to imply that what we consider to be an improved means of conceptualizing cardiac decompensation solves the problems of caring for patients with it. We must still ask why the heart fails to compensate at a certain point. Why are some patients refractory to treatment? How can we predict decompensation and intervene before that point?

In an attempt to answer some of the preceding questions, researchers have pointed to the vital role of the kidneys in maintaining fluid and electrolyte balance. It has been shown that under conditions of decreased renal perfusion, the ability of the kidneys to excrete sodium and water diminishes. Some researchers appear to feel that the subsequent fluid and electrolyte derangements are primary to the process that we most often call congestive heart failure.[37] It is certain that diuretics are a valuable tool in resolving the patients' symptoms. They and the digitalis preparations constitute a typical part of the treatment regimen for cardiac decompensation. Diuretics are extensively reviewed in Chapter 17; Table 12-9 presents a synopsis of the frequently used digitalis preparations.

The phenomenon of venous pooling which we mentioned earlier is readily apparent in the patient with decompensated heart disease and a source of much discomfort. Vital organs, such as the liver and the digestive tract in general, are hampered by venous congestion, often to the point of the destruction of cells and the onset of pain. It may be difficult for the nurse to help such a patient find a position of comfort. It is also difficult to differentiate the nausea and anorexia which often accompany this condition from that which is a warning signal that the upper limits of the digitalis preparation has been reached for that individual.

A small proportion of patients experience decompensation of only the right side of the heart, at least for a period of time. In this case, the underlying etiology is usually decreased pulmonary compliance—lungs with stiff, unyielding capillary beds. Right heart deterioration occurs after efforts to pump blood into an unyielding system and results in engorgement of the great veins. Eventually, the venous congestion effects generalized cardiac decompensation.

PULMONARY EDEMA

Pulmonary edema is said to be caused by a failure of the left ventricle to adequately pump blood. This failure results in the engorgement of the lungs with blood and the subsequent extravasation of fluid into the alveoli. It should be emphasized that a failure of the left ventricle rarely occurs alone. It has been estimated that it is capable of exerting seven times the pressure of the right. When the left ventricle decompensates, the patient is placed in double jeopardy. First,

TABLE 12-9
The Digitalis Preparations: Inotropic Agents for Patients with Poor Myocardial Contractility

PREPARATIONS AND COMMON SYNONYMS	ADULT DIGITALIZATION DOSE ORAL	INTRAVENOUS	ADULT MAINTENANCE DOSE (ORAL)	ONSET OF ACTION
Digitalis (Digitalis Purpura leaf)	Rarely used for digitalization.	No parenteral form.	0.5-2.0 mg	½ - 2 hrs
Digoxin (Lanoxin) (glycoside Dig. Lanata leaf)	2.0-4.0 mg	0.75-1.0 mg	0.25-1.0 mg	5 - 30 min
Digitoxin (Crystodigin) (purified Dig. Lanata leaf)	1.0-1.5 mg	1.0-1.5 mg	0.05-0.2 mg	5 - 30 min
Lanatoside (Cedilanid-D) (Deslanoside is the injection)	5.0-10.0 mg	1.2-1.6 mg	0.5-2.0 mg	10 - 30 min
(g-Strophanthin) Ouabain (injectable only)	Rarely used for digitalization.	0.25-0.5 mg	—	3 - 10 min
Gitalin (Dig. Purpura Glycoside)	4.0-8.0 mg	No parenteral form.	0.25-1.0 mg	½ - 2 hrs

there is a very narrow margin of safety between optimal pulmonary capillary pressure and a pressure high enough to cause pulmonary edema; transudation of fluid occurs with only a few millimeters of mercury increment. Second, the decreased oxygenation of blood, which results from the presence of fluid in the lungs, increases the heart rate, further compromising general tissue perfusion.

It should be stated that the discrepancy between the force of the right and left ventricle can be a handicap to the patient. In patients who have mitral stenosis (a common occurrence in those with rheumatic heart disease), the left ventricle propels blood backward into the atrium through the incompetent valve with every systole. Such patients are usually prone to pulmonary edema and subsequent cardiac decompensation.

Pulmonary edema is also an iatrogenic hazard of too generous or too rapid fluid administration. Frequent assessment of the patient which includes a check of his IV, his lung sounds, and his symptoms can prevent pulmonary edema from this cause. If the patient has a central venous pressure line, there is simply no excuse for overhydration!

The occurrence of severe pulmonary edema is a medical emergency. Efforts are directed toward reducing the blood flow to the lungs while promoting adequate ventilation and oxygenation of the tissues through the administration of oxygen. A reduction of the blood flow to the lungs is often effected with the use of rotating tourniquets, which when used correctly, serve to pool blood in the extremities, thus reducing the pulmonary hydrostatic pressure. Adjunctive diuretic therapy may be ordered by the physician. Analgesics are usually given, both to reduce pain and for their additional action in reducing cardiac and respiratory work caused by stress. Some, such as morphine, have a direct action in depressing respirations. If bronchospasm is evident, aminophylline will probably be ordered and given IV in an infusion. Digitoxin is also usually used if the patient is not already receiving it. Both drugs increase cardiac output.

After emergency treatment, close surveillance is necessary. Not only can the nurse prevent or modify another episode, but her physical presence tends to reassure the understandably apprehensive patient. Since the patient has usually diaphorized profusely, he will need to be bathed and changed as soon as his physical conditions allows it. We remind the reader that edematous skin is prone to necrosis!

In summary, cardiac decompensation may be regarded as a "complication" of several more proximate etiologies. These include arrhythmias, valvular defects, hypertension, and myocardial infarction. Cardiac decompensation, particularly following myocardial infarction, may be a signal of impending shock. In any case, the condition is more readily prevented than cured. Prevention is only possible if premonitory signs are recognized and the patient is treated to minimize his cardiac workload. The responsibility of assessing the patient and alerting the medical staff to an ominous change in the patient's condition is most often the nurse's. Here, she is truly an agent of primary prevention.

Cardiac Effects of Electrolyte Disturbances

SODIUM.   Since the serum level of sodium as assessed by current methods merely reflects the concentration of sodium to water as they exist in the plasma, the value obtained can be misleading. It does not reflect the absolute amount of sodium in the body. Either hypernatremia or hyponatremia can be present when the patient is clinically dehydrated or when he is edematous. The most reliable assessment of the patient's sodium balance includes both the patient's history and his clinical symptoms, in conjunction with laboratory data.

Dehydration (volume depletion) may exist in the presence of sodium balance, hyponatremia, *or* hypernatremia. When fluid depletion is not accompanied by a concurrent loss of sodium, laboratory data will reveal hypernatremia, despite no real increase in total body sodium. Similarly, the patient can lose sodium in excess of fluid and have what is called "dilutional hyponatremia." In both instances, it is the balance that is faulty. However, when the patient suffers concurrent fluid and electrolyte loss and his needs are not met orally or with adequate IV therapy, he will become both dehydrated and hyponatremic, despite remaining "in sodium balance." In addition to the signs of hypotension and tachycardia which occur from volume depletion, the hyponatremic patient is prone to seizures and other severe mental disturbances.

The patient with pre-existing kidney disease, and/or congestive heart failure is particularly prone to dehydration due to excessive loss of sodium and water from the kidneys. His volume and sodium depletion may occur despite the presence of edema. In fact, the use of diuretics in an attempt to decrease edema and mobilize fluid from the extravascular compartment may be the cause of the condition.

On the other hand, the dehydrated patient who has lost water in excess of salt demonstrates hypernatremia. Reduced extracellular volume in conjunction with reduced plasma volume decrease cardiac output. Poor tissue perfusion results. However, the reader will probably be most familiar with hypernatremia associated with water retention: the condition giving rise to edema.

Edema is a classic sign of decompensated cardiac disease. The increased extravascular fluid volume is usually (although not always) associated with an increased intravascular fluid volume. The latter imposes an additional workload on the heart. Although severe edema is usually generalized, the nurse can observe it most quickly by looking at and palpating the dependent portions of the body: the pretibial areas of the ambulatory patient and the presacral area of the patient in bed. Good skin care, including the systematic relief of pressure is most important for this patient. Care must also be taken to prevent constriction of the circulation. Tight clothing and sharply flexed extremities should be avoided.

CALCIUM. Hypercalcemia leads to decreased muscular contractility. ECG recordings reveal prolonged Q-T intervals which reflect the slower transmission of impulses during ventricular depolarization. Cardiac output drops due to decreased systolic force and rate decreases in most instances. Since hypercalcemia usually occurs secondary to conditions which cause bone deterioration, primary conditions are the focus of treatment rather than reduction of serum calcium.

Hypocalcemia is reflected in the condition known as tetany. It most often occurs after accidental damage to the parathyroid glands or their inadvertent removal during a thyroidectomy. The myocardium and skeletal muscles react to the low serum calcium with spastic, ineffectual contractions. There is a risk of fibrillation and the development of ectopic foci in the myocardium. The usual treatment is the administration of calcium intravenously. After the emergency, treatment is directed to correcting the primary condition.

POTASSIUM. Hyperkalemia produces tall peaked T waves on the ECG in the very early stages. The heart is extremely sensitive to fluctuations of potassium. In the case of hyperkalemia, the repolarization process is retarded. If the potassium continues to increase, P waves disappear and the QRS complex widens. Cardiac standstill is the final outcome. The heart stops in diastole as the high amount of potassium does not permit the sodium influx (accompanied by calcium) that is necessary for repolarization. Intravenous sodium bicarbonate injection will rapidly diminish serum potassium levels. Intravenous calcium injection will immediately antagonize the effects of hyperkalemia on the cardiac muscle.

Hypokalemia causes an increased electrical potential across the cell membrane. The tendency for sodium to move into the cell in the case of reduced serum potassium causes the increased irritability. The cell is hyperpolarized. Ventricular fibrillation is a hazard to the patient. The electrocardiogram will show low amplitude T waves and, in some cases, U waves. U waves are thought to be the result of retrograde depolarization attempts. Intravenous potassium is administered to the patient with hypocalcemia. Many patients who demonstrate the condition have been digitalized. The digitalis may be temporarily discontinued until the potassium level is restored, since patients often manifest symptoms of digitalis intoxication when their potassium level is low.

ACIDEMIA. Acidemia is the result of excess hydrogen ion in the blood. Acidemia contributes to the movement of potassium out of the cell. Sodium and calcium tend to replace it, giving rise to a hyperirritable state with its risk of ectopic impulse formation and fibrillation. This situation necessitates the administration of base during resuscitation attempts. Unless the acidemia is corrected, an effective heartbeat may not occur. Since many of the patients prone to cardiac disease also have diabetes, the role of acidemia in leading to derangements of the heartbeat should not be forgotten when a person is admitted with diabetic acidosis.

CORONARY ARTERY DISEASE AND MYOCARDIAL ISCHEMIA

Perhaps the most important concept to remember with regard to myocardial ischemia is that it can occur from a *relative* lack of blood flow through the coronary system. Ischemia may occur when there is a sudden decrease in the blood flow to a portion of the myocardium: this most often occurs when a thrombus occludes a major vessel but it can occur because of vessel spasm. More frequently, symptoms of ischemia occur because there is an increase in the metabolic demands of the tissue which cannot be met by the available supply of blood. Either of these situations is most likely to occur in the presence of coronary atherosclerosis.

Atheromas have been found in the coronary vessels of children in this country. Autopsies of young men in their late teens and early twenties have shown extensive atherosclerotic plaque formations. Contrary to popular belief, the early stages of coronary artery disease do not necessarily involve lipid deposits. Atherosclerotic plaques are now thought to develop through the following stages: 1) fragmentation of the internal membrane and thickening of the intima, 2) lipid collection, particularly at the junction of the intima and media, 3) degeneration of areas within the plaque, and 4) hyalinization and calcium deposition replacing normal tissue.[38]

Atheromas present three hazards to the function of the myocardium. They decrease the size of the vessel lumena. They cause rough areas on the surface of the intima which predisposes the person to thrombus formation. And, they may break off from the intima, thereby acting as em-

boli. It has been postulated that vessel spasm is an additional mechanism of coronary circulation deprivation. Although the gradual and insidious nature of plaque formation allows time for the development of collateral circulation, it is obvious from the number of people who have angina pectoris (if not an acute myocardial infarction) that the body's natural defenses cannot effectively combat the problem. One factor that mitigates against an effective degree of collateral circulation is the generalized nature of plaque formation. Another is the life style of most sufferers of acute ischemic attacks. Regular but moderate exercise is purported to retard myocardial impairment by hastening the development of collateral branches over areas where blood flow is moderately restricted. However, there is still great controversy over the role of exercise in the prevention and rehabilitation aspects of coronary disease.

Other researchers have investigated other possible primary causes of ischemic heart disease. Raab observed the fact that potassium depletion leading to an influx of sodium and calcium is associated with myocardial ischemia.[39] He postulates that myocardial hypoxia leads to potassium depletion. The hypoxia is a consequence not only of narrowed lumena, but also of neurogenic reactions and hormonal factors. Figure 12-13 shows Raab's three-faceted model.

The reader can readily see the postulated roles of stress and sedentary living as well as those of others of the demonstrated coronary risk factors in this model. Stress has been implicated in several theories about the pathogenesis of coronary artery disease through its relationship to increased adrenergic activity and the concomitant need for greater oxygen and nutrients. Despite the implication of stress as an etiologic agent in myocardial infarction, it is still not determined *how* stress acts; therefore it is not possible to predict the effects of a given kind and amount of stress on a given individual. As most nurses will have observed, we are not particularly effective in reducing stress, despite a growing armory of drugs and regimens for doing so.

The possibility that electrolytic shifts are responsible for permanent ischemic damage has also been explored by Sodi-Pollares, et al.[40]

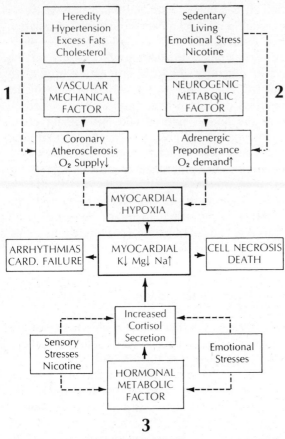

FIGURE 12-13.
"Structural Formula" of pluricausal pathogenesis of so-called coronary heart disease. Three basic pathogenic elements interfere in crucial myocardial ionic balance: Coronary atherosclerosis (1), in conjunction with adrenosympathetic overactivity (2) causes myocardial hypoxia (discrepancy between vascular O_2-supply and metabolic myocardial O_2-consumption), which, in turn, deranges ionic equilibrium. Adrenocortical overactivity (3) intensifies catecholamine cardiotoxicity, presumably by further equidirectional electrolyte displacement. (All details are clinically and or experimentally documented.) Source: After Raab, W.: Dis. Chest 53: 629-631, 1968.

They have published laboratory and clinical research data regarding their "polarizing" treatment which is based on correcting intracellular hypokalemia. The essence of their treatment is provision of dietary and intravenous potassium and restriction of potassium-depleting drugs and sodium. Since thiazides, quinidine, digitalis, and several other medications usually employed in this country are among those which would be subjected to close scrutiny rather than typically prescribed, the polarizing treatment and its theoretical background have aroused a great deal of controversy.

We will begin discussing the nursing care of the person with coronary heart disease under the topic of angina pectoris. Unfortunately, it is not until the point of chest pain that most people are known to have coronary artery disease. However, we are beginning to routinely screen some groups of the general population to discover risk-prone individuals. It is hoped that this effort will be extended in conjunction with research to determine factors which lead to coronary disease and how they may be controlled and prevented. It is also hoped that nurses will involve themselves in the preventive and teaching aspects of this widespread problem as well as in the care of acutely ill patients.

Angina Pectoris

Precordial pain, angina pectoris, is the most common subjective complaint related to myocardial ischemia. It is often accompanied by a feeling of tightness, fullness, or constriction. Some people describe a burning sensation; others a dull aching pain. People may locate the pain over the heart, although in many, it radiates to the left shoulder and arm. However, there is a documented entity called the "silent coronary" in which the person has suffered permanent myocardial damage without acute pain. In retrospect, some of this group will remember pain that they had interpreted as "indigestion."

There are several theories related to the referred pain which is so typical of myocardial ischemia. The interest in the mechanism of pain is particularly keen at the present time as medical scientists attempt to understand the old oriental practice of acupuncture. In the current hypotheses regarding pain, there are several which bear relating. One states that the visceral impulses act as an irritable focus in the segment of the spinal cord at which the nerves enter.[41] Another suggests that the visceral and somatic impulses converge in the spinal cord, causing afflicted people to interpret as the offending part, the one served by the somatic nerve.[42] Studies have also shown that myocardial ischemia produces chest muscle spasm as a result of a visceromotor reflex.[43] Whatever the precise mechanism of pain may be, the patient who suffers anginal pain needs relief. The ability to gain relief from anginal pain through the use of coronary vasodilators and/or the cessation of activity usually signals the fact that permanent myocardial damage has been avoided.

Pain, whatever its location and characteristics, serves as a protective device for the body. The nurse is so frequently called upon to administer analgesics, that the protective and signalling aspects of pain ("physical" or "psychic") are often not heeded. Anginal pain alerts the patient, the physician, and the nurse to the presence of myocardial ischemia. Its pattern of occurrence can reveal which of the patient's activities and reactions place an added burden on his heart. This information is necessary to the process of effective teaching and counseling. Anginal pain rarely occurs without the presence of atherosclerotic plaques; however, despite the preexisting disease, assessment of precipitating factors and prompt intervention may delay or even preclude permanent myocardial damage.

The patient with chronic anginal pain may be treated medically, surgically, or both. Medical treatment usually consists of counseling and the administration of one or more of the coronary vasodilators. Acute or severe episodes may require the use of analgesics. Some people appear to profit from the use of tranquilizers routinely or "ad lib." The agents noted above are summarized in Table 12-10, p. 336.

It should be emphasized that medications should be considered supplemental therapy to the processes of counseling and teaching as well as to the relief of anxiety. Counseling must be directed to helping the patient to reduce or control factors in his life which appear to precipitate "attacks." Changing these conditions, which often represent the habits of a lifetime, is no easy task. Patients and therapists must appreciate this at the outset if they are to succeed. While it is

rarely admitted, the nurse should appreciate the fact that a patient has the right not to change. Patients are put under such societal pressure to follow our rational regimens that they often feel they must at least pretend to agree with them. As most nurses know, patients who say yes in the hospital may act out NO! in their home environment.

Through the teaching of health professionals and the programming of the mass media, the American public has been made aware of many coronary risk factors: smoking, high-cholesterol diets, obesity, and sedentary living have been highly publicized and popularized. However, it may be that this zeal for "educating" has some unfortunate sequelae. The extent of misinformation and the degree of "cardiac anxiety" in the public approaches epidemic proportions. Whether this is due to the mixture of health information and advertizing campaigns or to less apparent sources of confusion is not known. It is apparent, however, that nurses must find out what patients think about their diseases and symptoms and work from there in presenting information and ways of intervention.

It should be emphasized that the so-called coronary risk factors often presented have not all been validated. Table 12-11 (p. 337) separates established hypotheses from those which are only partially supported at this point.

While Table 12-11 was published in 1968 and may, therefore, appear to be out of date, we wish to emphasize the point that the roles of exercise and stress as well as personality patterns are *not yet established,* despite the publicity they receive.

The nurse dealing with patients who have had symptoms of angina or evidence of coronary artery disease should emphasize the deleterious effects of smoking, high-cholesterol diets, and uncontrolled hypertension. She should also supply positive information regarding the benefits of moderate and consistent exercise, sensible eating patterns, and means of reducing tension. Giving information is not necessarily effective teaching. The individual needs also to exchange his view of his illness, to have help in formulating a plan for reducing his coronary risk that is "cus-

TABLE 12-10
Chemotherapeutic Agents for the Relief of Pain Due to Myocardial Ischemia

AGENT	PRINCIPAL EFFECTS	DOSAGE	MAJOR PRECAUTIONS AND SIDE EFFECTS
Coronary Vasodilators			
Nitroglycerin	Coronary and cerebral vasodilatation.	1 sublingually	Frequently accompanied by headaches. Tachyphalaxis occurs.
Amyl nitrite	Some systemic vasodilatation occurs with all these drugs.	Ampule held under the nose.	Some patients complain of dizziness.
Peritrate (penta-erythrityl tetra-nitrate	Beta-adrenergic blockade allows reflex vasodilatation.	10 mg q.i.d. p.o.	Cross tolerances develop.
Inderal (propranolol) beta receptor blocking agent	Used for intractable angina. Relief may be provided from blocked perception of pain or reduction in myocardial metabolic needs.		Myocardial depressant. Not used in heart block or heart failure.
Isordil (isosorbide dinitrate)			
Sedatives			
Chloral hydrate	Sedatives promote rest and decrease heart work.	0.5 Gm hs. p.o.	All sedatives may be habituating. Barbiturates are particularly so.
Phenobarbital		¼ gr g. 4 hr. p.o.	
Tranquilizers			
Valium (diazepam) Librium (chlordiazepoxide)	Reduction of anxiety promotes rest. Relief of apprehension is direct.	5-10 mg q.i.d. p.o. 5-10 Gm q.i.d. p.o.	The tranquilizers may be habituating. Tachyphylaxis occurs.
Analgesics			
Morphine	Analgesics relieve pain, thereby decreasing apprehension, stress, and heart work.	Dosages to equal morphine 8-5 mg s.c. p.r.n.	All narcotic analgesics may be addicting and are respiratory depressants. The synthetic narcotics tend to decrease blood pressure. Nausea and vomiting may occur especially in upright positions.
Dilaudid (hydromorphone)		2 mg s.c., I.M. or p.o.	
Levo-Dromoran		2 mg s.c., I.M. or p.o.	
Prinadol (phemazocine) Demerol (meperidine)		2 mg I.M. or p.o. 75-150 mg s.c. or I.M.	
Nisentil (alphaprodine)		40-60 mg s.c.	

TABLE 12-11
Coronary Risk Factors

ESTABLISHED RISK FACTORS	POSTULATED RISK FACTORS
Hypercholesterolemia: 250 mg/100 ml (including lipoproteinemia and increased blood triglyceruide levels).	Hyperuricemia. Decreased vital capacity. Thyroid dysfunction (hypothyroidism predisposes to atherosclerosis; hyperthyroidism causes increased cardiac work.)
Hypertension: diastolic pressure over 95 mm/Hg before the sixth decade.	
Cigarette smoking.	
Diabetes.	Renal disease.
Overweight: weight 110% over normal.	Sedentary living.
Family history of premature death from heart disease (under age 60).	Personality patterns (high degree of drive, overly ambitious).
ECG abnormalities: bundle branch block, L. ventricular hypertrophy, and other changes indicative of ischemia or strain.	Diet high in calories, total fat content, cholesterol, saturated fats, refined carbohydrates, and salt.*

*The diet may be considered a major risk factor because it could contribute to obesity, hypertension, hyperlipidemia, and diabetes.
From: Stamler, J., et al. Coronary risk factors. *Med. Cl. N. Am.* 50:229-254, 1968. Used with permission.

tom fitted," and to have support through the difficulties of changing basic patterns. Not the least of the positive health habits to be established is that of having regular medical checkups. People will tend to make and keep such appointments when they feel it is in their best interests to do so. Obviously, there is a great need for health teaching in this area.

In summary, the principles basic to teaching and counseling the patient and his family about coronary heart disease are derived from three sources:

1. Knowledge of the coronary risk factors in general and for a given individual.
2. Understanding of factors which increase heart work and sensible alternatives for reducing the increase.
3. Knowledge of the person to be taught, his life style, and how he views it.

Currently, surgical amelioration of coronary heart disease has become common. For a brief discussion of this relatively new procedure, see pp. 343 to 346.) Since the care necessary for the patient who undergoes myocardial revascularization is derived from the same general principles involved in all cardiac care, we will first discuss myocardial infarction and then cardiac surgery and the nursing care of patients who undergo it.

MYOCARDIAL INFARCTION
The ultimate result of recurrent myocardial ischemia is usually permanent myocardial damage—a myocardial infarction. Local tissue changes in the infarcted area include sudden loss of contractility, necrosis of myocardial fibers, and congestion, hemorrhage, and edema in the connective tissue stroma. An area around the infarct also demonstrates loss of contractility. In this marginally deprived zone there appears to be enough to permit normal functioning. The prompt administration of oxygen in conjunction with analgesic and other methods of work reduction may prevent subsequent permanent damage to this area.

The emphases for the nursing care needed for the patient who has just suffered a myocardial infarction are: assessment, prompt intervention in the case of increasing pathology, assistance to the patient to help conserve his energy, and maintenance of optimal cardiac function. The patient's family is often in great need of attention during such a crisis. The nurse can do a great deal to allay their apprehension and to set the stage for a supportive family visit to the patient.

One of the greatest challenges to the nurse is dealing with the overriding sense of doom presented by many patients and their families. "Everything will be all right," is not always a reassuring statement and it is never enough. Even if the physician does not want to inform the patient of what has occurred, the nurse can allay apprehension by explaining the protective features of the patient's environment. She can also help him regain his sense of control by explaining how he can participate in his treatment and his recovery. Although the nurse must help to allay fear and apprehension, she must also be aware that building false hopes may undermine the patient's confidence in her. She should also remember that the patient will probably be encouraged to modify his life style in the future and that he will undergo some rather onerous restrictions during his hospitalization. For a patient to be motivated to cooperate in his treatment, he must have some understanding of the seriousness of his condition and the relationship of his treatment regimen to his welfare. Therefore, it is not wise to share in pretending that everything is all right. Although it is difficult, we must neither build false hopes nor undermine denial if that is the only defense the patient can muster.

If there are no contraindications imposed by the patient's behavior, the physician's plan of treatment, or institutional policies, the nurse may wish to share the information regarding an MI—what it is and what it means—with the patient and his family. He should be briefly informed of the plan of care for him and the reasons for it. During this time, any objections the patient has or any other source of modifications to the usual course of treatment can be worked out. It is usually reassuring to patients to know that they will be watched carefully and that the frequency of monitoring is a routine rather than an indication that they are becoming more sick. Most patients respond well to information about the ways in which they can help themselves to recover: by resting as much as possible, by allowing the staff to help them, and by alerting the staff to their feelings and general needs. The nurse may help a patient feel more relaxed by inquiring about any imperative matters that need to be taken care of at home or at work and then facilitating the process.

Since one of the most serious sequelae of a myocardial infarction is an extension of the ischemic area, we will present a functional grouping of the signs and symptoms of an infarction as presented by Rushmer.[44] This grouping is also helpful in distinguishing between anginal pain and an infarction. For the patient with chronic angina pectoris, this marks the difference between supplying his medication and alerting the medical staff.

I. Pain
    *When the pain reported by a patient who has angina is not relieved by the usual amount of medication, or if it is of more severe intensity or of more ominous quality than that which the patient usually experiences, the physician should be alerted.

II. Autonomic effects
    Pallor
    Sweating
    Tachycardia *or* bradycardia
    Hypotension or other signs of impending shock
    Syncope
    Vomiting
    Disturbed sensorium

III. Effects resulting from diminished myocardial contractility
    A. "Congestive heart failure"
        1. Left ventricular failure
            Dyspnea
            Othopnea
            Cough
            *Hemoptysis
        2. Right ventricular failure
            Peripheral congestion
            Enlarged, tender liver
            Edema
            Cyanosis
    B. Cardiac signs
        Weak heart tones
        Gallop rhythm
        Systolic murmers
        Pulsus alternans
        Ventricular enlargement
        paradoxical pulse
        Pericardial friction rub
        ECG alterations

*C. Shock
    Cold, clammy skin
    Hypotension (compared to patient's norm)
    Tachycardia
    Oliguria
    Disturbed sensorium

---

*Writer's additions

The above outline also indicates a sequence of events that frequently occurs after a myocardial infarction and which may contribute to the extension of the infarcted area. The loss of myocardial contractility which inevitably follows a myocardial infarction often leads to decompensation of the heart because it can not meet the systemic demands for nutrients. Although bradycardia may occur initially, it is usually followed by compensatory tachycardia. Shock is a frequent complication.

Pain is usually the first symptom of a myocardial infarction. It is usually followed by the signs of autonomic response. These signs—pallor, sweating, and vomiting—are often partly a result of the emotional as well as the physical impact of the experience. Syncope, or disorientation, reflects both the emotional reaction and the diminished cardiac output which result in poor cerebral perfusion. Peripheral resistance may decrease due to the reflex vagal hypertonicity, further compromising tissue perfusion.

In addition to the preceding effects of an infarction, arrhythmias often occur. The hyperirritable state of the ventricles often leads to life-threatening arrhythmias such as ventricular fibrillation. Coronary care units were first established to detect and treat such arrhythmias. They have made a significant impact in reducing the mortality rate from arrhythmias *for hospitalized patients*. Since so many people die before they reach the hospital, some communities are teaching ambulance attendants to detect and treat life-threatening arrhythmias as a first aid procedure.

The major classes of chemotherapeutic agents which are traditionally utilized for patients with myocardial infarctions have been dis-

cussed previously (see Tables 12-9 and 12-10). Here we will briefly discuss the use of anticoagulant therapy.

The use of anticoagulants for the treatment of patients after a myocardial infarction has been controversial for two reasons: 1) It has been documented that many persons who suffer myocardial ischemia do not have thrombi[45] and the available preparations are known not to dissolve formed clots anyway. 2) Anticoagulants impose iatrogenic hazards on people which some physicians feel are not outweighed by demonstrable benefits.[46] It is readily apparent to nursing practitioners that some physicians feel that the use of anticoagulants is justified, at least for some patients. It appears that fewer patients are put on long-term anticoagulant therapy, but many are heparinized for the period immediately following the infarction. Some patients are retained on heparin therapy while others are gradually switched to an oral anticoagulant.

Heparin is usually administered for initial anticoagulation. It may be given subcutaneously or intravenously, but due to the speed of action that is desired and the local tissue reaction to subcutaneous injection, the intravenous route appears currently to be more commonly ordered. Heparin acts directly to neutralize the thrombin and to inhibit factors IX and XI. The desirable level of the drug is assessed by the Lee-White clotting time. The action of intravenously administered heparin is nearly immediate. The dose is usually calculated on the basis of body weight. Should severe bleeding occur, the antidote is protamine sulfate. The latter is given intravenously in a dose that matches the dose of heparin, milligram for milligram *if the bleeding occurs within a half hour after the heparin was given.* Heparin has a short half-life; the nurse should remember that in relation to giving the medication on time. Failure to do so entails the risk of a rebound phenomenon and is a great hazard to the patient. Since the duration of action of heparin is so short, the dosage of the antidote is reduced by half if hemorrhage occurs after a half hour has elapsed. It has been found that the most dangerous side effects of protamine sulfate occur from too rapid infusion. It is suggested by Goodman and Gilman that no more than 10 mg per 5 minutes to be given and that no more than 100 mg be given unless there is certain knowledge that more is required to neutralize the heparin. The patient should be watched for signs of bradycardia and hypotension during a protamine infusion. If they occur, the physician should be notified immediately.[47]

Oral anticoagulants require 24 to 48 hours before adequate blood levels are usually attained. The dosages of these agents are highly individualized and the effects are assessed with the use of the prothrombin time. Should an antidote be required, aquaMEPHYTON is administered intravenously. The dosage range is between 10 and 50 mg, depending on the dosage of the anticoagulant that was given.

All anticoagulant therapies require that the patient be closely observed for bleeding. In addition, there are several frequently used drugs which interact with anticoagulants to produce synergistic or antagonistic effects. The nurse should be alert to the possibility of an inadvertent prescription and should teach the patient not to take the following drugs without his physician's specific directions. The oral contraceptives and some sedatives such as the barbiturates, chloral hydrate, and glutethimide have an antagonistic effect to that of some anticoagulants. Salicylates, tolbutamide, phenylbutazone, indomethacin and many other drugs potentiate or act synergistically to them.

In conclusion, we wish to summarize our statements regarding the supportive and teaching aspects for the patient after a myocardial infarction. In the acute phase, the emphasis should be on close observation and on the provision of rest and comfort measures. We do *not* find intervention in denial or systematic attempts to teach the patient useful at this time. Instead, supplying information that is asked for and that directly relates to the patient's care is usually enough. The critically ill patient does not retain much of the information given right after admission. His senses are so bombarded with stimuli and his anxiety level so high that he is particularly vulnerable to the distortion of information. Therefore, information of a supporative nature is most

helpful. The nurse will probably find that she will have to repeat explanations given earlier as the patient attempts to understand the meaning of what has happened to him. There is time later in the patient's hospitalization to develop a plan of teaching. By this time also, there will have been an opportunity to assess the patient's coping mechanisms, his general reaction to the illness, and his assets and limitations relative to rehabilitation. All of the preceding factors should be considered in the processes of teaching and counseling.

CARDIAC TRAUMA

Accidental Cardiac Trauma

Wounds of the heart caused by accidents are generally of two types: 1) those in which the heart has been penetrated by a foreign object, such as a bullet or a knife; and 2) those resulting from an impact to the chest such as a blast injury or an impact with the steering column of an automobile. In the latter case, the heart is bruised against the rib cage by the force of the impact.

The bruised heart may bleed into the pericardial sac to the extent that the pressure of the blood in the small space impinges on the heart. Having less musculature, the great veins are most vulnerable to compression. The result is reduced cardiac filling and, consequently, reduced cardiac output that may lead to shock. A "classic" sign of pericardial tamponade is a reduced pulse pressure. Patients with trauma to the chest should be watched closely for this as well as for muffled heart sounds, falling blood pressure, and signs of cardiovascular decompensation (shock). The treatment of such a patient may consist of a pericardial tap or surgery for cardiac suturing, depending on the estimated amount and severity of hemorrhage.

Penetrating wounds of the heart, although they may be amenable to surgical repair, are particularly dangerous due to the rapid exsanguination that may occur and the disorders of the heart beat they often produce. If the patient lives long enough to get to surgery, repair of the torn muscle is usually possible.

Cardiac tamponade and ventricular rupture are also complications of a myocardial infarction. The treatment is essentially the same as that outlined above, but the patient suffers increased risks due to his underlying condition.

"CARDIAC" SURGERY

There are many more similarities than differences in the nursing care of the "medical" cardiac patient and the "surgical" cardiac patient. The act of surgery, although it is ostensibly therapeutic, imposes a trauma to the heart. The nurse must add the principles of care of the surgical patient to those applicable to any patient with cardiac disease; then all of these must be modified to meet the needs of the particular individual to be cared for.

The most far-reaching distinction in the various forms of cardiac surgery that is important to the nurse, is whether or not the patient required extracorporeal circulation during surgery.

Intracardiac Surgery

With the exception of some mitral commissurotomies, intracardiac surgery requires the use of a cardiopulmonary bypass technique. Several of the complications patients experience are a direct result of having extracorporeal circulation. We will discuss three of the machines so that the reader may appreciate their complexity as well as the common processes through which the blood is treated. Any of these may cause postsurgical complications. The pumping mechanism, which so often traumatizes cells, is crucial to the maintenance of tissue perfusion.

The blood is first pumped into some kind of oxygenator (Fig. 12-14). Although several types of oxygenators exist (screen, film, membrane, and variations on each type) each damages the blood cells which travel through it to some extent. Figure 12-15 illustrates the problems which arise from the destruction of the various blood components. In addition, there is the possibility of anemia and a compensatory increase in cardiac work. While the latter is readily treated, the nurse must observe the patient in order to pick up the early signs.

Blood reactions are another potential source of problems to the patient undergoing cardiac surgery. Pump-oxygenators vary in the amount they require for priming. Some of the larger models require as many as 15 to 20 units of blood. A mixture of these units remains in the patient's body after surgery. We have not yet perfected matching techniques for all of the blood components. Both of these facts lead to more rapid hemolysis of donor blood.

The kidneys are particularly vulnerable to damage under conditions of an increased rate of hemolysis. If hemolysis results from a reaction to foreign proteins, it will be almost immediate. If it is due to the decreased life of transfused cells which then die off over a shorter period of time, or to cellular damage from the pump, it will occur postoperatively, and increase over a period of several days. The nurse is most likely to observe the patient who is suffering excessive cell death of donated blood because of the time element stated. The patient who becomes jaundiced, easily fatigued and who reports dark-colored urine is likely to be experiencing massive hemolysis which should be reported at once. When massive hemolysis occurs, the liver cannot possibly process all of the liberated hemoglobin. The hemoglobin may remain free in the bloodstream until it reaches the capillaries of the glomeruli. There it precipitates in the tubules and causes obstructions. Acute renal failure may result.

In addition to potential renal damage, the patient will be anemic and, depending on the extent of damage, could develop the shock syndrome. The usual medical therapy consists of the administration of isotonic saline and mannitol. The fluid helps increase the glomerular filtration rate and mannitol produces an osmotic diuresis which helps prevent precipitation and sludging of the hemoglobin. Depending on the patient's hemoglobin level, he may also receive blood or packed cells. He should receive very close monitoring by the nurse at this time. We should emphasize the fact that the kidney is also extremely vulnerable to a diminished blood flow and the heart to an increased workload, both of which may occur under these circumstances. Accurate observation of urine output is mandatory!

The threat to the lungs during extracorporeal circulation is an additional problem for many patients, as is the effect of anesthesia which may be

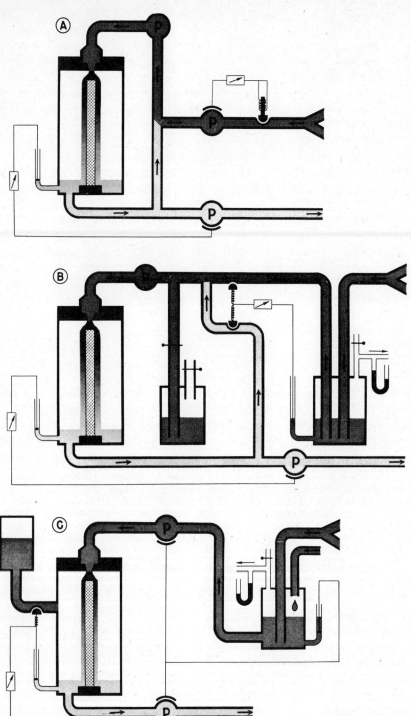

FIGURE 12-14.

Blood circuit schemes in various stationary screen oxygenators (screen symbolized by diagonal crosshatching in rectangular box on left of each scheme).

(A) Gibbon's original oxygenator. The venous line includes a segment of soft resilient tubing provided with a diameter-sensing device based on the principle of the differential transformer. If the venous pump generates too much suction, fluttering of the soft rubber tube actuates an electrical circuit which slows down the pump before actual caval collapse occurs. The recirculation pump (top P) is set at a constant flow rate which is always higher than that of the venous and arterial pumps. Thus, there is always an upward flow of blood in the recirculating line (vertical connection between arterial and venous line). The rate of arterial pumping is automatically controlled by a level-sensing device in the collecting chamber, which tends to maintain a constant volume of blood in the extracorporeal circuit (electrical circuit acting on pump P, lower right).

(B) Gibbon-Mayo oxygenator. Venous blood is transferred in a closed reservoir by the action of a controlled vacuum. The recirculation pump, set at a constant flow rate, aspirates, in varying proportions, blood from the venous arterial lines in such a way that the levels in the venous reservoir and in the oxygenator remain constant.

(C) Oxygenator described by Greisser (1958). Venous and coronary return are obtained by a controlled vacuum. The venous pump serves solely to transfer blood from the venous reservoir into the artificial lung. The output of both the venous and arterial pumps is under the control of level-sensing devices in the venous reservoir and in the artificial lung. Source: Galletti, P. M. and Brecher, G. A.: Heart-Lung Bypass. New York, Grune and Stratton, 1962, p. 84. Used by Permission.

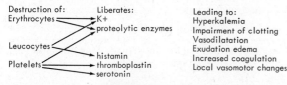

FIGURE 12-15.
Physiologically active substances which can be liberated by destruction of formed blood elements in an extracorporeal unit. Source: Adapted from Galletti, P. M. and Brecher, G. A.: Heart-Lung Bypass. New York, Grune and Stratton, 1962, p. 271.

administered for a relatively long period of time. The effect of the pump is thought to be related to a decrease in pulmonary compliance and to changes in surfactant (the surface tension of the alveoli). To aid the compromised respiratory system, most patients receive oxygen and some form of mechanical ventilation after surgery.

Patients who appear well oxygenated and ventilated may receive intermittent therapy with a pressure-controlled ventilator. Others, who have evidence of reduced pulmonary compliance and/or pulmonary hypertension prior to surgery or those who decompensate during the immediate postsurgical period, are likely to have tracheotomies. Volume-controlled respirators have several advantages for these patients. They provide for full ventilation despite the natural tendency to "splint" the chest against full inspiration which is often painful. The nurse may help the patient by the judicious use of analgesia and by reporting any signs that the machine has not been properly set for the patient. (See Chapter 14 for a more detailed discussion of the nursing care required.) We feel, however, that many of the patient's problems with ventilatory assistance can be prevented by thorough preparation prior to surgery. This preparation should include practice in the techniques of deep breathing and coughing.

The heart itself and the blood vessels may also suffer from the effects of surgery. Many operations require cessation of the heartbeat. Cannulations of the vessels and clamping inevitably traumatize them. If they are friable, either insidious bleeding or dramatic rupture may occur. Therefore, chest drainage supplies an index of cardiovascular integrity as well as the maintenance of negative thoracic pressures. Measurement of drainage and observations for patency of the drainage system are most important for the patient's welfare.

The last and most generalized trauma imposed during surgery occurs from the necessity of cutting into the body. Through the surgery itself, maintenance of vital systems (such as chest drainage, IV therapy and tracheotomies) and monitoring devices, the patient is susceptible to infections from several portals. Temperature elevations should be watched closely. They may yield information about the locale of an infection. They also impose an increased cardiac workload. Very early elevations may be a reaction to the profound hypothermia which the patient underwent. However, pulmonary infections can develop in a very short time. They should be ruled out even in the first postoperative day. The second common source of infection is the urinary bladder. Temperature elevations usually occur after 48 hours and tend to be low grade. Wound infections develop most slowly. They are rarely demonstrable in less than five days. A chronic, low-grade infection beginning well into the recovery phase may signal the onset of "postpericardotomy syndrome." Table 12-12 provides a summary of specific kinds of cardiac surgery.

Myocardial Revascularization

It is estimated that of the nearly one million people who sustain myocardial infarction each year, nearly one-half die, and one-half of these never reach the hospital.[48]

A nationwide pilot program is now underway to reduce this figure. Training courses for some police, firemen, and a new professional group called, "emergency medical technicians" who can then render cardiopulmonary resuscitation, provide cardiovascular support or difibrillate patients *at the scene* are now instituted in several cities.

For those who reach the hospital, improved coronary care, inseparable from the development and proliferation of coronary care units, has reduced the mortality rate from nearly 30 percent to approximately 15 percent.[49] The un-

TABLE 12-12
Common Types of Open-Heart Surgery in the Adult and Attendant Complications

Mitral commissurotomy	Systemic embolism; traumatic mitral incompetence. (May be done with or without extracorporeal circulation.)
Mitral prosthesis	Systemic embolism; sepsis, prosthetic dislodgement and thrombosis.
Aortic prosthesis for stenosis or insufficiency	Generally the same risks. Prosthesis may be more prone to thrombus formation because of increased turbulence. Also increased force increases the risk of displacement.
Aortic valve homografts for stenosis	General operative risks. In addition, rejection responses. Fewer problems from thrombotic and hemorrhage phenomena.
Congenital Defects in Adults Atrial septal defects Tetralogy of Fallot Ventricular septal defects Pulmonary stenosis Patent ductus arteriosis	Severe pulmonary hypertension leads to increased risk in most patients. Other risks are attendant upon cardiac surgery in general.

fortunate people who are represented in the latter statistic usually die from shock or "power failure" of the heart.

The mortality rate of patients who never reach treatment has given rise to emphasis on both primary and secondary prevention of coronary artery disease (see pp. 333 to 337). Myocardial revascularization, since it is usually performed after the appearance of severe angina pectoris combined with a history of infarction or other such factors or in recent treatment of myocardial infarction, may be considered as a means of secondary, or (in the last instance because it attempts to prevent shock and/or death) tertiary prevention.

Surgical treatment for pronounced and incapacitating coronary artery thrombosis was first clinically utilized by Vineburg almost three decades ago.[50] Since then, the idea that myocardial revascularization constitutes an efficacious treatment for people suffering from coronary artery insufficiency as well as a prophylactic measure against myocardial infarction has received widespread recognition. (Such surgery was performed for an estimated 25,000 patients in 1973). Subsequently, several methods of improving the blood supply to the myocardium have been advocated and a large number of people have undergone some form of surgical myocardial revascularization techniques.[51] A more recently developed procedure features a form of grafting

with a saphenous vein with carbon dioxide gas endarterectomy of the coronary arteries.[52] Less popular have been attempts to promote better coronary circulation by "medical" means: combinations of pharmacological therapy and advocation of judicious exercise and "more healthy" living habits.[53] These therapies have been directed toward promoting circulation through the existing vasculature (coronary vasodilators and the like) and promoting the development of collateral circulation (exercise programs). The prevention of further atherosclerotic formations by dietary modification, physical fitness, and, in some cases, anticoagulants or experimental agents designed to lower serum cholesterol levels have also been attempted.[54]

The original Vineburg procedure consisted of freeing a portion of omentum (without interrupting its blood supply) and wrapping it around the anterior portion of the ventricles after they had been denuded of epicardium.[55] Collateral vessel formation soon penetrated into the myocardium under ideal conditions. Currently, two other surgical methods of improving myocardial circulation are more frequently practiced.

A second type of procedure entails using autogenous graft (usually a length of saphenous vein turned inside out) which may be anastomosed to the thoracic aorta and inserted into a tunnel formed in the posterior left ventricle.[56] Alternatively, the length of vein may be anastomosed to a still potent portion of coronary artery and a distal portion of the left or circumflex coronary arteries thus bypassing narrowed or impotent portions of coronary artery.

Third, the left internal mammary artery may be used as a pedicle graft and implanted in the myocardium or anastomosed to existing vasculature supplying the ventricle to bypass nonpotent or compromised vessels. This method appears to be used most frequently at present.[57] Patients are subjected to less surgical trauma, are under anesthesia for less time, and have the advantage of only one anastomosed site. The latter consideration is particularly important since the most frequent immediate complication of this surgery is bleeding and the hazards to the patient of pro-

longed time under extracorporeal circulation and anesthesia have been reviewed.

The indications considered by surgeons to warrant surgical myocardial revascularization have been extended over the past five years. They now include not only patients with "intractable" angina and demonstrable coronary insufficiency (usually demonstrated by coronary angiography) with symptoms of impending myocardial infarction, but also patients who have recently suffered overt myocardial infarction and those who are undergoing cardiac valve prosthesis insertions. Myocardial revascularization has also been performed in conjunction with other forms of treatment for patients suffering cardiac arrest or cardiogenic shock (Fig. 12-16).

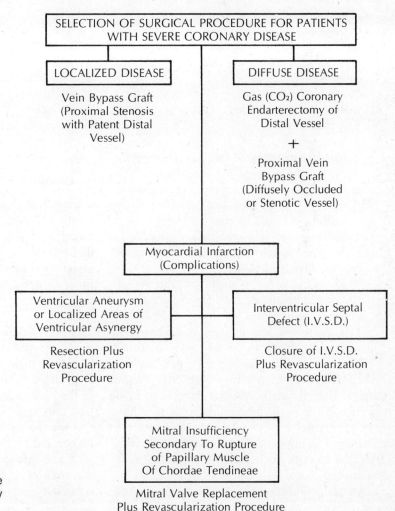

FIGURE 12-16.
Selection of surgical procedure for patients with severe coronary disease.

The reported success (in terms of improved patient function and low operative or perisurgical mortality) of revascularization is extremely varied. Obviously, factors such as general health of the candidate, extent of coronary artery disease and presurgical preparation have a great deal to do with the outcome. Other factors depend on the extensiveness of the surgery and the expertise of the surgical team. The third factor influential in patient recovery is postoperative care; in this area, the nurse may be most influential.

The nursing care of these patients has been generally reviewed. Specific care will depend on the procedure the patient underwent (e.g., extracorporeal circulation or not; saphenous vein removal or not, and so on.) There are, however, specific risks associated with the procedures of which the nurse should be aware:

1. Patients may have received curare; all autonomic innervation will be suspended until it is reversed or metabolized (patients are, therefore, more prone to shock).
2. Patients will usually be receiving mechanical respiratory assistance through endotracheal tubes or a tracheotomy.
3. Patients are particularly prone to extreme shifts of blood pressure and to cardiac arrhythmias.
4. Patients have received heparized donor blood and should be watched for posttransfusion reactions, bleeding, and the usual signs of depressed pulmonary or renal function.
5. Patients will receive extensive pharmalogical support and monitoring, each of which carries hazards already discussed.
6. Perisurgical cases of death include emboli, myocardial infarction, and "power failure."
7. "Late" causes of death include pulmonary emboli, septicemia, hepatitis, myocardial infarction, and cardiac failure.[58]

Obviously, despite every precaution, myocardial revascularization represents a major surgical risk. Recently charges have been made that it is being performed on patients who have not been treated by more conservative means in an attempt to improve their conditions. Considering the risks of such surgery, a public outcry has ensued.

Another factor currently receiving widespread attention is the demonstrated graft closures which may occur within a few months. The return of symptoms *does not* always accompany graft closures. One can only speculate that the reason is enhanced collateral circulation or that it rests with subjective elements.

It is quite obvious that several constraints are important with respect to imposing surgical risks. Foremost is the necessary condition that the anticipated benefits to the patient should outweigh tha probable risks. Second, the privilege to perform such surgery should be limited to experienced and otherwise qualified surgical teams who operate in settings with adequate personnel and facilities. Third, nurses should contribute to preventive measures which could diminish the necessity of such procedures and its attendant risks.

Nurses care for patients. That care may include the pre- or postoperative patient. However, if more attention were paid to the primary and secondary aspects of prevention by all types of health care providers, it is doubtful that nurses would need to deploy so many of their resources to the acute situation. We advocate that nurses set an example in this respect.

Cardiogenic Shock

Cardiogenic shock results from factors which directly decrease the ability of the heart to pump blood; the most common of which are myocardial infarction, congestive heart failure and persistent major arrhythmias. The term "power failure" actually reflects the poor perfusion of the coronary vessels which is the precipitating factor in most forms of myocardial inefficiency. The precipitating factor to the shock state is the resultant reduced ability to pump the blood which in turn results in poor tissue perfusion. Poor tissue perfusion to vital organs often results in the vicious cycle of progressive decompensation illustrated in Figure 12-17. Mortality statistics for the patient in profound shock approach 90 percent.[59]

Cardiogenic shock is a complication in approximately 15 percent of patients *who are treated* for myocardial infarction and precedes

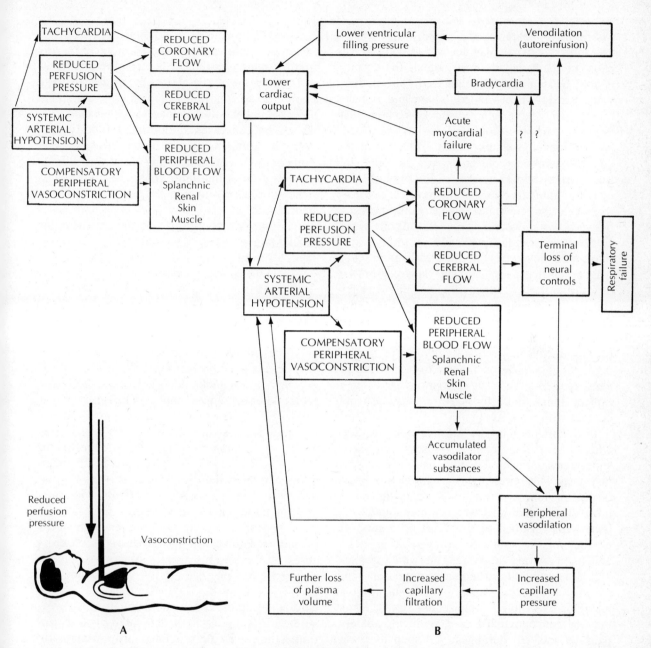

FIGURE 12-17.
Systemic arterial hypotension with vicious cycles. (A) Effects of systemic arterial hypotension, including reduced coronary and cerebral blood flow as well as peripheral blood flow through important visceral organs. (B) Vicious cycles in terminal circulatory collapse. Severe and prolonged hypotension can induce vicious cycles which tend to further depress cardiac output or to induce vasodilation rendering the hypotension progressively more intractable.

"congestive heart failure," many arrythmias, and surgery as a cause of death.[60] Obviously, the cause of deaths which occur outside the hospital cannot be definitively established. The patient, who by history is presumed to have had a "heart attack," may have suffered shock as a complication of the insult. About one third of the treated patients develop shock within six hours of the onset of symptoms, one half within 24 hours, and two thirds within 35 hours. An additional 13 percent are "late reactors," and develop shock after one week; the remaining one fifth fall somewhere between two days and one week.[61] While shock is an understandably dreaded complication, those who develop symptoms early fare somewhat better than those who are "late reactors" in terms of mortality. However, since there are few survivors of profound shock, it is obvious that the key to better patient care lies in early detection and treatment. Patients must be treated before poor tissue perfusion results in further myocardial damage or damage to other vital organs. Nurses have a key role in the early detection of shock since they are in more constant contact with patients.

The patients who are most at risk are those who have had large infarctions (shock rarely supervenes until about 40 percent of the myocardial tissue is disabled), those who have a previous history of myocardial damage, or those who have other conditions which either demand an increased workload of the heart or reduce the efficacy of the systemic compensating mechanisms.[62] Among the conditions which demand greater heart work are endocrine conditions such as pheochromocytoma or myxedema, valvular insufficiencies, hypovolemia, and stress. Stress may be conceptualized as excitement, anxiety, pain, or internal derangements such as fever. The shock state itself results in increased heart rate (through the mediation of the sympathetic division of the autonomic nervous system). The increased work of the heart may jeopardize the "border zone" of marginally underperfused myocardium which initially surrounds the ischemic area. A vicious cycle of an increasing tissue need and a decreasing supply of oxygenated blood is set in motion.

Underlying conditions such as hypertension, congestive failure, and previous myocardial infarction decreases the cardiac reserve and leads to further myocardial injury under stress. Extra-cardiac conditions such as pre-existing diabetes, renal and liver damage, and, particularly, chronic lung diseases, undermine the body's attempt to compensate for underperfusion. Patients with these underlying conditions, who develop myocardial infarctions, are more likely to manifest shock and to fail to react to treatment.

The classical picture of the cardiogenic shock state includes:
1. Cold, clammy skin
2. Altered level of consciousness
3. Oliguria
4. Hypotension

There are three reasons that reliance on the classic picture is misleading. Low peripheral blood pressure, traditionally the most relied upon index of shock, is itself prone to three sources of error in terms of the quick and effective prevention of profound or decompensated shock. 1) Low blood pressure is a sign of *decompensation:* it occurs when the increase in vasomotor tone is no longer effective in implementing adequate perfusion pressures. 2) Low blood pressure is an index relative to the patient's norm; what is low for one patient is not for another. Patients with pre-existing hypertension may be decompensated at what appear to be normal or even high blood pressures. People who usually have blood pressures at the lower extremes of normal have a reduced safety margin in terms of the blood pressure reading itself. They usually have greater cardiac reserves as indicated by the low pressure. 3) Blood pressure as indicated by auscultation at the extremity is, at best, an approximation of the central perfusion pressures. Under the circumstances of increased vasomotor tones (which is most pronounced in the extremities) and a decreasing pulse pressure, the indirect peripheral reading is even less indicative of the effective blood pressure to the vital organs. Therefore, the patient may be dangerously underperfused before overt signs of hypotension as measured by the usual auscultatory methods occur.

The second problem in accepting the classic picture of shock occurs because all patients in shock, even all patients with shock arising from cardiac inefficiency, do not manifest the classic signs. In a study of 547 patients who had myocardial infarctions, 73 developed shock according to measures of their central perfusion pressures and their overall clinical picture. The findings with respect to the signs they manifested are shown in Table 12-13:

TABLE 12-13
Physical Findings in Patients with Cardiogenic Shock

PHYSICAL FINDINGS	PERCENTAGE OF PATIENTS
Skin:	
Cool and moist	87
Warm and dry	13
Brain:	
Normal mental status	46
Depressed (with confusion, lethargy, or agitation)	37
Frank coma	17
Urine Output:	
Oliguria (< 20 ml/hr)	71
Normal (> 20 ml/hr)	16
Anuria (None for > 1 hr.)	13
Pulmonary edema:	
None	54
Overt	46

S. Schedit, R. Ascheim and T. Killip: Shock after acute myocardial infarction. 26: 557. Am. J. Cardiol.

It is obvious that the nurse at the bedside must have the knowledge and skill to evaluate the *total* picture of patient status if she is to fulfill the role of alerting the physician to significant changes in the patient's condition. As an additional illustration of that point, it must be emphasized that shock is *not* necessarily associated with ar-

rhythmias. One cannot rely on the now common bedside monitor to detect shock in its early stages.

The last problem in detecting shock in its early stages has been discussed previously but deserves special emphasis: the classic signs occur when the body is at least on the verge of *decompensation*. Treatment is then already too late for many patients. The finding of oliguria, without concurrent hypotension, may indicate compensation mediated by an increase in ADH which acts on the renal tubules to effect a conservation of water. The production of renin (in response to baroreceptor stimulation and intrarenal sensors) acts to maintain renal perfusion by local vasoconstriction which raises the blood pressure within the arterial tree to maintain effective filtration pressures. Aldosterone also is instrumental in maintaining effective cell perfusion. By instigating the reabsorption of sodium, the blood becomes hyperosmotic tending to mobilize the shift of water from the interstitial compartment into the bloodstream. (Concurrent peripheral vasoconstriction exists in the case of dropping intra-arterial pressure so oliguria may exist without clinical hypotension demonstrable by indirect auscultatory methods.) When clinical hypotension is demonstrable, chances are that not only the vasoconstrictive compensation is falling, but that the kidney is reacting to insufficient perfusion and must subsequently fail in its effort to effect compensation. To reiterate: the patient has already progressed past the stage of effective compensation by the time the classic symptoms of shock appear. Figure 12-18 illustrates this point.

Meltzer suggests four methods for the early

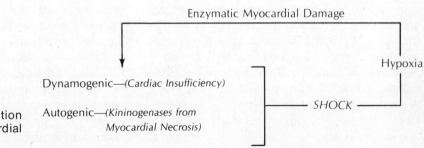

FIGURE 12-18.
Shock of myocardial infarction (double etiology of myocardial infarction shock).

detection of "power failure" which he considers nonintimidating:

1. Daily radiographic films: examination for the appearance of interstitial edema, increased heart size, and volume.
2. Physical examination by the nurse.
3. Circulation time (determined by an oxymeter on the ear which registers the time a dye—usually Evans Blue—takes to travel from the right atrium (after injection through the CVP catheter) to the right ear. The normal time is about eight seconds.
4. Continuous phonocardiography with assessment of the third and fourth sounds, the frequency of sounds and the time between electrical and mechanical systole.[63]

We will focus here on the physical assessment by the nurse because it should be a routine part of assessment by *any nurse*. The other methods will depend on the physician's philosophy and hospital facilities. However, the technique of phonocardiography is disputed by Weil and Shubin as a reliable index.[64] We question that it is nonintimidating.

There are four indices of the failing heart in addition to changes of rhythm and changes in the other areas of assessment of circulatory status. They include: 1) gallop rhythms and rates, 2) neck vein distention, 3) hepatojugular reflux, and 4) liver tenderness. Meltzer states that when these occur in conjunction with restlessness and increasing pulse, they are signs of incipient heart failure.[65] The patient should be closely observed and the physician alerted.

To avoid redundancy, we refer the reader to Chapter 13 for the pathophysiology of the shock state and the general nursing and medical care for patients in shock. Here, we will focus on the problem of the patient with cardiogenic shock as a basis for developing a model of nursing care and for discussing the alternatives of medical therapy in which the nurse may participate. However, it must be emphasized that the following materials make much more sense if they are understood on the basis provided by knowledge of normal functioning and the compensatory mechanisms of the body; particularly those most relevant to shock.

Cardiogenic shock differs from other forms in that it is not associated with the *loss* of body fluids, nor is it associated *initially* with the shift of fluids out of the vascular compartment, or with the loss of vasomotor tone. The primary problem lies with the heart's failure as a pump.

The several reactions of body mechanisms to restore what the body perceives as reduced effective blood pressures, are the same in all cases of shock. However, the effective reaction of the body defenses may not be possible, depending on the underlying cause of shock. In the case of shock precipitated by increased vascular capitance from the loss of vasomotor tone (which may occur from ganglionic blocking agents, high spinal anesthesia as in reaction to endotoxins or cellular metabolites) the vasoconstrictive compensatory mechanism is not effective. In the case of shock superimposed on an underlying pulmonary deficit, the hyperventilation observed in most patients in shock (which occurs in reaction to the lactic acidemia imposed by poor tissue perfusion) is not effective. These are just a few examples.

In the case of cardiogenic shock, heart damage is the precipitating factor in the development of hypotension. The stimulus to increased heart rate and force mediated through both the central and autonomic nervous system can only elicit effective cardiac compensation *if* the cardiac perfusion is adequate and *if* enough cardiac reserve exists to do the work without further damage. The generalized vasoconstrictive response further threatens the heart because it must exert more force to overcome increased peripheral resistance. Given these facts, the reader can see that the augmentation of a generalized vasoconstrictive response (as its maintenance) even if the coronary vessels are spared, is of doubtful therapeutic use because of the corresponding increase of heart work demanded of the already damaged myocardium. This fact, coupled with the failure of vasoconstrictive agents to effect a reduction of the death rate and their potent toxic effects have precipitated a great controversy regarding their use.[66] In addition, it has been documented that profound vasoconstriction existing over eight hours is incompatible with life.[67] These are major arguments against the use of

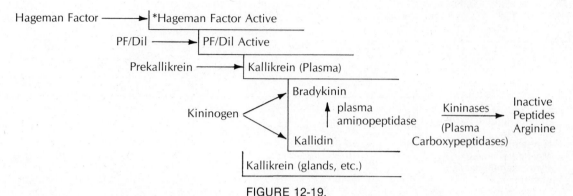

FIGURE 12-19.
Factors in the formation and destruction of plasma kinins, bradykinin, and kallidin.
*Hageman factor activated by various physical and chemical means.

vasopressors except in unusual cases or as an intermediate measure while cardiac efficiency is being augmented.

Since the major precipitating event in cardiogenic shock is myocardial damage, the goals of therapy are to: 1) protect the heart from further damage, 2) augment its function by whatever means are available, and 3) mobilize other compensatory mechanisms to improve tissue perfusion which will combat hypotension with (hopefully) no increase in heart work. In pragmatic terms, these goals are reflected in: 1) the reduction of external stress by the relief of pain, reassurances, sedation, and temperature moderation; 2) the use of inotropic drugs when indicated by reduced contractility, anti-arrhythmic agents when arrhythmias exist, and/or beta adrenergic blocking agents when the heart rate is too high to permit adequate filling and coronary perfusion; and 3) oxygen and IV fluids are used with caution. In experimental circumstances, glucagon is being used to improve the nutrient value of the blood which is delivered, thereby reducing the stimulation for increased heart work in conjunction with an attempt to raise the level of tissue perfusion.

Recent work postulates a second etiology pertinent to cardiogenic shock. It has been found that cardiac output is normal in 70 percent of patients with myocardial infarction, yet some of these patients also develop shock.[68] It is evident that other factors must be relevant to the instiga-

tion of the shock state. Several writers have discussed their search for naturally occurring hypotensive factors;[69] others have looked for a mechanism that produces the observable shift in fluid and electrolytes.[70]

A growing body of research demonstrates the significance of the plasma kinins in producing or augmenting cardiogenic shock.[71] Figure 12-19 portrays the relationship. These substances had already been implicated in shock precipitated by hemorrhage, trauma and anaphalactoid reactions. The plasma kinins of importance here are bradykinin and kallidin. Their precursors—kinogen and kallikrein—exist naturally in copious amounts. Plasma kinins may be activated under many circumstances, including cell necrosis, increased capillary permeability, and edema formation and evoke pain. The mechanism of pain production is thought to be by an effect—especially the effect of bradykinin—on the pain receptors (nocio receptors) which renders them more sensitive to ischemic damage. Kinins also act directly on smooth muscles to cause dilatation, an action not blocked by ganglionic blocking agents or atropine. Experimentation with the drug Trasylols (which inhibits the conversion of kallikrein to kallidin) has demonstrated the potent pain-producing effects and vasodilatation of these substances. The action of prostaglandins is also under investigation; they have a hypothesized role as vasodilators.[72]

Another substance investigated for the

TABLE 12-14
Effects and Uses of Sympathomimetic Drugs

	EFFECTIVE DOSES IN ADULT MAN (MG)	HEART RATE REFLEX ACTIVITY	
		NORMAL	BLOCKED
Epinephrine	0.5–1.0 s.c.	+ or −	+
Norepinephrine (Levarterenol)	0.002–0.008/min i.v. infusion	−	+
Ephedrine	15–50 s.c., i.m., 8–10/min i.v.	+ or −	+
Methamphetamine	10–30 i.v., i.m.	+or −	+
Mephentermine	10–30 i.v., i.m.	+ or −	+
Hydroxyamphetamine	5–10 i.v., 10–20 s.c.	+ or −	+
Metaraminol	5–10 i.v., i.m.	+ or −	+
Phenylephrine	0.5–1.0 i.v., 5–10 s.c.	−	0
Methoxamine	5–10 i.v., 10–20 i.m.	−	0 or −
Dopamine	100–1000 μg/hr i.v. drip	+	0
Isoproterenol	0.2 i.v., 0.5 i.m. 0.25 Solution as inhalant	+	?

0 no effect	Alpha activity (α receptors)	Beta activity (β receptors)	CNS—central nervous system
+ increased	A = Allergic reactions	B= Bronchodilator	O= Anorectic
− decreased	N= Nasal decongestion	C= cardiac	
N.A. not available	P= pressor (may include β activity)	M = muscle vessel dilatation	
	V= other local vasoconstriction		

treatment of patients in cardiogenic shock and refractory congestive failure is glucagon. Glucagon is supposed to be liberated by the alpha cells of the pancreas. Its "natural" action appears to be the stimulation of hepatic glycogenolysis and gluconeogenesis. However, large amounts stimulate the adrenal medulla to release catecholamines, the most prevalent of which, epinephrine, causes both some vasoconstriction and positive inotropic and chronatropic effects on the heart. In addition, glucagon stimulates the production of insulin. It has been used effectively in doses of 1 mg (IV, IM, or s.c.) in conjunction with IV glucose to reverse hypoglycemic states. A recent study employed glucagon as treatment in 50 patients, 40 of whom had refractory heart failure and/or cardiogenic shock.[73] It was felt that glucagon administered IV in doses of about 5 mg per hour (in 5 percent dextrose and combined with prochlorperazine to prevent nausea) had a definite role in improving the condition of myocardial depression and reversal of bradycardia in these patients. It is sometimes used adjunctively with traditional therapies.

The agent dopamine, an immediate precursor of epinephrine has passed the experimental stage and is now frequently employed in the treatment of patients with cardiogenic shock. It has a particular asset in that it dilates the splanchnic and renal arterials, thus better protecting those vital organs. In addition, it acts to stimulate the myocardium and increases cardiac output. It is an adrenoceptive agent and has some vasoconstrictive effects also.

Before discussing the wide array of drugs utilized in the therapy of these patients, it might be well to make the point that the sympathomimetic drugs may be visualized as a continuum (Table 12-14). All have some alpha and some beta stimulant properties; however, they range in activity from almost purely alpha effects—as in phenylephrine—to almost purely beta effects—as in isoproterenol. Another factor which influences their activity is their relative availability for action and the substances available to antagonize their action or to obliterate them. There are also differing numbers of alpha and beta receptors. The importance of visualizing the body as a system lies in implication of the concept of *system*. Through the use of feedback mechanisms, the body monitors and reacts to alterations in any one component of the system. The variety of subsystems and the rich supply of communication devices is fortunate for the normal individual but often detrimental under the impact of severe pathology. This complexity is

TABLE 12-14
Effects and Uses of Sympathomimetic Drugs (continued)

FORCE OF CARDIAC CONTRACTION		CARDIAC OUTPUT	CORONARY BLOOD FLOW	TOTAL PERIPHERAL RESISTANCE	BLOOD PRESSURE SYSTOLIC/ DIASTOLIC	MAIN CLINICAL USES		
SMALL DOSES	LARGE DOSES					α RECEPTOR ANAV	β RECEPTOR BCM	CNS O
+	+	+	+	−	+/−	A, P. V,	B, C,	
+	+	0 or −	+	+	+/+	P,		
+	−	+	+	+ or −	+/+	N, P,	B, C,	
+	−	+		0, +, or −	+/0	P,		CNS, O
+	−	+	+	+	+/+	N, P,		
+	−	+	+	+	+/+	N, P,	C,	
+	−	0 or −	+	+	+/+	P		
0	+	−	+	+	+/+	N, P		
0	−	0 or −	0	+	+/+	N, P		CNS, O
+	+	+	?	0	+/+	P		
+	+	+	0	−	0/−		BC	CNS

Compiled and amended from Tables 24-1 and 24-3 (pp. 485 and 506) in Goodman, L. S., and A. Gilman: *The Pharmacological Basis of Therapeutics,* ed. 4. New York: Macmillan Co., 1970. Used with permission.

the daily burden of both the researcher and the clinician.

Treatment of the patient in cardiogenic shock is first directed to the improvement of cardiac output. If cardiac decompensation has occurred, the patient is digitalized—digitalis may be used in conjunction with other agents—lidocaine, procaine amide (Pronestyl) or quinidine to control cardiac arrhythmias, and in some cases with isoproterenol (Isuprel), metaraminol (Aramine) or phenylephrine (Neo-synephrine) to improve vasomotor tone. The latter agents cause an increase in peripheral resistance and a concomitant increase in the necessary systolic ejection force. Consequently, therapy directed toward the alleviation of the underlying cause requires delicate adjustment between further fatiguing the heart and maintaining vital cell viability.

The second goal of treatment (which in the practical situation will probably be implemented concurrently) is directed toward augmenting compensatory mechanisms. The therapy consists of 1) oxygen administration which both better oxygenates the blood and reduces respiratory work; 2) positioning for maximal respiratory ease *and* protection of cerebral perfusion; and 3) in many cases—certainly if vasodilating agents are used—plasma volume expansion. The latter

therapy is usually monitored by the use of central venous pressure measurements. Readings above 15 cm/water indicate an inability of the heart to handle the increased volume load. Serial ECG recordings will probably be utilized if the patient is not continually monitored. Signs of increasing irritability are particularly relevant as are the appearance of U waves or dichrotic QRS complexes.

Nursing care in case of incipient or overt shock may be divided into four areas, the details of which have already been discussed:

1. Surveillance, assessment and judicious referral.
2. Support and reassurance of the patient with respect to the administration of any therapies for which orders have been written.
3. Preparation for and the assistance in delivering medical therapy.
4. Observation of the patient specifically for his reactions—improvement or toxic—to the therapies employed.

Of particular note following therapy are any indices of further cardiac decompensation because blood flow to the heart has diminished with the need for greater heart work. Hemoconcentration is another problem which occurs if cardiac shock (as well as several other types of shock) is allowed to progress. There is leakage of plasma into extravascular spaces. (It is felt that the increased venous pressure promotes the leakage.) In addition, the poorly nourished vascular walls may become more permeable. The increased viscosity of the blood predisposes the patient to thromboembolic episodes as well as increasing the workload. Elevated serum potassium occurs because of cell damage and may have a deleterious effect on the heart. Acidemia also occurs in the hypoxic state. There are many potentials for a vicious circle of decreasing cardiac efficiency as cardiogenic shock progresses. Blood coagulation time is prolonged, perhaps due in part to extravasation of blood proteins. Decreased metabolic processes occur initially and become progressively worse as the severity of tissue deprivation increases. Consumption coagulopathies also occur. The reasons for these changes are explained in more detail in Chapter 13.

Nurses may be most instrumental in alerting the physician specifically to patient responses to drug therapies. While some physicians advocate the utilization of alpha receptor antagonists, such as phenoxy-benzamine (Dibenzyline) for selected patients, others will administer a vasopressor agent such as levarterenol (Levophed) or metaraminol (Aramine). As previously stated, levarterenol is similar to norepinephrine. Metaraminol acts to release norepinephrine as well as having a direct pressor effect. Both agents are most effective in IV drips. The nurse must observe patients receiving these agents very closely. Blood pressure must be maintained at a level delicately balanced between maintenance of vital tissue perfusion and prevention of the undue cardiac stress which occurs from high doses of the alpha receptor antagonists (stimulators) which result in vasoconstriction. A second hazard to the patient is present if the drug is allowed to extravasate. Severe localized tissue sloughing will occur. In such a case, the nurse should notify a physician immediately and facilitate treatment by having antagonistic agents such as phentolamine (Regitine) or tolazoline (Priscoline) available for a local infiltration.

Since the majority of infarcts occur in the left ventricle, the resulting impairment frequently causes pulmonary congestion and right ventricu-lar failure. Initially the increased sympathetic activity usually allows the body to compensate and the patient remains normotensive. However, large infarctions damage the heart to the extent that the ventricles are so compromised in their function that compensation is incomplete at best. Such complications as extension of the area of infarction, arrhythmias, or ventricular rupture hasten the advent of shock and exaggerate its severity.

Several other conditions may precipitate myocardial injury and shock, but are less common than those discussed previously. They include pericardial tamponade, hemorrhagic pericarditis, ventricular aneurysms, myocardial neoplasms and valvular diseases. Pericardial tamponade and hemorrhagic pericarditis both impinge on the heart and restrict ventricular filling. Paradoxical pulses, an increasingly narrow pulse pressure and muffled, dull heart sounds are diagnostic signs. The nurse should be conscious of their increased risk after cardiac surgery, trauma to the chest, or, infrequently, massive myocardial infarction. Surgical intervention is usually necessary, either to remove the fluid or to repair the bleeding site. The pericardial sac may also need repair if a traumatic chest wound has occurred.

Ventricular aneurysms decrease the systolic ejection force. They jeopardize the patient's life because they may render him prone to shock and consequent death. In selective cases, successful resection of the aneurysm and myocardial grafting have been performed. Unless the aneurysm ruptures, the patient is likely to present signs and symptoms of increasing shock and requires extensive examination before the cause is apparent.

Chronic conditions such as valvular defects and myocardial tumors also may cause myocardial strain. Treatment of the underlying condition should be instituted long before shock occurs. Occasionally decompensation does occur rapidly and the patient needs emergency maintenance and immediate treatment of the underlying condition.

While the mortality rates for the patient in cardiogenic shock have not been appreciably diminished over the past decade, many avenues of research are being undertaken to change this. The emphasis in dealing with shock still must be on prevention. Coronary and/or cardiac care units are rapidly becoming more numerous, and the concept of coronary care which began as a small experiment has grown to a viable entity. Alone, these units cannot replace close and sensitive observation of cardiac patients which allows intervention in the earliest stages of shock or, ideally, before shock occurs, thereby reducing the mortality rates.

"NONCARDIAC" CAUSES OF REDUCED CARDIAC OUTPUT

Pulmonary embolism may also give rise to cardiogenic shock. The embolism obstructs the flow of blood to the left atrium, leading to a reduced output to the system. In addition, blood is backed up by the resistance to flow in the lung and right heart engorgement results; congestive failure of the right heart may ensue. Signs and symptoms of shock, chest pain, tachypnea (fast respiratory rate) hemoptysis, cyanosis, and increased venous pressure are suggestive of pulmonary embolism and pulmonary edema.

After pulmonary angiography to localize the clot, the patient may have to undergo an embolectomy. Medical treatment includes the provisions for optimal oxygenation and dilatation of the bronchial tree and vasculature. Vasopressors are also frequently used to maintain systemic tissue perfusion. Morphine may be ordered to reduce pain and to decrease respiratory work; however, its respiratory depressant effect may preclude its use in some patients. Although heparin will not resolve the existing clot, its use is indicated when a predisposing condition such as thrombophlebitis, phlebothrombosis or traumatic injuries—especially of the pelvis or legs—exists.

Hypoxia, in addition to causing certain metabolic derangements, leads to chemical imbalances and acidemia. Increased vascular permeability and the reduction of blood volume may result. Starvation or diabetes mellitus may directly decrease cardiac contractility, thereby decreasing the cardiac output. Thyrotoxicosis also

jeopardizes the heart because it increases the need for cardiac output beyond the cardiac reserves. In all cases, treatment of the underlying condition prevents the possibility of shock.

Hyperinsulinism produces insulin shock. Its counterpart, hypoinsulinism, also presents "shocklike" signs. This apparent contradiction is explicable because at blood levels of 50 to 70 mg of glucose, there is increased neural activity and hormonal augmentation of the sympathetic system. Below this level, shock symptoms occur due to the decreased nutrition of cells. Poor cell nutrition is also the primary etiology of shock in hyperinsulemic conditions. Treatment consists of therapy to balance the insulin and glucose content of the blood (see Chapter 15). Whether the pathology is that of insulin excess or diabetes mellitus, mobilization of utilizable glucose is diminished. Correction of acidemia and reduction of concurrent hyperkalemia must take place to aid the re-establishment of circulation. Despite the need for quick treatment, diagnosis is extremely difficult in the late stages of either condition. The nurse should not state a diagnosis, however familiar she may be with the condition, but should check the chart, promptly call for a physician, and prepare equipment for a blood sample and for IV injection. It is wise to have both glucose and regular insulin ready for the physician's use as well as saline, an alkalizing agent, and potassium chloride.

MECHANICAL DEVICES FOR CIRCULATORY AUGMENTATION

Mechanical devices utilized in the treatment of cardiogenic shock are generally called circulatory augmenters and currently exist in three forms.

1. Left ventricular partial bypass of blood with an external pump. The theory is that the impaired heart will recover when its work load is reduced by this means and that better myocardial nutrition and oxygenation is provided while the heart recovers its strength.

2. Intra-aortic balloon assist. A catheter with a balloon pump at its end is inserted in a retrograde direction into the aorta. It is actively expanded with helium during diastole and passively deflates

during systole. The pulse is then conveyed by the pump. The left ventricle then has only to perform the work of pushing blood past the balloon since the bulk of the blood has been pushed by the pump.

3. Intracardiac pump. This device collects and pumps blood from within the left ventricle (under experimentation at present).

While these machines have proven effective, they require extensive operative procedures and are difficult to "wean" the patient from. The patient must be subjected to a major surgical procedure and its attendant risks. The devices are of limited practicality both because of risks to the patient, and because a skilled team and time to prime and prepare them are required (see bibliography).

However, the procedure of intra-aortic balloon pumping which has received the most extensive clinical trials appears promising. To this point patients have received this kind of assistance after the judgment has been made that they would die of shock. Obviously candidates who have less chance of irreversible changes would be more likely to survive. Some surgeons advocate the use of circulatory augmentation in addition to emergency bypass autografts with a length of saphenous vein anastamosed to the descending aorta and the distal portion of a coronary vessel, thus bypassing occluded parts.[74]

During the past few years, we have seen the assent and rapid descent of cardiac transplantation. The primary reason is obvious: most of the patients have survived for a very short time. Pending the development of immunological research and/or the improvement of mechanical hearts, a virtual moratorium has been declared on cardiac transplantation.

References

1. U.S. Department of Health, Education, and Welfare: Mortality Trends in the United States, 1964-1973. Pub. Health Service Series 30, #2.
2. See American Hospital Association guide issues to emergency services. JAMA 29, 8, 1955; 45, 15, 1971; and 49, 6, 1974. See also Report of the Emergency Services Task Force of the Philadelphia Department of Public Health, Feb. 1972.
3. Coronary Risk Handbook. Am. Heart Assoc., 1973.
4. Rushmer, R. F.: Cardiovascular Dynamics, ed. 3. Philadelphia, W. B. Saunders, 1970.
5. Schlesinger, M. J.: Relationship of anatomic pattern to the pathologic condition of the coronary arteries. Arch Pathol. 30:406, 1940.
6. Wiggins, C. J.: The functional significance of the coronary arteries. Circulation 5:609, Apr. 1952.
7. Russek, H. I. and Zohman, B. L. (eds): Changing Concepts in Cardiovascular Disease. Baltimore, Williams & Wilkins, 1972.
8. Rushmer, *op. cit.*
9. *Ibid*. See also Rushmer, R. F.: Structure and Function of the Cardiovascular System. Philadelphia, W. B. Saunders, 1972.
10. Janis, I. L.: Psychological Stress. New York, John Wiley & Sons, 1958.
11. *Ibid*.
12. Best, C. H. and Taylor, N. B.: The Psychological Basis of Medical Practice, ed. 9. Baltimore, Williams & Wilkins, 1974.
13. See McCaffery, M.: Nursing Management of the Patient with Pain. Philadelphia, J. B. Lippincott, 1972; Renzler, S. H.: Cardiac Pain. Springfield, Ill.: Charles C Thomas, 1951; and Wehrmacher, W. H.: Pain in the Chest. Springfield, Ill.: Charles C Thomas, 1964.
14. Schnaper, N.: The psychological implications of severe trauma: emotional sequelae to unconsciousness. J. Trauma 15:100-194, Feb. 1975.
15. Gunroth, W. G.: Electrical activity of the heart. *In* Rushmer: Cardiovascular Dynamics, *op. cit.*, pp. 355-417.
16. Koch-Wegen, J.: Drug interactions in cardiac therapy. Am. Heart J. 90, 1:93ff., July 1975.
17. Harvey, A., et al. (eds.): The Principles and Practice of Medicine. New York, Appleton-Century Crofts,
18. Duggan, J. J., et al.: Unheeded signals of fatal coronary-artery disease. RN 36:1-2, Aug. 1973.
19. Adgey, A. A.: Domiciliary management of cardiogenic shock in myocardial infarction. *In* I. M. Ledingham and T. A. MacAllister (eds.): Conference on Shock. Proceedings of the Conference of the Royal College of Physicians and Surgeons, Glasgow. St. Louis, C. V. Mosby, 1972.
20. See Bergman, S. A., Urschel, H. C., and Blumquist, G.: Pre- and postoperative testing in pa-

tients undergoing direct myocardial revas-cularization. Abstract presented before the Am. Heart Assoc. meeting, Nov. 1971. Najmi, M., et al.: Results of aortocoronary artery saphenous vein bypass surgery for ischemic heart disease. Am. J. Cardiol. 33:42-48, Jan. 1974. Urschel, H. C. and Ruzzuk, M. A.: Surgery for coronary artery disease. *In* J. C. Norman (ed.): Cardiac Surgery, ed. 2. New York, Appleton-Century Crofts, 1972, pp. 447-472. Mundith, E. D. and Austin, W. G.: Surgical measures for coronary heart disease. New Eng. J. Med. 293, 1:13-19, July 3, 1975; 293, 2:75-79, July 10, 1975; and 293, 3:124-129, July 17, 1975.

21. Mundith and Austin, *ibid*.

22. See Bergman, Urschel, and Blumquist, *op. cit.* See also Flemma, R. J., et al.: Is vein bypass here to stay? Adv. in Cardiol. 9:124-153, 1973; and Moss, A. J., et al.: Overdoing heart surgery? Time 4 Mar. 1974, p. 60.

23. Russek, H. I.: The "natural" history of severe angina pectoris with intensive medical therapy alone: a five year prospective study of 133 patients. Chest 65:46-51, Jan. 1974.

24. Woytowich, R. M.: Information viewed helpful to patients undergoing cardiac catheterization. Unpublished research project submitted to the University of Pennsylvania School of Nursing, 1969.

25. Redman, B. K.: Client education therapy in treatment of cardiovascualr disease. Cardiovas. Nurs. 10:1-6, Jan.-Feb. 1974.

26. Rushmer, Cardiovascular Dynamics, *op. cit.*

27. Grossman, B. J.: Chemotherapeutic prevention of rheumatic fever. Med. Clin. N. Am. 50:273-281. 1966.

28. Brown, J. C. and Epstein, W. V.: Pathogenic mechanisms of rheumatic disorders. Postgrad. Med. 45:75-81, Jan. 1969.

29. *Ibid.*

30. See Doyle, E. F.: Rheumatic fever, a continuing problem. Cardiovas. Nurs. 10:17-21, July-Aug. 1974; and Kunin, C. M., Tupasi, T., and Craig, W. A.: Overuse of antibiotics. Annals Intern. Med. 79:555-560, Oct. 1973.

31. See Cohn, K. E. and Kelly, J. J.: Congenital heart disease in adults. Postgrad. Med. 46:103-109, Sept. 1969. See also Barnharst, D. A., et al.: Isolated replacement of the aortic valve with the Starr-Edwards prosthesis: a nine year re-view. J. Thor. and Cardiovas. Surg. 70:113-119, July 1975.

32. Aagaard, G. N.: Treatment of hypertension: the hypertensive patient, his drug therapy and his life style. Circulation 45:660-669, June 1972.

33. *Ibid.*

34. Wilber, J. A. and Barrow, J. G.: Hypertension: community problem. Am. J. Med. 52:653-663, May 1972.

35. See Alderman, M. H. and Schoenbaum, E. E.: Detection and treatment of hypertension at the worksite. New Eng. J. Med. 293:65-68, July 10, 1975. See also Oakes, T. E., et al.: Social factors in newly discovered blood pressure. Nurs. Digest 3:33-35, Jan.-Feb. 1975.

36. Caldwell, J. R., et al.: The dropout problem in hypertension treatment. J. Chronic Disease 22: 579-592, Feb. 1970.

37. See Raab, W.: Prevention Myocardiology: Fundamentals and Targets. Springfield, Ill.: Charles C Thomas, 1974. See also Flear, C. T. G.: Disturbances of volume and composition of body fluids in congestive heart failure. *In* E. Bajusz (ed.): Electrolytes and Cardiovascular Disease. New York, Karger, 1966, pp. 357-385.

38. Guyton, A. C.: Textbook of Medical Physiology, ed. 4. Philadelphia, W. B. Saunders, 1971.

39. Raab, W.: Myocardial electrolyte derangements. *In* Raab, Preventive Myocardiology, *op. cit.,* pp. 34-59.

40. Sodi-Pollares, D., et al.: The polarizing treatment in cardiovascular conditions. *In* Bajusz, Electrolytes and Cardiovascular Disease, *op. cit.,* pp. 198-238.

41. Wehrmacher, *op. cit.*

42. Rinzler, *op. cit.*

43. *Ibid.*

44. Rushmer, Structure and Function of the Cardiovascular System, *op. cit.*

45. Russek, Changing Concepts in Cardiovascular Disease, *op. cit.*

46. Goodman, L. S. and Gillman, A.: The Pharmacological Basis of Therapeutics, ed. 5. New York, Macmillan, 1970.

47. *Ibid.*

48. Noble, J. H., Jr. (ed.): Emergency Medical Service, Behavior and Planning Perspectives. New York, Behavioral Publications, 1974.

49. See Sabiston, D. C.: Cardiogenic shock: surgical management. Cardiovas. Review 44-46, 1973;

and Weil, M. H. and Shubin, H.: Cardiogenic shock. Cardiovas. Review 32-34, 1973.

50. Vineburg, A. M.: Development of anastamosis between coronary vessels and transplanted internal mammary artery. Can. Med. Assoc. J. 55:117-132, 1946.

51. Mundith and Austin, *op. cit.*

52. Urschel and Ruzzuk, *op. cit.*

53. See Hartley, L. H., Jones, L. G., and Mason, J.: The usefulness of exercise therapy in the management of coronary heart disease. Adv. Cardiol. 9:174-179, 1973. See also Moss, A. J., et al.: The hospital phase of myocardial infarction: identification of patients with increased mortality risk. Circulation 99:460-466, Mar. 1974; and Majmi, et al., *op. cit.*

54. Moss, *op. cit.* Najmi, et al., *ibid.*

55. Vineburg, *op. cit.*

56. Norman, *op. cit.* and Sabiston, D. (ed.): Christopher's Textbook of Surgery, ed. 19. Philadelphia, W. B. Saunders, 1972.

57. See Hutchinson, J. E., III, Green, G. E., Mekhjian, H. E., and Kemp, H. G.: Coronary bypass grafting in 376 consecutive patients with three operative deaths. J. Thor. and Cardiovas. Surg. 67:7-13, Jan. 1974. See also Lambert, C. J.; Mitchell, B. R., Adam, M., and Geissler, G. E.: Emergency myocardial revascularization for impending myocardial infarction. Chest 61: 474-481, Mar. 1969.

58. Norman, *op. cit.;* Sabiston, Christopher's Textbook of Surgery, *op. cit.*

59. Sanders, A. A., Buckley, M. J., and Leinbach, R. C., et al.: Mechanical circulatory assistance. Circulation 45:1292-1301, June 1972.

60 Weil and Shubin, *op. cit.*

61 Lang, T., Vyden, J. K., and Corday, E.: Therapy of power failure of the heart. *In* Russek and Zohman, *op. cit.,* pp. 245-261.

62. Moran, N. C.: Evaluation of the pharmacologic basis of the therapy of circulatory shock. Am. J. Cardiol. 26:250-258, Dec. 1970.

63. Scheuer, R.: Coronary nurse training program: an evaluation. Nurs. Research 21:22-32, May-June 1972.

64. Weil and Shubin, *op. cit.*

65. Scheuer, *op. cit.*

66. Moran, *op. cit.*

67. Shires, G. T., Carrico, C. J., and Canizaro, P. D.: Shock. Maj. Prob. in Clin. Surg. 13, 1973.

68. Lang, Vyden, and Corday, *op. cit.*

69. See Guyton, *op. cit.;* Goodman and Gillman, *op. cit.* See also McCann, W. D. and O'Donovan, T. P.: Acute circulatory failure secondary to myocardial infarction. Postgrad. Med. 49:74-79, May 1971; Shurlis, L.: Pathophysiology of Shock. *In* F. D. Ownby (ed.): Advanced Cardiac Nursing. Philadelphia, Charles Press, 1970; and Sicuteri, F., DelBianco, P. L., and Fanciulli, M.: Kinins in the pathogenesis of cardiogenic shock and pain. Adv. Exper. Biol. and Med. 22:315-322, 1972.

70. See Russek, *op. cit.;* Sodi-Pollares, *op. cit.;* and Wood, J. E., Barrow, J. G., and Kries, E. D., et al.: Guidelines for detection, diagnosis and management of hypertensive populations. Circulation 44:A263-A272, Nov. 1971. See also Weil, M. H. and Shubin, H.: Changes in venous capitance during cardiogenic shock. Am. J. Cardiol. 26:613-614, Dec. 1970.

71. See Guyton, *op. cit.;* Goodman and Gillman, *op. cit.;* Sicuteri, DelBianco, and Fanciulli, *op. cit.*

72. See Cuthbert, M. F.: The Prostaglandins. Philadelphia, J. B. Lippincott, 1973. See also DePalma, J.: Aspirin-like drugs and prostaglandins. Am. Fam. Phys. 12:120-121, July 1975.

73. Loff, R., and Wilcken, D. E. L.: Glucagon in heart failure and in cardiogenic shock. Circulation 45:534-542, Mar. 1972.

74. Sanders, Buckley, and Leinbach, *op. cit.*

Bibliography

Cardiovascular Function

Braunwald, E. (ed): Cardiovascular function. *In* The Yearbook of Medicine—1973. Chicago, Yearbook Medical Publishers, 1973, pp. 7-9.

Brest, A. N. and Moyer, J. H. (eds): Cardiovascular Disorders. Philadelphia, F. A. Davis, 1968.

Chiong, M. A., West, R. and Parker, J. O.: Myocardial balance of inorganic phosphate and enzymes in man. Circulation 49:283-290, Feb. 1974.

Coates, K.: Non-invasive cardiac diagnostic procedures. Am. J. Nurs. 75:1980-1985, Nov. 1975.

Conn, H. L. and Horowitz, O.: Cardiac and Vascular Diseases. Philadelphia, Lea & Febiger, 1971.

Conover, M. H. and Zalis, E. G.: Understanding Electrocardiography: Physiological and Interpretive Concepts. St. Louis, C. V. Mosby, 1976.

Corr, P. B. and Gillis, R. A.: Role of the vagus nerve in the cardiovascular changes induced by coronary occlusion. Circulation 49:86-97, Jan. 1974.

Curran, R. L. and Harnden, D. G.: The Pathological Basis of Medicine. Philadelphia, W. B. Saunders, 1972.

Federspiel, B.: Renin and blood pressure. Am. J. Nurs. 75:1462-1465, 1975.

Gould, L., Zahiv, M., DeMartino, A. and Gomprecht, R. F.: Cardiac effects of a cocktail. JAMA 218:1799-1802, Dec. 20, 1971.

Henry, J. P. and Meehan, J. R.: The Circulation: An Integrative Study. Chicago, Yearbook Medical Publishers, 1971.

Hurst, J. W., et al. (eds.): Heart, Arteries and Veins, ed. 3. New York, McGraw-Hill, 1974.

MacBryde, C. M. (ed): Signs and Symptoms, ed. 5. Philadelphia, J. B. Lippincott, 1970.

Matheny, N. M. and Snively, W. D., Jr.: Nurses' Handbook of Fluid Balance. Philadelphia: J. B. Lippincott, 1967.

Multi-Media Systems for Nursing Education.: Physical Diagnosis in Patient Assessment; Cardiopulmonary Anatomy and Physiology; Electrocardiography; Arrhythmia Recognition. Livonia, Mich., Medical Electronic Services Inc. (cassettes).

Nassau, M. G.: The coronary system. *In* R. F. Rushmer: Cardiovascular Dynamics. Philadelphia, W. B. Saunders, 1970.

Page, I. H., et al. (eds.): Hypertension and the Cardiovascular System. Minneapolis, Modern Medicine Publications, 1972.

General Medical, Surgical and Pharmacological Therapy

Andreoli, K. G., Fowkes, V. H., Zipés, D. P., and Wallace, A. G.: Comprehensive Cardiac Care, ed. 3. St. Louis, C. V. Mosby, 1975.

Asperheim, M. R. and Eisenhauer, L. A.: Pharmacologic Basis of Patient Care, ed. 2. Philadelphia, W. B. Saunders, 1973.

Beeson, P. B. and McDermott, W.: Cecil-Loeb Textbook of Medicine, ed. 13. Philadelphia, W. B. Saunders, 1971.

Bergensen, B. S. (in consultation with Goth, A.): Pharmacology in Nursing, ed. 13. St. Louis, C. V. Mosby, 1976.

Falconer, M. W., Patterson, H. R., and Gustafson, E. A.: Current Drug Handbook, 1976-78. Philadelphia, W. B. Saunders, 1976.

French, R. M.: Nurses' Guide to Diagnostic Procedures, ed. 3. New York, McGraw-Hill, 1971.

Haimovici, H. (ed): Surgical Management of Vascular Diseases. Philadelphia, J. B. Lippincott, 1970.

Kosik, J. and Thompson, J.: Allergic reactions to antibiotics. Med. Clin. N. Am. 54:1-6, Jan. 1970.

Noble, R. J., Dickerson, L. S. and Fisch, C.: The use and abuse of digitalis in acute myocardial infarction. Heart and Lung 1:762-775, Nov.-Dec. 1972.

Rinear, C. E. and Rinear, E. E.: Recognition and management of life-threatening emergencies. Pennsylvania Nurse part I—April 1975, part II—June 1975.

Selzer, A.: The use and abuse of quinidine. Heart and Lung 1:755-761, Nov.-Dec. 1972.

Strand, M. M. and Elmer, L. A.: Clinical Laboratory Tests. A Manual for Nurses. St. Louis, C. V. Mosby, 1976.

Schoche, P. A. (ed.): Mosby's Comprehensive Review of Critical Care. St. Louis, C. V. Mosby, 1976.

General Nursing Care

Abdellah, F. G., et al.: New Directions in Patient-Centered Nursing. New York: Macmillan, 1973.

Beland, I. L.: Clinical Nursing: Pathophysiological and Psychosocial Approaches, ed. 2. New York, Macmillan, 1970.

Bernard, J. S. and Thompson, L. F.: Sociology: Nurses and Their Patients in a Modern Society, ed. 8. St. Louis, C. V. Mosby, 1970.

Blumberg, J. E. and Drummond, E. E.: Nursing Care of the Long Term Patient, ed. 2. New York, Springer, 1971.

Brunner, L. S., and Suddarth, D. S.: Textbook of Medical-Surgical Nursing, ed. 3. Philadelphia, J. B. Lippincott, 1975.

Capell, P. T. and Case, D. B.: Ambulatory Care Manual for Nurse Practitioners. Philadelphia, J. B. Lippincott, 1976.

Capuzzi, C. F.: Blood Transfusion Reactions and Complications: A Programmed Text. N.Y., Tivesias Press, 1975.

Chung, E. K. (ed.): Cardiac Emergency Care. Philadelphia, Lea & Febiger, 1975.

Cosgriff, H. and Anderson, L.: The Practice of Emergency Nursing. Philadelphia, J. B. Lippincott, 1975.

Downs, F. S.: Bedrest and sensory disturbances. Am. J. Nurs. 74:434-438, Mar. 1974.

Driefus, L.: Hazards of tranvenous catheters. Chest 65:2-7, Jan. 1974.

Forrester, J. S., Diamond, G., McHugh, T. J. and Swan, H. J. C.: Filling pressures: a reappraisal of CVP monitoring. New Eng. J. Med. 285:190-195, July 1971.

Fox, D. J.: Fundamentals of Research in Nursing, ed. 2. New York, Appleton-Century Crofts, 1970.

Gentry, W. D. and Williams, R. B.(eds.): Psychological Aspects of Myocardial Infarction and Coronary Care. St. Louis, C. V. Mosby, 1975.

Howe, P. S.: Basic Nutrition in Health and Diseases, ed. 6. Philadelphia, W. B. Saunders, 1976.

Hudak, C. M., Gallo, B. M. and Lohr, T.: Critical Care Nursing. Philadelphia, J. B. Lippincott, 1973.

Hudak, C. M., Redstone, P. M., Horanson, N. L. and Suziki, I. E.: Clinical Protocols—A Guide for Nurses and Physicians. Philadelphia, J. B. Lippincott, 1976.

Johnson, M. M., Davis, M. L. C. and Bilitch, M. J.: Problem Solving in Nursing Practice. Dubuque, Iowa, W. C. Brown, 1970.

King, I. M.: Toward a Theory for Nursing: General Concepts of Human Behavior, New York, John Wiley & Sons, 1971.

Krause, M. V. and Hunscher, M. A.: Food, Nutrition and Diet Therapy. Philadelphia, W. B. Saunders, 1972.

Krueger, S.: Monitoring Central Venous Pressure: A Programmed Sequence. Springfield, Ill, Springer, 1973.

Lee, J. M.: Emotional reactions to trauma. Nurs. Clin. N. Am. 5:577-588, Dec. 1970.

Lee, R. E. and Ball, P. A.: Some thoughts on the psychology of the coronary care unit patient. Am. J. Nurs. 75:1498-1501, Sept. 1975.

Lewis, G. K.: Nurse-Patient Communication. Dubuque, Iowa, W. C. Brown, 1973.

(The) Lippincott Manual of Nursing Practice. Philadelphia, J. B. Lippincott, 1974.

Medical Programs Incorporated: Patient assessment: taking a patient's history (programmed Instruction). Am. J. Nurs. 74:293-324, Feb. 1974.

Neilson, M. A.: Intra-arterial monitoring of blood pressure. Am. J. Nurs. 74:48-53, Jan. 1974.

Pain and suffering (Supplement). Am. J. Nurs. 74:489-523, Mar. 1974.

Petty, T. L.: Intensive and Rehabilitative Respiratory Care, ed. 2. Philadelphia, Lea & Febiger, 1974.

Redman, B. K.: Process of Patient Teaching in Nursing, ed. 3. St. Louis, C. V. Mosby, 1976.

Reickle, M. J.: Psychological stress in the intensive care unit. Nurs. Digest 3:12-16, May-June 1975.

Robinson, L.: Psychological Aspects of the Care of Hospitalized Patients, ed. 3. Philadelphia, F. A. Davis, 1976.

Rodbard, S.: The clinical utility of the arterial pulses and sounds. Heart and Lung 1:776-784, Nov.-Dec. 1972.

Skillman, J. J. (with nursing implications by P. J. Woolridge): Ethical dilemmas in the care of the critically ill. Nurs. Digest 3:26-29, Sept.-Oct. 1975.

Smith, D. W., Germain, G. P. H., and Gips, C. D.: Care of the Adult Patient, ed. 4. Philadelphia, J. B. Lippincott, 1975.

Stryker, R. P.: Rehabilitative Aspects of Acute and Chronic Nursing Care. Philadelphia, W. B. Saunders, 1972.

Woolley, A.: Excellence in nursing in the coronary care unit. Heart and Lung 1:785-792, Nov.-Dec. 1972.

Xura, H. and Walsh, M. B.: Nursing Process: Assessment, Planning, Implementation, Evaluating, ed. 2. New York, Meredith, 1973.

Focus on Prevention

Ames, R.: How to recognize—and survive—a heart attack. Readers Digest 103:110-114, Nov. 1973.

Biorck, G.: Early diagnosis of coronary heart disease—what is it good for? Adv. in Cardiol. 8:27-37, 1973.

————. Computers, Electrocardiography and Public Health. Washington, D.C., U.S. Department of Health, Education and Welfare, Pub. Health Service Publication #1644, 1967.

Boyle, M. J. and Kaufman, A.: Strip screening to prevent rheumatic fever. Am. J. Nurs. 75:1487, Sept. 1975.

Cox, M. and Wear, R. F., Jr.: Campbell soups program to prevent atherosclerosis. Am. J. Nurs. 72:253-259, Feb. 1972.

Dack, S.: Too little, too late? Cardiovasc. Rev. 13-14, 1973.

Duncan, J. J., et al.: Symposium: education of patients—a program for teaching of cardiovascular patients. Heart and Lung 2:508-525, July-Aug. 1973.

Eleck, S. R.: How to spot the coronary-prone patient. Consultant 13:19-20, July 1973.

Fox, S. M.: A national program for cardiovascular health. Adv. in Cardio. 9:212-219, 1973.

Grace, W. J., Crockett, J. E., Weinberg, S. L. and Soffer, A.: Intermediate care after myocardial infarction. Heart and Lung 1:818-824, Nov.-Dec. 1972.

Hellerstein, H. K.: Rehabilitation in coronary artery disease. *In* F. D. Ownby (ed): Advanced Cardiac Nursing, Philadelphia, Charles Press, 1970. Chapter 19.

Hirshfeld, J. W., et al.: Reduction in severity and extent of myocardial infarction when nitroglycerin and methoxamine are administered during coronary occlusion. Circulation 49:291-297, Feb. 1974.

Hymovich, D. P. and Barnard, M. U.: Family Health Care. New York, McGraw-Hill, 1973.

Julian, D. G.: The natural history of ischemic heart disease. Adv. in Cardiol. 9:38-48, 1973.

Kannel, W. B. and Dauber, T. R.: Contributors to coronary risk, implications for prevention and public health: the Framingham study. Heart and Lung 12:797-809, Nov.-Dec. 1972.

Maki, D. G., Goldman, D. A., and Rhame, F. S.: Infection control in intravenous therapy. Nurs. Digest 3:5-11, May-June 1975.

Meltzer, L.: Detection of early heart failure. *In* F. D. Ownby (ed.): Advanced Cardiac Nursing, Philadelphia, Charles Press, 1970, Chapter 15.

Report of The Criteria Committee of the New York Heart Association: Nomenclature and Criteria for Diagnosis of the Heart and Great Vessels. Boston, Little, Brown, 1974.

Schimmel, E. M.: The hazards of hospitalization. Annals Intern. Med. 279:1321-1325, 1968.

Nursing in Specialized Areas

Behrendt, D. M. and Austin, W. G.: Patient Care in Cardiac Surgery. Boston, Little, Brown, 1972.

Beth Israel Hospital: Respiratory Intensive Care Nursing. Boston, Little, Brown, 1973.

Brainbridge, M. V.: Postoperative Cardiac Intensive Care, ed. 2. New York, Oxford Press, 1972.

Burrell, L. O. and Burrell, Z. L.: Intensive Nursing Care, ed. 2. St. Louis, C. V. Mosby, 1973.

Fleming, J. M.: Effect of pre-operative intervention on altered sensory perception in cardiac surgical patients. Unpublished thesis, School of Nursing, University of Pennsylvania, Phila., Pa, 1973.

Frank, M. H. and Alvarez-Mena, S. V.: Cardiovascular Physical Diagnosis. Chicago, Yearbook Medical Publishers, 1973.

Fuhs, M., Rieser, M. and Brisban, D.: Nursing in a respiratory intensive care unit. Chest 62:14S-18S, Aug. 1972. (Supplement)

Hamilton, W. P. and Lavin, M. A.: Decision Making in the Coronary Care Unit. St. Louis, C. V. Mosby, 1976.

Jacoby, F. G.: Nursing Care of the Patient with Burns. St. Louis, C. V. Mosby, 1972.

Lewis, C. E. and Resnik, B. A.: Nurse clinics and progressive ambulatory patient care. WEJM 277:1236-1241, Aug. 17, 1967.

Lewis, E. P.: Nursing in Cardiovascular Diseases. New York, Am. J. Nurs. Co., 1971.

Meltzer, L. E., Abdellah, F. G. and Kitchell, J. R. (eds.): Concepts and Practices of Intensive Care for Nurse Specialists. Philadelphia, Charles Press, 1969.

Meltzer, L. E., Kitchell, J. A. and Pinneo, R.: Intensive Coronary Care, A Manual for Nurses. Philadelphia, Charles Press, 1970.

Modell, W., Schwartz, D. R., Hazeltine, L. S. and Kirkman, F. T.: Handbook of Cardiology for Nurses, ed. 5. New York, Springer, 1966.

Nelson, R., et al.: Care of a man with a partial artificial heart. Am. J. Nurs. 73:1580-1585, Sept. 1973.

Ownby, F. D.: Advanced Cardiac Nursing. Philadelphia, Charles Press, 1970.

Pitorak, E. F., et al.: Nurses Guide to Cardiac Surgery and Nursing Care. New York, McGraw-Hill, 1969.

Powers, M. and Storlie, F.: The Cardiac Surgical Patient; Pathophysiologic Considerations and Nursing Care. New York, Macmillan, 1969.

Sanderson, R. G.: Cardiac Patient: A Comprehensive Approach. Philadelphia, W. B. Saunders, 1972.

Secor, J.: Coronary Care: A Nursing Specialty. New York, Appleton-Century Crofts, 1971.

———. Patient Care in Respiratory Problems. Philadelphia, W. B. Saunders, 1969.

Sharp, L. and Rabin, B.: Nursing in the Coronary Care Unit. Philadelphia, J. B. Lippincott, 1970.

Sobel, B. E.: The cardiac care unit in 1973. Hosp. Proceed. 8:115-124, Feb. 1973.

Storlie, F.: Double entendre in a C.C.U. Am. J. Nurs. 74:666-667, Apr. 1974.

Storlie, F., Rambousek, E. and Shannon, E.: Principles of Intensive Nursing Care. New York, Appleton-Century Crofts, 1969.

Sowton, E.: Physical parameters during resuscitation. *In* F. D. Ownby (ed.): Advanced Cardiac Nursing. Philadelphia, Charles Press, 1970, Chapter 16.

Wagner, D.: Nursing in a H.M.O. Am. J. Nurs. 74:236-240, Feb. 1974.

Walt, A. J. and Wilson, R. F. (eds.): Management of Trauma: Pitfalls and Practice. Philadelphia, Lea & Febiger, 1975.

Patients with Congenital Heart Disease, Valvular Defects, Arrhythmias and Congestive Heart Failure

Brause, N. L.: Current thoughts on thromboembolisms. Surg. Clin. N. Am. 54:229-238, Feb. 1974.

Castinada, A. R.: Surgical treatment of cardiac valvular disease. Clin. Sympos. 21, 1:19-31, 1969.

Chung, E. K.: Introduction: cardiac arrythmias—a burning fuse. Post. Grad Med. 53:21-22, Apr. 1973.

Davidson, D. M., Braak, C. A., Preston, T. A. and Jacobson, R. D. J.: Permanent ventricular pac-

ing: effect on long-term survival, congestive heart failure and subsequent myocardial infarction and stroke. Annals Intern. Med. 77:345-351, Sept. 1972.

Farman, S. and Norman, J. C.: Pacing and pacemakers. *In* J. C. Norman (ed.): Cardiac Surgery, ed. 2. New York, Appleton-Century Crofts, 1972, pp. 489-531.

Griffin, F. M., Jr., Jones, G. and Cobbs, C. G.: Aortic insufficiency in bacterial endocarditis. Annals. Int. Med. 76:23-28, Jan. 1972.

Hinkle, L. E., Carver, S. T. and Plaken, A.: Slow heart rates and increased risk of cardiac death in middle aged men. Arch. Intern. Med. 129:732-748, May 1972.

Kennedy, J. H.: Support of the Failing Circulation: The Use of a Pump Oxygenator in Clinical Cardiac Failure. Springfield, Ill, Charles C Thomas. 1967.

Narula, O. S., Samet, P. and Javier, R. P.: Significance of the sinus node recovery time. Circulation 45:140-158, Jan. 1972.

Sauvage, L. R., Berger, K. E. and Mansfield, P. B.: Future directions in the development of arterial prosthesis for small and medium caliber arteries. Surg. Clin. N. Am. 54:213-227, Feb. 1974.

Wallace, A.: Cardiac pacing. Med. J. Australia 2:55-63, Aug. 12, 1972.

Winslow, E. H. and Powell, A. H.: Sick Sinus Syndrome. Am. J. Nurs. 76:1262-1265, Aug. 1976.

The Patient with Hypertension

Brunner, H. R., et al.: Essential hypertension: renin and aldosticone, heart attack and stroke. New Eng. J. Med. 286:441-449, Mar. 2, 1972.

Ferrario, C. M., Gildenbarg, P. L., McCubben, J. W.: Cardiovascular effects of angiotensin mediated by the central nervous system. Circulation Research 30:257-262, Mar. 1972.

Foster, J. H. and Dean, R. H.: Changing concepts in renovascular hypertension. Surg. Clin. N. Am. 54:257-269, Feb. 1974.

———: Hypertension and renal disease. (Special Issue) Post. Grad. Med. 52:66-131, Sept. 1972.

Gottlieb, T. B., Katz, F. H. and Chilsey, C. A.: Combined therapy with vasodilator drugs and P-adrenergic blockade in hypertension . . . Circulation 45:571-582, Mar. 1972.

Griffith, E. W. and Madero, B.: Primary hypertension: patients' learning needs. Am. J. Nurs. 73:624-627, Mar. 1973.

Gross, F.: Renin-angiotension system and hypertension. Annals Intern. Med. 75:777-787, Nov. 1971.

Sheps, S. G.: Hypertensive crises. Post. Grad. Med. 49:95-104, May 1971.

United States Veterans Administration Cooperative Study Group on Antihypertensive Agents, Part II: Effects of treatment on morbidity in hypertension. JAMA 213:1143-1152, Aug. 17, 1970.

———. Influence of age, diastatic pressure and prior cardiovascular disease on morbidity in hypertension. Circulation, 45:991-1004, May 1972.

Patients with Coronary Artery Disease and Myocardial Infarction

Aronow, W. S. and Stemmer, E. A.: Bypass graft surgery versus medical therapy of angina pectoris. Am. J. Cardiol. 33:415-420, Mar. 1974.

Berlotasi, C. A., et al.: Unstable angina—prospective and randomized study of its evaluation, with and without surgery. Am. J. Cardiol. 33:201-208, Feb. 1974.

Cannon, D. S., Miller, D. C. and Shumway, N. E., et al.: The long term follow up of patients undergoing saphenous vein bypass surgery. Circulation 49:77-85, Jan. 1974.

———: Coronary risk handbook. American Heart Association, 1973.

Dietrich, E. B. and Prian, G. W.: A proposed classification for analysis of the results of aortocoronary bypass grafts. Adv. in Cardiol. 9:101-118, 1973.

Friedberg, C. K.: The early diagnosis of coronary heart disease: critical review. Adv. in Cardiol. 9:1-24, 1973.

Gott, V. L.: Outlook for patients after coronary artery revascularization. Am. J. Cardiol. 33:431-437, Mar. 1974.

Graham, A. F., et al.: Heart transplantation: current indications and long term results (Nursing Im-plications by M. J. Aspinall). Nurs. Digest 3:25-29, Nov.-Dec. 1975.

Greene, A., Goldstein, S. and Moss, A. J.: Psychosocial aspects of sudden death: preliminary report. Arch. Intern. Med. 129:725-731, May 1972.

Rose, L. B. and Press, E.: Cardiac defilbrillation by ambulance attendants. JAMA 219: 63-68, Jan. 3, 1972.

Rose, M. R., Glassman, E., Isom, O. W., and Spencer, F. O.: electrocardiographic and serum enzyme changes of myocardial infarction after coronary artery bypass surgery. Am. J. Cardiol. 33:215-220, Feb. 1974.

Ross, J., Jr.: Introduction to the symposium on the effects of surgical treatment on the natural history of acquired heart disease, Part I: coronary artery disease. Am. J. Cardiol. 33:421-430, Mar. 1974.

Shepherd, R. L., Itscoitz, S. B., and Clancy, D. L., et al.: Deterioration of myocardial function following aorto-coronary bypass operation. Circulation 49:467-478, Mar. 1974.

Tyzehouse, P. S.: MI—its effect on the family. Am. J. Nurs. 73:1012-1013, June 1973.

Smith, A. M., Thurir, J. A. and Huang, S. H.: Serum enzyme in myocardial infarction. 73:277-279, Feb. 1973.

Vineburg, A. M., Pifarre, J. and Criollos, R., et al.: Myocardial revascularization by omental graft without pedicle: experimental background and report on 25 cases followed 6-16 months. J. Thoracic Cardiovasc. Surg. 49:103-115, 1965.

Shumer, W. and Nyhus, L. M.: Treatment of Shock: Principles and Practice. Philadelphia, Lea & Febiger, 1974.

Surgery and Sequelae of Cardiac Problems

Ayers, Stephen M., Miller, H., Giannelli, S., and Fleming , P., et al.: The lung in shock . . . Am. J. Cardiol., 26:588-594, Dec. 1970.

Baldwin, L.: Symposium: pulmonary embolism. Heart and Lung 3:207-218, Mar.-Apr. 1974.

Barnhorst, D. A.: Extracardiac thoracic complications of cardiac surgery. Surg. Clin. N. Am. 53:937-944, Aug. 1973.

Engle, M. A., McCabe, J. C., Ebert, P. A., and Zabriskie, J.: The post pericardotomy syndrome and antiheart antibodies. Circulation 49:401-409, Mar. 1974.

Gilbert, R., Auchingloss, J. H., Peppi, D. and Ashatosh, K.: The first few hours off a respirator. Chest 65:152-157, Feb. 1974.

Neilson, M. A.: Intra-arterial monitoring of blood pressure. Am. J. Nurs. 74:48-53, Jan. 1974.

Rynearson, R. R. and Stewart, W. L.: Dependency problem: the most common surgical risk. Surg. Clin. N. Am. 52:459-467, Apr. 1972.

Selecky, P. A.: Tracheotomy: a review of indications, complications and care. Heart and Lung 3:272-283, Mar.-Apr. 1974.

The Patient with Cardiogenic Shock

Amsterdam, E. A., et al: Evaluation and management of cardiogenic shock: drug therapy. Heart and Lung Part I, 1:433-442, Part II, 1:663-671, 1972.

Hardaway, R. M.: Emergency management of the patient in shock. Hosp. Med. 9:62-69, Oct. 1963.

Kennedy, J. H.: Preferred mechanisms for temporary circulatory support. Adv. in Cardiol. 9:152-167, 1973.

Scheidt, Ascheim, S. R., and Killip, T.: Shock after acute myocardial infarction. Am. J. Cardiol. 20:556-564, Dec. 1970.

13

The Patient in Shock: mechanisms of shock and related therapy, nursing goals and functions for patients in shock

WEALTHA COLLINS MCGURN

Principles of Anatomy, Physiology, and Biochemistry • *Pathophysiology of the Shock Syndrome* • *General Care of the Patient in Shock* • *Specific Conditions Underlying the Shock Syndrome: Pathophysiology, Nursing Care, and Nursing Functions Adjunctive to Medical Treatment* • *The Shock Research Unit: Its Use and Abuses*

During the past few years, the literature on the pathophysiology of the shock syndrome, the biochemical alterations in the shock state, and the care of the patient in shock has proliferated. Part of this literature is the result of patient studies done in clinical research units. These units are staffed with specialized personnel who utilize sophisticated surveillance equipment for treating patients with extensive trauma and shock. Such units have generated a growing body of data concerning specific underlying mechanisms leading to shock and individual reactions to them.

While the development of "shock units" and the increasing sophistication regarding biochemical alterations and potential corrective therapies have not yet appreciably improved the mortality statistics of patients in profound shock, inroads into the problem have been made. It is hoped that the "software" represented by the understandings of nursing and medical personnel caring for patients for whom shock could have been prevented or who are still in compensated stages of shock, will continue to improve. It is also hoped that such software will be increasingly augmented by improved technology for the service of *all* patients, including those who now have refractory or irreversible shock which leads to their deaths.

The magnitude of the problem is staggering. Trauma is the leading cause of death in the first three decades of life and the fourth overall cause of death in America. Shock is the most frequent cause of death from trauma.[1] It may occur because of neurogenic trauma (such as from head or spinal injuries) or from massive fluid and electrolyte losses which typically occur when people are burned or suffer crush injuries. It may also occur from loss of blood, pain, or undue manipulation after the injury. Infection often supervenes from other causes, leading to shock from a combination of several etiologies. The point is that only recently has general exposure in the literature been in even approximate proportion to the occurrence of shock after traumatic injuries.[2]

Numerous studies have led to a growing body of literature on the shock syndrome arising after myocardial injury, or "cardiogenic shock." Despite this fact, mortality ranges between 75 percent and 90 percent, depending on the study read. Approximately one million people suffer myocardial damage in the United States each year and approximately 15 percent or *150,000* people develop shock.[3] This country is losing well over a hundred thousand people, many in the prime of life, to death from cardiogenic shock. In addition to this dismal picture, an increasing number of people die from "septic" shock. The mortality rate from septic shock approaches 75 percent.[4] This entity is probably the most preventable since its underlying etiology is infection, many cases of which could have been arrested if they had been detected and treated early. A distinctive characteristic of septic shock is that, in a significant number of cases, it is directly attributable to iatrogenic bases, ranging from cross-contamination of patients by hospital personnel to the abuse of antibiotics. This subject will be pursued in greater detail later in this chapter.

A word about the format of this chapter is in order. In response to the constructive suggestions made about the first edition, the normal physiology of the autonomic system and its chemical mediators have been included in this chapter. The general compensatory changes which occur as the body tries to maintain tissue perfusion will be discussed in depth with reference to normal function.

Next, the effects of failing compensation which produce the classic signs of profound shock will be presented in conjunction with the general medical and nursing regimens of care. As mentioned previously, there is a growing body of knowledge regarding underlying mechanisms of shock. These will be discussed in detail as a basis for the nursing and medical care specific to the conditions.

Finally, a discussion of the specialized care in clinical research units designed for the treatment and study of patients in shock and the new and experimental techniques of therapy will be presented. It is hoped that nurses will be provoked to think about the present and potential roles they may undertake in caring for patients who are prone to or suffering from shock.

Principles of Anatomy, Physiology, and Biochemistry

ANATOMY OF THE AUTONOMIC NERVOUS SYSTEM

The sympathetic nervous system and the thoracolumbar division of the autonomic nervous system are synonymous. The general action of this system, when it is in a position of dominance, is to ready the organism to react to stress-producing stimuli. The cell bodies of the preganglionic fibers lie in the lateral horn of the spinal cord between T1 (thoracic intravertebral space 1) and L2 (lumbar intravertebral space 2). Short myelinated fibers leave the cord to synapse with a postganglionic fiber. The ganglion is formed by the cell bodies of the second fiber and by the end fibers of the preganglionic fiber. They usually lie within the paravertebral chain of ganglia on either side of the spinal cord or, in a few instances, in the prevertebral (unpaired) ganglia.

There are many more postganglionic fibers than ganglia or preganglionic fibers. The latter are matched with the intravertebral spaces. There are three cervical ganglia—the superior, middle, and inferior—from which arise the superior, middle, and inferior cardiac nerves. These and postganglionic fibers from T1 to T4 are most important in the stimulation of the heart, lung, trachea and bronchi, and the carotid artery. Fibers from the superior ganglion also innervate the eye and salivary glands.

Postganglionic fibers from T5 to T12 reach to

the large celiac ganglion (in the area of the solar plexus), and from there, still another large mass of fibers innervates the viscera and the abdominal blood vessels. One preganglionic fiber departs from the celiac ganglion to synapse with its postganglionic fiber at the superior mesenteric ganglion. The reader can avoid confusing pre- and postganglionic fibers by remembering that a fiber is preganglionic until it has passed through its terminal ganglion (the last cell body). Postganglionic fibers terminate at the effector site (Fig. 13-1, p. 368). An inferior mesenteric ganglion receives preganglionic fibers from cells at locations L1 and L2 and distributes postganglionic fibers to the lower colon, kidney, bladder, sex organs, and genitals.

Because this discussion concerns the postganglionic distribution in relation to the phenomenon of shock, all of the distribution has not been included. The most important remaining site of action of the sympathetic nervous system in this regard is on the adrenal medulla. There is a preganglionic fiber directly routed to supply this site. Secretion of the catecholamines from the adrenal medulla, whose effects on the body are very similar to sympathetic stimulation, will result from predominance of the sympathetic system.

The parasympathetic or cranial-sacral division of the autonomic system has its inception either in the spinal cord at S1 or S2 (sacral segments 1 and 2) or in several of the motor nuclei in the brain or medulla. Usually the preganglionic fibers synapse with cell bodies within the organ, but there are a few postganglionic fibers associated with the vagus nerve. The vagus nerve (cranial nerve XII) is particularly important in determining breathing and heart rates and in the force of cardiac contraction. Its postganglionic fibers lie within heart and lung tissues, with particularly rich supplies of fibers around the S-A (sinoatrial) and A-V (atrioventricular) nodes in the heart.

PHYSIOLOGY

The physiology of the autonomic nervous system requires an understanding of neural transmission and of the action of several humoral agents. In general, a sequential shift of ions along the course of a nerve fiber (depolarization) propagates an impulse. However, at the synapses and at the neuromuscular, or neuroeffector, junctions, chemical mediation is particularly important to impulse transmission. A more detailed discussion of the anatomy and physiology of the nervous system will be found in Chapter 20. Here the intent is to focus on the chemical mediators in order to provide a basis for an understanding of vasoactive substances—both those naturally occurring and those used as pharmacological therapy for patients in shock.

In terms of motor activity, the two divisions of the autonomic system act both antagonistically and as complements to each other. Table 13-1 demonstrates their relationship to body functions. In general, it is the sympathetic system which responds to either external or internal stimuli which threaten homeostasis or systemic integrity. It prepares the individual for flight or fight and mediates adaptive efforts. In the case of falling blood pressure, there is dominance of the sympathetic division of the system which, among other alterations, causes an increase of heart rate and force of contraction and the constriction of the peripheral vasculature in an attempt to protect the vital organs and re-establish generally effective arterial pressure (Table 13-1, p. 369).

Once the stimulus is removed, the parasympathetic division acts to re-equilibrate the system, providing for the return to and maintenance of the homeostatic state and for general functions such as digestion.

However, within physiological limits, sympathetic dominance will persist as long as the stimulus is present. In studying the mechanisms of shock, we observe that the sympathetic reactions may be effective in re-establishing effective blood pressure with or without intervention. But, if hypotension persists, the mechanism of vasoconstriction will also persist—even to the point where its potentially compensatory and life-protecting effects deprive vital organs of nutrients, and lead to death. The physiological mechanisms which act to re-establish adequate blood pressure are shown in Figure 13-2. The stimulus of hypotension which activates the

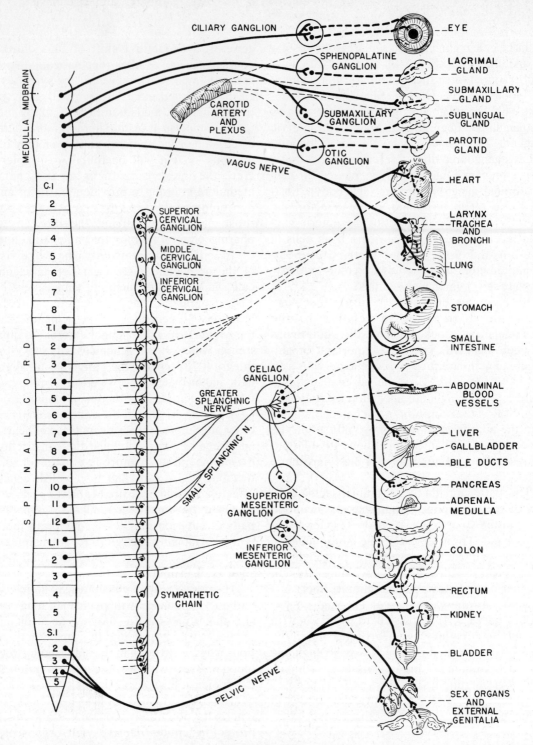

FIGURE 13-1.

Diagram of the efferent autonomic pathways. Preganglionic neurons are shown as solid lines, post-ganglionic neurons as dotted lines. The heavy lines are parasympathetic fibers; the light lines are sympathetic. Reproduced, with permission, from: Fundamentals of Human Physiology, ed. 2, by W. B. Youmans. Copyright © 1962, Yearbook Medical Publishers, Inc. Used by permission of Yearbook Medical Publishers, Inc.

TABLE 13-1
The Effects of Sympathetic or Parasympathetic Dominance on Specific Target Tissues

ORGAN	SYMPATHETIC—THORACOLUMBAR	PARASYMPATHETIC—CRANIOSACRAL
Eye	Dilates pupils. Permits accommodation for far vision.	Constricts pupils. Permits accommodation for near vision.
Heart	Increases rate and force of contraction.	Decreases rate; maintains systolic ejection force.
Lungs	Contracts smooth muscle—provokes bronchial constriction.	Contracts smooth muscle; thereby dilates bronchi.
Digestive canal	In general decreases blood supply and thereby decreases secretions and motility.	Maintains or regulates secretions. Controls blood supply and motility according to digestive needs.
Liver	Converts more glycogen to glucose.	Regulates secretion and synthesis.
Blood vessels	Dilates those of brain, lungs, and heart. Constricts others.	Dilates those of nose, pharynx, and digestive system and its accessory organs.
Adrenals	Increased adrenocortical secretion.	None demonstrated.
Pituitary	Stimulus from cortex is mediated here and in reticular system, activating all sympathetic fibers and adrenals.	Indirectly controls secretion in posterior lobe.
Sweat glands	Controls secretion; increases with stress.	None demonstrated.
Spleen	Contracts muscular capsule, forcing blood into circulation.	
Bladder	Inhibits contraction.	Stimulus elicits contraction.
Vessels of kidney	Constricts muscles of blood vessels and provokes renin-angiotensin mechanism activation leading to initial increase then decrease in urine output.	None demonstrated.
Heart and brain	Relaxes (greater blood supply results).	Maintains homeostasis.
Skeletal	Relaxes (blood is shunted to those in use).	
Viscera	See digestive canal.	Aids in digestion by increasing motility.

Adapted from Stackpole, C. E. and Leavell, L. C.: Textbook of Physiology, pp. 109, 110. New York, Macmillan; and Guyton, A. C.: Function of the Human Body, ed. 2. Philadelphia, W. B. Saunders, 1964.

sympathetic system is not different in *effect* from many other internal or external stimuli. *Any* situation which threatens systemic integrity stimulates sympathetic response. The person who perceives an external threat will undergo the same general physiological responses as the person who hemorrhages. In either case, if the situation is not remedied, there will be deleterious effects. Problems as varied as "stress" ulcers,

"psychogenic" asthma, and psychoses illustrate the point (Fig. 13-2, p. 370).

BIOCHEMISTRY
As most readers will remember, in order to relay impulses to muscle, the autonomic system requires that at least three conditions be met: 1) anatomical integrity of the nerve system, 2) concentration of several ions—particularly of

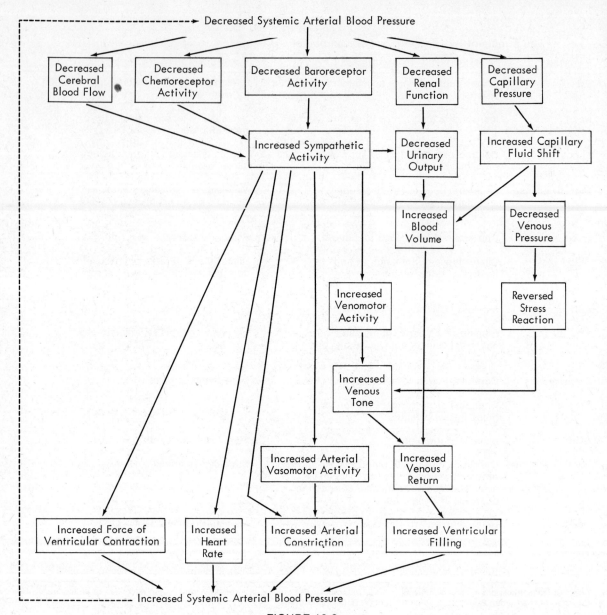

FIGURE 13-2.
Cardiovascular negative feedback mechanism. Source: Guyton, A. C.: Textbook of Medical Physiology, ed. 4. Philadelphia, W. B. Saunders, 1971.

sodium, potassium, calcium, magnesium, and chloride—within physiologically normal limits, and 3) neurohumoral transmitters—most notably acetylcholine and norepinephrine—and their appropriate antagonists. The following description of the action and effects of the biochemical and pharmacological agents most pertinent to the shock syndrome (and those caring for patients with it) is abstracted from the work of Goodman and Gilman.[5]

Biochemistry and Associated Physiological Principles

Goodman and Gilman provide a useful distinction between the *conduction* of an impulse (more accurately an action potential) and its *transmis-*

sion. Conduction refers to the wave of sequential ionic changes preceding the arrival of the action potential and following its passage along a nerve fiber. Simply put, these are represented by depolarization, repolarization (coinciding with the "resting" potential during which another impulse cannot be perpetuated), and hyperpolarization. The latter is required at the arrival of an action potential if it is to be conducted along the fiber. *Transmission* refers to the perpetuation of the action potential across synaptic spaces and neuroeffector junctions. The transmission of action potentials requires the presence of neurohumoral agents in addition to nervous system integrity and normal concentrations of ions; with the notable exception of the heart, conduction does not.

Acetylcholine is the most pervasive neurohumoral transmitter. It is required for the function of all pre- and postganglionic fibers of the parasympathetic system and for some postganglionic fibers of the sympathetic system, including those innervating the heart. The fibers requiring acetylcholine for transmission are cholinergic fibers, and the postjunction sites acted upon by the transmitter are cholinoceptive.

Similarly, most of the sympathetic or *adrenergic* fibers require norepinephrine for transmission. The inconsistency of terms results from their historical context. The existence of the chemical norepinephrine (with its metabolite epinephrine) was postulated long before it was chemically isolated. "It" was named sympathin. Then the names adrenalin and noradrenalin were in vogue because research allowed the extraction of these catecholamines from the adrenal gland. It was demonstrated that this substance also activated certain nerve fibers which were then called adrenergic fibers, a term which is still used. Correspondingly, the target sites are adrenoceptive. Quite recently, it has been discovered that there are at least two types of adrenoceptors: alpha and beta. Alpha adrenoceptors are sites on smooth muscle where adrenergically sympathetic activation produces excitation. Beta adrenoceptors are sites where sympathetic activation produces inhibition.

Table 13-2 will help to clarify the effects of cholonergic and adrenergic mediation. Where target organs have both receptor types, one usually predominates. For instance, adrenergic stimulation causes generalized dilatation of coronary vessels despite the presence of alpha receptors. There is still much to be learned in this area, not only in terms of the other substances which affect autonomic system activity, but also with regard to the conditions under which response to a known chemical mediator is variable.

With reference to sympathetic stimulation of blood vessel musculature and the heart, it can be seen that the release of norepinephrine will cause an increase in heart rate—a *chronotropic* effect—and increased force of cardiac contraction—an *inotropic* effect. Because of their prevalence of beta adrenoceptors, the coronary arteries dilate in response to sympathetic or adrenergic stimulation as do those of the brain (slightly). Most other blood vessels have a predominance of alpha receptor sites which effect vasoconstriction.

Unfortunately, the reaction of tissues to sympathetic stimulation is not as straightforward as the preceding paragraph suggests. Table 13-3 shows that such factors as the type and amount of catecholamine present and the availablity of adenosine triphosphate (ATP) for neural innervation and muscle work (dependent partially on the rate of glycogenolysis and the blood transport system) are important. The presence of still other chemical substances which influence the production, liberation, and metabolism of both acetylcholine and the catecholamines mentioned also determines the systemic response to sympathetic and parasympathetic stimulation. The following is a discussion of the production, action, and metabolism of the neurohumoral transmitters and their antagonists. Once a thorough understanding of the factors is achieved, the task of dealing with numerous pharmacological agents (which is intensified by the often imaginative but rarely informative trade names drug companies apply to them) is immeasurably easier, and patient care can be improved accordingly.

Current theorists postulate that the neurohumoral transmitters are synthesized and stored near the axonal terminals. The arrival of

TABLE 13-2
Responses of Effector Organs to Autonomic Nerve Impulses

EFFECTOR ORGANS	ADRENERGIC IMPULSES		CHOLINERGIC IMPULSES
	Receptor Type	Responses*	Responses*
Eye			
Radial muscle: iris	α	Contraction (mydriasis) ++	——
Sphincter muscle: iris		——	Contraction (miosis) +++
Ciliary muscle	β	Relaxation for far vision (slight effect)	Contraction for near vision +++
Heart			
S-A node	β	Increase in heart rate ++	Decrease in heart rate; vagal arrest +++
Atria	β	Increase in contractility and conduction velocity ++	Decrease in contractility, and (usually) increase in conduction velocity ++
A-V node and conduction system		Increase in conduction velocity ++	Decrease in conduction velocity; A-V block +++
Ventricles	β	Increase in contractility, conduction velocity, automaticity, and rate of idiopathic pacemakers +++	Slight decrease in contractility claimed by some
Blood Vessels			
Coronary	α,β	Constriction +; dilatation +++	Dilatation ±
Skin and mucosa	α	Constriction +++	Dilatation
Skeletal muscle	α,β	Constriction ++; dilatation ++	Dilatation +
Cerebral	α	Constriction (slight)	Dilatation
Pulmonary	α,β	Constriction +; dilatation +	Dilatation
Abdominal viscera	α,β	Constriction +++; dilatation +	——
Salivary glands	α	Constriction +++	Dilatation ++
Lung			
Bronchial muscle	β	Relaxation +	Contraction ++
Bronchial glands		Inhibition (?)	Stimulation +++
Stomach			
Motility and tone	β	Decrease (usually) +	Increase +++
Sphincters	α	Contraction (usually) +	Relaxation (usually) +
Secretion		Inhibition (?)	Stimulation +++
Intestine			
Motility and tone	α,β	Decrease +	Increase +++
Sphincters	α	Contraction (usually) +	Relaxation (usually) +
Secretion		Inhibition (?)	Stimulation ++
Gallbladder and Ducts		Relaxation +	Contraction +
Urinary Bladder			
Detrusor	β	Relaxation (usually) +	Contraction +++
Trigone and sphincter	α	Contraction ++	Relaxation ++
Ureter			
Motility and tone		Increase (usually)	Increase (?)
Uterus	α,β	Variable	Variable
Sex Organs		Ejaculation +++	Erection +++

TABLE 13-2
Responses of Effector Organs to Autonomic Nerve Impulses (continued)

EFFECTOR ORGANS	ADRENERGIC IMPULSES Receptor Type	Responses*	CHOLINERGIC IMPULSES Responses*
Skin			
Pilomotor muscles	α	Contraction + +	——
Sweat glands	α	Slight, localized secretion +	Generalized secretion + + +
Spleen Capsule	α	Contraction + + +	——
Adrenal Medulla		——	Secretion of epinephrine and norepinephrine
Liver		Glycogenolysis	——
Pancreatic Acini		——	Secretion + +
Salivary Glands	α	Thick, viscous secretion +	Profuse, watery secretion + + +
Lacrimal Glands		——	Secretion + + +
Nasopharyngeal Glands		——	Secretion + +

*Responses are designated 1+ to 3+ to provide an approximate indication of the importance of adrenergic and cholinergic nerve activity in the control of the various organs and functions listed.

From Goodman, L. S. and Gilman, A.: The Pharmacological Basis of Therapeutics, ed. 4. New York, Macmillan, 1970, p. 406. Used with permission.

TABLE 13-3
Effects and Uses of Sympathomimetic Drugs

	EFFECTIVE DOSES IN ADULT MAN (MG)	HEART RATE REFLEX ACTIVITY NORMAL	BLOCKED
Epinephrine	0.5–1.0 s.c.	+ or −	+
Norepinephrine (Levarterenol)	0.002–0.008/min i.v. infusion	−	+
Ephedrine	15–50 s.c., i.m., 8–10/min i.v.	+ or −	+
Methamphetamine	10–30 i.v., i.m.	+or −	+
Mephentermine	10–30 i.v., i.m.	+ or −	+
Hydroxyamphetamine	5–10 i.v., 10 –20 s.c.	+ or −	+
Metaraminol	5–10 i.v., i.m.	+ or −	+
Phenylephrine	0.5–1.0 i.v., 5–10 s.c.	−	0
Methoxamine	5–10 i.v., 10 –20 i.m.	−	0 or −
Dopamine	100–1000 µg/hr i.v. drip	+	0
Isoproterenol	0.2 i.v., 0.5 i.m. 0.25 Solution as inhalant	+	?

0 no efffect   Alpha activity (α receptors)   Beta activity (β receptors)   CNS—central nervous system

+ increased   A = Allergic reactions   B= Bronchodilator   O= Anorectic

− decreased   N= Nasal decongestion   C= cardiac

N.A. not available   P= pressor (may include β activity)   M = muscle vessel dilatation

V= other local vasoconstriction

Compiled and amended from Goodman, L. S., and Gilman, A.: The Pharmacological Basis of Therapeutics, ed. 4, New York: Macmillan Co., 1970, pp. 485, 506.

TABLE 13-3
Effects and Uses of Sympathomimetic Drugs (continued)

FORCE OF CARDIAC CONTRACTION		CARDIAC OUTPUT	CORONARY BLOOD FLOW	TOTAL PERIPHERAL RESISTANCE	BLOOD PRESSURE	MAIN CLINICAL USES		
SMALL DOSES	LARGE DOSES				SYSTOLIC/ DIASTOLIC	α RECEPTOR ANAV	β RECEPTOR BCM	CNS O
+	+	+	+	−	+/−	A, P. V,	B, C,	
+	+	0 or −	+	+	+/+	P,		
+	−	+	+	+ or −	+/+	N, P,	B, C,	
+	−	+		0, +, or −	+/0	P,		CNS, O
+	−	+	+	+	+/+	N, P,		
+	−	+	+	+	+/+	N, P,	C,	
+	−	0 or −	+	+	+/+	P		
0	+	−	+	+	+/+	N, P		
0	−	0 or −	0	+	+/+	N, P		CNS, O
+	+	+	?	0	+/+	P		
+	+	+	0	−	0/−		BC	CNS

an action potential at a junctional point triggers the release of either the transmitter acetylcholine or norepinephrine. The neurotransmitter is then thought to combine with postjunctional fibers to produce an action potential in the distal nerve fiber. When an action potential is of sufficient strength to be propagated, all competing potentials are temporarily inhibited. The time required for repolarization is variable (depending mainly on the physiological limits of the tissue). In essence, a fiber which has just conducted an impulse will not accept another. The resting period necessary to the fiber therapy acts to inhibit competing stimuli. The rate of impulse transmission is also limited by the very rapid destruction of the neurohumoral transmitters by their antagonists.

In summary, five events of impulse propagation can be delineated. Each event requires a set of preconditions and each represents a potential point of inhibition of the action potential.

1. Neuronal conduction requires nerve fibers of anatomical integrity, a stimulus above their threshold of response, and adequate concentrations of ions to permit depolarization.
2. Release of the transmitter which may result in propagation or inhibition of the impulse at a synapse or neuroeffector function.
3. Combination of the transmitter with postsynaptic fibers which perpetuates the action potential, provided that the fiber was in a resting state.
4. Action potential conduction along the postjunctional fiber.
5. Destruction or dissipation of the neurohumoral transmitter once the impulse has passed.

These events *each* represent a potential mechanism and site of action for enhancing or inhibiting motor reaction to autonomic nervous system stimuli.

Acetylcholine has been mentioned as the necessary agent for the transmission of action potentials by the parasympathetic system and to mediate transmission at some postganglionic fibers of the sympathetic division. In the latter case, it is hypothesized that acetylcholine initiates the release of norepinephrine. Additionally, in the case of the cardiac muscle and conduction system (in contrast to skeletal muscle and all other neurons), acetylcholine acts only to enhance the intrinsic activity rather than to initiate it. Acetycholine is rapidly destroyed after its release from vesicles near presynaptic sites by the specific enzyme *acetylcholinesterinase*, which circulates freely in the blood and other fluids.

Norephinephrine is the effective neurotransmitter for most sympathetic postganglionic fibers. It is synthesized from the amino acid, phenylalanine in the following manner: phenylalanine → tyrosine → dopamine → norepinephrine → epinephrine. It should be noted that each step of the preceding conversion requires highly specific enzymatic activity. Therefore, the production of norepinephrine (or epinephrine) can theoretically be modified at several points in its synthesis by agents which enhance or inhibit the synthesis or activity of the enzymes.

Norepinephrine is the catecholamine which predominates in the storage granules in the postganglionic fibers of the sympathetic nerves. Epinephrine predominates in the adrenal medulla. The synthesis of the two agents preceding the formation of dopamine takes place in the cellular cytoplasm. Dopamine then may enter granules located in the adrenal medulla where it is converted first to norepinephrine, then to epinephrine, and finally bound to protein. Or, it may enter granules in the sympathetic axions where it is mainly converted to norepinephrine and then stored in protein-bound form. The storage of these catecholamines acts as a reserve pool which is augmented by the ability of the cytoplasm to recapture circulating catecholamines. The reserve pool enables adrenergic fibers to sustain an output of norepinephrine for prolonged periods of time.

How nerve impulses trigger the release of catecholamine and how it is eventually metabolized is not known. However, the enzymes monoamine oxidase (MAO) and catechol-o-methyltransferase (COMT) have been implicated. The processes of oxidation and subsequent conversions of catecholamines by methods not completely known produce the substance VMA ("Vanillymandelic acid") familiar to nurses as an agent assayed to determine myocardial damage.

Research has now demonstrated that these agents of neurohumoral transmission—acetylcholine, norepinephrine, and dopamine—act in basically the same ways with respect to the central and peripheral-somatic nervous systems as they do with respect to the autonomic nervous system. In addition, these substances are generated by *both* the nervous and endocrine systems, the difference being one of duration of release and action. The release and action of neurotransmitters by the autonomic system is nearly instantaneous. It occurs in reaction to stimuli originating from either the cortical, subcortical, or spinal portions of the central nervous system. The cortical and subcortical stimuli are integrated at the hypothalamus. The release and action of the neurohumoral transmitters from the endocrine system is slower and more sustained but it is initiated by the same (or similar) conditions.

The purpose of presenting this formulation of neural transmission is to allow the nurse to understand the purpose and action (including toxic reactions) of the many drugs utilized in the regulation of blood pressure. A review of Table 13-3 will demonstrate the point that the action of large groups of drugs may be understood if one understands the part of impulse propagation they affect and their site of action. At this point the action and reaction of the central nervous, somatic, and autonomic systems in relation to hypotension and shock can be conceptualized, and it is time to discuss the "classic picture" of shock and its general pathophysiology.

Pathophysiology of the Shock Syndrome

THE CLASSIC PICTURE OF SHOCK

The main defect of homeostasis giving rise to the classic clinical signs of shock is that of poor tissue perfusion. Tissue perfusion requires: 1) an adequate supply of blood, 2) blood that is oxygenated and contains other vital nutrients, 3) blood that is free of lethal toxins, 4) blood that is delivered to cells at a pressure adequate to permit cellular exchange of metabolites and waste products. Two points emerge from the above requirements. First, there are a host of etiologies which may inhibit any one of the requirements; these are the underlying mechanisms of shock. Second, hypotension, the most immediate antecedent of shock, can be influenced by several factors, namely, hypovolemia, myocardial work deficiency, and/or increased vessel capacity. Since the first two factors were first known, and the auscultatory measurement of blood pressure was an early diagnostic technique (and also probably because of the prevalence of research on heart disease), a disproportionate amount of attention has been given to "cardiogenic" shock.

First, we will present the general clinical picture of shock, its most proximate etiologies, and general regimens of care. Then we will deal with specific and predictable causative agents.

Classically the clinical signs of shock are:

1. Hypotension*
2. Weak, rapid, and thready pulse
3. Cold clammy skin
4. Mental confusion (or other signs of altered sensorium, such as agitation or lethargy).
5. Urine output reductions to under 20 cc per hour.

While the above signs include only moderate reductions in urine output and cerebration, we may assume that the body is effectively compensating to protect the kidney and brain. The increased cardiac and respiratory rates, as well as water conservation, are in themselves effective compensation. However, should all the signs be present and progressive, the patient's compensatory mechanisms will fail and the stages of refractory, irreversible shock are imminent. Frank coma and prolonged anuria herald decompensation. Figure 13-3 presents a schematic representation of refractory shock. It is easily seen as a vicious cycle within which several feedback mechanisms serve to augment the progression of underperfusion of vital organs rather than to protect those organs. Also shown are several interrelationships which in themselves may trigger hypotension. One such relationship is that of toxin release and vasodilatation.

Unfortunately, the classic picture has many variants. Failure to know that a patient in shock may not demonstrate all of the signs of shock or that he may, in fact, have completely antithetical signs (such as warm dry skin and a bounding pulse which may be observed in a patient who manifests an early stage of "endotoxic" shock) jeopardizes the chances for recovery of the patient. Few people recover from profound shock. Current therapies are most effective in the early stages. Better yet, the alert nurse may *prevent* shock by alerting the medical team to special

*Hypotension is usually defined as a diastolic blood pressure under 70 mm per Hg and/or a systolic pressure under 90 mm per Hg. However, the definition advanced more recently is: hypotension is blood pressure reduction of more than 25 percent of its "normal" reading for that person.[6]

hazards or suspicious signs that patients in her care may manifest.

Table 13-4 was compiled from data presented by 73 patients who manifested cardiogenic shock. It illustrates the variability of the signs of shock syndrome, *even shock syndromes with the same underlying etiology*.

TABLE 13-4
Overt Signs of Shock in 73 Patients with
Cardiogenic Shock

PHYSICAL FINDINGS	PERCENT OF PATIENTS
Skin:	
Cool and moist	87
Warm and dry	13
Brain:	
Normal mental status	46
Depressed brain function (confusion, lethargy, or agitation)	37
Frank coma	17
Urine output:	
Oliguria (< 20 ml/hr)	71
Normal (> 20 ml/hr)	16
Anuria (no urine for one hour)	13
Pulmonary edema:	
None	54
Overt	46

Scheidt, Stephen, Ascheim, Robert, and Killip, Thomas: Shock after acute myocardial infarction. A. J. Cardiology, 26:557, Dec. 1970. Used with permission of the authors.

We have briefly reviewed the early general pathophysiology of shock; a brief outline of the body changes which make the shock state irreversible is in order. Again, the reader is urged to consult Figures 13-2 and 13-3 for better conceptualization of the mechanisms of compensation and decompensation. The commonality of the stages of irreversible shock is tissue necrosis to the point that vital organs cannot function. Actually, the release of histamine from dead cells, whether they are vital or not, will lead to vasodilatation and a further decrease in blood pressure. That further compromises tissue perfusion unless the blood volume is adequate and can be mobilized. One might implicate generalized cellular necrosis as the common beginning of refractory shock.

Most commonly, the heart is the first organ to be irretrievably damaged. Although the kidney appears to be the first vital organ to respond to hypotension when insufficiency occurs, the kid-

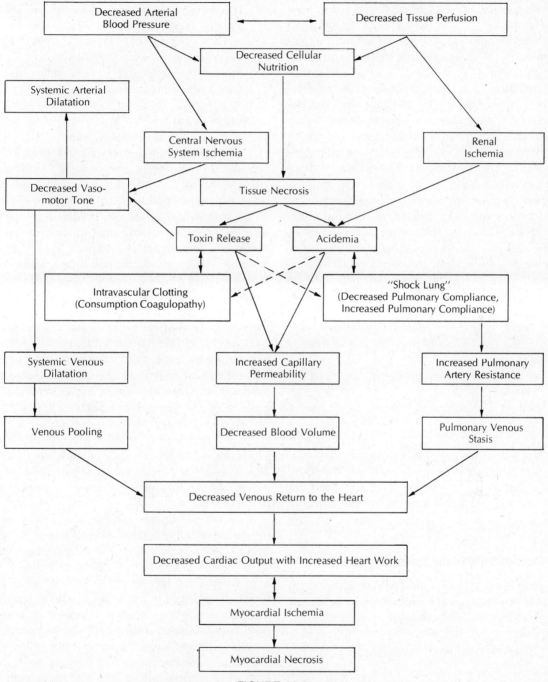

FIGURE 13-3.
Schematic representation of refractory shock.

ney may withstand lack of perfusion for at least 15 minutes and return to adequate function. It has been demonstrated to be viable for as long as 90 minutes.[7] The heart drops markedly in effective function if its arteries are even marginally underperfused for 15 to 20 seconds. Its vulnerability is compounded by the fact that the demands on it are great under the conditions which cause underperfusion in other organs.

Brain death occurs in most cases after four minutes, sometimes sooner. The brain is perhaps the most vulnerable of all organs to marginal underperfusion, and irreversible damage may occur before other signs alert the onlooker to the severity of the situation. Both societal expectations and "medical" ethics are undergoing the ordeal of change with respect to definitions of life and death. However, the tragedy of the resuscitation of a physically functional person minus most of his former personal capacities still occurs.*

Three major research questions are paramount if progress in preventing and treating shock is to be made.

1. Is there a naturally occurring hypotensive factor? How is it mobilized?
2. Where is blood pooled in episodes of hypotension?
3. What pharmacological agent would selectively aid the perfusion of vital organs?

Current progress in research on these questions and others that are more specific to underlying etiologies of shock will be discussed later in this chapter.

General Care of the Patient in Shock

In general, there are four goals of care of the patient in shock toward which the physician and nurse share joint and complementary functions. They are:

1. Maintenance of tissue perfusion.

---

*Recently an entity called "shock lung" has been added to the list of changes in vital organs brought about by shock. It is postulated that its components include: 1) increased arteriovenous shunting, 2) microemboli, and 3) increased pressure in the vascular tree leveling to a loss of surfactant and decreased compliance.

2. Discovery of the underlying mechanism of the shock syndrome and the administration of therapy.
3. Physiological and psychological support.
4. Surveillance: ongoing assessment of the patient's condition and his needs.

NURSING CARE

The functions of assessment, support, and the planning and administering of nursing care are reciprocally dependent and ongoing. However, while there are routinized actions taken for patients who are hypotensive, even these are based on the assessment of the occurrence of hypotension in conjunction with other signs and symptoms. Some patients are especially prone to develop a shock syndrome due to age, illness, or therapy. They require vigilant observation and assessment. For these reasons, we will consider the nursing function of assessment first. Assessment includes both the observation of relevant parameters of the patient's condition *and* the more complex process of interpreting data in a manner that provides a basis for intelligent and thorough nursing care. (See Chapter 4 for a discussion of the general principles and practices involved in assessment.)

Nursing care also includes the responsibility of judging when to alert other health team members, particularly the physician, to changes in the patient's condition which warrant re-evaluation or treatment.

Several of the parameters need to be assessed only occasionally, some at hourly intervals, and others more frequently. Hospitals frequently have preset nursing routines for the frequency of assessments and rely on physicians to "write orders" for changes in the routine. This is a questionable practice at best: it wastes physicians' time to write prescriptions for nursing care, it wastes someone else's time to transfer the orders, and it wastes nurses. (In the opinion of this author, any nurse who doesn't know enough to closely monitor a postsurgical patient, or any other patient who has suffered a severe insult to his system, shouldn't be practicing.) There is also an insidious effect that arises out of such orders. They tend to lend a false sense of security when they have been followed. The patient's condition and the risks of complications should dictate what parameters are monitored and how frequently. At most, orders or routines are only a guideline and represent *maximal* intervals between assessments.

It has been mentioned that several of the above parameters will be used or not used according to the patient's condition, and according to practices in the hospital or on the patient unit. If the patient in shock is placed in a coronary care unit or a shock unit, his ECG will generally be monitored continuously. If he is not, that data may not be available except as his physician orders it. Central venous pressure lines are now very commonly inserted but they are not part of standard treatment in many hospitals. Arterial catheters for serial determinations of blood gases (or, in specialized units, for continuous monitoring of "central" arterial pressure), are rarely part of standard care for the patient in shock outside of teaching and research-oriented institutions.

The disparity in practices of patient care reflects considerable differences in the philosophies of physicians regarding the efficacy of different treatments, the risks *versus* benefits of several monitoring devices and the general prognosis of the patient in shock. It also reflects the primary purpose of the hospital, its size, and the sources of funding of the institution (e.g., "teaching" versus "community"). Another factor is the lack of knowledge of what causes shock, what defines its progress, or what will predictably influence its outcome. The need for minimal standards of care for the human being—who is after all at the center of this controversy—is apparent.

Dr. Robert Hardaway, from his experience as chief of the shock research unit at Walter Reed Army Medical Center implies such minimal standards.[8] He advocates minimal *facilities* for monitoring any patient in shock, the addition of other equipment for monitoring which he feels is "highly desirable," and equipment (which implies techniques) for teaching or specialized treatment-research units. They are listed below.

Minimal facilities include basic monitoring devices: 1) sphygmomanometer and stetho-

scope, 2) intravenous fluid administration equipment, 3) equipment for monitoring central venous pressure, 4) facilities for the administration of oxygen, and 5) an indwelling urethral catheter to determine hourly urine output.

Very desirable shock treatment facilities include 1) capability to perform arterial and venous blood gas, electrolyte, enzyme and lactate studies and blood-clotting time, and specific organ function studies at any time of day, 2) an effective volume-cycled respirator with oxygen concentration controls, 3) defibrillation equipment, 4) electrocardiograph and oscilloscope for continual monitoring, 5) hyperthermia and hypothermia administration equipment, 6) x-ray services and radiological and other specialists available for consultation, and 7) suitable flowsheets (forms for recording data).

Optional facilities. (The implication is that these facilities should be available in teaching and/or research institutions): 1) facilities for determining red cell mass, plasma volume, and total body water, 2) metabolic scale, and 3) apparatus for cardiac output studies.*

Shock research facilities. 1) Several channel recorders (for continuous records of parameters such as peripheral and central arterial pressure, central venous pressure, temperature, and so on, 2) cardiac catheterization facilities and associated equipment for determining intracardiac and pulmonary pressures, and 3) a computer and facilities for data processing.

It becomes obvious that much of the patient's treatment will be governed by the nature of the equipment in the hospital to which he is taken rather than his condition *per se*.

Dr. Hardaway lists several qualities as important for nursing personnel. These include interest, intellect and intellectual freedom, manual dexterity, and knowledge of electronic equipment. We can concur that these attributes are important, but we take exception to his "shifting" application of "professional" in his opening remarks.

It would be interesting to hear what qualities

---

*We feel that a metabolic scale should be listed as a desirable piece of equipment for determining the resolution of edematous states associated with congestive heart failure.

patients would desire. Several studies demonstrate that patients are concerned that the nurse demonstrate "caring" attitudes, kindness, and friendliness. Some studies report that patients desired these qualities *more than* such qualities as skill, efficiency, and so on. With these thoughts in mind, let us return to the subject of nursing assessment of the patient prone to or manifesting shock. Several of the parameters require comments and clarification. To simplify the matter, they will be discussed in the order in which they were listed in Table 13-5.

PULSE. The pulse rate of the hypotensive pa-

TABLE 13-5
Parameters for Assessment of the Hypotensive or
Shock-Prone Patient

Cardiovascular:
  Pulse: Rate   Quality   Area monitored*
  Blood pressure: Reading   Remarks:
  Heart sounds: Normal (   )   Muffled (   )
                  Irregular (   )   Change (   )
  Neck veins: Flat (   )   Distended (   )
                  Pulsations?
  Peripheral veins: Flat (   )   Engorged (   )
  Nail beds: Normal (   )   Pale (   )
                  Refill: Good (   )   Poor (   )
  *Central venous pressure: Reading   Site
checked (   )
  *Intra-arterial blood pressure: Reading   Site
checked (   )
  *Electrocardiograph: Rate   Rhythm   Change?
Respiratory:
  Respiration: Rate   Character
  Lungs: Clear (   )   Rales (   )
              Cough (   )
Renal:
  Hourly output   *Specific gravity
Sensorium:
  Mood: Unremarkable (   )   Anxious (   )
            Depressed (   )   Agitated (   )
  Alertness: Responsive (   )   Slowed (   )
                  Obtunded (   )   Coma (   )
Skin and mucous membranes:
  Color: Normal (   )   Pale (   )
            Flushed (   )   Cyanotic (   )
            Mottled (   )
  Temperature: Normal (   )   Hot (   )
                    Cold (   )   Disparity?
  Moisture: Dry (   )   Moist (   )
                Diaphoresis (   )   Skin Turgor?
Change of habits:
  Rest/Activity   Eating   Elimination
Patient complaints:

*These parameters may or may not be monitored according to the condition of the patient and the facilities available.

tient is usually rapid. Unless myocardial damage is present, the pulse should be regular until the point of extreme or prolonged tachycardia (more than 120 beats per minute). At that point, or if the patient is hypovolemic, the character of the pulse is likely to be weak and thready. In the first case, this happens because the heart does not have the time to fill. In the second case, venous return is impaired and the blood arrives at the right atrium in a lesser amount and under less pressure. When the system begins to decompensate, myocardial ischemia occurs. Ischemia may precipitate arrhythmias and/or a group myocardial infarction. Ventricular arrhythmias may be detected in the pulse. In this, as in all other assessments, it is important to refer to the patient's preexisting and/or underlying condition. For instance, if the patient has sclerosed arteries, his pulse will typically feel weak: a weak, thready pulse alone does not reflect decompensation. An important exception to the general case is the patient who has an underlying infection; his pulse may feel full and bounding despite relatively severe shock.

Pulsus paradoxicus is a condition in which the normal slight diminishing of the pulse beats during inspiration is greatly exaggerated. The patient is aware of a rebound of pulse on expiration in this condition, when normally it would not be noticeable. Cardiac tamponade frequently causes this symptom. The increased intrathoracic negative pressure decreases the blood flow into the left ventricle and when the chamber is impinged upon there is even less blood available for output into the system. The net result is very weak pulse during inspiration. In other conditions in which the ventricle does not fill adequately, the heart beats but the cardiac output is not great enough to be transmitted as a radial pulsation. A weak myocardium beats ineffectually and the systolic ejection force is not great enough to overcome the peripheral resistance, so that a radial pulse is not felt. Other conditions may also predispose to a pulse deficit. It is always wise to use the apical pulse to count heart beats, but peripheral pulses are a better indication of the tissue perfusion.

BLOOD PRESSURE. Traditionally, the most important measure of the ratio between vascular capacity and blood volume has been the arterial blood pressure. However, the blood pressure recording is subject to several types of errors. 1) Reader errors may occur both in determination of the height of the column of mercury and through faulty technique. 2) Equipment for taking the blood pressure is subjected to punishing treatment in most institutions and should be frequently inspected for leaks in the bladder, cracks or punctures of the tubing, partial disconnections, or other signs of an inoperative condition or one that can lead to inaccuracies. 3) Blood pressure by the auscultatory method is an indirect measure of arterial pressure at best. Vasoconstriction of the peripheral beds tends to cause a deceptively high reading. In addition to the problem of inaccurate blood pressure readings, there is the problem of frequent relegation of the blood pressure taking to personnel who may not have been trained to observe the overall pattern of changes. The professional nurse, even if she has confidence in her ancillary personnel, must not abdicate the responsibility of observing the patient. She should periodically review the signs of the patient and provide a check on blood pressure reading and recording both for herself and for any other personnel.

The hypotensive patient may not proceed to shock, while patients who do not have preliminary hypotension may relatively suddenly manifest signs of severe shock. The anaphylactic reaction illustrates the latter point. It cannot be overemphasized that those who read and assess blood pressure levels should do so in the light of the patient's norm. Many individuals are fully functional with blood pressures of 90/70 and others are in severe shock at 140/90.

HEART SOUNDS. Although many nurses have not been trained to listen to the chest, all professional nurses should be able to determine when abnormal sounds are present. Nurses should also be able to detect unusually loud or soft (muffled) heart sounds and irregularities as minimal requirements for the care of acutely ill patients.

NECK VEINS. Neck veins are normally flat when the patient's head and shoulders are raised above a 30° angle. If they are not, and if they pulsate, venous congestion is indicated. If the

patient did not demonstrate these signs before, or if they are appreciably more distinct with a concurrent deterioration indicated by other measurements, a physician should be notified *immediately*.

PERIPHERAL VEINS. Many people have bulging veins in their extremities (without varicosities); however, they should flatten when the extremity is at heart level. If they do not, they demonstrate the presence of venous congestion.

NAIL BEDS. The color of the nail bed reflects both circulation and oxygenation of blood in the capillary beds. Paleness is indicative of poor perfusion. Cyanosis is a relatively late and ominous sign, since it reflects a very high degree of unoxygenated blood. The nail bed should blanch when pressed and rapidly return to its normal color if perfusion is adequate.

CENTRAL VENOUS PRESSURE (CVP). The method of taking CVP is too detailed to record here. It is readily available with the equipment and the learner should make her first readings after a demonstration and with *supervision*. The hazards to the patient with a centrally positioned catheter are not so readily seen. They necessitate nursing observations to rule out the following problems: 1) bleeding at the site of insertion, 2) bleeding through the catheter from malpositioning of the stopcock, 3) inflammation or infection (detectable from swelling, redness, tenderness, and abnormal warmth at the site of insertion or along the course of the catheter), and 4) malpositioning of the catheter (the nurse should alert the physician if the level of fluid does not fluctuate with breathing, if the patient complains of pain when fluid is administered, or if fluid does not flow *readily* through the line). Figure 13-4 shows the correct placement of the CVP catheter.

The limits of a "normal" CVP are variable within institutions and the nurse should report readings beyond those limits. However, as general guides, the nurse should *certainly* report 1) variations beyond 5 cm/water on serial recordings, 2) CVP below 2 cm/water which indicates inadequate venous return to the heart, and 3) CVP above 15 cm/water which indicates congestive heart failure. Thal notes that a gross rise in CVP is preceded by a rise in left atrial pressure

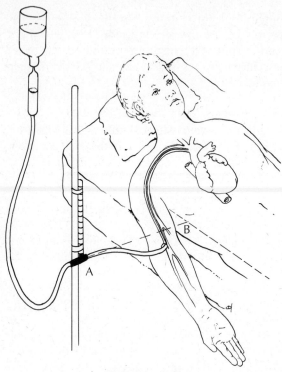

FIGURE 13-4.
A basilic or brachial vein cut down at the elbow is performed and a large polyethylene catheter is passed as far as the superior vena cava or until wide excursions in central venous pressure occur with each breath. Zero reference point for measurements is the middle of the anteroposterior diameter of the chest. Central venous pressure can also be measured by direct puncture into the subclavian vein under and parallel to the first portion of the clavicle.

minutes or even hours earlier.[9] Therefore, the nurse should familiarize herself with the more subtle signs of incipient failure (see Chapter 12).

INTRA-ARTERIAL BLOOD PRESSURE. This parameter is increasingly monitored, even intermittently for patients who are not in specialized units. The nurse should be aware that the intra-arterial catheter carries all the hazards of a central venous catheter as well as the following: 1) The catheter is far more rigid than that used to give IV fluids; that fact, in addition to catheter position, creates increased risks of stimulating arrhythmias and inadvertent trauma to tissues. 2) The catheter is in the arterial system; if bleeding occurs it will be more rapid and therefore more

dangerous. Patients with any kind of arterial catheter should be closely watched. 3) There is a hazard of injecting air into the arterial tree since the system must be flushed under relatively high pressure to overcome the resistance provided by the counter force of the arterial blood pressure.

One advantage of arterial catheters to the patient is the avoidance of repeated vessel puncture for laboratory studies. For the patient whose blood pressure is monitored intra-arterially, the advantage rests in the physician's ability to monitor the patient's condition more accurately and a correspondingly more precise course of treatment, resulting, one hopes, in recovery. However, at present, the majority of patients in profound shock, for whom such advantages would most logically outweigh the risks, rarely recover. For most, the benefit lies in contributing to research for better methods of treatment.

The basic components of an intra-arterial monitoring system are: 1) an arterial catheter, 2) a flushing system, 3) a transducer, and 4) a monitor. The transducer replaces the sphygmomanometer as the indicator of pressure; it converts the pressure to an electrical signal on the monitor. The monitor may be connected to a recorder for graphic records. The screen of the monitor is scaled so that the nurse may "take" a blood pressure by recording, mentally if not physically, the level of the topmost and lowest portions of the waves produced by heart action. In addition to increased precision, this method of measurement reflects changes in heart rhythm. The direct method of blood pressure measurement more closely reflects the extent of perfusion to vital organs. It will be higher than the indirect (sphygmomanometer) reading in cases of vasoconstriction and lower when arteriolar dilatation is present.

ELECTROCARDIOGRAPHIC MONITORING. This principle of nursing care for the patient with continual monitoring is presented in Chapter 12. *All* nurses should be able to detect life-threatening arrhythmias. An oscilloscope or a serial ECG printing provides a more sensitive detection device; it is not a substitute for human intelligence and does nothing for the patient unless it is interpreted. The major advantage of these instruments is that they indicate heart action more quickly, more precisely and less obtrusively than does the pulse or the heart sound.

RESPIRATORY STATUS. The respiratory rate also reflects poor tissue perfusion. The patient is usually tachypneac and may demonstrate air hunger. Fast, shallow, or labored breathing places a great demand on the muscles of respiration so that they require much more oxygen than usual. Conscious patients usually experience anxiety about the character of their respiration. Oxygen therapy is usually employed and mechanical respiratory assistance may also be necessary. The nursing role is to observe the quality and number of respirations. The nurse must also know the principles involved in the use of oxygen and the equipment for administering it.

All too frequently the humidifying apparatus for oxygen therapy is not functioning properly, causing the patient discomfort and a greater risk of pulmonary problems. Whether or not the patient is seen by an inhalation therapist, the nurse retains the responsibility for insuring his comfort, safety, and general welfare.

RENAL STATUS. Renal shutdown may occur when the effective blood pressure in the renal arteries is below the level of 70 mm mercury. Therefore, the production of adequate amounts of urine, above 30 ml an hour, rules out a hypotensive state (except in the case of endotoxin shock, in which urine volume production is adequate, although the BUN still rises). Accurate, frequent monitoring of urinary output remains a vitally important index to the patient's physical status. Many patients have a urinary catheter inserted so that a greater accuracy of measurement of the urinary output may be obtained. The risk of bacterial contamination by careless techniques in obtaining the drainage cannot be overemphasized. Standardization of the procedure and the time for the collection of urine is also important to prevent errors in assessments. Specific gravity is a rough index of renal effectiveness. It should be between 1.002 and 1.028. These are *maximal* limits; high or increasing specific gravity is a rough bedside index of water conservation, a protective and compensatory mechanism for hypovolemia or hypotension in general.

SENSORIUM. Despite the increasing emphasis on quantitative data, there remains in nursing a place for the general assessment, "the patient looks sicker." The patient may also voice vague feelings of becoming worse. While there is no way to communicate either case on paper, the concerned and observant nurse develops skill in recognizing that something is "going wrong" for the patient. Sometimes there is a definite deterioration in the patient's mental condition, or he may complain of tingling or numbness in his extremities, of blurring vision or tinnitus as cerebral perfusion diminishes, or of feeling cold. While general vasodilatation in the skin is not desirable, warm blankets may be supplied.

Although sensorial changes (particularly with respect to mental alertness) do occur, they do not necessarily proceed from alertness, to confusion, to coma, to death. Although he may be weak, the patient often remains relatively alert until the time of death. Others are confused, agitated and/or apprehensive, with minimal or borderline shock. The hemorrhaging patient is particularly likely to exhibit apprehension. It is difficult to determine whether it is the blood loss or the conscious recognition of it (and what it means) which causes the patient to become anxious. In any case, the nurse must be alert to the fact that something is wrong when sensorial changes are evident. The patient in pain may present himself in much the same manner as the patient in shock. Astute assessment is required to determine how to intervene: should a medication be given? Should the physician be called? Or, does the patient need only reassurance or emotional support?

SKIN AND MUCOUS MEMBRANES. Except in cases of shock featuring vasodilatation (such as those occurring after anaphylactic reactions, overdoses of vasodilators or anesthesias, or other "neurogenic" causes), the patient in shock usually exhibits pallor, mottling, or cyanosis. His skin is usually moist and cold and he *feels* cold. This occurs as a result of the body's attempts to compensate for decreased perfusion with peripheral vasoconstriction. In addition to the assessment and reporting of changes, the nurse should supply extra blankets and, unless it is contraindicated, the patient should be helped to assume a position of optimum comfort.

The traditional Trendelenburg's position is now rarely recommended because it necessarily compromises the patient's respiratory status.[10] The position of comfort implies that the respiratory status is maintained at the optimal level and attention also is given to the effect of gravity on cerebral perfusion. Even in shock, the patient should not remain in one position. Poorly perfused tissues are jeopardized further by undue or prolonged pressure. In hospitals where there is a written policy or opinion regarding the treatment of the patient in shock, the nurse is, of course, responsible for observing it. But, she is also responsible for effecting needed changes in outdated policies and procedures, and for doing so through the "proper channels."

The nurse should be especially alert to the conditions of patients who are most prone to hypotension because of their age, underlying disease, or from artifacts of intended therapy. The following list is only suggestive of patients prone to hypotension.[11]

Patients with multiple injuries
Profound emotional stress
Pain
Paracentesis; any rapid decompression
Visceral instrumentation
Elderly surgical patient
Infants, especially after surgery
Deep general anesthesia
Maintenance on hypertensive agents
Extensive spinal anesthesia
Urinary obstructive disease
Peritoneal dialysis
Hypoglycemias

The majority of patients who are apt to develop shock are readily identified by the nurse. However, shock is a complex phenomenon. Even the healthy young person who is suffering intense anxiety may develop shock, even after a relatively minor procedure. Pain may also intensify the risk of shock. Visceral instrumentation, such as cystoscopy, may provoke shock due to the stimulation of the vagal reflexes. The mechanism of shock is the same when the abdomen is rapidly decompressed, (whether it is because of withdrawal of gastric contents, urine, or ascitic fluid). Such patients also have a risk of bac-teremia which can lead to shock. Patients with an intestinal obstruction or ascites usually suffer decreased effective blood volume and have even greater risks. Peritoneal dialysis done with hypertonic glucose solutions provokes the withdrawal of large amounts of fluid into the abdominal cavity. This fluid loss from the interstitial spaces is reflected in blood vessel volume and may result in shock. Because the nurse is responsible for monitoring the vital signs of her patient, both during and after the procedures, it is particularly important that she recognize the signs of shock and know the risks of its occurrence.

When a patient has been subjected to deep general anesthesia, he is usually kept in the recovery room for a prolonged period of time, where nurses are continually alert for symptoms of shock. The patient who has spinal anesthesia becomes mentally alert very quickly and may be returned to the general care area. However, because these patients have been subjected to drugs which curtail sympathetic influence on vasomotor tone, they may react with symptoms of shock from profound pooling of blood in the lower extremities. Therefore, they must be watched closely *beyond* the period of apparent stabilization of blood pressure, until the effects of the anesthetic are no longer detectable.

Infants as well as the elderly have decreased tolerance for most forms of stress, have a small safety margin with respect to blood volume alterations, and easily become dehydrated. The elderly have sluggish adaptation mechanisms and do not respond readily to blood volume alterations. Both groups need particularly close observation after surgery or other potentially shock-producing therapies. The elderly are more frequently hypertensive; their blood pressure readings are often unreliable and a poor index to their welfare, unless they are compared with their individual norm.

In the case of an emergency, the nurse may need to begin therapy. This will depend on the policy of the institution and her own level of expertise. Table 13-6 was compiled from several sources as a general guide to aid the nurse who is most likely to be preparing the patient and gathering equipment for the physician's administration of therapy. It combines the parameters of assessment with the clinical features of common conditions (Table 13-6, pp. 386-387).

THE NURSING ROLE IN THE DELIVERY OF MEDICAL THERAPIES

The most immediate goal of medical therapy is to provide for the maintenance of good tissue perfusion or to restore perfusion to the best possible level. A concomitant goal is the discovery and correction of the evocative agent or primary etiology of the shock syndrome. In general therapy, the patient usually receives medications, oxygen, and intravenous fluids or blood (or its derivatives). They will be briefly discussed in that order. Additional efforts are directed toward maintenance and support as needed or restoration of any suboptimal vital function if it exists. The latter measures are specific to underlying pathophysiologies and will be discussed in the next section.

MEDICATIONS. The controversy over the use of vasopressor agents, versus vasodilator agents in conjunction with blood volume expansion, rages on. The basis for using these two general classes will be briefly discussed here. Table 13-7, pages 388-389, compiles the pertinent data about the commonly used agents of both types.

Vasopressors are used in an attempt to improve blood pressure and, thereby, tissue perfusion by maintaining or augmenting vasoconstriction. Actually, drugs acting directly to cause vasoconstriction such as methoxamine or phenylephrine and similar agents are the only true vasopressors. Currently, drugs which improve circulation by directly acting on the heart, such as levarterenol or metaraminol, or by mobilizing pooled blood (dopamine) are also classed generally as vasopressors when their primary action may not be vasoconstriction.

The general disenchantment with vasopressors centers on their failure to reduce mortality in shock patients with the *possible* exception of those in cardiogenic shock.[13] Second, the primary need of shock patients is the improvement of tissue perfusion in vital organs, not the improvement of blood pressure per se. Vasopressors have several side effects which may ultimately jeopardize tissue perfusion: 1) the myocardium is forced to pump against a greater peripheral resistance; 2) often an even greater rate of heartbeat and respiration is induced; 3) the patient often develops a tolerance to the drug (higher and higher doses are required to prevent hypotension *tachyphylaxis*); and 4) it is often difficult to withdraw the drug after prolonged use (withdrawal, even in minute decrements, may induce hypotension). In addition, there are several very dangerous toxic or untoward effects of therapy with vasopressors:

1. Hypertension with danger of CVA pulmonary edema, cardiac decompensation, and acute cardiac dilatation.
2. Arrhythmias are especially frequent when alpha receptor agonists are given; such as epinephrine, isoproterenol, hydroxyamphetamines, and ephedrine.
3. Central nervous system stimulation.
4. Local reactions—tissue necrosis and ulceration from capillary constriction.
5. Ischemic necrosis of the liver.

Vasodilators used in conjunction with plasma volume expansion are purported to protect the vital organs from underperfusion or to restore perfusion to them, thus reversing the effects of generalized vasoconstriction. There are several studies which report beneficial effects from the use of beta adrenoceptor blocking agents; propranolol (Inderol) is the only drug of this class currently in widespread clinical use.[14] More recently, researchers have reported beneficial effects from the use of dopamine.[15]

Vasodilatation could be induced by several means. It is possible to virtually eliminate autonomic activity—and that may inadvertently occur with anesthesia. Second, the ganglionic blocking agents, such as mecamylamine (Inversine) and pentolinium (Ansolysen), induce vasodilatation. Hypotension is a frequent complication of inadvertent overdosage of patients treated with these agents for hypertension. Obviously they represent a nonspecific or "shotgun" approach to obtaining vasodilatation for patients with poor tissue perfusion from shock states. Alpha receptor agonists or beta receptor agonists

TABLE 13-6

Common Clinical Conditions Preceding Shock: Summary of Physiology, Clinical Features and Prevalent Initial Therapy[12]

	PHYSIOLOGY	CLINICAL FEATURES	USUAL INITIAL THERAPY
		DECREASED CARDIAC OUTPUT	
Myocardial disease Valvular disease Arrhythmias	Depressed myocardial contractility	Decreased or irregular heart sounds; gallop rhythm, murmurs, ECG changes, perhaps signs of CHF.	Vasopressor in IV infusion. Treatment of underlying disease. (Digitalis, antiarrhythmic drugs.)
Pericardial tamponade	Fluid-filled sac restricts heart filling	Elevated venous pressure, narrowed pulse pressure, dull heart sounds.	Pericardial tap; may require surgery for sutures or ligature of bleeding vessels.
Pulmonary embolism	L. atrial filling restricted—left ventricular failure	Pain, tachypnea, cyanosis, venous distention; clinical setting for thromboembolism.	Oxygen therapy; vasopressor infusion; surgery may be performed.
Metabolic derangements: Hypoxia acidosis Diabetes mellitus	Decreased myocardial contractility due to hypoxia and/or acidosis	Kussmaul's respirations, cyanosis; evidence of chronic lung disease, pronounced hypoxia or diabetes.	Alkalizing agent, treatment of underlying conditions, oxygen therapy (usually with IPPB); vasopressor.
		DECREASED CIRCULATING BLOOD VOLUME	
Blood loss	Decreased venous return—decreased cardiac output	Evidence of occult or front bleeding; most difficult if into body cavity.	Transfuse with whole blood, pressure to external wounds, ice water lavage to GI tract; may require surgery.
Plasma loss	As above	Burns, dermatitis, intra-abdominal fluid accumulation.	Transfuse with plasma or plasma volume expander; may remove fluid or perform gastrointestinal decompression.
Fluid and electrolyte loss	As above	History of copious vomiting, diarrhea or polyuria; signs of salt depletion or intestinal or pylar obstruction.	Saline then electrolyte-rich intravenous infusion according to blood chemistry; a vasopressor may be used.

		NEUROGENIC	
Vagal reflex	Pain or visceral instrumentation	Bradycardia and decreased arteriolar resistance; nausea, sweating and sometimes syncope.	Discontinue precipitating procedure, relieve pain; allay apprehension; atropine to combat bradycardia.
Anesthesia or drugs	Decreased sympathetic response	Toxic effects of drugs manifest evidence of parasympathetic dominence; often peripheral manifestations not apparent because of sympathetic blocking.	Vasopressor may be used; treatment will depend on causative agent; antidote prepared if existent; keep patient warm and dry and in position of comfort or in Trendelenburg's position.
Sympathectomy	Decreased sympathetic innervation		
Anaphylaxis	Decreased vascular resistance from antigen-antibody reaction.	Abrupt onset, history of antigen administration, laryngeal edema.	Aqueous epinephrine 1/1000; respiratory assistance; corticosteroids may be used.
		SEPTIC	
Gram-negative bacteremia or septicemia	Decreased vascular resistance	Often accompanied by chills and fever. History of precipitating event.	Antibiotic therapy, prevention of further infection, vasopressor.
Perforated viscus	As above	As above	As above, plus corrective surgery.

TABLE 13-7

Drugs Relevant to the Treatment of Shock

CLASS OF DRUG	GENERIC NAME	TRADE NAME IN USA	MODE OF ACTION	COMMENTS
Ganglionic blocking agents	Hexamethonium	Hexamethonium	Decreases transmission at autonomic ganglia. All drugs act in essentially the same way.	Patients with hypertensive encypalopathy low sodium intake or thiazides are particularly sensitive. Dosages must be highly individualized; overdosage or bolus absorption may lead to shock. Trimethaphan causes histamine release.
	Mecamylamine	Inversine		
	Pentolinium	Ansolysen		
	Trimethaphan Camsalate	Arfonad		
Alpha receptor agonists: direct action (Alpha-mimetic effect)	Methoxamine	Vasoxyl	Direct action on smooth muscle of arterioles producing vasoconstriction. Reflex heat slowing; venous pooling occurs.	Constricts veins and arteries. Increases workload of myocardium. No direct inotropic or chronotropic effects.
	Phenylephrine	Neo-Synephrine	Similar to methoxamine.	Some inotropic and chronotropic effects in very large doses.
Alpha receptor agonists: dual actions	Levarterenol	Levophed	Marked constriction of arteries and veins. Direct stimulant effect on cardiac receptors. (Inotropic and chronotropic effects)	May be used in cardiogenic shock since volume is not usually depleted and it improves cardiac output. However, myocardial work is also increased.
	Metaraminol	Aramine	Sustained vasoconstriction; inotropic effects in some patients but marked reflex bradycardia.	Decreases net cardiac output unless heart is prevented from slowing; Reduces renal and cerebral perfusion.
Alpha receptor agonists	Phentolamine	Regitine	Depresses responses at alpha receptor sites resulting in vasodilatation.	Acts at some intermediate point of catecholamine synthesis. No beta effects. Slow onset and prolonged action.
	Phenoxybenz-amine	Dibenzyline	Relaxes smooth muscle of arteries and veins. Marked increase in vascular volume though fluid mobilization.	Same as above.

Category	Generic name	Trade name		
Beta receptor agonists (Betamimetic effects)	Epinephrine	Adrenaline	Both alpha and beta receptor effects. In doses used in man the beta effects are dominant.	Usually reserved for anaphylacuc shock. Stimulates anaerobic metabolism and causes metabolic acidosis which must be corrected.
	Isoproterenol	Isuprel	Decreases systemic and pulmonary vascular resistance. Marked direct inotropic and chronotropic effects. Short duration of action.	Useful in Stokes-Adams attacks. Elicits myocardial stimulation without vasoconstriction. Effective in cardiac resuscitation.
	Nylidrin	Arlidin	Causes smooth muscle relaxation in all vessels. Inotropic and chronotropic effects.	Increases cardiac output for more than one hour.
Beta receptor antagonist	Propranolol	Inderal	Little action on "normal" heart but profound effect in reducing response to sympathetic activity. Directly affects sodium concentration in cells.	Both beta receptor antagonism and direct effects on myocardial cells. Can be effective in inhibition of ventricular arrhythmias.
Other vasoconstrictors	Angiotensin II	Hypertensin	Stimulates smooth muscles of arteries. Does not constrict veins, causes venous pooling. Reduces heart rate reflexibility.	Does not stimulate heart. Probably should not be used in cardiogenic shock.
	Dopamine	Dopamine	Increased blood pressure through inotropic effects. No increase in peripheral resistance. Renal blood flow and performance improve.	Immediate precurser of adrenaline causes renal artery dilatation that is not blocked by alpha or beta stimulation.

Compiled from: Goodman, L. S. and Gilman, A.: The Pharmacological Basis of Therapeutics. New York. Macmillan, 1970; Marshall, R. J., and Darby, T. D.: Pharmacological Principles in Treatment. Springfield, Ill., 1966; and Weil, M. and Shubin. H.: Diagnosis and Treatment of Shock. Baltimore, Williams & Wilkins, 1967.

are more specific, more readily regulated, and have fewer dangerous side effects for the patient in shock.

The major problem in the use of vasodilators is insuring adequate plasma volume and cardiac efficacy to fill the dilated vessels. The effects of not doing so are obvious! Betamimetics may cause tachycardia and increased myocardial work and oxygen need. Other toxic reactions are drug specific. Weil suggests that the so-called vasopressors and vasodilators are not entirely antagonistic in their effects on all components and suggests conceptualizing a spectrum of agents in terms of hemodynamic effects.[16] It is likely that either class of drugs may be used profitably *depending on the underlying condition and the stage of tissue perfusion.*

OXYGEN. The uses and abuses of oxygen and its various modes of administration are discussed in detail in Chapter 14. The administration of oxygen generally reduces heart work and provides more oxygen to cells per unit of blood delivered. Both are important for the patient in shock. The delivery of well-humidified oxygen at the highest safe concentration is a primary measure in emergency treatment and for maintenance of the patient.

INTRAVENOUS FLUIDS. As an emergency measure, Ringer's solution is an adequate plasma volume expander. Further fluid needs will be determined on the basis of serum electrolytes and precipitating conditions, for example, blood loss, serum loss, and so on. Indwelling IV catheters are usually inserted for hypotensive patients. Catheters should be changed at regular intervals *or if any one of the following signs are present*: 1) undue tenderness, swelling, inflammation, purulence, or odor at the site of insertion; 2) swelling, tenderness, discoloration, or lumps along the course of the catheter or at its terminal end; 3) a "dry" fluid bottle has been up for an undetermined or prolonged period of time; or 4) there is air in the system or the fluid drips intermittently or very reluctantly.

One of the hazards of IV therapy, particularly in emergencies, is the administration of incorrect or incompatible substances. Multiple types of infusions hung piggy-back compound this problem.

Nurses should know the basic list of incompatible solutions and routinely inspect the tubing and container for precipitate, discoloration, agglutination, or air.

The IV administration of medications carries an additional hazard to the patient who receives the wrong drug or the wrong dose: there is very little time to correct the mistake! Some solutions are locally irritating. Levarteronol is particularly notable for the widespread tissue damage it causes if it is injected or leaks into skin or subcutaneous tissue. Infiltration of a wide area around the site with a solution of 5 to 10 mg of phentolamine will minimize the effect. For intermittent or continuous administration of levarteronol with a drip apparatus, some clinicians recommend that 5 mg of phentolamine for each 1 mg of levarteronol be present in the infusion.[17] The key nursing activity if such a substance is being infused is intelligent and constant surveillance. Nurses reading this text are familiar enough with IVs to appreciate the many extraneous factors which affect infusion rates.

A FINAL NOTE. The patient in shock, wherever he is, has the usual human needs: physical and emotional comfort, meaningful interpretations of what is going on around him (and *perhaps* its implications for him), a judicious diversion, and *rest*! To all her other activities, the nurse must add these. The more dire his situation, the more these functions are needed by the patient. We include this note here as well as in the general nursing care section because the functions of a nurse as a caring person—a patient advocate—encompass these activities in terms of both good nursing and her role adjunctive to the physician. The need is often multiplied and the function is all too infrequently observed, in the process of doing . . . things.

In summary, the general points necessary to the nursing care of patients in shock have been reviewed. These have included the nurse's functions in delivering medical therapy and in contributing to the physician's care of the patient. We would like to emphasize that current research demonstrates that shock, like many of its historical antecedents, is a state which encompasses very diverse underlying antecedents. It is *not* a disease.[18] Like dropsy, shock will one day be regarded as a handy label for the symptom-turned, syndrome-turned several "diseases" united by a common sign: arterial hypotension.

We can now turn to what we have termed "underlying mechanisms of shock"—but with a word of caution. Medical research has demonstrated that the improvement of certain kinds of antecedent states will improve tissue perfusion and subsequently resolve the shock state. This does not necessarily mean that a primary etiology has been unraveled. A case in point is congestive heart failure which leads to myocardial damage which leads to shock. Or is it that myocardial damage leads to congestive failure and *then* to shock? The *primary* etiology of congestive failure is not known; nor is the primary etiology of myocardial infarction, nor are the basic underlying mechanisms of shock!

Still, caring for patients presupposes that, within the limits imposed by the notion of "a quality of life," we attempt to preserve lives, a purpose to which nurses as well as physicians devote themselves. To bring as much knowledge as possible to bear on patient care, nurses must give up simplistic ideas about complex phenomena and must concurrently tolerate the knowledge that there is no "right way." In the case of shock, we can only discuss current methods of care. Even then, the methods employed are, in part, dependent on the facility in which the patient lies. Care of the patient in shock in a small general hospital differs greatly from that of a similar patient in a large teaching/research/care facility. There are differing opinions as to whom is receiving the better care. This controversy inspired the format of this chapter: We have reviewed a general model of care; We will now discuss primary mechanisms which are thought to lead to shock (if not to cause it) and the care necessitated by those mechanisms.

Underlying Mechanisms of Shock

In the first edition of this book, we discussed a classification of the major types of shock which included: 1) cardiogenic, 2) hypovolemic, 3) neurogenic, and 4) septic. More current thinking indicates that while several of the underlying states which lead to myocardial damage and thus to shock *could* be classified as cardiogenic, to do so obscures the real picture and is not directive. For example, pheochromocytoma, myxedema, and myocardial infarction may all result in myocardial damage and then in shock, but only myocardial infarction is a proximate cause. The endocrine pathologies may lead to myocardial damage, but their early treatment may arrest increased demands on the heart, thus avoiding the whole process. Should myocardial damage and shock occur in addition to a pathology such as myxedema, the underlying pathology must be treated before resolution of the shock state and myocardial healing will occur.

The cardiogenic classification has also been used for such conditions as pericardial tamponade and pulmonary embolism. These conditions share the common pathology of obstructing the flow of blood, to which the heart reacts secondarily. Dissecting aneurysm of the aorta and thrombi of mechanical valves might also be more logically classified as obstructive shock.

Similarly, neurogenic shock includes diverse pathologies ranging from autonomic nervous system paralysis (as a result of drug overdoses, high spinal anesthesia or spinal cord transsection) to anaphylactoid reactions. We now feel that more attention given to the underlying mechanism will promote more individualistic and effective nursing care.

Weil and Shubin proposed a reclassification of shock which is useful for developing principles of nursing care.[19] They state its purpose to be (to) " . . . help pinpoint the priorities of management of shock states."[20] The classification is presented in an amended form in Table 13-8. The major types proposed will subsequently be utilized to discuss underlying mechanisms of the shock state, prevalent medical therapies, and nursing care.

The major advantage to the reader of presenting the material in this way is parsimony. The care of patients manifesting any of these underlying mechanisms is complex and must be *superimposed* on the general nursing care re-

TABLE 13-8
Reclassification of Shock States

TYPE OF SHOCK	CAUSE
Hypovolemic shock	
Exogenous	Blood loss Plasma loss Protein loss Electrolyte loss
Endogenous	Extravasation
Cardiogenic shock	Myocardial infarction Cardiac failure Arrhythmia
Distributive shock	
High or normal peripheral resistance (increased venous capitance; selective or general)	CNS injury Bacillary shock Barbiturate intoxication Ganglionic blockade
Low peripheral resistance (Arteriovenous shunt)	Inflammatory vasodilation, abscess, active hyperemia
Obstructive shock	Vena caval compression Pericardial tamponade Ball-valve thrombus Pulmonary embolism Dissecting aortic aneurysm

Amended from Weil, M. H. and Shubin, H.: Proposed reclassification of shock states with special reference to distributive defects. Adv. Exp. Med. & Biol. 23: 16, 1973. Used with the permission of the authors.

quired by the patient who is in shock. We hope that understanding of the underlying mechanisms, the signs manifested by patients who are subject to them, and of assessment skills may be combined by nurses to effect not only better care of patients in shock, but the prevention of some cases of profound shock by alerting physicians to the patient's condition before he becomes so ill.

Therefore, we have adopted a format which utilizes the reclassification scheme and which will entail only a brief description of those underlying mechanisms that are discussed in detail in other chapters. In such cases, the reader will be referred to the specific chapter. In other cases, we will discuss nursing care in detail. Patients with shock arising from trauma or from underlying infections have complex needs and we will discuss their care in depth.

HYPOVOLEMIC SHOCK
As presented by Weil and Shubin, the exogenous types of hypovolemic shock include hemorrhage, plasma loss due to burns or inflammation, and fluid loss associated with electrolyte losses such as those caused by extensive vomiting or diarrhea.[21] Endogenous conditions resulting in vascular hypovolemia (and *potentially* shock) are those which entail extravasation of fluid: inflammation, trauma, tourniquet application, anaphylaxis, and pheochromocytoma. We would add that group of conditions in which extravasation occurs as a result of protein loss through the kidney or skin, or from increased capillary permeability such as that arising from cirrhosis.

We will discuss the care of patients with hypovolemia resulting from 1) hemorrhage, 2) plasma loss, and 3) water and electrolyte loss; and we will discuss in depth the care of the patient with trauma who may suffer from all these primary etiologies of hypovolemia.

HEMORRHAGE. Shock resulting from an actual reduction in blood volume is one of the most common forms. Symptoms of hemorrhagic shock do not occur, however, until approximately 25 percent (5 units) of the blood volume is lost. In addition to the real blood loss, wounds produce local vessel dilatation, a particularly serious consideration in the case of large wounds, however well bleeding vessels are ligated. If blood loss is the primary factor and the source of bleeding can be controlled, the condition should be amenable to blood replacement. When blood replacement does not improve the patient's condition, other factors may have been primarily responsible. Concomitant plasma loss, increased vascular capacity (neurogenic shock), or cardiogenic factors may coexist in the underlying disease process. Treatment of the latter is then necessary before the patient responds.

A common example of the interplay of factors causing shock is that of the patient who has had a D and C (dilatation and curettage). Blood loss is usually minimal, or it is replaced; however, a patient may suffer persistent hypotension after surgery. Many factors should be considered: the anesthetic and preanesthetic, the length of time the patient's legs were in stirrups (and the amount of blood pooling in them when she is later placed in a supine position), the state of hydration, her emotional reaction to the surgery (it is often done after a miscarriage and the patient may be mourning), chronic blood loss and the amount of pain she feels. All of these factors are magnified in major surgical procedures. A single or stereotyped assessment, treatment, or measure of supportive care is often ineffective.

Arterial catheters pose an iatrogenic hazard of hemorrhage, particularly if patients who have them are on units where close surveillance is not possible or usual. Nurses who know that quality care for a patient will be impossible under any circumstances should make that clear. For example, if a unit is staffed with a nurse and a minimally trained aide, no one can observe any one patient very closely. There is no resolution possible for that nurse; if she attends the very sick patient as he deserves, others will (and often do) suffer lack of attention. If nurses consistently and strongly report such situations on the basis of facts, and place the responsibility for lack of care with whom it belongs in that situation, in strong terms more planning on the basis of nursing time needed by specific patients rather than on nurse-to-room assignments *will* ensue.

Similarly, patients with a possibility of internal bleeding need very close surveillance. Here, the bleeding must be deduced from the pattern of signs and symptoms the patient manifests. The mode of correction may be replacement of blood loss or surgical intervention. The decision will also rest on the signs the patient presents (and in many cases radiological consultation). The nurse's close observation is of particular importance. Figure 13-5 presents a schematic representation of probable internal bleeding sites after trauma.*

The primary result of hemorrhage is reduction of the venous return causing reduction in cardiac output. The decrease in arterial pressure then evokes sympathetic reflexes, so that most of the arterioles constrict to raise blood pressure (those of the coronary and cerebral circulations are initially exempted). The veins and venous reservoirs constrict, helping to maintain venous return. The heart and respiratory rates increase, helping to compensate by delivering more and better-oxygenated blood to vital tissues. According to Guyton, the sympathetic reflexes permit a reduction of blood volume up to 30 to 35 percent (or about 3 to 5 units) of the blood volume. Without such protection, a 10 to 20 percent blood loss (1 or 2 units) would lead to death.[22] In addition to the sympathetic responses, a slower response is effected by the absorption of fluid from the intestinal tract and renal conservation of salts and water. The conscious individual experiences thirst and ingests large quantities of fluids. Should bleeding continue, however, the compensatory mechanisms can no longer effect adequate tissue perfusion and the condition becomes progressively worse. Cardiac deterioration, vasomotor tone loss and the release of toxins by ischemic tissues occur, causing a vicious cycle from which there is little hope of recovery. Table 13-9 provides a capsule view of the cardiorespiratory compensations evoked by hemorrhage.

The therapeutic goal is prevention of the decompensation phase of shock. Adequate fluid replacement during surgery and close monitoring of operative sites are important measures. In the emergency situation, prompt occlusion of bleeding wounds and surgical closure may prevent shock. Situations in which closure of wounds is impossible (some gastric and intestinal hemorrhages and diseases such as hemophilia which involve bleeding into tissues) usually require prompt and frequent whole blood administration. Hopefully, blood replacement will enable the organism to eventually repair itself and forestall the development of shock. Bleeding of operative wounds may be obscured by bandages or by the patient's position. The area *under* the patient and nearby body crevices should always be checked. Close observation of any patient particularly prone to bleeding is important in the early detection and treatment of hemorrhage.

---

*We should add that bleeding is also likely after cardiac surgery necessitating artificial perfusion.

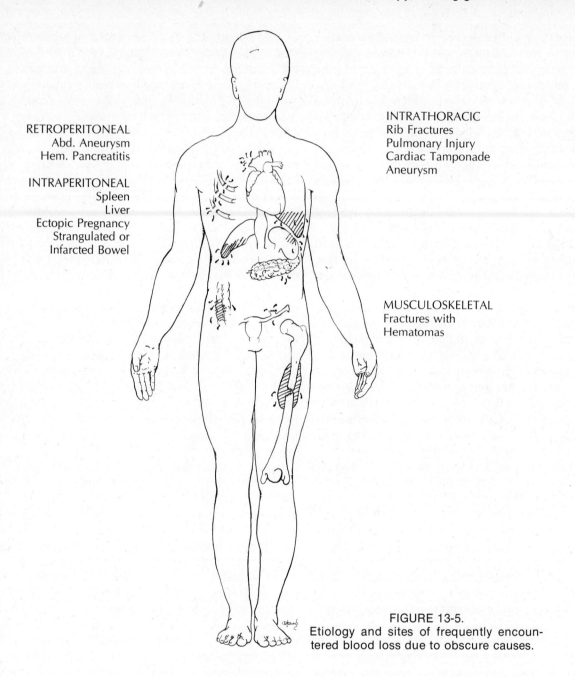

RETROPERITONEAL
Abd. Aneurysm
Hem. Pancreatitis

INTRAPERITONEAL
Spleen
Liver
Ectopic Pregnancy
Strangulated or
Infarcted Bowel

INTRATHORACIC
Rib Fractures
Pulmonary Injury
Cardiac Tamponade
Aneurysm

MUSCULOSKELETAL
Fractures with
Hematomas

FIGURE 13-5.
Etiology and sites of frequently encountered blood loss due to obscure causes.

PLASMA LOSS. Several relatively common conditions allow the loss of plasma into the extravascular tissues. Burns cause local vasodilatation, grossly increased capillary permeability, and, depending on their extent and depth, massive amounts of fluid may be lost. Careful assessment and administration of fluids for patients having burns cannot be overemphasized. Extensive dermatological diseases, such as exfoliative dermatitis, also cause plasma loss. The signs and symptoms associated with this type of shock are identical to those occurring when hemorrhage is

TABLE 13-9
Cardiorespiratory Alterations After Hemorrhage

PHYSIOLOGIC EFFECTS	COMPENSATORY RESPONSES	PHYSIOLOGIC CHANGES WITH DECOMPENSATION
Primary effect	Increased heart rate	Further decreased arterial pressure
Decreased blood volume	Increased systemic vascular resistance	Decreased heart rate
Secondary effects		
Decreased mean arterial pressure	Increased pulmonary vasc. resist.	Further decreased cardiac output
Decreased cardiac output	Redistribution of blood volume	Increased central venous pressure
Decreased central venous pressure	Increased myocardial contractility, tendency to increased cardiac output	Increased mean transit time
Increased mean transit time		Decreased systemic vascular resistance
Decreased central blood volume	Increased O_2 extraction	Decreased stroke index
Decreased left ventricle stroke work	Hyperpnea, tachypnea, respiratory alkalosis	Decreased left stroke
Decreased O_2 availability		Decreased myocardial contractility
Decreased O_2 consumption		Decreased art. pO_2
Metabolic acidosis		Decreased oxygen availability
		Decreased oxygen consumption
		Metabolic acidosis

From Shoemaker, William C.: Physiologic mechanisms in clinical shock. Adv. in Exp. Med. & Biol. 23:66, 1972. Used with permission of the authors.

the precipitating factor. However, emotional shock, pain, increased blood viscosity, and the danger of septicemia compound the problem and must also be dealt with.

Intestinal obstruction is a potential source of hypovolemic shock. Surgical intervention is often necessary. Rupture of the intestine is avoided at all costs and poses a hazard of shock, both in general terms and because of the release of gram-negative organism toxins, which in themselves may lead to shock.

The nephrotic syndrome, cirrhosis of the liver, and nutritional deficiencies of protein all result in a decreased serum protein. The result, whatever the cause may be, is a decreased col-loidal blood pressure, which allows fluid to escape the vascular compartment. Hypovolemic shock may then result. In the case of nephrotic syndrome, protein is also lost into the urine. Cirrhosis poses a double threat to fluid loss; hypoproteinemia (from decreased protein synthesis) occurs and there is an escape of protein into the abdominal cavity. Both tend to enhance the fluid loss from the vascular compartment into the abdomen and into the pleural space. Acute problems may be treated with salt-poor albumin. Another goal is the prevention of further damage to the involved organ.

WATER AND ELECTROLYTE LOSS. Dehydration is the predominant clinical syndrome associated with nonprotein fluid loss. MacBryde and Guyton provide comprehensive lists of predisposing conditions.[23]

1. Excessive sweating.
2. Severe diarrhea or vomiting.
3. Vigorous diuretic therapy.
4. Inadequate intake of fluid and electrolytes.
5. Inefficacy of adrenal cortices with failure to reabsorb NaCl and H_2O.
6. Decreased amounts of antidiuretic hormone by the supraoptic-hypophyseal system.

Several of these conditions combine to produce the effects of heat prostration or shock from cold exposure. These conditions are found outside of the hospital and should be immediately treated by attempts to return the body temperature to normal by putting the victim at rest and, if he is conscious, by administering lukewarm salty liquids. Children, especially infants, and elderly people are especially prone to dehydration and hypovolemic problems because of their decreased body compensatory powers.

Emergency Treatment of Hypovolemic Shock

1. Replacement of vascular volume
   a. blood
   b. plasma or albumin
   c. fluid and electrolytes
2. Position patient comfortably; aid respiration if necessary.
3. Vasodilators are purported to mobilize extravasated fluids back into vascular chambers. Other regimens advocate vasopressor therapy.
4. Attempts to forestall further loss of vascular fluid must take first priority, especially in the case of hemorrhage.

The principles of nursing care for these patients are derived from a few commonalities:

1. These are critically ill, usually frightened people who have undergone severe stresses in terms of both the illness and its therapy.
2. Most of these patients have a ready portal of entry for infection from the incision or denuding of skin. In the case of the surgical patient, pathogens may have been inadvertently introduced in an excellent culture media! All of these patients tend to be debilitated and weak.

3. The hypovolemia may result from a.) hemorrhage b.) plasma loss, or c.) water and electrolyte loss.

Patients are likely to receive whole blood or packed cells, albumin, or hyperalimentary solutions in addition to the usual variety of IV therapy. Each of these solutions should be viewed as a medication, with attendant risks of dangerous side effects.

For a more comprehensive understanding of the care of patients with specific conditions the following chapters should be consulted. Chapter 11 gives a detailed review of the care necessary for the patient with burns. Chapter 16 discusses the care of the patient with fluid and electrolyte losses. Chapter 17 reviews fluid and electrolyte losses resulting from kidney disease. Chapter 23 discusses anaphylaxis.

The Patient with Trauma

Trauma is the most prevalent antecedent of shock. Not only is trauma a frequent occurrence in itself—primarily through automobile accidents and construction accidents—but the patient who suffers from trauma is prone to hypovolemia from several routes, to infection of his wounds, and to pain and other occurrences which induce emotional stress. Traumatic shock represents a convergence of potential shock-producing influences on the patient:

1. He has suffered an unexpected insult to his systemic integrity. Often he has perceived the event as a life threat and suffers emotional shock.
2. He is usually in pain, and may have been for a prolonged time.
3. He usually has open wounds allowing hemorrhage.
4. He frequently has internal injuries caused by the impact of solid instruments (or his impact on them) or the effects of G-forces.
5. His open wounds and the usual circumstances of traumatic shock (e.g., automobile and construction accidents, battlefield casualties, extremes of heat or cold exposure) combine to vastly increase his risk of systemic infection.
6. He has suffered the destruction of large amounts of tissue which liberates vasoactive substances into his body and cause massive electrolyte shifts and water and plasma loss.

Factor 6 is the common denominator of traumatic shock. Massive cell destruction evokes several homeostatic mechanisms as the body attempts to compensate for the insult. Shoemaker presents a clear and comprehensive list of cardiorespiratory reactions after trauma (Table 13-10). Added to these is the additional workload imposed on the heart by the loss of whole blood, which causes a decreased cardiac output and evokes vasoconstriction and a redistribution of blood volume. Both of the latter add to the workload of the heart and lungs in the attempt at compensation.

The brain is doubly jeopardized in trauma. Not only is there a high incidence of head injuries and resulting loss of blood, but hypoxemia frequently results from associated chest injuries or the pulmonary damage known as shock lung which frequently occurs after traumatic and hemorrhagic shock. Figure 13-6 presents a hypothetical sequence of events which occur to produce it. The most effective therapy for either lies in good emergency care, oxygenation and fluid volume replacement.

PREVENTION. Nurses as well as physicians are called upon to give emergency first aid measures after trauma. Table 13-11 is a guideline which is conveniently set up to imply a triage of priorities. Nurses may be called upon to make these physical assessments at the scene of an accident or other situation where there is no physician immediately available. For nurses in the hospital, the table constitutes a list of signs which should impel the nurse to: 1) perform emergency measures, 2) call a physician stat, or 3) call a physician to report changes and continue to observe the patient.

It should be emphasized that nurses *must* be the guardians of patients who arrive at the hospital emergency room or on the patient unit after trauma (accidental *or* surgical). These people are too often moved abruptly from litter to table or bed thus causing pain, a chance of more trauma, and the possibility of precipitating hypotension from one or both conditions.

The condition known as anaphylactic shock or anaphylactic reaction is described in Chapter 23. We wish to point out that anaphylactic shock and massive trauma, such as burns or crush injuries, share a common response with endotoxic shock. In both there is a liberation of vasoactive substances from necrosed tissue, specifically his-

TABLE 13-10
Cardiorespiratory Alterations After Trauma

PHYSIOLOGIC EFFECTS	COMPENSATORY RESPONSES	PHYSIOLOGIC CHANGES WITH DECOMPENSATION
Primary effects		
Tissue injury	Increased heart rate Increased cardiac output	Further decreases in art. press.
Breakdown of damaged tissues, release of breakdown products and intracellular components into the circulation	Increased stroke work Increased left vent. stroke work Increased myocardial contractility	Decreased heart rate Further decreases in cardiac output Increased central venous press. Increased mean transit time
Secondary effects		
Decreased mean art. press. Increased O_2 requirements Propagation of afferent neural (pain) stimulation	Increased pulmonary vasc. resist. Hyperpnea and tachypnea Respiratory alkalosis Increased O_2 consumption	Decreased systemic vasc. resist. Decreased stroke index Decreased left vent. stroke Decreased myocardial contractility
		Decreased art. pO_2
		Decreased O_2 avail.
		Decreased O_2 consumption
		Metabolic acidosis

From: Shoemaker, William C.: Physiologic mechanisms in clinical shock. Adv. in Exp. Med. & Biol. 23:67, 1973. Used with permission of the author.

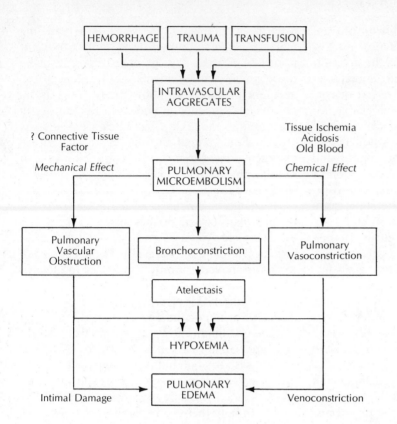

FIGURE 13-6.
Hypothetical sequence of events in the development of pulmonary insufficiency after shock and trauma.

TABLE 13-11
Checklist for the Emergency Situation

A. Emergency conditions demanding nursing "first aid."
   1. Insure adequate ventilation
      a. Patent airway
      b. Integrity of the chest wall
   2. Insure adequate circulation
      a. Heartbeat
      b. Hemorrhage control
   3. Splint fractures (if nurse is at scene of accident)
B. Imminently life-threatening conditions
   1. Signs of pericardial tamponode
   2. Signs of air or fluid in the pleural cavity
   3. Paradoxical motion of the chest wall
   4. Presence of dyspnea and cyanosis
C. Conditions requiring intervention
   1. Clinical signs of low perfusion
   2. Rising venous pressure
   3. Decreasing urine flow
   4. Signs of occult hemorrhage

tamine, bradykinin from mast cells and "slow reacting substance" (SRS) which is stored in lipoid tissue and could be released in case of trauma or as an effect of necrosis after poor tissue perfusion. These substances appear to effect widespread vasodilatation when they are liberated. They may also contribute to microemboli formation which has the dual effect of blocking blood flow to tissues (of particular import to the lung and kidney) and of "using up" the clotting components of the blood. In the latter case, a consumption coagulopathy results which will further predispose the patient to hemorrhage. The nurse should be particularly alert to the possibility of occult bleeding. It can be readily seen that the traumatized patient is prone to shock from any one of several pathophysiological processes.

We wish to make one additional point. The nurse who cares for the patient after trauma should be acutely aware that antibiotics and blood are two common causes of an anaphylactic reaction: The trauma patient is likely to receive both. Therefore, we have compiled this checklist of nursing action necessitated in the event of the following signs: 1) tracheal spasm, 2) rising heart rate, and 3) falling or "low" blood pressure:

1. Discontinue precipitating agent (blood, antibiotic, procainamide, and so on).
2. Position patient for optimal cerebral perfusion *and* respiration.
3. Provide for a patent airway; note respiratory qualities.
4. Oxygen (usually by mask because it is quickest).
5. Prepare 0.2 ml epinephrine 1:1000 in water s/c. stat.
6. Diphenhydramine (Benadryl) 50 mg IV (or other antihistaminic of choice).
7. IV—5 percent glucose and water (monitor urine output later).
8. Hydrocortisone succinate 200 to 300 mg IV (or high dose of other rapid-acting corticosteroid.
9. Aminophyllin 500 mg in 200 ml IV over 1 to 2 hours (or tracheostomy, if laryngeal edema is severe or persistent, or if spasms occur).

Numbers 1 to 4 should be immediately performed by the nurse in addition to calling the physician, stat. The nurse may give epinephrine in an emergency or if it is hospital policy. The other items represent guidelines of medical care. It should be noted that the patient who is having a transfusion reaction may complain of flank pain prior to other symptoms or signs of a reaction. Too often, it is assumed that this is a result of trauma and the early symptom is ignored.

Patients who have suffered trauma are in particular need of rest. In addition to reassurance and the provision of comfort measures, the patient should receive enough pain medication to be comfortable (short of jeopardizing vital functions). The action of pain as a stressor is frequently overlooked; it is such a constant oppressor in a hospital. However, in the case of severely injured people it is even more important than usual to prevent such avoidable insults.

CARDIOGENIC SHOCK

Cardiogenic shock has, until recently, received a lion's share of the research on and literary treatment of shock. However, as research has progressed to provide a better understanding of the shock state, the classification "cardiogenic" has been more sharply delineated and is circumscribed to include only the conditions which demonstrably produce shock as a result of poor cardiac performance, that is, myocardial infarction (MI), cardiac failure, and arrhythmias.

The mortality from MI *per se*, and from arrhythmia has been sharply reduced by the use of coronary care units to provide rest and early treatment for the patient who reaches them. Similarly, the incidence of death from heart failure has been reduced by the improvement of medical-pharmacological treatment. But, once a patient is not able to profit from the application of these standard treatments and develops profound underperfusion, the mortality from shock approaches 90 percent.[24]

Many patients arrive at the hospital in shock, or worse, are found dead and never receive treatment. We have so far only been able to improve the chances of patients who have the less severe insults and who make it long enough to get to the hospital.* This factor is an index of their stamina as well as the degree of heart damage. We do not really know the "cause of death" in *most* other victims, but tend *to assume* that a heart attack has taken place in the case of sudden death in a man age 35 to 65 or in the patient who has had a history of congestive heart disease. We have examined these points and others pertinent to nursing care of the patient with heart disease more thoroughly in Chapter 12.

DISTRIBUTIVE SHOCK

The classification distributive shock implies a primary problem which results in an increased venous capitance (although other vessels *may*

---

*This situation is fast improving under the impact of the emergency services programs and the development of training centers for police, firemen, and ambulance attendants. The programs train personnel to administer CPR, defibrillation, and other life-supporting techniques at the scene and during transport.

also be affected) leading to poor tissue perfusion. There are two types: 1) distributive shock with a high or normal *general peripheral* resistance in which there is either a selective or generalized increased *venous* capitance which acts to sequester great pools of blood; and, 2) distributive shock with low peripheral resistance, vasodilatation, and resulting multiple arteriovenous shunting (See Table 13-12).

The reader can see that this category subsumes the entities usually grouped as neurogenic shock as well as several others. The advantage of this classification is that it points out more basic etiology that is, poor delivery and/or poor oxygenation of blood and reduced oxygen extraction from blood by the cells. With the exception of central nervous system injury and vasovagal syncope there is nothing inherently wrong with the nervous system in any of the conditions usually listed under neurogenic shock. Except in the two cases mentioned, the classification of neurogenic is misleading and not prescriptive of either nursing or medical care. For a discussion of the patient with central nervous system injuries, see Chapter 20.

Vasomotor deficits result in the sudden loss of vasomotor tone which results in a hypotensive state and may eventually progress to shock. The more benign forms of the condition simply cause fainting, with a resultant return to consciousness in the recumbent position. There is a closely associated form of temporary circulatory collapse called vasovagal syncope. There is not vasomotor failure but, instead, stressful circumstances produce excitation of the vagal mechanism with reflex slowing of the heart and vasodilatation in skeletal muscle. The net result is a reduced arterial blood pressure and poor cerebral perfusion in the upright posture. It is not known under what circumstances this condition leads to shock or what initiating mechanisms provoke the initial deficit.

To return to distributive shock, we find that pooling of venous blood and some arteriovenous shunting commonly occur associated with endotoxic shock. Here we refer specifically to shock preceded by infection with gram-negative organisms; the enteric coli are the most common offenders. Patients suffering from septic abortions, trauma (general types), or perforation of the gut are particularly prone to this problem.

The reader is probably familiar with the term septic shock which has generally meant shock associated with sepsis-infection. However, gram-positive (e.g., staphylocci, streptococci, and pneumococci) organisms account for less than one third of the cases of septic shock. The mortality rate is estimated to be about 50 percent.[25] The manifestations and the underlying mechanisms (and of course the treatment) of shock resulting from infections with gram-negative bacteria—which produce endotoxins—is quite different. Endotoxic shock results from a toxin produced by gram-negative bacilli which is released into the bloodstream when the bacteria die or are damaged. The mortality rate is about 75 percent.[26]

The incidence of shock arising from infections with gram-negative organisms is increasing. This finding may well represent several general trends of interest to nurses: 1) the increased numbers of surgical procedures—particularly of genitourinary instrumentation; 2) the increased numbers of older patients in hospitals; 3) a reservoir of resistant organisms resulting from the

TABLE 13-12
Types of Distributive Shock and the Conditions
Associated with Them

1. High or normal resistance (increased venous capitance)
   A. Bacillary shock (particularly from gram-negative organisms resulting in bacteremia)
   B. Barbiturate intoxication
   C. Central nervous system injury
   D. Ganglionic blockade
2. Low resistance with arteriovenous shunting and generalized vasodilatation
   A. Inflammatory vasodilatation (this occurs in gram-positive bacteremias such as those caused by pneumococci, streptococci and staphylococci resulting in pneumonitis or peritonitis).
   B. Abscesses
   C. Reactive hyperemia

Adapted from Weil, M. A. and Shubin, H.: Proposed reclassification of shock states with special reference to distributive defects. Adv. in Exp. Med. & Biol. 23:15, 1972.

abuse of antibiotics; and 4) the harboring of pathogens in hospitals. Patients in the hospital with open wounds and tracheotomies are prone to staphyloccocal infections. Patients with indwelling catheters in blood vessels (such as those used for IV's, CVP, and hyperalimentation) or urinary catheters are also more prone to infection, and the rate is increasing. However, it is the gram-negative type of sepsis which is increasing most rapidly.

Death from these endotoxic bacteremias particularly occurs in people who have underlying diseases which limit the operation of their compensatory mechanisms in response to the vasodilatation which occurs. Death from gram-negative bacteremia is becoming more prevalent because of the resistance of many organisms to the antibiotics available.

Nurses could play an important role in reducing those infections and the subsequent deaths occurring as iatrogenic hazards of hospitalization and medical therapy by attending to the hand-washing techniques of personnel and by working to reduce other forms of breaks in medical asepsis. Nurses may also play an important role in the potential prevention of shock by closely observing patients at risk (patients medicated with cytotoxic agents and immunosuppressives should be included) and by reporting the early signs of impending shock. These include mild hyperventilation, falling blood pressure, full pounding pulse, increased temperature, flushed face, and warm extremities.

Some writers contend that the underlying mechanism is a beta adrenergic response which leads to pronounced A-V shunting in the splanchnic and pulmonary capillaries.[27] This is compensated by hyperventilation initially, but it may progress to metabolic acidemia and eventually to signs of poor tissue perfusion. They advocate treatment specific to the infection, plasma volume expansion, and beta adrenergic blockade to forestall the noncompensatory changes.

Other writers feel that A-V shunting is particular to infection with the gram-positive organism and that the changes associated with gram-negative organisms emanate from the liberation of vasoactive materials from dead cells,

endogenous and bacterial. Or, that the primary antecedent to shock is microembolism of the lung caused by an aggregation of platelets in response to the liberation of heparin and histamine by dead mast cells.[28] This results in a consumption coagulopathy which also leaves the patient prone to bleeding (as nurses have also observed him to be).

We have mentioned previously that the liberation of histamine—a potent vasodilator—also occurs in endotoxic shock.

Other potentially hypotensive factors have been discovered which may operate to produce shock. Circulating in the plasma are the precursors of several polypeptides which have been shown to exert a potent vasodilator effect. They are called kinins, of which bradykinin and kallidin are two of the most thoroughly investigated. The Hageman factor (factor XII) is at least partly responsible for conversion of the precursor substance kallikreinogen to kallikrein and, likewise, conversion of kininogen to kinin.

Although the kinins are destroyed very quickly by kininase, several other proteolytic enzymes, and chelating agents, their action simulates an early inflammatory response and has a profound relaxing (dilatory) effect on smooth muscle. They have also been proven to cause the release of catecholamines (epinephrine and norepinephrine) by direct stimulation of the adrenal medulla and indirectly through the basoreceptor reflexes. Epinephrine enhances the destruction of kinins by kininase, so the two factors are antagonists in the maintenance of a normotensive system.

The study of the kinins is particularly relevant to endotoxic shock, because it is thought that endotoxins activate the Hageman factor. This factor, in turn, may be responsible both for the presence of kinins and for the multiple small thrombi in the peripheral capillaries which are demonstrable in this kind of shock. Since prolonged clotting times are common to patients in endotoxic shock, it is postulated that the consumption coagulopathy is produced because the clotting factors are activated; thrombi that form in the microcirculation use up these factors and a deficit of them is discernible in the general circu-

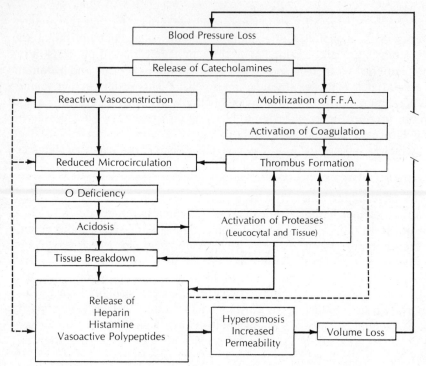

FIGURE 13.7.
The effect of trisylol in shock.

lation. A general model of the process is presented in Figure 13-7.

While intensive research goes on, a few points may summarize the clinical care of these patients. There is a significant mortality risk for patients manifesting *any* kind of septic shock. The presenting signs are at first those of bacteremia, rigors (hard, shaking chills) and a rise in temperature. Approximately one third of these patients then go into shock with hypotension, respiratory distress, and a warm dry skin. Frequently the condition is accompanied by gastrointestinal disturbances. Cyanosis and cold clammy skin are late symptoms. Their sensorium is variable, ranging from alertness to disorientation, to lethargy. Often there is minimal physical discomfort. Unlike most patients in shock, their urinary output may be adequate, but blood chemistry studies reveal a rising BUN because of tubular necrosis.

The most prevalent causative organisms of gram-negative bacteremias include *Escherichia coli*, *Proteus*, *Salmonella* and *Aerobacter aerogenes*, all commonly found in the intestinal

tract. Ports of entry include surgical incision, instrumentation (especially of the genitourinary tract), septic abortion, parturition, and open skin lesions. Older men and women of childbearing age are particularly susceptible, if only because of their propensity for the above-stated conditions.

Medical therapy is directed toward identification of the site of infection, control of the bacteremia and the usual treatment for shock. Unfortunately, for treatment to be effective it must be instituted long before culture and sensitivity tests are available. Among the antibiotics usually effective against gram-negative organisms are: cephalothin (Keflin), colistin (Coly-Mycin), kanamycin (Kantrex), ampicillin (Ampicin), and gentamicin (Genticin). One or more is usually given until culture and sensitivity tests can be made to determine the offending organism and effective antimicrobial therapy.

Table 13-13 presents antimicrobial therapy specific to the control of gram-negative infections which are the most common causative agents of septic shock. In addition to antibiotic

TABLE 13-13
Specific Antimicrobial Agents for Use in Gram-Negative Bacterial Infections

AGENT	ANTIBIOTICS	DAILY I/M DOSE	PRECAUTIONS
Escherichia coli	Ampicillin	3.0-12.0 gm	All those associated with penicillin. GI disturbances.
	Tetracyclines	2.0-4.0 gm	
Aerobacter	Kanamycin (Kantrex)	1.0-2.0 gm	Ototoxicity—nephrotoxicity, agranulocytosis
	Chloramphenical (Chloromycetin)	2.0-3.0 gm	
Pseudomonas	Colistin (Coly-Mycin)	2.5 mg/kg	Neurotoxicity—nephrotoxicity (minimal)
	Polymyxin B	2.5 mg/kg	Neurotoxicity, local irritation
Klebsiella	Cephalothin (Keflin)	12-16 mg	Pain or infection, blood dyscrasia
	Kanamycin (Kantrex)	1.0-2.0 gm	Ototoxicity, nephrotoxicity
Proteus	Kanamycin (Kantrex)	1.0-2.0 gm	Ototoxicity, nephrotoxicity

Adapted from Petersdorf, R. G. and Sherris, J. C.: Methods and significance of in vitro testing of bacterial sensitivity to drugs. Am. J. Med. 39:766-769. Nov. 1965. Used with permission.

therapy, replacement of fluid and electrolytes (or blood) is indicated if the patient is suffering from hypovolemia, whether it is due to the loss of blood, extravasation of fluids, or severe vomiting and diarrhea. Respiratory assistance may be required, particularly for the elderly patient.

Staphylococci and streptococci, as well as many other gram-positive organisms, may also cause septic shock. These organisms secrete an exotoxin. The penicillins and the semisynthetic and synthetic analogues are still the drugs of choice for patients with gram-positive infections. For the resistant or allergic patient, drugs such as lincomycin (Lincocin), erythromycin (Ilotycin, Erythromycin, Erythrocin), or cephalothin (Keflin) may be employed. Despite its toxicity, streptomycin may be employed for these critically ill patients. The nursing care of such a patient should be modified according to his needs, but usually the care is the same as that for a patient with a given infection who is in shock.

The nursing care of patients with shock resulting from sepsis is complicated by the presence of communicable disease. These patients often require admission to intensive care facilities in which there are frequently other patients with surgical incisions and urinary and various other types of catheters, making it imperative that *all* the staff be careful to avoid cross-contamination. The nurse may have to turn part policeman to effect asepsis.

Patients who suffer gastrointestinal disturbances as a result of their infection need meticulous attention to hygiene. They are frequently too ill to retain bowel control or to ask for an emesis basin. Vomitus and diarrheic stools are extremely irritating and quickly cause skin breakdown. Another portal of entry for organisms is then open if diligent nursing care is not given. Renal failure is also a particularly serious complication for these patients and close monitoring of the urine output is very important. Accurate fluid balance sheets must be kept, notwithstanding the difficulty caused by incontinence and frequent emesis.

Controversy remains regarding the relative merits of vasopressors versus vasodilators for these patients. The latter are becoming more commonly used. Some receive large doses of corticosteroids, antihistaminics and/or antiserotonin agents as adjunctive therapy. Their use *still* depends on the physician's philosophy and is not well substantiated by the literature.[29]

The remaining conditions leading to problems

in the distribution of oxygenated blood relate to the misuse or abuse of drugs. Table 13-14 demonstrates the wide range of agents which may lead to hypotension. Nurses need to be particularly cautious in the administration of ganglionic blocking agents to elderly people. This group at risk also usually needs particularly detailed and thorough teaching and practice in self administration of medications for hypertension.

Barbiturate intoxication is frequently self-inflicted. In addition to the risks of hypotension and severe respiratory depression, the patient is in need of a great deal of emotional support. Whether his overdose was "accidental" or deliberate, he needs the service of skilled counselors as well as medical care and support. Nurses are often alert to these needs but fail to take an active role in seeing that they are met.

TABLE 13-14
Drugs Whose Toxic Effects Include Hypotension

DRUG	UPPER LIMITS OF DOSE	CLASS	ACTION, ANTIDOTES, OTHER INFORMATION
Phentolamine (Regitine)	Varies with purpose	Alpha adrenergic blockade	Drugs are competitive with adrenergic catecholamines; their effects may be counteracted by using them.
Phenoxybenzamine HCl (Dibenzyline)	60 mg		Leverterenol is the antidote of choice.
Hexamethonium Pentolinium (Ansolysen)	60 mg	Ganglionic blockage	Venous dilatation—peripheral pooling—decreased cardiac output—hypotension. Transmission across both symp. and parasymp. ganglia occurs. Therefore, decreased GI motility, loss of pupillary accommodation, urinary retention and impotence may occur. Latter may be ameliorated with neostigmine etc.
Mecamylamine (Inversine)	20 mg	Used with reserpine 50 mg in 500 ml IV	
Trimethaphen (Arfonad)	variable		
Thiazides		Diuretics	Often used as conjunctive therapy for hypertension.
Reserpine	.25-50 mg	Sympatholytic (Allows parasympathetic dominance)	Tranquilizer. Depletes body of norepinephrine and serotonin. Used with ganglionic blocker and diuretic.
Crude root (Raudixin, etc.)	100 mg		
Alseroxylon (Rauwiloid, etc.)	2 mg		
Guanethedine sulfate (Ismelin)	50 mg	Adrenergic neuron blockade	Acts as the ganglionic blocking agents without parasympathetic blockage. The latter system predominates. Interrupts norepinephrine and serotonin synthesis. Intensifies beta sympathomimetic effects. Used with other hypotensives.
Methyldopa (Aldomet)	2000 mg		
Hydralazine (Apresoline)	200 mg	(Also an MAO-inhibitor)	
Veratrum Alkaloids (Veriloid)	4 mg IV	Sympathetic inhibition	Inhibition of sympathetic tone and vagal augmentation by baroreceptor sensitivity. Prevent resultant bradycardia with atropine.
Protoveratrines A & B (Veralba)	0.5 mg IV		
Caffeine	20 gm	Xanthines	Stimulation of CNS. Relaxes smooth muscle, especially bronchiolar. Acts on the kidney to produce diuresis. Stimulates cardiac muscle, increases blood pressure and intensifies effects of narcotic analgesics and anesthetics.
Theophylline (Quibron)	0.5 gm		
Aminophylline	1.5 gm		

Adapted from Meyers, F. H., Jawetz, E. and Goldfein, A.: Review of Medical Pharmacology. Los Altos, Medical Publications, 1969.

OBSTRUCTIVE SHOCK

Obstructive shock has a clearly implied etiology; it occurs when obstructions to the flow of blood reduce the blood supply to distal tissues. Not only are these tissues then underperfused, but the amount of blood returning to the heart is reduced. The compensatory mechanisms medicated by the sympathetic system are called into play by the physiological alterations caused by both factors.

Patients at risk include: 1) those with chest trauma who may suffer compression of the heart or great vessels; 2) patients with pulmonary emboli; 3) patients after heart surgery who may have bleeding into the pericardial sac and resulting pericardial tamponade; 4) patients who have had heart valve replacements (thrombi may form on or around the prosthesis); 5) patients with dissecting aneurysms of the aorta.

The care of patients with these specific entities is discussed in Chapter 12.

The Shock Research Unit

Shock research units subsist with the dual purpose of providing patient care and collecting data about the underlying mechanisms of shock and the agents which are or may be generally employed to combat them. The human patient is thus both the object and the subject of research—a situation which has somewhat antithetical components.

The primary justification for the research on shock is the high mortality rate associated with shock. We have assumed that better understanding and more technology will produce better results. Yet, a report from an investigator in another country purports to demonstrate results as good or better from the management of the patient *in cardiogenic shock in the home* rather than in the hospital. We cannot assume that the same results would occur in America, where faith in technology is extreme. Faith is probably one of the patient's greatest assets. However, studies like this, and many others, are rarely found in American literature and they not only deserve, but require the attention of nurses and other health care providers.

C. M. MacBryde, well known to legions of medical and nursing students through his text, *Signs and Symptoms*, states, "Man's technological skills have exceeded his judgment . . ."[30] He goes on to express the opinion that of the myriad of drugs available, a few are essential, many are highly useful, but a great majority could be dispensed with.[31] This is a point pertinent to a situation where the most current writers can find little or no evidence that the drugs being used do any real good and probably do harm in some instances; yet the use of vasopressors is widespread in the care of every type of patients with shock—as are glucocorticoids. Either may mask the underlying deficits in tissue perfusion and even perpetuate the acute problems. The shock research unit may generate data which will have a positive impact on patient care generally, but it poses practical as well as ethical dilemmas in the use of human subjects as well as human resources.

Doctor Hardaway was quoted at length in a preceding section regarding his views of the training of nurses. We also utilized his estimates of the costs of equipping and staffing a shock research unit.[32] An approximation of the cost of hardware for such a unit was $73,000 in 1968. This is equipment in addition to usual equipment. He also estimated the cost in nonprofessional (i.e., nonmedical) manpower to be $50,000 per patient. These costs are far too low for today's purchasing power but they demonstrate the great expense of research. The unit at Walter Reed Army Medical Center required the full time services of at least five professional nurses and five nursing assistants. We do not know how many people could receive care there.

We wish to make the point that the drain of money and human resources that these units impose is formidable when it is multiplied by the many units across the country. This is particularly noteworthy when it is recognized that several units can and do exist in some cities, even side by side and collecting the same types of data on the same types of patients. In other areas of the country there is no specialized facility for hundreds of miles.

To the extent that such facilities as clinical

research units are desirable for the care of some patients, they should be available to them. It is apparent that no such criterion is met. How do we then defend these units in terms of patient care? Should the public monies be utilized to support so many units and units which are so maldistributed in terms of their accessibility to patients? Aren't we perpetuating the maldistribution of health care personnel by failing to establish specialized facilities for their education and research and their employment on a more sensible basis? Our patients suffer from problems both entering into the system and physically getting to the type of facility they need. If they don't have to risk city traffic they have to travel many miles—there is little in between.

We feel that the great disparities in the care given to patients in shock cannot be allowed to persist. It is apparent that the care depends on where the patient is; not on what he needs. This fact demonstrates a failure of human compassion as well as human intellect—there is no technological device that adequately substitutes for either.

Case Study of a Patient in Shock

A. Mr. Malone's admission was routine. His chief complaint was that of abdominal pain, accompanied by nausea and vomiting. His past medical history revealed that he had been hospitalized previously for symptoms of rheumatic fever and congestive heart failure. One year previously, he was hospitalized for the implantation of a Starr-Edwards valve to replace a poorly functioning mitral valve. The significant findings upon physical examination were:

> apparently well-functioning mitral Starr-Edwards valve replacement; B/P: 110/88; Pulse: 90; Respiration: 18; Temperature: 99.8; Weight: 130; Height: 5′4″; Liver enlarged 3 cc below the right costal margin
> Pain and abdominal tenderness localized in the right lower quadrant
> > Impressions:
> > 1. Appendicitis

LABORATORY FINDINGS:
  Leucocytosis (20,000)
  Hemoglobin 9.8
  Hematocrit 30
  Prothrombin time 38 sec., 41% activity

TREATMENT REGIMEN:
  Vitamin B$_{12}$
  Ferrous gluconate
  Discontinue Coumadin
  1 unit whole blood
  Procaine penicillin
  House diet
  Up ad lib

PRESURGICAL LABORATORY TESTS:
  Prothrombin time
  Hemoglobin, hematocrit and CBC
  Bilirubin: direct and indirect
  Urinalysis

The patient was 45, married, had two children (boys, 15 and 17), and owned his home. He was currently employed, full time, as an accountant for a large firm. He liked his job and was glad of the company's medical benefits. With his wife working too, he felt the family "had their heads above water" financially after his previous surgery. He said that it was just in time, because his oldest boy had been admitted to college. He had really begun "to feel like a whole man again."

B. A day later, an appendectomy was performed under general anesthesia, with no unusual incidents. The appendix was inflamed and a fecalith was found occluding the proximal portion. Mr. Malone was admitted to the recovery room, remained there until he was responsive and was then taken to a general care area in the early afternoon.

C. Mrs. Handy, head nurse on the general care unit, reviewed the postoperative orders for Mr. Malone and then went in to see him. He was sleepy but easily aroused. His speech was a bit slurred. He complained of some pain but said it was not bad. His temperature was 99.6, pulse 94, blood pressure 100/84. He was pale but his extremities were warm. He had an IV of 5% D/W running and had absorbed 450 cc since surgery. Nothing remarkable occurred in his postoperative course for the next three days.

D. Saturday morning, Mr. Malone seemed very groggy when he was awakened. His speech was slow and slurred, but appropriate. He was paler than usual and perspiring slightly. His pulse was 102/minute, blood pressure 94/68, temperature had risen to 100.2° F and respirations were

24. He was transferred to the intensive care unit. Stat diagnostic measures were ordered:

    Lumbar puncture
    CBC
    Protein electrolytes studies, Po_2, Pco_2 and bilirubin assessments
    Neurological consult
    Electrophoresis
    ECG
    Prothrombin time

STAT TREATMENTS:
    Central venous pressure line inserted. First reading 5 cm water
    Isoproterenol (Isuprel) in 500 cc D/W 80 microdrips elevated the blood pressure to 94 millimeters of mercury. To be maintained at 90-100 mm/kg systolic.
    Foley catheter inserted. Hourly readings and specific gravity recorded.

Mr. Malone remained in essentially the same condition until Monday morning.

THE RESULTS OF LABORATORY TESTS WERE:
    ECG—Sinus tachycardia. Nonspecific ST segment changes, signs of left ventricular hypertrophy and strain.
    Lumbar puncture—No cells. (Opening and closing pressures normal)

NEUROLOGICAL CONSULT:
    R pupillary reflex sluggish
    R pupil questionably dilated
    Questionable R Babinski reflex
    Intact reflexes

SENSORIUM:
    Responses slow, words slurred, affect slightly flat.
    Responses appropriate.
    Findings consistent with L. cerebral vascular accident of small vessel or multiple small emboli.

SERUM ELECTROLYTES:
    Na 130 mg per 100 ml
    Cl 100 mg per 100 ml
    K 3.2 mg per 3.2 ml
    Bilirubin direct 0.2, indirect 0.8
    Prothrombin time 14.6 sec., 85%
    Po_2 100 mg per 100 ml
    Pco_2 18 mg per 18 ml
    BUN 20 mg per 20 ml
    Electrophoresis—within normal limits excepting slightly decreased albumin

COMPLETE BLOOD COUNT:
    Hemoglobin 9.6
    Hematocrit 31
    RBC—normal 4.250 million
    Leukocytes—42,000 many immature cells
    Platelets—200,000

THE PHYSICIANS WERE CONSIDERING:
1. Cerebral vascular accident leading to neurogenic shock
2. Embolus to adrenal gland—hypovolemic shock from mineralocorticoid deficiency
3. Gram-negative or endotoxin shock from peritoneal contamination with bowel contents

E. Mr. Malone's condition was deteriorating. The nurses increased the rate of Isuprel infusion to 140 drops per minute. The physicians later doubled the amount of drug in the solution, in order to reduce the rate of flow, when his central venous pressure climbed within one hour to 22 cm water. His heart rate increased to 120 beats a minute. A stat ECG demonstrated a right bundle branch block. Urine output fell sharply until no output could be measured, despite treatment first with mannitol (Manicol), then ethacrynic acid (Edecrin), then Fursemide (Lasix). With each agent employed, urine output increased for the next hour then diminished to 0 to 10 an hour. Norepinephrine (Levophed) was substituted for Isuprel. A supplemental dose of digitalis was ordered and given IV. No signs of digitalis toxicity appeared. Serum potassium remained at 4.4 mEq, BUN climbed to 58. Mr. Malone was made more comfortable with a heat blanket and oxygen 5 L per minute by nasal catheter. His heart rhythm had been monitored since early morning but showed no arrhythmias other than sinus tachycardia.

F. Mr. Malone's blood pressure began falling again about 8 A.M., despite vigorous vasopressor therapy. At this time the nurses' notes read: T. 98.0, P 124, R 24, B/P 72/? Levophed in 500 cc 5% D/W at 96 gtt/min. Pulse very weak and thready. Respirations deep and labored. CVP 12. Urine output 7-8 PM 4 cc sp gv 1.008. Patient responds only to shouted name, although without provocation he rouses and mumbles confused sentences. Pupillary responses sluggish. Color is ashen, extremities very cold. Moderate ankle edema; abdomen distended. Incontinent of feces once. Family members are here; wife visits for about five minutes every hour or so. She is not apparently recognized now.

At 9 P.M. that same evening, Mr. Malone died, despite all efforts.

The reader may test himself for knowledge of the pathophysiology of shock, its treatment and the associated nursing care by answering the following questions:

1. What parameters constitute a clinical picture of shock?

2. What classifications of shock are appropriate to the signs and symptoms manifested by Mr. Malone?

3. What is the dosage range for the following agents; what is their desirable effect; what special considerations on the part of the nurse does each agent entail?
   a. Cedilanid
   b. ferrous gluconate
   c. vitamin B_{12}
   d. isoproterenol
   e. norepinephrine
   f. procaine penicillin
   g. cephalothin
   h. mannitol
   i. fursemide
   j. ethacrynic acid
   k. Coumadin
   Justify the change from Isuprel to Levophed in terms of the physiological action of both drugs.

4. What comfort measures are most appropriate for Mr. Malone at each stage of his illness? (Sections A to F)

5. What additional assessment should have been made and recorded at each stage (other than those presented in the case study)?

6. What special considerations are involved in each of the following assessments?
   a. pulse
   b. blood pressure
   c. urine volume measurement
   d. cardiac monitoring
   e. central venous pressure measurement

7. What could Mr. Malone's nurse do with respect to the family during each stage of his illness; at the time of his death?

8. What are the staff's needs in a situation such as

this? What special considerations should be given to patients in close proximity to Mr. Malone?

Unfortunately, an autopsy permission was not granted by Mr. Malone's family. A definite diagnosis of the underlying condition could never be established. The case presented demonstrates both the complexity of the syndrome of shock and the difficulty in treating it effectively.

In conclusion, the care of the patient in shock requires the synthesis of knowledge of the functions of several body systems. It requires the exercise of sensitive assessment and close attention to carrying out the physician's prescribed regimen. Finally, the patient needs to perceive the nurse as a person who cares about him and who will competently minister to his needs.

References

1. Hruza, Z.: Resistance to Trauma. Springfield, Ill., Charles C Thomas, 1971.

2. Weil, M. H. and Shubin, H.: Proposed reclassification of shock status with special reference to distributive defects. Adv. Exp. Med. & Biol. 23: 13-24, 1972.

3. Scheidt, S., Ascheim, R. and Killip, T.: Shock after acute myocardial infarction. Am. J. Cardiol. 20: 556-564, Dec. 1970.

4. See MacLean, L. D., Mulligan, W. G., MacLean, A. P. H. and Duff, J. H.: Patterns of septic shock in man. Ann. Surg. 166: 543-562, Oct. 1967. See also McCabe, W. R., Kreger, B. E. and Johns, M.: Gram-negative bacillary infections. New Eng. J. Med. 287: 261-267, Aug. 10, 1972.

5. Goodman, L. S. and Gilman, A.: The Pharmacological Basis of Therapeutics, ed. 4. New York, Macmillan, 1965.

6. Shoemaker, W. C.: Physiologic mechanisms in clinical shock. Adv. Exp. Med. & Biol. 23: 57-73, 1972.

7. Forland, M. and Talley, R. C.: Treatment of renal abnormalities accompanying shock. Postgrad. Med. 49: 128-138, Sept. 1970.

8. Hardaway, R. M.: Clinical Management of Shock. Springfield, Ill., Charles C Thomas, 1968.

9. See Forrester, J. S., Diamond, G., McHugh, J. J. and Swan, H. J. C.: Filling pressures: a reap-

praisal of CVP monitoring. New Eng. J. Med. 285: 190-195, July 1971; and Thal, A.: Shock: A Physiologic Basis of Treatment. Chicago, Yearbook Medical Publishers, 1971.

10. Shirls, G. T., Carrico, C. J. and Canizano, P. C.: Shock—Major Problems in Clinical Surgery, vol. 13. Philadelphia, W. B. Saunders, 1973.

11. *Ibid*. See also Best, C. H. and Taylor, N. B.: The Physiological Basis of Medical Practice, ed. 9. Baltimore, Williams & Wilkins, 1973. Harrison, T. R. (ed.): Principles of Internal Medicine, ed. 7. New York, McGraw-Hill, 1974. Harvey, A., et al. (eds.): The Principles and Practice of Medicine, ed. 17. New York, Appleton-Century Crofts, 1969.

12. Best and Taylor, *ibid*.; Harrison, *ibid*.; and Harvey, et al., *ibid*. Collins, V. J.: Principles of Anesthesiology. Philadelphia, Lea & Febiger, 1966. Drapenas, T. and Litman, L. S.: Trauma and the management of the acutely injured patient. *In* D. Sabiston (ed.): Christopher's Textbook of Surgery. Philadelphia, W. B. Saunders, 1972, pp. 351-397. MacBryde, C. M. (ed.): Signs and Symptoms, ed. 5. Philadelphia, J. B. Lippincott, 1970. Marshall, R. J. and Darby, T. D.: Shock: Pharmacological Principles in Treatment. Springfield, Ill., Charles C Thomas, 1966. Guyton, A. C.: Textbook of Medical Physiology, ed. 4. Philadelphia, W. B. Saunders, 1971. Henry, J. P. and Meehan, J. P.: The Circulation: An Integrative Physiologic Study. Chicago, Yearbook Medical Publishers, 1971. Weil, M. H. and Shubin, H. Symposium on shock and syncope. Am. J. Cardiol. 26: 553-555, Dec. 1970.

13. Guyton, *ibid*. Shoemaker, *op. cit*. See also Mayer, J. H. and Lewis, G. M.: Vasopressor agents in shock. Am. J. Nurs. 75: 620-625, April 1975. Shoemaker, W. C.: Introductory remarks on shock. Adv. Exp. Med. & Biol. 23: 11-12, 1972.

14. Goodman and Gilman, *op. cit*. Ballet, S. and Kastes, J. B.: Recent advances in the therapy of cardiac arrhythmias: a symposium. Springfield, Ill., Charles C Thomas, 1972.

15. Goodman and Gilman, *op. cit*. Shanbour, L. L.: Dopamine in the treatment of shock. Adv. Exp. Med. & Biol. 23: 245-251, 1972.

16. Weil and Shubin, Symposium on shock and syncope, *op. cit*. Weil, M. H. and Shubin, H.:

Diagnosis and Treatment of Shock. Baltimore, Williams & Wilkins, 1967.

17. *Ibid*.

18. Shoemaker, Introductory remarks, *op. cit*. Weil and Shubin, Proposed reclassification, *op. cit*.

19. Weil and Shubin, *ibid*.

20. *Ibid*.

21. *Ibid*.

22. Guyton, *op. cit*.

23. MacBryde, *op. cit*.

24. Lutz, H.: Forms of shock. Minerva Med. 64: 2630-2633, 1973. Meltzer, L.: Detection of early heart failure. *In* F. C. Ownby (ed.): Advanced Cardiac Nursing. Philadelphia, Charles Press, 1970.

25. MacLean, Mulligan, Maclean and Duff, *op. cit*.

26. Ibid. Guyton, *op. cit*.

27. Curran, R. C. and Harnden, D. G.: The Pathological Basis of Medicine. Philadelphia, W. B. Saunders, 1972. Jacobson, E. D.: Are adrenergic overactivity and splanchnic vasoconstriction prime physiological events in shock? Adv. Exp. Med. & Biol. 23: 107-111, 1972. Weil, M. H. and Shubin, H.: Changes in venous capitance during cardiogenic shock: a search for the third dimension. Am. J. Cardiol. 26: 613-614, Dec. 1970.

28. Weil and Shubin, *ibid*. Wilson, R. F. and Robb, H. J.: Platelet, hemodynamic and respiratory changes in shock, sepsis and trauma. Adv. Exp. Med. & Biol. 23: 145-147, 1972.

29. Jacobson, *op. cit*.

30. MacBryde, *op. cit*.

31. *Ibid*.

32. Hinkhouse, A.: Craniocerebral trauma. Am. J. Nurs. 73: 1714-1922, Oct. 1973.

Bibliography

Abbot, W. E.: Nutrition, body fluid, shock and burns. Surg. Gyn. Ob. 116: 1-14, Feb. 1963.

Adgey, A. S. Jennifer: Domiciliary management of cardiogenic shock in acute myocardial infarction. *In* I. M. Ledingham and T. A. MacAllister (eds.): *Conference on Shock* (proceedings of Conference of Royal College of Physicians and Surgeons in Glasgow). St. Louis, C. V. Mosby, 1972.

Altmeir, W. A., Todd, J. C., and Inge, W. W.: Gram

negative septicemia a growing threat. Ann. Surg. 166: 530-542, Oct. 1967.

Artz, C. P. and Moncrief, J.: The Treatment of Burns, ed. 2. Philadelphia, W. B. Saunders, 1969.

Ayers, Stephen M., Miller, H., Giannelli, S., and Fleming, P., et al.: The lung in shock. Am. J. Cardiol. 26: 588-599, Dec. 1970.

Bachman, F., et al.: The hemostatic mechanism after open heart surgery. J. Thor. and Cardiovasc. Surg. 70: 76-85, July 1975.

Berman, I. R.: The lung lesion in shock. Adv. Exp. Med. & Biol. L. B. Hinshaw (ed.) 23: 51-56, 1972.

Bertelli, A. and Beck, N.: Shock: Biochemical, Pharmacological and Clinical Aspects. New York, Plenum, 1970.

Campbell, E. B.: Nursing problems associated with prolonged recovery following trauma. Nurs. Clin. N. Am. 5: 551-562, Dec. 1970.

Cuthbert, M. H.: The Prostaglandins. Philadelphia, J. B. Lippincott, 1973.

Driefus, L.: Hazards of transvenous catheters. Chest. 65: 2-8, Jan. 1974.

Frey, C. F.: Initial Management of the Trauma Patient. Philadelphia, Lea & Febiger, 1976.

Gentry, W. D., Foster, S. B., and Froehling, S.: Psychologic response to situational stress in intensive and non-intensive nursing. Heart and Lung 1: 793-796, 1972.

Hershey, S. G., Del Guerco, L. R. M., and McConn, R. (eds.): Septic Shock in Man. Boston, Little, Brown, 1971.

Jenneti, B.: Head injuries and shock. *In* A. Bertelli and N. Beck (eds.): Shock: Biochemical, Pharmacological and Clinical Aspects. New York, Plenum, 1970, pp. 134-138.

Johnson, A. R.: Liberation of vasoactive materials from mast cells in anaphylactic shock. Adv. Exp. Med. & Biol. 23: 365-375, 1972.

Jude, J. R. and Elam, F. O.: Fundamentals of Cardiopulmonary Resuscitation. Philadelphia, F. A. Davis, 1965.

Kosik, J. and Thompson, J.: Allergic reactions to antibiotics. Med. Clin. N. Am. 54: 1-6, Jan. 1970.

Kellermyer, R. W. and Graham, J. R.: Kinins—Possible Physiologic and pathologic roles in man. New Eng. J. Med. 279: 754, 802, 859, 884, 1968.

Kretchman, L. A. and Schronts, J. S.: The adult respiratory distress syndrome. Postgrad. Med. 54: 63-76, July 1973.

Lee, J. M.: Emotional reactions to trauma. Nurs. Clin. N. Am. 5: 577-588, Dec. 1970.

McGehee, W. G. and Rapaport, S. I.: Systemic hemostatic failure in the severely injured patient. Surg. Clin. N. Am. 48: 1247-1261, Dec. 1968.

Muirhead, M. A.: Vasoactive and antihypertensive effects of prostaglandins and other renomedullary lipids. *In* M. F. Cuthbert (ed.): The Prostaglandins. Philadelphia, J. B. Lippincott, 1973, pp. 236-250.

Nielson, M. A.: Intra-arterial monitoring of blood pressure. Am. J. Nurs. 74: 48-53, Jan. 1974.

Noble, J. H., Jr., et al. (eds.): Emergency Medical Services, Behavioral and Planning Prospectus. New York, Behavioral Publications, 1974.

Rush, B. F.: Irreversibility in the post-transfusion phase of hemorrhagic shock. Adv. Exp. Med. & Biol. 23: 215-234, 1972.

Schimmel, E. M.: The hazards of hospitalization. Ann. Intern. Med. 279: 1321-1325, 1968.

Schnaper, N.: The psychological implications of severe trauma. J. Trauma 15: 100-104, Feb. 1975.

Schumer, W.: Histamine release in endotoxin shock. Adv. Exp. Med. & Biol. 23: 235-243, 1972.

Sherry, S. and Coleman, R. W.: Observations on the plasma kallikreinogen (pre kallikrein)—kalikrein enzyme system. Trans. Assoc. Am. Phys. 81: 40-48, cit. no. 405 2360.

Shillingford, J. P.: Syncope. Am. J. Cardiol. 26: 609-612, 1970.

Shoemaker, W. C. and Walker, W. F.: Fluid and Electrolyte Therapy in Acute Illness. Chicago, Yearbook Medical Publishers, 1970.

Shumer, W. and Nyhus, L. M.: Treatment of Shock: Principles and Practice. Philadelphia, Lea & Febiger, 1974.

Tinker, J. H. and Wehner, R. J.: Postoperative recovery and the neuromuscular function. Am. J. Nurs. 74: 74-76, Jan. 1974.

Vissher, M.: Introduction: an overview of the shock problem. Adv. Exp. Med. & Biol. 23: 3-7, 1972.

Watt, A. J. and Wilson, R. F. (eds.): Management of Trauma: Pitfalls and Practice. Philadelphia, Lea & Febiger, 1975.

14

The Gaseous Exchange Process: the nature of the problem and nursing goals

MARY EARLY

Prevention • The Process • Assessment • Client Problems and Nursing Intervention • Rehabilitation

The increasing prevalence of chronic obstructive pulmonary disease (COPD), as well as rising death rates from this disorder, has served to identify a major public health problem in the United States. COPD was ranked as ninth in the causes of death in 1970, and was second only to heart diseases in worker's disability allocations under the Social Security Administration.[1] Further evidence of the epidemic proportion of COPD has been obtained from a physician's survey which indicates that 60 percent of those surveyed (324,000 cases) gave chronic bronchitis as the reason for the first visit.[2] These statistics reveal only a small portion of the iceberg of COPD, not to mention the invalidism, discouragement, suffering, and health care problems associated with it. The magnitude of the problem has become one of the major concerns of citizens and health care professionals.

The high incidence of carcinoma of the lung, recognition of the acute respiratory distress syndrome resulting from shock and trauma, greater understanding of the genetic factors involved in pulmonary disease, and newly discovered functions of the lung in maintaining homeostasis, are all factors which have had their impact on the education and research of respiratory diseases and care of patients suffering with these disorders.

Today every facet of health-life style is being examined in terms of the relevancy of what is occurring in relation to the quality of the life lived. This necessitates consideration of health care results versus cost. Prevention of disease, promotion of health, and care of distributive and episodic illnesses are services thought to be the right of each individual-family in our society. Consideration of the scope of services required prompts the realization that consumers and health care professionals must work together in addressing themselves to the future health of the nation. Thus, nursing as a profession must be responsible for a meaningful role in the health care of the patient-client-family. This role in respiratory care begins with viewing man, man's internal and external environment, and the dynamic equilibrium maintained between the two for survival.

The first step is to identify factors in the environment which retard good respiratory health, result in pathophysiological changes, promote illness rather than health, or, as Dunn has suggested, act as interferences in high-level wellness

411

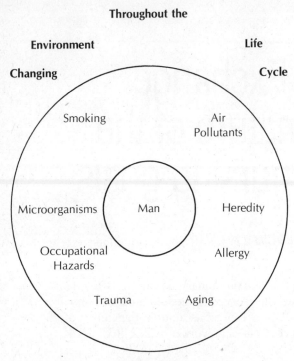

Figure 14-1.
Contributing factors in the occurrence of respiratory pathophysiological processes.

or functioning. Figure 14-1 illustrates what are presently known from epidemiological studies to be contributing factors in the occurrence of respiratory pathophysiological processes.

Prevention

Prevention is one of the most unique and challenging roles of the nurse in respiratory care. Often the nurse has heard such comments as, "Is there really anything to smoking cigarettes and cancer?" "or emphysema?" Or, "if it's all that bad for you, why doesn't it show up until later on in life?" "What about all those around you that continue to smoke when you've managed to quit?" The nurse must be alert and ready to respond at this "teachable" moment, for the Surgeon General's Committee report on smoking has provided the fact that a nonsmoking population is the single most significant factor in the prevention of lung diseases. Other major findings

of the Committee and additional research supports were:

1. Close relationship between smoking and the development of pulmonary emphysema, lung cancer, and coronary heart disease.
2. Decided increase in the number of smoking-related deaths.
3. Correlation between the number of cigarettes smoked and the mortality rate.
4. Increased recurrent illnesses among smokers.
5. Cigarette smoking as the most important cause of chronic bronchitis, increasing the risk of dying from chronic bronchitis and pulmonary emphysema.
6. Autopsies show destruction and/or shortening of cilia, increase in the number of goblet cells and hypertrophy and hyperplasia of bronchial mucous glands. Such alterations interfere with the cleansing mechanism of the respiratory tract.[3]

Fletcher commented that, "Many meticulous studies, using a wide variety of pulmonary function tests, have demonstrated that not only is the ventilatory function of the lungs impaired by airway obstruction in the cigarette smoker, but gas-transfer ability, the ability to get oxygen from the air into the arterial blood, is also reduced even in the young, apparently undisabled smoker."[4] Unfortunately, it has been found that the damage to the bronchioles and alveoli which occurs in chronic bronchitis and pulmonary emphysema is usually irreversible. The disregard of the long-range danger of cigarette smoking is a problem to surmount in persuading people to give up smoking. Fear has not been a strong motivating factor in most instances. Statistics and facts have been helpful, primarily with the moderate cigarette smoker.

The World Conference on Smoking and Health suggested a pragmatic approach to the problem.[5] Their first recommendation involves prevention—not initiating the patterns of smoking. The exemplary role is one of the important factors in creating a heathful milieu. The nurse, as well as parents, teachers, heroes, and other significant persons in the life of the young adolescent, must serve as an example. Ira Gordon suggested applying the positive concepts of virility, beauty, and sex prowess to the nonsmoker.[6]

Making places to smoke less available and less desirable, and not having ashtrays at hand are other recommendations.

Numerous antismoking programs and clinics have been initiated based upon the same concept as Alcoholics Anonymous and Weight Watchers. One such clinic postulated "that altering smoking behavior initiates a process of relearning, characterized by a reordering of psychological mechanisms, wherein emotional states formerly modulated by smoking become tolerable in a cigarette-free state."[7] Strong emotional support is necessary if nonsmoking behavior is to be achieved. More recent has been the use of behavior modification techniques.

The introduction of marijuana smoking among segments of society has caused concern among respiratory physiologists. At this time, little is known about its biological effects on the lung. A recent study demonstrated that a "water-soluble component of the gas phase of marijuana smoke is toxic to the alveolar macrophages and impairs the bactericidal activity of this key cell in the host defense network of the lung in a dose-dependent manner."[8] Increased use and potential legalization of marijuana will possibly result in a need for more definitive research in this area.

The highly industrialized society of the 20th century has brought with it new occupational hazards as by-products of technological innovations and achievements. The nurse recognizes that some of these by-products are associated with materials that directly damage the lung. Continuous and repeated exposure to air pollution and irritant dust, particularly among the cigarette-smoking population, damages the defense mechanisms of the lungs. Lungs are made incapable of carrying out their primary function of gas exchange because of recurrent infections and scarring.

The occupational health nurse is most familiar with the important passage of the Federal Coal Mine Health and Safety Act of 1969. This act spelled out certain health and safety standards to be maintained in the mines, including maximum levels of respiratory dust exposure. It was this law which laid the groundwork for the Occupational Safety and Health Act of 1970 which provided for health and safety of workers in other occupations.

In discussing air pollution and the lung, Bates has identified five statements which he believes can be made from epidemiological data:

1. Where air pollution is sufficiently great, episodes of increased sulfur dioxide and particulate pollution result in increased mortality rates among those with chronic lung disease and some increased morbidity rates.

2. Concentrations of sulfur dioxide greater than approximately 0.08 parts per million as an annual average, particularly when accompanied by particulate pollution of the order of more than 150 micrograms as an annual average, are accompanied by increased morbidity rates from chronic bronchitis in the adult city population.

3. Threefold increase in morbidity rates from lower chest infections in infants, and children younger than two years, in moderate and high pollution regions as compared to very low pollution areas.

4. Cigarette smoking and air pollution seem to lower the forced expiratory volume (FEV_1) in one second. The exact relationship between the two factors remains an area for further definitive study.

5. Reports from Japan suggest increased symptoms and affect on pulmonary function in the grossly polluted regions. Reseachers in the United Kingdom showing lowered economic status being more of a factor.[9]

Gareth Green has stated that small particles, 1 to 5 microns in size, may penetrate deeply into alveoli of the lung and cause direct injury.[10] The combination of these particles, water, and toxic gases (nitrogen oxide, ozone, and industrial chemicals) can be extremely dangerous. The defense mechanism of the lung, however, is remarkable in its mucociliary secretory powers and the macrophage's ability to phagocytize inhaled particles. This process has been demonstrated by a new technique developed for scanning electron microscope.

Our industrialized society has made materials that have improved our health, welfare, and safety in some spheres, while at the same time adding to our illnesses in other spheres. The solution is not simple, but problems must be viewed analytically to determine which materials are most damaging to the lung and the degree of exposure which is damaging. Trade-offs may be necessary, eliminating some and reducing others to an absolute minimum.

Progressive massive fibrosis and carcinogenicity resulting from continuous exposure to air pollutants and irritating dust is and should be of great concern to all consumers and health professionals alike. This concern must start with the provision of excellent health care in childhood and continue throughout the life cycle. Repeated respiratory illnesses, particularly in the formative years, may establish the continuing destructive lung disease process.

This leads to the consideration of another factor influencing the occurrence of lung disease, the individual's genetic makeup. Genetically determined differences exist in the cells and tissue of the lung, the immune system of the body, and the protective antienzyme systems of the blood which alter the normal response to injurious agents. Cystic fibrosis and alpha$_1$ antitrypsin (AAT) deficiency are examples of the more common genetic defects presently known. (See Chapter 6 concerning hereditary health problems.)

Homozygous deficiency of serum alpha$_1$ antitrypsin, a deficiency of the major serum alpha$_1$ globulin (alpha$_1$ antitrypsin), is transmitted by a single autosomal recessive gene. Homozygotes may develop panlobular emphysema in early adult life while heterozygotes appear predisposed to the development of centrilobular emphysema related to cigarette smoking. Mittman, et al., studies demonstrated large lung volumes (mainly loss of alveolar walls predominantly in the vascular portion), low diffusing capacities, and arterial hypoxemia without carbon dioxide retention in individuals with severe and intermediate AAT deficiency.[11] The mechanism involved is not definitely known; however, specific and characteristic lesions have been seen in patients with lung disease and AAT deficiency. Mittman has suggested that the following evidence might be a plausible explanation:

AAT inhibits a wide array of proteases but most evidence implicates the leukocytic proteases and specifically of leukocytes in the pathogenesis of emphysema. We have demonstrated that proteases of leukocytic origin are capable of digesting human and hamster lungs and that this proteatysis is inhibited by the AAT of human serum.[12]

This theory suggests that a severe absence of AAT may result in a rapidly fulminating COPD while the triad of smoking, pollution, and AAT intermediary deficiency might result in a slower development of the disease process.

It is now possible to laboratory test for AAT deficiency, suggesting the feasibility of establishing screening centers such as those for sickle cell anemia. Eventually, substitution therapy may become possible, using endogenous antiproteases. Earlier detection will hopefully prevent the occurrence of the emphysematous process and identify needs for genetic counseling in some, and strong encouragement to discontinue smoking in others.

Genetic counseling programs have been concerning themselves with the problem of mucoviscidosis (cystic fibrosis). Children homozygous for the recessive mucoviscidosic gene secrete abnormally tenacious bronchial mucus which obstructs air passages, predisposes to lower respiratory infection, bronchiectasis, and progressive lung destruction.

As part of the aging process, it is common to see reduction of physical fitness, decrease in ventilatory capacity (as a result of decreased compliance and elastic recoil), uneven distribution of ventilation, decreased diffusing capacity, increased residual volume and a slightly greater ratio of physiological dead space to tidal volume. With the shift of the population curve to approximately 14.1 percent (1970) in the age group 60 and over, it can be anticipated that the number of individuals with COPD will increase in addition to that of the group with potential pulmonary implications secondary to other long-term illnesses. This will cause demands for a program of primary preventive care, and place emphasis on good respiratory care in long-term health facilities. Already there have been interesting physical fitness programs initiated for the older individual, with positive results in terms of subjective improvement.

Severe trauma, thoracic and nonthoracic injury, hemorrhagic shock, fat embolism, overwhelming septicemia, diffuse intravascular coagulation, aspiration, and near drownings are known entities to every emergency treatment center and ICU. A partially understood phenomenon, the adult respiratory distress syndrome (ARDS) characterized by severe oxygen transport impairment, decreasing lung compliance, and pulmonary infiltration, has occurred among this high-risk group. Many names have been given to this pathological process—"the Da Nung lung," "traumatic wet lung," "hemorrhagic wet lung syndrome," to mention a few. Speed of travel, alcoholism, and drugs have been identified as contributing factors to the severity of trauma. Better means of transporting the severely injured and ill and specially prepared health personnel have increased the number of clients surviving the initial insult—a most vulnerable group for the development of ARDS. Nursing support and participation in the development of sound safety programs, legislation to insure safety measures in various modes of transportation, further development of effective emergency care systems, and an attack on the problem of alcoholism and drugs would go a long way in reducing the incidence of ARDS. There is a need to develop additional educational programs for physicians and nurses in the early recognition and treatment of ARDS, as well as further research for greater understanding of this syndrome.

Allergies are another major cause of pulmonary symptomatology and disease. No attempt will be made to discuss these problems since they will be discussed in greater detail in Chapter 23 of this text.

It seems prudent now to focus attention on the vast number of clients with pre-existing pulmonary problems. Therefore, a brief review of the breathing process and medical and nursing interventions will be presented.

The Process[13]

Asleep or awake, the complex process of breathing goes on unrelentingly, maintaining a normal blood and tissue level of oxygen, carbon dioxide, pH, and various electrolytes.

To achieve these essential end results, this complex process requires:

1. Suitable oxygen and carbon dioxide concentrations in the inspired air.
2. Adequate ventilation and perfusion of the alveoli.
3. Permeable alveolar-capillary membrane.
4. Adequate pulmonary and systemic circulation.
5. Ability of the blood to transport oxygen and carbon dioxide between the lungs and tissues.
6. Ability of the cells to utilize oxygen and eliminate carbon dioxide.

Each of the parameters in the process will be discussed, with consideration of the role of each in health and pathophysiological states, along with goals for appropriate nursing intervention.

SUITABLE OXYGEN AND CARBON DIOXIDE CONCENTRATIONS IN THE INSPIRED AIR

The ambient air supporting human life on this planet is greatest within the first 10,000 feet from the earth's surface. Figure 14-2 shows that the percentage of oxygen variation is small even as high as 35,000 feet. However, the barometric pressure, or atmospheric pressure, and the partial pressure of oxygen in alveolar air are altered significantly at this distance. The atmospheric gaseous mixture exerts a pressure at sea level of 760 mm Hg (Standard Temperature Pressure Dry), which scientists use as a reference point in discussing pressures. Pressures less than those of ambient air are called negative or subatmospheric, and those greater than ambient air pressure are designated positive. Since air is a mixture, according to the law of partial pressure, its total pressure is equal to the sum of all the partial pressures of the individual gases. If the altitude and percentage concentration of a gas are known, the partial pressure (tension) can be calculated:

Partial Pressure = Percentage of Gas (dry) ×
Total Barometric Pressure (dry)

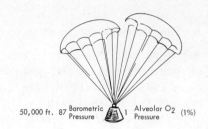

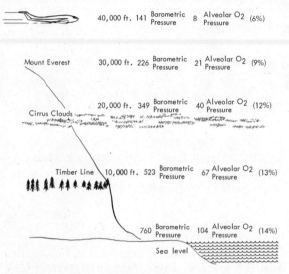

tial pressure of 158 mm Hg. By the time the oxygen mixes with gases already in the air passages which do not undergo exchange, and becomes saturated with water vapor at body temperature, the intra-alveolar oxygen tension is approximately 104 mm Hg. Blood entering the capillary has an oxygen tension of 40 mm Hg, providing a

FIGURE 14-2.
Relationship of altitude in feet—barometric pressure—Po_2 in aveoli (mm Hg)

The actual movement of the air into the airway passages depends upon the pressure differential between ambient and alveolar air. Approximately 300 to 500 ml of air is involved with each normal quiet inspiration and expiration. This volume is called tidal volume. Figure 14-3 illustrates the tidal volume and reserve volumes found in the lungs under normal physiological conditions.

The exchange of gases between the alveoli and the blood capillaries involves a partial pressure differential. However, it is important to note that the partial pressures of gases in the alveoli are not identical to the partial pressures of the same gases in ambient air. At sea level, under standard dry conditions, oxygen concentration of ambient air is 20.93 percent and exerts a par-

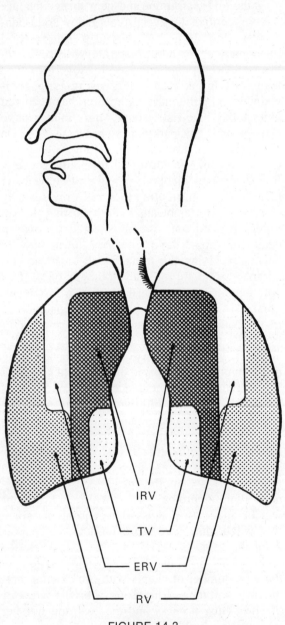

FIGURE 14-3.
Lung capacity volumes.

pressure gradient of 64 mm Hg between the alveoli and blood capillaries; thus, oxygen moves from the alveoli into the blood. By the time the blood reaches the other end of the pulmonary capillary, the oxygen tension is approximately 104 mm Hg. The "time integrated" average tension during normal respiration, however, is approximately 11 mm Hg. That is, equilibration of pressures between the alveolar oxygen and the red cell takes place within an 0.8 second interval, with a pressure gradient of less than 11 mm Hg, existing for a relatively large part of this time.

Carbon dioxide makes up approximately 0.04 percent of the inspired tidal volume. Intra-alveolar carbon dioxide tension is normally 40 mm Hg. The blood entering the pulmonary capillaries has a carbon dioxide tension of 45 mm Hg, but the tension has decreased to 40 mm Hg by the time it leaves these capillaries. Being approximately 40 mm Hg, the alveolar carbon dioxide pressure provides a diffusion gradient of 5 mm Hg between the alveoli and blood, considerably less than the diffusion gradient for oxygen. Carbon dioxide is 20 to 30 times more diffusible than oxygen, so that less pressure is needed to drive the gas. The alveolar P_{CO_2} depends upon the P_{CO_2} in the blood and the rate and depth of breathing. The respiratory centers in the pons and medulla control the rate and depth of breathing in order to maintain the optimum elimination of carbon dioxide and the pH of the blood.

The body's defense mechanisms can make adjustments to changes in oxygen and carbon dioxide tensions, particularly if they are gradual processes. These include such changes as an increase in the rate and depth of breathing, increased production of red blood cells, and acceleration of the heart and circulatory action. There are limits to this adjustment in both time and tensions. Therefore, one can appreciate the need for pressurized cabins for high-altitude flying and space travel, as well as pressurized suits with adequate oxygen and carbon dioxide exchange in extravehicular space maneuvers. A milieu compatible with human survival is necessary also for those whose work is done at great depths below sea level, such as oceanographers and submariners.

ADEQUATE VENTILATION

The achievement of adequate ventilation depends upon the bellows function of the thorax and maintenance of a patent airway. Adequate ventilation is important because the body has little ability to store oxygen, and the cells of the brain, myocardium, and kidney are extremely sensitive to hypoxia.

The thorax is a closed cavity in which the lungs are encased in a highly elastic serous membrane called the visceral pleura. The visceral pleura is directly adherent to the lung surface. At the point where the main bronchus and pulmonary vessels enter the lung (the hilum), the pleural membrane is reflected onto the interior chest wall and the upper surface of the diaphragm and is called the parietal pleura. The two pleural surfaces lie adjacent to each other and provide only a potential space. A few millimeters of fluid lie between the pleurae, creating surface tension (a pulling or drawing action), and allowing the lungs to glide or move along the inside of the chest wall as they expand and contract. This pulling action helps to prevent the collapse of the lung during expiration and creates a subatmospheric pressure within the pleural cavity. This subatmospheric pressure ranges from − 8 mm Hg during inspiration to − 2 mm Hg during expiration.

Interference with the integrity of the thoracic cavity becomes a problem that demands immediate intervention in order to re-establish subatmospheric intrapleural pressure. For example, trauma to the chest wall, or pulmonary or cardiac surgery may result in the admission of atmospheric air into the intrapleural space, causing collapse of the lung. Increased fluid, pus, or air in the intrapleural space may result in a similar effect.

The lung substance and bronchial tree are richly endowed with elastic tissue. As the inspiratory muscular force is alerted to contract, the lungs expand, filling the cavity so that the elastic fibers are stretched. During the expiratory phase, the elastic fibers tend to recoil to their original size. Subambient intrapulmonary pressure is created by the volumetric changes in the lungs during inspiration, causing atmospheric air to move into the airway. This atmospheric air moves in rapidly at the beginning of inspiration and more slowly as intrapulmonic pressure begins to approximate that of the atmosphere. It is important to remember that the lungs play only a passive role during the usual respiratory cycle.

PATENT AIRWAY

The maintenance of a patent airway—the nose, pharynx, trachea, bronchioles, alveolar ducts, atria, and approximately 350 million alveoli—is vital to adequate ventilation. The patency of the airways is facilitated by the C-shaped cartilaginous structures of the trachea and bronchi. A fibroelastic membrane exists between the cartilaginous rings, allowing flexibility and movement of the trachea and major bronchi. These rings and the strong fibroelastic membrane eventually become irregular in the similar bronchioles, and are completely replaced by circular smooth muscle fibers in the terminal bronchioles. Since the terminal bronchioles contain only smooth muscle, which is regulated by autonomic nervous control, the patency of the lumen of the airway in this section depends upon the pressure gradient between the lumen and the walls of the bronchioles. The intraluminal pressure must exceed the intramural pressure in order to maintain the patency of these minute air passages.

A ciliated columnar epithelium (mucous membrane) lines the respiratory tract and is accompanied by secretory goblet cells in all except the bronchioles. Approximately 100 ml of fluid (mucus) is produced in 24 hours. This mucus acts to moisten and filter out particles larger than 10 microns from ambient air. The hairlike projections called cilia continually sweep the mucus toward the oropharynx to be either expectorated or swallowed. This process is often called the self-cleansing or sterilizing process, and may be seriously impaired in the cigarette smoker and individuals exposed to air pollutants. One of the categories in fibrotic pulmonary disease (pneumoconiosis) may result from prolonged exposure to microparticles (silicon, coal dust and asbestos, and the like).

A mixture of lipoproteins, surfactant, is produced by the large alveolar epithelial cells. The surfactant decreases surface tension uniformly throughout the lung and adds to the stability of the smaller alveoli, thus protecting them against collapse and atelectasis. It decreases the effort of breathing by lowering the pressure required to inflate the lung. Also, the leakage of blood and fluid into the alveolar spaces is inhibited by pulmonary surfactant. Normal production of surfactant depends upon sufficient lung perfusion and intact metabolism of the large alveolar cells. There are questions still unanswered about it, but experimental and clinical evidence points to certain conditions that may be associated with inactive or insufficient surfactant—immaturity of infant lungs, hyaline membrane disease, pneumonia, pulmonary edema, lung pathology associated with prolonged use of the cardiopulmonary bypass, and immunological reaction.

PERFUSION OF THE ALVEOLI

Perfusion of the alveoli refers to the normal pulmonary circulation which provides the means for the gaseous exchange between the capillary and the alveoli. The thin-walled right ventricle pumps the blood into the pulmonary artery as efficiently and in the same volume as the left ventricle does, but at lower pressure. The right ventricular pressure varies from 22 mm Hg during systole to around 0 mm Hg during diastole. Within physiological limits, the heart is capable of adjusting its rate and stroke volume to pump all the blood delivered to it, and to do so in such a way that ventricular pressure does not rise excessively. The stroke volume may vary from a few ml to about 160 ml. Not until the rate reaches 150 beats per minute, however, is stroke volume compromised (see Chapter 12).

The pulmonary artery receives the total amount of blood from the right ventricle and has a similar systolic pressure. After the pulmonic valves close, the systolic pressure in the pulmonary artery drops more gradually and to a lesser degree than the right ventricle, namely to 8 mm Hg. The pulmonary artery branches into right and left main branches which carry blood to the right and left lungs for the exchange. The terminal branches enter a widely anastomosed alveolar capillary network. This network is so dense that the space between capillaries is less than their diameter, which is 8 microns. Considering the great number of alveoli, one can appreciate the magnitude of the capillary system. Because of changes in the cardiac output and the desirability for maintenance of a normal pulmonary artery pressure, a network of reserve capillaries is either collapsed or dilated to make this accommodation.

DIFFUSION THROUGH THE RESPIRATORY MEMBRANE

Diffusion, the gaseous exchange, occurs in the pulmonary unit which consists of the respiratory bronchiole, alveolar duct, atria, and the alveolar sac. The respiratory membrane is extremely thin, making it possible for the alveolar gases to come into close proximity to the capillaries. Figure 14-4 shows the structure of the respiratory membrane, which consists of a uninuclear layer of surfactant, a very thin layer of fluid, a layer of alveolar epithelial cells, an interstitial space containing elastic and collaginous connective tissue fibers plus a small amount of fluid, and the capillary endothelial cells. Despite the number of layers, the overall thickness of the respiratory membrane is less than 1 micron.

As noted above, on the average, the pulmonary capillaries are only 8 microns in diameter, which means that the surface membrane of the

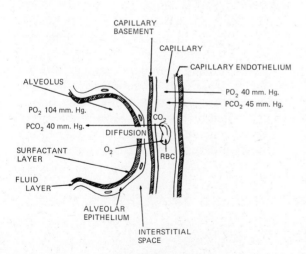

FIGURE 14-4.
Ultrastructure of respiratory membrane.

red blood cells actually contacts the capillary walls as they squeeze through them. This makes it possible for diffusion of oxygen and carbon dioxide to take place between the red blood cells and alveoli without passing through the plasma, facilitating the rate of diffusion.

The rate of gaseous diffusion through the respiratory membrane depends on the thickness of the membrane, the amount of surface area for diffusion, the diffusion coefficient for each gas through the membrane, and the pressure gradient. Any condition that alters these factors affects normal gas exchange. Such conditions as pneumonia, pulmonary edema, fibrosis, emphysema, and surgical removal of lung tissue may adversely affect the diffusing capacity of oxygen and carbon dioxide.

ADEQUATE PULMONARY AND SYSTEMIC CIRCULATION

An adequate systemic circulation is essential for the maintenance of an adequate oxygen and carbon dioxide exchange between the tissues and blood, and for returning blood to the heart. Only if sufficient blood returns to the heart can it be conveyed to the lungs for gas exchange. Adequate blood drainage from the lungs supplies the blood, which is pumped into the systemic circulation. The pulmonary and systemic circulations are dependent upon each other for adequate tissue respiration.

The regulation of the pulmonary and systemic circulation lies primarily with the heart and buffer mechanisms, which act reflexly to control blood pressure and to maintain circulation. In tissues, however, autoregulation plays a prominent role in regulating blood flow through the capillaries. In capillaries in the systemic circulation, decreased Po_2 or increased Pco_2 produces vasodilatation which slows the blood flow and permits more time for gas exchange to take place. On the other hand, this local hyperemia produces decreased peripheral resistance, and venous return to the heart may be decreased if the local reaction is widespread. Decreased venous return may decrease cardiac output and blood pressure, further decreasing blood flow. At this time nervous buffer mechanisms come into

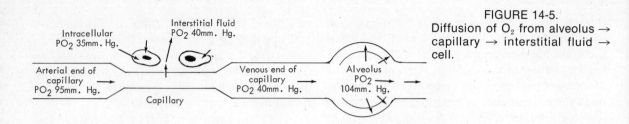

FIGURE 14-5.
Diffusion of O_2 from alveolus → capillary → interstitial fluid → cell.

play. In the pulmonary circulation, decreased P_{O_2} produces vasoconstriction of capillaries and blood is shunted to capillaries in the better-ventilated areas of the lung. In these ways, the tissues make every attempt to utilize the oxygen that is available.

In hemorrhage, shock, impaired venous return, and heart failure, there may be interference with this normal process. Systemic blood pressure decreases because of impaired venous return. If the buffer mechanisms cannot restore the blood pressure, blood flow to tissues is slowed and decreased in volume. The autoregulatory mechanism slows the blood flow even more in order to permit exchange of gases to take place. But with decreased blood volume, the tissues may not receive sufficient oxygen and nutrients to maintain metabolic activities in the cells. Autoregulatory vasodilatation may be a further hindrance, because of the local decrease in peripheral resistance and subsequent decrease in venous return to the heart. The mechanism then becomes one of positive feedback rather than the normal negative feedback system.

UTILIZATION OF OXYGEN AND ELIMINATION OF CARBON DIOXIDE

ABILITY OF THE BLOOD. Oxygen is transported in two forms in the blood. A small amount is dissolved in the plasma and exerts a corresponding partial pressure. However, the major portion of oxygen is transported in loose associa-tion with hemoglobin in the red blood cells. The dissociation of oxygen from the hemoglobin is accelerated by increased P_{CO_2} in the plasma. In the tissue capillaries, the P_{CO_2} increases because carbon dioxide diffuses from the tissues into the blood; oxygen is dissociated from the hemoglobin and diffuses into the tissues. This diffusion is achieved down a pressure gradient.

Figures 14-5 and 14-6 show intracellular interstitial capillary (arterial end and venous end), and alveolar P_{O_2} and P_{CO_2}. The diffusion gradient for P_{CO_2} is much smaller than for P_{O_2}, but carbon dioxide diffusion is not hampered. Carbon dioxide is 20 to 30 times more diffusible than oxygen and can move rapidly down a small gradient. Thus, patients will have a serious problem with oxygen diffusion sooner than with carbon dioxide diffusion.

The oxygen-carrying ability of the cells is affected when the number of red cells is greatly reduced or the hemoglobin concentration is below normal levels. Such a condition is found in carbon monoxide poisoning, in which the combination of carbon monoxide with hemoglobin renders the hemoglobin unavailable for use by oxygen.

Carbon dioxide is an important gas which is formed as the result of cellular metabolism. Large quantities are continually being formed and eliminated by the lungs. Most of the carbon dioxide taken in undergoes chemical transformation into four different forms: 1) dissolved carbon

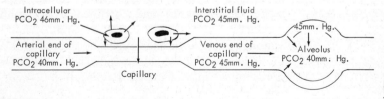

FIGURE 14-6.
Diffsion of Co_2 from cell → interstitial fluid → capillary → alveolus.

dioxide (approximately 10 percent); 2) combined with water to form carbonic acid (approximately 4 percent); 3) dissociation of carbonic acid resulting in bicarbonate and hydrogen ion formation (approximately 60 percent); and 4) carbamino compounds resulting from combination with hemoglobin (approximately 30 percent). Obviously the latter two forms are the most significant.

Although carbon dioxide and oxygen do not combine at the same point on the hemoglobin molecule, they interfere indirectly with one another's combination with hemoglobin. Hemoglobin bound with oxygen combines poorly with carbon dioxide; therefore, the release of oxygen to the tissues increases the carbon dioxide uptake, which is of physiological import. Although hemoglobin bound with carbon dioxide causes less oxygen to be taken up, the influence on oxygen uptake is only slight and, therefore, not significant.

The following reaction of carbon dioxide within the red blood cell happens within 0.1 second, while in the plasma this reaction is only half completed in 10 seconds. The enzyme carbonic anhydrase is abundant within red blood cells and accelerates the reaction.

$$CO_2 + H_2O \longrightarrow H_2CO_3 \longrightarrow HCO_3^- + H^+$$

The rapidly dissociated hydrogen ion combines with the hemoglobin, which is also an acid-base buffer. In the absence of hydrogen ions, the hemoglobin combines with intracellular potassium, but it gives up the potassium for a hydrogen ion when there is an excess of the latter, due to carbonic acid dissociation. As the bicarbonate ion concentration within the red blood cell increases over that in the plasma, bicarbonate ions move out of the cells. To maintain electrical balance, the chloride ion then moves into the red blood cell. Because potassium cannot pass through the cell membrane as rapidly as the bicarbonate ion, the surplus positive charge must be neutralized. To restore osmotic equilibrium between the red cell and plasma, water also moves into the cell. The reverse of this split-second reaction takes place in the pulmonary capillaries and carbon dioxide, under higher tension, moves to the area of lower tension, namely the alveoli.

ABILITY OF THE CELLS. Under normal conditions, approximately 5 ml of oxygen is utilized by the tissues from each 100 ml of blood which passes through the pulmonary capillaries. During increased demands on tissue utilization, such as strenuous exercise, 77 percent of the hemoglobin can give up its oxygen. This is about the highest utilization coefficient that can attained for the overall body when tissues are in extreme need of oxygen. As much as 100 percent has been recorded in local areas where the blood flow is slow and the tissue demands are high.

To determine the total oxygen uptake, one must consider the total cardiac output per minute as well. Normally the cardiac output is 5,000 ml per minute, accounting for a delivery of 250 ml of oxygen to the tissues per minute. This can be increased tenfold by greater tissue utilization and another fivefold as the result of increased cardiac output. Higher levels may be attained, in such situations as athletic training, by increasing the total hemoglobin concentration and achieving maximum cardiac output. However, with an increased hematocrit there is a reduction in the cardiac output, resulting from the increased viscosity of the blood, nullifying the increased oxygen-carrying power of the concentrated blood. The reverse is not true and, therefore, for optimal physiological functioning, the hematocrit needs to remain close to normal level.

Hemoglobin performs a function in maintaining the tissue Po_2. It is able to buffer a decreasing tissue Po_2 by its ability to release additional molecules of oxygen to the tissues, preventing the tissue Po_2 from falling much below 15 mm Hg. It also serves to buffer ambient changes in the Po_2. Partial pressures of atmospheric oxygen varying from 60 to more than 500 mm Hg cause the tissue Po_2 to vary only a few ml from normal. If all the oxygen needed by tissues was carried in the dissolved state in the blood, the oxygen tension would be excessively high and oxygen poisoning would occur. At pressures greater than 100 mm Hg, chemical reactions within cells are accelerated to the point of actual tissue destruction. The central nervous system is particularly

TABLE 14-1

STUDY	NORMAL VALUES	COMMENTS
CAPACITIES		
TLC (Total lung capacity)	Residual volume plus vital capacity. (RV + VC = TLC) Approx.—6L	Diminishes in restrictive disease such as interstitial fibrosis; normal or decreased in obstructive disease.
VC (Vital capacity)	Maximal volume of air exhaled after maximal inspiration. Approx.—4-5L	Decreased in chronic obstructive lung disease and other lung disorders to a lesser extent.
TVC (Timed vital capacity)	Maximal volume of air exhaled after a maximal inspiration per unit of time.	Decreased in chronic obstructive disease.
VOLUMES		
TV (Tidal volume)	Volume of air breathed in and out during quiet respiration. Approx.—350-500 ml	
IRV (Inspiratory reserve volume)	Maximal volume of air which can be inspired after completing a normal tidal inspiration. Approx.—3,000 ml	
ERV (Expiratory reserve volume)	Maximal volume of air which can be expired after a normal tidal expiration. Approx.—1,000 ml	
MVV (Maximum ventilation volume; also known as MBC, maximum breathing capacity)	Greatest volume of air that can be ventilated on command during a given interval.	Reduced in obstructive lung disease and may be in neuromuscular orders. Normal in restrictive disease. Note: The patient is asked to breathe as hard and as fast as possible, usually a 15-second interval.
RV (Residual volume)	Gas remaining in lungs at the end of a forced expiration. Approx.—1.0-1.5 L	
FEV (Forced expiratory volume in 1, 2, 3, seconds) FEV$_1$ FEV$_2$ FEV$_3$	Usually 70-85% of VC 83% 94% 97%	Reduced FEV$_1$ indicates obstructive lung disease. Normal FEV$_1$ in restrictive diseases. Note: The patient inspires as deeply as possible and then exhales as rapidly and completely as he can. The spirometer measures the volume of exhaled air.
MEF (Maximal expiratory flow	Measures total amount of expired air, breathing as rapidly as possible. Approx.—400 L/min.	Reduced in air trapping.
MIF (Maximal inspiratory flow)	Measures total amount of inspired air, breathing as rapidly as possible. Approx.—300 L/min.	

The above set of symbols, abbreviations, and definitions has been agreed upon by the American Pulmonary Physiologists and are commonly used in reporting the results of the studies.

sensitive, but pulmonary membranes are no exception.

A more recent development has been interest in the role of organic phosphates in respiration, long known but little appreciated. The two most significant are 2-3-diphosphoglycerate (2-3 DPG) and adenoisine triphosphate. The former is found in the erythrocyte, is formed as one of the chief end products of glucose metabolism, and is bound to unsaturated hemoglobin. High levels of DPG, such as in states of hypoxia and anemia, expedite oxygen availability to the tissues, with lower levels in the normal state. Further investigation is under way to better understand the role of the organic phosphates.

Pathophysiological conditions may alter the usual effectiveness of these parameters of oxygen and carbon dioxide exchange. Recently, there has been a decided increase in the number of patients having interference in one or more of these parameters. To the professional nurse, the newly developed diagnostic aids and guides to therapy have important implications for nursing care. Table 14-1 lists symbols and definitions commonly used in reporting study results.

DIAGNOSTIC AIDS AND GUIDES IN THERAPY

Pulmonary Function

Pulmonary function studies are an integral part of the diagnosis and management of persons with cardiopulmonary diseases. These studies include gas volumes and capacities, chemical analyses of pulmonary and blood gases, and other biochemistry. Respiratory physiologists encourage greater use of simple screening devices in mass screening centers and in physicians' offices. Selected patients are referred to hospital cardiopulmonary and research laboratories for more definitive studies. The nurse may either assist with or do some of these studies in mass screening centers, physicians' officies, or hospitals. However, laboratory personnel are usually available in hospitals.

These studies require the cooperation of the patient to the best of his ability. The nurse must be aware of the patient's fear or anxiety because of a simple lack of knowledge about what is to be done and why it is necessary. A simple explanation of the purpose of the test, the patient's role during the procedure, and what is happening, may do much to allay apprehension. The apparatus in the cardiopulmonary laboratory is often formidable in appearance and frightening. Many patients ask, "How am I going to be able to breathe?" "I'm not used to breathing through my mouth." "Do I have to use the clip on my nose?" At times explanations must be repeated numerous times, because the high level of anxiety may cause loss of memory in the more hypoxic patient.

Arterial Blood Gases, Oxygen Saturation, and pH Measurements

BLOOD GASES, pH, HCO_3^- AND BASE EXCESS MEASUREMENTS. These studies are important in treatment and diagnosis. They reflect ventilatory sufficiency, ability of hemoglobin to carry oxygen and carbon dioxide, rate of cellular metabolism and the status of the buffer system. Blood samples may be obtained from arteries, or a central venous catheter located in the vena cava, right atrium or ventricle, and the pulmonary artery (mixed venous blood) or "capillary stick" of an extremity.

Table 14-2 shows normal blood values, and these parameters seem to provide adequate information for intervention and evaluation. Nurses in intensive care situations should acquire the knowledge, understanding, and technical expertise to obtain these blood samples as indicated by the client's status.

The conscious client is often upset by the

TABLE 14-2
Normal Blood Values

	ARTERIAL	MIXED VENOUS
P_{CO_2}	35-45 mm Hg	41-51 mm Hg
P_{O_2}	80-100 mm Hg	35-40 mm Hg
pH	7.35-7.45	7.31-7.41
O_2 saturation	96-98%	70-75%
HCO_3^-	22-26 mEq/L	22-26 mEq/L
Base excess	− 2 to + 2	− 2 to + 2

need for frequent sampling and must be reassured. Knowledge, understanding, and proficiency in the skill is vital; this procedure is not to be carried out on a trial-and-error basis.

Small blood gas analyzers are available for use in intensive care settings. Careful selection should be based upon accuracy, speed, simplicity, and durability. Personnel utilizing the equipment should thoroughly understand how the equipment functions to provide reliable data.

Assessment[14,15,16,17]

Since the maintenance of a homeostatic blood and tissue level of oxygen, carbon dioxide, pH, and various electrolytes has the highest priority among the basic needs for survival, recognition of the client's status with respect to these parameters becomes an important nursing intervention. The approach to the assessment process is contingent on the status of the client when first encountered in the health care system. This naturally will range from absence of or vague subjective symptoms on one end of the health-illness continuum to apnea such as results from cardiopulmonary arrest. Therefore, for the purpose of discussion, the family profile will be followed by the client respiratory profile and, lastly, the physical assessment of the thorax and lungs.

The family profile obtained through the nursing interview is a most valuable tool, particularly for clients with a long-term illness. It is also an ongoing process which can be utilized to include additional information, status of existing problems with action taken and results, and identification of new problems. This provides for individual-family, goal-directed care, with planning, implementation, and evaluation of the care process.

FAMILY PROFILE

Name of client: _____

Individuals present at time of interview and their relationship to the client: _____

_____

_____

Health problem which caused client-family to seek assistance (description of problem and its history by client and contributions of others present at interview):

_____

_____

_____

What things have been done by client and others before seeking assistance? _____

_____

Systems review (identify cues for later validation): _____

_____

_____

_____

Occupation: _____

Level of education: _____

Economic status: _____

Family structure (include kinship and present structure):

_____

_____

Roles of immediate family structure: _____

_____

Decision-making patterns: _____

_____

Attitudes toward health and illness: _____

_____

Positive factors in the family constellation:_____

_____

Problem areas: _____

_____

Progress notes (include status of problem and identify other problems occurring throughout contact): _____

_____

_____

_____

Client Respiratory Profile

A more detailed individual respiratory profile may be helpful in gathering data regarding the present crisis and the progress in the hospitalized client. Nursing personnel may want to extract or elaborate on portions of this profile to develop a checklist appropriate to the health care setting. It may have potential in computer data collection and retrieval in the future.

Name_____Age_____

Sex_____Height_____Weight_____

Temperature: _____

Respirations:

Neck

Trachea in midline_____

Neck veins_____

Rate _____

Interval (inspiration vs. expiration) _____

Degree of chest expansion—Barrel chest _____

Muscular contraction:
  Diaphragmatic _____
  Abdominal _____
  Use of accessory muscles _____
  Rib retraction _____
Breathing:
  Mouth _____
  Nasal _____
Quality:
  Eupnea _____
  Bradypnea _____
  Tachypnea _____
  Dyspnea _____
    Bed rest _____
    Sitting in chair _____
    Movement about room _____
    Free movement _____
  Orthopnea _____
  Biot _____
  Cheyne-Stokes _____
  Apnea _____
  Kussmaul's _____
  Pursed lip breathing _____
Cough:
  Persistent _____
  Chronic _____
  Hacking _____
  Feeble _____
  Productive _____
  Nonproductive _____
  Activities inducing cough _____
  Time of day increased or decreased _____

Sputum
  Absent _____
  Present _____
  Color
    Clear _____
    Yellow _____
    Green _____
    Hemoptysis _____
  Consistency
    Thin _____
    Thick _____
  Amount
    Small _____
    Moderate _____
    Copious _____
  Odor
    None _____
    Foul _____
Circulation:
  Pulse _____
  Blood pressure _____
Skin:
  Color
    Normal _____
    Flushed _____
    Cyanotic _____
  Temperature
    Red and warm _____
    Warm and pale _____
    Cold and clammy _____

Nailbeds:
  Normal _____
  Cyanotic _____
Clubbing of fingers:
  Absent _____
  Present _____
Neurological:
  Level of consciousness
    Alert and awake _____
    Oriented to time, place, and person _____
    Restless _____
    Sleeplike state _____
    Responds to verbal stimuli _____
    Responds to painful stimuli purposefully _____
    Responds to pain in nonpurposeful manner _____
    No response, no gag or cough reflex _____
    Size, shape, and equality of pupils _____
  Reflexes
    Corneal _____
    Gag _____
    Joint _____
  Impaired judgment _____
  Psychological disturbances _____
  Neuromuscular irritability, weakness, ataxia _____
Kidneys:
  Anuria _____
  Oliguria _____
    Amount per hour _____
Tenderness: _____
Scars: _____
Deformities of the spine:
  Kyphosis _____
  Scoliosis _____
Medications:
  Cough _____
  Mucolytic agents _____
  Bronchodilators _____
  Antibiotics _____
  Antituberculosis _____
Respiratory aids:
  Endotracheal tube (cuffed type) _____
    No. of cc _____ Deflation schedule _____
  Tracheotomy
    Regular _____ Cuffed type _____
    No. of cc _____ Deflation schedule _____
  Oxygen L/min. and % O_2
  Nasal catheter _____
  Nasal cannula _____
  Mask (%) _____
Ventilator:
  Assisted _____
    Type _____
    Settings _____
  Controlled _____
    Type _____
    Settings _____
  T-Tube _____
Pulmonary function tests:
  FEV_1 _____
  Tidal volume _____
  Others _____
  FIo_2 _____

Laboratory tests:
  Arterial blood gases
    Pao_2 _____
    $Paco_2$ _____
    pH _____
    % O_2 saturation _____
  Hemoglobin _____
  Hematocrit _____
  Standard bicarbonate _____
  Base excess _____
Electrolytes:
  Sodium _____
  Potassium _____
  Chloride _____
Red blood cell count: _____
Sedimentation rate: _____
White blood cell count: _____
  Neutrophils _____
  Eosinophils _____
  Basophils _____
  Lymphocytes _____
  Monocytes _____
Serum enzymes:
  SGOT _____
  LDH _____
  CPK _____
Skin tests:
  PPD _____
  Histoplasmin, blastomycin, coccidoidin
Sputum analysis: _____
Nose and throat culture: _____
Direct visualization procedures (i.e., bronchoscopy, biopsy, fibroscopy): _____

Radioactive studies (i.e., lung scientography): _____

PHYSICAL ASSESSMENT

The client's welfare has been greatly enhanced by the professional nurse's ability to carry out a systematic bedside assessment through the use of palpation, percussion, and auscultation. (See Chapter 4 for a discussion of assessment techniques in respiratory and other body systems.)

Palpation involves evaluation for areas of tenderness, masses, scars, crepitus, and deformities of the spine. It also includes evaluation of vibratory sensations of the chest wall. Vocal fremitus utilizes the voice as a medium for setting up these vibrations in the bronchial tree which are felt by the hands of the nurse. The client is asked to say, "ninety-nine," "one, two, three," or "ee-ee," comparing the vibrations felt on either side of the chest wall. Palpation tends to identify gross changes. Vocal fremitus may be increased, decreased, or absent, or altered due to

the intensity and pitch of the voice, thickness of the chest wall, and area assessed. It is more pronounced in the parasternal region in the right second interspace and in the interscapular area because of the bifurcation of the bronchi directly beneath these areas. Increased vocal fremitus occurs in consolidation of the lung around the bronchial tree. Decreased fremitus may occur in blockage of airways and when fluid or air is located in the pleural space. The nurse will find the palmar surfaces or tips of the fingers most sensitive to these vibrations. Crepitus is a crackling sensation which may be felt over areas which have been infiltrated with air (subcutaneous emphysema).

Percussion is a sound produced by striking the distal interphalangeal joint of the middle finger as it is placed in a palmar position on various areas of the chest wall. Much practice is necessary in utilizing this method of physical assessment since the vibrations elicited are described in acoustical terms such as resonance, tympany, dullness, and flatness. For example, the sounds from an air-filled lung are described as resonant; gastric air bubbles are called tympany; the sounds heard over the cardiac area are described as a dull thud; and the extreme of dullness is called flatness. Nurses beginning to develop this skill will do well to practice percussing a variety of surfaces as a means of training the ear to sound changes. It must be remembered that only the middle finger should touch the surface. The nurse's fingernails should be short to avoid discomfort in the striking process. The striking finger should be flexed and rigid with no movement of the shoulder or elbow. With the wrist relaxed, two or three staccato strikes will be adequate before moving to another area.

In auscultation of the chest a stethoscope is used to listen to the vibrations created by the movement of a bronchotracheal air column throughout the entire respiratory tract. It is one way of determining the adequacy of ventilation. The nurse's selection of a quality stethoscope for this purpose, and practice in listening to normal, as well as abnormal, breathing sounds will often determine the nurse's effectiveness in utilizing this method of physical assessment. Continuous use and development of expertise is critical and the availability of a knowledgeable mentor for collaboration and validation is imperative. A stethoscope with two types of chestpieces is indispensible, each receiving a different range of sound. The bellpiece transmits all sounds from the chest, but the low-pitched sounds come through particularly well.The diaphragm serves as a filter to exclude low-pitched sounds, therefore amplifying the isolated high-pitched sounds. The diaphragm should be pressed tightly against the chest wall in contrast to the rim of the bell which should touch the chest wall lightly. The entire rim of the bell must touch the skin; otherwise, a roaring sound from extraneous noise will indicate a leak.

Effective auscultation of the chest depends upon communicating to the client the way in which you want him to breathe, that is, through the mouth or more deeply and forcefully than normal. The nurse begins listening at the lung apices anteriorly and works downward, comparing symmetric points, followed by the same procedure on the posterior and midaxillary wall of the thorax. At all points on the chest, breath sounds should be identified.

The quality of breath sounds varies from region to region, even in normal individuals, depending upon the proximity of the larger bronchi to the chest wall. Several types of breath sounds produce distinctive qualities. All are characterized by a rising pitch during inspiration, and a falling pitch during expiration. The distinguishing feature of the various breath sounds is the duration of the two phases of respiration. The longer the phase, the louder the sound in that phase.

The breath sounds heard during quiet respiration produce a whishing noise that can be heard over the entire lung surface except beneath the manubrium sternum and in the upper interscapular region. They are called vesicular breath sounds, have a longer inspiratory phase and a shorter expiratory phase, and are considered normal vesicular breathing.

Bronchovesicular breathing is characterized by the equality of the respiratory phases, although expiration is frequently a bit longer. Normally it is heard at the manubrium sternum and in the upper interscapular region. Bronchovesicular breathing is pathological if located in other parts of the lung and indicative of a small degree of pulmonary consolidation or compression that transmits sounds from the bronchial tree with greater facility.

Bronchial breathing does not occur in the normal lung. When present, it indicates pathology and results from consolidation or compression of pulmonary tissue that facilitates transmission of sound from the bronchial tree. Bronchial breath sounds have a short inspiratory phase; and a long expiratory phase.

Table 14-3 lists normal and abnormal breath sounds.

Sounds in the lungs that are not modifications of breath or voice are called adventitious sounds. They are not normally heard over the chest and have a variety of origins. Table 14-4 utilizes the pulmonary nomenclature of ACCP-ATS Joint Committee on Pulmonary Nomenclature to simplify the understanding of the adventitious sounds. In listening to these sounds, the nurse must remember to listen to a number of respiratory cycles. When rales or rhonchi are present, listening to determine in what portion of the respiratory cycle they occur is significant.

It is vitally important for the nurse to frequently assess the adequacy of ventilation. The nurse plays an important role in maintaining a patent airway, free of obstructing secretions. Evaluation, through utilizing the techniques of assessment, will provide this information which is a determining factor in the caring process.

Loss of lubricating fluid resulting from inflammation of the pleura, with the opposing pleural surfaces rubbing together, produces a sound similar to that made when rubbing two dry pieces of leather together. The sound may be emulated by firmly rubbing the thumb against the forefinger near the ear.

The client profile and physical assessment has identified other problems not necessarily noted in the family profile. Still others may have been validated through this process. The following section will focus on some of the common problems and salient interventions to assist the clients to cope with their illness.

TABLE 14-3
Breath Sounds

NORMAL	ABNORMAL	ABNORMAL	
		CAUSES	PATHOLOGICAL PROCESS
—	Absence	Massive obesity, complete obstruction of larynx, trachea or bronchi (due to foreign body, excessive bronchial secretions, bronchial tumor, edema, or laryngeal spasm), malposition of endotracheal tube, pneumonectomy, paralyzed diaphragm, severe pulmonary fibrosis, pleural effusion, pneumothorax, atelectasis.	Loss of ventilating lung.
Bronchovesicular (heard over manubrium and interscapular area)	Other than normal areas	Atelectasis, solid without complete obstruction, pneumonia, pulmonary infarction, compression of alveoli resulting from pleural effusion, acute respiratory distress syndrome.	Degree of pulmonary consolidation or compression.
Vesicular (heard over most of chest except where trachea and bronchi are near the surface)	—	—	—
Not occurring in normal lung	Bronchial	Atelectasis, solid without complete obstruction, pneumonia, pulmonary infarction, compression of alveoli resulting from pleural effusion, acute respiratory distress syndrome.	Alveoli filled with fluid, collapsed or replaced by solid mass.
—	Asthmatic	Bronchial asthma.	Result of obstructed airways requiring more time for expiration to be completed.

Client Problems and Nursing Intervention

HYPOXIA

Hypoxia is the ultimate problem involved in interferences with the various parameters of the breathing process. It simply means an inadequate supply of oxygen to the tissue cells. Figure 14-7 provides an analysis of the effects of hypoxia on all body systems. It may appear in varying degrees, from an acute insufficiency to a slowly developing state (see Fig. 14-7, p. 430).

Inadequate ventilation resulting from the lack of a patent airway is one of the most common client problems encountered by the health care team. Mr. B. is an example of the many clients seen in the emergency room in an episodic respi-

TABLE 14-4
Adventitious Sounds

The American College of Chest Physicians-American Thoracic Society Committee on Pulmonary Nomenclature have sought to simplify and clarify the terms utilized in describing the adventitious breath sounds. They have suggested the following:

Rale: Crackling or bubbling (discontinuous) sounds or vibrations, crackles.

Rhonchus: Musical (continuous) sound or vibration, usually of longer duration; wheezes: May vary in pitch, quality, and intensity.

Other adventitious sounds or vibrations:

Mediastinal crunch: A course crackling sound or vibration synchronous with systole, heard over the precordium in the presence of mediastinal emphysema.

Plural rub: A grating sound or vibration associated with breathing and unaffected by cough.

Pericardial rub: A regular to and fro grating sound or vibration associated with the heartbeat which persists in the absence of breathing and is affected by cough.

Pleurapericardial rub: A sound or vibration with some features of both pleural and pericardial rub.

A Report of ACCP-ATS Joint Committee on Pulmonary Nomenclature. Chest 67, 5:586, May 1975.

ratory crisis. He gave a long history of smoking, alcoholism, arrested tuberculosis, upper respiratory infections, pulmonary emphysema and cor pulmonale. It was not until dyspnea became apparent, in carrying out simple activities of daily living, that Mr. B. sought medical attention. His major problem when first seen was thick tenacious tracheobronchial secretions resulting from a superimposed respiratory infection. The efforts of the health care team concentrated on providing respiratory support until the secretions became liquified and more compatible with Mr. B.'s self-cleansing excretory process. It was hypothesized that many cilia of the columnar epithelium lining of the respiratory tract had been destroyed. There was hyperplasia of the goblet cells resulting in an increase in the usual amount (100 cc per 24 hrs.) of mucus produced, secondary destruction of many alveolar septa,

and the presence of mucous plugs obstructing the gas flow to the existing diffusing surfaces. This assumption was validated by the $Paco_2$ of 65 mm Hg, Pao_2 of 31 mm Hg, and a pH of 7.34. Auscultation detected expiratory wheeze, rhonchi, and diminished breath sounds. The nurse's role was to assist Mr. B. in achieving and maintaining an adequate fluid intake. Mr. B.'s preoccupation with breathing, decreased ventilatory sufficiency, and age provided a real challenge to the nursing care team. A schedule was worked out by the nursing care team by which adequate fluid intake could be achieved during the daytime hours, providing more rest, relaxation, and sleep during the night. The plan provided smaller, more frequent non-gas-forming feedings, thus reducing the pressure on the diaphragm and facilitating chest expansion. It was to his advantage that Mr. B. enjoyed any type of liquids at room temperature, since iced drinks may cause reflex bronchospasm. An accurate intake and output was necessary for assessing the effectiveness of the plan, as was the degree of urinary concentration indicated by the specific gravity.

Humidification of the room air contributed to the liquification of Mr. B.'s secretions. Atmospheric air is totally humidified before it reaches the alveoli, either by water vapor in the inspired air or by the fluid present in the respiratory passage. How this could be accomplished for Mr. B. without creating fear or increased anxiety was the problem. Commercial humidifiers, vaporizers, ultrasonic nebulizers and temperature-humidity controlled rooms are available in most hospital settings. Although it is not the most effective means of providing higher levels of humidity, in this instance a steam inhalator was placed at Mr. B.'s bedside. Whatever method is used, an attempt is made to provide additional moisture in the inspired air at a comfortable temperature, with the water particles being small enough to reach the lower respiratory passages. The nurse discussed the use of the inhalator with Mr. B.'s wife and described how it could be applied in the home situation.

Mr. B. had found that the Fowler's or semi-Fowler's position provided him the greatest degree of chest expansion. The nursing care team,

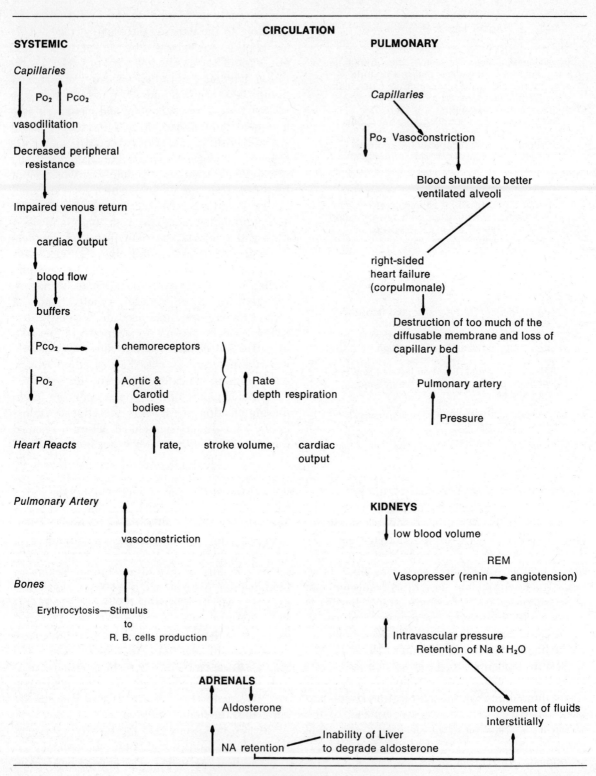

FIGURE 14-7.
The effects of hypoxia on the various body systems.

however, worked diligently to see that he was turned from side to side, altering the thrust of the upper chest from a semiprone and semisupine position, to facilitate the gravitational drainage of mucus from the various segments of the lung. Chest clapping, vibration, percussion, and postural drainage have been utilized effectively in some care regimens. Although bed rest makes less demands for oxygen, activity is more valuable in ventilatory and circulatory improvement. Judicious use of oxygen can often be helpful in supporting the client in such situations.

Effective coughing is vitally important for the expulsion of the accumulated mucus. To begin the laborious task of helping the client remove the night's accumulation, the nurse needs to provide a great deal of encouragement. A deep breath immediately preceding the coughing efforts not only improves ventilation, but also provides a greater volume of air for forward propulsion of the mucus during expiration. A cough is usually a reflex action resulting from some form of stimulation to the sensitive epithelium of the larynx, trachea, or bronchi. Coordinated neuronal activites result in: 1) movement of a column of air into the airway passage; 2) closure of the epiglottis and vocal chords; 3) buildup of pressure in the lungs followed by 4) the sudden opening of the vocal chords and epiglottis with expulsion of air at high velocity.

Expectorants, such as guaiacolate and potassium iodide, have been used for many years to assist in the liquifying process. However, there is some controversy among physicians as to their value because mild toxicity from the iodides is not uncommon.

Retained tenacious secretions, which may be aggravated by bronchospasm and/or edema of the bronchial wall, frequently result in inadequate or unequal ventilation of the alveoli. Intermittent positive pressure breathing (IPPB) is a popular form of treatment used to improve ventilation, reduce the physiological dead space, and move secretions up the tracheobronchial tree. Intelligent nursing care for Mr. B. and for others with problems of retained tenacious secretions (e.g., following cardiac surgery, neurosurgery, stroke, pulmonary surgery, or high abdominal surgery) demands the understanding of the principles of IPPB and skill in the use of the equipment. This understanding is reflected in remarks to clients such as, "It will make it easier for you to get air in and out of your lungs—it will help you do a more effective job of breathing." Through the nurse's skillful handling of the equipment, the patient's anxieties can be markedly decreased and can even be replaced by feelings of confidence and security.

IPPB machines have been designed either to augment the patient's inspiratory effort (assisted ventilation) or to assume complete control (controlled ventilation) of his ventilation. The machines provide air or oxygen-enriched air, at increased pressure to the tracheobronchial tree during inspiration, with expiration occurring automatically by release of the pressure. Assisted ventilators are triggered by the inspiratory efforts of the client and produce a flow of gas resulting in a greater tidal volume than can be achieved by the client himself. Controlled ventilation is utilized in the absence of respiratory efforts, or in other instances when the physician judges such control to be important.

Artificial Ventilatory System

There are two types of machines in use: volume-preset and pressure-preset ventilators. The former delivers a specific volume of air to the lungs, irrespective of lung compliance or resistance, and is considered a volume-control and pressure-variable apparatus (Bennett MA-1, Engström, Emerson, Ohio, Airshields, and Morch models are available). The pressure-preset ventilators are spoken of as pressure-limited and volume-variable. This means that when a certain pressure is reached, the machine cycles off no matter how much air is delivered. With increased compliance, a large volume of air is delivered, although the apparatus has been set at 20 cm H_2O pressure which delivers 500 ml in a normally compliant lung. It is important to recognize that the tidal volume may change when utilizing the pressure-preset ventilator. (Pressure-preset machines include most of the Bird, Bennett, and Mine Safety models.)

IPPB is frequently given periodically rather

than continuously. The treatment is usually done three or four times a day for 15 to 20 minute intervals, utilizing pressures of 10 to 20 cm H_2O. Inhalation therapists are often available to supervise this treatment, but in many situations the nurse is responsible. The success of the treatment usually depends on the manner in which it is introduced to the client. Opportunities should be provided for the client to ask questions, handle the equipment, and participate as much as possible in assembling and disassembling the apparatus. This serves two functions: it gives the individual a sense of control, and it provides a teaching modality for those who must continue the treatments at home. Individual differences such as motivation, ability to learn, and the client's pathophysiological condition have a bearing upon what the nurse can expect from each client. For example, Mrs. C., a middle-aged schoolteacher, admitted for an elective cholecystectomy, mastered the skill in a few days, while Mr. W., who suffered from a slowly progressive state of hypoxia, continued to need a great deal of assistance with each treatment. (The nurse must fully appreciate the effect of chronic hypoxia on the brain cells. Nursing care personnel have sometimes thoughtlessly and superficially classified these patients as "uncooperative, senile, and ungrateful.")

The nurse should ask the patient to practice breathing through the mouthpiece before attaching it to the machine. Breathing through the mouth may be accomplished more easily if the individual has been instructed to say "Ah" while at the same time closing off the nasal airway with his hand or a nose clip.

While the client is practicing, the nurse prepares the proper solution and/or medication that must be an adjunct to any artificial ventilatory system. This may include use of normal saline, detergents, mucolytic agents, proteolytic enzymes, and bronchodilators. Mucolytic agents such as acetylcysteine (Mucomyst) have a rapid onset and may be administered in aerosol form or as instillation into the tracheobronchial tree. The nurse should be aware of the disagreeable odor of these agents, their corrosive effect on both rubber and metal, and their incompatability with certain antibiotics. Proteolytic enzymes, for example, pancreatic dornase (Dornavac) or pancreatic trypsin (Tryptan), are reserved for use when mucus is purulent and fibrinous, since they do not affect the mucus itself. Bronchodilators such as isoproterenol (Isuprel) may be used effectively in the presence of bronchospasm. The nurse must recognize that these drugs are also cardiac and central nervous system stimulants and should be given in diluted form.

Whatever the aerosol used, the amount of medication or solution must last for the entire treatment. It must be synchronized with the length of treatment time. If this is not possible, the nurse, in collaboration with the physician, may add additional normal saline. Heated solutions may also be used in some instances to increase the humidity content. Nebulization should produce a spray of small particles which tend to precipitate farther down the bronchial tree.

Lower pressures are tolerated best upon initiation of the first treatment. Pressure settings of 10 to 12 cm of H_2O may be maintained until the client has adjusted to the treatment, and then it can be successfully increased to the desired setting by small increments. Sensitivity settings are determined by the quality of the client's inspiratory effort, while the rate of flow regulates the speed at which the gas is delivered. Clients should be encouraged to breathe slowly and to allow time for the flow of air into their lungs. This will result in hyperventilation of the alveoli that have good communication with the airway and good compliance. Areas having poor compliance but good communication need the increased pressure to fill. Alveoli with imperfect communication, due to obstruction, fill after the others are ventilated. When problems occur with both communication and compliance, higher pressures and lower flow rates must pertain before these alveoli will ventilate. The hyperventilation occurring in the more expandable areas contributes to a more expanded bronchial lumen, which opens still other airways to alveoli. As the result of better ventilation, a greater volume of air moves out of the alveoli on expiration, contributing to the movement of secretions up the tracheobronchial tree. The pause after inspiration allows additional time for better distribution of the gases, and also makes it possible for aerosol particles to precipitate in the lower tracheobronchial tree. A postexpiratory pause should be encouraged to permit adequate right atrial filling and cardiac output.

Clients on long-term treatment must be encouraged to maintain a ratio of 1:2 (inspiration, expiration, and rest) inspiration to expiration. Incisional pain in the chest and abdomen of the postoperative client often results in an unwillingness to allow the chest to expand adequately during the inspiratory phase. The nurse's skillful timing of the prescribed analgesic prior to treatment will enhance the value of this therapeutic modality.

It is important that the nurse make an assessment of the client's respiratory status, apical pulse and blood pressure before, during, and after treatment. This evaluation is particularly significant because of the need to assess the effectiveness of the therapy and to be alert for potential untoward effects.

The nurse is responsible for providing a safe and healthy environment, most imperative for the hypoxia client. This begins with proper handwashing to prevent the spread of microorganisms to a very high-risk group of clients. Reinarz, et al recommend daily sterilization of the ventilatory apparatus, and it has been found that restricting particular equipment to one client is a satisfactory means of reducing the chance of contamination.[18] Most observers attribute superimposed infections to bacterial growth in the humidifying or nebulizing reservoir.

Monitoring the effectiveness of the cleaning method should be encouraged, particularly with respect to the hard-to-eradicate Pseudomonas species and other gram-negative rods. Sanford suggests that proper handwashing is by far the most effective means of controlling iatrogenic infections.[19] He suggests a one-a-week monitoring of the equipment to determine the effectiveness of the sterilizing method. Sanford and Bendixen refer to the little understood mechanism of the unusual vulnerability of the critically ill individual to iatrogenic infections.[20]

DYSPNEA

Dyspnea is another common problem. No definition seems to adequately tell the story; however, it is agreed that it is a conscious or unconscious increase in the work of breathing. The underlying cause of dyspnea varies as to the cardiopulmonary status, the pathophysiological disease involved, and the patient's interpretation of it. The significance of the symptom is important to the physician, and, therefore, important for the nurse to observe, report accurately, and assist in alleviating.

The necessity for air is manifested by the patient's often unrelenting struggle and preoccupation with breathing. Perception of the patient's needs tends to dilute the anxiety, apprehension, and fear which prevail in the presence of dyspnea. Talking or responding to questions is very irritating to the patient and makes additional demands upon him. The nurse should work calmly and efficiently in carrying out the measures which provide the greatest relief. It is helpful when the nurse gives clear, simple explanations of the techniques and procedures being carried out. Family members are also comforted by the nurse's presence. Their emotional reactions, as well as those of the patient, must be understood and considered in the total plan of care.

Dyspneic patients are often more comfortable in an upright position, although this may depend upon the patient's body fluid. Some find sitting in a firm, comfortable chair satisfying. Patients often find leaning forward on a pillow on the overbed table a welcome relief for short periods. These positions may provide comfort by increasing the size of the thoracic cavity. The abdominal contents cause less compression of the diaphragm during inspiration; however, expiratory flow can be facilitated by a forward movement of the body as the result of the opposite effect.

Dyspnea caused by the chronic obstructive diseases (i.e., bronchial asthma, pulmonary fibrosis and emphysema) may sometimes be alleviated through initiation of more adequate breathing patterns. Studies have been done to determine the effectiveness of breath training, with varying results. However, exercise programs carried out over a period of time seem to result in subjective improvement-responses by patients. Miller purports that the aim of breath training is to assist the patient to breathe with minimal effort and with maximum efficiency at any given level of physical activity. He stresses slow and relaxed controlled breathing at all times.[21] Inspiration should occur through the nasal passage to allow for the moistening, filtering, and warming effect of the inspired air. Expiration through the mouth, by placing the teeth together and producing a hissing sound, allows the person to monitor the length of the expiratory effort. This method reduces the pressure gradient in the airway and acts as an inhibitory factor to airway collapse.

Oxygen Therapy

Dyspnea may be relieved by the addition of oxygen to the inspired air. The value of oxygen therapy to a patient depends upon the underlying cause of the dyspnea. However, as Meltzer, et al., indicated, an adequate arterial oxygenation is essential, particularly to the brain and myocardium, and prevents the compensatory response to hypoxia from occurring.[22]

Oxygen therapy is probably one of the most common methods of treatment instituted by members of the health care team. "It requires just as much understanding and precision in dosage as any other form of drug therapy" and unfortunately is sometimes given in a haphazard fashion.[23] It should never be discontinued without collaboration with the physician, even though on low liter flow per minute. Sudden discontinuation of oxygen may be catastrophic to the cardiovascular system due to the sudden drop in arterial saturation. Through addition of oxygen to the inspired air, the percentage of oxygen can be increased from 30 to 100, although the latter percentage is used infrequently and then only for short periods. The nasal catheter, cannula, mask, tent, and ventilators are all familiar methods of administration. The nurse finds that patients can usually accept the nasal catheter and cannula most easily. These methods allow for greater freedom of movement, do not seem to interfere with eating or talking, and are less expensive than other routes of administration.

The nurse should insure the proper placement of the nasal catheter (catheter tip below the soft palate and just above the uvula) to avoid undue drying and gastric distention. Catheters should be removed and cleaned and reinserted into the opposite nostril every six to eight hours. Cleaning of the nares is important in removing the secretions, maintaining a patent airway, and reducing irritation. The nurse will administer frequent mouth care to alleviate the drying effect, remove secretions, and prevent superimposed infections. Taping the catheter securely to the tip of the nose, bringing it across the zygometic arch, and then attaching it to the patient's gown keeps the catheter out of the patient's direct view and causes less irritation to the nares. Perspiration and skin oils may cause the tape to loosen; therefore, it must be checked frequently.

Plastic oronasal masks have been utilized in the care of some patients; however, it is difficult to provide both a comfortable and a tight-fitting mask to fit the various facial contours. The nurse will find the mask a quick way of supplying oxygen, and concentrations up to 100 percent can be achieved, depending upon the type of mask. Masks should be removed every one or two hours to prevent skin irritation.

Plastic hoods and oxygen tents may be used to provide high-humidity environments. The nurse will find it difficult to maintain the desired concentration of oxygen in a tent even at flow rates of 10 to 12 L, because oxygen is heavier than air and is readily diffused whenever the tent is opened.

Oxygen may also be given through an endotracheal tube, a tracheostomy, or a cuffed tracheostomy, utilizing a positive pressure apparatus. Whatever method is used, humidification of inspired gases is essential, because gases tend to be extremely dry. For example, compressed air usually has a humidity of 4 percent at normal ambient pressure.

The nurse, in collaboration with the physician, may be responsible for adjusting the oxygen concentration depending upon the patient's Pa_{O_2}, O_2 saturation, FI_{O_2}, and Pa_{CO_2}. In the presence of hypercapnia, both physician and nurse must work closely to provide the patient with supplemental oxygen for the tissue cells and, at the same time, improve the ventilatory status. Carbon dioxide, being a potent stimulant of the respiratory center in the medulla, exerts the major chemical control of alveolar ventilation. However, if the Pa_{CO_2} increases beyond certain limits, it begins to depress rather than to excite the respiratory center. The respiratory drive may then depend upon the lowered Pa_{O_2} stimulus of the chemoreceptors located in the carotid and aortic bodies. As a result, respiratory arrest may follow the removal of this hypoxic effect if supplemental oxygen is administered injudiciously in the presence of hypercapnia.

The nurse should be constantly alert for clues which might suggest carbon dioxide retention—headache, dizziness, muscle twitching, progressive decrease in consciousness, or convulsions. Deep coma and death follow if the situation is not corrected.

The retention of carbon dioxide may result in a compensated or uncompensated respiratory acidosis. The nurse can sometimes assist the patient to achieve more effective breathing patterns, as described earlier, to facilitate the elimination of the carbon dioxide. However, more drastic measures may need to be taken (such as endotracheal intubation and aspiration, bedside bronchoscopy, tracheostomy, and use of the mechanical ventilator) to achieve a patent airway and provide adequate alveolar ventilation. The nurse should have Ringer's lactate, an electrolyte solution, available as a buffering agent and a means of providing hydration to liquify the secretions. Sodium bicarbonate may also be given intravenously.

Careful monitoring of the ventilatory status of the patient is another vital function of the nurse. The assessment guide is helpful in evaluating the respiratory and cardiac status. Too rapid a conversion of the hypoxia has resulted in ventricular fibrillation and death.

Endotracheal intubation may not be suitable for the conscious patient and the nurse assists the physician in performing a tracheostomy. The cuffed tracheostomy procedure is advantageous because it allows for easier removal of tenacious secretions, reduces the dead air space and provides for effective use of the assisted or controlled ventilators. Although the patient seems preoccupied with each breath, the nurse needs to explain in simple, concise terms the purpose of the tracheotomy and how it will be accomplished. Reassurance and constant vigilance by the nurse are of utmost importance, particularly in the first hours following the procedure. A major fear of patients is being unable to remove the mucus or make their needs known.

One of the care objectives for the tracheostomized patient is the maintenance of a patent airway. This involves endotracheal aspiration as necessary. The catheter should be approximately half the size of the tube to prevent irritation or trauma to the walls of the air passages, but it must also be large enough for secretions to enter into the catheter. It is introduced to the desired level, approximately 10 to 50 ml of normal saline instilled, and suction is applied as the catheter is gently rotated to facilitate aspiration. Suction should be applied for approximately five to ten seconds, then released. When possible, a three-minute lapse of time between suctioning is a good practice. It must be remembered that air as well as mucus is being aspirated during the suctioning procedure, and oxygen may be indicated prior to and after the procedure.

The results of numerous studies have provided conclusive evidence supporting the use of sterile technique with tracheal aspiration. This involves the use of a sterile catheter for suctioning and sterile gloves worn by the nurse in handling the catheter. Having the conscious patient cough or auscultating with a stethoscope will assist the nurse in determining the effectiveness of the suctioning.

The cuffed tracheostomy tube is advantageous in that it provides a closed system and contributes to better ventilation with the positive pressure ventilators. Approximately 7 to 10 ml of air is used to inflate the balloon. The nurse should plan the schedule of balloon deflation with the physician to prevent tracheal edema and necrosis. (Double-cuffed and low-pressure tubes are available which reduce the chance of this complication.) Tracheal aspiration should be carried out prior to deflation of the cuff to remove the secretions above the cuff. The deflation should be done slowly to allow the secretions to be forced upward by the positive pressure. The small test balloon on the distal end of the tubing remains inflated as long as the cuff is inflated.

Inflation of the cuff is also done slowly and with just enough air to produce a leak-free system. This may be determined by the production of aphonia in the conscious patient or absence of air flow from the nose, mouth, and around the tracheal tube when the tube is temporarily occluded. Rodman and Sterling recommend temporarily increasing the pressure or flow of the ventilator to accentuate the air leakage as the cuff is slowly inflated;[24] a self-inflating bag may be utilized for the same purpose. (Using the latter technique, one person listens with a stethoscope placed just below the patient's chin [submental region] and determines the point at which no leak, or better still an inconsequential leakage, is heard.) Since the inflation volume is reproducible, the nurse records the amount of air used in proper inflation of the cuff. Disposable plastic tracheostomy tubes which contain two adjacent built-in inflatable cuffs have eliminated the danger of herniation of the cuff downward over the distal end of the tracheal tube; these tubes have been left in place for two to four weeks without difficulty. The double-cuffed tube is highly desirable for the apneic person. Periodic checking of cuff pressures has been strongly suggested by many authorities to insure that cuff pressures do not exceed 20 mm Hg pressure. (Above this level capillary blood flow is occluded.) Crosby and Parson's study suggests that as little as 1 ml, 5 ml definitely, over the amount suggested for inflation will exceed the 20 mm Hg pressure.[25] Lack of knowledge about the product and too small tracheostomy tubes have also been involved in the occurrence of tracheal stenosis. Hyperventilation prior to, during, and after deflation and inflation prevents the serious hazards of inducing hypoxia.

To maintain the patency of the airway, aspiration beyond the trachea may be necessary. Entry of the catheter into the left bronchus is achieved by turning the patient's head to the right, elevating the chin and turning the chest to the left, and vice versa for the right bronchus. As with tracheal aspiration, liquefaction of the secretions may be augmented by instillation of 5 to 10 ml of normal saline (up to 50 ml has been used in some instances but only upon specific request of the physician). Normal saline may be injected directly into the catheter prior to aspiration.

Ventilatory Therapy

Once the health care team has established the patency of the airway, a decision is made whether to institute ventilatory therapy. Ventilators, commonly spoken of as respirators, are based upon the principles of negative or positive pressure. Presently, the negative pressure apparatus is utilized more frequently in the short- or long-term management of neuromuscular disorders resulting in respiratory failure. However, in more common use are the positive pressure machines—to augment the individual's respiratory efforts, to control respiration in the apneic patient, or to correct an undesirable breathing pattern. Mr. L. was unable to provide adequate oxygen or eliminate carbon dioxide to maintain adequate cellular metabolism. His loss of diffusion and perfusion surface, as well as a superimposed bronchitis, made the cost of breathing excessive; thus, he was unable to sustain himself without ventilative assistance.

Ventilatory assistance or controlled ventilation may be used for patients such as Mr. L. and for a myriad of others suffering from chronic or acute respiratory insufficiency and/or failure. According to one source, respiratory insufficiency exists when the individual's lung is unable to meet the body's demand for gaseous exchange during effort, and failure occurs when this is not possible, even in a resting state.[26] There is general agreement among authorities that respiratory failure exists when the partial pressure of oxygen falls to 50 to 60 mm Hg or the carbon dioxide tension exceeds 50 mm Hg; unless ventilation is improved, the condition becomes worse and is incompatible with life. For example, the patient with chronic obstructive lung disease, pulmonary fibrosis, or progressive neuromuscular disease, may experience a slowly progressive insufficiency, resulting in cardiopulmonary disease and respiratory failure. In contrast, acute respiratory insufficiency occurs abruptly and may occur during an acute asthmatic episode of bronchospasm, an overwhelming pulmonary infection, acute ventricular failure, upper airway obstruction, or conditions resulting from paralysis of the respiratory muscles, such as results from drug poisoning.

The nurse's role in providing ventilatory support varies among hospital settings and the types of units that are provided for the respiratory care of patients. The health care team members—the nurse, physician, inhalation therapist, anesthesiologist—must work closely together in developing and implementing an effective course of action. Presently, the nurse's role varies from one of observation, reporting, and assisting to one of assessment, initiation, evaluation, and adjustment of ventilatory therapy in close collaboration with the physician. In the case of Mr. L., the assistive type, pressure-preset, mechanical positive pressure ventilator was attached to his cuffed tracheostomy to augment his own respiratory efforts and to achieve a more adequate ventilation. A simple explanation was given to Mr. L. and his wife. Mr. L., being hypoxic, needed this information repeated over and over again, often trying the patience of the health care members and the family. His wife also needed much reassurance and support, for she saw the use of the mechanical ventilator as an undesirable change in his condition. Tracheal and bronchial aspiration preceded the institution of the ventilatory support. Constant vigilance by attendant personnel was essential in initiating and providing safe and effective ventilatory support to Mr. L., who was extremely apprehensive, restless, and irritable. However, the use of sedation with assistive ventilation is fraught with dangers; it would have been unwise to mask his level of consciousness or orientation since it may have interfered with determining improvement or deterioration in his ventilation. Moreover, many of the drugs utilized for sedation have a depressant effect upon the respiratory center.

After Mr. L. was on the ventilator, adjustments were made in the response to his rate and depth of respiration. The goal was a slower rate with increased depth, bringing about more adequate alveolar ventilation. The nurse noted that periodically he took in a larger volume of the oxygen-air mixture. This appeared adequate to simulate the usual sighing pattern of the "normal" patient, and was important in preventing the phenomena of microatelectasis (leading to macroatelectasis) experienced by persons with a consistent rate and tidal volume. Although Mr. L. was on the ventilator, the nurse applied the principles of good respiratory hygiene and tracheostomy care (i.e., change of position, humidification of the inspired air, and so on). The heated humidifier was essential to maintaining liquefaction of the tracheobronchial secretions and preventing irritation of the tracheobronchial tree; however, it did pose a potential hazard for bacterial growth. The removable parts of the ventilator, including the humidifier, were thoroughly cleaned to remove mucus and were sterilized every 24 hours, making it necessary to have additional equipment on hand. Monitoring of the FIO_2, arterial blood gases, O_2 saturation, pH, sodium bicarbonate level, and base excess gave good indices of the effectiveness of the therapy and indicated whether adjustments were necessary. Continuous use of assistive ventilation calls for adjustments of the ventilator to synchronize it with the patient's breathing patterns, and to prevent overcorrection of the existing problem.

Control of ventilation may need to be assumed by the members of the health care team. This can involve everything from mouth-to-mouth resuscitation in respiratory arrest, followed by use of the hand ventilator, to institution of controlled ventilation with an IPPB apparatus. The latter may be achieved through use of either the volume- or pressure-preset machines. Institution of controlled respiration in the apneic patient obviously does not pose the same problems as those with existing respiratory efforts. Rodman and Sterling found that the major problem in the use of the volume-cycled respirator is to assist the conscious patient to abandon all respiratory efforts, including coughing.[27] They have "talked a patient into" allowing the machine to take over, while at the same time increasing the patient's respiratory rate with the use of large volumes at the initiation of therapy. Hyperventilation by use of a self-inflating bag has been suggested as a means of diminishing the patient's respiratory drive. Counting the respiratory rate of the tachypneic patient and then setting the rate ten respiratory cycles higher, with a shallow tidal volume, has sometimes proved successful in initiating therapy. Adjustments in rate and tidal volume may be made after patient acceptance is insured. Use of narcotics such as meperidine (Demerol), promethazine (Phenergan), and morphine sulfate, or curarelike drugs (e.g., succinylcholine), may be used if the other methods fail in depressing a patient's own respiratory efforts. The experienced specialist nurse may be called upon to work closely with the physician in utilizing this latter technique.

Controlled ventilation provides what the individual cannot do or do well enough to maintain adequate alveolar ventilation and arterial oxygenation. Rate, tidal volume, airway pressure, ratio of inspiration to expiration, inspiratory and expiratory flow patterns, and end-expiratory pressure can be controlled. It must be remembered that a change in one parameter affects another. The physician bases his judgment on the appropriate settings, the nature of the problem, and the individual. Frequent evaluations are made at first and followed later as indicated by the client's status. A form placed at the bedside with the ventilatory settings, FIO_2, blood gases, O_2 saturation, pH, HCO^-, and base excess gives a concise picture of the individual's status at all times.

Though the astute nurse recognizes the life-saving qualities of ventilatory therapy, she also appreciates the potential hazards of its use. Prevention of complications is essential, and the nurse must be constantly alert to changes in the individual's condition. Oxygen toxicity is possible when the mechanical ventilator is driven by an oxygen-air mixture rather than by compressed air or room air since the amount of air drawn into the system is related to the velocity of oxygen flow. Individuals with stiff lungs or obstructed airways, where the velocity is low, may receive high concentrations of oxygen, which may in turn result in hyalinized changes in the respiratory membrane, and perhaps in an interference with the production of pulmonary surfactant to meet the demands. The lung tends to become less compliant and requires greater pressure to deliver the same tidal volume. The Pao_2 decreases because poorly ventilated or nonventilated alveoli are being perfused, increasing the venous admixture. Early recognition of this condition by the health care team will prevent an ensuing critical state of hypoxia. Monitoring of the oxygen concentration and of the temperature of the inspired air at the tracheal stoma, as well as observing the nature of the tracheobronchial secretions, are important assessments. A sudden rise in $Paco_2$ may be another indication of oxygen toxicity, especially when the individual's respiratory rate is depressed and the machine is not set to assume a satisfactory rate.

The use of ventilators increases dead air space; therefore, adjustments must be made to accommodate for this or there may be an aggravation of an existing alveolar hypoventilation. The nurse works in close collaboration with the physician and other members of the health care team in monitoring the Pco_2, which hopefully will show a gradual decrease when adequate alveolar ventilation occurs. Too rapid a dissipation of carbon dioxide may result in alkalosis, and the patient's pH may become excessively high before the Pco_2 has reached the desired level of 40 mm Hg. Clients with normal lungs may have the opposite problem, a low $Paco_2$ during artificial ventilation. Additional tubing in small increments may need to be added to increase the dead space, thereby elevating the $Paco_2$. This technique must also be carefully monitored. The nurse recognizes the necessity for the renal excretion of sodium bicarbonate to accompany the dissipation of the carbon dioxide by the lungs. Evidence points to the fact that there is a lag in this process in the brain and spinal fluids, which must be considered in aggressive hyperventilation. Moreover, rapid changes in the hydrogen ion concentrations may cause a large movement of potassium at the myocardial cellular level, resulting in ventricular arrhythmias. An accompanying hypochloremia may exist, making it increasingly difficult for the kidney tubules to excrete sodium bicarbonate. Administration of potassium chloride and carbonic acid anhydrase inhibitors may be given to augment the elimination of sodium bicarbonate. Hourly urine specimens are measured, with an accompanying pH determination to evaluate the effectiveness of the therapy.

The nurse must be very diligent in her observation of the inspiratory-expiratory rate and the time interval ratio of each phase. This should be carried out over a full 60-second interval, along with the pulse rate. Frequent blood pressure readings are also important. Prolonged inspiration, utilizing the positive pressure machines, can result in a decrease in venous return to the right side of the heart. Central venous pressure readings are usually instituted to determine blood volume and, when intravenous fluids are ordered, careful regulation must be maintained in close collaboration with the physician. Most recent has been the introduction of the cardiac catheter (Swan-Ganz) for use in bedside monitoring. Through the use of the cardiac catheter and its placement, the pulmonary artery (PA) and pulmonary artery occluded (PA_o) pressures are available. It is felt by its advocates to be superior to the CVP in reflecting the left heart hemodynamics and detecting alterations in the cardiopulmonary status before clinical manifestations occur. Nurses working in intensive care settings need to become well versed in this technique. Particularly the early hours of treatment involve constant vigilance to achieve desired results (e.g., proper correction while avoiding excesses in either direction).

When ventilatory assistance is no longer needed, the process of weaning from the machine may often be achieved with ease. More difficulty may be encountered when the patient has been long dependent upon the machine's support. The establishment of confidence, security, and good rapport with the health care team greatly enhances the process. Withdrawal may be initiated by allowing short periods (two or three minutes) of spontaneous respiration every half-hour to an hour, depending on the patient's reaction. The nurse should remain with him during this time to provide the necessary emotional support. Monitoring must continue, in order to assess the patient's ability to assume his role.

Daytime is the most desirable time to initiate the withdrawal, and, at first, machine support may be necessary during the night to have the patient achieve adequate rest. The time off the machine is increased as the patient responds favorably, and the ventilator is eventually discontinued. Tyler and Nett suggest the importance of supplemental oxygen and mist during the weaning period through use of a tracheostomy collar or T-tube, nebulizer, and large-bore tubing.[28] Should the individual need oxygen support after removal of the tracheostomy or endotracheal tube, it can be provided by nasal cannula. Kistner tracheostomy buttons can be used for a portal for sectioning, if secretions continue to be a problem. Leaving the equipment close at hand may provide additional emotional support to the patient's efforts. Plugging of the tracheostomy and gradual removal of the tube ensue as the patient's condition improves and the rehabilitation process proceeds.

Other techniques in ventilatory support have been introduced, namely PEEP (positive end-expiratory pressure), and inspiratory hold. These techniques have been especially effective in the treatment of individuals with distributive hypoxia. Distributive hypoxia may occur as the result of small airway or alveolar inspiratory obstruction, producing a microatelectasis or the lack of surfactant. The inspiratory hold provides time for air distribution throughout the lung. Greater than normal force may be necessary to open and inflate the small air sacs when there is a tendency of alveolar collapse or reduction in the volume of the alveoli in the absence of effective surfactant. If these air sacs are partially inflated it will take less pressure to provide effective tidal ventilation. This is often referred to as CPPV or CPPB (continuous positive pressure ventilation or breathing). As Bendixen has well stated there is no "free lunch" and determinations must be made as to the cost versus benefit to the client.[29] These techniques are not without dangers, as this maneuver disturbs normal physiology. The principle involved can be accomplished with or without the use of a ventilator and is particularly useful in the much discussed adult respiratory distress syndrome.

There is usually a preferred ventilator in each hospital setting and the members of the health care team become very familiar with its use. This is highly desirable in enhancing the skill of the personnel in the machine's therapeutic use. Also, understanding the nature of the patient's problem for which the ventilator was indicated is of utmost importance in the effective use of the machine. The literature provided by the manufacturer provides valuable information for the health care team.

HYPOXEMIA AND CARDIAC DYSFUNCTION

Another problem which sometimes plagues individuals and the health care team is the alteration in cardiac function resulting from impaired lung functioning. Gray stated that hypoxemia is the single most important cause of pulmonary hypertension and cor pulmonale (right ventricular failure), and results from unequal distribution of the ventilation-perfusion ratio.[30] Some areas of the lung may be quite well ventilated, while others have poor ventilation in relation to the amount of perfusion. Therefore, mixing of well-oxygenated and poorly oxygenated blood occurs (in emphysema, bronchitis, interstitial fibrosis, or obstruction to pulmonary blood flow).

The problem of hypoxemia and cardiac dysfunction may be illustrated by the case of Mr. J., well known to the health care team because of his frequent admissions for acute exacerbation of pulmonary infections. On this admission, Mr. J. exhibited dyspnea, dependent edema, and tachycardia. It was evident that his long-standing pulmonary emphysema had resulted in undesirable changes in cardiac functioning, culminating in right ventricular failure. The objectives of Mr. J.'s care involved: 1) reducing the demands of his body for oxygen; 2) providing a slightly increased oxygen environment during the acute phase of his illness; 3) assisting in alleviating the existing infections; 4) dispersing Mr. J.'s anxieties; and 5) providing emotional support to his wife during this period of stress. Many of the general principles of respiratory care were brought into play in the nursing team's implementation of intervention to meet these objectives. An additional dimension of his care in-volved the nursing implications resulting from the effect of his primary lung disease on other body systems.

There is controversy among authorities concerning the effectiveness of digitalis therapy in the treatment of right ventricular failure. However, most physicians, as did Mr. J.'s, digitalize and maintain a dosage slightly less than that usually given. The nurse understood that dramatic improvement in cardiac functioning could not be expected as the result of digitalization because of Mr. J.'s primary irreversible pulmonary disease. Particular alertness for early signs of digitalis toxicity was important because of the potential hazard resulting from flux of potassium out of the cell in the presence of acidemia, secondary to ventilatory insufficiency. Also, excesses of potassium can make the heart less susceptible to the action of digitalis, while paradoxically the two factors taken together can exert an additive effect on the A-V node, resulting in heart block. In this case, furosemide (Lasix) was preferred for diuretic therapy because of its effectiveness in the prevention of sodium and chloride reabsorption over the entire length of the nephron. Excessive losses of potassium do not usually occur because the effect is independent of the body acid-base balance. Frequent monitoring of the electrolytes plays an important role in effective diuretic therapy.

The nursing care team was prepared to assist with periodic phlebotomies if the increased viscosity of the blood, secondary to erythrocytosis, superceded the value of the additional oxygen-carrying power (usually when the hematocrit is above 55 percent). Had left ventricular failure occurred, with an accompanying pulmonary edema, the nursing care team was prepared to apply mechanical rotating tourniquets to reduce the venous return and dilute the work of the heart. In this procedure, the cuffs, resembling those utilized in taking arterial blood pressure, are applied as high on the extremity as possible, to facilitate pooling of the blood in the extremity. The nurse collaborates with the physician to determine the amount of pressure to be applied on each extremity—the degree of pressure is usually midway between the individual's systolic and diastolic pressure. It is important to monitor the arterial pulse below the cuff after application, to ensure an arterial blood supply beyond the point of application. At the conclusion of the procedure, the cuffs are removed one at a time, following the rotation schedule, to prevent a sudden strain on the heart, due to rapidly increased blood volume. This procedure was unnecessary in the care of Mr. J.; his condition improved by reducing the demands for oxygen, supplying a slightly increased oxygen concentration in his environment for a short period of time, providing good bronchial hygiene, maintaining supportive antibiotic therapy, and the addition of digitalis and diuretic therapy.

It was important to reassure Mr. J. that discontinuation of special therapies was an indication of improvement. One morning he was found to be extremely apprehensive and dyspneic. He breathlessly said that it was because the oxygen had been removed from his room during the night, for what he believed to be no apparent reason. He was quickly made aware that this was an indication of improvement, but that the equipment was readily available for his use if he felt the need for it. The episode points up the importance of working with both patients and their families in the gradual assumption of independence. Too dramatic a change from the role of dependence to independence may be overwhelming to patients and to their families.

RESTORATION OF SUBATMOSPHERIC INTRAPLEURAL PRESSURE

No discussion of respiratory care problems is complete without consideration of the nurse's role in restoration of the normal subatmospheric intrapleural pressure. This pressure, established with the first breath of life, is essential to producing the volumetric chest drainage system. This provides for the removal of air and/or fluid, by gravitational flow, from the pleural space into a drainage container devised so that the reverse of this flow is prevented. A catheter may be placed near the apex of the lung for the removal of air, since air tends to rise. For removal of serosanguineous fluid, a catheter is placed at the base of the lung. The catheters are attached to larger

pieces of tubing which are connected directly to water-sealed drainage bottles. Should the surgeon desire the addition of negative suction to facilitate lung reexpansion, a source and control of the amount of suction must be provided in the drainage system. The surgeon usually utilizes a negative pressure of between 10 to 20 ml of water, which is only slightly higher than the pressure existing in the pleural cavity during normal inspiration.

Such drainage systems were needed in the cases of Mr. V. and Mr. R., patients who required chest surgery. Each patient, in his own way, conveyed feelings of anxiety and fear of the upcoming surgery. Janis found patients' fears to be a combination of imminent dangers prior to a major surgical operation—possibility of suffering acute pain, undergoing serious body damage, and dying.[31] He has suggested that patients are capable of behaving in a more organized way if they have a concrete picture of what they will experience. Preparation of patients for upcoming surgery has become a vital role of the nurse. Mr. V. was more concerned about the pain he would experience following his chest surgery than about the potential seriousness of his diagnosis. The nurse discussed with Mr. V. his effective use of the analgesic, the importance of deep breathing, coughing, and changing of positions. At subsequent conferences, she discussed the breathing exercise program which was designed to strengthen and encourage more effective postoperative use of his muscles of respiration. Mr. V. and his wife asked many pertinent questions about the chest drainage system, IPPB, and oxygen therapy. The establishment of good communications among Mr. V., his wife, and the nurse was an essential ingredient for meaningful nursing intervention and personalized care.

The particular nursing requirements of Mr. V's immediate postoperative period included maintenance of the drainage system's patency, proper functioning of the apparatus, and monitoring and evaluating Mr. V's response. Use of a clear plastic chest catheter and tubing made it easier for the nurse to observe the gravitational flow and the nature of the drainage. Milking or stripping the tube away from Mr. V's body, using short overlapping strokes was helpful in maintaining the tube's patency. The extra tubing was coiled and secured to the bottom sheet to prevent undue tension on the chest tubes. It also allowed greater freedom of movement and prevented accidental disconnection. It is wise to place adhesive tape around the connections to ensure a closed system. Care was taken that the water seal in the drainage bottle was maintained on both inspiration and expiration. The nurse was alert for early signs of hemorrhage and monitored the character and amount of the drainage. Mr. V's drainage tended to be a cherry-red color during the first few hours, followed by a more serosanguineous drainage as the hours progressed. The drainage bottle was calibrated, making it possible for the nurse to monitor the amount of drainage, always determined at eye level. Constant assessment of the character of the respirations, pulse, and blood pressure provided information concerning Mr. V's cardiopulmonary status, and was a helpful adjunct to early detection of unforeseen postoperative complications.

Adequate alveolar ventilation was maintained by utilizing good bronchial hygiene measures, such as coughing, deep breathing, and changing body positions every hour. Adequate fluid intake, humidification of the oxygen-air mixture and use of the IPPB ventilator with nebulization of Mucomyst, aided in maintaining liquid, productive mucus. Had Mr. V. been unable to handle expectoration of his own mucus, aspiration of the tracheobronchial tree would have been considered by the health care team. The use of a hydrojet with a mucolytic agent could contribute to the liquefaction of the secretions. The health care team felt that Mr. V's cessation of smoking had contributed to a clearer airway by reducing the irritation of the tracheobronchial tree, decreasing the secretions, and improving the ciliary action. Mr. V's chest x-rays, taken on the afternoon following surgery and again the following day, indicated good lung expansion. It seemed that the deep inspiratory efforts had not only contributed to better ventilation, but had also caused the lung to expand toward the chest wall, forcing the accumulated fluid into the catheter.

Care was taken to maintain strict asepsis in handling the drainage equipment, to prevent entry of microorganisms into the pleural cavity. Large clamps were available to place on the tubes whenever they were disconnected. The drainage bottles were always kept below the levels of the chest to prevent drainage from reentering the pleural cavity.

Mr. V. needed to be encouraged to become increasingly active in the postoperative period, and the nurse noted that he had to be reminded to maintain as good a posture as possible, to facilitate chest expansion and preserve the muscle tone of the upper extremities. Mr. V's tubes were removed on the fourth postoperative day and plans were soon initiated with him and his family for discharge to his home, with follow-up health supervision in the chest clinic.

The principles of Mr. V's respiratory care could have been applied equally to Mr. R's care following an insertion of a prosthetic aortic valve. Ventilatory control was deemed necessary by the members of the health care team in the early hours of his care. This was achieved through the use of a volume-preset ventilator. In addition to the patient's ventilatory care, the nurse determined whether the ventilator had a built-in "sighing mechanism," since it was vitally important in preventing atelectasis and equally important in stimulating the usual production of pulmonary surfactant. Periodic cycling with increased tidal volumes was provided as well as a bleed-off system, in the event of excessive pressure to deliver the necessary tidal volume. Monitoring of the blood gases and pH made it possible to maintain the 1:20 ratio of carbonic acid to base bicarbonate. Nursing intervention directed toward diligent respiratory care is a major role of the nurse in caring for the patient following open heart surgery.

EVALUATION OF THE INTERVENTIONS[32]

Frequent reference has been made to the use of blood gas analysis, fractional inspiratory oxygen, pH, bicarbonate, and base excess. Therefore, it seems appropriate for the nurse to be able to determine the client's state of oxygenation, ventilation, and acid-base balance utilizing these parameters as guides.

In analyzing these parameters, the first most

important question to ask is, "What is the state of oxygenation? The level of oxygenation is evaluated by looking at the Pao_2 and O_2 saturation. Reference was made earlier to the fact that oxygen which has diffused into the lung capillaries is transported in two forms. A small amount is dissolved in plasma and red blood cell water and exerts a corresponding pressure (80 to 100 mm Hg). The major portion of the oxygen is transported by the hemoglobin component of the red blood cell, acting as a reserve supply to be released to the red blood cell water, plasma, and tissues. Thus, the Pao_2 reflects the pressure component of the dissolved oxygen in the plasma.

The measure used to determine oxygen saturation of hemoglobin is the percentage of oxygen saturation compared with the total amount of oxygen which hemoglobin could carry (85 percent or better). The amount and rate with which oxygen combines with hemoglobin is influenced by the Po_2. Therefore, knowledge of the O_2 saturation gives a good estimate of the amount of oxygen being carried in the blood. It will be noted in reviewing the oxyhemoglobin dissociation curve that the relationship between Po_2 and O_2 saturation is not a linear one. Therefore, with a rise in a very low Po_2 will result in a much more rapid rise on O_2 saturation. A rise in a Po_2, in the presence of a normal or higher O_2 saturation, would show only slight increase in the oxygen saturation.

The relationship of Po_2 and O_2 saturation is affected by body temperature, pH of the blood, abnormal types of hemoglobin, and 2 to 3 DPG. This knowledge is utilized in the therapeutic use of oxygen. The fractional percentage of inspired oxygen should be analyzed with the Pao_2 and O_2 saturation. Laboratory studies should show the time samples taken, whether the individual was receiving oxygen or not, and if so by what method. Therefore, the relationship of FIO_2, Pao_2 and O_2 saturation gives reliable information as to the client's state of oxygenation.

The second question to be answered is, "How well is the individual ventilating?" In other words, "How well is the lung eliminating the carbon dioxide resulting from cellular metabolism?" This parameter is evaluated by knowing the $Paco_2$. It will be remembered that carbon dioxide enters the tissue capillaries and diffuses through the alveolar capillary membranes as the result of a relatively small pressure differential in the normal individual. Carbon dioxide is carried by the blood in three ways: 1) dissolved in the plasma (approximately 10 percent). 2) Hydrated in the red cell primarily to form carbonic acid which dissociates to HCO_3 and H^+ (approximately 60 percent). The HCO_3 leaves the red cell in exchange for the Cl^- ion (known as a chloride shift). Another interaction, the Haldane effect, limits the amount of carbon dioxide which can be carried in the form of carboaminohemoglobin in the presence of oxygen, but does not affect the other means of transport. The presence of carbonic anhydrase accelerates the cellular dissociation process. 3) Combines with the amino group of the hemoglobin molecule in contrast to oxygen which is attached to the iron. Carbon dioxide combined with hemoglobin and pH decreases hemoglobin affinity for oxygen (Bohr effect). The reverse steps occur when the blood passes through the lung capillaries.

The lungs are the most important and efficient means for eliminating carbon dioxide. The kidneys have a less important role in eliminating carbon dioxide by the dissociation of a hydrated CO_2, H_2CO_3, to H^+ and HCO_3^-. The H^+ may be eliminated in the form of NH_4^+ and the HCO_3^- may be retained or eliminated.

Measurement of the pH is the way of determining the acid-base balance of the blood. Homeostasis or proper functioning of the body systems is maintained best in the pH range of 7.35 to 7.45. Imbalances may result from respiratory, metabolic, or combined causes.

HCO_3^- and base excess are influenced by metabolic processes and represent the nonrespiratory component. Conditions in which there is an accumulation of acids (i.e., diabetic acidosis) or a loss of HCO_3^- will result in a lowered HCO_3^- and a negative base excess (as compared to normal HCO_3 levels or other bases). The opposite is the case when excessive acids are lost and excess bicarbonate accumulates (bicarbonate level is elevated and the base excess positive). The lung and kidneys attempt to compensate for these imbalances but the degree of imbalance will determine whether this is accomplished without therapeutic intervention.

It becomes evident that inadequate ventilation can result in respiratory acidosis and hyperventilation, respiratory alkalosis. It is also possible for metabolic acidosis to occur from an inadequate oxygen supply resulting in a lactic acidemia. The body consistently attempts to maintain the 20:1 ratio of HCO_3^- to PCO_2.

In summary, it can be simply stated that the relationship of FIO_2, PaO_2, and O_2 saturation gives reliable cues to the client's state of oxygenation, the $PaCO_2$, the level of ventilation or ability to eliminate CO_2 through the lungs; the pH gives the information on the acid-base balance and HCO_3^-, and base excess measures the metabolic processes. This information can provide additional cues to guide the care process.

Rehabilitation

THE PATIENT

Throughout the discussion of respiratory care problems, references have been made to the involvement of patients and their families in the plan of care. Such participation is essential to the effective rehabilitation of the patient's experiencing a chronic respiratory disease and can be applied equally to patients who have other breathing problems, secondary to another condition (e.g., paralytic diseases, skeletal problems, pre- and postsurgery).

Rehabilitation is viewed as a broad philosophical concept which "embodies the recognition of the dignity and importance of the individual and the need for a holistic approach in reintegrating the disabled person in his society."[33] It recognizes the uniqueness of the human experience, the necessity for purpose and meaning in life and places value on participation in activities affecting one's life. There have been an increasing number of special respiratory care units established, with additional special research projects directed toward rehabilitation of the "respiratory-disabled" individual. It has been exciting to observe the interest and enthusiasm shown by the nurse and other members of the

health care team in a dynamic rehabilitation program. Ingredients of a sound rehabilitation program are generally agreed on. However, the manner in which this can be accomplished most effectively is still in the embryonic state. The ingredients of such a program are that the patient acquire:

1. Knowledge of the nature of his disease.
2. Realistic view of the limitations placed upon him as the result of the disease, as well as those activities which are to be encouraged.
3. Knowledge of the preventive aspects of his illness (i.e., general good health measures, bronchial hygiene, breathing exercises, postural drainage, and so on).
4. Skill in carrying out the prescribed treatment regimen (progressive exercise program, correct use of the medihaler, drugs, and special equipment).
5. Ability to recognize early signs of exacerbation of the existing condition.
6. Knowledge of the importance of health supervision and where to seek assistance when necessary.

In viewing the teaching role in the rehabilitative process, the nurse is cognizant that often the first contact with the individual is during an acute phase of his illness. This is a time when his physical needs are many and special competency is required of all members of the care team. Once this phase has passed, the task of rehabilitation is in its infancy, and the movement of the patient from a dependent to a more independent role has just begun. As with other care problems, an initial assessment of the individual and his health problem provides a good starting point. This assessment often involves the expertise of numerous members of the professional team— physician, nurse, pulmonary physiologist, psychiatrist and/or psychologist, social workers, and so on. Hopefully, with the assistance of the patient and his family, the team provides the guidelines and direction for the development, implementation, and evaluation of a health care plan.

Mr. O., a 38-year-old father of four children, was admitted to the hospital in a state of respiratory failure, secondary to an acute bronchial asthmatic episode. While he was recovering, Mr. O. indicated to the nurse that he first became aware of his problem while he was in the armed services. Following his initial attack he had experienced other episodes, such as this one, and had traveled to various parts of the country in an attempt to free himself of his symptoms. He had never allowed himself to stay with any treatment regimen sufficiently long to determine its effectiveness. After traveling extensively, and finding himself without funds, he arrived with his family at the home of his father. Mr. O. had been forced to face the reality of his illness and could no longer seek only temporary relief of his symptoms. Unfortunately, the patient's feeling of hopelessness is sometimes shared by members of the health care team as well. However, this was not true in his instance. After a year of hospitalization Mr. O. returned to his home, knowing a great deal about his condition, how to live with it, and how to maintain his role within the family structure.

Such a successful program of rehabilitation is not always possible with every patient. Sometimes this failure is due to his inability, physiologically and psychologically, to participate in his own care program. Kass and Sheets reported an initial observation resulting from limited experience with emphysematous patients.[34] They found that over half of the patients treated in their rehabilitation center suffered from some form of brain damage, which interfered with visual integration, memory, and perception beyond that expected for the patient's age. Should this be true in the longer range studies, the nurse may need to alter what is taught these patients and how it is done. Information provided by psychological testing may be helpful in determining the individual's ability to assume the self-help role.

The patient's self-help ability may be influenced by the nature of his respiratory problem, his intelligence and education levels, his feeling toward health personnel, his attitude toward preventive measures, and his personal credo of life. For example, it took many months to get Mr. O's respiratory problem stabilized before he and the care team could focus attention on the details of a self-help program. His past experience with his disease and his previous short-term treatment programs resulted in acquisition of much information about his disease and the emergency measures to be taken during acute episodes. He felt dependent upon the health care team for lifesaving measures, although he knew that they could not "cure" his problem. Mr. O. valued his position as head of his household, particularly with respect to providing not only for the basic needs of the family, but also for some luxuries. It is during the assessment process that the nurse and other members of the health care team become increasingly aware of the way the individual may view his illness in relationship to himself and to his family. As Carlson suggested, "illness of any nature is usually accompanied by physical, emotional and social changes that are likely to interfere with a patient's ability to function as he did in health."[35] The possibility Mr. O. found most threatening was that of losing certain aspects of his roles as father and provider. Another patient, Mr. E., viewed his loss of personal freedom as unbearable. Although these two patients suffered from the same kind of physical problem, the personal meaning of the illness varied considerably and they reacted quite differently to threats to their self-esteem. The nurse and the care team often need to work very closely with patients and their families in solving such problems. Probably one of the most significant nursing contributions is that of supporting each patient in his efforts to cope with his illness.

Once an assessment is completed, the members of the health care team can share what has been learned about the patient, his family, and the nature of the respiratory problem. Recommendations may be a collaborative effort, and include realistic goals with a plan for their implementation, and specific guides for definitions of the role of the patient, his family, and the various care team members. The physician is usually ready at this time to present the recommendations to the patient and his family. Sometimes this is too much for the family unit to assimilate at one time and additional meetings must be planned. The nurse can create the right atmosphere for encouraging the patient to ask questions about future plans, to clarify certain areas of concern and to precipitate free expression of underlying feelings.

Once there is general agreement on the course to be taken, the program should get underway. Usually the patient is receptive to the helpful efforts of the care team. Some care teams, for instance, strongly insist on the discontinuation of any smoking habit. (Many of these patients are smokers of long-standing.) Other care teams, while supporting this view, nevertheless are willing to allow a gradual reduction of the habit. The nurse must recognize the difficulty such a redirection may pose for some patients as they begin to recover. A patient may demand a great deal of emotional support in organizing his own resources to give up smoking completely. The nurse must help the family also to understand the effects of smoking and why its discontinuance is essential to the patient's welfare. It may also be a time when questions concerning other environmental irritants are asked and discussed—methods of home heating, humidity, climatic changes, housecleaning methods, use of aerosols, and the presence of air pollutants.

Small interaction groups of patients are often effective vehicles for sharing common problems and solutions. Group members may talk about any problem—for example, the distress many of them feel when arising in the morning. Knowing that this condition results from an accumulation of mucus, helps patients to understand the rationale of treatment measures, such as hot drinks, postural drainage, judicious use of the medihaler, slow pacing of activities, effective coughing, and breathing exercises. Sharing of firsthand knowledge and ideas provides a strong impetus to effective adjustment.

THE FAMILY

Family sessions have also been helpful in solving some patients' problems. Families usually welcome the opportunity to express their feelings concerning the problem. Such sessions often help them to develop insight into the patient's problems and they are able to view more clearly their own role in dealing with the illness. The

care team member may prove a good resource for the answers to certain questions, and from time to time may contribute the latest information gained from recent research. Special discussions on such subjects as the value of flu vaccine, prevention of respiratory infections, how to recognize and handle an upper respiratory infection, the importance of good nutrition and adequate hydration, can be very helpful.

THERAPY

The patient also may be participating in a physical therapy program to improve his muscle tone, develop more effective means of breathing, with or without oxygen support, and make effective use of gravitational flow to enhance the removal of mucus (i.e., postural drainage). The inhalation therapist can assist with the use of special equipment in the home (e.g., medihaler, IPPB devices, portable oxygen supply).

The nurse works very closely with the patient and his family and may even be responsible for coordinating the activities of the various members of the care team, including the public health nurse coordinator or community nurse who provides a link in the continuity of care and the patient's adjustment to the activities of daily living. For example, the patient has learned to effectively utilize the muscles of respiration during expiration. Mr. M. began his exercises in a supine position, utilizing a drawsheet to facilitate the final phase of expiration. He was taught to slightly clench his teeth, make a hissing sound on expiration, and encourage a longer expiratory phase of respiration. He understood how this was helpful in keeping his breathing passages open during the expiratory phase, facilitating alveolar ventilative exchange. This procedure was then carried out in a sitting position, and finally on ambulation, during activities at home and on the job (Fig. 14-8).

FINANCES

Chronic respiratory illness can become a financial burden on family resources. Where needed, assistance can be given to enable families to work through this real problem. Moreover, direct aid may be necessary to meet the basic

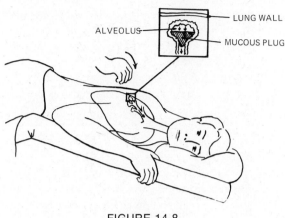

ALVEOLUS — LUNG WALL

MUCOUS PLUG

FIGURE 14-8.
Breathing exercises.

needs and those occurring as the result of the patient's illness. A successful preventive program depends on the ability of the patient and his family to carry out the program with as much independence as possible.

The vocational counselor prepares the patient to return to his job and reviews the activities involved in the patient's occupation. Whenever feasible, patients are helped to make the necessary adjustments to return to their former occupations. Should this be inadvisable, consideration is given to suitable alternatives. For example, Mr. O. was unable to return to his former occupation; after proper assessment, arrangements were made for him to take a short-term course in the operation of business machines. Mr. O. enjoyed his new occupation, found many opportunities for employment, and was able to assume the financial support of his family. He was able to maintain his self-esteem. Though employment may not be a realistic goal, the occupational therapist can encourage and assist the patient in having some interest other than his illness.

SUPPORTIVE HEALTH CARE

The nurse's role in providing emotional support in patient-family teaching, and in coordinating the patient's rehabilitation, extends beyond the hospital or rehabilitation center into the home, into other supportive health care agencies, and into the occupational situation. The program re-volves around the specific patient. Although every aspect of a total program of rehabilitation for the respiratory handicapped patient is not realistic or attainable, there is much value gained by the one who learns to maintain his personal integrity and independence.

Summary

The challenges presented by patients with respiratory care problems command the immediate attention of all members of the health care team. How well the team members meet this challenge depends on the use of all available knowledge, research, technology, and creativity. The nurse, probably more than any other team member, provides meaningful intervention to patients with respiratory care problems, participating in a dynamic process of rehabilitation and providing follow-up care in the home.

References

1. Chronic Obstructive Lung Disease: A Manual for Physicians, ed. 3. New York, National Tuberculosis and Respiratory Disease Association, 1972, p. 20.
2. *Ibid.*, p. 21.
3. Report of advisory committee to surgeon general, U.S.P.H.S. smoking and health. Washington, D.C., U.S. Dept. of Health, Education and Welfare, Pamphlet 2019, 1966.
4. Fletcher, C. J.: A paper—cigarettes and respiratory disease. Conference on Smoking and Health. Summary: World Conference on Smoking and Health, 1967, p. 78.
5. ———: Position papers. Summary: World Conference on Smoking and Health, 1967, pp. 258-284.
6. Gordon, I.: A paper—smoking education: when, where and how. Summary: World Conference on Smoking and Health, 1967, p. 153.
7. Fredrickson, D.: A paper—New York City smoking withdrawal clinic. Summary: World Conference on Smoking and Health, 1967, p. 192.
8. Green, G. M., In defense of the lung. Am. Lung Assoc. Bull. 4-16, Apr. 1974.

9. Bates, D.: Air pollutants and the human lung. Am. Review Respiratory Disease 105: 2, Jan. 1972.

10. Green, *op. cit.*, p. 4.

11. Mittman, C.: Chronic obstructive lung disease. Heart and Lung 2, 2:222-226, 1973.

12. *Ibid.*, p. 214.

13. Guyton, A.: Textbook of Medical Physiology, ed. 4. Philadelphia, W. B. Saunders, 1971, pp. 545-603.

14. DeGowin, E. L. and DeGowin, R. L.: Diagnostic Examination, ed. 2. New York, Macmillan, 1969, pp. 297-302.

15. Prior, J. A. and Silberstein, J. S.: Physical Diagnosis: The History and Examination of the Patient, ed. 4. St. Louis, C. V. Mosby, 1973, pp. 169-208.

16. Travers, G. A.: Assessment of thorax and lungs. Am. J. Nurs. 73, 3:466-471, 1973.

17. Druger, G.: The Chest: Its Signs and Sounds. Los Angeles, Humetrics Corp., 1973.

18. Reinarz, J. A., et al.: The potential role of inhalation therapy equipment in nosocomial pulmonary infection. J. Clin. Invest. 44:831, 1965.

19. Sanford, J. P.: Infection control in critical units. Crit. Care Med. 2, 4:211-216, July-Aug. 1974.

20. Bendixen, H. H.: Respiratory care. Anesthesiology 16, 2; Oct. 21, 1974. Los Angeles, Audio Digest Foundation.

21. Miller, W. F.: Rehabilitation of patients with chronic obstructive lung disease. Med. Clin. North Am. 51:349, 1967.

22. Meltzer, L., et al.: Concepts and Practices of Intensive Care for Nurse Specialists. Philadelphia, Charles Press, 1969, p. 1.

23. Hudson, L.: The acute management of the chronic airway obstruction patient. Heart and Lung 3, 1:93-96, 1974.

24. Rodman, T. and Sterling, F.: Pulmonary Emphysema and Related Lung Diseases. St. Louis, C. V. Mosby, 1969, p. 403.

25. Crosby, L. J. and Parson, L. C.: Management of lateral wall pressures exerted by tracheostomy and endotracheal tube cuffs. Heart and Lung 3, 5:797-803, Sept.-Oct. 1974.

26. Meltzer, et al., *op. cit.*

27. Rodman and Sterling, *op. cit.*, pp. 389-391.

28. Tyler, M. and Nett, L. M.: Intensive nursing and respiratory therapy. *In* T. Petty and L. M. Nett: For Those Who Live and Breathe with Emphysema and Chronic Bronchitis. Springfield, Ill., Charles C Thomas, 1967.

29. Bendixen, *op. cit.*

30. Gray, F. D.: Cardiac problems in obstructive respiratory disease—cor pulmonale. Mod. Treat. 6:2, 255, Mar. 1969.

31. Janis, I.: Psychological Stress. New York, John Wiley & Sons, 1958, pp. 411-412.

32. Keyes, J.: Blood-gases and blood-gas transport. Heart and Lung 3, 6:945-954, 1974.

33. Light, S.: Rehabilitation and Medicine. New Haven, Elizabeth Licht, Publishers, 1968, p. 30.

34. Kass, I. and Sheets, P.: Emphysema—a new approach to an old disease. NTRDA Bull. 55, 5: 6, May 1969.

35. Carlson, C. (ed.): Behavioral Concepts and Nursing Intervention. Philadelphia, J. B. Lippincott, 1970, p. 98.

Bibliography

Ayers, S. and Lagerson, J.: Pulmonary physiology at the bedside: oxygen and carbon dioxide abnormalities. Cardiovas. Nurs. 9, 1:1-6, Jan.-Feb. 1973.

Bartlett, R. and Allyn, P.: Pulmonary management of the burned patient. Heart and Lung 2, 5:714-719, 1973.

Bendixen, H. H.: Rational ventilator modes for respiratory failure. Critical Care Med. 2, 4:225-227, July-Aug. 1974.

Bendixen, H. H., et. al.: Respiratory care. St. Louis, C. V. Mosby, 1969.

Block, A. Jay, et. al.: Chronic oxygen therapy. Chest 65, 3:279-288, Mar. 1974.

Block, V.: Helping the patient to ventilate. Nurs. Outlook 31-33, Oct. 1969.

Bolognini, V.: The Swan Ganz pulmonary artery catheter: implication for nursing. Heart and Lung 3, 6:976-981, Nov.-Dec. 1974.

Broughton, J.: Chest diagnosis for nurses and respiratory therapists. Heart and Lung 200-206, Mar.-Apr. 1972.

Comroe, J. H., Jr., et al: The Lung, ed. 2. Chicago, Yearbook Medical Book Publications, 1968.

Dickie, H. and Chosy, L. W.: Some important occupational lung diseases. Disease-a-Month Chicago, Yearbook Medical Publishers, March 1972.

Dunn, R. C., et al: Determinants of tracheal injury by cuffed tracheostomy tubes. Chest 65, 2:128-135, Feb. 1974.

Dudley, D., et al: Psychosocial aspects of care in the chronic obstructive pulmonary disease patient. Heart and Lung 2, 3:389-393, 1973.

Duncan, O. D.: From social system to ecosystem. Soc. Inquiry 31:140-149, 1961.

Egan, D.: Fundamentals of Respiratory Therapy, ed. 2. St. Louis, C. V. Mosby, 1973.

Fagerbaugh, S.: Getting around with emphysema. Am. Lung Assoc. Bull. 12-16, June 1973.

Farber, S. M. and Wilson, R. H. L.: Chronic obstructive emphysema. Clin. Sym. (Cibia) 20, 2 Apr.-June 1968.

Fenn, W. O. and Rahn, H. (eds.): Handbook of Physiology. Sect. 3. Respiration. Vol. 1 Washington, D.C., American Physiology Society, 1964.

Filley, G.: Acid Base and Blood Gas Regulation. Philadelphia, Lea & Febiger, 1971.

Friedman, A.: The patient with chronic obstructive lung disease and his care at home. Nurs. Clin. N. Am. 3, 4:437-451, Sept. 1968.

Fuhs, M., et al: Nursing in respiratory intensive care unit. Chest 62, 2:145-185, Aug. 1972.

Gernert, C. and Schwartz, S.: Pulmonary artery catheterization. Am. J. Nurs. 73, 8:1182-1185, 1973.

Gibbon, J. H., et al (eds.): Surgery of the Chest, ed. 2. Philadelphia, W. B. Saunders, 1969, pp. 149-160.

Gilbert, R., et al: The first few hours off a respirator. Chest 65, 2:152-157, Feb. 1974.

Hanson, E. L.: Membrane oxygenator support for pulmonary insufficiency. Surg. Clin. N. Am. 54, 5:1171-78, Oct. 1974.

Hargreaves, A.: Emotional problems of patients with respiratory disease. Nurs. Clin. N. Am. 3, 3:479-487, Sept. 1968.

Helming, M. G.: Nursing of patients with chronic obstructive lung disease. Nurs. Clin. N. Am. 3, 4:413-428, Sept. 1968.

Hudak, C., et al: Critical Care Nursing. Philadelphia, J. B. Lippincott, 1973, pp. 131-209.

Jacoby, M. K.: The effect of nursing care on hospitalization of patients with chronic airway obstruction. Unpublished masters' thesis, University of Delaware, College of Nursing, Newark, Delaware, 1974.

Kass, I. and Sheets, P.: Emphysema: a new approach to an old disease. *NTRDA* Bull., pp. 14-16.

Kersten, L.: Chest-tube drainage system indications and principles of operation. Heart and Lung 3, 1:97-101, 1974.

Kilburn, K., et al: Byssinosis matter from lint to lungs. Am. J. Nurs. 73, 11:1952-1956, 1973.

King, T. K. C., et al: Oxygen transfer in catastrophic respiratory failure. Chest 65:405-445, Apr. 1974.

Krajna, K.: The relationship between upper and lower respiratory tracts in bronchial asthma. Ann. Otology 79:506-512, June 1970.

Larson, V.: The effect of preoperative teaching and specific nursing interventions on the postoperative pulmonary status of patients with chronic obstructive lung disease undergoing upper abdominal surgery. Unpublished masters' thesis, University of Delaware, College of Nursing, Newark, Delaware, 1973.

Lindeman, C.: Influencing recovery through preoperative teaching. Heart and Lung 2, 4:515-521, 1973.

Lyons, H. and Tabak, D.: Measurement of oxygen affinity of hemoglobin in hypoxemia in relation to acid-base status. Chest 61 2:265-395, Feb. 1972.

Luckman, J. and Sorenson, K.: Medical-Surgical Nursing. Philadelphia, W. B. Saunders, 1974, pp. 854-1038.

Marici, F.: The flexible fiberoptic bronchoscope. Am. J. Nurs. 73, 10:1176-1178, 1973.

Nett, L. and Petty, T.: Oxygen toxicity. Am. J. Nurs. 73, 9:1556-1558, 1973.

Petty, T. L.: A chest physician's perspective on asthma. Heart and Lung 1, 5:611-620, Sept.-Oct. 1972.

Petty, T. L.: Intensive and Rehabilitative Care, ed. 2. Philadelphia, Lea & Febiger, 1974.

Reister, B.: To identify the nursing action performed for selected adult patients in acute respiratory failure based on inferences relating to the clinical observations. Unpublished masters' thesis, University of Delaware, College of Nursing, Newark, Delaware, 1972.

Schell, P. and Campbell, A.: POMR—not just another way to chart. Nurs. Outlook 20, 8:510-514, Aug. 1972.

Scott, B.: Tensions linked with emphysema. Am. J. Nurs. 69, 5, Mar. 1969.

Secor, J.: Patient Care in Respiratory Problems. Philadelphia, W. B. Saunders, 1969, pp. 65-86; 164-180.

Sedlock, S.: Detection of chronic pulmonary disease. Am. J. Nurs. 72, 8, 1973. (Reprint distributed by the National League for Nursing.)

Selecky, P. A.: Tracheostomy: a review of present day indications, complications, and care. Heart and Lung 3, 3:272-281, Mar.-Apr. 1974.

Stichter, A.: A description of patient responses during the weaning process after prolonged artificial ventilation. Unpublished masters' thesis, University of Delaware, College of Nursing, Newark, Delaware, 1973.

Sutton, F.: Recognition and management of the adult respiratory distress syndrome. Chest 66:345-365, July 1974.

Traver, G. A.: Nursing the patient with respiratory insufficiency. League Exchange No. 96, New York, National League for Nursing, 1972.

Weiss, E.: Bronchial asthma. Clin. Symp. 27, 1 & 2. Summit, N.J., Ciba Pharmaceuticals, 1975.

Wilner, D., et al: Introduction to Public Health. New York, Macmillan, 1973, pp. 198-203, 217-219.

Yura, H. and Walsh, M.: The Nursing Process, ed 2. New York, Appleton-Century-Crofts, 1973.

15

Nursing Process in Providing Care for Patients With Diabetes Mellitus

PATRICIA A. LAWRENCE

The Process • Prevention • Case Finding and Diagnosis • Therapy and Control • Teaching the Diabetic Patient • Nursing Care • Summary

When the doctor called me in and told me I had diabetes I just looked at him. I couldn't believe it, and the first thing I said was "No, I don't either." I was shocked and upset, and I just couldn't believe that I had anything like that wrong with me. The first thing that came to my mind was, What am I going to do? I have diabetes, so my life is ended right now. I'm 18-years-old and I'm just as good as dead. It was as though he were telling me I had cancer and had only six months to live, or something.

I thought it meant I'd always be different. Wherever I went everybody was going to know that I was a diabetic, and I thought people would be afraid to be with me. I thought it was something to be ashamed of, and I was afraid to go anywhere. I felt I'd have to stay home and never see anybody.

We had studied about diabetes a little in biology in the tenth grade, but I had never *seen* anybody—you know, I thought they looked terrible, just like sticks and things. I just naturally assumed that a diabetic was like someone who had epilepsy or who had maybe one leg or something. I thought they would be sick all the time and look dead, and that anybody who was sick like that, who had a chronic disease, was just *doomed*—not doomed, really, but that they were just different from other people—that they couldn't date, or they couldn't go anywhere that other people went, like to the movies. I thought they were people who stayed at home a lot.

The preceding passage, quoted directly from a taped conversation with a 21-year-old diabetic patient, may seem surprising. Although the psychological and social needs of patients with many other types of chronic disability (epilepsy, facial deformity, paraplegia, and so on) are well documented and readily recognized, those of diabetics often tend to be overlooked because their disability is so much less overt.

Diabetes mellitus has all too often been considered a relatively "simple" chronic disease with which a person can live easily after learning a few basic facts and procedures. But the above patient and many others like her do not view diabetes as "simple," nor should health professionals. Diabetes is a complex disease, and its complexities have hardly begun to be understood. The diabetic's nursing needs are also complex, ranging from the intensive care and observation necessary for the patient in diabetic coma to the multiple teaching needs which must be met if the patient is to care for himself wisely. A diagnosis of diabetes also gives rise to many psychological, social, and family needs which the knowledgeable and understanding nurse can help the patient meet in a variety of ways.

To be able to give effective care to diabetic patients, the nurse must have a sound working knowledge of the current concept of the disease process and of the present-day philosophy of treatment. The following sections of this chapter provide such a framework, as well as a detailed discussion of the various aspects of nursing care which are relevant to the diabetic patient.

The Process

What is diabetes? For many years the disease was thought of simply as a malfunctioning of the islets of Langerhans in the pancreas. This attitude is understandable, both because of the overt derangement of carbohydrate metabolism and because the most apparent symptoms of diabetes respond dramatically to insulin therapy. However, such a concept is a gross oversimplification of a much more complex process which is now baffling the medical world, for research thus far has led to no convincing answers regarding the etiology or prevention of diabetes and its many chronic manifestations.

Thus, numerous theories are being explored and many questions are being asked: Is the malfunctioning of the pancreas the primary lesion in diabetes, or is it secondary to some disorder as yet unknown? Are the widespread abnormalities of the blood vessels (and a subsequent array of diabetic "complications") secondary to insulin lack and high blood sugar levels, or is the blood vessel disease a primary lesion in diabetes? What is the role of the pituitary, adrenal, and/or thyroid glands in the etiology of the disease? What part is played by glucagon? By proinsulin (the precursor to the insulin molecule)? Could diabetes be an autoimmune disease, or to what extent are viruses implicated?

The answers to these questions and many more await further research.

MANIFESTATIONS

IMPAIRED METABOLISM. Diabetes mellitus is characterized by an inadequate insulin supply and/or a delayed insulin response. Although it may seem contradictory, there are many diabetics who have above-normal insulin levels. However, this is explained by the fact that they are obese, for obese persons in general (nondiabetic as well as diabetic) have markedly increased insulin levels. Why this is true is not clearly understood, although there are several theories involving hormonal imbalances and insulin antagonists. Thus, the obese diabetic may have an above-normal insulin level when compared with nondiabetics in general, but insulin deficiency exists because the level is below normal when compared to nondiabetics who are obese.

When the supply of insulin is inadequate, metabolism is impaired on several levels. Insulin normally plays a major role not only in carbohydrate metabolism, but also in fat and protein metabolism. It is necessary in the synthesis of glycogen, fat, and protein; it plays a major role in the transport of glucose through cell membranes; it inhibits the breakdown of fat into fatty acids; and it increases amino acid transport. Thus insulin deficiency per se causes a vast array of symptoms.

The most well-known symptoms are the three "polys"—polyuria, polydipsia, and polyphagia. The explanation for this triad is simple. As the blood sugar level rises and the renal threshold is exceeded, the kidneys begin to excrete glucose. Because of the increased osmotic load in the urine, the kidneys must also excrete increased amounts of urine (polyuria). As a result of this fluid loss, the patient becomes thirsty (polydipsia), but the additional intake may not compensate for the loss of fluid, and dehydration results. Further dehydration occurs because the osmotic pressure within the bloodstream is increased by the high-glucose content, and fluid is thus drawn out of the cells. Therefore, the patient with advanced untreated disease exhibits marked intracellular and extracellular dehydration, and thirst may be severe. Increased appetite (polyphagia) is a result of the fact that the body is unable to obtain the nourishment it needs because of faulty metabolism. However, although the patient may consume additional amounts of food, he or she is unable to utilize it properly and, as a result, loses weight.

In addition to the three polys, other symptoms result from inadequate metabolism. When the body can no longer use carbohydrate as a major source of energy, it turns to a breakdown of fats and proteins (fats primarily) to meet its energy needs. In the diabetic, this process is speeded by the lack of insulin for, as stated above, insulin inhibits the breakdown of fat into fatty acids. The intermediary products of fat metabolism (acetone, acetoacetic acid and beta-hydroxybutyric acid) are thus increased. The patient begins to become acidotic, and acetone appears in the urine. As the body attempts to excrete these ketone bodies there is a loss of sodium, potassium, and other electrolytes. However, despite the net loss of potassium, the patient may be hyperkalemic, for, in the processes of dehydration and tissue breakdown, potassium moves from the cells to the extracellular fluid.

The patient in ketoacidosis may exhibit still other symptoms. Some of the most common are nausea, vomiting, and abdominal pain.

As ketoacidosis increases, the body attempts to compensate for the downward shift in pH by getting rid of excess hydrogen ions. This is accomplished as the acidemia stimulates the respiratory center, resulting in deep, labored respirations which blow off increased amounts of carbon dioxide ($H+ + HCO_3 - \leftrightarrows CO_2 + H_2O$). This type of breathing is known as Kussmaul's respirations and is accompanied by the fruity odor of acetone in the breath.

In advanced ketoacidosis, the accumulation of the toxic ketone bodies gradually results in a loss of consciousness. The patient then presents the typical symptoms of a person in diabetic coma: unconsciousness, dehydration, air hunger, acetone odor of the breath, hyperglycemia, glycosuria, acetone in the urine (ketonuria), and profound acidosis with electrolyte imbalances.

There is also a type of diabetic coma which is not associated with ketoacidosis. This is called nonketotic hyperosmolar coma, and occurs most frequently in older patients with a mild form of diabetes. Blood sugar levels are high and dehydration is marked. The reason for the lack of ketoacidosis is not entirely clear, but it is probably in large part due to the fact that these individuals have sufficient insulin production to prevent rapid fat breakdown. This type of coma usually follows a period of stress such as an illness, and it is associated with a relatively high mortality rate.

Fortunately, for many diabetics, coma and ketoacidosis are not imminent threats, except possibly under conditions of severe stress or infection. Ketoacidosis is a constant threat, however, to those who have the juvenile-onset type of diabetes for they generally produce no insulin endogenously, and their carbohydrate intolerance is thus severe. Some of these individuals experience little difficulty. However, for many the entire course of the disease is labile, and they must be constantly on the alert to avoid the acute symptoms of diabetes.

ATHEROSCLEROSIS AND MICROANGIOPATHY. Since the acute symptoms of diabetes can, for the most part, be controlled, and diabetics are thus living longer than they used to, we are now seeing an increasing incidence of the chronic manifestations of the disease. Considering the relatively large percentage of the total population which has diabetes, these chronic manifestations can truly be termed a major health problem.

Atherosclerosis and microangiopathy are among the most major of these chronic manifestations. A susceptibility to these diseases at an early age often causes such difficulties as hypertension, myocardial infarction, congestive heart failure, and slow wound healing. Blood vessel changes in the lower extremities are frequently severe, and it is not uncommon for an older diabetic with long-standing disease to require extensive amputation because of gangrene following a seemingly minor injury to the toe or foot. Vascular changes are also implicated in many of the other symptoms commonly associated with the disease (See below).

NEPHROPATHY. Several types of renal disease, such as infections and papillary necrosis, seem to occur more frequently in diabetics than in nondiabetics. Renal failure may then result. One of the most common types of renal involvement is a form of glomerulosclerosis, Kimmelstiel-Wilson syndrome, a disorder found almost solely in diabetics.

CHANGES IN THE EYES. Diabetic retinopathy, a result of aneurysms and hemorrhages of the capillaries within the retina, is one of the chief causes of blindness in the United States. Two major means of stopping its progression or bringing about its reversal are presently being used: photocoagulation (a method of coagulating and thus obliterating the microaneurysms) and pituitary ablation (a destruction of the pituitary gland by any of several methods). Just how pituitary ablation causes improvement in retinopathy is not entirely clear, although it is thought to be related to the level of growth hormone. This procedure is used much less frequently than photocoagulation, although both are currently considered to be experimental methods. Despite these advances, however, retinopathy still presents a major problem.

Diabetics also have other difficulties with their vision. For instance, cataract formation and glaucoma are both common and may occur at an earlier age than usual.

NEUROPATHIES. Neurological disturbances can affect so many parts of the body that diabetes often imitates other conditions. Cranial, spinal, and autonomic nerves may be involved. The symptoms vary in intensity from vague aches and pains or paresthesias to complete loss of sensation. Motor weakness, loss of bladder control, severe urinary retention, diarrhea or constipation, orthostatic hypotension, and delayed gastric emptying are but a few of the other varied symptoms which may occur. It also seems likely that the relatively high incidence of impotence among male diabetics is caused primarily by nerve involvement.

INCREASED SUSCEPTIBILITY TO INFECTION. Not only is the diabetic more susceptible to infection, but any infection is more prone to rapid extension and must be treated quickly and vigorously. It has been shown that phagocytosis is impaired in the presence of hyperglycemia, and, therefore, careful control of the blood sugar level can help prevent problems of this nature.

INCREASED DIFFICULTY DURING PREGNANCY. Although many diabetic mothers give birth to healthy babies, the likelihood of difficulty in pregnancy is greater for them than for nondiabetics. Rigid medical supervision and control are necessary. Common difficulties are toxemia, hydramnios, congenital anomalies, and perinatal mortality. To minimize the danger of intrauterine death, labor is generally induced or a cesarean section is performed in the thirty-fifth to thirty-ninth week of gestation. The optimal time for delivery is determined both by the mother's symptoms (occurrence of toxemia and so on) and by a combination of various types of monitoring. For instance, decreasing urinary estriol levels indicate placental failure and give warning of impending difficulty for the fetus, so these determinations are usually made frequently toward the end of pregnancy.

PRECIPITATING FACTORS

There are several precipitating or predisposing factors which influence the development of diabetes.

GENETIC PREDISPOSITION. It seems clear that heredity plays an important role in predisposing a person to diabetes. This has been a difficult area to research, however, and current data do not clearly fit any one theory. In the past, many felt that diabetes was transmitted as an autosomal recessive trait, but there is now strong evidence to support a multifactorial mode of inheritance. Although a consistently valid prediction of the development of overt diabetes is not yet possible on the basis of genetics alone, the hereditary nature of the disease must be taken into account in considering other determinants. (See Chapter 6 for further discussion of the role of heredity in diabetes.)

STRESS. The role that various types of stresses play in the course of diabetes is receiving considerable attention today, and the basis for their having a direct influence on blood sugar is sound. Adrenal hormones are liberated in varying amounts as a result of stress, and these hormones act to raise blood sugar even in the nondiabetic. (For example, one of the actions of adrenalin is to cause the liver to release its glycogen stores in the form of glucose. The glucocorticoids, which are also secreted by the adrenal glands in times of stress, have the promotion of glucogenesis as one of their major functions.) Thus, stress is sometimes seen as a precipitating factor in diabetes. It also often plays a major role in adversely affecting diabetic control.

OBESITY. Obesity seems to decrease the body's sensitivity to insulin, so larger amounts of insulin are needed to maintain normal metabolism. Thus, a diabetic who still has some pancreatic function may be able to produce enough insulin if body weight is within normal limits, and yet not be able to increase insulin production enough to meet the added demands of obesity. Many diabetics are able to attain satisfactory control of blood sugar merely by losing weight.

PREGNANCY. Not only does diabetes endanger the fetus, but pregnancy itself has a diabetogenic effect. The insulin needs of the diabetic mother usually increase markedly after the first trimester, probably due to the production of insulin antagonists by the growing placenta and to increased placental degradation of insulin. During pregnancy, a nondiabetic mother may also experience carbohydrate intolerance (gestational diabetes), although this effect is usually reversed following delivery. A woman who has had gestational diabetes should remain on the alert for the possible development of overt diabetes in later years.

DRUGS. There are two major types of drugs that are likely to precipitate diabetes in a person who is otherwise predisposed:

1. *Steroids*. The effect of the endogenous release of glucocorticoids has already been mentioned in relation to the role of stress in diabetes. The therapeutic administration of steroids has a similar effect. Upon withdrawal, the added glucose intolerance is usually reversible, but a response of even temporary hyperglycemia in a person thought to be nondiabetic may herald the development of overt diabetes at a later date. (See chapter 18 for additional material concerning the nature and action of steroid drugs.)

2. *Thiazide Diuretics*. This group of diuretics has been found to increase the body's need for insulin. The mechanism by which this occurs is not clearly understood. As with steroids, the effect is generally reversible upon withdrawal of the drug, but the patient who has had this response may later become diabetic.

OTHER FACTORS. Diabetes has also been found to be associated with other factors. It is much more common in women than in men, and the incidence varies from country to country and from race to race. The disease is increasing in the United States.* Although such trends may be partially related to diet and age, the exact reason for them is still unclear and probably awaits a more precise understanding of the true nature of the disease.

Prevention

The prevention of diabetes is a difficult topic to discuss because of the many unanswered questions regarding the etiology of the disease. However, several factors which may precipitate diabetes are known, and the occurrence of symptoms may be prevented or delayed by determining those who are potential diabetics and helping them avoid these factors. This help consists primarily of encouraging them to maintain normal weight or in helping those who are overweight to reduce.

Teaching and guidance during this phase of care are vital. Nurses play an important part in these aspects of care, for they are in a position to help disseminate information to the general public as well as to people whom they find to be within a high-risk group for the disease.

There are a number of high-risk groups toward whom preventive efforts should be aimed. Because of the genetic factor, anyone with a family history of diabetes is suspect. Those with two

*In quoting unpublished material from the 1973 Health Interview Survey, the Workgroup on Epidemiology for the National Commission on Diabetes reported that the current rate of diabetes is 20.4 per 1000 population.[1] This contrasts with a rate of 14.5 per 1000 population reported in 1968.[2]

diabetic parents are particularly susceptible. Women over age 40 are more susceptible than younger women or men, especially if they are obese. Women who have had gestational diabetes or those who have delivered large babies (over 9 pounds) are in a particularly high-risk group.

Another aspect of prevention is that of controlling the inheritance of the disease. Many feel that diabetics should not intermarry, but there is not total agreement on this. Regardless of the advice which is given, it seems unrealistic to think that this type of measure will significantly decrease the incidence of the disease when one considers the social forces which influence marriage and the numbers of people who are undiagnosed diabetics or who will become diabetic later in life. However, both diabetics and those with a family history of diabetes should be made aware of the risk of transmitting the diabetic predisposition to their children. They should also know that this risk is markedly increased if both parents have a positive family history. Nurses frequently have the opportunity for this type of counseling.

It appears that another method of preventing some cases of diabetes may be forthcoming, for viruses have now been implicated in causing diabetes in mice who have an inherited predisposition for the disease. Several reports over many years have also suggested that some cases of juvenile diabetes in man may be linked to virus infections. Thus it seems feasible that in the future some type of immunization may be possible to prevent those cases of diabetes which may be virus related.

Case Finding and Diagnosis

It is known that there are a great many undiagnosed diabetics. Although considerable attention is directed toward screening programs for diabetes, many are now questioning a major emphasis on this approach. Does a single negative test give a misleading and potentially harmful false security? Does present knowledge about the value (or lack of value) of early treatment justify a major effort to uncover asymptomatic cases of diabetes? Are medical resources sufficiently available to provide appropriate follow-up for those who have a positive screening test? Does the relatively small number of new diabetics who are found in a screening program justify the time and expense of the program? These questions are constantly being asked. However, screening is carried on in many places and by many groups, with the aim of minimizing some symptoms and avoiding others by instituting early treatment and teaching. (See pp. 459 to 461 for a discussion of the current concept of the value of treatment.)

When screening programs are held, participation by those who fall within one or more of the high-risk groups should be particularly encouraged. At the very least, such programs should focus primarily on adults over age 40, for this is the group in which the disease is most common and in which the onset is most likely to be insidious. Children and young adults generally have such an acute onset that they seek medical care immediately. Therefore, the traditional type of screening efforts within younger groups are largely nonproductive.

Although various screening methods are used, a blood sugar test taken two hours after a meal (two-hour postprandial blood sugar) is generally considered the most satisfactory test available for this purpose. It is a more useful screening tool than a fasting blood sugar test, for many diabetics exhibit normal values prior to food intake. Yet after eating, their blood sugars remain elevated for a longer period than normal.

Examination os the urine for sugar is another common test but is relatively unreliable. It has been used frequently in the past, for easy and inexpensive testing procedures have been developed. At best, this method constitutes a very rough screening device, for large numbers of false positives and negatives occur and may be misleading. The appearance of sugar in the urine depends upon the individual's renal threshold, which may vary markedly from person to person. This means that noniabetics may spill sugar in the urine despite normal blood glucose levels, or that it is entirely possible for a person to have clinical diabetes with an abnormally high blood sugar and yet evidence no glycosuria. Finally, there are occasional discrepancies in reading the results of these tests, even among trained personnel.[3] For these reasons, postprandial blood sugar tests have largely replaced urine testing in screening programs.

Although elevated postprandial or fasting blood sugars may be definitive enough to make a diagnosis possible, patients with positive single tests often must undergo further testing. A number of factors other than diabetes may cause abnormal results. Carbohydrate intolerance increases with age, and an elderly person with an elevated postprandial blood sugar should be tested carefully before a diagnosis is made. The time of day, previous dietary intake, certain drugs, activity, and emotional stress also influence carbohydrate tolerance and blood sugar levels. A fact which is all too frequently overlooked is that studies have shown that many hospitalized patients have elevated postprandial blood sugars, but not diabetes. Inactivity, stress, drugs, and other aspects of illness decrease glucose tolerance and may be responsible for these findings. Caution should be taken not to make a hasty diagnosis on such individuals, and they should be carefully retested when they are well.

GLUCOSE TOLERANCE TESTS

When postprandial or fasting blood sugar tests leave doubt as to the diagnosis, an oral glucose tolerance test is usually performed. This consists of drawing a fasting blood sugar, administering a specified amount of glucose (generally 100 Gm or an amount determined on the basis of weight and height), and obtaining hourly or half-hourly blood sugars for a total of from three to five hours. Typical normal and abnormal results are shown in Figure 15–1. Note that the diabetic's blood sugar level is not only higher, but also much slower in returning to the fasting level. Another interesting phenomenon is also pictured in Figure 15–1. *Hypo*glycemia several hours after ingesting glucose may be indicative of early diabetes. In fact, sometimes unknown diabetics first seek medical help because of the symptoms of hypoglycemia (see p. 481) several hours after meals. This occurs because insulin release is delayed and, therefore, the effect is continued even after the blood sugar has returned to normal.

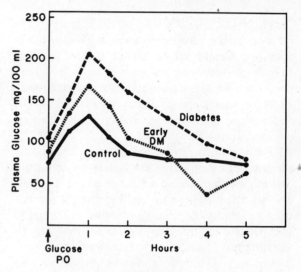

FIGURE 15-1.
Typical glucose responses to oral glucose tolerance testing in normal subjects, those with overt diabetes mellitus, and those with early diabetes with reactive hypoglycemia. Annals of The New York Academy of Sciences, Vol. 148, Art. 3, p. 780, Edward S. Horton, Bagher, M. Sheikholislam & R. Bressler. © The New York Academy of Sciences; 1968. Reprinted by permission.

Although the glucose tolerance test is generally accepted as the most definitive standard test for diabetes, variations in results of several tests on the same individual indicate that the test by no means yields 100 percent accuracy in diagnosis. Other factors which affect carbohydrate metabolism must still be considered, and the results must be viewed in light of other signs and symptoms of the disease. There has also been disagreement over the years as to how the test should be carried out and how the results should be interpreted. The American Diabetes Association has provided guidelines for the test's proper use,[4] although other sources establish slightly different criteria. A survey has also revealed the marked differences that exist in interpreting the results, even among diabetes specialists.[5]

Nurses frequently assist in carrying out glucose tolerance tests or in teaching patients what they must do. Unless the test is performed properly, the results will be misleading. There are several steps where difficulty is often encountered.

PREPARATION. Because of the effects of illness on carbohydrate tolerance, a glucose tolerance test should not be carried out for at least two weeks following an acute illness. It is best done on ambulatory patients, although strenuous exercise should be avoided for at least eight hours prior to the test. Smoking should also be avoided during this period.

Dietary preparation is extremely important, for any degree of starvation causes an abnormal and misleading glucose tolerance curve. In addition to being well nourished in general, the patient's carbohydrate intake must be *at least* 150 Gm per day for three days prior to the test. Although this consideration is extremely important, it is frequently forgotten by physicians and nurses administering the test. Patients must be specifically instructed regarding carbohydrate intake, and their intake carefully assessed before the test is done. It is equally important that the patient fast for eight hours immediately prior to the test. The results are invalid if the patient eats food at any time before the last blood specimen is drawn.

ADMINISTRATION OF GLUCOSE. Either commercial preparations of glucose may be used, or glucose powder may be dissolved in water. This beverage is so sweet that it tends to produce nausea in many patients, especially since they are in the fasting state. Adding unsweetened lemon juice to a glucose and water solution is allowed and is used routinely to decrease the sweetness and make the drink more palatable. Ice is added just prior to offering it to the patient, although warm water must be used initially to dissolve the glucose. Despite these precautions, some patients still vomit after drinking the solution. This, of course, makes the test invalid and is reason to terminate it for that day.

TIMING OF THE SPECIMENS. To assure meaningful results, the drawing of blood sugars must be timed accurately. This means the patient is encouraged to drink the entire glucose mixture within a very few minutes so that an accurate beginning time can be established. The actual drawing of the blood is generally not the nurse's responsibility, but she may be requested to obtain urine specimens at the same time intervals and test them for the presence of glucose.

OTHER DIAGNOSTIC TESTS

In addition to the standard glucose tolerance test, there are other types of tests which are sometimes used, including the two-dose glucose tolerance test, the tolbutamide response test, the intravenous glucose tolerance test, and the cortisone-glucose tolerance test. The latter test gives information which may be helpful in determining the prediabetic state.

IMPACT OF DIAGNOSIS

Although up to this point the emphasis has been on the mechanical aspects of diagnosis, the psychological effects of being diagnosed as a diabetic must not be overlooked. The patient who was quoted at the beginning of this chapter graphically indicates the impact that the diagnosis had on her, and such a response is by no means uncommon. Kimball[6] has presented a very vivid documentation of patients' feelings about the disease, and anyone who has contact with diabetics and allows them to express their feelings can readily supplement this documentation. Nor are such feelings limited to those who have a severe form of diabetes. An older woman who is completely diet controlled read the beginning of this chapter and stated, "I know exactly what she meant. I *really* felt doomed."

The feeling of doom or fright in patients and family members may stem from several causes, the most common of which are: 1) fear of the unknown; 2) knowing someone who suffered severe complications—amputation, renal failure, blindness, and so on; 3) fear of giving themselves daily injections; 4) realization of the need to diet, particularly for the obese person who "lives to eat" or for the youth who feels a need to "go along with the crowd"; 5) belief that it is contagious and/or cause for shame. One patient even thought diabetes was "caught" through intercourse and attributed to it the social stigma of venereal disease.

Not all patients, of course, experience this much fright or shame. But nurses must be aware of such a possibility and remain alert for indications of need. Patients should be given ample opportunity to air their fears. Misconceptions can be cleared up, and appropriate information supplied. The very act of disclosing their concerns to someone who demonstrates understanding and support may help them over the hurdle. It is interesting to note that after correlating diabetic control with many facets of care, Williams said "continued support for the patient may be as important and rewarding as teaching per se."[7]

In dealing with patients' concerns over the occurrence of complications, nurses frequently question how much patients should be told. Although many unjustified fears can be dispelled, it is also clear that the outlook is not wholly optimistic. However, since for many diabetics the course of the disease is relatively benign and since effective treatment is thought to decrease the severity of "complications," the truth can usually be told without causing undue alarm.

A diagnosis of diabetes also has a financial impact on the patient. The need for medications, supplies, and medical care on a continuing basis can be a financial drain, particularly when one considers that a large percentage of diabetics are in the lower income groups.[8] In addition, diabetics have been discriminated against in various ways, often without sound reason. Employment and educational opportunities have been closed to them, and various types of insurance have been difficult or impossible to obtain. Today employers are becoming more aware of the fact that most diabetics make safe and reliable workers, and although there is still discrimination, most jobs are available to well-controlled diabetics. Those who are likely to have insulin reactions should not be employed where such a reaction would be a potential hazard (flying airplanes, working at heights, and the like), and such jobs are understandably closed to them. Insurance is also becoming more available, although for many diabetics there are still severe limitations.

Therapy and Control

The numerous unanswered questions concerning the etiology and course of diabetes have caused present-day methods of treatment to be far from 100-percent effective. In the future, the answers to these questions hopefully will lead either to prevention or at least to more effective treatment. In the meantime, diet, exercise, and drugs (insulin and oral hypoglycemic agents) are used to keep the patient's metabolic disorders under control, while the other symptoms which may be connected with the disease are treated according to the pathology involved. New approaches to treatment are continually being sought, with transplantation and the development of an artificial pancreas currently taking the limelight. There is reason to be optimistic about both approaches, although there is a great deal more research to be done before either can be applied widely in the treatment of diabetes.

At present, diet and antidiabetic drugs are the main forms of therapy. Although basic information about these types of treatment is readily available elsewhere and a detailed discussion is beyond the scope of this chapter, there are several issues related to treatment which deserve discussion here.*

MAJOR ISSUES

THE DEFINITION AND VALUE OF CONTROL. Present-day control of diabetes generally implies the absence, or near absence, of glycosuria, the absence of ketonuria, and a fasting blood sugar at or near the normal level without frequent hypoglycemic episodes. However, no single definition of "good" control has been agreed upon, and physicians differ as to the importance they attach to rigid control. It is clear that an extreme lack of control with resultant ketoacidosis can be incapacitating or even life threatening. But what of the patient with a moderately elevated blood sugar who goes about his daily activities without apparent discomfort or ill effect? Is any harm being done?

It is now known that a lack of control increases the occurrence of some of the complications of diabetes, such as infections, neuropathies, and diabetic cataracts. But there is much less agreement about its effect on the vascular symptoms, which may be serious and life threatening. Many physicians are now convinced that these, too, are lessened when a diabetic remains in good control for, although studies to date have been somewhat conflicting, there is a

---

*For basic information about drug and diet therapy see pharmacology, diet therapy, and medical references. The remainder of this chapter assumes a basic knowledge of these components of treatment.

progressive accumulation of evidence that the chronic vascular manifestations of diabetes are related to the level of blood sugar. Therefore the trend is now for more rigid control than in the past, although not all subscribe to this philosophy of treatment.

One of the difficulties in getting a definitive answer to this question is that present-day treatment is, at best, far from ideal. One, two, or even three carefully planned insulin injections per day cannot begin to provide the fine control resulting from the constant monitoring of blood sugar and the subsequent adjustment of insulin release which takes place in the nondiabetic. Therefore, even diabetics who are in good control by the strictest present-day standards do not maintain *normal* blood sugars, and this lack of fine control may be responsible for the symptoms these patients develop. A final answer to the question probably awaits the perfection of a method of control which more nearly approximates normal, that is, transplantation or the artificial pancreas.

Meanwhile, patients can be told that their chances of developing complications will be less if they keep their diabetes under good control. Unfortunately, they cannot be promised an absence of such complications.

SAFETY OF THE ORAL AGENTS. In the late spring of 1970, statements were made in the news media concerning a study (the University Group Diabetes Program, or UGDP) ahich had shown that tolbutamide (Orinase) might lead to an early death from cardiovascular failure. Patients panicked and their physicians began receiving a flood of inquiries. Unfortunately, this information caught many physicians unaware, for the published report of the study did not appear in the medical literature until later that fall.[9] To add to the confusion, there was marked disagreement as to whether the study results were valid or not, and many noted diabetes specialists took stands in both professional and lay media as being strongly opposed to the implications of the study and its reported results. They cited numerous reasons for its lack of validity[10] and published statements saying that they would continue using the drugs. Even statisticians found justification for both sides of the argument.[11,12]

In the midst of this controversy, the Food and Drug Administration published a recommendation that "the use of Orinase and other sulfonylurea type agents . . . should be limited to those patients with symptomatic adult onset nonketotic diabetes mellitus which cannot be adequately controlled by diet or weight loss alone and in whom the addition of insulin is impractical or unacceptable."[13] The opponents of the study immediately took issue with the FDA, charging that its statement was premature and unjustified, that it was interfering with the practice of medicine, and that diabetics were thus being harmed.

Subsequently, the National Institutes of Health (which provided the funding for the UGDP) requested that the Biometric Society reanalyze the data and submit an opinion. Although in its report the Biometric Society agreed that there were some reservations about the conclusions of the study, they felt that the UGDP trial had "raised suspicions that cannot be dismissed on the basis of other evidence presently available."[14]

Thus, although several years have now passed since the study was published, and the din is not as loud as it was previously, the battle still rages. The overall outcome is that these drugs are still being used by many physicians, but with apparently more caution. It is, however, clear that the last chapter in the story has not yet been written.

COMPOSITION OF THE DIABETIC DIET. Another issue which has caused questions and misunderstanding is the recommended carbohydrate content in the diabetic diet. In September 1971, the Committee on Food and Nutrition of the American Diabetes Association published a statement entitled "Principles of Nutrition and Dietary Recommendations for Patients with Diabetes Mellitus: 1971."[15] In this report the statement was made that the usual proportion of carbohydrate in the normal diet (45 percent) was considered acceptable for most diabetics. This contrasted with the long-held theory that diabetics should restrict carbohydrates—a practice which necessarily raises the proportion of ingested fat and, therefore, is contradictory to the present-day concern about dietary fat, blood cholesterol, and atherosclerosis. Again the public press caused a furor. Not only did it report the recommendation regarding carbohydrate content, but in doing so it often implied that the use of sugar and concentrated sweets was therefore condoned. This, of course, was not the intent of the recommendation. As a matter of fact, elsewhere in the ADA report the authors specifically warned against using simple sugars.

Although there is still some disagreement regarding the optimal composition of the diabetic diet, the trend is strong toward decreasing the amount of fat. In the spring of 1976, both the American Dietetic Association and the American Diabetes Association revised their recommended exchange lists to emphasize the use of low-fat milk and meat products in contrast to those with a high-fat content.

FACTORS AFFECTING CONTROL

Despite the degree of control which is possible with the current drugs and with our knowledge of a diabetic's nutritional needs, diabetics are frequently not in good control. Why? Several of the most important factors are outlined below.

LABILE DIABETES. Some diabetics have an unstable form of the disease which is known as "labile" or "brittle." To some extent, all juvenile-type diabetics are in this category. However, a few have extreme difficulty in being controlled, and these are the individuals to whom the terms generally apply. Day-to-day blood sugars may vary greatly, and very small changes in insulin dosage, diet, exercise, or stress may cause profound symptoms of hyper- or hypoglycemia. Even at times when there is no apparent change in regimen, blood sugars can vary markedly. Labile diabetics must have an excellent understanding of their disease and the measures to be taken to avoid severe acidotic or hypoglycemic attacks. Close medical supervision is imperative.

INSULIN RESISTANCE. An occasional diabetic develops insulin resistance to the extent that hyperglycemia may not be controlled even with hundreds of units of insulin daily. The production of large numbers of antibodies is felt to be responsible for this problem of control. Although the antigenicity of beef insulin is relatively high, it is the major ingredient in most insulin preparations because of its availability. Pork insulin more nearly resembles human insulin in structure, and switching the insulin-resistant patient from beef to pork insulin may be the only action necessary. Some patients may require one of the modified forms of pure pork insulin (sulfated pork insulin, or the highly purified single-component insulin, both of which are investigational), which seems to be even less antigenic than the usual pork insulin. Others must be placed on large doses of steroids for a brief period of time in order to overcome the antibody response. Since insulin resistance can end abruptly, patients receiving any of the above treatments must be watched carefully in order to avoid severe hypoglycemia.

EMOTIONAL STRESS. The literature dealing with the role of the emotions in affecting diabetic control is abundant, and ranges all the way from descriptions of case studies in which stress has clearly been a major factor in repeated episodes of acidosis[16] to a discussion of a demonstrated placebo effect in some patients receiving oral hypoglycemic agents.[17] Most of this literature emphasizes the adverse effect of stress upon diabetic control. This effect may be due not only to the stress reaction itself, but also to inadequate performance of the methods of control (medication and diet) during such times.

SURGERY. Surgery creates a major source of emotional and physical stress. Patients are generally controlled by frequent doses of regular insulin rather than by their usual doses of long-acting insulin. Those who ordinarily receive oral hypoglycemic agents and those whose disease is controlled by diet alone usually require the addition of insulin at times of major surgery.

EXERCISE. Exercise is a helpful adjunct to other types of diabetic therapy, for exercise itself has an insulinlike effect, increasing the body's utilization of glucose without adding insulin. By the same token, it is easy for a diabetic to run into problems of control because of changes in activity. At any time when activity is expected to exceed the usual, the diabetic on medication must be prepared either to adjust the insulin or diet according to guide lines laid down by the physician, or to combat possible hypoglycemic attacks with a ready supply of carbohydrate. The reverse is true, of course, when activity is decreased.

INFECTION. When a diabetic develops an infection (which he easily does), his need for insulin is likely to increase markedly. The reason for this is not entirely understood, although an increase in the production of insulin antibodies with resultant insulin resistance may sometimes play a role. The stress of infection and the increased metabolism caused by fever can also increase insulin need. Thus, infection is frequently the primary cause when a diabetic's disease goes out of control.

DRUGS. There are numerous drugs which affect blood sugar, including some with synergistic or antagonistic actions in combination with either insulin or the oral hypoglycemic agents. As would be expected, diabetic control may be markedly influenced when these are taken. At times, the use of such drugs is contraindicated, while in other instances diabetic therapy may need to be altered. Two such groups of drugs—steroids and thiazide diuretics—have already been discussed (see p. 455). Other commonly used drugs which may increase a diabetic's blood sugar are diphenylhydantoin (Dilantin), thyroid preparations, and some of the oral contraceptives. On the other hand, alcohol is sometimes a major factor in cases of severe hypoglycemia.

Since there are many drugs which may have such actions, it is wise to check carefully before starting new drug therapy. Hansten's volume, *Drug Interactions,* is a particularly helpful reference for this purpose.[18]

FAILURE TO ADHERE TO THE PRESCRIBED REGIMEN. Since diet and hypoglycemic drugs have a direct relationship to one another and to the patient's disease, any failure to adhere to the prescribed regimen may influence control. This problem is much more critical for labile, ketosis-prone diabetics than for others, but it is certainly important for all. Unfortunately, the diabetic regimen is not necessarily as simple as it is sometimes thought to be. The types of dif-

ficulties which patients have in carrying out physicians' orders often seem almost endless. Many of these difficulties will be dealt with in the remainder of this chapter.

Teaching the Diabetic Patient

Everyone agrees that diabetic patients need teaching. However, it is not as easy to know which patients should be taught, and when. Certainly newly diagnosed diabetics need instruction, but the need of those who have lived with the disease for a number of years is not as obvious. Unfortunately it cannot be assumed that they are carrying out procedures properly or are basing their daily management on a sound informational base. For example, a study by Watkins et al in 1967 revealed some sobering findings. In analyzing the performance of 60 insulin-dependent diabetic patients who regularly attended the diabetes specialty clinics in two university medical centers, the following information was obtained:

33 percent had unacceptable equipment

77 percent sterilized their equipment in an unacceptable manner

18 percent did not sterilize their equipment

80 percent performed insulin administration in an unacceptable manner

52 percent made an error in insulin dosage, ranging from 5 percent to 100 percent error

45 percent tested their urine incorrectly and used the results in a way which was likely to be detrimental to their diabetic control

48 percent gave less than adequate foot care

Only one patient was found to perform acceptably in all five areas of management—diet, foot care, insulin dosage and administration, and urine testing.[19]

Further analysis of the data in the Watkins study revealed that there was a positive correlation between the length of time the patient had had diabetes and the number of errors made in insulin dosage.[20] Special note should be made of this, for all too frequently it is felt that because a person has lived with diabetes for a number of years he knows more about caring for his condition than do many of the health professionals. In some cases this is certainly true, but it is also very apparent that misinformation and a gross lack of information are prevalent among this group of patients. Nor do such shortcomings seem to be respecters of intelligence, educational level, or socioeconomic status.

Take, for example, the case of Mr. L., who is singled out here not because he is different, but because he is so similar to many other diabetics. He was from a lower-middle-class family, and seemed to be of average intelligence. He was able to read, he held a regular job, and he owned a small home.

> As far as Mr. L. was concerned, things seemed to be going along well. But he came into the clinic one day with a slightly elevated blood sugar and a history of positive urine tests, so his doctor decided to increase his insulin. In addition, when the doctor found out that in order to give his two kinds of insulin, Mr. L. was giving himself two injections each morning, he suggested that they both be mixed in one syringe. Mr. L. said he thought he could do that without any trouble, and was about to leave for home. Upon further questioning, though, it was found that he had considerable difficulty. He understood the increase in dosage adequately, and had no difficulty determining what the combined dose should be. But he ran into trouble when he tried to mix the two kinds of insulin in one syringe. He hadn't been in the habit of injecting air into the vial each time he withdrew a dose, so by the time the vial was half empty he had created a considerable vacuum. When he tried to mix the doses he found it almost impossible not to get one kind of insulin into the other vial . . . and he really didn't think this would make a great deal of difference as long as the total dose was accurate!

> Mr. L. was taught the proper method of mixing insulin, and he did well with it. Further questioning and a home visit revealed several other problems. First, Mr. L. never sterilized his syringe, and, although he was keeping his needle in alcohol, the alcohol was rarely changed. In addition, he was injecting only in his left arm, and this area was filled with hard knots. The fact that he was using a short intradermal needle resulted in a very shallow injection and probably contributed to the problem. And who would have thought that the bottles of insulin which he

had just bought were already outdated? The pharmacist hadn't been careful about checking his stock, and Mr. L. didn't know that he should look for the expiration date.

Further problems also emerged; a misunderstanding between Mr. L. and his doctor regarding how to determine the need for additional regular insulin at night; confusion in interpreting the urine-test results; and an improper method of storing his urine-test equipment.

ASSESSMENT OF KNOWLEDGE AND PERFORMANCE

Both the study findings quoted above and experiences with many patients like Mr. L. point out the fact that the knowledge of previously diagnosed diabetics needs to be carefully assessed. Failure to do so leads one to overlook important needs or, at the other extreme, to submit patients to the meaningless repetition of facts which they already know. Nothing is more deadly than the latter, and it may well lead to boredom and alienation from further teaching endeavors.

On the other hand, the new diabetic may know nothing about diabetes and its management, or he may have accumulated numerous facts and/or misconceptions about it as a result of contact with others who have the disease. So his knowledge also must be assessed in order to provide him with the sound background he needs to care for himself wisely.

Assessment of a patient's knowledge of diabetes and its management is not a simple task, and a few casually asked questions are not sufficient. In-depth information about both knowledge and the performance of procedures is essential. Furthermore, questions must be carefully worded in order to elicit meaningful information. Consider, for example, the different responses you might get from each of the following approaches:

"Let's see. You take NPH insulin, don't you?"

"What kind of insulin do you take?"

"Please pick out your kind of insulin from the bottles I have here."

"Please let me see your bottle of insulin."

A "yes" answer to the first question is what you expect—and what you are most likely to get.

But what does it mean? Has the patient understood what you said? Does he want to please you at all costs? Is he afraid to disagree with you? Does he really not know what kind of insulin he takes, but assumes you must be right? This yes answer really gives you little assurance that he is using the kind of insulin you think he is using.

The second and third approaches give you more information. By asking the patient to name his insulin you are at least finding out if he knows. However, this in itself is no guarantee that he is naming the kind he is actually using. Take, for example, the patient who said he was using NPH and regular insulins, which was what the physician had ordered. However, when he was asked to pick out his insulins from a variety of bottles he selected NPH and protamine zinc. Further investigation showed that he actually was making the mistake. Does it sound far-fetched? Unfortunately, it happens all too frequently.

The fourth approach, that of seeing the patient's own insulin bottle, sometimes uncovers errors not detected by the previous three. Not only can you be certain that it is the correct insulin, but you can check other points, such as the appearance of the insulin in the bottle and the expiration date on the label. Thus, whenever possible, this approach should be used. (The third approach is a good substitute when the patient's own equipment is not available, as illustrated above.)

The same principles can be applied to other aspects of the diabetic regimen. For example, which approach in each of the following sets will give you the most information?

"Are you sticking to your diet?"
"Please tell me what you ate yesterday. Start with when you got up in the morning, and go right through the day."

"Your urine tests are going OK, aren't they?"
"Please describe to me how you test your urine."
"Here is some Clinitest. Please show me how you test your urine."
"May I see your testing equipment? Now let me see you test your specimen with it."

"You rotate injection sites, don't you?"
"Tell me where you give your injections."
"Please let me see the places where you give your injections."

From the above examples, both the pitfalls of the yes-no type of question with an implied answer and the advantage of asking open-ended questions can easily be seen. In addition, whenever possible, direct observation of equipment and procedures is strongly advised. At times patients seem so confident in what they are doing that it may seem unnecessary to observe their actual procedures. However, such observation usually pays off, for often patients do not really know what errors they are making. As illustrated above, this type of assessment is best done using the patient's own equipment whenever possible. Home visits are ideal for this, but out-patients can be asked to bring their equipment and medicines with them to each visit, and in-patients can ask family members to bring them the next time they visit.

Assessment of knowledge and performance is important for another major reason: that of establishing priorities for teaching. A frequent error in diabetic teaching is trying to cover too much at once—with the end result of teaching nothing. Thus, teaching needs must be determined, and a decision made as to which needs are urgent and which can be delayed until a later time.

Although a skilled interviewer who is intimately familiar with the needed information can conduct an effective assessment of knowledge and performance without a written guide, a form is generally helpful for several reasons (Fig. 15-2). Not only does it help the interviewer to be thorough and provide a guide for wording the questions, it also facilitates communication among the various members of the health team. Another advantage of a standard written tool is that it can be used to measure teaching effectiveness by comparing the results of an assessment made both before a teaching program and at a later date.

In addition to questioning a patient and observing his techniques, other types of observations can be made which will provide clues to his

INSULIN ADMINISTRATION

Patient's Name _Jane Doe_
Interview Date _March 2, 1971_
Interviewed by _P. Smith, R.N._

Doctor's orders: _NPH insulin, 25 units q AM_

Date of order: _10/14/70_   Ordered by: _Dr. Q. Jones_

---

1. WHAT INSULIN DID THE DOCTOR TELL YOU TO TAKE? (kind, strength, number of units, timing)

   NPH U-80 — 25 units
   every morning

2. DO YOU EVER TAKE A DIFFERENT DOSE FOR ANY REASON?
   _no_

3. SHOW ME THE INSULIN YOU HAVE ON HAND.

	1.	2.
Kind(s)	_NPH_	
Strength(s)	_U-80_	
Expiration Date(s)	_8/71_	

4. SHOW ME THE SYRINGE(s) AND NEEDLE(s) YOU HAVE ON HAND.

   Syringe calibration: _U-80_   Needle length _1/2"_ and gauge _# 26_

5. SHOW ME HOW YOU GET THINGS READY TO TAKE YOUR SHOT.

   Boiled ✓   Soaked in alcohol   Disposable Needle _____   Syringe _____

   Technique adequate .... Yes (No)
   Assembled without contamination .... (Yes) No

6. WHAT INSULIN DID YOU TAKE THIS MORNING? (kind, strength, number of units, time)

   NPH U-80 — 25 units - 7:30 am

7. PLEASE DRAW UP THAT DOSE.
   Used correct withdrawal technique .... (Yes) No

8. Amount measured: _28 units_
   (If on more than one daily dose, observe measurement of each.)

9. Uses correct injection technique .... (Yes) No

10. Injection sites show evidence of good care and adequate rotation .... (Yes) No

11. WHAT DO YOU DO ABOUT TAKING YOUR INSULIN IF YOU ARE TOO SICK TO EAT?
    skip that dose

12. WHO KNOWS HOW TO GIVE YOU INSULIN IF YOU ARE TOO SICK TO GIVE IT TO YOURSELF?
    husband

Comments:

Water didn't cover equipment

Dose incorrect — has some trouble seeing numbers

Needs instruction re sick days

FIGURE 15.2. Assessment Guide: Insulin Administration.[21]
This guide is one of a series which has been prepared in order to help assess a diabetic patient's performance of various aspects of his care. Notice that an emphasis is put upon *observation*. Assessment based upon what a patient actually does rather than upon his description of what he does frequently reveals important teaching needs.

teaching needs. For example, the diabetic who has had an infection for a week, and has not been aware of progressively rising blood and urine sugars, undoubtedly needs an evaluation of his procedure in urine testing and guidance in the proper use of the results of these tests. As another example, knowledge of the fact that a patient's eyesight is failing should prompt reevaluation of his procedure in insulin administration, despite the fact that he has been successfully giving himself insulin for many years.

OTHER TYPES OF ASSESSMENT

Another important aspect of assessment prior to teaching is the consideration of the various psychological, social, and physical factors which will influence the teaching-learning process. This is a complex topic which deserves study far beyond the scope of this chapter, but a few observations about four of the major areas as they affect diabetic patients specifically are given here.

EMOTIONAL STATE. The emotional trauma which may result from a diagnosis of diabetes has already been discussed (see pp. 458 to 459). It may be unrealistic to expect a patient who is going through such turmoil to pay attention to even the simplest directions, much less absorb the quantities of detailed information with which he is sometimes bombarded. For this reason, the period immediately following diagnosis often is not a good time for detailed teaching. Letting the patient express his feelings, clarifying misconceptions, and providing basic information which will give him reassurance are, of course, appropriate. Certain procedures may also need to be taught at this time so that treatment can be started, but it may be only later that the patient is able to comprehend some of the more detailed or complex information.

SOCIOECONOMIC FACTORS. Just how much of a financial burden is a diagnosis of diabetes? This question has real significance in light of the fact that a large number of diabetics come from families with very limited financial means. Many of these patients, as well as many who are more financially secure, have difficulty meeting the additional costs of insulin, oral agents, syringes, needles, alcohol, urine-testing equipment, frequent physician visits, and the like. Therefore, all too frequently patients go without their medicines for a period of time because they feel they can't afford them, or they do such things as "fake" their urine sheets or neglect their diet in order to save money. Thus, a careful assessment of the financial burden which is being placed upon the patient may help health professionals plan with him more realistically and avoid some of the problems. For example, the required frequency of urine tests should be very carefully evaluated, the type of syringe (reusable versus disposable) should be recommended with thought to financial means, and the diet should be carefully individualized to contain not only the foods which the patient likes, but also those which are readily available to him.

EDUCATIONAL LEVEL AND READING ABILITY. A patient's educational level and reading ability must be assessed to serve as guides to the complexity of the content which should be presented and the teaching materials and methods which should be used. Although theoretically the grade of school completed should be indicative of a person's reading ability, this is not always true. If there is any question, it is best to have him actually read some of the material which he is being given before sending him home to use written diet lists or instruction booklets. As an example of the difficulty which can be encountered, Mary Mohammed studied the reading comprehension of 300 randomly selected patients in one medical center's diabetes clinic. She showed that only 22 percent of her study patients were able to profit from the written health information which was then being used at that clinic![22]

PHYSICAL FACTORS. The physical ability of a patient to carry out the procedures he is to be taught must be carefully assessed initially, and reassessed at intervals. With diabetics, the most common problem of this type is, of course, poor vision, and this changes as the years pass. Patients may not even be aware of the fact that they are reading their urine tests improperly or that they are drawing up the wrong insulin dose or getting their syringes half full of air. Once these difficulties are realized, they can be dealt with by such means as improving the lighting, changing the equipment, providing new glasses, or enlisting the help of a family member, and such considerations should be an integral part of the assessment of teaching needs.

CHOOSING APPROPRIATE TEACHING METHODS

A careful assessment of the areas just discussed will generally provide many clues regarding the appropriate teaching methods for meeting an individual patient's needs. For example, one must consider whether a particular newly diagnosed patient is emotionally ready to benefit from the content of a routine series of classes, or whether patients from vastly different socioeconomic and educational backgrounds can all benefit from the diet instruction in the same group. Many such decisions must be made in setting up a teaching program, and revisions should be made on the basis of an ongoing evaluation of patient learning.

A common question related to teaching methodology involves the selection of published materials to aid in the teaching process. These materials can be obtained through the American Diabetes Association, the American Dietetic Association, the U.S. Public Health Service, state health departments, many major drug companies, and various other sources. There are so many teaching materials readily available (and often free of charge) that selection can be confusing. Content is, of course, a major deciding factor. Equally important is the suitability of the material for the individual or group with whom it is to be used. Reading skills are one of the major factors. There is an abundance of material for good readers, but unfortunately very little is appropriate for use by patients who read poorly or not at all—and these may be just the patients who need them most! Because of the urgent need for this type of material, there have been a number of efforts to prepare some in recent years. One which is extremely effective is a pictorial representation of the diabetic diet entitled *Select-A-Meal*.[23] By a picture-matching technique, patients are helped to understand the exchange system and to select the proper foods in

the proper amounts. Since this is an area of confusion for patients who can read as well as for those who cannot, *Select-A-Meal* can help meet the needs of a large variety of patients. Several other aspects of diabetic management (insulin administration, foot care, and so on) have also been prepared pictorially and are available from the same source under the name of *Picture Pages*.[24]

Films about diabetes are also abundant, but these, too, must be carefully reviewed—not only for content, but for their appropriateness for the groups to whom they will be shown. Vocabulary, complexity of ideas, and cultural identification are all extremely important. For example, poor patients with little education are not likely to comprehend large words or complex ideas which are presented in a rapidly moving film sequence, nor will they readily identify with a film in which the foods and other customs are strictly middle class. On the other hand, such films may be perfectly appropriate for a better educated, middle-class audience with some knowledge of the topic.

Nursing Care

With the preceding introduction to the general teaching needs of diabetic patients, let us turn now to a detailed discussion of the major aspects of diabetic care which require teaching and/or other types of nursing intervention.

Before considering specifics, however, it might be well to point out the changing role which nurses are taking in providing diabetic care. Because of the chronic nature of the disease and the emphasis which must be put upon the teaching and supportive aspects of the care, this was one of the first areas in which nurses functioned as primary-care agents. This concept is growing rapidly, and is being met with great enthusiasm by the nurses, physicians, and patients who are involved.[25,26]

Although more and more nurses are now providing primary care to diabetic patients, most nurses are not functioning in this way. Therefore, the remainder of this chapter will focus on aspects of care which are needed by all nurses, without detailed discussion of the extended role.

FOOT CARE

Because of the strong tendency toward impaired circulation in the lower extremities, proper foot care is of utmost importance for all diabetics whether or not foot lesions are currently evident. Teaching proper foot care at the onset of the disease may prevent serious problems later, for even under medical management certain types of lesions may be difficult or impossible to heal. In fact, many physicians and nurses have considered the opportunity for foot-care instruction one of the prime benefits of early diagnosis.

The precautions which should be exercised by diabetics are, for the most part, identical to those recommended for any patient with peripheral vascular disease. Patients should bathe feet regularly, keep the skin soft with lotion, trim toenails carefully to avoid cuts and ingrown nails, keep feet warm without using hot water bags or other external sources of heat, and wear comfortable and properly-fitted shoes. They should avoid cutting out corns or using corn medicines, wearing round garters or other constricting clothing, and going barefoot, because of the risk of injury. One important difference between the diabetic and other patients with peripheral vascular disease is that, because of diabetic neuropathy, many diabetics have seriously impaired sensation. This means that they should be taught to examine all parts of their feet daily (using a mirror if necessary), and to inspect the insides of their shoes before putting them on. It also provides added reason for avoiding the use of heating pads, hot water bags, and hot foot soaks, for serious burns may easily result. Because their feet often feel cold, diabetics tend to use such heating devices; so they should be specifically cautioned against them.

The practice of good foot care should never be taken for granted. Patients sometimes have odd ideas about what constitutes "good" care, and some of their usual practices are dangerous. In addition to teaching good foot care, it is wise for a nurse or physician to observe diabetic patients' feet periodically. Poorly cut or ingrown nails, breaks in the skin, corns, calluses, and areas between the toes which are frequently sites of difficulty, all should be observed carefully.

More detailed information concerning other aspects of foot care are well outlined in general medical-surgical nursing texts. Any nurse not thoroughly familiar with this material should refer to it before caring for diabetic patients.

URINE TESTING

Urine testing is used widely by diabetics and can be an invaluable aid in regulating the disease. Twenty-four-hour specimens for glucose help to indicate overall control by showing the total amount of carbohydrate which is being lost. More commonly, single tests for sugar are done routinely both in the hospital and at home, with the frequency depending on the stability of the disease. Many diabetics also need to do a routine test for acetone, although those who have a stable form of diabetes and are not prone to ketoacidosis may need to test for acetone only if they start spilling large amounts of sugar.

In view of the wide use of urine testing and the judgments which may be made on the basis of the tests, it is important to understand the limiting factors and to realize that these tests can easily be misleading if not used and interpreted correctly. From the following discussion it is clear that it is unwise to vary treatment solely on the basis of small differences in urine-sugar readings. On the other hand, the presence of acetone in combination with large amounts of sugar is always an important warning signal and should not be ignored, providing the procedure has been done correctly and it is not a false positive, as described below.

The presence and percentage of sugar in the urine *reflect* the amount of blood sugar, but at best provide only a rough estimate. The percentage, for instance, is directly influenced by the dilution of the urine, so it will vary depending upon the amount a person has had to drink. To further complicate this matter, Feldman and Lebovitz have produced evidence to show that dilute urines may give falsely high readings on all the commonly used tests.[27] Even the meaning of the mere presence of sugar in the urine varies among individuals, for its appearance depends not only on the level of blood sugar, but also on the renal threshold—that is, the blood sugar level at which the kidney will allow sugar to "spill over" into the urine. Although the normal renal threshold is often quoted as approximately 180 mg per 100 ml, for many diabetics it is elevated. This means that the blood sugar can be considerably higher than normal and yet the patient continues to have negative tests for urine sugar. At the other extreme is the occasional diabetic patient who has an abnormally low renal threshold, resulting in a strongly positive urine sugar while the blood sugar is near or within the normal range. For such a patient, a negative urine test may indicate a blood sugar that is dangerously low. Therefore, it is helpful to check an occasional blood sugar at the same time as a urine sugar (from a second-voided specimen) in order to be better able to interpret the results.

There are also other factors which can lead to a misunderstanding of the results of these tests. Sometimes there is a warning that something is amiss, such as obtaining a color which does not match one on the color chart. Such a reaction can be caused when a patient who is using Clinitest is also taking cephalothin (Keflin) or has x-ray contrast media in the urine. At other times, however, the reading *appears* accurate but is not truly reflecting the level of glucose. For example, certain drugs such as ascorbic acid (in large doses), probenecid (Benemid) and nalidixic acid (NegGram) may cause false positives with Clinitest. A common misinterpretation of this type occurs near the end of pregnancy, when lactose normally appears in the urine. This will cause a positive reaction with Clinitest, but it has nothing to do with diabetic control. (The reagent strips—Tes-Tape, Diastix or Clinistix—are not affected by lactose.) False positives can also occur with reagent strip tests for acetone, most commonly with patients taking L-dopa or bromsulphalein (BSP).[28]

In addition, there are numerous substances which may cause false *negative* reactions with reagent strip tests for glucose.[29,30] To minimize the danger of a false negative test with these strips, a special technique can be used. This involves immersing only part of the test area. If glucose is present, color may appear in a thin line at the upper end of the wet area even in the presence of substances which otherwise inhibit the reaction.[31]

In addition to interpreting the tests correctly, it is also important that the procedures be carried out accurately. Patients are frequently asked to bring a record of urine tests with them each time they visit the physician. If these are incorrect, they may be not only useless but dangerously misleading. Accurate tests are also necessary if patients are to use their results in making judgments about the need for medical care or a change in regimen.

It may seem strange that emphasis is being placed upon performing the procedures accurately, for the products which are currently on the market for home use in testing urine sugar are accompanied by directions which appear very simple. However, one need not work closely with diabetic patients for very long to become aware of some of the difficulties which may arise. Nor is the inaccuracy necessarily confined to tests performed by patients. Several studies have pointed out marked discrepancies in the results of urine tests performed and recorded by trained personnel. Dobson, Shaffer and Burns analyzed the accuracy of urine testing by hospital ward personnel in a Texas hospital, and found it very common for the concentration of sugar and acetone to be reported in error. In this particular study, registered nurses were found to be the *least* accurate![32] Leifson, in analyzing the accuracy of tests performed by patients at home, found that not only were the patients frequently in error, but there were also discrepancies between the readings recorded by the trained persons who were carrying out the tests under standard conditions.[33] Not only may nurses become careless about the tests, but there are many subtleties which they frequently do not understand. Some of the more important of these are described. (Representatives from the drug companies which produce the tests can give additional help, and it is a good policy to take advantage of their availability to demonstrate to professional groups.)

AVOID USING INEFFECTIVE TEST MATERIALS. Though Tes-Tape and Diastix have an expiration date on each package, it is not uncommon to see an outdated package being used. And any of the materials, "outdated" or not, will become inactivated when left in high humidity. This frequently occurs because the bathroom, with its running water and steam, is where the materials are used and where they are most likely to be left. All jars should be closed securely when not in use, and Tes-Tape, which cannot be made air tight once it is opened, must be kept in a dry place. Materials which have become inactivated do not always change in appearance, although any such change is indication that they should not be used. (For example, when Clinitest tablets are too old to use they change to a dark blue-brown or blue-black color.) If there is doubt as to the effectiveness of the materials, they can be tested with a nondietetic cola beverage. (Ordinary table sugar, sucrose, should not be used.)

Another error which is commonly seen is allowing the color charts to become faded. Some of the colors are difficult to differentiate when the charts are new, but when they are faded an accurate comparison with the test material is impossible.

COLLECT THE SPECIMEN CORRECTLY. Many physicians request that, each time a urine specimen is checked for sugar, the patient use the second of two specimens voided about one-half hour apart (a "second-voided" specimen). This indicates the percentage of sugar which is being spilled into the urine at specified times, rather than the percentage in urine which has been collecting in the bladder over several hours. Since the physician bases the insulin order (kind[s], frequency, and amount) on the pattern in which the blood sugar varies during the day, the specific information obtained from second-voided specimens is generally more helpful. If this type of specimen is desired, it should be made clear to the patient and, at any time when a second-voided specimen for some reason is not obtained, the record should indicate this fact.

FOLLOW DIRECTIONS CAREFULLY. This word of caution sounds trite, for the directions accompanying all the tests are quite simple. However, the frequency with which directions are not followed is surprising, and incorrect procedure may change the results greatly. Common

errors include shaking the Clinitest solution while it boils, floating the reagent strips in the urine, and failure to read the color at the time specified in the directions. The problem of timing is an almost universal one, and patients and staff alike seem to treat it very lightly. Yet following this part of the procedure meticulously is essential for obtaining accurate readings.

Another common error is failure to observe the "pass-through" color change when using Clinitest. The directions specifically state that the tube must be watched as it boils, and that even a brief appearance of bright orange with a final color of greenish brown means a concentration of *over* the percentage indicated by bright orange. However, if only the final color is observed it probably will be mistaken for one of the colors lower on the scale. Because of the frequency of this error in using the more usual five-drop method (five drops of urine and ten of water), a two-drop method (two drops of urine and ten of water) has been made available. Because the concentration of the solution of urine is less, the test performed in this way is much more sensitive and urine sugar must be higher than 5 percent before the pass-through phenomenon occurs. Thus, for patients who run high urine sugars, this procedure not only decreases the danger of having pass-through occur and be misinterpreted, but it also provides more specific information about the amount of sugar present. The advantage of increased sensitivity is such that some groups have even gone a step further and use a one-drop method.[34]

Although the two-drop method decreases one source of error, it increases another: the danger of using the wrong chart. Because of the differing concentrations of the solution used in the two-drop and the five-drop methods, the color changes which represent varying percentages of urine sugar are somewhat different for each. Ames Company, the manufacturer of Clinitest, has published charts for use with both methods, and patients should be taught that they should use *only* the chart labeled for the procedure they are using.

The confusion between the two-drop and the five-drop color charts for Clinitest is not the only cause of having the wrong chart used. This can occur with any of the urine tests, particularly when patients switch from one test to another. They may not realize that a different chart must be used, and serious misinterpretations of the results may ensue. For example, try reading Tes-Tape against a Clinitest chart, and see what kinds of errors can occur!

Whatever test or method is used, caution must be taken to compare colors with the chart very carefully. Errors in reading colors are often made, particularly when one is trying to distinguish between two shades of the same basic color. Good lighting is important, but does not always overcome the difficulty. The diabetic whose eyesight is poor may need assistance with this part of the test. If so, it should be emphasized that he must read the chart at the proper time, and not lay it aside for another member of the family to check later.

MAKE THE SHEETS FOR RECORDING THE RESULTS AS SIMPLE AS POSSIBLE. This consideration is especially important for patients with low intelligence. Patients and their families sometimes keep records which seem totally incomprehensible. It is especially annoying when the person who has recorded the results does not accompany the patient when he visits the physician. The danger of confusion is increased when tests for both sugar and acetone are requested. However, it is usually not difficult to devise a simplified sheet to meet individual needs. This, of course, in no way safeguards against the occasional patient who will fill in his sheet at random without having tested his urine. Herein lies another value of frequent checks of blood sugar.

The record sheets should also specify what urine test is being used. Without having this information it may be impossible to know how much sugar is indicated by a particular symbol. For instance, ½ percent is indicated by "+" on Clinitest, but by "+++" on Tes-Tape.

Although these are among the most common mistakes that are made, it is impossible to enumerate all possible errors. Additional sources of confusion are elaborated elsewhere.[35,36] Any nurse who has worked closely with diabetic patients is able to add to the list. There is always the patient who urinates into the toilet bowl and sticks the Diastix into the resulting solution; or the one who thinks the tablets for testing acetone are for internal consumption; or the thrifty one who uses a single piece of Tes-Tape for several tests in a row. One patient, when told to test with "tape," was actually using adhesive tape and rejoicing in the fact it was always negative! Thus, it is clear that both the equipment and the actual procedure should, if possible, be observed at intervals, so that teaching can be based on observed difficulties. If the patient is being seen outside the home, it is often helpful to ask him to bring his equipment with him, for if he is given other equipment with which to demonstrate his procedure, such errors as an incorrect color chart or outdated materials will not be discovered.

Patients also need help in learning how to use the results of the tests. They should certainly be encouraged to seek medical help if a series of specimens shows a constant rise in sugar and/or acetone. Those who understand their disease well can be given instructions for altering their treatment according to certain urine test results and, depending upon their understanding, patients attain varying degrees of sophistication in doing this. Nevertheless, the caution should always be given, that patients not attempt to make their own judgments as to how the disease should be regulated, for it is not uncommon for them to get into serious difficulty by attempting to do so.

The question often arises regarding which of the several urine tests for sugar is the best. There is no one answer to this, for patients' needs vary. What may be best for one patient may be completely worthless for another. Therefore, each individual situation should be evaluated, and the test chosen on that basis. Some important considerations are as follows:

IS KNOWING THE PERCENTAGE OF SUGAR IN THE URINE IMPORTANT, OR WILL KNOWING THE MERE PRESENCE OR ABSENCE OF SUGAR BE SUFFICIENT? For example, Clinitest can give a high degree of specificity, especially with the two-drop procedure which has been described above. On the other hand, there is evidence that positive readings on Tes-Tape cannot be *differ-*

entiated with a high degree of accuracy,[37,38,39] but that it is certainly a sensitive indicator of the presence of glucose.

DOES THE PATIENT HAVE A PHYSICAL LIMITATION THAT MAKES HIM UNABLE TO PERFORM ONE OR MORE OF THE TESTS ACCURATELY? Manual dexterity is a consideration, particularly with older patients. For example, it is not uncommon for someone to have difficulty using a dropper properly or manipulating the Tes-Tape container without handling the test area of the strip. Eyesight is another factor, and certain of the color changes may be easier for an individual to differentiate.

DOES THE PATIENT HAVE ANY SUBSTANCE IN HIS URINE WHICH MIGHT CAUSE FALSE RESULTS WITH ONE OR MORE OF THE TESTS? Some of the more common of these substances have been discussed on pp. 468 to 469. Further detailed information can be obtained from the companies which manufacture the tests, or from their local representatives.

DOES URINE TESTING CAUSE A MARKED INCONVENIENCE FOR THIS PATIENT AT ONE OR MORE TIMES DURING THE DAY, AND WHICH TEST IS HE WILLING TO USE? This topic opens up a wide range of problems and points to the fact that patients should be included in the decision making. Doing so is certainly far preferable to having a patient fake his test results or use (and perhaps abuse) a test in which he has not been instructed or which will give him misleading results.

DIET

Although physicians hold differing philosophies regarding the dietary treatment of diabetics, and although individual patient needs dictate differences within these philosophies, almost all diabetic patients are given some type of dietary prescription. These diets may range from the carefully weighed diet to one with almost no restrictions. Most patients have a diet prescription which falls between these two extremes.

The difficulties which diabetic patients have in adhering to their diets are both widespread and well-known. For example, a study by Williams et al demonstrated that major dietary errors were being made by a large percentage of the study patients.[40] Yet diet is the cornerstone of current therapy for diabetes, and helping patients adhere to an appropriate dietary regimen is a major goal for the health team.

Although the nurse usually is not responsible for the calculation of the diet and the initial diet teaching, she does play a major role in giving support and guidance to patients. Thus, the focus here will be on the more common dietary problems which diabetics face and ways in which the nurse can help. At all times she should work very closely with the dietitian or nutritionist, when one is available.

Many diabetics, particularly those with adult-onset diabetes, are overweight, so one of the common goals in diabetic diet therapy is weight loss. Even if weight loss is not a goal, foods are restricted in quantity and in kind both to avoid weight gain and to balance caloric intake with available insulin. Thus, one of the more common problems faced by these patients is one which is of major health concern to society in general. For the diabetic, the need to maintain caloric restriction assumes greater importance than it does for many nondiabetics, but the job may not be any easier. For some the fear connected with the disease helps to provide motivation. But as the months and years pass, these patients, too, are likely to become careless about their food habits.

Much of the literature dealing with the problems of helping patients lose weight is discouraging. Many kinds of therapeutic regimens have been advocated, and some of these give good results. All too frequently, however, these reports are shadowed by two factors: either the long-term follow-up reports are discouraging or absent, or the same regimen used by a different therapist does not yield the same beneficial results.

When one considers the well-known social and psychological factors which help to determine a person's diet, it is clear that not only are food habits difficult to change, but that a person also needs considerable motivation before any lasting change is made. The nurse is in a position to develop a relationship with her diabetic patients which will help foster such motivation. In addition, after assessing the individual needs of a patient, it is often possible to suggest ways of helping him cope with the problems his diet creates.

Recently much has been written about the use of behavior-modification techniques as a way of helping people change behaviors of various types. The rationale behind this idea is that behavior changes according to the types of behavior which are rewarded and punished, and that persons can change their behavior (e.g., adhere to a weight-reduction diet) by cooperating with an individually planned reward system. For those who wish to explore this concept further, a book entitled *Behavior Modification and the Nursing Process* provides both the rationale and many striking examples.[41]

There are also a number of other ways to help patients adhere to prescribed diets. The following are a few such suggestions.

SEE THAT THE DIET FOLLOWS THE PATIENT'S USUAL FOOD HABITS AS CLOSELY AS POSSIBLE. This is perhaps the most important single guideline to follow in helping patients maintain diet therapy. To be fully aware of food habits, a careful diet history should be taken both before the diet is written and periodically thereafter.

SET REALISTIC, SHORT-TERM GOALS. It is discouraging to have to think of losing 50 or 80 pounds, but it is more tolerable to strive for a loss of one pound in a week. It also helps to avoid discouragement and feelings of guilt if the stated goals are realistic. Since energy output must exceed food intake by 3500 calories in order to lose a single pound, a goal of two or three pounds per week is usually maximum. For patients whose caloric maintenance requirement is low, even this amount is unreasonable.

PROVIDE FOR FREQUENT CONTACT WITH THE PATIENT. If the nurse-patient relationship is beneficial, it helps to provide a constant source of motivation, and return visits may be scheduled solely for this purpose. The same result may be accomplished by regularly scheduled meetings of groups of patients who are all trying to lose weight.

ENLIST THE HELP OF A FAMILY MEMBER OR FRIEND. These efforts may be more effective if this person is also trying to lose weight. However, be careful! This does not always work. Sometimes patients resist help from those who are closest to them, because they see it as "nagging." Consequently, they may do even worse with their diets. In these instances it is best to try to interpret the situation to the family members and encourage them to offer help in other ways.

USE GROUP SESSIONS. Several patients who are trying to lose weight can share problems and suggestions. Because of the social pressures of the group, individual commitments to lose a certain amount of weight each week or two helps to maintain motivation.

SUGGEST LOW-CALORIE FOODS TO ADD BULK TO MEALS. If meals have been planned carefully, keeping this point in mind, patients on low-calorie diets frequently marvel at the amount of food they may have for each meal. This can best be done by using quantities of those beverages and vegetables which have few or no calories. Specially prepared "diet" foods are also used to help achieve this, although they are expensive and must be carefully included in figuring the total number of calories. With few exceptions, they are far from being calorie free, as some patients seem to think.

HAVE PATIENTS KEEP WEIGHT CHARTS. This may be done either individually or as a group project.

HELP PATIENTS PLAN FOR USING DIVERSION APPROPRIATELY. The purpose here is to avoid situations in which the craving for food is likely to be the strongest.

Severe caloric restriction is not necessary for all diabetics. For example, those with juvenile onset diabetes are not likely to be overweight, and during childhood and adolescence, when energy expenditure and caloric needs are often extremely high, food intake may be quite liberal. This means that children, who do not like to be labeled as "different," are able to eat treat foods such as potato chips, ice cream or popcorn in moderation, if such foods are figured into their diets. Adults who are very active also may be allowed high caloric intakes for the same reason.

For the diabetic, and particularly for the one who is on medication, regularity and spacing of meals is as important as the total daily caloric intake. The type and dosage of medication are very carefully regulated with the expectation that a specific dietary prescription will be followed, and any deviation in amount or timing causes difficulty. The patient on long-acting insulin who skips his afternoon or evening snack, is in serious danger of a hypoglycemic attack. Or the one who decides to skip breakfast so that he can eat more at suppertime not only risks hypoglycemia in the morning, but also may forfeit diabetic control for the next two or three days. For this reason, employment which does not allow for regularity of schedule may be difficult or impossible for the severe diabetic, and frequently help is needed in making plans so that regularity of meals is maintained.

Eating away from home often creates problems for the diabetic, although this need not be true if he understands his diet and the foods that can be substituted for one another. Generally the only types of food which are completely omitted on a diabetic diet are those which contain concentrated sweets; (and possibly foods with a high fat content); therefore other foods may be eaten, provided the quantity is controlled. Familiarity with the common exchange lists helps a person know quickly what quantities of various foods should be eaten. Although it takes time to become thoroughly familiar with these lists, many patients are able to use them skillfully. Various types of teaching aids are available and are extremely helpful in gaining the skill that is needed to be able to substitute foods within food groups. When a person is unfamiliar with the content or method of preparation of certain items on a restaurant menu, the waitress can easily be questioned. For example, some restaurants routinely presweeten iced tea, whereas others do not. This type of information should be sought prior to placing an order. With these few precautions there is no need for a diabetic to avoid eating out.

MEDICATIONS

The necessity for having to take medication, and particularly injections, for the rest of one's life is sometimes a diabetic patient's major concern.

Some diabetics are controlled on diet alone or on oral medication; others may need considerable help in coping with the idea of taking daily injections. Most patients have heard that some diabetics can take pills instead of injections, and this usually prompts insulin-dependent diabetics to question their physicians or nurses about the possibility of switching to the pills. If they do not ask, a point should be made of explaining to them that the pills are *not* insulin and that their type of disease would not respond to oral medication. Without knowing this, some patients go so far as to obtain pills from a friend or relative and give them a trial on their own.

Despite the dislike for daily injections, most patients, when given the necessary help, are able to master the mechanics of the procedure and to accept it emotionally. It is gratifying to see even a very young child able to give himself an injection expertly. The thought of actually pushing the needle into one's own skin is usually the part of the procedure which causes the most anxiety, and it may be wise to help the patient overcome this anxiety by having him learn how to inject the needle before he tackles the rest of the procedure. When he finds out that this is not as impossible as he thought it would be, he will be able to concentrate on the rest of the things he needs to learn.

At least two people should be taught how to give the injection for every patient, for this safeguards against times when one person is temporarily ill or away from home. Except in occasional situations when for some reason it is deemed impossible, one of these two people should be the patient himself. The advantages of being able to give one's own injection rather than relying on someone else are so great that a decision not to teach the patient should be very carefully weighed. Even those with very poor eyesight have been able to do the procedure successfully with the help of a variety of syringe controls that can be set for the correct dose. Problems encountered with using this type of control are that they usually are not satisfactory for mixing two kinds of insulin, and it is very easy to give less than the ordered dose by getting air into the syringe. (The chances of getting air in the syringe can be minimized or avoided by having the patient keep track of the number of doses he has withdrawn, and discard the vial before it is entirely empty.) When eyesight is extremely poor, it may be necessary to have someone else withdraw the insulin or check the dose before it is administered.

AVOIDING MEDICATION ERRORS. Unfortunately as with urine testing, there are numerous pitfalls which can cause serious medication errors. Some institutions have found that the frequency of error in insulin administration warrants a policy that all insulin doses be checked by two people. Student nurses, even after having mastered the injection technique itself, often find that the selection and measurement of insulin is confusing. The large array of kinds and strengths of insulin, as well as types of insulin syringes, is largely responsible.

The following examples demonstrate some of the types of difficulties which patients may encounter.

Mrs. T. arrived in clinic with her urine tests showing, as usual, that her diabetes was not in good control. Her medication prescription was for 35 units of NPH insulin daily. She verbalized complete confidence in giving her own injections, for she had been giving them to herself for six years. The decision was made to observe her drawing up a dose of insulin. She was given a U-100 syringe and a vial of NPH insulin U-100—the same equipment she used at home. The first dose she drew up was about 43 units—it was quite apparent that she was unable to see the syringe plainly. The light was improved, and she tried again. This time the plunger arrived closer to 35 units, but the syringe was two-thirds full of air. She was unaware of it, and looked up at the nurse with complete satisfaction. A third try yielded a dose of close to 65 units. It was obvious that her morning doses of insulin might have been ranging anywhere between 0 and 100 units. When asked if she ever gave herself more or less insulin than the physician had ordered, she replied that if her urine were positive in the afternoon she would give herself "a little more."

Mrs. R. was brought into the emergency room unconscious and convulsing. She was in severe hypoglycemia. In trying to determine what had happened, the staff learned that she had changed from U-40 to U-100 insulin, but she

didn't want to throw away her old syringes. Thus she had used the U-40 syringe, and had given herself 2½ times her usual dose.

Mrs. F. had an order for 15 units of NPH insulin before breakfast and 15 units of regular insulin before supper. While interviewing her one day, it was discovered that she often took her regular insulin in the morning and her NPH insulin at night. She did not think it made any difference as long as she took both kinds. She had been wondering why she had so many "nervous spells" midmorning.

Again, as with urine testing, it is impossible to foresee all the potential errors and difficulties. However, familiarity with some of the more common ones helps the nurse avoid errors, both by improving her own practice and by helping her teach in such a way that her patients can avoid many of them.

One of the major sources of error in the past has been the availability of two strengths of insulin (U-40 and U-80) and a wide variety of corresponding syringes. To complicate this matter, the dual-scale syringe (Fig. 15-3) has been in common usage and has created a great deal of difficulty and confusion. In fact, this type of syringe has been so dangerous that at least one major syringe manufacturer has actively discouraged the use of its own product! To alleviate the confusion over two strengths of insulin, the American Diabetes Association, in cooperaion with the insulin and syringe manufacturers, developed a plan several years ago whereby there would be only one strength readily available to patients. U-100 was selected because of its compatibility with the decimal system. It was recognized that during the transition period, while all *three* strengths were on the market, there might be added confusion, but the benefits of eventually having almost all patients on only one strength of insulin are felt to outweigh these potential problems. As this book goes to press there are still the three strengths available, but it is hoped that before long all patients will be switched to U-100 insulin and the U-40, U-80 problem will be only history. Meanwhile, it is very important that patients who are using U-100 insulin know that they must use a U-100 syringe.

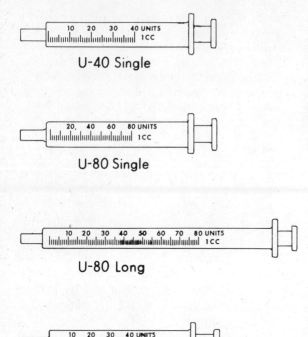

U-40 Single

U-80 Single

U-80 Long

U-40 – U-80 Dual

FIGURE 15-3.
This illustration shows two major sources of error in the U-40 and U-80 syringes: (1) In some instances each line in the scale represents one unit of insulin and in others it represents 2 units. This is particularly confusing to patients who learn on one type of syringe and then go home to use another type, especially if they are not accustomed to reading numbers and systems of measurements. (This source of confusion is not totally alleviated in the U-100 syringes.) (2) A person can be easily confused in using the dual-scale syringe, particularly when administering doses of 40 units or less.

Therefore, all U-40 and U-80 syringes should be discarded as soon as a patient starts using U-100 insulin, for using the wrong syringe could cause serious dosage errors.

In contemplating the change to U-100 insulin, a major concern of some physicians has been the question of accuracy in administering small doses of the more concentrated solution. This is particularly important for many pediatric patients, for often they receive very small doses of at least one type of insulin, and they may be extremely sensitive to minute differences in dose. The problem has been dealt with by manufacturing special U-100 syringes which have a high degree of accuracy in the low-dose range. Another option is to have the pharmacist dilute the insulin before dispensing it, using a special diluent which is available from the insulin manufacturers. Although this accomplishes the purpose well, it naturally increases the risk of confusion in using a syringe which is not made specifically for that strength of insulin.

In the past, the wide variety in the sizes and markings on the syringes has been a major source of error (see Fig. 15-3). The change to only one strength of insulin will minimize this, but the various U-100 syringes still have enough variation to cause confusion. Teaching patients with the same syringe they will use at home and encouraging them not to use other kinds without first checking with their nurse or physician will help avoid errors. Patients should also be taught to take an old syringe with them when they purchase new ones, and to insist on receiving identical syringes.

Patients who mix two types of insulin are likely to make a different kind of dosage error because of the "dead space" in certain types of syringes. This problem has become particularly significant with the advent of the more concentrated U-100 insulin. When a drug is drawn into a syringe with the conventional type of removable needle, there is a "dead space" within the tip of the syringe and the hub of the needle which may hold as much as 10 units of U-100 insulin.[42] This dead space is the cause of the large air bubble which must be removed before measuring the dose. When the air is expelled, it is replaced by medication which is in excess of the ordered dose. If a single type of medication is administered there is no problem, for the extra medication stays in the dead space after injection, and the correct dose is administered. But if two kinds of medication are withdrawn into the same syringe, difficulty may arise. Assume, for instance, that a diabetic patient is taking a dose of 5 units of regular insulin mixed with 25 units of NPH insulin, and that he draws the regular insulin into the syringe first. After getting rid of the air bubble, he has 5 units in the barrel of the syringe, and up to 10 units in the dead space. He then draws up 25 units of NPH insulin, making a total of 30 units of insulin in the barrel of the syringe and 10 units in the dead space. Although only 30 units will be administered (and 10 units will remain in the dead space), the proportion of the two types of insulin in the syringe is now 15/25 rather than 5/25. The dose received therefore contains more regular insulin and less NPH insulin than ordered. The problem is further complicated if on some days the NPH insulin is drawn up first, for the ratio could then change to 5/35. Patients may be regulated using this type of syringe, although the actual daily dose is somewhat different from that which is ordered. But if the procedure or equipment are changed, daily fluctuations can well make a difference in diabetic control. Thus patients using a syringe with dead space need to be careful to draw up the insulin in the same order each day. In contrast, some of the newer types of syringes have negligible dead space and therefore do not present this problem. But the availability of both types of syringes means that changing from one type to the other could cause difficulty in control. Therefore all patients who take insulin must be taught that they should not change the type of syringe they use without professional advice.

Another common source of insulin error is the large variety of preparations available. Having only one strength commonly used instead of two will decrease but not alleviate, this problem. Not only are there regular insulin, globin zinc insulin, NPH insulin, protamine zinc insulin, Lente insulin, Semilente insulin and Ultralente insulin, all with somewhat different lengths of action, but these come in various types of preparations (beef and pork, pure pork, and the like.) Add to this the facts that different strengths are available for special needs (such as U-500 for use by insulin-resistant patients) and that the different drug companies which produce the insulin use somewhat different labeling and trade names. It is no wonder that patients and health professionals alike become confused! Therefore, patients should be taught to check new bottles of insulin with older ones to be sure that they are the same, and nurses who are using insulin from a stock supply should read labels with extreme caution.

Because of the many types and strengths of insulin available, nurses must insist that orders be written very explicitly. Another potential source of error is in the way the dosage is written. Any time that an order is handwritten, either the word "units" should be spelled out or the abbreviation "U" should *precede* the figure. ("5 units" or "U5," not "5U.") It is too easy for a U written after a number to be mistaken for an 0. If it were, the dose administered would be ten times greater than that which was intended! Care must also be taken not to use insulin which has lost its potency or has been altered in any other way. For example, heat causes insulin to lose its potency; therefore, insulin should be kept at room temperature—75° F. (24° C.)—or below. Prolonged storage, even at room temperature or below, may cause a decrease in potency, so all bottles of insulin which are not in current use should be kept refrigerated and expiration dates should be heeded regardless of refrigeration. Freezing should also be avoided, for it, too, may cause loss of potency as well as changes in the suspensions which make it difficult or impossible to obtain uniform doses.

Patients often feel that traveling will present major problems if they are on insulin. Now that disposable equipment is available and insulin need not be refrigerated at all times, matters are simplified. However, when temperatures are extremely warm, insulin should be insulated. It is also wise to avoid carrying it in a pocket next to the body, for the temperature there can get very warm.

Although patients who are on insulin are more likely to experience difficulty in administering their medication, those on the oral agents are not immune to error. Such patients tend to feel that since they do not have to take injections, their disease is not severe. Therefore, they are more likely to forget to take their pills and to be less conscientious about them in general. Patients have also been known to take pills prescribed for another diabetic, reasoning that since they are all for diabetes one should do just as well as another. Dosages and actions of the various oral hypoglycemic agents vary markedly, and the patient who interchanges them may get into serious difficulty.

In view of the difficulties which patients have with their medications, the advice to *observe* patients' equipment, medicines, and procedures at intervals bears repeating. This is particularly important any time there is a change in the insulin order or in the type of equipment being used, but should not be limited to these occasions.

MAINTAINING STERILITY. The sterility of equipment is another major factor to consider. Surprisingly enough, some individuals have used a clean rather than a sterile technique for years and have not encountered a single infection. However, the possibility of infection always exists and has caused major difficulty often enough so that any technique which does not assure sterility is far from ideal.

The increasing use of presterilized disposable equipment has decreased the problems of contamination. However, patients using this need to be taught how to maintain sterility and that the equipment should be used once and thrown away. (Some patients try to economize by reusing disposable equipment, with the result that it may not be sterilized properly—if at all—or the marks may become so faded they are difficult or impossible to see.)

Of those who use glass syringes and reusable needles, some boil them once or twice a week and keep them in alcohol between injections. This technique is satisfactory, provided care is taken to remove all the alcohol from the barrel of the syringe before the insulin is drawn into it. It is also a very simple procedure to boil the syringe and needle immediately prior to each injection. Regardless of the technique used, the patient must know how to handle the equipment without contaminating it prior to injection.

AVOIDING TISSUE REACTIONS. To maintain the best possible tissue integrity, all patients giving multiple insulin injections should follow a number of recommendations. The most common of these is the rotation of sites. Although this is very widely known and most patients can verbalize the fact that it should be done, it frequently is not done with the care that the situation demands. Numerous sites may be used—the thighs; the upper arms; the upper, outer quadrant of the buttocks; and the abdomen. (Because of its vascularity, a 2-inch circle around the umbilicus should not be used.) Usually a patient prefers one or two sites (most often the thighs) and tends to use those more than the others. Many dislike the thought of injecting themselves in the abdomen, and yet, after they have done it several times, they find that it is no worse than doing it elsewhere. In fact, sometimes they discover, to their amazement, that they actually prefer this site. The arm is not as easy to use as the thigh because only one hand is available for actually giving a self-injection. Yet it is fairly simple to pinch up the tissue on the arm by supporting it against a wall or chair rather than having to do it with two fingers of the opposite hand (Fig. 15-4). It also takes practice for a right-handed person to give himself an injection in the right arm. The buttocks require a bit of twisting to be able to hit the proper site, but with a little practice most patients can manage this with ease. Therefore, patients need to be shown all the usable sites explicitly, and be given assistance in acquiring the skill necessary to use these sites. Rotation of the sites within each major injection area is also important. For instance, the area for injection in the upper thigh is large enough so that numerous injections can be given, while still keeping the sites fairly far apart. This means that by using all eight possible major areas, and rotating injections within these areas, the same tissue need not be used more than once every one or two months. It is often helpful to make out a chart or diagram that will assist the patient in accomplishing the rotation systematically. Otherwise it becomes haphazard, and the more preferred tissues are endangered.

In addition to the rotation of sites, there are other precautions which should be taken. It is now generally agreed that a deep subcutaneous injection should be given. The technique may, of course, need to be altered depending upon the amount of subcutaneous tissue available. For many diabetics, the use of a 90-degree angle with a subcutaneous needle (½ to ⅝ in. in length) will accomplish this, but for a very thin person a 45-

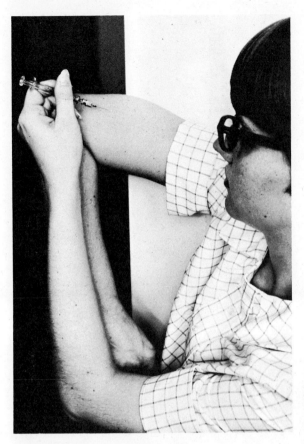

FIGURE 15-4.
Giving oneself an injection in the arm is not as difficult as it may seem at first. Patients who have been taught this technique do it easily. A person with considerable subcutaneous tissue often does not need to pinch up the skin in order to insert the needle. Source: Courtesy, Diabetes Education Center, Minneapolis, Minnesota.

degree angle may be sufficient. Depending upon the tissue, it may be either pinched up or stretched while inserting the needle. Occasionally patients obtain an intradermal rather than a subcutaneous needle, and use it, thinking that an injection will be less painful with a smaller needle. The short intradermal needle will *not* give a deep subcutaneous injection, and its use should be discouraged.

Another precaution that should be used is to avoid injecting cold insulin. Many physicians feel that this factor may contribute to tissue reactions. Although traditionally all insulin has been kept in the refrigerator, it is now known that the bottle in current use can safely be kept at room temperature—75° F. (24° C.). Keeping the bottle of insulin which is being used out of refrigeration is, therefore, now generally advised. (All extra bottles should be refrigerated. See pp. 477 to 478.

Although many patients can give themselves insulin year after year without showing evidence of major tissue reactions, there are some who have great difficulty. For instance, allergy, hypertrophy, or atrophy may occur in spite of the above precautions (Figs. 15-5 and 15-6).

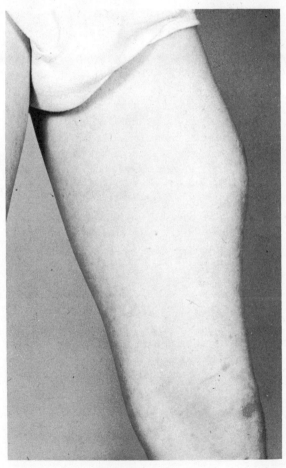

FIGURE 15-5.
Marked lipoid hypertrophy in the thigh of a 14-year-old boy who had had diabetes since the age of one year. His other three extremities had similar areas of hypertrophy.

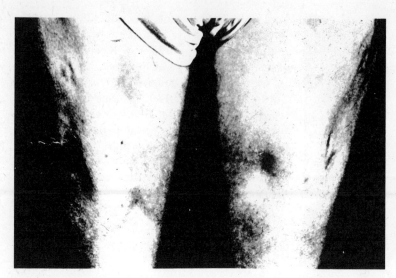

FIGURE 15-6.
Both hypertrophy and atrophy in a 28-year-old woman whose use of insulin extended over 16 years. Source: Waife S. O. (ed.): Diabetes Mellitus. ed. 7. Indianapolis, Lilly Research Laboratories, 1967, p. 107. Reprinted through the courtesy of Eli Lilly and Company, Indianapolis.

Most of the allergic reactions show the typical local signs: redness, swelling, itching, and so on. Fortunately these usually disappear spontaneously as the patient continues to use insulin. Sometimes changing the type and/or brand of insulin is helpful, and antihistamines, or occasionally corticosteroids, may both be used successfully. Very occasionally there are severe or even life-threatening allergic reactions, and these must of course be treated promptly as is done with any other severe allergy. Persons with such reactions may need to go through a course of desensitization.

Patients who develop either hypertrophy or atrophy are not caused as much discomfort as those with allergies, but the lesions may be unsightly and may even be so severe that there is difficulty deciding where to give the next injection in order to assure proper absorption. The causes of these two problems are poorly understood, so it is hard to know how to prevent or treat them. It is clear that the above-suggested approaches to avoiding tissue damage are not totally effective in preventing hypertrophy or atrophy, although they well may help. Fortunately, many cases of atrophy disappear spontaneously over a period of years. The most encouraging suggestions have come within the last few years, for it has been reported that the more purified type of insulin which is now being used

may cure or prevent many of the cases of atrophy.[43,44] The problem has not, however, been alleviated.

ADDITIONAL TEACHING. In addition to learning how to administer the medications, patients need to know why they are receiving them, how they work, their relationship to diet and exercise, and what to do if they receive an overdose. With this type of increased understanding comes the increased possibility of self-regulation of dosage. Since a diabetic must assume much of the responsibility for his own care, this type of decision making is often condoned *providing it is done on the basis of sound knowledge, is within the guidelines defined by the physician, and is accompanied by routine medical supervision.* Any other type of self-regulation should be strongly discouraged, for many diabetics have been in severe difficulty by trying to make their own judgments on the basis of insufficient knowledge or in situations which demanded medical attention.

HYPOGLYCEMIA

Because any patient who is receiving either oral hypoglycemic agents or insulin is likely to experience hypoglycemia at some time, he should be well acquainted both with the symptoms and the treatment. Since hypoglycemia can progress very rapidly to unconsciousness, those customarily in close contact with a diabetic should also be aware of the symptoms and of the appropriate course of action in case of emergency.

Symptoms of hypoglycemia differ somewhat from person to person, and each diabetic should become thoroughly familiar with the ones that indicate danger for him. Because of the speed and frequency with which children may have insulin reactions, it is often advised that every child who is placed on insulin be made to experience hypoglycemia so that he will readily recognize it. Some physicians also follow this practice with adults, although for many adults a thorough explanation is sufficient. In any case, experiences which diabetics have with hypoglycemia should be capitalized upon as teaching opportunities.

Many of the symptoms of hypoglycemia are related to the autonomic or central nervous system. This is true because nerves need a constant supply of glucose and because the autonomic nervous system plays a major role in the body's homeostatic response to a drop in blood sugar. Common early symptoms include tachycardia, palpitations, blurred vision, headache, muscle twitching, hunger pains or nausea, paresthesias, pallor, and feelings of apprehension, fatigue, weakness, dizziness, or drowsiness. Increased perspiration is frequently a cardinal symptom. Delirium, unconsciousness, and convulsions are more advanced symptoms as the blood glucose continues to fall and the supply to the central nervous system becomes more depleted. Permanent brain damage and even death are possible with a prolonged and severe episode of hypoglycemia.

Generally, if a diabetic has been properly instructed, he can be aware of an impending insulin reaction and ward it off with proper treatment. At times, however, a change in behavior accompanied by a loss of judgment may be the initial symptom, and to the casual observer the person seems drunk. The behavior change and judgment loss cause the diabetic to let the reaction progress without treatment; in fact, his attitude may even be such that he will resist help, insisting that nothing is wrong. Thus, those who are near him may be the ones best able to observe the warning signs and insist that the person eat. Family members, friends, and close associates of diabetics should be made aware of this possibility, and know the proper action to take if it should occur.

Following episodes of hypoglycemia, a rebound phenomenon may take place, causing the blood sugar to rise above normal. This is a result of the body's homeostatic defense mechanism, involving increased adrenal stimulation with subsequent liberation of glycogen stores and promotion of glucogenesis.

Prevention of hypoglycemia is, of course, a primary goal, and patients should be thoroughly familiar with the possible causes. An overdose of medication, excessive activity, and failure to eat scheduled meals are commonly at fault. Labile diabetics may experience such episodes with no apparent cause, and the unpredictable course for these persons makes it all the more important that they be constantly on the alert. Attacks of hypoglycemia, whether mild or severe, should be reported to the physician so that he may evaluate the prescribed therapy and make necessary adjustments in order to avoid further difficulty. Patients must be made aware of the importance of this, for otherwise they may feel that mild reactions are not worth mentioning.

For the person who has not lost consciousness, any rapidly absorbed form of carbohydrate is useful in treatment: hard candy, sugar cubes, fruit juice. Five to ten grams are usually sufficient. Diabetics on medication should carry some source of concentrated carbohydrate with them at all times. And, although it may seem obvious, it should be noted that diabetics need to understand the *variety* of foods which can be used to treat a reaction. Orange juice is the one which, for some reason, has traditionally been used, and it is surprising the number of people who think that it is the *one* specific remedy. One woman arrived in clinic with a gallon jug with about 500 cc of orange juice in the bottom, and it was difficult to convince her that she could use something a little easier to carry. Another diabetic made the front page of the newspaper by having a reaction while he was working in the crawl space under his house. His daughter went in with orange juice, but to no avail: the space was too low for him to sit up and drink. The family then called the rescue squad, who dragged him from under the house. He was still conscious, and was then able to drink the juice!

Following the initial treatment of hypoglycemia with a rapidly absorbed form of carbohydrate, foods containing carbohydrates which are absorbed more slowly (such as bread or milk) should be eaten in order to avoid another reaction. This often may be done merely by eating the next scheduled meal.

A word of caution should be used in relation to the amount of extra food which is eaten during an episode of hypoglycemia. Small or moderate amounts are usually sufficient. It should not be a signal to consume large amounts of food in addition to the prescribed diet. One patient used every hint of a possible insulin reaction as an excuse to consume large quantities of candy, cake and sandwiches, with the comment that "I'm a big woman, and when I get hungry, I get *hungry*!" Needless to say, this served only to increase her 220 pounds.

If a patient is unconscious at the time hypoglycemia is discovered, and if medical care is available, intravenous glucose is usually used. Food or fluid should *not* be given orally to an unresponsive person because of the danger of aspiration. If medical help is not available it should be obtained as quickly as possible. However, there are two other possible courses of action available if there is proper equipment. One is the injection of glucagon—a pancreatic extract which raises the blood sugar by causing liver glycogen to convert to glucose. This treatment is not to be used except under a physician's prescription. But for patients who are likely to go into rapid and severe insulin reactions, it is often advised. Members of the family who already know injection technique need to be taught primarily the indications for the use of glucagon, how to mix it (it is supplied in powder form with a separate ampule of solvent), and what to do following administration. If the patient responds, some form of oral carbohydrate should be given to assure an adequate supply of glucose. Whether the patient responds or not, the physi-

cian should be notified so that he can give treatment and/or adjust the insulin order as indicated.

The other "home" remedy for severe hypoglycemia is oral administration of one of the concentrated glucose preparations which have been developed for this purpose. They are thick, sticky substances which are squeezed into the mouth between the teeth and cheek, and are slowly absorbed or swallowed by reflex action; the danger of aspiration is considered negligible. As the sugar reaches the bloodstream, the patient slowly responds enough to eat, thereby avoiding the need for immediate medical help. At least two of these preparations are available at this time—Instant Glucose* and Reactose.†

Nocturnal hypoglycemic attacks are not uncommon when patients are on long-acting preparations of insulin, and such patients should be cautioned to eat prescribed bedtime snacks. Nurses working night duty should routinely check these patients and should arouse them slightly if there is any question as to their condition. A light flashed toward the face may not awaken them but will often be enough to make them squint or turn the head, thus assuring the nurse that all is well. Any diabetic who is perspiring as he sleeps or who wakens with a headache or other possible symptoms of hypoglycemia should be check very closely.

When a diabetic is found unconscious, it is not always easy to determine immediately whether or not the cause is hypoglycemia. Nor is it always possible for a diabetic to know whether or not vague symptoms are heralding hypoglycemia. If Dextrostix are available, they can be used to help determine the cause of the symptoms. A urine specimen, whether it is positive or negative, is not diagnostic. However, because of the speed with which a hypoglycemic reaction may progress, it is wiser to treat it as such if hypoglycemia seems a reasonable possibility, rather than to risk withholding treatment and being in error.

*Instant Glucose may be obtained only through the Diabetes Association of Greater Cleveland, 10205 Carnegie Avenue, Cleveland, Ohio 44106.
†Reactose is dispensed by C. R. Canfield & Co., 2744 Lyndale Avenue South, Minneapolis, Minnesota 55408.

KETOACIDOSIS

The following excerpts were taken from the chart of a diabetic patient who was hospitalized in severe acidosis:

> Mrs. J., age 54, was diagnosed with adult-onset diabetes 18 years ago. For the last several years she has been fairly well controlled on 35 units of NPH insulin daily. She has never before been in acidosis, although she has had some hypoglycemic attacks. She checks her urine "now and then," the last time being a week ago when it was negative. Several days ago her foot became infected, and she has been nauseated with intermittent vomiting for two or three days. She has taken her usual daily dose of NPH insulin despite decreased intake of food and fluids. She was brought to the hospital this morning because of fever and lethargy. Blood sugar—800 mg per 100 ml.

Many diabetics who have had the disease for a number of years with little fluctuation in urine sugars become extremely negligent in testing urine specimens. Mrs. J. is a good example. However, had she been testing even a single daily urine specimen, and assuming that she knew the significance of increased urine sugar and acetone, it is probable that she would have detected the danger signal considerably earlier than the point at which she finally obtained medical help.

It is of vital importance that diabetics understand the potential causes of ketoacidosis and be impressed with the absolute necessity for testing urine specimens at those times. Every diabetic should understand the relationship between ketoacidosis and infection, for infection is one of the most frequent causes of ketoacidosis. Periods of any other type of illness and times of particular stress should also indicate potential danger and make the diabetic more conscientious about his care.

The symptoms of ketoacidosis have been described earlier in this chapter (see p. 453). Usually this is a relatively slow process in which the patient develops progressive symptoms over a period of days or even weeks. However, the presence of infection speeds up the process so that it may progress to a severe state within a matter of hours. Diabetics should be well acquainted with the danger signals and be cautioned to seek immediate medical help.

Too frequently patients try to treat themselves when they start to develop glycosuria and/or symptoms of ketoacidosis. Such "home" remedy often takes three common but dangerous forms.

1. The patient who detects glycosuria may increase his insulin and, unless this is done under a physician's instructions, he may well do it incorrectly.

2. He may try to cut down on his food intake, with the thought that less food will cause less glucose to appear in the urine. This reasoning is fallacious, for the body's own glycogen and fat stores are released in the presence of any degree of starvation. By omitting food, body fats are broken down and acidosis is increased. Blood glucose also continues to rise.

3. He may omit insulin if he is nauseated and unable to eat normally. This too may lead to difficulty. Insulin is needed for the metabolism of glucose, whether it is obtained from food which is ingested or from the breakdown of body stores as a result of inadequate intake. In addition, nausea and vomiting themselves may be caused by an already far-advanced ketoacidosis. For example, Mrs. J.'s blood sugar was 800 mg per 100 ml. despite the fact that she had taken her usual doses of insulin but had eaten little. Had she omitted her insulin, acidosis would have progressed even more quickly. Most physicians advise patients to take their insulin, to keep a careful check of urine sugar and acetone, to eat a liquid diet if possible, and to seek medical advice. (Advice about taking insulin during episodes of nausea and/or vomiting may vary depending on whether or not infection and fever are present, whether or not the patient can keep food down, and the results of urine tests for sugar and acetone. Frequent doses of short-acting insulin may be advised instead of the usual longer-acting insulin.)

Medical treatment for ketoacidosis consists of the administration of insulin, fluids, and electrolytes to restore fluid and electrolyte balance as well as normal metabolic processes. The exact types and amounts are determined by clinical findings. During the acute stage, regular insulin is given subcutaneously and/or intravenously and it has traditionally been given in relatively large doses. More recently, however, very low doses of insulin have been advocated as effective and safer.[45,46] Sodium chloride and fluids are given to combat the dehydration, and sodium bicarbonate may be given to combat severe acidosis. Later in the course of treatment, the administration of potassium is usually indicated. Although before treatment potassium has left the cells and the serum potassium may be normal or even elevated (see p. 453), as the process of acidosis begins to reverse, potassium reenters the intracellular fluid compartment and hypokalemia becomes a serious threat.

Nursing care during acute acidosis consists largely of supportive care for a patient exhibiting common symptoms—dehydration, vomiting, coma. Observations related to changes in symptoms, including electrolyte imbalances, are vital. An indwelling catheter may be ordered, as well as frequent checks for urine sugar and acetone. A nasogastric tube may be put in place, particularly if the patient is vomiting or in coma with danger of aspiration. The appearance of small amounts of blood in the aspirated gastric contents may be noted and should be reported. However, it need not cause undue alarm, for this is not unusual as a result of the mild gastritis which often accompanies severe acidosis.

Amid the urgency of the physical care which must be given to the unconscious acidotic patient, it is of utmost importance that the patient's family not be forgotten. They often need considerable explanation, encouragement, and support, for the patient's symptoms seem extreme.

Because a diabetic may be found unresponsive, either from hypoglycemia or from acidosis, he should be strongly encouraged to have with him at all times something that will identify him as a diabetic. Such identification may take the form of a small card in a wallet and an identification bracelet or necklace. It is also helpful if the identification includes the type and dosage of usual medication and the name and address of the patient's physician.

Since episodes of ketoacidosis may be both severe and dangerous, diabetic teaching should aim toward their prevention. Frequently a careful history following an acidotic episode will reveal some type of negligence in the patient's care of himself. However, through careful assessment, skillful teaching, and a supportive relationship, the nurse is often able to help a patient care for himself wisely.

Summary

Neither diabetes nor the care it requires is simple. Yet most diabetics, if they have received the proper help, are able to live nearly normal lives. A few are handicapped almost daily by their disease.

Since it is a responsibility of the nurse to help the diabetic adjust to necessary changes for normal life, considerable research is needed. The care outlined in this chapter is based on the information available at present. But nursing studies which have been carried out have been in limited settings and have focused primarily on pinpointing areas of difficulty in diabetic care. They have raised many questions, most of which have gone unanswered in any systematic fashion. As medical research strives to make the true nature of diabetes known, it will be a challenge to the nurse to investigate not only the current questions in the field, but also those which will emerge as a result of a more accurate understanding of it.

References

1. Report of the Workgroup on Epidemiology, Report of the National Commission on Diabetes to the Congress of the United States, Volume III, Part 1, p. 71, U.S. Department of Health, Education, and Welfare, 1975.
2. Diabetes Source Book, p. 7, U.S. Department of Health, Education, and Welfare, 1968.
3. Leifson, J.: Glycosuria tests performed by diabetics at home. Pub. Health Reports 84:28-32, Jan. 1969.
4. Meinert, C. L.: Standardization of the oral glucose tolerance test. Diabetes 21:1197-1198, Dec. 1972.

5. West, Kelly M.: Substantial differences in the diagnostic criteria used by diabetes experts. Diabetes 24:641-644, July 1975.

6. Kimball, C. P.: The patient and diabetes: impressions from dialogues. JAMA 219:83-85, Jan. 3, 1972.

7. Williams, T. F. et al.: The clinical picture of diabetic control, studied in four settings. Am. J. Pub. Health 57:448, Mar. 1967.

8. Diabetes Source Book, *op. cit.,* p. 49.

9. Klimt, C. R., et al: A study of the effects of hypoglycemic agents on vascular complications in patients with adult-onset diabetes. Diabetes 19:747-830, Supplement 2, 1970.

10. Seltzer, H. S.: A summary of criticisms of the findings and conclusions of the University Group Diabetes Program (UGDP). Diabetes 21:976-979, Sept. 1972.

11. Schor, S.: The university group diabetes program—a statistician looks at the mortality results. JAMA 217:1671-1675, Sept. 20, 1971.

12. Cornfield, J.: The university group diabetes program—a further statistical analysis of the mortality findings. JAMA 217:1676-1687, Sept. 20, 1971.

13. Oral hypoglycemic agents. In FDA, Current Drug Information, Washington, D.C., Food and Drug Administration, Department of Health, Education, and Welfare, Oct. 1970.

14. Gilbert, John P. et al.: Report of the committee for the assessment of biometric aspects of controlled trials of hypoglycemia agents. JAMA 231:599, Feb. 10, 1975.

15. Bierman, E. L. et al: Principles of nutrition and dietary recommendations for patients with diabetes mellitus: 1971. Diabetes 20:633-634, Sept. 1971.

16. Schless, G. L. and von Laveran-Stiebar, R.: Recurrent episodes of diabetic acidosis precipitated by emotional stress. Diabetes 13:419-420, Jul.-Aug., 1964.

17. Singer, D. L. and Hurwitz, D.: Long-term experience with sulfonylureas and placebo. New Eng. J. Med. 277:450-456, Aug. 31, 1967.

18. Hansten, P. D.: Drug Interactions, ed. 3. Philadelphia, Lea & Febiger, 1975.

19. Watkins, J. D. et al.: A study of diabetic patients at home. Am. J. Pub. Health 57:453-454, Mar. 1967.

20. *Ibid.,* p. 455.

21. Watkins, J. D. et al: Diabetes Mellitus Assessment Guides. North Carolina, The Association for the North Carolina Regional Medical Program, 1971. (Currently distributed by The North Carolina Diabetes Association, 408 N. Tryon St., Charlotte, N.C. 28202.)

22. Mohammed, M. F. B.: Patients' understanding of written health information. Nurs. Research 13:107, Spring 1964.

23. Wason, C. D., Coyle, V. C. and Moss, F. T.: Select-A-Meal. North Carolina, The Association for the North Carolina Regional Medical Program, 1970. (Currently distributed by The North Carolina Diabetes Association, 408 N. Tryon St., Charlotte, N.C. 28202.)

24. Lawrence, P. A. and Coyle, V. C.: Picture Pages. North Carolina, The Association for the North Carolina Regional Medical Program, 1973. (Currently distributed by The North Carolina Diabetes Association, 408 N. Tryon St., Charlotte, N.C. 28202.)

25. Jordan, J. D. and Shipp, J. C.: The primary health care professional was a nurse. Am. J. Nurs. 71:922-925, May 1971.

26. Runyan, J. W. Jr.: The Memphis Chronic Disease Program. JAMA 231:264-267, Jan. 20, 1975.

27. Feldman, J. M. and Lebovitz, F. L.: Tests for glucosuria: an analysis of factors that cause misleading results. Diabetes 22:117-120, Feb. 1973.

28. Urine Constituents Reaction Chart. Elkhart, Ind., Ames Company.

29. Feldman, J. M., Kelley, W. N. and Lebovitz, H. E.: Inhibition of glucose oxidase paper tests by reducing metabolites. Diabetes 19:337-343, May 1970.

30. Gifford, H. and Bergerman, J.: Falsely negative enzyme paper tests for urinary glucose. JAMA 178:423-424, Oct. 28, 1961.

31. *Ibid.,* p. 423.

32. Dobson, H. L., Shaffer, R. and Burns, R.: Accuracy of urine testing for sugar and acetone by hospital ward personnel. Diabetes 17:281-285, May 1968.

33. Leifson, *op. cit.,* pp. 30-32.

34. McFarlane, J. and Nickerson, D.: Two-drop and one-drop test for glycosuria. Am. J. Nurs. 72:939, May 1972.

35. Lawrence, P. A.: Pitfalls in urine testing. ADA Forecast 25:1-4, Mar.-Apr. 1972.
36. Watkins, J. D. and Moss, F. T.: Confusion in the management of diabetes. Am. J. Nurs. 69:521-524, Mar. 1969.
37. Feldman and Lebovitz, *op. cit.*, p. 120.
38. Leifson, *op. cit.*, p. 30.
39. Leonards, J. R.: Evaluation of enzyme tests for urinary glucose. JAMA 163:260, Jan. 26, 1957.
40. Williams, T. F. et al.: Dietary errors made at home by patients with diabetes. JADA 51:19-25, July 1967.
41. Berni, R. and Fordyce, W. E.: Behavior Modification and the Nursing Process. St. Louis, C. V. Mosby, 1973.
42. Kochevar, M. and Fry, L. K.: Insulin and dead space volume. Drug Intelligence and Clinical Pharmacy 8:33-34 Jan. 1974.
43. Watson, B. M. and Calder, J. S.: A treatment for insulin-induced fat atrophy. Diabetes 20:628-632, Sept. 1971.
44. Wentworth, S. M. et al: The use of purified insulins in the treatment of patients with insulin lipoatrophy. Diabetes 22:290, Supplement 1, 1973.
45. Kidson, W. et al: Treatment of severe diabetes mellitus by insulin infusion. Brit. Med. J. 2:691-694, June 29, 1974.
46. Moseley, J.: Diabetic crises in children treated with small doses of intramuscular insulin. Brit. Med. J. 1:59-61, Jan. 11, 1975.

Bibliography

Albisser, A. M. et al: Clinical control of diabetes by the artificial pancreas. Diabetes 23:397-404, May 1974.
Albrink, M. J.: Dietary and drug treatment of hyperlipidemia in diabetes. Diabetes 23:913-918, Nov. 1974.
Allison, S. E.: A framework for nursing action in a nurse-conducted diabetic management clinic. J. Nurs. Admin. 3:53-60, July-Aug. 1973.
Bagdade, J. D. et al: Impaired leukocyte function in patients with poorly controlled diabetes. Diabetes 23:9-15, Jan. 1974.
Bennett, M.: The Peripatetic Diabetic. New York, Hawthorn Books, 1969.
Eaton, R. P. Evolving role of glucagon in human diabetes mellitus. Diabetes 24:523-524, May 1975.
Education and Management of the Patient with Diabetes Mellitus. Elkhart, Ind.: Ames Company, Division Miles Laboratories Inc., 1973.
Ellenberg, M.: Impotence in diabetes: the neurologic factor. Annals Intern. Med. 75:213-219, Aug. 1971.
Employment of diabetics: a statement of the Committee on Employment and Insurance, American Diabetes Association. Diabetes 21:834-835, July 1972.
Fulton, M. et al: Helping diabetics adapt to failing vision. Am. J. Nurs. 74:54-57, Jan. 1974.
Goodkin, G.: The truth about life insurance for diabetics. ADA Forecast 26:1-6, Sept.-Oct. 1973.
Graber, A. L. et al: Diabetes and Pregnancy: A Guide for the Prospective Mother with Diabetes. Nashville, Vanderbilt University Press, 1973.
Guthrie, R. and Guthrie, D. W.: Diabetes in youth: the use of U-100 insulin in children. ADA Forecast 26:8-11, Nov.-Dec. 1973.
Hamlin, C. R. et al: Apparent accelerated aging of human collagen in diabetes mellitus. Diabetes 24:902-904, Oct. 1975.
Kozak, G. P. et al: Skin disorders in diabetes. Hosp. Med. July-Aug. 1972.
Lawrence, P. A.: U-100 insulin: let's make the transition trouble free. Am. J. Nurs. 73:1539, Sept. 1973.
McFarlane, J.: Children with diabetes: special needs during growth years. Am. J. Nurs. 73:1360-1363, Aug. 1973.
McFarlane, J. and Hames, C. C.: Children with diabetes: learning self-care in camp. Am. J. Nurs. 73:1362-1365, Aug. 1973.
Miller, L. V. and Goldstein, J.: More efficient care of diabetic patients in a county-hospital setting. New Eng. J. Med. 286:1388-1391, June 29, 1972.
Moore, R. H. and Buschbom, R.: Work absenteeism in diabetes. Diabetes 23:957-961, Dec. 1974.
Nickerson, D.: Teaching the hospitalized diabetic. Am. J. Nurs. 72:935-938, May 1972.
Runyan, J. W. et al: A program for the care of patients with chronic diseases. JAMA 211:476-479, Jan. 19, 1970.
Salzar, J. E.: Classes to improve diabetic self-care. Am. J. Nurs. 75:1324-1326, Aug. 1975.

Schmitt, G. F.: Diabetes for Diabetics. Miami, The Diabetes Press of America, 1971.

Seltzer, H. S.: Drug-induced hypoglycemia. Diabetes 21:955-966, Sept. 1972.

Storvick, W. O. and Henry, H. J.: Effect of storage temperature on stability of commercial insulin preparations. Diabetes 17:499-502, Aug. 1968.

Sussman, K. E. and Metz, R. J. S. (eds.): Diabetes Mellitus, ed 4. New York, American Diabetes Association, Inc., 1975.

Tattersall, R. B. and Fajans, S. S.: A difference between the inheritance of classical juvenile-onset and maturity-onset type diabetes of young people. Diabetes 24:44-53, Jan. 1975.

Tetrick, L. and Colwell, J. A.: Employment of the diabetic subject. J. Occupational Med. 13:380-383, Aug. 1971.

Tyson, J. E. and Felig, P.: Medical aspects of diabetes in pregnancy and the diabetogenic effects of oral contraceptives. Med. Clin. N. Am. 55:947-959, July 1971.

U100 insulin: a new era in diabetes mellitus therapy. Diabetes 21:832, July 1972.

Walsh, C. H. and O'Sullivan, D. J.: Effect of moderate alcohol intake on control of diabetes. Diabetes 23:440-442, May 1974.

Watkins, J. D. et al: Observation of medication errors made by diabetic patients in the home. Diabetes 16:882-885, Dec. 1967.

Weinsier, R. L. et al: Diet therapy of diabetes: description of a successful methodologic approach to gaining diet adherence. Diabetes 23:669-673, Aug. 1974.

Williams, S. M.: Diabetic urine testing by hospital nursing personnel. Nurs. Research 20:444-447, Sept.-Oct. 1971.

16

Water and Electrolytes in Health and Disease

W. D. SNIVELY, JR., M.D. and DONNA R. BESHEAR

Basic Characteristics of Body Fluid • Dynamics of Water and Electrolytes • Acid-Base Disturbances • Alterations Produced by Disease • Nursing Observations • Therapy • Special Considerations

Basic Characteristics of Body Fluids

Body fluids consist chiefly of water and dissolved substances. Water is one of the most abundant and widely distributed substances on earth. No known form of plant or animal life can exist without it. In the development and maintenance of life, it has no substitute. Of all the planets in our solar system, only earth has enough water to support human life. Among the mysteries of water that have continuously baffled scientists are its unexpectedly high boiling point as compared to such closely related chemicals as hydrochloric acid and ammonia and the quantity of heat required to change water into vapor. The boiling point of water (212°F. or 100°C.) and its freezing point (32°F. or 0°C.) are ideally suited to the body's temperature. They enable us to withstand all but the most drastic changes of heat and cold. On the other hand, the freezing points of ammonia (−77.74°C.) and of hydrochloric acid (−114°C.), and their boiling points (−33.42°C. and −85°C. respectively), make them unsuitable as the basic liquid for human body fluids.

The mysteries of water's chemical characteristics have been partially solved by the finding that, while the molecules of most liquids are closely packed with twelve molecules as near neighbors, the molecules of water are far apart, with each molecule having only four or five near neighbors. This open chemical structure of water requires more heat for vaporization and boiling than the tighter chemical structure of the other substances. It might help to understand this if you picture a room in which a large number of people have gathered compared to a room containing only a few people. Clearly, it will take more time and heat to reach a specified temperature in the room with less people than in the tightly packed room.

Water is found both inside and outside the cells. Extracellular water consists of water found in both the blood vessels and the interstitial spaces, while cellular water is that portion within the cells. Water constantly and rapidly passes back and forth between all compartments of the body, exchanging through capillaries and cellular membranes in a state of dynamic equilibrium.

Infants and children contain a higher percentage of body water than do adults. During the first month of life, approximately 76 percent of the body weight is water. This drops to 63 percent by the ninth month. The relative water content of children continues to decrease gradually with age, reaching average values of 61 percent of the body weight for males and 51 percent for females by age 17. This slow decline of body water continues with age. Part of this decline may be related to an increase in body fat because the deposition of fat is accompanied by little water per gram fat, in contrast to approximately 4 grams water per gram protein. Extracellular fluid in the infant constitutes approximately 48 percent of the body weight. With maturity, this compartment decreases to about 15 percent of the body weight in males and 14 percent in females.

Plasma and interstitial fluid comprise the extracellular fluid, as contrasted to the fluid within the cells, the cellular fluid (intracellular fluid). Plasma, interstitial fluid, and cellular fluid each has its own normal composition of cations and anions. The cations of plasma and of interstitial fluid include sodium, potassium, calcium, and magnesium. Sodium is the chief cation of plasma and of interstitial fluid. The anions of plasma and of interstitial fluid include bicarbonate, chloride, phosphate, sulfate, organic acids, and proteinate, with chloride being the chief anion of both. The main difference between plasma and interstitial fluid is the much greater quantity of proteinate contained in plasma. This proteinate maintains the fluid volume of the plasma, offsetting its considerably greater hydrostatic pressure as contrasted with interstitial fluid.

Cellular fluid contains the cations sodium, potassium, calcium, and magnesium, with potassium being the important cation. Its anions include bicarbonate, sulfate, phosphate, and proteinate.

The total cations in any body fluid always equal the total anions of that same fluid because electrical balance must, in accord with physiochemical laws, be maintained. Electrolytes, however, exist in the body not as compounds, such as potassium chloride or sodium phosphate, but as independent cations and anions. They exist in electrical balance but not in union with one another. The composition of the body fluids is shown in Table 16-1. Gains and losses of body fluids are shown in Figure 16-1.

Various body secretions and excretions are derived from extracellular fluid. As they are depleted, the inevitable result is depletion of the extracellular fluid. As extracellular fluid is depleted, the cellular fluid gradually becomes depleted. However, cellular fluid is not available as an *emergency* replacement of losses of extracellular fluid. Interrelations of body fluids are presented diagrammatically in Figure 16-2. Electrolyte composition of various body excretions and secretions is shown in Figure 16-3.

Lymph may be regarded as a special form of interstitial fluid. Interstitial fluid enters the lymphatics after diffusing into microscopic lymph capillaries. It is nudged along by the kneading effect of muscle action and the sucking effect of breathing. Lymph vessels originate in nearly all the tissue spaces as microscopic capillaries. Plasma proteins continuously leak through pores in the capillaries, about 1/25 of the total proteins in the circulation each day. Probably the most important function of lymph is the return of plasma proteins to circulation after they leak out of the bloodstream. If these proteins were not returned to the body's circulation, death would soon follow; the lymphatics provide the only channel by which the restoration of plasma proteins can take place.

TABLE 16-1
Electrolyte Composition of Body Fluids

ELECTROLTYE	INTRAVASCULAR	INTERSTITIAL	CELLULAR
Cations			
Sodium	142	147	15
Potassium	5	4	150
Calcium	5	2.5	2
Magnesium	2	1	27
Total	154	154.5	194
Anions			
Chloride	103	114	1
Bicarbonate	27	30	10
Proteinate	16	0	63
Organic acids	5	7.5	0
Phosphate	2	2	100
Sulfate	1	1	20
Total	154	154.5	194

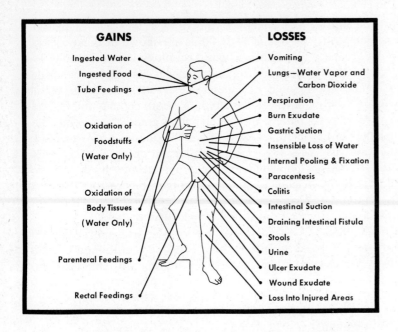

FIGURE 16-1.
Gains and losses of body fluids.

Dynamics of Water and Electrolytes

Since each body fluid has its own peculiar composition and purpose, it might appear that the various body fluids are totally independent and self-sufficient. However, there is a constant exchange of materials between the various fluids, occurring by means of diffusion, osmosis, active transport, and pinocytosis.

DIFFUSION

When diffusion occurs, all molecules and ions intermingle and are transported through either the pores or the matrix of the semipermeable cell membrane as a result of their random thermal movement. Their movement may be compared to the movement of balls in a pinball machine, which travel in one direction until they hit an obstacle and bounce off in another direction.

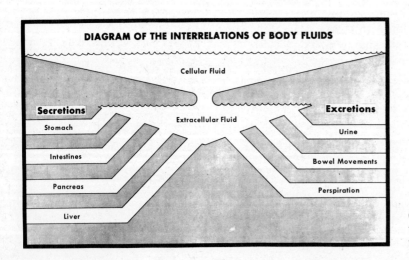

FIGURE 16-2.
Cellular fluid connects with extracellular fluid, which connects with secretions and excretions.

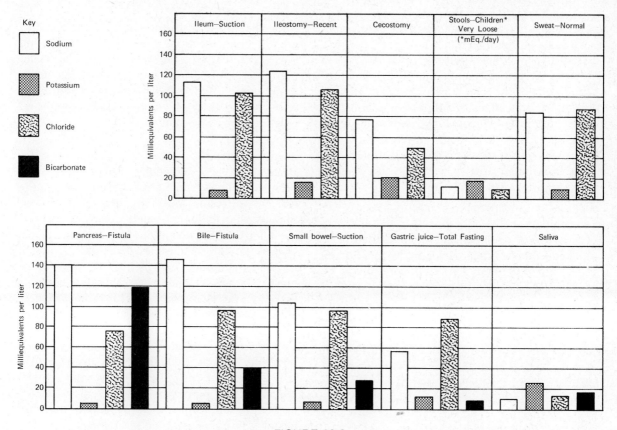

FIGURE 16-3.
Electrolyte composition of various body secretions or excretions.

When the molecules and ions strike against a pore, they pass through to the other side of the membrane, much as the pinball does when it reaches the lower end of the board and drops into a slot. Water and electrolytes move in this manner from areas of their higher concentration to areas of their lesser concentration until equilibrium is established.

Diffusion is limited only by the size of the pores in the different membranes. The water molecule and various ions, such as sodium, chloride, and lactate, are all much smaller than the membrane pores and can easily pass through them; other molecules, such as glucose, are larger than most pores and cannot cross the membrane in this manner.

Water, which can cross the membrane only by diffusion through the pores, is the most important substance that passes through the mem-

brane. Although pores represent only a tiny portion of the cell membrane, enough water to equal approximately 100 times the volume of the cell itself diffuses through the pores every second, illustrating how rapidly diffusion occurs.

The matrix of the cell membrane is composed of lipoprotein; hence, lipid-insoluble substances cannot diffuse through the matrix of the membrane. However, such substances as oxygen, carbon dioxide, and alcohol, which are important to the function of the cell, are lipid-soluble and can pass through the membrane by becoming dissolved in the matrix and then diffusing to the other side.

There are certain substances that cannot be diffused at all, such as protein molecules or lipoproteins. When the semipermeable membrane separates such a substance from those substances that can be diffused, the diffusible anions and cations are unequally distributed on the two sides of the membrane. However, the products of their concentrations are equal, and the total of the diffusible and nondiffusible anions on either side of the membrane is equal to the total of the concentrations of diffusible and nondiffusible cations. The unequal distribution of diffusible ions causes a potential difference between the two sides of the membrane (i.e., the outside may become positive as compared to the inside, thus upsetting equilibrium).

OSMOSIS

The body cells compensate for this difference in concentration through osmosis, the most important method the body uses to transfer fluids. Osmosis is the diffusion of more water molecules in one direction than in the other. This phenomenon occurs as a result of the pulling power of nondiffusible minerals when there is a higher concentration of these on one side of the membrane than on the other. For example, if pure water were on one side of the membrane and a solution of sodium chloride on the other, more water molecules would leave from the pure water side than from the sodium chloride solution (i.e., water goes where the salt is).

Except for very short periods of time, usually only a few seconds, osmosis maintains the cellular and extracellular fluids in constant balance (i.e., the concentrations of nondiffusible substances on the two sides of the membranes remain nearly equal). If the concentrations become unequal, osmosis of water occurs so quickly that balance will be re-established in only a few seconds.

ACTIVE TRANSPORT

Diffusion and osmosis do not fully explain the movement of all electrolytes. Sometimes it is necessary for ions to move from the lesser concentration to the higher concentration. This is accomplished by active transport, the only transfer mechanism that requires energy. The exact source of this energy is believed to come from certain cell enzymes that combine with the substance to be transported and release tremendous quantities of energy that move the substance

from the dilute concentration to the area of greater concentration. Sodium and potassium ions are actively transported through the membranes of all body cells, and some cell membranes actively transport chloride, hydrogen, phosphate, calcium, magnesium ions, and creatinine and uric acid.

PINOCYTOSIS

Particularly large molecular weight substances, such as proteins, can be transported through the cell membranes only by the process of pinocytosis, in which small quantities of surrounding fluid are taken into the cell by invagination of the cell membrane. After the surface of the cell membrane invaginates, the membrane closes, the vesicle disintegrates, and its contents disperse into the cytoplasm. This is an extremely slow process in comparison with direct diffusion of small molecules through the cell membrane. For example, water is diffused into the cell membrane about 1,000,000 times faster than it can be moved into the cell by pinocytosis. Nevertheless, pinocytosis is extremely important to the cell, for it is the only method the body has of transporting certain large molecules.

Acid-Base Disturbances

An *acid* is a chemical that can release hydrogen ions. A *base* is a chemical that can accept hydrogen ions. For example, carbonic acid can donate a hydrogen ion to the base bicarbonate. An alkali can produce OH ions in watery solutions—for example, sodium hydroxide (NaOH) or ammonium hydroxide (NH_4OH).

Any acid placed in water breaks up, in whole or in part, into its component ions. Thus, HCl breaks up into hydrogen and chloride. The strength of an acid depends on the degree to which it breaks up or dissociates and on the concentration of the hydrogen ions that it contains. In 1909, Sorensen introduced the symbol pH as a convenient way of expressing hydrogen ion concentration. The pH symbol was devised to express more easily the tiny amounts of hydrogen ions present in body water and other biological fluids. For example, the hydrogen ion concentration at the pH generally considered neutral, 7.0, is 1/10,000,000 Gm per L, while that of a pH of 8.0 is 1/100,000,000 Gm per L. The hydrogen ion concentration within the normal physiological pH range varies from approximately 1/22,000,000 to 1/28,000,000 Gm per L. In measuring quantities of electrolytes the milliequivalent (mEq) is used. If this term is used for hydrogen, the mEq of hydrogen in extracellular fluid range from 1/22,000 to 1/28,000 mEq of hydrogen ion per L.

Water dissociates into H and OH ions. Thus, H_2O breaks down into H plus OH. The equilibrium of this reaction at room temperature has been found to be $H \times OH = 10^{-14}$. Since pure water yields equivalent amounts of H and OH ions, it follows that the hydrogen ion concentration of pure water is 10^{-7}. Since pH is in reality the reciprocal of the logarithm of the hydrogen ion concentration, the pH of water is 7. Since acids have a greater hydrogen ion concentration than water, the pH of an acid is lower than 7. Bases have a lower concentration of hydrogen ions than water, so the pH of a base exceeds 7. Because the normal pH of blood and of body fluids lies between 7.35 and 7.45, body fluids normally have a faintly basic, or alkaline, reaction. In fact, if body fluids had the neutral reaction of 7, one would be near death.

Tiny though the concentration of hydrogen ion in the body fluids is, this concentration must be maintained within narrow limits of normal if one is to go on living, much less functioning normally. To maintain pH, three factors share the responsibility:

1. Chemical buffers of the body fluids themselves neutralize strong acids and bases which are produced within the body or which enter the body.
2. Respiratory regulatory mechanisms help eliminate and regulate the concentration of carbonic acid, the major acid end-product of metabolism.
3. The kidneys help eliminate excess acids and bases. The kidneys are the most important of the three mechanisms because they compensate for any defects in the action of the buffer salts or of respiratory origin.

THE BODY'S CHEMICAL BUFFERS

The term buffer describes a chemical substance that decreases the pH change caused by the addi-tion of an acid or of a base. A buffer is either a mixture of a weak acid and its alkali salt or of a weak base and its acid salt. The important buffers in the body are mixtures of weak acids and their alkali salts, such as carbonic acid and sodium bicarbonate, monohydrogen and dihydrogen phosphate salts, and the proteins with their alkali salts, such as hydrogen protein and base protein. All of the bases available for immediate neutralization of acids in the body are in the form of buffer salts. Salts of strong acids, such as sodium chloride, possess no neutralizing power. A strong alkali, such as sodium hydroxide, cannot exist in the living body.

There are four main buffer systems of the body which help in the important job of maintaining the constant pH.

1. The bicarbonate-carbonic acid buffer system, the largest and most important in the body, operates in the extracellular fluid.
2. The phosphate buffer system operates in the red blood cells and others, especially the cells of the kidney tubules where it enables the kidneys to excrete hydrogen ions.
3. The protein buffer system operates in the tissue cells and plasma.
4. The hemoglobin buffer system operates in the red blood cells.

The Bicarbonate-Carbonic Acid Buffer System

The most important of the various buffer systems is the bicarbonate-carbonic acid buffer system. During the course of the normal metabolic activities of the body, most of the organic and inorganic acids formed are stronger than carbonic acid. Thus, hydrochloric acid unites with sodium bicarbonate to form carbonic acid and sodium chloride. Carbonic acid breaks down in the body into water and carbon dioxide, a gas. The bicarbonate ion is not the only one that is able to neutralize acids, but bicarbonate is unique—its acid is volatile, that is, is a gas. When the bicarbonate salt reacts with an acid, the carbon dioxide set free by the reaction can be removed immediately by the lungs. Therefore, a foreign acid can be completely neutralized by bicarbonate, the acid being converted first into a neutral salt, then into carbon dioxide, which is expelled through the lungs.

On the other hand, when a base, such as sodium hydroxide, enters the body, or is formed within the body, it combines with carbon dioxide to form bicarbonate. Carbon dioxide is continuously produced in the body by the processes of metabolism. Any base that enters the body can be immediately and automatically converted into bicarbonate.

Because of the importance of bicarbonate and carbon dioxide in the regulation of acid or base excesses or deficits, the pH of the blood depends on the bicarbonate-carbonic acid ratio in the plasma. Under normal conditions, the bicarbonate-carbonic acid ratio is 20:1, and the pH is 7.35 to 7.45.

When the bicarbonate concentration of the blood rises, or the carbonic acid concentration falls, the bicarbonate-carbonic acid ratio increases. The pH becomes greater than the normal value of 7.35 to 7.45. The result is *alkalosis*.

When the bicarbonate concentration of the blood falls, or the carbonic acid concentration rises, the bicarbonate-carbonic acid ratio decreases, and the pH becomes less than the normal value of 7.35 to 7.45, resulting in *acidosis*, even though the pH is still more alkaline than the neutrality of water.

RESPIRATORY REGULATION OF pH

Both the chemical and the physiologic effects of a gas depend on its pressure (the partial pressure of the gas), usually represented by the symbol P. Thus, Pco_2 represents the partial pressure of carbon dioxide. The partial pressure of a gas, which depends on the number of molecules in the gas in a given volume and also on the temperature, is completely independent of other gases in the same space. The partial pressure may be determined by either chemical or physical means. When physical means are used, the result is given as millimeters of mercury pressure (mm Hg). When chemical means are used, the result is given as volumes percent. At the normal barometric pressure, 760 mm Hg, this formula is used to convert volumes percent CO_2 to mm Hg CO_2: 1 volume percent CO_2 = 7 mm Hg.

The respiratory center in the medulla of the brain responds with varying degrees of sensitivity to the Pco_2 in the alveolar air of the lungs, to the partial pressure of oxygen (Po_2) in the alveolar air, and to the pH of the blood. The rate and depth of respiration are also affected by chemoreceptors in the aortic arch and carotid sinus. These receptors also respond to lack of oxygen, to pH, and to the carbon dioxide content of the blood.

Either excess of carbon dioxide or lack of it stimulates the respiratory center. If the Pco_2 of alveolar air rises above 9 volumes percent, or 65 mm Hg, it depresses the central nervous system, resulting in carbon dioxide narcosis. This can occur in patients with severe respiratory acidosis. Oxygen does not normally stimulate the respiratory center, but if anoxemia occurs with the amount of available oxygen reduced, the decreased oxygen concentration of the blood stimulates respiration. If a patient with cor pulmonale is given excessive concentrations of oxygen—for example, more than 50 percent—inhaled oxygen can cause the respiratory center to stop functioning. Excessive carbon dioxide accumulates, and the patient may become comatose and die (see Chapter 12).

Changes in pH also affect respiration. The marked overbreathing that results from a fall of the pH to 7.2 does this. Hyperventilation becomes maximal with a pH of approximately 7; but when the pH falls below 7, hyperventilation disappears. This is why hyperventilation, usually present in acidosis, does not always occur in *severe* acidosis.

The Pco_2 in the alveolar air exists in equilibrium with the Pco_2 of the arterial blood. The latter equilibrates with the carbonic acid content of the blood. Therefore, a change in the Pco_2 of the alveolar air causes a corresponding change in the Pco_2 and the carbonic acid content of the blood. Normally, the Pco_2 of the alveolar air is about 40 mm Hg, or 5.5 volumes percent CO_2. Should the concentration of carbonic acid in the blood increase, an increase in the Pco_2 of the alveolar air results. The respiratory center is stimulated. Hyperventilation lowers the Pco_2 of the alveolar air by causing carbon dioxide to be blown off faster than it is produced. Extreme voluntary hyperventilation can lower the P_{CO_2} to about 15 mm Hg. (Hyperventilation can also lower the P_{CO_2} of the alveolar air by causing deeper breathing, even though the rate of respiration is not increased.)

The bicarbonate concentration of the blood can be regulated by the lungs. Suppose that a patient is given a massive dose of sodium bicarbonate so that the normal bicarbonate of 27 mEq per L rises to 54. The respiratory center responds by decreasing the rate and depth of breathing. Lung volume is decreased, P_{CO_2} increases from its normal value of 40 mm Hg to 80. The carbonic acid content of the blood, normally 1.35 mEq per L, rises to 2.7 mEq per L. Thus, the bicarbonate-carbonic acid ratio and the pH remain unchanged.

Should the bicarbonate concentration of the blood decrease, respiratory rate and depth increase, causing the lung volume to increase, and the P_{CO_2} of the alveolar air and the carbonic acid of the blood to decrease. The pH remains at its former level.

Both the buffer and respiratory conpensations represent temporary mechanisms. Frequently they do not succeed in restoring or maintaining the pH of the blood and extracellular water. It is the kidneys that are able to make permanent adjustments.

HOW THE KIDNEYS REGULATE pH
The kidneys regulate pH. In the course of normal metabolism, the body produces an excess of acids. The kidneys compensate for this by screening acids and returning bicarbonate to the plasma. Therefore, the pH of the urine is usually acid, ranging from 5.5 to 6.5, while the pH of plasma and extracellular fluid is alkaline, ranging from 7.35 to 7.45.

The kidneys regulate pH by reabsorbing bicarbonate. Normally, all the bicarbonate ions that pass through the glomeruli and enter the tubular urine are reabsorbed by means of an exchange of hydrogen ions from the renal tubular cells for sodium ions in the tubular urine. In the tubular urine, hydrogen ions combine with bicarbonate ions of the tubular urine to form car-

bonic acid. This, then, forms water and carbon dioxide. The water is excreted and the carbon dioxide reabsorbed by the tubular cells. At the same time, sodium ions pass from the tubular urine into the tubular cells, where they unite with the bicarbonate ions to form sodium bicarbonate. The bicarbonate then passes into the plasma.

A similar exchange mechanism operates between hydrogen ions of the renal tubular cells and the sodium salt Na_2HPO_4 (disodium hydrogen phosphate), which appears in the tubular urine. Ammonia (NH_3) forms in the renal tubular cells by oxidation of the amino acid glutamin by the enzyme glutaminase and by oxidation of other amino acids. Free ammonia is converted into an ammonium ion, NH_4, by uniting with a hydrogen ion and is excreted as ammonium chloride (NH_4CL). Thus, another hydrogen ion is removed from the body.

When acidosis occurs, all kidney regulatory mechanisms are exaggerated. The urine shows a pH that may be as low as 4.5. Bicarbonate excretion may diminish or disappear. Acid and chloride excretion increase. Excretion of ammonium salts increases. Excretion of cations, such as sodium and potassium, decreases.

In alkalosis, these regulatory mechanisms slow down or stop. The urine shows a pH that may rise to 7.8, although in alkalosis due to potassium deficiency, the urinary pH may remain low. Bicarbonate excretion increases. Ammonium salt excretion decreases, and excretion of cations, such as sodium and potassium, increases. Titrable acid and chloride excretions also decrease.

MEASUREMENT OF ACID-BASE DISTURBANCES
The plasma pH is of great use in telling whether the patient has acidosis or alkalosis. Plasma pH can be measured directly by a pH meter or by the use of a colorimeter. Either heparinized arterial blood or "arterialized" blood from a warmed earlobe or fingertip can be employed. Alternatively, blood from a vein can be used if it is carefully drawn and kept stoppered under oil. The plasma pH answers the basic question of whether the patient is in acidosis or alkalosis, but it does not explain how he arrived at this state,

whether from metabolic acidosis or alkalosis, respiratory acidosis or alkalosis, or from renal or pulmonary compensatory mechanisms. Only a careful analysis based on history, physical examination, and all lab findings can answer this crucial question.*

Carbonic acid measured by a Pco_2 meter, of course, represents CO_2 + HOH. From this value, the amount of carbonic acid can be determined by use of a nomogram. Normal Pco_2 values range from 35 to 38 mm Hg if arterial blood is used, and from 40 to 41 mm Hg if venous blood is used.

How is the bicarbonate content of the plasma determined? Bicarbonate cannot be measured directly, so it is measured indirectly by one of the following tests: CO_2 content, CO_2 capacity, or CO_2 combining power test. One should not be misled by the names fixed to these tests; *they are not done to determine the plasma CO_2, but rather, the plasma bicarbonate*.

*Additional complications cloud the diagnosis of acid-base disturbances when one is dealing with a mixed disturbance resulting from several primary and compensatory processes affecting the same blood gas values. For example, how does one differentiate between a metabolic acid-base disturbance with respiratory compensation and a metabolic acid-base disturbance plus a respiratory acid-base disturbance? Nomograms help, but more is needed. Clinical information concerning the specific patient is essential. McCurdy presents a "system for diagnosing clinical acid-base disorders [that is] easy to use and avoids most of the pitfalls of quick decisions based only on blood gas values and nomograms": 1) Scan the history for potential processes that lead to simple acid-base disorders. 2) Note findings on physical examination that suggest an acid-base disturbance. 3) Check the routine electrolytes for a) plasma bicarbonate (CO_2 capacity test or CO_2 combining power test); b) unspecified anions; to calculate the unspecified, or undetermined, anions, which include anionic proteins, phosphates, sulfates, and organic acids, subtract the sum of carbon dioxide and chloride from the serum sodium concentration. This undetermined, or unspecified, anion fraction, also described as the anion gap or delta, is normally less than 12 to 14 mEq per L. If the total is higher than 14, metabolic acidosis is present; c) plasma potassium, which usually moves opposite to arterial pH. 4) Examine other laboratory data for disease processes associated with acid-base disturbances. 5) Explain the blood gas values. If a change in Pco_2 or HCO_3 is attributed to compensatory mechanisms rather than to an additional primary acid-base disturbance, be sure it is within the physiologically possible range. How to make this determination is clearly explained in the splendid article by McCurdy. (McCurdy, D. K.: Mixed metabolic and respiratory acid-base disturbances: diagnosis and treatment. Chest 62:35S-44S, Aug. 1972 Supplement.)

In all of these tests, the plasma is treated with an acid (e.g., sulfuric or lactic), which causes the bicarbonate radical to release its CO_2, which can be measured. By measuring the CO_2 released from bicarbonate, one can determine the bicarbonate content. Inevitably, however, the CO_2 gas dissolved in the plasma, which represents the acid portion of the acid-base balance, is measured along with the CO_2 freed from the bicarbonate. The total CO_2 measured represents both the CO_2 released from bicarbonate and the CO_2 gas dissolved in the plasma. Their sum gives us the *CO_2 content*, which normally ranges from 24 to 33 mEq per L. For the most part, the CO_2 content represents bicarbonate, which represents the alkaline side of the acid-base balance. The contribution of the acid side—that is, H_2CO_3 + dissolved CO_2 gas—normally equals only .03 × Pco_2 expressed in mm Hg, and does not significantly affect the CO_2 content. But should a respiratory acid-base disturbance prevail, the plasma would not contain the normal concentration of CO_2, and the CO_2 content test would not represent an accurate measure of the bicarbonate. For example, in carbonic acid excess, or respiratory acidosis, the plasma CO_2 is elevated because of the CO_2 retention by the lungs. In this case, the CO_2 content would inaccurately indicate that the plasma bicarbonate is unduly high. In carbonic acid deficit, or respiratory alkalosis, CO_2 is blown off, so the plasma CO_2 is depressed. In this case, the CO_2 content would show the plasma bicarbonate as being too low. Obviously, the CO_2 content test leaves something to be desired, as it accurately reflects the plasma bicarbonate only when the level of CO_2 gas dissolved in the plasma is normal.

The *CO_2 capacity* test and the *CO_2 combining power* test give a more accurate measurement of the plasma bicarbonate, even when an acid-base disturbance due to respiratory factors is present. In these tests, the actual CO_2 concentration of the plasma being tested is adjusted to normal through a process called equilibration. In the CO_2 capacity test, equilibration is achieved by bubbling a 5.5 percent CO_2 gas mixture through the test plasma. In the CO_2 combining power test, the laboratory technician blows his own breath (assumed to be normal) through the test plasma. Thus, if the CO_2 level of the test plasma is elevated because of respiratory acidosis, bubbling a normal concentration of CO_2 gas through it will cause the excess to be blown off, thereby reducing the CO_2 concentration to normal. Should the CO_2 gas of the test plasma be depressed because of respiratory alkalosis, equilibration returns it to normal by supplying the needed CO_2. In either the CO_2 capacity or the CO_2 combining power test, the test plasma is, in effect, recirculated through the lungs of a healthy person and is thus enabled to achieve its normal CO_2 concentration. Once equilibration has been accomplished, the CO_2 measurement will give, with fair accuracy, the bicarbonate content of the test plasma, regardless of whether the patient has respiratory acidosis, respiratory alkalosis, or no respiratory acid-base disturbance. In the normal individual, the CO_2 capacity varies from 24 to 33 mEq per L, and the CO_2 combining power from 24 to 35 mEq per L.

The CO_2 content, bicarbonate, pH, Pco_2, and carbonic acid all can be determined by the use of a nomogram if any two of the values are known. When a straight line is drawn between the two known points, the unknown values can be read from the other three scales.

MECHANICAL ANALOGY OF ACID-BASE DISTURBANCES

To picture what actually happens in acidosis and alkalosis, a simple mechanical analogy of acid-base balance of the body fluids can be used. Whether the body fluid is acid, neutral, or alkaline depends upon its concentration of hydrogen ions. When the concentration rises above a certain level, the patient's body fluid is acid; he has acidosis. When the concentration of hydrogen ions falls below a certain level, the patient's body fluid is alkaline; he has alkalosis. The chief factor in determining the hydrogen ion concentration of the body fluid is the ratio of carbonic acid to base bicarbonate, the latter meaning the bicarbonates of sodium, potassium, calcium, and magnesium. Because carbonic acid is 20 times as powerful as base bicarbonate, body fluid is neutral as long as there is one part, or 1 mEq, of

carbonic acid to 20 parts, or 20 mEq, of base bicarbonate. Actually, the normal amount of carbonic acid is 1.35 mEq per L, with the normal amount of base bicarbonate 27 mEq per L. But the important determinant of acid-base balance is not the absolute amounts of these substances, but the ratio. As long as the ratio is one part of carbonic acid to 20 parts of base bicarbonate, the patient's body fluid is neutral.

Examine the mechanical acid-base balance in Figure 16-4. On the right end of the balance are four black blocks, representing the normal quantity of base bicarbonate in each liter of extracellular fluid. Each block has a value of 6.75 mEq. On the left side of the balance are four white blocks, representing the normal quantity of carbonic acid in the extracellular fluid. Each white block represents about .33 mEq of carbonic acid. The mechanical acid-base balance in Figure 16-4, A is level. The following disturbances can upset it.

Metabolic Acidosis (Primary Base Bicarbonate Deficit)

Suppose a baby develops a severe diarrhea with the production of acid metabolites. These neutralize half of the base bicarbonate of the extracellular fluid, so two of the base bicarbonate, or black, blocks can be removed. The balance tilts to the left, and acidosis is present (Fig. 16-4, B).

The body always tries to correct an imbalance. The lungs blow off carbon dioxide through deep, rapid breathing. This lessening of carbon dioxide reduces the amount of carbonic acid in the extracellular fluid. The lungs may blow off enough to partially restore balance—for example, the amount represented by the removal of one white block (Fig. 16-4, C). Or, they might blow off enough to restore balance, as shown when the second white block is removed (Fig. 16-4, D). The kidneys try to help the situation by retaining bicarbonate and excreting hydrogen. The urine becomes acid.

Suppose that pulmonary compensation was not adequate and that there was still an imbalance, as shown by the replacement of one white block (Fig. 16-4, C). By giving the patient bicar-

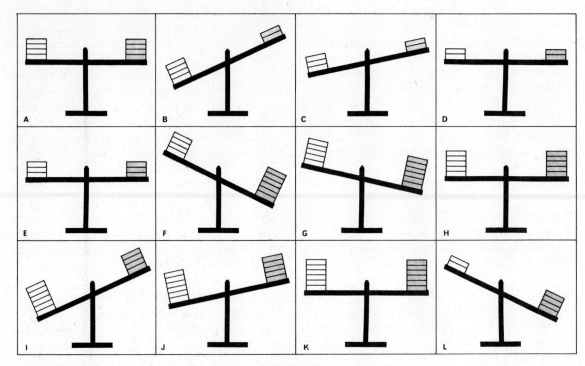

FIGURE 16-4.
Mechanical acid-base balance. (A) Level. (B) Acidosis is present, and balance is off. (C) Lungs may blow off enough carbon dioxide to partially restore balance. (D) Lungs blow off enough to restore balance. (E) Balance restored by giving patient bicarbonate or lactate parenterally, or alkaline solution orally. (F) Alkalosis is present. (G) Lungs hold back carbonic acid. (H) Chloride administered to reduce amount of bicarbonate. (I) Carbonic acid increased. (J) Kidneys hold back bicarbonate. (K) Balance restored by adding bicarbonate or lactate. (L) Carbonic acid in extracellular fluid reduced.

bonate or lactate parenterally, or by giving him an alkaline solution by mouth, symbolized by adding another black block (Fig. 16-4, E), the balance is restored to normal. Notice that there is not the same amount of carbonic acid and bicarbonate as there was at the beginning. That is not important; what is important is the ratio.

Metabolic Alkalosis (Primary Base Bicarbonate Excess)

Start again with four white blocks on the left and four black blocks on the right. Suppose the patient has vomited large amounts of chloride in his gastric juice. Chloride is an anion. As it is lost, bicarbonate increases, because the total anions lost must always equal the total cations. Bicarbonate adds up, so that two black blocks can be added (Fig. 16-4, F). The balance tilts to the

right; alkalosis is present. The lungs hold back carbonic acid, shown by adding a white block (Fig. 16-4, G). This does not restore the balance to normal, so chloride is given to reduce the amount of bicarbonate. This can be demonstrated by removing a black block (Fig. 16-4, H). The kidneys are also active in compensation. They excrete bicarbonate and hold back acid in an effort to restore the balance to normal.

Respiratory Acidosis (Primary Carbonic Acid Excess)

Again start with four black blocks and four white blocks. Suppose that the patient has pneumonia and cannot normally exhale carbon dioxide. Carbonic acid increases, symbolized by adding two white blocks (Fig. 16-4, I). The balance tilts to the left; respiratory acidosis is present. The lungs cannot participate in compensation because they are affected by the pneumonia; but the kidneys can, and they hold bicarbonate, symbolized by adding a black block (Fig. 16-4, J), helping restore the balance to normal. The balance could be further restored by giving bicarbonate or lactate, as symbolized by the additional black block (Fig. 16-4, K). But the most important measure is to cure the primary pulmonary disease. Suppose this is done, as shown by removing two white blocks (Fig. 16-4, F). The compensatory increase in bicarbonate is then reduced by the body, as symbolized by removing two black blocks (Fig. 16-4, A).

Respiratory Alkalosis (Primary Carbonic Acid Deficit)

Now suppose that the patient has overbreathed because of hysteria. Excessive quantities of carbon dioxide are blown off from the lungs. The carbonic acid in the extracellular fluid is reduced, symbolized by removing two white blocks (Fig. 16-4, L), and alkalosis occurs. The lungs cannot participate in compensation, but the kidneys can and do. They permit bicarbonate to pass through the urine, symbolized by removing two black blocks (Fig. 16-4, D). The balance returns, or tends to return, to normal. Restoration to the initial quantities of carbonic acid and base bicarbonate is achieved only when normal retention of carbon dioxide occurs with the relief of the hysteria. This is symbolized by adding two white blocks (Fig. 16-4, B). The kidneys then permit bicarbonate to return to normal, as symbolized by adding two black blocks (Fig. 16-4, A).

COMMENT

By the use of the mechanical analogy, one can reproduce any acid-base disturbance that can occur. Not only can metabolic acidosis or metabolic alkalosis, respiratory acidosis or respiratory alkalosis, be reproduced but also combinations of the two types of imbalances. The balance is also useful in helping to evaluate the results of laboratory findings. But it must be remembered that the *absolute* quantities of carbonic acid or bicarbonate make no difference; it is the *relative* quantities. As long as one increases base bicarbonate—for example, by doubling it—and at the same time increases carbonic acid by the same factor, the acid-base balance is maintained. It is also maintained when one divides both quantities by two. Acid-base imbalances occur, then, when one increases carbonic acid or base bicarbonate, or decreases carbonic acid or base bicarbonate, without a corresponding change in the other. Note that metabolic or systemic (nonrespiratory) conditions affect the right side of the balance, while pulmonary, or lung, conditions affect the left side.

For the history, symptoms, and laboratory findings of the four basic types of acid-base disturbances, see Table 16-2, pp. 500 to 502, subheads 9, 10, 11, and 12.

Alterations Produced by Disease

To understand the alterations in body fluids produced by disease, the clinical picture approach is employed. In doing this, one must first recognize that disturbances of water and electrolytes result from a fairly small number of mechanisms, most of which are readily understandable. Some disturbances are primary—for example, the sodium deficit that occurs when one sweats excessively and drinks only water. Other disturbances occur secondary to disease—for example, the base bicarbonate deficit, or metabolic acidosis, that occurs in uncontrolled diabetes mellitus. Although produced by a wide variety of etiologic factors, these disturbances can be divided into 16 clinical entities. Understanding the entities helps one understand the combinations, as well as the interrelationships, between these fluid balance disturbances and other diseases (Table 16-2). In examining this table, an understanding of which is essential for mastery of body fluid disturbances, the reader should remember the following: extracellular fluid volume represents the *total volume in ml* of extracellular fluid present in the body. Obviously, there is no precise means of measuring this, although acute gain or loss of weight is the best measure of a volume deficit or excess. Compositional changes relating to sodium, potassium, and so on, refer *not* to total

TABLE 16-2

Diagnostic Entities of Body Fluid Disturbances

IMBALANCE	HISTORY	SYMPTOMS	LABORATORY FINDINGS
1. Extracellular fluid volume deficit	Decreased water intake Diarrhea Draining fistula Intestinal obstruction Systemic infection Vomiting	Acute weight loss—in excess of 5 percent Body temperature drop Dryness of skin and mucous membranes Longitudinal wrinkles or furrows of tongue Oliguria or anuria	Packed cell volume or hemoglobin increase Red blood cell count increase
2. Extracellular fluid volume excess	Congestive heart failure Excessive adrenocortical hormones Excessive ingestion of sodium chloride Hyperaldosteronism Parenteral infusion of isotonic solution of sodium chloride Renal disease	Acute weight gain—in excess of 5 percent Edema Edema of tissues at operation Moist rales in lungs Puffy eyelids Shortness of breath	Packed cell volume or hemoglobin decrease Red blood cell count decrease
3. Sodium deficit of extracellular fluid	Excessive sweating, plus drinking water Gastrointestinal suction, plus drinking water Inhalation of fresh water Parenteral electrolyte-free solution Potent diuretic Water enema	Abdominal cramps Apprehension Convulsions Fingerprinting on sternum Oliguria or anuria	Chloride of plasma below 98 mEq/L Sodium of plasma below 137 mEq/L Specific gravity of urine below 1.010
4. Sodium excess of extracellular fluid	Decreased water intake Diarrhea Excessive ingestion of sodium chloride Inhalation of salt (ocean) water Tracheobronchitis Unconsciousness	Dry, sticky mucous membranes Flushed skin Oliguria or anuria Thirst Tongue rough and dry	Chloride of plasma above 106 mEq/L Sodium of plasma above 147 mEq/L Specific gravity of urine above 1.030
5. Potassium deficit of extracellular fluid	Burn after third day Diabetic acidosis Diarrhea Draining fistula Parenteral potassium-free solution Potent diuretic Ulcerative colitis Vomiting	Anorexia Gaseous distention of intestine Silent intestinal ileus Soft, flabby muscles Weakness	Electrocardiograph shows low voltage, flattened T wave, depressed S-T segment Potassium of plasma below 4 mEq/L

	Causes	Symptoms	Laboratory findings
6. Potassium excess of extracellular fluid	Adrenal insufficiency Burn, early Excessive parenteral administration of potassium Massive crushing injury Mercuric bichloride poisoning Oliguria or anuria Oral intake of potassium exceeding renal tolerance Renal disease	Diarrhea Intestinal colic Irritability Nausea	Electrocardiograph shows high T wave, depressed S-T segment Potassium of plasma above 5.6 mEq/L
7. Calcium deficit of extracellular fluid	Acute pancreatitis Excessive administration of citrated blood Massive infection of subcutaneous tissues Parenteral administration of calcium-free solution Primary hypoparathyroidism Recent correction of acidosis Sprue	Abdominal cramps Carpopedal spasm Muscle cramps Tetany Tingling of ends of fingers	Calcium of plasma below 4.5 mEq/L Sulkowitch's test on urine: no precipitation
8. Calcium excess of extracellular fluid	Excessive administration of vitamin D Hyperparathyroidism Multiple myeloma Parathyroid tumor Pathologic fracture Prolonged immobilization Renal disease	Bone cavitation Deep bony pain Flank pain Kidney stones Muscle hypotonicity	Calcium of plasma above 5.8 mEq/L Sulkowitch's test on urine: heavy precipitation
9. Primary base bicarbonate deficit of extracellular fluid	Decreased food intake Diabetic acidosis Ketogenic diet Parenteral infusion of isotonic solution of sodium chloride Renal disease Salicylate intoxication (not early) Systemic infection	Deep, rapid breathing (Kussmaul's) Shortness of breath on exertion Stupor Weakness	Bicarbonate of plasma below 25 mEq/L in adults; below 20 mEq/L in children pH of plasma below 7.35 pH of urine below 6
10. Primary base bicarbonate excess of extracellular fluid	Excessive adrenocortical hormones Excessive ingestion of sodium bicarbonate Gastrointestinal suction Parenteral potassium-free solution Potassium deficit Potent diuretic Vomiting	Hypertonic muscles Tetany Decrease in rate and depth of respiration	Bicarbonate of plasma above 29 mEq/L in adults; above 25 mEq/L in children pH of plasma above 7.45 pH of urine above 7.0 Potassium of plasma below 4 mEq/L

11. Primary carbonic acid deficit of extra-cellular fluid	Anxiety Early salicylate intoxication Extreme emotion Fever Hysteria Intentional overbreathing Oxygen lack Rapid breathing (not Kussmaul's)	Convulsions Tetany Unconsciousness	Bicarbonate of plasma below 25 mEq/L in adults; below 20 mEq/L in children pH of plasma above 7.45 pH of urine above 7.0
12. Primary carbonic acid excess of extra-cellular fluid	Asthma Barbiturate poisoning Breathing excessive carbon dioxide Emphysema Morphine poisoning Occlusion of breathing passages Pneumonia	Coma Disorientation Respiratory embarrassment Weakness	Bicarbonate of plasma above 29 mEq/L in adults; above 25 mEq/L in children
13. Protein deficit of extracellular fluid	Burn after third day Decreased food intake Decubitus ulcers Fracture Loss of whole blood Severe trauma Wound drainage	Chronic weight loss Emotional depression Pallor Ready fatigue Soft, flabby muscles	Albumin of plasma below 4 Gm/100 ml Packed cell volume, hemoglobin, or red blood cell count decreased (significant only if iron stores are adequate)
14. Magnesium deficit of extracellular fluid	Chronic alcoholism Diarrhea Enterostomy drainage Impaired gastrointestinal absorption, surgical Parenteral administration of magnesium-free solution Vomiting	Chvostek's sign positive Convulsions Disorientation Hyperactive deep reflexes Positive therapeutic response to magnesium sulfate Tremor	Magnesium of plasma below 1.4 mEq/L
15. Plasma-to-interstitial fluid shift of extra-cellular fluid	Acute occlusion of major artery Burn, early Intestinal obstruction Massive crushing injury Perforated peptic ulcer Severe trauma	Cold extremities Low blood pressure Pallor Tachycardia Weak to absent pulse Weakness	Packed cell volume or hemoglobin increased Red blood cell count increased
16. Interstitial fluid-to-plasma shift of extracellular fluid	Burn after third day Excessive infusion of large molecular solution (plasma, dextran, etc.) Fracture Loss of whole blood	Air hunger Bounding pulse Cardiac dilatation Engorgement of peripheral veins Moist rales in lungs Pallor Ventricular failure Weakness	Packed cell volume or hemoglobin decreased Red blood cell count decreased

body electrolyte, but to *concentration* of the electrolyte in question in *mEq per L*. An individual with greatly expanded extracellular fluid volume can have more than the normal body content of sodium and still have a dangerously low sodium content in terms of mEq per L. Conversely, an individual with less than the normal body content of sodium can die of sodium excess if his extracellular water is severely depleted. The crux, then, is mEq per L, not total body content, when composition of electrolytes is involved.

A fascinating relationship holds for the total water and the sodium concentration per liter, for with few qualifications, body water content depends upon sodium, and sodium concentration depends upon water. For example, an individual ingesting sufficient water can deplete his body sodium, and an individual who is severely dehydrated will suffer from excessive body sodium concentration. Conversely, ingesting sufficient sodium can kill through water retention. Indeed, an ancient method of execution consisted of forcing the victim to eat a cup of salt. But the individual depleted of sodium (e.g., through heavy sweating with ingestion of water only) will be unable to retain sufficient water for normal physiology. So bear in mind that what is being discussed here is not *total water content*, but *sodium concentration per liter*.

Following are examples of frequently seen imbalances.

LOW-SODIUM SYNDROME

The low-sodium syndrome can develop as a result of decreased intake or increased loss of sodium or as a result of excessive intake or decreased loss of water. It can be preceded by several different clinical situations. There may have been excessive sweating plus drinking of water; gastrointestinal suction plus drinking of water (a fairly common occurrence in hospitals); administration of a potent diuretic, usually in excess; repeated administration of enemas of water; parenteral infusion of an electrolyte-free solution; or inhalation of fresh water, as occurs in fresh water drowning.

The symptoms include apprehension, a bizarre, indefinable feeling of impending doom; abdominal cramps; convulsions; oliguria or anuria. Other symptoms are that of vasomotor collapse, including hypotension; rapid, thready pulse; cold, clammy skin; and cyanosis. The fluid volume of the extracellular fluid, both plasma and interstitial, is decreased. For this reason, tissues tend to retain any shape caused by pressure deformation—that is, they become more plastic than normal. Thus, when the thumb is pressed firmly over the sternum, a visible thumb-print may be apparent.

Laboratory findings reveal a plasma chloride usually below 98 mEq per L, and a plasma sodium below 137 mEq per L, although it may be much lower. The specific gravity of the urine is characteristically below 1.010.

Treatment of a well-developed deficit consists of administration of a hypertonic solution (3 percent or 5 percent) of sodium chloride.

POTASSIUM DEPLETION

Potassium depletion is another body fluid disturbance that occurs frequently. Although potassium is present in both cellular and extracellular fluid, its chief role is played within the cells. Since the body conservation mechanism for potassium is at best inefficient, potassium deficit inevitably occurs when there has been no ingestion of potassium for several days. But a deficit can occur when there are excessive losses of potassium, such as may result from destruction of cells, as in burns or crushing injuries; in diarrhea or ulcerative colitis; severe vomiting; following administration of a potent diuretic, such as one of the thiazides. The latter cause is probably by far the most common. Many physicians believe that half the patients receiving thiazides will sooner or later develop potassium deficit.

The first symptom of potassium deficit is usually malaise, just not feeling well. But as the deficit develops, symptoms relating to muscle systems appear. Some of these, such as generalized weakness or flabby muscles, relate to the skeletal muscles. Some, such as weak pulse or faint heart sounds, relate to the heart muscle. Others, such as vomiting or paralytic ileus, refer to the muscles of the gastrointestinal tract. Some, such as shallow respiration and difficulty in breathing on exertion, relate to the muscles of respiration.

Laboratory findings include a plasma potassium below 4 mEq per L. Since metabolic alkalosis frequently occurs, the chloride may be below 98 mEq per L, and the plasma bicarbonate above 29 mEq per L. An electrocardiogram characteristically shows evidence of potassium deficit.

Prophylactic treatment includes administration of a salt of potassium. Ingestion of high potassium foods, such as bananas and orange juice, also helps forestall deficits. Treatment includes oral administration of potassium salts, which does not necessarily have to be a chloride salt, or, if the patient is unable to take nourishment by mouth, parenteral infusion of potassium.

HYPERCALCEMIC CRISIS

The causes of hypercalcemia include tumor of the parathyroid glands, excessive vitamin D in arthritis therapy, overactivity of the parathyroid glands, or multiple myeloma.

Hypercalcemic crisis is the most critical syndrome of calcium. It is an emergency situation that must be treated or the patient will die of cardiac arrest.

Symptoms of hypercalcemic crisis include intractable nausea and vomiting, dehydration, stupor, coma, and azotemia.

Medical management has generally been unsatisfactory, since none of the regimens utilized has been consistently successful, because of slow action or inherent toxicity. There is currently a renewed interest in the inorganic phosphate treatment of hypercalcemia. It appears to be effective in rapidly lowering serum calcium levels, beginning within three minutes of the start of an infusion, with a return to normal calcium values within 24 hours. It is thought that phosphate acts by deposition of a calcium phosphate salt into the bones or soft tissues.

The main concern in the use of phosphate is the risk of producing metastatic extraskeletal calcification, particularly when serum phosphorus is persistently elevated during treatment or when renal function is impaired. Hypotension, as well as thrombophlebitis or calcium deposits, or both, at the infusion site can occur. But even with these possible complications, prompt relief of hypercalcemic crisis by this treatment appears to justify its use.

Sulfate solutions have also been shown to be effective in lowering serum calcium levels. Although sulfate preparations act more slowly than phosphate preparations, metastatic calcification has not been a problem. However hypomagnesemia may develop with sulfate therapy; for this reason, magnesium supplements should be available when a patient is being treated with a sulfate solution.

PROTEIN DEPLETION

Protein depletion can follow repeated or chronic loss of whole blood, decreased food intake, a burn, trauma, or fracture. It can also result from wound drainage or decubitus ulcers.

Its symptoms include emotional depression; ready fatigue; pallor; and soft, flabby muscles. The protein-deficient patient frequently appears to have decreased resistance to infection. He shows chronic weight loss. The plasma albumin is sometimes, though not necessarily, below 4 Gm per 100 ml. The packed cell volume, hemoglobin, and red blood cell count are decreased. The decrease in red cell count is significant only if the iron stores of the patient are adequate. (Otherwise the anemia and hypohemoglobinemia may be due to iron deficiency.)

Protein deficit is best treated by a well-balanced nutritional program. This can be given in the form of high-protein tube feedings or by the use of a well-balanced diet, if tolerated, or both.

MAGNESIUM DEFICIT

While not common, magnesium deficit must be considered. The history frequently reveals chronic alcoholism, vomiting, or diarrhea. There may be impaired gastrointestinal absorption, either because of disease of the small intestine or surgical removal of portions of the intestine. Magnesium deficit may follow enterostomy drainage or parenteral administration of magnesium-free solutions. It frequently occurs in conjuction with potassium deficit. *Magnesium deficit should always be considered when a potassium deficit does not respond to appropriate therapy.*

Treatment consists of administration of magnesium as magnesium sulfate or other salt.

Magnesium deficit should be considered in patients with primary aldosteronism.

Nursing Observations

Prompt and astute nursing observations are just as important in the field of fluid balance as in any other clinical area. Many body fluid disturbances can be anticipated and thus prevented by early treatment. The nurse is in an excellent position to assess the patient's state of fluid balance and make a tentative diagnosis if she knows what to look for. As a first step to making such an evaluation, the nurse should answer the following questions.

1. Is there a disease state present that can disrupt body fluid balance? If so, what imbalances usually result from this condition? See Table 16-3.
2. Is any medication or treatment being given that can upset fluid balance? If so, how? See Table 16-4, p. 508.
3. Are there unusual losses of any body fluid? If so, what imbalances usually result from the loss of the particular body fluids? See Table 16-5, p. 509.
4. Is the patient on a restricted diet? If so, can this affect fluid balance?
5. Is the patient taking adequate amounts of water and other nutrients orally or by some other route? If not, how long has the intake been inadequate?
6. How does fluid intake compare with output?

If the answers indicate that a fluid imbalance is likely to occur, the nurse should then set up a program of planned observations. When she discovers significant symptoms, she should report them to the physician and ask for specific orders, thus making early diagnosis and treatment possible.

Among the observations that should be made are TPRs, which may reveal the state of the patient's fluid balance. Fever causes an increased loss of body fluids, so it is highly important that temperature elevations be reported. Pulse, usually checked at the same time the temperature is taken, should be evaluated in terms of rate, volume, regularity, and ease of obliteration. Varying pulse rates are seen in many fluid balance disorders. Changes in respiration rate, depth, and regularity should be reported, because respiratory changes accompany not only respiratory alkalosis and respiratory acidosis, but also metabolic alkalosis and metabolic acidosis as well. TPRs are usually taken at least four times a day, more often if indicated. All should be evaluated carefully, taking into consideration any extraneous variables that may affect the accuracy of the readings.

Blood pressure should be checked frequently when there is an actual or potential fluid imbalance. When the reading is abnormal, pressure should be checked in both arms. Variables that affect blood pressure, such as activity, emotional upsets, or position changes, should be considered in evaluating the significance of blood pressure changes.

Peripheral veins can be observed to help evaluate the patient's plasma volume. When the hand is elevated, the veins usually empty in three to five seconds; they fill in the same amount of time when placed in a dependent position. A decreased plasma volume, which may be secondary to an extracellular fluid volume deficit or a shift of fluid from the plasma to interstitial space, causes the hands to take longer than three to five seconds to fill when in a dependent position. When plasma volume is reduced, the veins are not readily apparent. The slow filling of the veins often precedes hypotension when the patient is in early shock. An increased plasma volume, which may be secondary to extracellular fluid volume excess, or a shift of fluid from interstitial space to plasma, causes the hand veins to take longer than three to five seconds to empty when the hands are elevated. The veins may be engorged and are clearly visible with increased plasma volume.

Skin elasticity and mucous membrane moisture should be checked and evaluated in relation

TABLE 16-3
Various Clinical Conditions and Resultant Fluid Imbalances

CONDITION	IMBALANCES APT TO RESULT	CONDITION	IMBALANCES APT TO RESULT
Adrenal insufficiency	Potassium excess	Inhalation of salt water (drowning)	Sodium excess
Alcoholism, chronic	Magnesium deficit	Massive crushing injury	Potassium excess Plasma-to-interstitial fluid shift
Asthma	Respiratory acidosis		
Burn, early	Potassium excess Plasma-to-interstitial fluid shift	Massive infection of subcutaneous tissues	Calcium deficit
Burn, after third day	Potassium deficit Protein deficit Interstitial fluid-to-plasma shift	Meningitis	Respiratory alkalosis
		Multiple myeloma	Calcium excess
Congestive heart failure	Fluid volume excess	Occlusion of breathing passages	Respiratory acidosis
Diabetes mellitus, uncontrolled severe	Metabolic acidosis Potassium deficit	Occlusion of major artery, acute	Plasma-to-interstitial fluid shift
Emphysema	Respiratory acidosis		
Encephalitis	Respiratory alkalosis	Oxygen lack with hyperpnea	Respiratory alkalosis
		Pancreatitis, acute	Calcium deficit
Fever	Fluid volume deficit Respiratory alkalosis	Peptic ulcer, perforated	Plasma-to-interstitial fluid shift Respiratory acidosis
Fractures	Plasma-to-interstitial fluid shift Protein deficit	Pneumonia	Respiratory acidosis
		Pulmonary edema	Respiratory acidosis
Gastric disease, repeated vomiting	Potassium deficit Metabolic alkalosis	Renal disease	Potassium excess Fluid volume excess Metabolic acidosis Calcium deficit
High external temperature with physiologic hyperpnea	Respiratory alkalosis		
Hyperaldosteronism	Fluid volume excess	Systemic infection	Metabolic acidosis Fluid volume deficit

Condition	Associated imbalance(s)
Hyperparathyroidism	Calcium excess
Hypoparathyroidism, primary	Calcium deficit
Inhalation of fresh water (drowning)	Sodium deficit
Administration of adrenocortical hormones	Fluid volume excess; Potassium deficit; Metabolic alkalosis
Administration of potent diuretics	Potassium deficit; Sodium deficit; Metabolic alkalosis
Barbiturate poisoning	Respiratory acidosis
Early salicylate intoxication	Respiratory alkalosis
Excessive administration of citrated blood	Calcium deficit
Excessive administration of vitamin D	Calcium excess
Excessive infusion of large molecular solution	Interstitial fluid-to-plasma shift
Excessive ingestion of sodium bicarbonate	Metabolic alkalosis
Excessive ingestion of sodium chloride	Sodium excess; Fluid volume excess
Excessive parenteral administration of calcium-free solutions	Calcium deficit
Excessive parenteral administration of magnesium-free solutions	Magnesium deficit
Tracheobronchitis	Sodium excess
Trauma, severe	Plasma-to-interstitial fluid shift; Protein deficit; Potassium excess
Excessive parenteral administration of potassium	Fluid volume excess; Metabolic acidosis
Excessive parenteral infusion of isotonic solution of sodium chloride	Sodium deficit; Metabolic alkalosis; Potassium deficit; Respiratory alkalosis
Gastrointestinal suction plus drinking water	Respiratory acidosis
Mechanical respiratory inaccurately regulated (causing too deep or too fast breathing)	Potassium excess
Mechanical respiratory inaccurately regulated (causing too shallow or too slow breathing)	Respiratory acidosis
Mercuric bichloride poisoning	Potassium excess
Morphine or meperidine (Demerol) in excessive doses	Calcium excess
Oral intake of potassium exceeding renal tolerance	Calcium deficit; Metabolic acidosis
Prolonged immobilization	Sodium deficit; Potassium deficit
Recent correction of acidosis	
Salicylate intoxication (not early)	
Water enemas	

TABLE 16-4
Imbalances Resulting from Medical Therapy

THERAPY	IMBALANCES APT TO OCCUR	THERAPY	IMBALANCES APT TO OCCUR
Administration of adreno-cortical hormones	Fluid volume excess Potassium deficit Metabolic alkalosis	Excessive parenteral administration of potassium	Potassium excess
Administration of potent diuretics	Potassium deficit Sodium deficit Metabolic alkalosis	Excessive parenteral infusion of isotonic solution of sodium chloride	Fluid volume excess Metabolic acidosis
Barbiturate poisoning	Respiratory acidosis	Gastrointestinal suction plus drinking water	Sodium deficit Metabolic alkalosis Potassium deficit
Early salicylate intoxication	Respiratory alkalosis	Mechanical respirator inaccurately regulated (causing too deep or too fast breathing)	Respiratory alkalosis
Excessive administration of citrated blood	Calcium deficit		
Excessive administration of vitamin D	Calcium excess	Mechanical respirator inaccurately regulated (causing too shallow or too slow breathing)	Respiratory acidosis
Excessive infusion of large molecular solution	Interstititial fluid-to-plasma shift	Mercuric bichloride poisoning	Potassium excess
Excessive ingestion of sodium bicarbonate	Metabolic alkalosis	Morphine or meperidine (Demerol) in excessive doses	Respiratory acidosis
Excessive ingestion of sodium chloride	Sodium excess Fluid volume excess	Oral intake of potassium exceeding renal tolerance	Potassium excess
		Prolonged immobilization	Calcium excess
Excessive parenteral administration of calcium-free solutions	Calcium deficit	Recent correction of acidosis	Calcium deficit
Excessive parenteral administration of magnesium-free solutions	Magnesium deficit	Salicylate intoxication (not early)	Metabolic acidosis
		Water enemas	Sodium deficit Potassium deficit

to fluid balance disturbances. Poor skin turgor and dry mucous membranes are indicative of fluid volume deficit. In addition, pallor; flushed, dry skin; cold, clammy skin; pitting edema; fingerprinting on sternum, longitudinal wrinkles on tongue; and rough, red, dry tongue are all symptoms of various fluid imbalances and should be watched for.

A severe extracellular fluid volume deficit causes the patient to have a drawn facial expression; the eyes are sunken and feel much less firm than normal. When there is an excess of extracellular fluid, the patient may exhibit puffy eyelids and cheeks that appear fuller than usual.

Even variations in speech may be significant in evaluating a patient's state of fluid balance, and the nurse should be alert for subtle changes in quality, content, and formation of speech. Difficulty in forming words may result from dry mucous membranes or generalized muscle weakness. Potassium deficit may be responsible for hyperactive, irrelevant speech, and extracellular fluid volume excess can cause hoarseness.

Various behavior changes, such as lassitude, emotional depression, impaired mental function, apprehension, giddiness, irritability, restlessness, excitement, disorientation, hallucinations, stupor, unconsciousness, and carphologia, are important symptoms of fluid balance disorders and should be considered in making the diagnosis. In addition, the patient's fatigue threshold should be observed for day-to-day changes, with careful note being made of muscle weakness, easy fatigue, and diminished stamina and endurance. Weakness or cramping of skeletal muscles should be noted.

TABLE 16-5
Imbalances Resulting from Fluid Loss of
Specific Body fluid

FLUID BEING LOST	IMBALANCE LIKELY TO OCCUR
Gastric juice	Extracellular fluid volume deficit Metabolic alkalosis Sodium deficit Potassium deficit Tatany (if metabolic alkalosis is present) Magnesium deficit
Intestinal juice	Extracellular fluid volume deficit Metabolic acidosis Sodium deficit Potassium deficit
Bile	Sodium deficit Metabolic acidosis
Pancreatic juice	Metabolic acidosis Sodium deficit Calcium deficit Extracellular fluid volume deficit
Sensible perspiration	Extracellular fluid volume deficit Sodium deficit
Insensible water loss	Water deficit (dehydration) Sodium excess
Wound exudate	Protein deficit Sodium deficit Extracellular fluid volume deficit
Ascites	Protein deficit Sodium deficit Plasma-to-interstitial fluid shift Extracellular fluid volume deficit

Symptoms include hyperirritability of the muscles and central nervous system. Other findings include tremor, hyperactive deep reflexes, positive Chvostek's sign, and convulsions; confusion, even hallucinations, may occur, as well as elevated blood pressure and tachycardia. Therapeutic response to magnesium sulfate is helpful in diagnosis. Laboratory findings reveal a plasma magnesium below 1.4 mEq per L.

Sensation changes, such as light-headedness, abdominal cramps, tingling of ends of fingers and toes, circumoral paresthesia, muscle cramps, numbness of extremities, nausea, tinnitus, abnormal sensitivity to sound, deep bony pain, and flank pain, frequently occur in patients with water and electrolyte imbalances. Their presence should be reported.

Anorexia and thirst are also important symptoms in assessing a patient's body fluid status, since they occur in many imbalances.

In addition, the nurse must maintain accurate intake-output records on any patient who has a real or potential water and electrolyte balance problem, for most fluid imbalances result from differences between gains and losses of body fluids. To evaluate them, it is necessary that the amount and kind of fluids lost and the amount and kinds of fluids taken in be recorded on the intake-output record. Intake of solids must be considered in keeping the record, since they consist largely of water. In addition, bowel movements and any significant facts concerning them should be recorded. Liquid stools should be estimated as to volume and recorded. The importance of keeping exact intake-output records cannot be overemphasized, because an accurate record can be a major tool for the physician in diagnosing and planning therapy for patients with fluid imbalances.

Daily weighing of patients with actual or potential fluid imbalances is also important, because rapid fluctuations in weight closely reflect changes in fluid volume. Since physicians often gauge the administration of fluids and diuretics by the recorded weight changes, it is important that the same procedure be followed each time the patient is weighed in order to obtain accurate measurements. However, fluids that are lost inside the body, such as the pooling that occurs in intestinal obstruction, are not reflected by weight changes.

When nursing observations indicate an imminent fluid balance disorder, the nurse should, of course, present her findings to the physician and ask for further directions. However, the nurse can do much to prevent potential imbalances. For example, if the patient is taking a thiazide diuretic, his need for potassium will increase. If the physician has not prescribed a specific diet, the nurse can encourage the patient to eat foods high in potassium. Patients with fever should be given additional water, as well as extra amounts of all nutrients. The heavily perspiring patient should be given liquids containing both water and electrolytes freely, since great amounts of these are lost in sweat. The patient who is vomiting should not drink water since gastric electrolytes are lost with vomited water. Nor should the patient who is receiving gastrointestinal suction be given water or ice chips, since water washes electrolytes from the stomach, causing metabolic alkalosis, sodium deficit, and potassium deficit. Corticosteroid therapy—especially if prolonged, employing high doses—causes retention of sodium and excretion of potassium. Therefore, sodium intake should generally be restricted and potassium intake encouraged when these hormones are given (see Chapter 11).

Therapy

When water and electrolyte imbalances occur, they must be treated as soon as detected. The goals of therapy in planning the treatment of a patient with an actual or potential fluid balance disturbance are: 1) to repair any pre-existing water and electrolyte deficits; 2) to provide water and electrolytes to maintain the needs of the patient; and 3) to replace water and electrolytes being lost through such routes as vomiting, diarrhea, dialysis, tubular drainage, wound or burn exudate, and so forth.

Before therapy is started, one should determine whether renal function is adequate. Otherwise, parenteral solutions—particularly those containing potassium—can be hazardous. Renal function can be impaired because of renal impairment, because of disease, or because of a deficit in extracellular fluid volume, which prevents adequate blood from flowing through the kidney glomeruli. The latter functional renal de-

pression can be readily corrected, after which one can proceed with administration of potassium-containing solutions. On the other hand, depression of renal function caused by partial or complete renal failure requires careful diagnosis by experts in kidney disease and should be followed by replacement therapy based upon precise calculations of the need.

How does one distinguish between renal depression (due to extracellular fluid volume deficit) and organic impairment of the kidneys? If any of the following conditions exists, functional renal depression *or* organic renal impairment may be present:

- Specific gravity of urine above 1.030 (indicates functional renal depression, not renal impairment)
- Less than three voidings in 24 hours (could be due either to functional renal depression or renal impairment)
- Absence of urine in the bladder (could be due either to functional renal depression or renal impairment)

If there has been massive acute loss of extracellular fluid, functional renal depression is almost certainly present. The therapeutic test described below often corrects it.

Functional and organic renal depression can be differentiated by administering an initial hydrating solution, which typically provides sodium, 51 mEq per L, chloride, 51 mEq per L, and glucose, 5 Gm per L (actually, that is one part isotonic solution of sodium chloride in 5 percent glucose and two parts of 5 percent glucose in water) at the rate of 8 ml per square meter of body surface per minute for 45 minutes. The therapeutic test reestablishes urinary flow if the suppression is due to volume deficit. The initial hydrating solution is discontinued if kidneys begin to function, and therapy is started with other appropriate solutions, However, if urinary flow is not restored, the infusion is continued for another hour at the rate of 2 ml per square meter of body surface per minute. If urination fails to occur at the end of this time, the physician must assume that the problem is renal impairment rather than volume deficit.

Once the kidneys have proven functional, the physician can begin his program of repairing pre-existing deficits and providing water and electrolytes for maintenance. He may use a single solution of the type devised by Butler and his associates at the Massachusetts General Hospital and used with great success in many parts of the world. When a Butler-type solution is used to meet the patient's fluid volume requirement, it provides electrolytes in amounts balanced between the minimal needs and the maximal tolerances of the patient. Therefore, it may be called a balanced solution. A hypotonic solution, it is only one-third to one-half as concentrated as plasma. In addition to providing both cellular and extracellular electrolytes, it provides free water to form urine and to carry out metabolic functions. The Butler-type solution also contains 5 or 10 percent carbohydrate to reduce tissue destruction, to counteract ketosis, and to spare protein. The body homeostatic mechanisms select the electrolytes that are needed and reject those not required. When used properly, the Butler-type solution has a great margin of safety. It can be administered by mouth, by nasogastric tube, or intravenously, but not subcutaneously. The usual rate for administering the solution intravenously is 3 ml per square meter of body surface per minute for all age groups.

The proper dosage for correcting a moderate pre-existing deficit and meeting maintenance needs is 2,400 ml per square meter of body surface per day. If the pre-existing deficit is severe, the correct dose is 3,000 ml per square meter body surface per day.

Continuing abnormal losses, as in vomiting or diarrhea, are corrected by administration of a solution with a composition similar to the fluid being lost. Replacement solutions are usually administered at the rate of 3 ml per square meter body surface per minute and are generally used for treating disturbances that result from differences between intake and output, such as fluid volume deficit, sodium excess, potassium deficit, base bicarbonate deficit, and base bicarbonate excess. Other imbalances require therapy specifically tailored to the imbalance, such as shown in Table 16-6.

Since it is often difficult to obtain specific orders from the physician as to how rapidly fluids should be administered, the nurse should be able to accurately determine the correct flow rate. Factors to be considered in determining correct flow rate include type of fluid, need for fluids, cardiac and renal status, age, body size, reaction of the patient to the infusion, and vein size.

Infusion rates vary with the type of fluid being used; therefore, the nurse should be familiar with the recommended rates of infusion for the various solutions. These are listed in Table 16-7. However, the other variables must be considered: if a patient is in great need of fluids, as in hypovolemic shock, the infusion is much faster than usual. If the heart or kidneys are not functioning normally, too rapid administration of fluids can cause a dangerous fluid excess. Elderly patients are likely to have renal or cardiac impairment, so fluids should be administered to them more slowly than to younger persons. If the usual flow rate of 3 ml per square meter body surface per minute must be altered or does not apply to the type of solution being used, one can assume that if all other factors are equal, a large person can tolerate a larger amount of fluid per minute than can a smaller person.

Patients respond differently to parenteral fluid administration just as they do to other medications; therefore, the patient's reaction to the infusion is one of the best guides to safe flow rate. The patient should be checked at least every 15 minutes during an infusion, with the nurse being alert for symptoms associated with improper administration of various solutions. Complications that may occur with intravenous fluid administration are listed in Table 16-8.

The nurse should also be aware that even though the desired flow rate may have been established, there are several mechanical factors that may alter it.

1. Change in needle position (needle lumen might be lodged against wall of vein).
2. A change in the height of the bed or infusion bottle can increase or decrease the flow rate since infusions flow in by gravity.
3. Patency of needle (a small clot can occlude the needle lumen and decrease the rate of flow; the rate increases when the clot is released).
4. Limb movement or exercise.

TABLE 16-6
Imbalances Requiring Specific Therapy

IMBALANCE	THERAPY
Plasma-to-interstitial fluid shift	Relieve condition causing shift. Localized shifts may be restricted by the application of a binder. Maintain or restore plasma volume by the parenteral administration of dextran, plasma, or a plasma-like electrolyte solution.
Interstitial fluid-to-plasma shift	Phlebotomy or tourniquets may be used if shift is caused by remobilization of edema fluid. If shift is caused by loss of whole blood, blood transfusions should be given.
Whole blood deficit	Administer whole blood. If volume of extracellular fluid is excessive, only red cells should be given.
Sodium deficit	Provide sodium chloride in such concentration as to return to normal the sodium level of extracellular fluid without causing fluid volume excess. If fluid volume is normal or elevated, administer 3 or 5 percent solution of sodium chloride. If volume is decreased, administer an isotonic solution of sodium chloride.
Protein deficit	Administer high protein foods or supplements or administer intravenously amino acids with provision of generous quantities of calories in the form of alcohol, or dextrose, or both. It may be necessary to use all three expedients.
Calcium deficit	If deficit is acute, administer intravenously a 10 percent solution of calcium gluconate; if tetany or convulsions have occurred, this is particularly important.
Calcium excess	Treat underlying condition. If other imbalances are being treated, use only calcium-free solutions.
Extracellular fluid volume excess	Withhold all liquids for a period.
Potassium excess	Avoid additional potassium either orally or parenterally. If kidneys are impaired, any of the following methods may be used to remove excess potassium from the extracellular fluid: administration of carefully measured replacement fluids, supplying fats and carbohydrates but no protein materials; administration of carbonic anhydrase inhibitors; administration of insulin and dextrose; use of ion exchange resins; peritoneal dialysis; use of artificial kidney.

The conscientious nurse checks the flow rate every time she checks the patient.

Special Considerations

In addition to the general subjects discussed, which apply to patients of all ages and conditions, there are special considerations applying to specific groups of patients.

THE ELDERLY PATIENT

Basic differences between the elderly patient and the younger adult contribute to the specific cluster of problems that may confront him. With aging, various structural changes occur. Muscles lose their elasticity; bones become rarefied, often shortened. The general pace of body functions slows. The kidneys, heart, intestines, and brain operate on a lower key. Body homeostasis tends to be impaired. Rapid recuperation is the exception, not the rule. (The Bible accurately describes the aging process in Ecclesiastes 12:1-7. It portrays impairment of vision, mental depression, tremors, loss of teeth, impairment of hearing, loss of libido, development of fears, loss of nervous coordination, and urologic problems.)

The nurse's observations of the geriatric patient should include his behavior, circulatory integrity, breathing, general state of his nutrition, and condition of the skin with particular regard to turgor. In addition, intake and output and various key laboratory tests, including urinalysis, hemoglobin, red blood cell count, and plasma sodium, potassium, and bicarbonate are important.

Complications prone to occur in the elderly include extracellular fluid volume deficit, sodium excess, atelectasis, pulmonary edema, hypoxia, osteoporosis, protein and potassium deficit—especially if the patient has been receiving a diuretic, digitalis, or has a cardiovascular ailment.

INFANTS AND CHILDREN

Fluid imbalances occur with far greater frequency in children than they do in adults. Factors responsible for this difference include: 1) the infant's body surface area, which is several times greater than that of the adult in relation to weight or volume; 2) his daily fluid exchange, which is greater than the adult's; 3) his metabolic rate, which exceeds that of the adult.

Because of these considerations, children cannot be treated as miniature adults. And since they cannot adequately describe their symptoms, the nurse must be particularly observant. She should bear in mind the following facts: 1) the skin turgor in the obese infant with fluid volume deficit may appear deceptively normal; 2) infants or children with fluid excess may present elastic, firm tissue turgor and have flushed cheeks and bright eyes—and still be in mortal danger; 3) respiration is not the helpful clue to metabolic alkalosis or acidosis in children as it is in adults; 4) slow respiration does not necessarily mean metabolic alkalosis, nor does rapid respiration always mean metabolic acidosis; 5) the absence of tearing and salivation may indicate fluid volume deficit; 6) pinched skin that fails to spring back to the normal position indicates fluid volume deficit; 7) fingerprinting over the sternum indicates sodium deficit; 8) and an acutely ill infant has a higher pitched, less energetic cry than the normal infant.

THE SURGICAL PATIENT

As an aftermath of surgery, fluids may be lost abnormally, as in vomiting, gastric or intestinal suction, or drainage from a colostomy or ileostomy. Accurate, detailed intake-output records and daily weight measurements should be kept to help the physician determine whether replacement fluids are needed, and if so, how much.

In the early postoperative period, while the water retention from a stress reaction is still present, water excess (sodium deficit) may occur, especially in the aged and in the very young. During the stress period, the fluid intake should not exceed body fluid losses; the normal 24-hour intake should be about 1,500 to 2,000 ml. A mild water excess can be corrected by withholding fluids. If it is allowed to continue, serious illness or death can occur.

Many surgical patients develop respiratory acidosis for one or more of the following reasons:
- Depression of respiration by anesthesia
- Blockage of oxygen-carbon dioxide exchange in the

TABLE 16-7
Recommended Flow Rates for Various Solutions

TYPE OF SOLUTION	RECOMMENDED MAXIMAL RATES OF ADMINISTRATION
Electrolyte solutions	3 ml/M² body surface/min
Dextrose 5%, 1,000 ml	1½ hrs
Dextrose 10%, 1,000 ml	3 hrs
Dextrose 20%, 1,000 ml	6 hrs
Invert sugar 5%, 1,000 ml	1½ hrs.
Invert sugar 10%, 1,000 ml	2 hrs
Fructose 10%, 1,000 ml	1½ hrs
Protein hydrolysate 5%, 1 L	1½ to 2½ hrs
Alcohol 5%, 200-300 ml	1 hr
Levophed	2 to 4 μg/min
Dextran, 500 ml	20 to 40 ml/min

To calculate drops per minute, the following equation may be used:

$$\text{GH/min} = \frac{\text{Total volume infused} \times \text{Drop factor (GH/mil.)}}{\text{Total time of infusion in minutes}}$$

TABLE 16-8

Complications of Intravenous Infusions

COMPLICATION	CAUSE	SYMPTOMS	ACTION TO BE TAKEN
Local infiltration	Dislodging of needle	Edema at injection site; no blood return when bottle is lowered below needle; discomfort around injection site; significant decrease or complete stop in flow of fluid	Stop infusion immediately
Pyrogenic reaction	Pyrogenic substances in infusion solution or in administration apparatus	Abrupt temperature elevation (from 100 to 106°F.), severe chills, usually occurring about 30 minutes after start of infusion; backache; headache; general malaise; nausea and vomiting; vascular collapse with hypotension and cyanosis (if reaction is severe)	Stop infusion immediately; check vital signs; notify physician; save solution so it may be cultured if necessary
Speed shock	Too rapid administration of solutions containing drugs	Syncope and shock may occur; symptoms vary with type of drug used	Reduce flow rate
Thrombophlebitis	Clot formation in an inflamed vein; irritating solutions, such as alcohol, hypertonic solutions, carbohydrate solutions, and solutions with alkaline or acid pH are frequently associated with thrombophlebitis	Pain along course of vein; redness and edema at site of injection; if severe, systemic reactions to the infection (tachycardia, fever, and general malaise) may occur	Stop infusion immediately; apply cold compresses to thrombophlebitic site; later, apply warm, moist compresses to relieve discomfort and promote healing. Physician may change the infusion order so other veins will not be lost; further infusions should be started in another vein to permit healing of the traumatized vein
Circulatory overload	Excessive administration of intravenous fluids; patients with cardiac decompensation particularly prone to develop symptoms of circulatory overload	Increased venous pressure; venous distention; increased blood pressure; shortness of breath; increased respirations; coughing; pulmonary edema with severe dyspnea and cyanosis	Stop infusion immediately; notify physician; patient may be raised to sitting position to aid breathing
Air embolism	Entrance of air into vein; as little as 10 ml may be fatal to some patients	Cyanosis; hypotension; weak, rapid pulse; elevated venous pressure; unconsciousness	Stop infusion immediately; notify physician; patient may be placed on left side with head down, on theory air will rise into the right atrium and permit some blood to empty into the left side of heart from right ventricle; administer oxygen

lungs because of pneumonia, bronchial obstruction, or atelectasis

- Excess breathing of carbon dioxide during anesthesia
- Shallow respiration because of abdominal distention and crowding of the diaphragm
- Depression of respiration because of frequent or excessive sedation
- Shallow respiration because of pain in the operative site or binding dressings

Respiratory acidosis may be avoided by encouraging the patient to cough and breathe deeply at regular intervals, unless contraindicated by the type of surgery. Narcotics should be given in such doses as to allow the patient to tolerate coughing without producing shallow respiration. If the dose prescribed does not seem proper for the patient, the nurse should ask the physician for new orders. Pneumonia and atelectasis can be discouraged by turning the patient at regular intervals.

Severe hemorrhage and hypovolemic shock are also complications of surgery, and symptoms should be reported immediately. To prevent irreversible shock, it is mandatory that the hemorrhage be stopped and the fluids lost be replaced immediately. The period of hypotension must be kept at a minimum, because damage can occur to the vital organs as a result of decreased blood flow.

Acute renal insufficiency frequently complicates surgery and is usually secondary to the reduction of renal blood flow (as occurs in shock), or to a hemolytic reaction to a blood transfusion. The nurse can help prevent acute renal insufficiency by observing the patient for early symptoms of shock and reporting their presence to the physician.

THE BURNED PATIENT

Burns lead to a series of fluid balance disorders for which the nurse must be alert.

Burn shock, for example, is one complication that may occur, beginning with such symptoms as extreme thirst, restlessness, tachycardia, pallor (the skin *may* be pink, however), cold perspiration (the skin *may* be warm or dry), disorienta-tion, oliguria, vomiting of blood, and sleepiness. If the body is not too extensively burned to permit application of a blood pressure cuff, blood pressure should be checked at least once an hour and may vary considerably. TPRs should be checked hourly. Behavior changes, such as restlessness or disorientation, may indicate the onset of burn shock.

An accurate intake-output record is extremely important in the burn patient. Absent or decreased urinary output should be reported to the physician since it may be indicative of inadequate fluid replacement, gastric dilatation, or renal failure. It is important to irrigate the indwelling catheter at regular intervals with a carefully measured solution to prevent clogging. A clogged catheter can falsely indicate oliguria. The amount of irrigating solution used, as well as the amount recovered, should be recorded on the intake-output record.

Because of the possibility of water intoxication, water should not be given to the burned patient until the second or third postburn day. The patient may be given an oral electrolyte solution prescribed by the physician. Electrolyte solutions are not given, however, in the presence of acute gastric dilatation, frequent vomiting, sodium excess, peripheral vascular collapse, or mental confusion.

Remobilization of edema fluid, which represents an interstitial fluid-to-plasma shift, begins on the second or third postburn day and continues for 24 to 72 hours. During this phase, patients should be observed for symptoms of pulmonary edema. In addition, the nurse should be alert for increased urinary flow. If diuresis does not occur, the kidneys may be damaged.

Whether or not the severely burned patient survives may depend upon nutritional replacement. The replacement program usually includes a high-protein supplement between meals, and it is up to the nurse to see that the patient takes the full amount prescribed. Patients who cannot or will not take oral replacement can be fed by nasogastric tube. When tube feedings are used, the nurse should be alert for gastric bleeding or other indications of Curling's ulcer.

The patient's emotional attitude is also important, and the nurse should make every effort to keep his morale high (see Chapter 11).

THE UROLOGIC PATIENT

The indispensable function of the kidneys is to retain needed water, electrolytes, and organic materials and excrete the rest. Kidney malfunction, therefore, subjects the patient to a cluster of water and electrolyte disturbances, including:

- potassium excess
- fluid volume excess
- metabolic acidosis
- sodium deficit
- calcium deficit
- anemia
- uremia

When symptoms of any of these conditions are detected, the nurse should notify the physician and ask for instructions (see Chapter 17).

Patients with ureteral transplants (ureterosigmoidostomy or ureteroileostomy) may develop metabolic acidosis and potassium deficit. To help minimize or prevent such disturbances, the patient should be encouraged to drink about 3,000 ml of fluids daily, unless intake is restricted, to insure frequent emptying of the intestine. Since activity favors emptying of the intestine, the nurse should encourage the patient to walk. In addition, the patient with a ureteral transplant into the intact bowel should be encouraged to evacuate every few hours to limit the absorption time of urine. If the patient has an ileal-bladder, the ileostomy bag should be emptied before it is completely full so that urine drainage will not be obstructed or back up into the ureters. Teaching the patient to dilate his stoma will prevent poor urine drainage due to stricture. Any symptoms of electrolyte disturbances should be reported to the physician.

THE PATIENT WITH NEUROLOGIC DISEASE

Since many metabolic functions are controlled by the hypothalamus and the brain stem, brain infections, tumors, or trauma can cause a number of fluid balance problems. Water and electrolyte balance frequently is the difference between life and death in the neurologic patient; hence, it is important that the nurse be acutely aware of problems that commonly occur.

The body heat control center is located in the hypothalamus, and so injuries in this area, pressure from edema, or masses in other areas of the brain can cause an elevation in body temperature. In general, the extent of the temperature elevation gives a good indication of the severity of the injury—the higher the temperature, the worse the injury. A temperature rise in a neurologic patient is an ominous sign.

Fever, of course, speeds up body metabolism and increases the need for food and water. Unfortunately, however, patients with brain damage are sometimes unable to recognize thirst or hunger. In addition, impaired motor function may interfere with the mechanics of eating and drinking, and so the patient may be unable to respond with increased intake. Since the fever may continue for weeks or months, it is highly important that his need for food and fluids be fully met. The nurse can help assess the patient's nutritional needs and aid the physician in determining which replacement route is best. Accurate intake-output records should be maintained on all confused or unconscious patients, and weight should be recorded daily.

Pathologic conditions of the central nervous system can cause stimulation or depression of the respiratory neurons, altering plasma pH. Therefore, the nurse should be alert for respiration changes and watch for symptoms of respiratory acidosis or alkalosis. Some symptoms, such as convulsions, coma, weakness, blurred vision, and disorientation, may be caused by tumors or cerebrovascular accidents and should be evaluated according to the patient's history and neurologic status. The physician may order frequent pH and bicarbonate tests to help distinguish between symptoms of electrolyte disturbances and those of neurologic origin.

Sodium excess often occurs following brain injury. It is usually caused by decreased water intake, stress reaction, and fever. When symptoms of sodium excess are detected, efforts should be made to supply sufficient water by mouth, if possible. The physician may give specific instructions as to the patient's fluid intake. If a specific intake is not prescribed, fluids should be given in adequate amounts to keep the tongue moist and the skin turgor normal.

If excessive water has been given following brain injury, sodium deficit may occur, especially if the patient is perspiring heavily or vomiting. It may be corrected by withholding water until the excess water is excreted. However, sodium deficit may occur as a result of cerebral salt-wasting, which involves the urinary excretion of large amounts of sodium, even if there is an existing sodium deficit. The mechanism of cerebral salt-wasting is not known, nor is its frequency. The nurse should always consider the possibility of its presence and be alert for symptoms of sodium deficit if the patient is losing large amounts of sodium and drinking large amounts of sodium-free fluids. An accurate intake-output record is extremely important in the patient with cerebral salt-wasting.

Polyuria and polydipsia in patients with brain tumor, head injury, vascular disease, or cerebral infection may indicate diabetes insipidus, because these conditions interrupt the supra-optico-hypophyseal pathway so that the posterior pituitary gland does not adequately secrete antidiuretic hormone. If the patient is found to have diabetes insipidus, his fluid balance is remarkably well maintained, provided he has access to as much water as he wants.

All patients with cerebral abnormality should be observed for symptoms of elevated intracranial pressure, such as slowed pulse and respiratory rates, persistent dull headache (most severe in the morning), dimming of vision, change in consciousness level, projectile vomiting (often *without* nausea), and progressive rise in blood pressure. When such symptoms are observed, the physician should be alerted so that treatment can be started immediately (see Chapter 15).

THE PATIENT WITH ENDOCRINE DISEASE
Disease of the endocrine homeostatic controls (the adrenals, the parathyroids, and the anterior and posterior pituitary glands) leads to numerous fluid imbalances.

Adrenocortical insufficiency leads to sodium deficit, potassium excess, extracellular fluid volume deficit, mild metabolic acidosis, and hypercalcemia. When patients with decreased adrenal function are exposed to stress, such as surgery, trauma, emotional upset, or prolonged medical illness, the nurse should be alert for acute adrenocortical insufficiency, or adrenal crisis, and report symptoms to the physician. Symptoms include nausea, vomiting, hypotension, thready pulse, confusion, circulatory collapse, and fever (up to 105°F.). After therapy has been started, the nurse should maintain a close watch on vital signs. In addition, she should shield the patient from further stress.

Hypoparathyroidism results in decreased plasma calcium concentration and increased plasma phosphate concentration. Symptoms are primarily those of neuromuscular irritability caused by the calcium deficit. The patient who has undergone thyroidectomy should be observed carefully for signs of calcium deficit so that appropriate calcium and vitamin D therapy can be started before the onset of laryngeal spasms and convulsions.

Hyperparathyroidism results in increased plasma calcium concentration and decreased plasma phosphate concentration. The major symptoms of hyperparathyroidism are primarily those of calcium excess. Treatment consists of the surgical removal of the overactive parathyroid tissue.

Patients with diabetes mellitus may develop diabetic acidosis, which occurs when insulin lack interferes with glucose metabolism, and body fats and proteins are catabolized to meet body energy needs. The onset of diabetic acidosis is often associated with the omission of insulin, overeating, lack of carbohydrate, or failure to increase insulin dosage during infections, trauma, pregnancy, surgery, and thyrotoxicosis, when insulin needs are greater. The nurse should be alert for the symptoms of diabetic acidosis in any diabetic patient.

Since lack of insulin precipitates diabetic acidosis, it is necessary to administer insulin to correct it. After therapy is started, the nurse should observe the patient for signs of hypoglycemia. She must also perform urine sugar and acetone tests accurately, as well as check insulin orders and carefully measure insulin dosage.

After the initial dose of insulin has been given, blood volume is restored and the extracellular and cellular fluid deficits repaired by administration of 2 to 3 L of hypotonic solution of sodium chloride or hypotonic electrolyte solutions during the first 2 to 6 hours. In this early phase, the plasma potassium level is usually elevated, and signs of potassium excess may occur. After about 4 to 8 hours of therapy, the patient is usually greatly improved, and the rate of intravenous infusion can be slowed. Oral solutions can usually be tolerated by this time.

Approximately 8 to 24 hours after therapy begins, plasma potassium decreases for the following reasons:

1. The previously administered fluids have diluted the plasma.
2. The return of plasma volume to normal increases potassium excretion through improved renal function.
3. Some of the extracellular potassium enters the cells as they take up glucose as a result of the administered insulin.
4. Further potassium is withdrawn from the extracellular fluid because of the formation of glycogen within the cells.
5. Potassium enters the cells to repair the cellular potassium deficit.

During this phase, the nurse should be alert for symptoms of potassium deficit. Potassium replacement should be started as soon as renal function improves and the plasma potassium concentration falls to normal.

The nurse should teach the patient and his family to recognize symptoms of diabetic acidosis so that future episodes can be prevented. She should impress upon the patient the importance of taking his prescribed amount of insulin daily, reporting conditions that may alter insulin needs, adhering to the prescribed diet, performing urine sugar and acetone tests accurately, and seeking medical checkups as indicated (see Chapter 15).

THE PATIENT WITH DIGESTIVE TRACT DISEASE

Because of the large amount of fluids in the gastrointestinal tract and the many ways in which they can be lost from the body, loss of gastrointestinal fluids is the most common cause of water and electrolyte disturbances. Loss of large amounts of fluids through vomiting or gastric suction may result in fluid volume deficit; metabolic alkalosis; potassium, sodium, and magnesium deficits. In addition, ketosis of starvation occurs unless the patient with prolonged vomiting or gastric suction is provided with adequate parenteral nutrition. Ketone bodies accumulate in the blood and convert metabolic alkalosis into metabolic acidosis. Loss of fluids from the gastrointestinal tract through diarrhea, intestinal suction, or ileostomy can result in fluid volume deficit, metabolic acidosis, sodium and potassium deficits.

The nurse should watch for symptoms of the above imbalances and report their occurrence to the physician. In addition, she can take steps to keep at a minimum the loss of water and electrolytes by vomiting, diarrhea, and gastric or intestinal suction. If vomiting, or diarrhea, or both, are persistent and frequent, oral intake—particularly of water and irritating foods apt to stimulate peristalsis—should be discouraged; p.r.n. medications may be administered as prescribed to relieve nausea or diarrhea. The amount of vomitus and feces lost from the body should be measured or estimated as accurately as possible and recorded on the intake-output record to aid the physician in ordering replacement fluids. Daily weight measurements should also be recorded.

The physician should be alerted early if there is substantial improvement in the patient's condition so that the patient can be returned to an oral diet as soon as possible.

The nurse also has important duties in caring for the patient with gastric or intestinal suction. The suction tube should be irrigated with an isotonic electrolyte solution, such as isotonic solution of sodium chloride, or still better, a mixture of extracellular and cellular electrolytes, such as Lytren. Water or electrolyte-free solutions should not be used for irrigation purposes. The volume of irrigating solution instilled should be recorded as input; the quantity recovered should be noted as output. Water and other electrolyte-free solutions should not be given by mouth. Ice chips made from a suitable electrolyte solution, such as isotonic solution of sodium chloride or Lytren, may be given if prescribed by the physician.

Prolonged use of laxatives and enemas predisposes to serious water and electrolyte disturbances, especially potassium deficit. In addition, sodium deficit and fluid volume deficit may occur. Patients should be instructed to avoid repeated use of cathartics and enemas. An isotonic electrolyte solution should be used when frequent bowel irrigations are employed.

Drainage from fistulas can cause deficits of sodium, potassium, chloride, or bicarbonate, depending on the viscus in which the fistula is located. The nurse should measure or estimate as accurately as possible the amount of fluid lost through a fistula, even to the extent of stating how thoroughly the dressing, gown, and linens were saturated.

THE OBSTETRIC PATIENT

Several characteristics of the obstetric patient, including circulatory stress (chiefly overload), increased nutritional requirements, nausea and vomiting, and the tendency to develop toxemia of pregnancy, make her peculiarly prone to the development of body fluid imbalances. These same characteristics lead quite naturally to cardiac decompensation, hypertension, malnutrition, pernicious vomiting, potassium deficit, and toxemia of pregnancy, including eclampsia.

Particular emphasis should be placed on providing the pregnant patient with adequate protein, calcium, and vitamins. Pernicious vomiting of pregnancy is treated by appropriate parenteral fluid therapy.

Symptoms of toxemia of pregnancy should be reported to the physician as soon as they are detected so that treatment may be started immediately. Magnesium sulfate has proven useful in the treatment of toxemia.

THE PATIENT WITH CONGESTIVE HEART FAILURE

Congestive heart failure is a complex illness involving the heart, the adrenal cortex, the central nervous system, the kidneys, the vascular network, and the liver. Imbalances associated with the disease and its treatment are sodium deficit, potassium deficit, respiratory acidosis, metabolic alkalosis, metabolic acidosis, and fluid volume excess. The nurse should be alert for symptoms of these imbalances.

Whenever possible, treatment of congestive heart failure consists of eliminating the underlying condition causing it. If this is impossible, the only alternative is to use the remaining cardiac function as efficiently as possible. Rest, low-sodium diet, digitalis, and diuretics are commonly prescribed to improve cardiac function. The keeping of accurate intake-output records and daily weighing are especially important for the patient whose physician wishes to adjust the dose of a diuretic drug or the degree of sodium restriction.

If the patient has been ordered to "Rest," "Don't overdue it," or "Take it easy," the nurse should encourage him to ask his physician for specific instructions regarding activity. She may aid the physician in determining the degree of activity by observing the patient's response to it and reporting any untoward symptoms, such as alterations in pulse and respiration rates, dyspnea, or chest pain.

If the patient is receiving digitalis, the nurse should be alert for signs of digitalis toxicity. Before administering digitalis, the nurse should check the resting radial pulse. If it is below 60, she should check the apical pulse. If it is below 60, the digitalis should not be given. The physician should be notified immediately, because the slow pulse may indicate an impending heart block due to digitalis overdose (see Chapter 12).

THE PATIENT WITH HEAT DISORDERS

Exposure to high temperatures predisposes to heat cramps, syncope, exhaustion, and stroke.

Heat stroke, the most serious heat disorder, occurs the world over and has a high mortality rate. Its exact pathology is not understood but the production of sweat seemingly fails. Central nervous system symptoms, failure of sweat formation, and high body temperature (above 105°F.) are usually present in this disorder. Various factors, such as obesity, recent alcohol intake, inadequate acclimatization, recent use of atropinelike drugs, pre-existing acute or chronic illness, high relative humidity, inadequate water and salt intake, extremes in age, diuresis, potassim deficit, and strenuous physical exercise in hot environments, contribute to heat stroke.

The onset of heat stroke usually is sudden. Symptoms include disorientation; absence of sweating; hot, dry skin; complaint of feeling hot; rectal temperature of 105°F., or more; involuntary limb movements; projectile vomiting; convulsions; rapid pulse and respiration; systolic pressure elevation, incontinent liquid feces; red, blotchy face; petechial hemorrhages in the brain, heart, kidneys, or liver; circulatory collapse; and coma. Respiratory alkalosis and potassium excess may occur, the latter causing sudden death. Most heat stroke victims are comatose at the time they receive medical treatment, and often they are mistaken for stroke victims because of the presence of neurological symptoms resembling those seen in stroke.

In treating heat stroke, it is essential the body temperature be reduced quickly to prevent irreversible brain damage. No matter how high the temperature is, it should be reduced to 102°F. during the first hour of treatment. The most effective method of cooling is immersion in a tub of ice water. The patient should be reassured and watched constantly during the immersion period to prevent drowning. Body temperature should be taken every five minutes, usually orally. The patient should be removed from the ice water after the temperature has decreased to 102°F., since too much cooling could result in subnormal temperature and shock. Temperature should be checked frequently so that any subsequent temperature rises may be detected and reduced promptly. Blood pressure should also be checked frequently. Until adequate renal function is established, replacement of salt and water losses must be done slowly. Sweat glands will again become functional after one to three days of intensive treatment, but it may take as long as six months for them to secrete normally. The patient should stay at bedrest for one to two weeks after body temperature has been reduced to normal.

Bibliography

Artz, C. and Moncrief, J.: The Treatment of Burns. Philadelphia, W. B. Saunders, 1969.

Carey, R. W., Schmitt, G. W., Kopald, H. H. and Kantrowitz, P. A.: Massive extraskeletal calcification during phosphate treatment of hypercalcemia. Arch. Intern. Med. 122:150-155, Aug. 1968.

Dutcher, I. E. and Fielo, S. B.: Water and Electrolytes: Implications for Nursing Practice. New York, Macmillan, 1967.

Goldberger, E.: A Primer of Water, Electrolyte and Acid-Base Syndromes, ed. 3. Philadelphia, Lea & Febiger, 1965.

Guyton, A. C.: Function of the Human Body. Philadelphia, W. B. Saunders, 1964.

Metheny, N. M. and Snively, W. D.: Nurses' Handbook of Fluid Balance, ed. 2. Philadelphia, J. B. Lippincott, 1974.

Peirce, E. C.: Is acid-base balance important? Med. Times 95:1231-1256, Dec. 1967.

Snively, W. D. and Becker, B.: Minerals, macro and micro: dynamic nutrients—part I, the macro-minerals. Ann. Allergy 26:167-176, April 1968.

———: Minerals, macro and micro: dynamic nutrients—part II, the micro-minerals. Ann. Allergy 26:233-240, May 1968.

Snively, W. E. and Brashier, B.: The ABCs of acid-base disturbances. J. Ind. State Med. Assoc. 64:23-32, Jan. 1971.

Snively, W. D. and Dick, R. G.: Computer approach to diagnosis of body fluid disturbances. J. Ind. State Med. Assoc., 59:233-246, Mar. 1966.

Snively, W. D. and Sweeney, M. J.: Fluid Balance Handbook for Practitioners. Springfield, Charles C Thomas, 1956.

Snively, W. D. and Thuerbach, J.: Sea of Life. New York, David McKay, 1969.

———: Voluntary hyperventilation as a cause of needless drowning. J. Ind. State Med. Assoc. 65:493-497, June 1972.

Stedman's Medical Dictionary, ed. 21. Baltimore, Williams & Wilkins, 1966.

Weisberg, H. F.: Water, Electrolyte and Acid-Base Balance, ed. 2. Baltimore, Williams & Wilkins, 1962.

17

The Insulted Kidney: medical and nursing intervention for patients with renal failure

JAMES E. KINTZEL, ELIZABETH M. CAMERON and HOWARD SILBERMAN

Acute Renal Failure • Chronic Renal Failure • Renal Homotransplantation

During the past 30 years, tremendous progress has been made in the treatment of patients with acute and chronic renal failure. The first clinical applications of the artificial kidney were carried out during World War II. In the early 1950s, kidney transplantation was being performed with some success, and, in 1960, maintenance hemodialysis became a reality. In the early 1970s, various state agencies began providing funds for patients with chronic renal failure, and, in 1973, the federal government, through its Medicare program, began supporting almost all patients with endstage renal failure.

Kidney disease is perhaps the one major disease that can be adequately controlled by current therapeutic modalities. In the recent past, kidney disease was responsible for approximately 60,000 deaths per year, a number exceeded only by heart disease, cancer, and stroke. The magnitude of its importance is evidenced by the recent comprehensive Medicare program to treat all patients with endstage renal failure, regardless of age, either by transplantation or chronic dialysis. In September 1967, the Gottschalk Committee on Chronic Kidney Disease reported that some 27,345 persons died of primary renal disease in 1964.[1] In addition, some 70,000 patients died of hypertension-related renal disease. Studies in Seattle have suggested that perhaps as many as 50 people per million population per year will be afflicted with endstage renal disease.[2] With a population of 220 million in the United States in 1974, the magnitude of the situation can be readily appreciated. This figure of 50 per million per year may be an underestimate. In the population area of one of the authors of this chapter, which is close to 500,000, 41 new patients who developed endstage renal disease were referred during the course of one year.

The role of the nurse in the care of the patient with both acute and chronic renal disease is a highly important one, since it is the nurse who handles the day-to-day care of the transplant patient and the patient on chronic dialysis. As therapeutic approaches to renal failure continue to evolve, the nurse's role undergoes concomitant extension and change. In addition, understanding the problems and intervening in the variety of health and life-threatening situations experienced by patients with acute and chronic renal failure requires a working knowledge of the basic physiology of the kidney and of uremia. Thus, the nurse who would effectively care for patients with renal failure must be thoroughly familiar with specific modes of current therapy as well as the pathophysiology of uremia and the impact of the disease process on patients and families. In this chapter, the care of people undergoing dialysis and homotransplantation will be discussed, along with the characteristics and management of acute and chronic renal failure. Because of its complex nature, the chapter will be divided into three parts: 1) Acute Renal Failure, 2) Chronic Renal Failure, and 3) Transplantation.

PART ONE.
Acute Renal Failure

JAMES E. KINTZEL and ELIZABETH M. CAMERON

Etiology of Acute Renal Failure • Conservative Management of the Patient with Acute Renal Failure • Extracorporeal Dialysis • Management of the Patient with High Output Acute Renal Failure • Hyperalimentation

A sound understanding of the basic functional characteristics of the normal kidney is essential in order to appreciate the problems encountered by the patient with either acute or chronic renal failure.*

Acute renal failure may be defined as the sudden cessation of renal function with a fall in urine output, producing oliguria of less than 400 ml of urine per day or anuria of less than 50 ml of urine per day. After ruling out pre- and postrenal factors, the exact nature of the intrinsic renal dysfunction must be sought in order to institute prompt and proper treatment. So-called acute tubular necrosis is probably the most common cause. However, vascular, glomerular, and interstitial damage can appear as acute renal failure.

Sudden vascular occlusions will often present with anuria and hematuria and may be associated with flank pain. Emboli from bacterial endocarditis vegetations, as well as traumatic thrombosis, may obstruct renal artery flow. Severely dehydrated infants may develop bilateral renal vein thrombosis. Trauma and vena cava thrombosis may produce a similar picture in the adult. Hemorrhagic infarction may result.

Extensive obstetrical hemorrhage may be complicated by bilateral renal cortical necrosis, involving an irreversible necrosis of the glomeruli and tubules. Drug-induced acute interstitial nephritis or a fulminating glomerulonephritis of diverse etiologies may appear as acute renal failure.[3]

Iatrogenic acute renal failure remains a significant problem today. In recent years, certain lifesaving antibiotics, when administered improperly, have been associated with acute renal failure. Kanamycin and gentamicin, as well as cephaloridine, have definitely been associated with nephrotoxic reactions and must be administered with this possibility in mind. The recommended daily doses must not be exceeded, and renal function should be measured with serum creatinines on at least an every other day basis. More recently, serum levels of gentamicin can be determined, which is also a useful guide to its therapy. (Gentamicin is an excellent bacterioci-

*For a detailed review see Pitts, R. E.: Physiology of the kidney and Body Fluids, ed. 2. Chicago, Yearbook Medical Publishers, 1968; Wesson, L. G., Jr.: Physiology of the Human Kidney. New York, Grune & Stratton, 1969; and Meuhrcke, R. C.: Acute Renal Failure: Diagnosis and Management. St. Louis, Mosby, 1969.

dal drug against Pseudomonas, but in the experience of one of the authors of this chapter it has been associated with the majority of acute renal failure episodes seen by him in the last two years.) A complicating factor in patients receiving antibiotics is the very nature of the disease being treated. These patients have episodes of septicemia with hypotension which can cause acute renal failure. It is often impossible to pin down the exact etiological agent. Unfortunately, all too often these drugs are administered without careful monitoring of renal function, and acute renal failure is discovered when routine electrolyte abnormalities and oliguria develop. These patients often have high output as opposed to oliguric acute renal failure. Recovery from antibiotic-induced acute renal failure is often markedly prolonged as compared to other common etiologies.

Methoxyflurane (Penthrane) anesthesia has been associated with high output acute renal failure and even severe renal failure without recovery.[4] Renal biopsy in these cases often showed characteristic oxalate crystals in the cortex. For example, an 80-year-old lady received Penthrane anesthesia for surgery and also had been getting nephrotoxic antibiotics. Approximately ten weeks after her operation when she expired from an episode of heart block, she had not yet recovered renal function and had to be maintained on hemodialysis. Approximately six weeks after the operation, renal biopsy showed characteristic oxalate crystals in the cortex. It is recommended that patients with any degree of impaired renal function or patients who are obese not be given Penthrane anesthesia.

In a study of 15 patients observed over a three-year interval, rhabdomyolysis with myoglobinuria from nontraumatic causes was the sole cause of acute renal failure.[5] The myoglobinuria resulted from seizures, prolonged coma, strenuous exercise, viral illnesses, and myopathies. It has an excellent prognosis.

Methicillin and other pencillins have been associated with acute, interstitial nephritis associated with renal failure.[6] Sulfonamides, and, in certain cases, furosemide have caused acute interstitial nephritis producing acute renal failure.[7] This has occurred in patients who were being treated for the idiopathic nephrotic syndrome. Acute renal failure can occur after pregnancy and is probably related to renal vascular disease.[8] A fulminant, fatal course is typical, but patients have been described with only mild transient abnormalities.[9] Pathological examination showed changes suggestive of fibrin deposition in the renal vasculature. Last to be considered is systemic arteriolitis, such as seen in polyarteritis nodosa, scleroderma, or malignant nephrosclerosis.

Etiology of Acute Renal Failure

The nature of of acute renal failure was first appreciated during World War I. Interest was renewed during World War II, when Bywaters, et al, studied air raid casualties with a crush syndrome who died with acute oliguric renal failure.[10] Focal tubular necrosis, interstitial edema, and inflammation with hemoglobin casts in the tubules were seen predominately in the distal nephron. This gave rise to the term "lower nephron nephrosis." Mechanical obstruction of the tubules was a popular concept proposed by Oliver, who stated that "water can't flow through stuffed pipes."[11] In his microdissection studies of individual nephrons in rats treated with bichloride of mercury, he demonstrated generalized destruction of proximal tubular cells with basement membranes remaining intact. With ischemic injury there was also focal destruction of nephrons, which was thought to lead to leakage of tubular fluid causing compression of the afferent capillaries. Meanwhile, other investigators identified renal arteriolar changes and felt that renal ischemia and decreased glomerular filtration rate might have been responsible. Since the late 1950s, studies have been carried out in rats using potassium dichromate and human globin to produce acute renal failure.

Three main etiological theories have been explored: 1) tubular obstruction, 2) passive backflow or leakage, and 3) intrarenal vascular factors.

Oken and other investigators have demonstrated that intrarenal vascular factors are probably the most important and have proposed the term ''vasomotor nephropathy.''[12] In rats treated with bichloride of mercury, they used tubular micropuncture techniques to analyze intratubular pressures and fluid. The decreased proximal tubular flow rates were felt to be due to decreased glomerular filtration rate. It was felt that intratubular obstruction was not important since pressure would rise in the tubules if obstruction were present.

The possible role of the renin-angiotensin system was demonstrated when it was found that rats previously salt-loaded were protected from acute injury.[13] Salt-loading is known to deplete renin. It is an oversimplification to look for one single cause for acute renal failure. In the experimental model, vasomotor changes with failure of glomerular filtration are frequent. Tubular obstruction is sometimes important.

The idea of passive backflow (tubular leakage) was proposed by Richards in the 1930s.[14] The principal recent works supporting this are the studies by Bank, et al, which showed increased permeability to lissamine green dye injected into animals.[15] After treatment with bichloride of mercury, the proximal tubular epithelium became abnormally permeable to the dye. Prior to the injection of mercury, the dye could first be seen in the proximal and, after a time interval, in the distal segment. After poisoning, the dye could not be followed into the distal tubular segments.

Hollenberg, in a discussion of renal hemodynamic changes in acute renal failure, showed that renal cortical blood flow is reduced by approximately 70 percent using the Xenon washout technique.[16] It does not matter if the acute renal failure is induced by nephrotoxins, shock, or hemolysis; the decrease in blood flow is identical. Using microsphere injections and supravital stainings in rats, it has been shown that the diameter of microspheres that get trapped in the afferent glomerular arteriole is 23.1 microns in the normal rat, as compared to 18.9 microns in the rat with mercuric chloride-induced acute renal failure. This decreased arteriolar diameter represents a threefold increase in glomerular vascular resistance. It must be remem-

bered that, according to Pouisielle's law, resistance varies with the fourth power of the radius.

After inducing hemorrhagic shock in experimental animals, Flores, et al, found that ischemic changes persist after replacement of the vascular volume.[17] This is partially reversed by the administration of solute, either mannitol or dextran, as judged by Xenon wash-out and silicone rubber techniques. The recovery was correlated with shrinkage of cells and opening of capillary lumens. The mannitol prevented swelling of the cells and kept the capillary lumens open. The basic etiology of the nephropathy was felt to be anoxia of the cells with breakdown of the sodium-potassium exchange pump which allowed sodium to diffuse into the cells, causing cell swelling, subsequent pressure on the vessels, and decreased blood flow.

A detailed review of acute renal failure can be found in the Proceedings of the Conference on Acute Renal Failure.[18] Alexander Leaf states:

Today it seems most likely that acute renal failure almost always involves multiple pathogenetic factors including obstructing casts, catecholamines, angiotensin, each in varying degrees. To this list I would like to add cell swelling with its consequent secondary obstruction of the renal microvasculature sustaining a patchy ischemia of the kidney after correction of the initial systemic hypotensive or hemorrhagic episode, i.e., ''no-reflow.'' The contribution of cell swelling to acute renal failure may be a common final pathway through which each of the other factors (at least hypotension, anoxia, catecholamine, and angiotensin) may create a sustained renal ischemia.[19]

(Figure 17-1 shows a proposed scheme for the development of acute renal failure.)

The syndrome of acute tubular necrosis is a well-defined and predictable entity. Multiple etiologies can produce the classical syndrome with all gradations of length and severity. Hemorrhagic shock, ischemia, endotoxemia, nephrotoxic chemicals such as carbon tetrachloride, and acute hemolytic transfusion reactions are some of the more common causes. In a certain percentage of cases, no clear-cut etiology can be discerned. The mortality rate varies from 25 percent in uncomplicated medical causes to

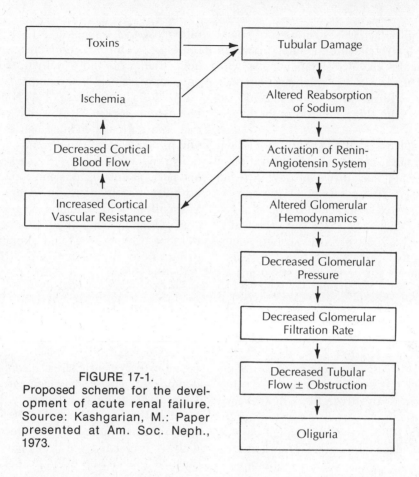

FIGURE 17-1.
Proposed scheme for the development of acute renal failure. Source: Kashgarian, M.: Paper presented at Am. Soc. Neph., 1973.

close to 70 percent when extensive trauma and infection are present. The syndrome derives its name from necrosis or other histologic alterations of the epithelial cells of the renal tubules, with the glomerular basement membrane remaining intact. These highly metabolically active cells are much more susceptible to injury than are the glomeruli and interstitial elements. Given enough time, the cells regenerate on the intact basement membrane and gradually resume normal functional capabilities. Loughbridge, et al, defined five distinct stages through which the patient progresses—onset, oliguric, diuretic, recovery, and finally convalescent.[20]

Acute derangement of the kidneys' regulatory function results in severe metabolic disturbances which may cause death within a few days. However, if the patient can be maintained by supportive means until the renal tubular

epithelium regenerates (usually 10 to 14 days, but may be as long as 47 days or longer), complete recovery is the rule.[21] The patient's azotemia will disappear in a matter of days, but his kidneys' concentrating ability may take several months to regain maximum levels.

Conservative Management of the Patient with Acute Renal Failure

Perhaps the most life-threatening derangement in acute renal failure is the development of hyperkalemia, which may be severe enough to cause myocardial depression to the point of asystole. The hyperkalemia is aggravated by the occurrence of acidemia. Hydrogen ions accumulate because the kidney is unable to excrete them or to neutralize the excess with regenerated bicarbonate ions, causing a metabolic acidosis. This acidemia provokes increased liberation of potassium from the body cells into the interstitium. In turn, the patient's elevated catabolic rate with breakdown of muscle cells, which accompanies the renal failure, further increases the acid load and aggravates both the acidosis and the hyperkalemic state.

Calcium antagonizes the action of potassium on the myocardium, so that the administration of calcium gluconate may prove lifesaving in an acute emergency. The sodium-potassium ion exchange resin, kayexalatate, can also be administered, both prophylactically and therapeutically. If given orally, it is dissolved in sorbitol, since this nonresorptive cathartic hastens the resin's transit through the gut. In extreme situations, as much as 50 Gm of kayexalatate per hour can be given rectally by means of high colonic enemas, thus removing a considerable amount of potassium. (Refer to Chapter 16, concerning fluid-electrolyte balance.)

Since patients with acute renal failure are unable to produce any significant amount of urine, they are prone to overhydration. In the early hours of oliguria, it is critically important for the physician to decide whether the patient has suffered acute tubular necrosis (ATN) or is merely severely dehydrated, as vigorous attempts to hydrate the patient with renal failure may lead to hyponatremia or congestive heart failure. In fact, ATN is characterized by an isotonic or hypotonic urine with a sodium concentration of greater than 20 mEq per L, whereas the dehydrated patient excretes a concentrated urine containing almost no sodium. The normal kidney, faced with a decreased glomerular filtration rate, reabsorbs almost all of the filtered sodium in the proximal tubule and maximally concentrates the urine. However, when damage to the tubular epithelium occurs, no concentration is possible and little if any of the filtered sodium which entered the tubule at the normal serum concentration (140 mEq per L) is absorbed. Examination of a concomitant urine and serum osmolality by means of an osmometer greatly aids the physician in making the distinction between ATN and dehydration, as an elevated urine-to-plasma osmolality ratio points to dehydration, while a ratio close to 1.0 suggests ATN. In addition, obtaining a central venous pressure may also help—the profoundly dehydrated patient will have an extremely low reading.

As the oliguric phase of ATN progresses, the blood urea nitrogen (BUN) and serum creatinine rise, the patient becomes nauseated and often vomits, and cerebroneuromuscular complications produce irritability, altered consciousness, and perhaps convulsions and coma. Dilantin may be given prophylactically to prevent seizures. Susceptibility to infection is greatly increased and, especially when the failure occurs in conditions of trauma or wound contamination, may bring about the patient's death. The use of catheters should be avoided in the alert patient in order to eliminate a possible source of infection. This is a time of waiting and watching, as a significant number of patients may be managed without resorting to dialysis.

Acute renal failure may be complicated by bleeding from gastric stress ulcers, which greatly complicate patient management, with the elevated BUN being aggravated by the presence of blood in the gastrointestinal tract not to mention the problems caused by the bleeding. If hemodialysis is carried out, regional heparinization must be utilized to prevent further bleeding. (See pp. 531-533 for studies on serum gastrin levels.)

The patient's diet is one rich in calories but contains no sodium or potassium. If tolerated, butterballs and sourballs alone may provide enough calories to prevent the body from catabolizing protein. Accurate daily weight measurements are mandatory, and fluids are carefully calculated, taking into account the patient's insensible water loss (about 600 to 800 ml per day in the average adult male without fever or respiratory distress). Urine output, if any, is of course also recorded. The patient usually loses about a pound of body weight per day, and losses of 30 to 40 pounds during the course of the illness are not unusual. Electrolytes administered include bicarbonate to combat the acidemia; keeping the acidosis under control aids in treating the hyperkalemia.

Glucocorticoids such as hydrocortisone,

prednisone (as well as all of the tetracyclines) greatly increase the body's catabolic rate and should not be administered in this situation. Should significant infection develop, antibiotics are chosen with full knowledge of their pharmacology and mechanism of excretion. For example, kanamycin, streptomycin, colistin, vancocin, amphotericin B, and gentamicin are excreted exclusively by the kidney, and although these drugs may be indicated, they must be given in reduced doses to be certain of preventing ototoxicity and resultant deafness. Aqueous penicillin is likewise excreted by the kidney, and aside from the cerebral irritant qualities of the drug, which may cause convulsions, every 10 million units contains 21 mEq of potassium.

Should all these conservative measures fail to prevent uremia, or if the patient's clinical condition has markedly deteriorated by the time he is first evaluated, peritoneal or hemodialysis is indicated. Peritoneal dialysis is preferred, since it requires a minimum of patient preparation and corrects the uremia gradually over several days. Hemodialysis is indicated if recent abdominal surgery or abdominal injury is present. Commonly, it is the young healthy patient with extensive trauma who has such a massive and rapid catabolic rate that peritoneal dialysis is not fast enough. Some of these patients may require daily or every other day six-hour hemodialysis.

Extracorporeal Dialysis of the Patient with Acute Renal Failure

Caring for patients in acute renal failure is a demanding but challenging experience.

Preparing the acutely ill patient for extracorporeal dialysis can require a great deal of equipment. In general, a dialysis unit is used if available, since it is specially equipped for the task. However, the equipment may be moved to the patient's bedside, and the authors have found this advantageous in providing continuity of patient care without technical disadvantages.

The area must be clean and essential emergency drugs and resuscitation equipment must be immediately available, including suction, oxygen and electrocardiogram equipment.

Before dialysis is started, the patient is carefully weighed. It is preferable to use a bed scale so that the patient's weight may be followed closely throughout the dialysis; ultrafiltration, the technique by which excess fluid is removed, may lead to a significant weight loss. A predialysis electrocardiogram is obtained and frequently the patient is monitored continuously.

For the patient with acute renal failure the following access routes are generally utilized. An accessible vein and artery (usually in the patient's forearm) are sought for cannulation. A modification of the Scribner technique of vessel cannulation with Teflon tips and silicone rubber is often used (see Fig. 17-9, p. 557). Usually the physician implants the cannula surgically in the forearm, under local anesthesia, in the unit, just prior to dialysis. Some units prefer to have this placement done by specially trained surgeons. The nurse should briefly explain the procedure to the patient. She should also record vital signs at this point and accurately note the patient's level of consciousness. (See Chapter 20 for a detailed description of the evaluation of consciousness.) If only a single dialysis is required, as in the case of a drug overdose, Shaldon catheters can be inserted into the femoral vein. At the end of the procedure they are withdrawn and firm pressure is applied over the area.

As the patient is being cannulated, the dialyzer is prepared. The coil dialyzer is most often used for acute extracorporeal dialysis (see Fig. 17-7, p. 557). The membrane is rinsed with normal saline and primed with albumin or blood when the shunt insertion is completed. It is important that the priming blood be loaded into the coil membrane under pressure of at least 100 mm of mercury; thus the blood path is not distended by the patient's own blood volume as the procedure commences. Inadequate priming pressure is a cause of hypotension in the early minutes of dialysis. (See Part 2 for a detailed explanation of the principles of extracorporeal dialysis.)

After the patient's connection to the dialyzer has been established, the nurse takes continuous blood pressure readings until his vital signs are stable and an initial dialysis flow rate of at least 100 ml per minute is obtained. As the patient's well-being is now directly related to the smooth performance of the dialyzer, it is monitored visually and automatically throughout the procedure. Venous and arterial pressures in the dialyzer are observed, and high and low limits are set. The dialysate is observed for the presence of hemoglobin, which indicates a leak from membrane to bath and necessitates the discontinuance of the dialysis until a new dialyzer can be prepared. In the event of a mechanical or electrical failure, the dialysis is stopped; therefore, it is desirable to have emergency power available for the dialysis room. If there is more than a ten-minute interruption in the procedure, the patient must be taken off the dialyzer in order to prevent clotting of his shunt.

When the dialysis is begun, the patient is heparinized, unless there is a contraindication (i.e., recent bleeding). Dosage is roughly calculated according to body weight, usually ½ to 1 mg per kg of body weight. This is supplemented in small doses throughout the dialysis, as proven necessary by serial clotting times. If the patient has undergone surgery recently or there are sources for bleeding, systemic heparinization cannot be used. In these cases, regional heparinization may be substituted. By means of a constant infusion pump, heparinized normal saline is infused into the blood as it enters the dialyzer, and then normal saline with protamine is infused into the blood before it returns to the patient. Additional small amounts of protamine and heparin are given, as necessary to maintain the patient's clotting time, at control levels of approximately ten minutes and the dialyzer clotting time more than sixty minutes. Table 17-1 shows one type of sheet used for frequent serial clotting times (every ten minutes). The phenomenon of heparin rebound has been reported by Hampers, et al.[22] Apparently, this occurs as a result of more rapid degradation of protamine than of heparin. This results in effective anticoagulation of the patient approximately one to three hours after dialysis. To counteract this reaction, 25 mg of protamine sulfate is given at the close of the procedure and the patient's clotting time is checked four to six hours afterwards. An additional dose of protamine is given if the clotting time is prolonged at that time, and the clotting time is rechecked. An alternative method is the use of a low-dose infusion of heparin with careful monitoring of clotting times.

TABLE 17-1
Regional Heparinization Record Used During Hemodialysis

TIME DRAWN	PATIENT TIME CLOT	TIME	TIME DRAWN	MACHINE TIME CLOT	TIME

The physiological response to dialysis of the acutely ill patient is unpredictable. For this reason, a physician experienced in the care of patients undergoing hemodialysis should be present or immediately available at all times.

The patient is continuously observed for bleeding from any source, respiratory difficulty, cyanosis, twitching, convulsions, or change in sensorium. Vital signs must be monitored frequently and any change reported. Often the patient may become hypovolemic on the basis of ultrafiltration, which is usually indicated by a lowering of blood pressure and an increased pulse rate. At this time the alert patient may also complain of feeling light-headed, agitated, and nauseated. As volume is being replaced, the nurse should explain to him the reasons for the sensations he is experiencing and continually reassure him.

During dialysis, the patient is given intensive nursing care. Mouth and skin care is particularly necessary. His position is changed at least once every hour, though mobility is limited by the connection of his shunt to the dialyzer. He is encouraged to cough and breathe deeply. Tracheal aspiration and positive pressure breathing apparatus are used as necessary. Scheduled medications and treatments are given with the knowledge of the physician conducting the dialysis. A continuous flow sheet is made up and returned to the patient's unit. All intake and output observations, plus medications and treatments, are recorded on it. The record is frequently lengthy. For example, in the case of drug intoxication, dialysis is continued until the patient's vital signs are spontaneous and stable (as long as 24 hours). In this circumstance, return of reflexes and changes in sensorium and orientation must be noted and recorded.

When dialysis is terminated, postdialysis blood samples are drawn and the patient's shunt closed. The patient and the nursing staff on his floor are then instructed in maintaining the shunt. (Figure 17-2 shows an instruction sheet to be at-

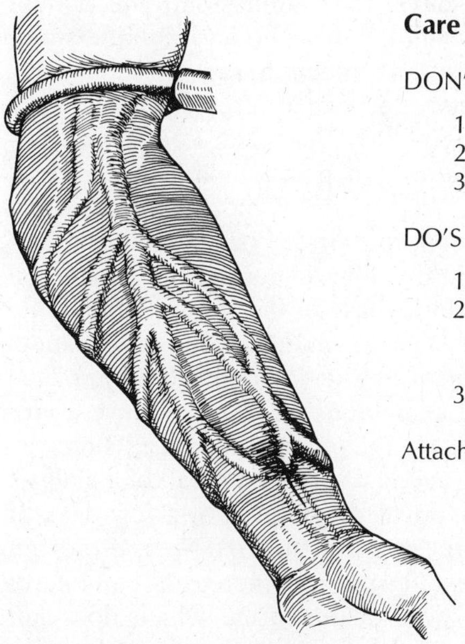

Care of the patient with arteriovenous fistula:

DON'TS on the fistulized arm:

1. No BP's
2. No IV's
3. No tourniquets or venipunctures

DO'S

1. Notify Renal-Electrolyte Team for *profuse* bleeding
2. For profuse bleeding, apply tourniquet or blood pressure cuff above the bleeding site and inflate to 20 mm Hg above the patient's arterial pressure and deflate every ten minutes for 30 seconds to one minute.
3. Check arm for hematoma and swelling postoperatively q 1 h x 4.

Attach this reminder sheet to patient's bed.

FIGURE 17-2.
Instructions for care of A-V fistula. Note that the tourniquet applied in the illustration is for demonstration of hypertrophied veins only.

HOUR

_____ **SUMMARY**   **DATE & TIME** _____

Predialysis   **Postdialysis**

      Wgt. _____   Wgt. _____

      B/P _____   B/P _____

    Temp. _____   Temp. _____

Intake PO _____   Output PO _____

      IV _____   Other _____

Medications _____   Comments _____

_____   _____

_____   _____

_____   _____   **FIGURE 17-3.**

  Held _____   _____   Hemodialysis summary.

tached to the patient's bed with a chart outlining the necessary measures.) If the electrocardiogram has not been used for continuous monitoring, a tracing is often taken at the close of the dialysis. The patient's intake and output are totalled and the staff nurse is given a detailed verbal report of the dialysis as the patient is returned to his room. A stamp may be useful in summarizing the dialysis course of the patients cared for in the dialysis unit (see Fig. 17-3). If the patient is not dialyzed every two or three days for a time, the dialysis staff changes his shunt dressings at his bedside between dialyses.

Maintenance of patients in acute renal failure requires a great investment in time and energy on the part of the dialysis staff. Most of these patients have serious complications in their hospital course, such as sepsis and bleeding. They may require daily dialysis, such as in cases of acidosis and/or increased catabolic rates which cannot be controlled by conservative means. They may need to be maintained for as long as six weeks before diuresis is sufficient to sustain life.

J.N., a 32-year-old male in previous good health, was transferred to the Hospital of the University of Pennsylvania after a subtotal gastrectomy was performed at another hospital. At the time of transfer, his BUN was 150 mg per 100 ml, and oliguria was present. Acute tubular necrosis probably occurred as a result of hypotension during his original episode of gastrointestinal bleeding at the outlying hospital.

Gastrointestinal bleeding occurred immediately after his admission and again later in his hospital course. On both occasions, surgical intervention was necessary. In preparation for his operation, a six-hour, twin-coil dialysis was carried out with regional heparinization. Other problems included sepsis from a left, lower lobe pneumonia, congestive heart failure, and liver disease. Oliguria persisted for six weeks during which time 13 twin-coil dialyses were performed. Despite his many problems, J.N. recovered and was discharged 96 days after admission. The patient with acute renal failure, who has multiple surgical procedures and infection, runs a 70 to 80 percent mortality rate.[23] Therefore, it is particularly gratifying to follow patients like J.N. to successful rehabilitation. In posttraumatic acute renal failure in the Vietnam war, mortality rates averaged 66 percent in four dialysis facilities.[24]

Following the oliguric period, the patient enters the diuretic phase of the syndrome of acute renal failure. The magnitude of diuresis is somewhat dependent on the state of hydration of the patient. The edematous patient may have a profuse diuresis. On the other hand, diuresis may be aborted for several days as the result of a dialysis with fluid removal. During the first few days of the diuretic phase, the BUN and serum creatinine rise despite the increasing volume of urine flow—poor-quality urine which does not contain the usual solutes. In the diuretic phase, the fine adjustment mechanism for solute excretion functions poorly. Large quantities of electrolytes, such as sodium and potassium, may be lost in the urine; and if the patient is not followed closely, severe sodium and potassium depletion may result. It is often advisable for the physician to monitor the daily urinary sodium losses on a quantitative basis in order to avoid this difficulty. The serum urea and creatinine begin to fall and within a week to ten days the patient's uremic symptomatology abates, and he is able to adjust to gross changes himself. However, six months to a year may be required to restore tubular function completely to normal.

Management of the Patient with High Output Acute Renal Failure

Not all patients with acute renal failure manifest the classical stages of oliguria followed by a diuretic period. A number of patients do not develop oliguria and have been designated as high output acute renal failure, which is a syndrome characterized by a rise in BUN and creatinine in the absence of oliguria. Fluid balance and hyperkalemia are minimized in these patients and recovery is often possible without dialysis.

A typical example is M.W., a 59-year-old male admitted with a two-week history of right upper quadrant pain, who presented in shock secondary to gram-negative sepsis in the emergency room. After vigorous treatment of the shock with large volumes of intravenous fluids regulated by means of a central venous pressure catheter and the administration of antibiotics and intravenous Decadron, the patient developed a gradual rise in BUN and creatinine. His urine output was in excess of 1,000 ml per day. Problems with hypokalemia and metabolic alkalosis developed because of the presence of a nasogastric tube which removed potassium and hydrogen ions. Within a week's time, the patient's BUN had gradually risen to 200 with a serum creatinine of approximately 15. The patient's acid-base balance presented no significant problems other than those mentioned and he, at no time, developed any signs of metabolic encephalopathy. Within ten days the BUN and creatinine gradually began to drop. Since the patient's mental status did not deteriorate and fluid and electrolyte balances were no problem, the patient did not require peritoneal dialysis or hemodialysis and eventually made a complete recovery with return of renal function to normal.

The state of hydration at the time of insult to the kidneys is of primary importance in determining the patient's subsequent clinical course. A well-hydrated patient with good renal blood flow and good glomerular filtration rate may not develop much oliguria as compared to a dehydrated patient undergoing the same insult. Sodium restriction sharply reduces the cortical component of renal blood flow. An oliguric patient with all the attendant problems of fluid and potassium balance is a far more difficult patient to manage than one who is voiding adequate amounts of urine.

Good examples of the influence of the state of hydration at the time of the insult are illustrated by two patients who developed acute renal failure after receiving mismatched blood transfusions. T.S., a 67-year-old female with an abdominal mass, was surgically explored and found to have an early but inoperable carcinoma of the pancreas. Because of intraoperative bleeding she was given 1 unit of whole blood at the conclusion of the procedure. In the postoperative period her urine was noted to be scant in amount and reddish in color, but this was felt to be due to some irritation of the bladder by the catheter. The following morning it became apparent that the patient was severely oliguric, and, on further investigation, it was learned that she had received the wrong unit of blood at the time of surgery. At no time did she develop shock or hypotension or receive any nephrotoxic antibiotics or anesthetics. At the time of the mismatched blood transfusion she was obviously volume depleted, having been dehydrated in the preoperative period, and no attempt was made at significant hydration during the postoperative period. She was transferred to another hospital and did well until the seventh oliguric day when mental confusion was noted by the nurses. On closer examination asterixis was obvious, and she underwent insertion of cannulas in preparation for hemodialysis. This metabolic flap is a very early and sensitive indicator of uremic encephalopathy. The patient underwent two hemodialyses on the eighth and tenth oliguric day, at which time she started her diuretic phase and required no further dialysis. However, her uneventful recovery was complicated by a massive retroperitoneal hematoma which developed during intravenous heparin therapy for treatment of her clotted A-V shunt. She was discharged from the hospital with normal renal function and lived out the remaining nine months of her life without any evidence of renal dysfunction.

In contrast, H. K., a patient in the intensive care unit, developed what was thought to be acute pulmonary edema during a transfusion of packed red cells. He was initially treated for his pulmonary edema with 50 mg of intravenous ethachrynic acid, was digitalized, and had marked improvement in his symptomatology. After the transfusion was completed, it was realized that the patient had received the wrong unit of blood. He was immediately given 50 ml of 25 percent mannitol IV and no oliguria developed. His BUN and creatinine rose to a maximum of 82 and 8.0 in ten days and gradually returned to normal. At no time did he become oliguric. He did not develop any uremic symptoms, did not require dialysis, and made a complete recovery.

T. S., who was dehydrated at the time of mismatched blood transfusion and who did not receive any diuretic or mannitol treatment or fluid replacement, developed severe oliguria which lasted approximately ten days, and she required two hemodialyses with significant morbidity from her heparin-induced hematoma. On the other hand, H. K. had no symptoms at all and recuperated from his initial surgery with nothing more than close monitoring of his renal function.

In recent years, investigators have employed large doses of loop diuretics such as ethachrynic acid and furosemide (Lasix) in patients who developed oliguric acute renal failure. Furosemide has the additional advantage of having no ototoxicity and can be given in doses ranging from 20 to 1,000 mg. Under certain experimental conditions, it can increase renal cortical blood flow.[25] It is the practice of one of the au-

thors of this chapter when encountering an oliguric nondehydrated patient to administer 25 Gm. of mannitol and 100 ml of 25 percent solution, if there is no evidence of fluid overload. If there is adequate hydration with compromised cardiac function, mannitol may very well precipitate pulmonary edema, since it will draw fluid into the vascular space. A central venous pressure catheter is often extremely helpful in evaluating patient's fluid needs since what was thought to be a well-hydrated patient may have a central venous pressure of only 2 to 3 and large volumes of fluid can be given and the oliguria corrected.

If 25 Gm. of mannitol has no effect in a well-hydrated patient with producing increased urine volume, 400 mg of intravenous furosemide may be given slowly over 20 minutes. If overhydration is present, mannitol cannot be used and furosemide is given alone. If any degree of reversibility exists, the patient may be able to generate a significant urine output. On the other hand, if no increased urine output is generated, further doses are probably of no value. Repeated large doses of furosemide every six to eight hours have generated urine in the face of severe oliguria in some patients. An example is P. M., a 32-year-old female who developed disseminated intravascular coagulation syndrome with acute renal failure following a saline-induced abortion. She was initially oliguric but responded to 200 mg of furosemide IV. This dosage was repeated every eight hours for three days which enabled her to generate greater than 1,000 ml of urine every day. It must be emphasized that, before furosemide is given, the patient should have all volume defects corrected.

Furosemide was studied prospectively by Muth, using either induced acute renal failure in dogs, or clinical observations in patients with acute renal failure.[26] He was unable to demonstrate a significant delay in the need for dialysis between patients with diuresis alone, and patients who had no response to furosemide. Except in prerenal failure patients with cardiogenic shock and cardiac decompensation, he was unable to substantiate a significant therapeutic effect from furosemide.

Hyperalimentation

Recently, hyperalimentation has been found to be very valuable in patients with acute renal failure. Abel, et al, treated acute renal failure patients with intravenous essential-L-amino acid and hypertonic glucose.[27] The survival rates for these patients were better than those for patients treated with glucose solutions alone. In the treated group, the BUN decreased and the daily creatinine rise was less. Prior to the advent of hyperalimentation, emphasis was placed on providing adequate calories in a nonprotein form to prevent the patient from breaking down his own protein by gluconeogenesis. This, of course, would result in a rise in BUN. Many patients with acute renal failure have had previous surgery and, therefore, a problem with wound healing, fighting infections, and so on. Essential amino acid infusions are carried out in the same way as if a person did not have renal failure. Rather than postponing hemodialysis until the patient needs it, it is the policy of one of the authors to vigorously hemodialyze the patient three or four days a week and continue hyperalimentation as if no renal failure existed. In this way the BUN and creatinine can be kept under control and the wounds and proximal tubular epithelium will hopefully heal more quickly.

Hyperalimentation is also helpful in chronic renal failure. Yeager, et al, evaluated the effects of parenteral essential amino acids in hypertonic 46 percent dextrose therapy in patients with chronic renal failure undergoing bilateral nephrectomy in preparation for eventual transplant surgery.[28] In the postoperative period, patients were divided into three groups—those receiving essential amino acids and 46 percent dextrose, those receiving 46 percent dextrose alone, and those receiving 10 percent dextrose. The latter two groups received no amino acid therapy. Patients receiving essential amino acids with 46 percent dextrose therapy had a significantly lower postoperative BUN than those patients receiving 10 percent dextrose alone. In addition, the postoperative BUNs were lower than the preoperative values in those patients receiving essential amino acids and 46 percent dextrose.

The serum creatinine levels were no different in the two groups. All groups manifested some degree of negative nitrogen balance. The group receiving essential amino acid and 46 percent dextrose had the least degree, and those receiving 10 percent dextrose and water had the most severe degree of negative nitrogen balance. The essential amino acid and hypertonic glucose therapy blunted the catabolic response and demonstrated that urea nitrogen may be reutilized in patients receiving parenteral nitrogen therapy.

In an attempt to study the value of more vigorous dialysis in patients with acute renal failure, Conger carried out a prospective study in 18 patients with traumatic acute renal failure.[29] Eight patients were hemodialyzed on a daily basis to keep the BUN less than 70 and the creatinine less than 5. Ten patients were dialyzed when clinically indicated only, that is, pulmonary edema, hyperkalemia, BUN greater than 150, and so on. The first group received a mean of 13.5 dialyses, and the second 4.3 dialyses for the duration of their acute renal failure. The mortality rate was 36 percent in the daily dialyzed group vs. 80 percent in the control group. Gram-negative sepsis was the most common cause of death. In the daily dialyzed group, the magnitude of sepsis and refractoriness to treatment was much less severe.

References, Part 1

1. Report of the Committee on Chronic Kidney Disease, Carl W. Gottschalk, Chairman. Prepared for Bureau of the Budget, Washington, D.C., Sept. 1967.

2. Kirby Cooper, M.S. and Blagg, C. R., M.D.: Modified Markov chain analysis in long term planning of treatment programs for chronic renal failure. Clin. Dialysis & Transplant Forum Program & Abstracts, p. 161, 1973.

3. Chazan, J. A., et al: Acute interstitial nephritis. A distinct clinico-pathological entity? Nephron 9:10, 1972.

4. Panner, B. J., et al: Toxicity following methoxyflurane anesthesia: I. Clinical and pathologic observations in two fatal cases. JAMA 214:86, 1970. Hollenberg, N. K., et al: Irreversible

acute oliguric renal failure: A complication of methoxyflurane anesthesia. New Eng. J. Med. 286:877, 1972. Churchill, D. and Knaack, J., et al: Persisting renal insufficiency after methoxyflurane anesthesia. Report of two cases and review of literature. Am. J. Med. 56:575, April 1974.

5. Grossman, R. A., et al: Nontraumatic rhabdomyolysis and acute renal failure. New Eng. J. Med. 291:807, Oct. 1974.

6. Baldwin, D. S., et al: Renal failure and interstitial nephritis due to penicillin and methicillin. New Eng. J. Med. 279:1245, 1968.

7. Lyons, H., Pinn, V. W., Cortell, S., Cohen, J., and Harrington, J. T.: Allergic interstitial nephritis causing reversible renal failure in four patients with idiopathic nephrotic syndrome. New Eng. J. Med. 288:124, Jan. 1973.

8. Robson, J. S., et al: Irreversible postpartum renal failure. Quart. J. Med. 37:423, 1968.

9. Finkelstein, F. O., Kashgarian, M., and Hayslett, J. P.: Clinical spectrum of postpartum renal failure. Am. J. Med. 57:649, Oct. 1974.

10. Bywaters, E. G. L., and Beall, O.: Crush injuries with impairment of renal function. Brit. Med. J. 1:427, 1941.

11. Oliver, J., MacDowell, M., and Tracy, A.: The pathogenesis of acute renal failure associated with traumatic and toxic injury: Renal ischemia, nephrotoxic damage and the ischemic episode. J. Clin. Invest. 30:1307, 1951.

12. Oken, D. E., M.D.: An overview of the pathophysiology of vasomotor nephropathy. Proc. Conf. on Acute Renal Failure. DHEW (NIH) 74-608, 1973, p. 89.

13. Thiel, G., McDonald, F. D., and Oken, D. E.: Micropuncture studies of the basis for protection of renin depleted rats from glycerol induced acute renal failure. Nephron 7:67, 1970.

14. Richards, A. N., Westfall, B. B., and Bott, P. A.: Insulin and creatinine clearances in dogs, with notes on some late effects of uranium poisoning. J. Biol. Chem. 116:749, 1936.

15. Bank, N., Mutz, B. F., and Aynedjian, H. S.: The role of 'leakage' of tubular fluid in anuria due to mercury poisoning. J. Clin. Invest. 46:695, 1967.

16. Hollenberg, N. K.: Presentation at Am. Soc. Neph. Conference on Acute Renal Failure, 1973.

17. Jorge, E. Flores, et al: The role of cell swelling in ischemic renal injury. Proc. Conf. on Acute Renal Failure, 1973, p. 19.

18. Proc. Conf. on Acute Renal Failure. DHEW Publication #74-608, 1973.

19. Leaf, A.: Cell swelling and renal ischemia. Proc. Conf. on Acute Renal Failure, 1973, p. 13.

20. Loughbridge, L. W., et al: Clinical course of uncomplicated acute tubular necrosis. Lancet 1:351, 1960.

21. Siegler, R. L. and Bloomer, H. A.: Acute renal failure with prolonged oliguria. JAMA 225:133, July 1973. Maher, J. F., et al: Regional heparinization for hemodialysis: Technical and clinical experience. New Eng. J. Med. 268:451, 1963.

22. Hampers, C. L., Blaufox, M. D., and Merrill, J. P.: Anticoagulation rebound after hemodialysis. New Eng. J. Med. 275:776, 1966. Kjellstrand, C. M. and Buselmeier, T. J.: A simple method for anticoagulation during pre- and postoperative hemodialysis, avoiding rebound phenomenon. Surgery 72:630, 1972.

23. Bluemle, L. W., Jr., Webster, G. D., Jr., and Elkinton, J. R.: Acute tubular necrosis; analysis of 100 cases with respect to mortality, complications and treatment with and without dialysis. Arch. Int. Med. 104:180, 1959.

24. Whelton, A.: Post-traumatic acute renal failure in Vietnam combat injuries: incidence, morbidity and mortality. Proc. Conf. Acute Renal Failure. D1-19W 74-608, 1973. Hollenberg, N. K., Adams, D. F., and Solomon, H. S., et al: What medicates the renal vascular response to a salt load in normal man? J. Applied Physiol. 33:4, 1972.

25. Birtch, A. G., Zakheim, R. M., and Jones, L. G., et al: Redistribution of renal blood flow produced by furosemide and ethacrynic acid. Circ. Res. 21:869, 1967.

26. Muth, R. G.: Furosemide in acute renal failure. Proc: Conf. on Acute Renal Failure, 1973, p. 245.

27. Abel, R. M., Beck, C. H., Jr., and Abbott, W. M.,

et al: Improved survival from acute renal failure after treatment with intravenous essential L-amino acids and glucose. Results of a prospective, double-blind study. New Eng. J. Med. 288:14, 1973.

28. Yeager, H. C., et al: Parenteral essential amino acids (EAA) and hypertonic dextrose (D50) in anephric humans. Abstracts Am. Soc. Neph. 115, 1973.

29. Conger, J. D.: A controlled evaluation of daily dialysis in post-traumatic acute renal failure (ARF). Abstracts Am. Soc. Neph. 18, 1974.

PART TWO.
Chronic Renal Failure

ELIZABETH M. CAMERON and JAMES E. KINTZEL

Etiology and Histology • Pathophysiology and Characteristics • Conservative Management of the Uremic Patient • The Patient Undergoing Dialysis • Dialysis Disequilibrium Syndrome • Pediatric Hemodialysis • New Approaches to Hemodialysis • Hepatitis • Air Embolism • Home Dialysis • Psychological/Sociological Aspects of Care of the Patient on Chronic Dialysis • Limited-Care Facilities • Projected Dialysis Needs in the Future • Rehabilitation

The other aspect of renal failure to be considered is the chronic form, in which the patient gradually experiences the effect of progressive loss of nephron function, culminating in the uremic syndrome. To understand the clinical characteristics of gradual functional deterioration, it is important to be aware of the several underlying pathological processes.

Etiology and Histology

Chronic renal failure is diverse in its etiology and histology. Immunologic insults, hereditary afflictions, and chronic drug ingestion can all result in progressive nephron destruction with the resultant uremic symptomatology characteristic of endstage kidney disease. By far the largest percentage of patients with endstage renal disease are those with chronic glomerulonephritis. The time course of the disease varies from a few months to several decades. For example, so-called rapidly progressive glomerulonephritis (subacute glomerulonephritis) first presented in a 22-year-old architectural student as weakness and a hemoglobin of 8.0 on examination at the school infirmary. When he failed to improve on oral iron therapy within three weeks, he was transferred to his local hospital and underwent an emergency peritoneal dialysis when his BUN was recorded as 250, serum creatinine 15, and serum potassium 8.2. He had never complained of polyuria, nocturia, or dysuria. After his initial peritoneal dialysis, his urine volume was approximately 100 ml per day, was grossly bloody, contained 4+ protein, and was loaded with red cell casts. A renal biopsy performed within the next week revealed that all glomeruli were almost completely destroyed with extensive inflammation, crescent formation, and scarring. The patient had no prior symptomatology but recalled that approximately three months before developing uremia, he had what was described as flu with upper respiratory tract symptoms which lasted two to three days and required no therapy.

At the other end of the spectrum is a 51-year-old salesman in whom red cells and proteinuria were discovered at age 18. Today he is hypertensive, but his renal function reveals a creatinine clearance of 40 ml per minute. The proteinuria persists, as does microscopic hematuria and an occasional red cell cast.

With the extensive use of percutaneous renal biopsy techniques, many histologic and immunologic patterns of glomerular involvement have emerged.

GLOMERULONEPHRITIS

If urines are examined, all patients with chronic glomerulonephritis have some degree of proteinuria or hematuria. It should be emphasized that most patients who develop terminal glomerulonephritis have never had any symptoms of their disease and do not recall any acute illness. Proteinuria and hematuria may go undetected for years. In glomerulonephritis, light microscopic examination of renal tissue may reveal no abnormalities in the glomerulus or may show a diffuse increase in the number of endothelial and epithelial cells, so-called proliferative glomerulonephritis. A diffuse thickening of the glomerular basement membrane without accompanying increase in cellularity may be present in what is called membranous glomerulonephritis. In the more rapidly progressive glomerulonephritis, inflammatory crescents originating in Bowman's capsule may develop. Various degrees of glomerular scarring may be present. Immunologic studies have revealed two basic types of glomerular involvement—a so-called linear pattern and a lumpy-bumpy pattern.[1] These have been demonstrated with fluorescein-labeled antibodies against gamma globulin.

ANTI-GLOMERULAR BASEMENT MEMBRANE NEPHRITIS

In Goodpasture's syndrome and in rapidly progressive glomerulonephritis, a linear staining pattern may be observed. Goodpasture's syndrome is characterized by rapidly progressive glomerulonephritis associated with pulmonary hemorrhage. In this syndrome linear staining can be seen along the glomerular basement membrane, and along the alveolar capillary basement membrane in the lung as well. This pattern is identical to that found in the experimental animal model in which specific antibodies are formed against, and react with, the glomeruluar basement membrane. The important point is that antibodies have been formed against the glomerular basement membrane of the kidney. Lerner, et al, studied a patient with rapidly progressive glomerulonephritis and found circulating antibodies in the serum once bilateral nephrectomy had been performed in preparation for transplant surgery.[2] Within a day of the transplant surgery, the antibodies were no longer detectable in the serum, but on biopsy examination of the transplanted kidney, linear staining of the glomerular basement membrane was identified. When the kidney eventually had to be removed because of rejection, these antibodies were eluted from the kidney tissue, injected into monkeys, and caused an identical histologic pattern of the glomeruli in the injected monkeys.

The other type of immunologic insult (immune complex nephritis) is the result of antigen-antibody complexes that are not related to the kidney, but are filtered at the glomerulus and subsequently cause damage. DNA and anti-DNA antibodies in systemic lupus erythematosus can be found on the epithelial side of the glomerular basement membrane where they set up an inflammatory response. Using electron microscopic techniques, one can see these antigen antibody complexes as electron dense deposits, or humps, along the glomerular basement membrane. This, along with the nodular immunofluorescent staining observed, gives rise to the term "lumpy, bumpy disease." The lumpy, bumpy glomerular pattern has been demonstrated in systemic lupus erythematosus, post beta streptococcal glomerulonephritis, and the glomerulitis associated with viral hepatitis, malaria, and heroin addiction. (See Chapter 22 for discussion of immunologic mechanisms in health and disease.)

THE NEPHROTIC SYNDROME

The initial manifestation of glomerulonephritis may be the nephrotic syndrome. This is defined as proteinuria in excess of 3.5 Gm per 24 hours, hypercholesterolemia, hypoalbuminemia, and edema. Proteinuria should always be documented by a quantitative 24-hour collection with the number of Gm per 24 hours being recorded. A simple dipstick measurement is only a crude estimate, since it measures only protein concentration. Two Gm of protein in 500 ml of urine will give a higher dipstick reading than 2 Gm in a 3 L specimen. Proteinuria has diverse etiologies, but proteinuria in excess of 2 Gm per day is almost always indicative of glomerular involvement. The glomerular basement membrane in some ways becomes leaky, allowing the passage of predominately albumin, and sometimes globulins, into the glomerular filtrate and, thus, into the final urine.

The nephrotic syndrome has many etiologies. Systemic lupus erythematosus may present this way. Diabetes mellitus with intracapillary glomerulosclerosis may cause the nephrotic syndrome. Amyloidosis, Henoch-Schoenlein purpura, proliferative glomerulonephritis, and membranous glomerulonephritis are some of the more common causes. The first manifestation of multiple myeloma may be proteinura. All of these disease entities can eventually cause renal failure.

Treatment of the nephrotic syndrome is directed against the underlying disease process and sodium and water retention. As a result of proteinuria, hypoalbuminemia develops with a low-circulating plasma volume triggering a secondary hyperaldosteronism with resultant sodium retention. The mainstay of treatment is sodium restriction with aldosterone antagonists such as spironolactone, supplemented by a thiazide and/or the more powerful loop diuretics. Treatment of the edema in no way affects the underlying disease process causing the proteinuria. Treatment of the increased glomerular permeability obviously depends upon the disease entity. There is no specific treatment for diabetic glomerulosclerosis. Early in the course of idiopathic nephrotic syndrome caused by either membranous or proliferative lesions, or no lesions on light microscopy, high doses of steroids can be used. At least 60 mg per day should be used on a daily basis, or an equivalent dosage should be administered on an alternate day basis. These regimens have often proved beneficial in reducing the magnitude of proteinuria most characteristic of so-called lipoid nephrosis in which no demonstrable lesion is seen on light microscopy. There

are, however, no data to show that steroids delay or prevent any progressive nephron destruction. In addition to prednisone (Deltasone), certain immunosuppressive drugs such as azathioprine (Imuran) and cyclophosphamide (Cytoxan) have been tried. At the present time azathioprine is probably not useful in glomerulonephritis, but there are several prospective double-blind studies showing that cyclophosphamide may be of some use. Drummond, et al, showed that cyclophosphamide can cause remission in steroid-dependent, minimal lesion nephrotic syndrome in children.[3] Azathioprine and cyclophosphamide have been beneficial in some patients with lupus nephritis, with some more success being obtained with cyclophosphamide on short-term studies.[4] All of these agents are obvious two-edged swords. The side effects of steroids are well known, and most clinicians apply alternate day therapy first, rather than beginning with high doses of steroids daily. Sometimes as long as nine months to a year may be required before proteinuria is affected. In addition to causing bone marrow suppression, cyclophosphamide also has the complications of hemorrhagic cystitis, alopecia, and gonadal scarring.

POLYCYSTIC KIDNEY DISEASE

Polycystic kidney disease has been described as a rare disease by medical and nursing texts, but patients affected by it make up a significant percentage of the chronic dialysis population. It is a gratifying experience to treat a patient who has lost a mother and four brothers and sisters in the last ten years of this disease. Every nephrologist has had the experience of treating at least two generations of the same family for this disease. Polycystic kidneys may remain asymptomatic for years with the gradual development of lumbar pain, hematuria, and appreciation of palpable kidneys, and, finally, uremia. For example, a 43-year-old patient presented in terminal uremia and gave a history of having had a "hydro-nephrotic-pyelonephritic" kidney removed at the age of 18 following the development of hematuria from a football injury. In retrospect, the kidney removed 25 years earlier was a polycystic one; at autopsy the typical multicystic enlarged renal mass was identified. Copious urine volume is a feature of this disease even as terminal uremia sets in. A previously healthy 67-year-old woman presented with a six-month history of uremia without clear-cut etiology. Massive hematuria became a problem terminally and at autopsy, typical polycystic kidneys were found.

INTERSTITIAL NEPHRITIS

Interstitial nephritis (e.g., analgesic abuse nephropathy) has received an increased amount of attention in the last several years.[5] Patients with a long history of analgesic abuse can have radiographic evidence of a renal papillary necrosis with renal failure. For example, chronic renal failure, associated with papillary necrosis, was found in a number of patients with a long history of phenacetin ingestion, most noticeably in the employees of a Swiss watch factory who were accustomed to taking phenacetin pill breaks instead of coffee breaks.

Renal histology demonstrates interstitial round cell infiltration and sloughing of the papillary tips. Patients may present with classical symptoms of kidney stone with flank pain radiating to the groin. However, the material passed is not a calculus, but a necrotic renal papillary tissue. Phenacetin, when fed in large amounts over a long period of time to laboratory animals, produces a similar histologic picture. N-acetyl paraminophenol, which is the active metabolyte of phenacetin, has a structural similarity to urea. Dogs fed large amounts of phenacetin develop a very high tissue level of Napap in the renal medulla. A prospective study was carried out by Meyers, et al, who demonstrated that water-deprived rats, when fed phenacetin and aspirin, developed papillary necrosis.[6] The implication is obvious: indiscriminate use of phenacetin-containing analgesics, APC tablets, Darvon compound, and so on, can lead to renal failure. In the last few years a number of drug companies have marketed acetaminophen as a nonaspirin pain reliever. Acetaminophen is really n-acetyl paraminophenol. (One of the authors of this chapter has observed a patient who ingested eight to ten Daprisal tablets per day for approximately ten years, and presented with a creatinine clearance of less than 20 ml per minute. Four years later she began chronic hemodialysis therapy.)

Certain other drugs, such as penicillin and methicillin, have produced acute interstitial nephritis. Border, et al, presented a patient who developed renal failure while receiving methicillin therapy.[7] Renal biopsy revealed immunoglobulin G, C3 and a methicillin antigen present in a linear pattern along the tubular basement membrane, but not along the glomerular basement membrane. Antitubular basement membrane antibody was found in the serum. The immune process may be associated with interstitial and tubular injury as a primary process.

DIABETIC NEPHROPATHY

The management of a patient with endstage renal disease as a result of diabetic nephropathy presents certain challenging problems. In May 1974 at Minneapolis, the Symposium on Diabetic Nephrology and Endstage Renal Disease was held to review this problem in depth.[8] It was found that endstage renal failure is most often associated with juvenile onset diabetes, but may complicate maturity onset diabetes as well. It was estimated that there are 300,000 juvenile diabetics in the United States alone, and that 50 to 60 percent of these will eventually die in renal failure. It was conservatively estimated that 30 to 40 diabetics per million population per year will die of endstage renal disease. The malignant nature of renal failure was evidenced in one study of 23 patients in which azotemia (a BUN of greater than 30) developed. Within one year, 16 patients had died, and the remaining seven died within two years.

The survival statistics for diabetics on chronic dialysis are not as good as those for nondiabetics with renal failure. The diabetic has far less tolerance for the uremic state than does the nondiabetic. In a study of 58 diabetic patients on hemodialysis, the survival rate was 62.9 percent at one year and 41.7 percent at two years. The most common cause of death was cardiac problem in 13 patients and uremia in 5 patients who had discontinued dialysis. The poor survival rate of diabetics was shown in the statistics of deaths per thousand treatment months. The figure for diabetics was 37; for nondiabetics over the age of 60 it was 23.6; for nondiabetics under the age of 60 it was only 12.9. Interestingly, blind patients had much better survival on dialysis program, since it was felt that they had become adjusted to their blindness before going on hemodialysis. At the University of Minnesota, from 1969 until May 1974, 74 transplants were carried out in diabetic patients. Of this number, 29 percent or 18 died, and 71 percent or 45 lived. Their average age was 34. Compared to nondiabetic patients, they had a significant number of urologic complications. It was the overall feeling that transplantation from a related living donor was the most favorable form of therapy. The three-year survival rate was 65 percent in these patients, as compared to 30 percent in patients with cadaver transplants, and 24 percent in those on hemodialysis alone. Gotch presented biopsy findings in transplant kidneys in which some basement membrane changes characteristic of diabetes were found in the very early stages in these transplanted kidneys.[9] With regard to the problem of failing vision in the diabetic, some of the patients' ocular lesions progressed on dialysis, but, in general, their vision tended to stabilize after the first year of treatment.

Nutritional problems can be significant in the diabetic patient. Aside from swings of hyper- and hypoglycemia, they may have severe malnutrition. It is well known that as renal failure develops, the diabetic patient requires less and less insulin, since the kidneys no longer metabolize the insulin to a great degree. In one study, patients required more insulin after they had been on dialysis for two months. Problems of intractable nausea and vomiting with hypomotility of the stomach have been treated empirically with corticosteroids with some success.

One of the common problems in diabetics is the diabetic peripheral neuropathy with its bladder involvement. The diabetic bladder becomes more and more distended with less and less appreciation of distention by the patient, and this may progress to massive bladder enlargement with back pressure and hydronephrosis and resultant kidney damage. Any infection that is present, of course, is a severe complicating factor.

Another problem in diabetics is that the vascular access devices are fraught with many complications including an undue rate of infection from the classic Scribner type of external shunt. Bovine grafts have become extremely valuable on these patients, as have A-V fistulas. Because of the possibility of an ulnar steal syndrome, it is recommended that, especially in the diabetic, an end-artery to side-vein anastomosis be made at the wrist when creating an A-V fistula. If this is not done, the blood from the ulnar artery often comes down the palmar arch and runs off through the A-V fistula, thus depriving the fingers of needed blood supply with resultant problems of ischemia.

Simmonds reported 74 diabetics who had received transplantation since 1968.[10] He again emphasized the advantages of transplantation, citing that 30 percent of the patients could not walk pretransplant due to peripheral neuropathy, and that one year posttransplant all of the patients could walk. His total survival statistics were 75 percent with a related living donor, 63 percent with a cadaver donor, and 53 percent on dialysis. Compared to 38 of 54 patients alive at 5 years after a related living donor transplantation in a nondiabetic population, 31 of 46 kidneys are functioning at 5 years in the diabetic related transplants, and 12 of 22 are functioning at 3 years in the diabetic cadaver transplants. (See Chapter 15 for a discussion of other problems associated with diabetes mellitus.)

Heroin addiction may be a cause of chronic renal failure. Friedman, et al, described 14 heroin addicts with massive proteinuria.[11] These patients' renal biopsies revealed focal and segmental glomerulosclerosis. Deterioration of renal function was rapid so that in all 8 patients with follow-up, uremia developed in 6 to 48 months. Friedman believed that this glomerular lesion was specific for heroin addiction, since other patients with a nephrotic syndrome did not have this renal biopsy picture and their clinical course of renal deterioration was not as rapid.

Pathophysiologic Characteristics of Chronic Renal Failure

One of the classic hallmarks of uremia is the elevation of the BUN. However, the serum creatinine and the creatinine clearance are much more reliable than the BUN in evaluating renal function, as the constancy of creatinine production is related only to the amount of the body's muscle mass. On the other hand, the BUN is directly related to hepatic production and dietary protein intake. Decreased renal perfusion (as may occur in congestive failure and vascular collapse), as well as bleeding into the gastrointestinal tract, urinary tract obstruction, and the catabolic effect of glucocorticoids and tetracycline may also elevate the BUN out of proportion to the serum creatinine. As shown in Figure 17-4, the BUN does not rise above normal until the glomerular filtration rate as measured by the creatinine clearance falls to 50 percent of normal. As creatinine clearance falls, the BUN rises more steeply, so that it can be appreciated why a 50 percent decrease in renal function will have a much greater effect on the patient with an already compromised glomerular filtration rate as measured by creatinine clearance.

One of the earliest regulatory functions of the kidney to fail is the maximal urine concentrating

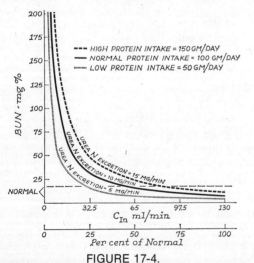

FIGURE 17-4.
Relation of BUN to glomerular filtration rate at different levels of protein intake. Source: Strauss, M. and Welt, L.: Disease of the Kidney. Boston, Little, Brown, 1963.

ability. This subtle impairment develops long before significant azotemia ensues. The kidney is still able to excrete the solutes presented to it, but to do so, it must excrete large urine volumes—up to 3,000 ml per day. It is during this period that dehydration can rapidly develop following fluid restriction, as may occur during an injury or the simple procedure of catharsis and fluid deprivation preceding an x-ray contrast study. Copious poor quality urine is passed. Thus, one of the earliest symptoms of chronic renal failure may be polyuria accompanied by polydipsia and nocturia. Normally two to three times as much urine is produced during the waking hours as at night. The loss of normal diurnal variation in urine production often deludes the patient into thinking that his kidneys are working well, since many people equate renal function with urine volume.

The tubules gradually lose their ability to conserve electrolytes as well as water. Because of the loss of the fine adjustment to regulate the final urine sodium content, sodium retention or depletion may occur. If sodium intake is restricted, the inability to reabsorb all of the filtered sodium may result in severe sodium depletion and further compromise of renal circulation and kidney function. Some forms of chronic renal disease, such as pyelonephritis and interstitial nephritis, may be characterized by salt wasting. As much as 200 to 300 mEq of sodium per day may be lost in the urine. If it is recalled that 1 Gm of sodium contains 43 mEq, the need for supplemental sodium for these patients is appreciated. Conversely, overzealous ingestion or administration of sodium may precipitate congestive failure. It is during this time, when renal function is 20 to 25 percent of normal, that any acute stress may precipitate frank uremia. Dehydration, any acute febrile illness, the stress of surgery, or severe diarrhea may precipitate the uremic syndrome. When glomerular filtration rate decreases to less than 10 ml per minute, the typical clinical picture of chronic uremia manifests itself. Chronic fatigue, insomnia, anorexia, or even intractable nausea and vomiting are often the first symptoms experienced by the patient. Hypertensive symptoms with headaches and visual difficulties from retinal hemorrhages may cause the patient to seek medical advice.

Chronic renal failure exerts its effect on the metabolism of the entire body. It is obvious that fluid and electrolyte balance becomes extremely delicate in these patients. The ability of the distal tubule to secrete potassium is well maintained until the urine volume drops below 1,000 ml per day. It is not until the final stages of the renal disease that problems related to potassium retention become evident. Serum inorganic phosphorous levels rise above normal once the glomerular filtration rate has decreased to 25 percent of normal. Serum calcium level is depressed as the result of an acquired vitamin D resistance which decreases gastrointestinal reabsorption of the ion. Serum uric acid is elevated also, though the incidence of cases of secondary gout is low.

The typical laboratory electrolyte picture when the patient reaches endstage renal failure is one of hyperkalemia, normal or low serum sodium, normal or high serum chloride and a low serum carbon dioxide. The low total CO_2 content is the result of a decreased serum bicarbonate, so that the blood pH drops into the acidemic range. Bicarbonate is depressed secondary to the tubule's failure to excrete hydrogen ion and to regenerate more bicarbonate. Ammonia production is likewise impaired as a result of decrease in the total functional renal mass, and acid excretion diminishes. The urine remains acid, however, because the few remaining nephrons produce enough hydrogen ions to acidify the tubular contents. It is the total reduction of functional renal mass and the kidney's failure to excrete large acid loads and regenerate bicarbonate that results in the chronic metabolic acidosis of the uremic patient. The respiratory compensatory response to this derangement, hyperventilation, may produce subjective dyspnea. (See Chapter 16 for further discussion of acid-base imbalances.)

Perhaps one of the greatest errors committed by the average physician taking care of a patient with chronic renal failure is the administration of unnecessary blood transfusions. Patients with chronic uremia may well tolerate hematocrits of 16 to 20 percent without life-threatening symptoms. As the uremia progresses, the anemia becomes more severe and will only be corrected by adequate dialysis. Transfused blood has a very short lifespan and only serves to further suppress the patient's own bone marrow and, most important, expose him to the risk of serum hepatitis. Patients in whom transplantation is a possibility are exposed unnecessarily to leukocyte antigens which may interfere with subsequent attempts to tissue matching.

ANEMIA

According to Fisher, et al, factors postulated to play a role in the anemia of chronic renal insufficiency include hemolysis, erythropoietin deficiency, decreased erythroid cell responsiveness to erythropoietin, and the presence of serum and plasma inhibitors of hemesynthesis or erythroid cell proliferation.[12] Utilizing a radioimmunoassay system for erythropoietin, they found that serum levels were actually higher in patients with the anemia of renal insufficiency than in normal subjects. However, this increased level was not sufficient to meet the demand for new red cells created by increased red cell destruction in the uremic state. An inhibitor of heme synthesis was demonstrated which was felt to possibly play an important role in anemia. This inhibitor had a molecular weight of between 21,000 and 50,000. It was partially removed by peritoneal dialysis.

The uremic patient's bone marrow often is suppressed to the point of pancytopenia. The decreased white cell count is usually of little significance other than that of decreased resistance to an infection. Decreased platelet counts usually present no clinical problems. The anemia of uremia has received considerable attention and contributes to the lethargy and lack of energy that is so common with severe uremia. The severity of the anemia closely parallels the degree of renal functional impairment. Ferrokinetic studies have revealed decreased incorporation of labeled iron 59 into red cell precursors. The uremic marrow is rich in iron if no blood loss has occurred. The T½, or half life, of the erythrocyte is significantly reduced. In some forms of rapidly progressive uremia with vasculitis, the red cells may actually be torn apart by passage through damaged blood vessels with schistocytes found in the peripheral circulation. A progressive decreased production of erythropoietin by the shrinking scarred kidney is felt to be a prime factor in the decreased red cell production. The patient with polycystic kidney disease, in which shrinkage and scarring do not occur, usually has a higher hemoglobin than the patient with comparable compromise of renal function as, for example, in chronic glomerulonephritis. In a polycystic patient, however, considerable blood loss may occur when an intrarenal cyst bursts, tearing a blood vessel and resulting in blood loss. Episilon aminocaproic acid (Amicar) can be used in an attempt to stop bleeding in the polycystic patient. However, before this therapy is used, preparation should be available for dialysis. Polycystic kidneys stop bleeding but also stop producing urine with clots in both ureters. For example, in an elderly, obese patient with chronic renal failure, polycystic kidney disease was not suspected. Amicar was administered. The patient became oliguric, and, at autopsy, huge polycystic kidneys were found with bilateral obstructing clots in both ureters. A polycystic patient who begins bleeding should have his uremia controlled as quickly as possible with either peritoneal dialysis or hemodialysis to correct the bleeding tendency of uremia itself. All attempts should be made to keep the kidneys in the patient since nephrectomy will invariably lead to severe anemia with increased blood requirements.

It is the practice of one of the authors of this chapter to evaluate each chronic uremic patient with bone marrow determination to appraise the state of his iron stores. Typical bone marrow is rich in iron, and only control of uremia will result in improvement in anemia. However, if absent iron stores are found, a search must be made for the iron loss and the total body iron stores must be repleted. Often no gastrointestinal source of blood loss can be identified, and it is suspected that, with the bleeding tendency of uremic patients, small amounts of blood may be lost over a long period of time producing the iron deficiency. Many polycystic patients have diverticulosis and associated diverticulitis. The quickest way to correct the anemia is with the use of intramuscular or intravenous Imferon, since oral iron is absorbed very slowly.

A well-dialyzed patient with adequate iron stores who still has his own kidneys usually needs no blood transfusions, since the hemoglobin and hematocrit will start to rise within several months after a regular dialysis program has begun. Several patients with chronic glomerulonephritis have been observed who required an 18-to-24-month period before their hematocrit returned to the normal range of 36 to 40 percent. This was without androgenic steroid stimulation of the bone marrow. It is important not to give transfusions and to let the patient's bone marrow recover at its own rate. The obvious exception to this rule is the patient who develops severe angina pectoris which will, of course, be aggravated by the anemia; or the patient in whom there is an obvious acute source of blood loss.

Androgenic steroids stimulate erythropoiesis, and a number of centers employ these agents to significantly raise the hematocrit of their patients on chronic dialysis so that female patients may experience uncomfortable masculinizing side effects.

In the older literature it was taught that, once uremia developed, gastric acid secretions decreased and very few uremic patients had evidence of acid secretion. However, this theory has been disproved. A well-dialyzed patient, and even some uremic patients, will produce an inordinate amount of free acid and may develop peptic ulceration. Some authorities have found an increased incidence of peptic ulceration in patients on chronic dialysis which may be partly due to the decreased inactivation of gastrin by the diseased kidneys.[13] A typical example is the 49-year-old man with chronic glomerulonephritis whose hematocrit gradually began to drop after one year on hemodialysis. Initially, his bone marrow stores of iron had been adequate. Repeat bone marrow revealed absent iron stores. An upper gastrointestinal series revealed a small peptic ulceration. The patient was treated with intramuscular Imferon and his hematocrit, which had been in the range of 20 to 23 percent for the previous year, in a matter of four to six weeks had increased to 40 percent and remained so for two years without transfusions.

There are numerous other problems encountered in the terminal phases of uremia. The pruritis of uremic patients is poorly understood, but may be related to the high concentrations of urea and other ill-defined metabolic end products deposited on and in the skin. The combination of anemia and the deposition of urochrome (lipochrome) pigment in the skin is responsible for the yellowish, sallow appearance of the typical patient. The dyspnea which is frequently present can result from congestive failure, respiratory compensation for the acidosis, and the anemia. Pericarditis is a common accompaniment of terminal uremia, is often painful, and may be hemorrhagic and cause the patient's demise through cardiac tamponade. A qualitative platelet defect is responsible for the patient's bleeding tendency, which can be measured clinically as an abnormal prothrombin consumption. Neuropathy is yet another problem, affecting primarily the peripheral nervous system, but also the autonomic system. Footdrop, impotence, dysaesthesia, anaesthesia, motor weakness, and paralysis are all well known. The cause of the enhanced neuromuscular irritability is unknown, since correction of the hypocalcemia has no effect. Cerebral symptoms such as disorientation, agitation, stupor, and convulsions can be distressing problems.

Conservative Management of the Uremic Patient

Conservative management of the uremic patient primarily involves careful adjustment of fluids and electrolytes and restriction of dietary protein intake. The patient's thirst is an unreliable guide to the state of his hydration, necessitating daily weight measurements as the critical parameter. If not controlled, the patient's inordinate thirst can rapidly lead to overhydration and hyponatremia. On the other hand, a rapid weight gain may be due to sodium or water retention. The elimination of dietary protein removes the patient's primary source of exogenous potassium. Salt substitutes are usually strictly avoided since

they contain either potassium or ammonium as the cation. If hyperkalemia develops, despite protein restriction, or if the patient's urine volume falls below 400 ml per day, kayexalatate therapy is utilized.

A 24-hour urine specimen may be analyzed for determining the total volume excreted, as well as the amount of sodium excreted in it, since this helps to determine the daily intake of both fluid and sodium. In severe salt-wasting disease, supplemental sodium chloride may be needed, while excess sodium accumulation usually manifests itself in aggravated hypertension before peripheral edema develops. The patient's fluid requirements usually exceed the volume of daily urine output by 600 to 1,000 ml, depending on environmental conditions. However, the best gauge for replacement is still that of accurately determined daily weights.

DIET

Dietary protein restriction in the earlier stages of uremia, after the glomerular filtration rate has dropped below 10 ml per minute, is often accomplished by means of a modified Giordano-Giovanetti diet. This diet contains about 20 Gm of protein and all the essential amino acids. The low-protein—high amino-acid combination facilitates the induction of a desirable positive nitrogen balance. Further, the reduction of protein results in a diet which is also low in potassium, sulfates, and phosphates, an aid in obviating the hyperkalemia and acidosis. Deficiencies of the B vitamins and vitamin D in this sort of diet require supplemental multivitamin treatment. However, the diet plus vitamins can keep patients healthy and asymptomatic for much longer periods of time than had been possible previously. Indeed, if the patient is cooperative in following his diet and adhering to fluid and electrolyte restrictions, he may be able to be maintained for a year or more with a supplementary peritoneal dialysis every two or three months.

In addition to the value of the low-protein Giordano-Giovanetti diet in the early stages of chronic renal failure, a new dietary approach was advocated by Walzer, et al, in 1973.[14] They presented data, using essential amino acids and their keto and hydroxy derivatives as the sole source of nitrogen intake in patients with chronic renal failure. The group demonstrated a more positive nitrogen balance with the administration of essential amino acids compared to high biological quality protein alone. They used ketovaline, ketoleucine, ketoisoleucine, ketomethianine, phenolpyruvic acid, L-threonine, L-lysine monohydrochloride and L-tryptophan and L-histidine. This mixture can be made up, frozen, and administered in gelatin capsules. Hydroxy acids may also promote nitrogen conservation. The group also compared the essential amino acid diet with a ketoacid diet. In 11 of 13 subjects, the grams of urea appearing per day markedly decreased in the subjects when they were changed from an amino acid to a ketoacid diet. Hypophosphatemia appeared, as it does in patients on parenteral hyperalimentation, and was thought to represent increased protein anabolism.

Patients may experience inordinate thirst in the final stages of chronic failure, probably as a result of the osmotic effect of the increased amounts of retained urea. They may even drink themselves into congestive heart failure or hyponatremia. It is interesting to note that anorexia may be one of the earliest symptoms of the latter problem.

Those caring for the patient with chronic renal failure have probably had the experience of the patient suddenly becoming confused, even to the point of having seizures. Any patient with chronic renal failure who suddenly exhibits bizarre mental behavior should be a prime suspect for hyponatremia. For example, some patients, through injudicious fluid intake, have become severely hyponatremic. (See Chapter 16 for further detail concerning fluid and electrolyte imbalances.) One patient has had a temporal lobe focus triggered and he has "counting" seizures every time he develops hyponatremia. Patients usually respond to fluid restriction and mental abnormalities will improve, but it may take several days. A most severe life-threatening example was a patient with endstage renal failure who became extremely thirsty following his meperidine (Demerol) and atropine preoperative sedation for creation of his A-V fistula. The following morning the patient's spouse noted that he sounded very unusual over the telephone. The patient was examined by the clinician several hours later. He was found to be moribund and was experiencing a respiratory arrest. The patient, fortunately, was resuscitated and it was found that his serum sodium was 105. Careful calculation revealed that the patient had probably ingested up to 10 L of fluid in the preceding 12 hours. He became exceedingly thirsty, ingested more and more fluid, and became more and more confused.

RENAL OSTEODYSTROPHY

One of the major problems responsible for long-term morbidity of chronic hemodialysis patients is bone disease. So-called renal osteodystrophy can develop early in uremia or may not become manifest until several years after the beginning of dialysis. Acidosis, parathyroid hyperactivity, defective intestinal calcium reabsorption, failure of the kidney to convert vitamin D to its active form, and skeletal resistance to parathyroid hormone all play a role. As progressive renal destruction develops, medullary tissue is gradually destroyed with a loss of bicarbonate regeneration. Buffers in the bone help to prevent the onset of metabolic acidosis, but even these are not enough to prevent lowering of the systemic pH. Partially, as a result of the acidosis, a negative calcium balance develops. The active form of vitamin D (1,25-dihydroxycholecalciferol, $1,25\text{-}(OH)_2D_3$) is responsible for intestinal reabsorption of calcium. It has recently been found that the kidney is the only organ capable of converting the inactive form of vitamin D to the active form.

In 1972, DeLuca suggested that the parathyroid hormone could be considered a trophic hormone for the production of $1,25\text{-}(OH)_2D_3$.[15] More recently Rasmussen, et al, in a symposium on the parathyroid hormone, calcitonin, and vitamin D, discussed the interactions of the substances in mineral and skeletal homeostasis.[16] It was their feeling that not only does parathyroid hormone control the renal synthesis of $1,25\text{-}(OH)_2D_3$, but also that $1,25\text{-}(OH)_2D_3$ acts as a feedback inhibitor of parathyroid hormone secretion. Therefore, the plasma concentrations of both $1,25\text{-}(OH)_2D_3$ and calcium are controlled by the action of parathyroid hormone and both of these metabolites operate as feedback inhibitors of parathyroid hormone secretion. Rasmussen also discussed the effects of these hormones on their three second messengers—cyclic adenosine monophosphate (AMP), calcium ion and monohydrogen phosphate—within the cell. Garabedian, et al, demonstrated that thyroparathyroidectomized animals do not synthesize $1,25\text{-}(OH)_2D_3$, and that exogenous parathyroid hormone given to these animals restores the synthesis of $1,25\text{-}(OH)_2D_3$ to normal.[17]

With the destruction of renal tissue, less and less $1,25\text{-}(OH)_2D_3$ is available which contributes to defective calcium reabsorption. However, failure of $1,25\text{-}(OH)_2D_3$ synthesis is not the entire explanation for intestinal malabsorption of calcium. Avioli discussed many of the metabolic derangements of calcium metabolism at a conference of The American Society of Nephrology in 1973.[18] Intestinal alterations in calcium reabsorption are demonstrable long before there is a defect in $1,25\text{-}(OH)_2D_3$ synthesis by the kidney which may possibly be caused by an alteration in the synthesis of a calcium-binding protein in the gut. In the uremic animal, there is an alteration in mitochondrial activity not only in the gut, but also in myocardial muscle, the liver, and the brain. The following factors adversely affect calcium absorption in the uremic animal:

1. Decreased intestinal protein synthesis.
2. Decreased mitochondrial activity—the mitochondria play a key role in the transcellular migration of calcium, and it has been demonstrated that a release calcium is not picked up normally in the uremic animal.
3. Increased luminal potassium concentration.
4. Metabolic acidosis.
5. Defective $1,25\text{-}(OH)_2D_3$ synthesis by the kidney.

It has been demonstrated that calcium reabsorption is abnormal, with serum creatinine levels above 3.0 representing only a 70 percent loss of renal function. At a time when the bone is responding to vitamin D, the gut is not. In some experimental rat studies, the synthesis of $1,25\text{-}(OH)_2D_3$ is impaired when the renal cortical phosphate level rises above the critical point. The hyperphosphatemia and increased cortical phosphate concentration may play a key role in the impaired $1,25\text{-}(OH)_2D_3$ base of the kidney.

That the kidney may still produce small amounts of $1,25\text{-}(OH)_2D_3$ and play a role in calcium absorption from the gut in endstage renal failure was suggested by Oettinger, et al.[19] They studied seven patients with endstage renal failure before and after bilateral nephrectomy, who were awaiting renal transplantation. Using a double isotope method to measure calcium absorption from the gut, they demonstrated a marked fall in calcium absorption after bilateral nephrectomy. The mean percent calcium absorption in the seven patients was 20.2 percent; postnephrectomy it dropped to 12.7 percent. In all patients the percent of calcium absorption declined.

It can be demonstrated very early in the course of renal deterioration, even before uremia develops, that parathyroid gland hyperactivity is present. Bricker, et al, postulated that as functional renal tissue is lost, a small rise in plasma phosphate occurs causing a slight, but significant, hypocalcemia.[20] In response to this hypocalcemia, parathyroid hormone secretion rises to produce phosphaturia by causing decreased renal phosphate reabsorption. As phosphaturia develops, plasma phosphate drops back to normal and serum calcium is again returned to normal. This continues in a step-wide fashion as progressive renal damage develops and is thought to be responsible for the hypersecretion of parathyroid hormone. When approximately 75 percent of renal function is destroyed, the serum phosphate level rises permanently. Hyperphosphatemia may play a role as has been demonstrated by Slataposky, et al, who fed a group of dogs a progressively decreased phosphate in their diet as renal function was experimentally progressively destroyed.[21] By decreasing the phosphate intake of the animals, hyperparathyroidism did not develop. Hypocalcemia eventually developed and this prolonged hypocalcemia acted as a continuing stimulant for parathyroid gland hypersecretion. The parathyroid hormone, of course, enhances bone reabsorption and causes osteitis, fibrosis of which can lead to progressive fractures, and so on.

Llach presented evidence to show that even at mild levels of renal failure with creatinine clearances of 35 to 93 ml per minute there was a definite skeletal resistance to the calcemic action of endogenous parathyroid hormones.[22] In mild renal failure, basal parathormone levels are increased in comparison to normal levels; the patient responds to an experimentally induced hypocalcemia with an exaggerated parathormone release. Brickman, et al, presented a paper in which he treated eight patients with oral administration of 1,25-$(OH)_2D_3$ for their skeletal disease, for a total of seven to fifteen weeks. Of the eight patients, four had osteomalacia and four had osteitis fibrosa as proven by bone biopsy.[23] With the aid of microradiographic techniques and biopsies, they were able to demonstrate significant benefit in the patients with osteitis fibrosa, but no beneficial effect was found in those with osteomalacia. In osteitis fibrosa the abnormally elevated percentage of bone reabsorbing was reduced to normal in all four patients with the disease, and the percent of mineralized bone rose to normal levels and was associated with rises in serum calcium. Brickman and his colleagues postulated that the orally administrated 1,25-$(OH)_2D_3$ increased gut calcium reabsorption which prompted a rise in serum calcium, reducing the elevated parathormone levels which led to decreased bone reabsorption.

Most authorities feel that patients with progressive chronic renal failure should be given aluminum hydroxide or aluminum carbonate to bind phosphate in the gut and keep the serum phosphate at a normal level, thus preventing, to a certain degree, hypocalcemia. Some authorities also feel that giving large amounts of calcium in the form of either calcium carbonate or calcium gluconate can enhance intestinal calcium reabsorption in the face of a reabsorption defect and keep the calcium at a near normal range. This would theoretically prevent the parathyroid hormone from becoming secreted in large amounts. Once the patient is on a regular hemodialysis program, the plasma phosphate level should be kept within the normal range using aluminum hydroxide or aluminum carbonate since the inorganic phosphate is a large middle molecule that travels across the cellophane membrane poorly. Calcium carbonate itself may keep the phosphate level normal, as well as cause a rise in serum calcium level to normal. A serum calcium of approximately 12 to 12½ mg per 100 ml should theoretically suppress parathyroid hormones secretion. As demonstrated by Fournier, et al, the concentration of calcium in the dialysis bath is also important.[24] Their home patients who dialyzed against a calcium bath of 5 mEq per L had more bone disease than those in whom the bath calcium concentration was 7 mEq per L. Goldsmith and Johnson showed that dialysis-induced bone disease can be prevented by increasing the dialysate calcium concentration to maintain a normal or slightly increased concentration of calcium in the serum.[25] Johnson, et al, found that the level of plasma phosphate concentration was a major factor in influencing the parathormone concentration.[26] In one patient intolerant of oral phosphate binders, there was a remarkable parallelism between parathyroid hormone levels and phosphorus variations, despite a high normal plasma calcium concentration controlled by the dialysate calcium level.

Kaye, et al, have utilized oral administration of dihydrotachysterol to enhance intestinal calcium reabsorption and repair some of the skeletal defects of uremia.[27] Obviously, long-standing uremia with poorly controlled secondary hyperparathyroidism is to be avoided. In patients in whom conservative medical management failed to halt the progression of the bone disease, or in patients in whom metastatic calcifications have developed, or who have severe intractable pruritus, parathyroidectomy can be carried out without significant morbidity. If the patient is considered a transplant candidate, usually three and one-half glands are removed so that there is some residual parathyroid hormone function when transplantation occurs. However, if there is no hope for a transplant, total parathyroidectomy can be carried out. Relief of bone pain, the increased well-being of the patient, and dramatic relief of pruritus make this a mode of therapy that should not be overlooked. For example, A. M. is a patient who had a long history of polycystic kidney disease when first evaluated in February 1972. At that time she had obvious secondary hyperparathyroidism with some hypercalcemia. Within six months she was on maintenance dialysis, but, despite keeping her serum calcium at high normal range, 11 to 11½ mg per 100 ml, and keeping the phosphate level well within the normal range and a calcium-phosphorus product below 50, she continued to have progressive bone pain, and had three spontaneous rib fractures. Seven months after beginning regular hemodialysis, she underwent a subtotal parathyroidectomy with three and one-half glands being removed. Since then, the patient has had complete relief of her bone pain and pruritus and healing of her bone lesions. Follow-up films one year later revealed complete healing of the subperiosteal changes in the bones of the hands.

To prevent metastatic calcification, the patient's calcium-phosphorus product—the product of calcium in mg per 100 ml multiplied by the phosphorus in mg per 100 ml—should not exceed 60. Above this level metastatic calcification can be a problem. Its presence around joints can be uncomfortable and disabling, but its presence in the myocardium and blood vessels can pose a real threat to life.

In another study by Hruska, et al, attention is focused on the role of the kidney per se in the increased levels of parathyroid hormone found in uremia.[28] By examining parathyroid hormone metabolism in uremic dogs, it was found that, in the healthy state, the kidney extracts 18.4 percent of infused parathormone with a renal clearance of parathormone of 55.7 ml per minute. In the normal animal, the kidney accounts for 67 percent of the total metabolic clearance rate. In uremic dogs, only a 20.6 percent extraction with

clearance of 11 ml per minute, or a 33.6 percent of the total metabolic clearance rate was carried out by the kidneys. It was postulated that perhaps the decreased metabolic clearance by the kidneys may have some relevance to the elevated parathyroid hormone levels in uremia. Stella, et al, have demonstrated, for the first time, impaired $1,25$-$(OH)_2D_3$ metabolism in rats made acutely uremic by ureteral ligation so that acute renal failure, per se, may cause impairment in the active metabolite of vitamin D.[29]

HYPERTENSION

In recent years more attention has been given to vigorous control of hypertension in the renal patient. Cardiovascular catastrophes—myocardial infarction and stroke—are the leading causes of death in the chronic dialysis population. Hypertension is the greatest risk factor in both strokes and myocardial infarctions. Before adequate dialysis and transplantation facilities were available, reduction of blood pressure often reduced renal function with aggravation of the uremia. Thus, vigorous control of blood pressure was not always carried out. In a recent California study, patients with primary hypertensive disease made up the second largest proportion of the chronic dialysis population.[30]

Malignant hypertension is a good example of a disease which causes rapid deterioration of renal function. Untreated, the disease was consistently fatal in four or five years with an 80 percent mortality rate in the first year.[31] In 1967, Woods and Blythe reported the results of vigorous therapy treating 20 patients with a BUN level of 50 mg per 100 ml or higher, noting a 55 percent one-year survival, 35 percent two-year survival, and 25 percent longer term survival.[32]

In the most recent follow-up study, one patient was still alive beyond eight years, two for seven and one-half years, four for five years and eleven for one year, after the original study began. Eleven of the patients died in uremia. Of the four patients who survived five years or longer, two had significant improvement of the glomerular filtration rate, and two had a decrease in the rate. The obvious conclusion is that aggressive reduction of blood pressure does not necessarily result in the deterioration of renal function and may prolong survival.[33]

Schwartz has described a 32-year-old Black woman who presented with severe hypertension (230/156) and endstage renal failure with a creatinine of 11 mg per 100 ml and a BUN of 109 mg per 100 ml.[34] Initial drug therapy consisted of methyldopa (Aldomet) and furosemide. Hydralazine (Apresoline) was later added. Within five days, the creatinine and BUN had increased to 15.3 mg per 100 ml and 193 mg per 100 ml respectively, and a 48-hour peritoneal dialysis was carried out. An open renal biopsy revealed malignant vascular changes with fibrinoid necrosis of the afferent arterioles. The glomeruli were nonspecifically thickened with minimal proliferation. Vigorous treatment of the hypertension by maintaining normal blood pressure with medication alone eventually resulted in improved renal function. Thirteen months later the renal function had stabilized with a serum creatinine of 2.9, and the creatinine clearance was recorded as 35 ml per minute.

Alpha-methyldopa and hydralazine have been useful drugs in the treatment of the hypertensive patient with chronic renal failure, since they are not associated with decreased renal blood flow, as is the case with guanethedine (Ismelin). The beta adrenergic blocker, propranolol (Inderal), has been used recently in combination with hydralazine to control hypertension with good results. Side effects are minimized and the antihypertensive effects of both the agents is augmented by furosemide. Much larger doses of furosemide, of course, are needed in patients with compromised renal function.

Most hypertension can be brought under control in the chronic dialysis population by means of vigorous ultrafiltration and sodium restriction. However, in one author's experience, about one third of the patients require oral antihypertensives, and, in an occasional patient with malignant hypertension, all these modalities fail. At this point bilateral nephrectomy must be carried out. Patients who undergo bilateral nephrectomy have a more readily increased blood requirement on chronic dialysis, most likely due to the absence of erythropoietin.

The Patient Undergoing Dialysis

PERITONEAL DIALYSIS

Peritoneal dialysis involves the instillation into the peritoneal cavity of a normal electrolyte solution rendered isosmotic to uremic plasma by the addition of glucose. This solution is known as the dialysate. Plasma molecules and ions move across the highly vascular semipermeable peritoneal membrane by a process of simple diffusion down a concentration gradient. Urea and creatinine are absent from the dialysate and are present in high concentrations in the uremic plasma, so that they readily diffuse from the plasma into the dialysate, filling the peritoneal cavity. On the other hand, the net transfer of sodium is less, since it is present in nearly equal concentration on either side of the peritoneal membrane. The clearance of any given substance depends upon particle size and charge. According to these criteria, Boen has shown the relative clearance rates as follows: urea > potassium > chloride > sodium > creatinine > phosphate > uric acid > bicarbonate > calcium > magnesium.[35] This is why the BUN is lowered much more than the serum creatinine during a peritoneal dialysis.

Solvent drag is another process by which substances are removed from the plasma by moving across the peritoneal membrane when hypertonic (4.5 percent) dialysate is used. Henderson and Nolph showed enhanced peritoneal permeability using 7 percent dialysate, which they attributed to enlargement of the intracellular channels that are present in the capillary wall and peritoneum.[36] Water (the solvent) moves through these pores in the membrane in response to an osmotic gradient by bulk flow rather than by diffusion, dragging along other molecules and ions in the stream of flow. Henderson demonstrated the force of solvent drag by showing a 38 percent enhancement of urea clearance when 7 percent dialysate was used. The contribution of solvent drag was almost 7 times greater than that which could be accounted for by diffusion.

Other factors must be considered if dialysis efficiency is to be maximal. Since clearance is directly dependent upon capillary area, it is axiomatic that dialysate be warmed to body temperature, as any vasoconstriction reduces capillary membrane area. Gross and McDonald found a 35 percent increase in urea clearance when dialysate temperature was raised from 20° C. to 37° C.[37] Fluid in the peritoneal cavity eventually equilibrates with plasma; therefore, the dialysate must be periodically drained and replenished. At the start of inflow, the concentration gradient between plasma and dialysate is maximal. It then decreases as a function of time as equilibrium approaches. Drainage time must be sufficient to remove all of the dialysate but not at the expense of efficiency. A practical compromise is a rapid inflow rate which usually takes 10 minutes, a 20-minute dwell time and a 20-minute drainage period, so that each exchange takes a total of 50 minutes.

Nursing Implications

The care of the patient undergoing peritoneal dialysis is entirely within the province of the nursing staff, although the physician usually inserts and removes the patient's peritoneal catheter. This form of dialysis is used extensively today because it is rapidly instituted and applicable for use in the community hospital. In addition, it does not require the specially trained personnel, priming blood, or expensive equipment necessary for extracorporeal dialysis. Nevertheless, it is not a procedure to be undertaken lightly. Safe and successful peritoneal dialysis requires a continuous monitoring by competent nursing personnel and supervision by a physician who has received training in the technique.[38]

There are a number of situations (which are discussed in more detail later) in which peritoneal dialysis is the treatment of choice. It is most widely used for supporting patients with acute renal failure, for certain drug ingestions, or during the evaluation of patients with chronic renal failure. Although it has been employed as an alternative to maintenance of extracorporeal dialysis, certain complications have been the limiting factor in its application in this manner. For example, in the series by Henderson, et al, experiences are reported with twelve patients on chronic peritoneal dialysis. Though two patients were maintained as long as eight months, ultimately the major complication was infection with subsequent fibrous exclusion of the peritoneal cavity.[39] J. P., an 18-year-old white woman underwent peritoneal dialysis for a year prior to acceptance on a chronic extracorporeal hemodialysis program. A year later she expressed a distinct preference for the latter. She disliked the insertion of the dialysis catheter, the fluid drainage following the procedure, and the multiple "scars on my abdomen." Some institutions, however, have found that properly performed, intermittent peritoneal dialysis is a satisfactory alternative procedure to conventional extracorporeal dialysis for a limited time.

Tenckhoff and his colleagues in Seattle have devoted most of their effort toward developing practical chronic peritoneal dialysis in recent years. In a paper presented at the American Society of Nephrology in November 1973, Tenckhoff described the current thoughts concerning this technique.[40] Chronic peritoneal dialysis has been made feasible by the development of a special catheter which is surgically placed in the abdomen and owes its success to two Dacron cuffs—one at the skin and the other at the peritoneal end of the catheter—which allow for the ingrowth of fibrous tissue and provide a water-resistant, bacteria-resistant barrier separating two compartments. Patients range in age from 3 to 76 and have undergone treatments for 3 months to over 6 years. The lifespan of a catheter is approximately 9 to 10 months, but one catheter has remained in place for 6 years and 3 months. Full activity, including swimming, is permitted. Automated equipment using the reverse osmosis principle for water purification has led to adaptation to home use. Following water purification, a proportioning pump mixes sterile dialysate concentrate with the water in the ratio of 2:1. The dialysis solution then flows past a conductivity meter into the patient and drains by gravity. The treatment schedule is usually 12 hours 3 times a week, or about 36 to 42 hours a week. With children a more frequent alternate day schedule is employed. The cost is currently $15 to $20 per dialysis with three quarters of the expense being the sterile concentrate. In the state of Washington, patients on chronic peritoneal dialysis make up 18 percent of the dialysis population. To date, their experience includes 107 patient years with approximately 15,000 dialyses. The infection rate is 0.56 percent with 1 per every 180 dialyses performed. Bone disease in these patients is no different from that in patients on chronic hemodialysis. High-protein diets have to be given to prevent hypoalbuminemia from albumin loss across the peritoneal membrane. The average patient's hematocrit is 24 percent without blood transfusions. Tenckhoff feels that safety and simplicity are the primary advantages of this system. Patients with limited intelligence and those living alone can adopt this form of therapy, whereas they could not undertake home hemodialysis. The chronic peritoneal approach is ideally suited for children, since vascular access devices are often difficult to obtain, children do not adapt well to repeated venipunctures, and shunt care problems are often difficult. Pediatric patients with chronic renal failure are treated on chronic peritoneal dialysis until they have attained adult height and weight. Only after this has been accomplished will transplantation be carried out. A well-dialyzed patient on an adequate protein intake can grow almost normally. With its avoidance of exaggerated changes in blood and volume shifts, peritoneal dialysis is suited to the elderly, patients with cardiovascular disease and instability, as well as the pediatric population. It is also useful where systemic heparinization is dangerous, as in the patient with multiple bleeding ulcers.

In addition, there is considerable advantage in the simplicity and convenience of the procedure. For example, T. J., a six-year-old boy, is dialyzed at home by his mother. Every other night at bedtime, his mother begins the procedure using an automatic peritoneal dialysis machine. The dialysis is completed by the time the boy awakes in the morning. His mother finds this method extremely convenient—it requires little preparation, almost no monitoring, and causes but slight disruption in family routine, as she is also able to sleep during the dialysis in her son's room.

Although only a short period of time is required to institute peritoneal dialysis, a certain amount of equipment is utilized. The choice of materials may vary, but patient care is greatly facilitated if these supplies are standardized and prearranged for use within a given institution. O'Neill provides one such list of equipment.[41] The composition of the usual dialysis fluid is:*

Sodium—140.5 mEq/L
Potassium—none (added as required)
Chloride—101.0 mEq/L
Calcium—3.5 mEq/L
Magnesium—1.5 mEq/L
Lactate—44.5 mEq/L
Dextrose—15.0 Gm/L (1.5%) or 40.5 Gm/L (4.5%)
Osmolarity—372 mOsm/L (1.5%) or mOsm/L (4.5%)

Preparation for Dialysis

Because it often sounds frightening to the patient, it is important for the nurse, in conjunction with the physician, to reinforce the explanation given the patient, and to elaborate on pertinent details, in order to provide an additional measure of reassurance. For example, the nurse can reduce the patient's anxiety by stressing the simplicity of the treatment and its advantages to him, such as allowing him a liberalized diet and fluid intake during the procedure. The specific approach, of course, varies from one patient to another. The patient needs further explanation and reassurance as the procedure progresses. Advance planning should take into account the necessity for teaching and support as ongoing nursing measures. This is as much a vital part of the procedure as the maintenance of aseptic technique and the evaluation of fluid balance.

Prior to the initiation of dialysis, the patient's weight and vital signs are obtained and recorded. These provide valuable parameters against which to check his fluid balance as the procedure progresses. If a great deal of fluid is withdrawn, as is often the case, relative hypotension is easily detected and the predialysis weight provides a check on the fluid cumulative balance figures.

---

*Commercially available as Inpersol (Abbott Laboratories), Dianeal (Baxter Laboratories), Peridial (Cutter Laboratories).

The patient should empty his bladder just prior to the time of dialysis in order to avoid perforation of the bladder during the insertion of the trochar through the abdominal wall. If the bladder is perforated, the patient may well have an immediate desire to urinate—the amount of the "urine" passed may be large, and, in fact, almost equal to the amount of dialysis solution just introduced. When tested, the composition of the urine is found to be similar to the dialysis solution.

The "blind" introduction of the trochar also carries with it the risk of bowel perforation—a risk which is increased when the operator is inexperienced in the technique. In one series of 1,400 dialyses performed on 40 patients, three such perforations occurred. Perforation was easily recognized in these cases by observation of cloudy dialysate drainage, obvious fecal contamination of the tip of the peritoneal catheter, and signs and symptoms of peritoneal irritation.

The patient is more cooperative during this lengthy treatment if he is as comfortable as possible at the outset of the procedure. In most circumstances, the position of choice for the initiation of dialysis is the modified semi-Fowler's. It is preferable that the patient be attired in a hospital gown. Meperidine and a barbiturate are generally administered one-half hour prior to the insertion of the peritoneal catheter, in order to provide analgesia and sedation. If the patient is lethargic, the dosage of these medications is adjusted accordingly.

Prewarming the dialysis solution in a constant temperature bath is effective. Infusion at body temperature is more comfortable for the patient and is, therefore, better tolerated. It also increases the peritoneal clearance and prevents hypothermia. The temperature of the bath must be checked frequently to avoid accidental infusion of fluid that is too hot or too cold. Other errors in administration may be avoided by placing rubber bands around each bottle to prevent loosening of the labels when wet and marking each bottle with a glass marking pencil to indicate the percentage of glucose concentration. Medications to be added to the dialysate are collected on a tray in a clean area, near the patient's bed. Just before the bottles are hung for infusion, medications are added. The addition of particular medications is more or less standard. Heparin is added in a dosage that is sufficient to prevent fibrin clots, but not adequate for systemic heparinization of the patient. The dosage of potassium is regulated according to the individual patient's needs. The addition of potassium is particularly important for the digitalized patient, since rapid lowering of serum potassium levels may accompany dialysis. When hyperkalemia has reached cardiotoxic levels, a potassium-free dialysate may be used for the first few hours, followed by raising of the concentration toward normal plasma levels. Conversely, if severe, prolonged vomiting has induced potassium depletion, a greater than normal concentration of potassium in the dialysate may be employed. Antibiotics are added to the dialysate only when specifically indicated.

There are a number of ways in which the nurse can reduce the possibilities for bacterial contamination of the dialysate. The use of single 2-liter bottles will reduce the opportunity for contamination during the addition of medications.* Dialysate solutions (with a high-dextrose content) are less likely to become contaminated if they are warmed before they are opened. Immersion of the necks of bottles in the warming solution must be avoided, because this allows for contamination. Coughing or talking over open bottles must be prohibited.

These simple precautions assume considerable importance when one reflects that *the most frequent serious complication of peritoneal dialysis is peritonitis*. The necessity for strict aseptic technique in the handling of solutions, and throughout the entire dialysis procedure, cannot be overemphasized. Dialysate is infused directly into the peritoneal cavity. Therefore, any contamination of the solution carries the threat of peritonitis—a threat which is substantial in the case of the uremic patient, who has limited ability to fight infection.

As a result of peritonitis, adhesions form within the peritoneal cavity separating it into sec-

---

*Available from Abbott Laboratories.

tions, and thus preventing free flow of dialysate fluid and adequate dialysis. In addition, such a peritoneal infection may preclude using this route for further dialyses for some time, if not permanently.

Initiation of Dialysis

The nurse assists the physician in beginning the dialysis. Since the introduction of the trochar actually constitutes a minor operative procedure, the physician wears a mask and sterile gloves. The patient's abdomen, which is shaved and scrubbed, is draped sterilely. The trochar is introduced following local anesthesia, about an inch below the umbilicus in the abdominal midline, and the peritoneal catheter is inserted through it (Fig. 17-5). The catheter is then sutured into place and the exchange tubing is connected. (Air-vent filters, if present, should be taped in place to prevent their becoming dislodged; if this occurs, the entire set must be changed.) The dialysate is then suspended about four feet above the patient's bed (Fig. 17-6). A sterile dressing is applied securely around the catheter, and it is well taped with the connecting set to the abdominal wall to avoid dislodging or kinking by the patient. Using a blunt trochar for catheter insertion has the advantage of minimizing the chance of bowel perforation. Also, the rigidity of the trochar allows the physician to direct the catheter into any position desired. The disadvantage of the trochar is that a firm purse-string suture is required to prevent leakage. Even this may not be effective, especially in obese patients. The direct introduction of the catheter with an inner removable stylet has the advantage of ease of insertion and infrequent leakage problems, but carries with it an increased risk of bowel perforation, due to the smaller diameter. Also, catheter placement in different abdominal quadrants may not be as easy as with the trochar; and in thin patients the catheter tip itself or the dialysate stream may come in contact with the rectum and cause rectal spasms.

The dialyzing solution is allowed to run into the patient's abdomen as rapidly as possible. The infusion period should not take more than 15 minutes and, as the bottles empty, the tubing

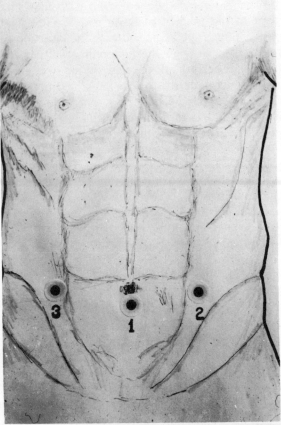

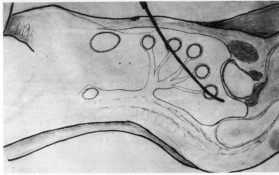

FIGURE 17-5.
(A) Sites for catheter placement in peritoneal dialysis. Site #1 is the preferred location. (B) Side view of abdominal cavity, showing peritoneal dialysis catheter in place in pelvic gutter.

should be clamped just before air enters it. The patient may complain of abdominal pain with the rapid infusion of fluid; if so, the rate of infusion may be temporarily decreased and then resumed.

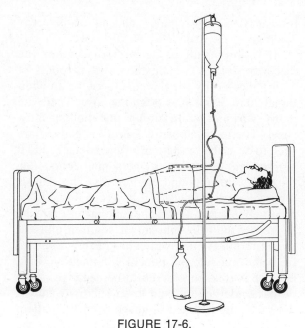

FIGURE 17-6.
System for fluid cycle in peritoneal dialysis.
Source: Abbott Laboratories. Used by permission.

The physician should be notified if the patient suffers persistent or severe pain. Lidocaine may be given (50 mg added to the dialysis fluid) for severe pain. If the pain persists, the physician may find it necessary to change the location of the peritoneal catheter, or administer a narcotic analgesic.

The infused fluid is allowed to remain in the peritoneal cavity for a period determined by the physician, usually 30 to 60 minutes. This is known as the equilibration or dwell period and is the time when the maximal amount of transport of solutes and fluid is taking place. It is the critical time to check the patient's vital signs, in order to ascertain that hypotension is not occurring secondary to fluid shifts. If the patient complains of feeling full, generally simple reassurance that this is a frequent occurrence may help him to adjust to the discomfort, although measures to reduce this discomfort, such as changing the patient's position, should be instituted. The nurse should remember that respiratory embarrassment can occur as the fluid volume pushes the diaphragm upward. Pneumonia and atelectasis may often occur secondary to prolonged

(three to four days) dialysis; thus, the nurse must encourage the patient to deep breathe and cough.

The first infusion should be drained immediately to determine whether the outflow path is obstructed. The drainage end of the exchange set is unclamped and the fluid is allowed to flow out of the abdominal cavity by gravity. A steady forceful stream of fluid is seen initially. (Figure 17-6 shows that the drainage system is closed and, therefore, sterility is maintained.) A drip chamber in the outflow tubing prevents ascending bacterial contamination.

The first drainage is often blood-tinged, due to the trauma of the insertion of the trochar; but if considerable blood is present, the nurse saves serial samples of the drainage and notifies the physician. The drainage period should not last longer than 30 minutes. Prolonged drainage periods slow down dialysis, decreasing the number of exchanges that can take place within the prescribed total time allotted for the treatment. If the outflow is slow, it may be improved by applying gentle pressure on the patient's lower abdomen, changing the patient's position from side to side, and checking the tubing system for kinks and clamps. Continued faulty drainage is probably due to poor catheter placement in the peritoneal cavity, and requires relocation by the physician. Cloudy drainage often indicates infection; it should be reported and a sample saved for culture. Generally a culture of the fluid is obtained every 12 exchanges. When needed, appropriate antibiotics may be instituted, either by addition to the dialysate, systemic administration, or both. The nurse is frequently responsible for saving serial samples of dialysate drainage in order to compare the appearance of the fluid in successive exchanges.

The fluid introduced in the first exchange may not be entirely recovered, due to sequestration of solution in and around the abdominal viscera. Subsequent drainage periods generally recover the amount infused plus 100 to 200 ml; however, the individual drainage period should not be unduly prolonged simply to recover all the fluid that was introduced during that period, as it may well be recovered in later drainage periods. If there is no outflow at all, it may be that the omentum has become adherent to the catheter, occluding the multiple small holes along its length. Using sterile technique, 50 ml of dialysis solution may be forced through the catheter with the aid of a large syringe, relieving the situation. Another reason for complete failure to recover infused fluid may be that internal bleeding has taken place and clots are blocking the catheter. At the end of the drainage period, when there is no more fluid dripping from the drainage tubing and most of it has been recovered, the tubing is clamped, more dialysate hung, and the infusion process repeated.

For each patient, the physician determines the amount and type of dialysate, the exchange timing, and the medications to be added. In some hospitals, a special order sheet has proved to be helpful to the nursing staff (Table 17-2).

The fluid balance must be measured accurately and recorded. Measurement errors of as little as 50 ml per exchange can lead to an error of 2,400 ml in the usual 48-hour dialysis.

It is important to determine whether the dialysate bottles contain the exact amounts of fluid indicated by the manufacturer, or an additional 20 to 50 ml as is often the case. There are many ways of maintaining the dialysis flow sheet. The terms "positive" and "negative" are used to describe the patient's fluid balance, and it is most important that the personnel conducting the dialysis understand these terms. The dialysis record shown in Table 17-3 has been found to be relatively simple. When the amount of drainage is greater than the amount of solution infused, the extra fluid is that which has been withdrawn from the patient; the patient's cumulative fluid balance is thus considered to be negative, since he has undergone a fluid loss. This is usually a desirable state. When drainage from the patient is less than the amount of solution infused, he

TABLE 17-2
Representative Physician's Order Sheet for Peritoneal Dialysis

1. Type and amount of fluid for each dialysis exchange.

    1.5% dextrose _____ml

    4.5% dextrose _____ml

2. Add to each 2,000 cc bottle

    a) _____mEq KCl

    b) _____units Heparin

    c) _____

3. Allow fluid to enter abdomen as rapidly as possible.

4. Fluid to remain in abdomen for total time of _____
    minutes.

5. Allow _____minutes for fluid to drain from abdomen.

6. A single dialysis exchange should be about_____
    minutes in length (or _____per 24 hours).

TABLE 17-3
Fluid Balance Sheet for Peritoneal Dialysis

DIRECTIONS

Positive or Negative Balance Column:
  Balance *Positive* when drainage is *Less* than infusion.
  Balance *Negative* when drainage is *Greater* than infusion.
Cumulative Balance Column:
  Positive or negative figure of each exchange is brought over to this column; *larger* number on top.
  If signs are alike, add figures, e.g., +1200 (+) +600 = +1800.
  If signs are different, subtract figures, e.g., +1800 (−) −900 = +900.
  Sign of result is *always* that of *larger* figure, e.g., −1200 (−) +600 = −600.

EXCH. NO.	TIME INFUSION STARTS STOPS	TIME DRAINAGE STARTS STOPS	VOLUME IN OUT	BALANCE (+ or −)	DIALYSATE 1.5% 4.5%	HEP.	KCl	ANTIBIO.	CUM. BAL.	COMMENTS OTHER MED.

has retained some of the infused fluid; he has gained fluid and is thus said to be in positive balance. The physician sets the limits of positive and negative balance that are considered desirable for each patient. In general, however, it should be reported if positive balance exceeds 500 ml or negative balance exceeds 1,000 ml. If hypertonic dialysate (greater than 1.5 percent glucose) is used, the amount of drainage may exceed the amount of infusion by as much as 500 ml per exchange. Thus, when using such a hypertonic dialysate, it is particularly important to monitor the patient's vital signs carefully, being alert for and reporting any symptoms or signs of hypovolemia or shock. The nurse should be aware that hypertension or hypotension may oc-

cur. Blood pressure readings must be compared to the particular patient's predialysis readings. Hypertonic glucose solution sometimes causes discomfort, due to irritation of the peritoneum, which may be alleviated, with the addition of 100 mg of lidocaine to the dialysate. The efficiency of dialysis is increased with the use of hypertonic solutions (glucose 4.5 percent) on the basis of solvent drag. Solutions hypertonic to plasma enhance the transfer of solutes in the bulk flow of fluid across the porous peritoneal membrane. Solute removal in this instance occurs more as a result of solvent drag than by simple diffusion. This procedure must be monitored with great care.

Dressings must be checked frequently for

leakage of dialysate or blood from the incision. The physician is notified if either occurs, and the dressings are changed by the use of a strict aseptic technique. Occasionally, additional sutures are necessary at the catheter site. Dressings should not be allowed to remain wet, since the peritoneal cavity may become contaminated and severe peritonitis result.

Nursing measures are best carried out concomitantly with dialysis during drainage periods. Frequent comfort measures are indicated, including skin care, oral hygiene, and changes in the patient's position. If his condition permits, the patient may sit in a chair or walk about the unit. During his dialysis, food and fluid restrictions may be liberalized without the danger of overhydration or potassium intoxication. Ideally, the patient's meals should coincide with drainage periods. If necessary, small, frequent feedings might be arranged. At the termination of the dialysis, the peritoneal catheter is removed and the incision is covered with a dry, sterile dressing.

During the course of peritoneal dialysis, the patient's urine volume usually diminishes. The exact cause of this phenomenon is unknown, but probably reflects a combination of fluid shifts, decreased solute load, volume depletion, and consequent decreased renal blood flow. This oliguria can be undesirable, since in many patients (particularly those with severe chronic renal insufficiency of any cause) urine volume may not return to predialysis levels. The addition of oliguria to the clinical picture further complicates the patient's medical management, as sodium, potassium, and water retention may rapidly develop if proper steps are not taken. The duration of a single dialysis varies from one patient to another, but a time of 36 to 48 hours is usual. Beyond that, oliguria may worsen and become refractory, and the risk of peritonitis increases significantly.

Infection, bleeding, compromise of pulmonary function with dyspnea or pneumonia, abdominal discomfort, and protein depletion are all potential complications of peritoneal dialysis. During prolonged hypertonic dialysis, hypernatremia with water depletion may occur.

Hyperglycemic, hyperosmolar, nonketotic coma may also develop from the high glucose concentration in the dialysate, if the body cannot metabolize the excess glucose load.

The individuality and independence of the patient must be continually supported and encouraged by the medical personnel. It is important for the nurse to develop good rapport with the patient, encouraging him to ask questions and answering them as frankly as the circumstances permit. The patient's family should also be reassured and the procedure explained to them as well as to the patient. In selected instances, patients may indeed be taught how to carry out the procedure themselves.

The ease with which peritoneal dialysis can be carried out is in direct relationship to the understanding, motivation, and conscientiousness of the nurse in attendance. It is a procedure which is often conducted at an emotionally trying time for the patient (i.e., acute onset of distress, recent discovery of chronic disease, during evaluation for an extracorporeal hemodialysis program, or renal transplantation). The understanding and support which the nurse offers is invaluable in helping the patient cope with these stresses.

HEMODIALYSIS

Hemodialysis Techniques

Abel, Rowntree, and Turner coined the term "artificial kidney" in 1913, when they reported the removal of diffusable substances from canine blood by the use of celloidin tubes surrounded by a glass cylinder containing dialysate.[42] In 1943 in the Netherlands, the first practical artificial kidney was built by Willem Kolff, who first dialyzed a patient with cellophane tubing wrapped around a rotating drum which was immersed in dialysate. In 1953, at the University of Pennsylvania, Inouye and Engelberg published their results with cellophane tubing wrapped around a plastic mesh support placed in a pressure cooker.[43] Kolff refined this apparatus, which led to the development of the first twin-coil dialyzer (Fig. 17-7). Skeggs and Leonards, in 1954, had approached the problem differently by using flat sheets of cellophane through which blood and

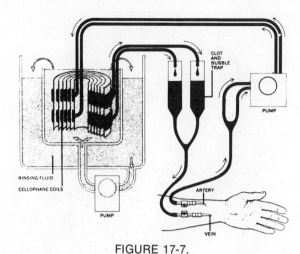

FIGURE 17-7.
Twin-coil dialyzer.

dialysate were circulated in opposite directions; and Kiil, in Norway, refined this approach of parallel-flow dialysis. Here dialysate circulated between ridged resin boards bolted together which supported two sheets of cellophane, creating a path for the blood (Fig. 17-8).

Up to this point, hemodialysis had not been successful in keeping an endstage uremic patient alive for any significant length of time. Teschan pointed out the importance of early and frequent dialysis, in order to prophylactically treat the patient rather than waiting for severe symptoms to develop.[44] Finally, in 1960, Scribner reported the first patients successfully treated for chronic renal failure. Thus, successful chronic dialysis

was dependent on the development of a circulatory access device which eliminated the need for performing a surgical cutdown for each dialysis. In 1960 Quinton, Dillard, and Scribner described such a device—a Silastic–Teflon external arteriovenous shunt which is now used in many dialysis centers[45] (Fig. 17-9).

Blood Access Devices

The same type of shunt as that developed in 1960 is still used today when rapid blood access is required (e.g., in a patient with acute renal failure who needs immediate hemodialysis). The greatest drawback with the external A-V shunt is its propensity for thrombi formation. If a clotted shunt is not detected within the first one or two hours, it may be impossible to declot it, and a new surgical procedure must be carried out. By using a straight shunt instead of the curved type, which was placed under the skin, a Fogarty catheter can often be used to remove a thrombus, a procedure that was not possible with the earlier shunt. Occasionally, bovine fibrinolysin can be instilled to try to dissolve the clot. However, this is not without pain on the arterial side and often may not work. Occasionally the intima of the vessel grows around the Teflon vessel tip resulting in progressive narrowing of the lumen which, if it occurs on the arterial side, can reduce the arterial blood flow and, if on the venous side, can increase the venous resistance. If proper

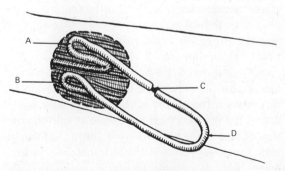

FIGURE 17-9.
Arteriovenous shunt. (A) Venous loop as it would come from vessel onto skin. (B) Arterial loop as it would come from vessel onto skin. (C) Teflon connector. (D) Section of shunt exposed for observation.

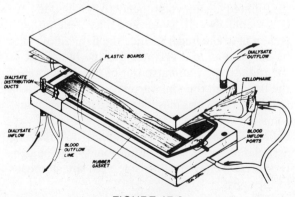

FIGURE 17-8.
Kiil dialyzer.

care of the shunt is not maintained—which includes keeping it wrapped at all times, keeping it clean, and keeping it dry—the shunt can become infected, resulting in sepsis, erosion of the blood vessels and even in cases of acute bacterial endocarditis. Even with the most meticulous care, shunt life may not exceed several months with a maximum of one or two years in the majority of patients. It is important to instruct the patient in meticulous shunt care to prevent infections and also to listen frequently for the bruit to pick up any early clotting. Nurses should be aware that bruits often cannot be heard, so nurses and patients alike should be taught to feel for a thrill and to observe the appearance of the area and evaluate warmth of skin. Small shunt clips should be included in the elastic bandage covering the dressing so that they are readily available to clamp off the shunt should accidental disconnection occur. Death from exsanguination can occur in minutes with a blood flow of 400 ml per minute.

Vascular access devices and techniques have received considerable attention in research efforts in the ensuing years. In 1966, Brescia, et al, described the creation of a chronic A-V fistula in the forearm of a patient by anastomosing the radial artery in an adjacent vein in a side-to-side fashion (Fig. 17-10).[46] In this way, the vein, after a few days, weeks, or months, gradually became dilated and enlarged making repeated needle punctures easy. In practice, 14-gauge needles filled with heparinized saline are placed in the dilated vein, one for arterial flow and the other for a returning venous line. The veins can be punctured almost indefinitely with some variation of the puncture site, and fistulas rarely clot off. They do, however, occasionally thrombos if the needle is placed too close to the actual fistula, but the failure rate is only a fraction of that of the external A-V shunt. Some centers teach patients self-venipuncture, which many patients can master quite easily. It is the practice in one center not to use any intradermal procaine or lidocaine, since this often is attended by some oozing, and many of the patients feel the discomfort of the lidocaine injection is more than that of the actual venipuncture.

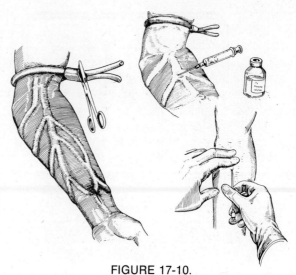

FIGURE 17-10.
Arteriovenous fistula. Source: Nose, Y.: The Artificial Kidney. St. Louis, C. V. Mosby, 1969, p. 192.

The disadvantages of the A-V fistula include at least a two-to-three-week waiting period for the vessel to mature, and an ideal waiting period is usually several months. A patient who arrives in endstage renal failure and who cannot be peritoneally dialyzed, will need an external A-V shunt for immediate use while the A-V fistula is undergoing maturation. This sacrifices a group of vessels, surgically creating the external shunt. Swelling of the distal extremity may become a problem in the first week after surgery and occasionally may persist for several months. This can often be remedied by a tight bandage, or by keeping the arm elevated, but occasionally some of the dilated distal veins need to be ligated. An occasional ''steal'' syndrome may develop with ischemia of the fingers, since the fistula flow may be so great as to divert most of the blood out of the radial artery and also out of the deep loop of the hand from the ulnar artery into the vein; as a result, the fingers may develop ischemic symptoms. In the patient with severe peripheral vascular disease, such as a diabetic, this may be associated with significant morbidity. Some centers create end-artery-to-side-vein anastomoses in the wrist.

Where vessel size precludes a good A-V fistula, an autogenous saphenous vein graft in the form of a U-shaped loop can be placed sub-cutaneously in the forearm and can be used quite well for a long period of time. However, meticulous care must be used in the operative site, since patients have often become infected from surgical wounds of the groin. For example, one patient who had a draining lymph duct in the groin which persisted for several months eventually developed a gram-negative sepsis. Occasionally a saphenofemoral loop can be created so that the dilated vein is in the thigh. Thomas, et al, described a large Dacron-cuffed external shunt which could be placed in a femoral artery and adjacent vein when no further peripheral sites were available.[47] A more recent procedure uses a bovine carotid artery graft placed in the appropriate extremity and anastomosed to the artery and vein. After a two-to-five-week waiting period, enough fibrous tissue has surrounded the artery graft so that repeated punctures can be made without difficulty. The thickened wall of the artery compared to a vein often prevents false aneurysm formation and dilatation. Dacron grafts have also been used; however, fibrous tissue must cover the graft so that no bleeding occurs when needles are removed. Some centers employ an external A-V shunt in the leg so that the patient is able to have both hands free, can operate the machine himself, and can connect and disconnect himself to the machine without assistance. This has obvious advantages, but a surgical creation of a leg shunt usually requires the patient to be off his feet for two weeks and full weight bearing may not be permitted for three to four weeks. If shunt difficulties develop which require further surgery, the patient again has to be off his feet for ten days to two weeks. This can result in considerable loss of time from one's employment.

Care of Vascular Access Routes

Care of access routes varies greatly from unit to unit. Some techniques which may be taught nurses (and patients) are set forth in Tables 17-4 and 17-5.

In general, the most important factors in increasing the life of access (thereby increasing the life of the patient) are meticulous care, limited usage, and avoidance of extra-long Silastic tubing loops. The area must be cleaned with regularity and with great care. At the first sign of infection or clotting, the staff will institute the appropriate therapy. The patient should use the extremity in a normal way, but it should not be subjected to venipunctures or blood pressures which may compromise flow and increase the chance of clotting.

REPEATED EXTRACORPOREAL DIALYSIS OF THE PATIENT WITH CHRONIC RENAL FAILURE

With the development of various hemodialysis techniques, treatment centers were set up in many areas of the United States, Europe, and Japan. The use of a central dialysate delivery system allowed for the efficient treatment of many patients in one dialysis center. Various criteria were set up for the acceptance of a terminal uremic patient into a chronic dialysis program. Attempts to judge emotional stability, predicted success in the program, and rehabilitation potential were carried out by various review boards for patient selection. Later, because of space and personnel limitations, high cost, and the large number of patients who could not readily commute to a large dialysis center, hemodialysis in the home was instituted. Center dialysis remains fairly static; there is little turnover of patients and it imposes rigid time restrictions on the patients.

In 1964, Merrill in Boston, Scribner in Seattle, and Sheldon in England began training patients and their spouses to dialyze themselves at home.[48] The advantages were reduction in cost, a saving of time and greater flexibility of scheduling, lesser incidence of hepatitis, and, perhaps most valuable, the marked increase of patient independence. Dialysis could be carried out in the evening so that it would not interfere with work schedules and it could be carried out with suitable frequency to meet the individual's metabolic needs. Simplified machines with built-in safety monitors, and the placement of shunts in the lower leg enabled the patient to connect himself to the machine and dialyze while sleeping.

An appreciation of the efficacy of chronic in-

TABLE 17-4
Instructions For Patient Self-Care of A-V Fistula

1. Check incisional area every three hours for a bruit using a stethoscope (Listen for a swishing sound).
2. Feel for the thrill over the incision every three hours using your fingers.
   a. Immediately notify the physician if unable to obtain the bruit or feel the thrill.
3. *Do not* allow anyone to use this extremity for any purpose.
   NO IV's   NO BLOOD PRESSURES
   NO BLOOD SPECIMEN
4. Do not redress or cleanse the extremity until the sutures are removed.
   a. If you notice any excessive bleeding, notify physician immediately.
5. For the first two weeks, keep the extremity elevated on one or two pillows.
6. Wear a sling for arm fistulas for two weeks when you are walking around, always remove sling to sleep.
7. After the sutures have been removed, keep that extremity clean. There is no special care required and there will be no limitation to the use of that limb.
8. Exercises for increasing the size of the vessels in the fistula:
   a. After the wound is healed, place the affected arm in water warm enough to turn the skin pink without causing a burn. Then, while the arm is in the water, apply a tourniquet above the fistula site. Open and close the hand (clenched into a fist and relaxed) for three to five minutes during the first attempt. The time is gradually increased at the discretion of the physician.
   b. A similar exercise can be performed as described, except that the arm is not immersed in water.
   c. Practice squeezing a firm rubber ball, increasing the exercise period as indicated.
   d. A tourniquet may be applied above the fistula site

for short periods of time each day. The time may be gradually increased at the discretion of the physician.
   e. Buy a hand exerciser at a sporting goods store and use it eight times a day increasing the length of time each day.
9. Check the fistula after the sutures are removed:
   a. Check the fistula at least every four hours to be sure it is still functioning.
   b. Listen to it with a stethoscope and feel it with your fingers.
   c. If you cannot feel the thrill at the fistula site or hear the bruit with a stethoscope *immediately* notify your physician and come to the hospital. Remember, if a clotted fistula is discovered immediately, there is a possibility that the fistula can be reopened. If it is not discovered, a new one will have to be created in your other arm. Then what do you use after that!
10. Warm wet soaks:
   a. Whenever you have infiltrated a needle, developed a hematoma, or had difficulty inserting the fistula needles, you should apply wet soaks to the area. It is best to apply the soaks for as long as possible. Overnight is helpful.
   b. Take a towel and soak it in warm water. Ring it dry and apply it to the entire arm.
   c. Wrap the arm with plastic to keep the moisture and heat inside.
   d. Place a heating pad on top and turn it to *low*.
   e. Keep on as long as possible.
11. After dialysis wrap the limb with an elastic bandage, very securely, starting at the hand or the foot and keep the bandage on securely for four hours. Loosen the bandage and reapply, keeping the bandage on for twelve hours.

termittent hemodialysis can be gained by examining not only survival statistics, but also the type of dialysis facilities and patient selection criteria. With a carefully selected group of 22 patients who were treated in a large dialysis center, and whose emotional stability and other factors were used as criteria for admission to the program, three deaths occurred during treatment ranging up to 50 months.[49] In sharp contrast, indigent patients were treated in a large city hospital. Of eight patients, seven died during a treatment time ranging from 1.5 to 22 months. Treatment was terminated for several reasons, including the inability of these patients to accept the quality of life on chronic dialysis with all its attendant regimentation and restriction.[50]

Lewis, et al, compiled survival data on 302

patients in 14 dialysis centers up to July, 1967.[51] Survival rates were as follows: of 133 patients 87 percent survived one year; 77.3 percent of 53 patients survived 2 years; 67.4 percent of 20 patients survived 3 years; and 63.6 percent of 14 patients survived 4 years. The study included 3 patients followed for 7 years with a 57.8 percent survival rate. Males and females did equally well in such programs. Survival rates were not statistically different under or over the age of 45. (Thus, age was an invalid criterion for selection on chronic dialysis programs.)

Of 2660 patients on chronic dialysis in December 1969, Ginn counted 36 percent who were supported by federal funds, 885 on home dialysis programs as compared to about 10 percent in 1967.[52] Since January 1967, the survival rate has

TABLE 17-5
Instructions for Patient Self-Care of A-V Shunt

For your shunt to function, the blood must flow freely through the plastic tubing. Here are a few simple, but *very* important instructions for care of your shunt.

1. Feel for a pulsation (thrill) above the venous shunt side every three hours.
2. Using a stethoscope, listen for a swishing sound (bruit) above the venous shunt site every three hours.
3. Check the appearance of the blood in the plastic tubing. The blood should be red.
4. DANGER SIGNS.
   a. If you cannot feel the thrill, or if you cannot hear the bruit, or the blood in the tubing has clotted and the blood appears separated into two layers. NOTIFY THE PHYSICIAN IMMEDIATELY.
   b. If you discover a clotted shunt immediately, probably the physician can declot it. The sooner you call, the sooner you can be helped.
5. *Do not* allow anyone to use this extremity for any purpose.
   NO IV's   NO BLOOD PRESSURES
   NO BLOOD SPECIMENS
6. It is essential to maintain cleanliness with your shunt.
   a. Keep extremity wrapped at all times.
   b. If shunt dressing should become wet, remove wet dressings, apply sterile dry dressings and rewrap.
7. Check extremity for signs of bleeding. Notify physician immediately if bleeding occurs.
8. If the shunt should separate, immediately apply a tourniquet above the shunt, unwrap extremity, clamp both sides of shunt, reconnect shunt, remove clamps, and remove tourniquet.
   a. Rewrap extremity and notify the physician.
   b. *This is an emergency.*
   c. Keep clamps on shunt dressing at all times.
9. If one of the shunt sides should pull out of the skin, immediately apply a tourniquet above the shunt. Notify the physician and come to the hospital. *This is an emergency.*
   a. If you do not have a tourniquet apply enough pressure to the area to stop the bleeding.
10. In general, the function of the shunt is related to the amount and type of activity done with that extremity.
   a. Avoid strenuous exercise.
   b. Do not bowl if shunt is in dominate arm.
   c. Use a golf cart if shunt is in the leg.
   d. Never cross the legs if shunt is in the leg.
   e. Do not sit or stand in one position for a long period of time. Move about with a leg shunt.
   f. Never put pressure against the shunt leg.
   g. Never sit in a chair that puts pressure against the underside of the thigh.
   h. Swimming is impossible.
   i. Tub baths and showers may be taken if a plastic cover is placed over the shunt area and the shunt area does *not* get wet.
11. If you notice any drainage from the shunt sites, notify your physician.

showed no differences from earlier studies, although the patients on home dialysis facilities since January 1967 did show a higher one- and two-year survival and rehabilitation rate than those treated by center dialysis.

Johnson, et al, compared several approaches to chronic dialysis over a five and one-half year period at the Mayo Clinic.[53] Of 24 men and 19 women, 17 men and 16 women were partially or wholly rehabilitated, in that they returned to their jobs or household duties. The incidence of complications requiring hospitalization was lowest in the patients on home dialysis. (Home dialysis was also much less expensive.) In contrast to a $19,760 annual fee for twice weekly center dialysis, thrice weekly dialysis could be carried out at home for $3,848. (See Part 3 of this chapter on Renal Transplantation in which current long-term [more than five years] survival rates are shown for the various forms of therapy for these patients.)

In conclusion, it would appear that age criteria in patient selection are unfair—indeed the older, less metabolically and physically active individual who often is more emotionally stable outdoes his younger counterpart on a chronic intermittent hemodialysis program. Home dialysis for a well-motivated patient allows for maximum rehabilitation at minimum cost.

Principles of Extracorporeal Dialysis

The basic principle involved in hemodialysis is the same as that of peritoneal dialysis—diffusion of substances through a membrane from the plasma to a dialysate, in response to a concentration gradient. Although the diffusion takes place through an artificial membrane outside the confines of the body, the dialysis concept remains unaltered. The dialysate composition is similar to that used in peritoneal dialysis, containing sodium, potassium, calcium, magnesium, acetate, chloride, and glucose in amounts determined suitable for the particular patient's situation. However, in hemodialysis several other variables must also be considered, including blood flow, membrane permeability, and membrane surface area.

The clearance of any substance from the body (dialysance) is directly proportional to the blood flow rate in ml per minute through the dialyzer. For example, dialysance of urea increases as blood flow rates increase and tends to level off at rates above 300 ml per minute. In addition, the clearance of smaller molecules, such as urea, is more rapid than that of larger molecules, such as creatinine, when flow rates are identical. The classical membrane used for hemodialysis is cellophane, which is approximately 250 times thicker than the kidney's glomerular basement membrane.

KINETICS OF HEMODIALYSIS

The efficiency of hemodialysis per unit time is primarily dependent upon three variables: 1) membrane permeability, 2) membrane area, and 3) blood flow rates. The more permeable the dialysis membrane, the more solutes and water will move across it. There is a limit to porosity, or the larger protein molecules would traverse the membrane and be lost in the dialysate. Strength is often inversely proportional to permeability. A very porous membrane that cannot tolerate high pressures is unsuitable because of frequent ruptures. The more rapid the blood flow rate, the greater the amount of net transfer of solutes from blood to dialysate. The curve for water movement across the membrane is directly proportional to the flow rate and moves in a straight line. The greater the blood flow, the greater the amount of water removed across the membrane. For small molecules, this curve is similar, with a maximum being reached. As molecular size increases, the curve becomes flatter, and for large and middle-sized molecules, such as inulin and vitamin B_{12}, dialysance, or transfer rate across the membrane, is only proportional to membrane size, and blood flow rate has little influence.

In the last few years much as been written about the so-called middle molecule and its role in the pathogenesis of uremia. Middle molecules have a molecular weight from 300 to 2,000 and, because of their size, are very slowly dialyzable across an artificial membrane when compared to urea. According to Babb, et al, evidence for speculation of a middle molecule comes from two clinical observations.[54] First, it has been noted that patients on chronic peritoneal dialysis, when compared to patients on chronic hemodialysis, often remain well and free of uremic neuropathy, despite significantly higher BUN and creatinine levels. Therefore, the peritoneal membrane may be passing some toxic molecules better than cellophane. Second, the prevention of peripheral neuropathy is dependent upon an adequate number of hours of dialysis per week, rather than on maintaining certain predialysis levels of BUN and creatinine. Small molecules, such as urea and creatinine where the molecular weight is 60 and 113, move across the membrane quite easily, whereas a middle molecule such as inulin, with a molecular weight of 5,200, moves across the membrane very slowly. The greater dialysance reflects a greater movement across the membrane. These figures are for the artificial kidney. The human kidney clears creatinine and inulin at identical rates. The peritoneum itself has been shown to be approximately ten times more permeable to large solutes than currently used membranes in the artificial kidney.

Since the small molecules move across the membrane quite easily, most of their clearance occurs at the beginning of a six-hour dialysis when their plasma concentration is high and their diffusion gradients are the steepest. Toward the end of a six-hour dialysis, not much urea and creatinine are moving across the membrane. However, a middle molecular weight substance which diffuses poorly across the membrane will have approximately the same clearance at the beginning as at the end of dialysis. This is why the total time on dialysis is important.

Recently, Henderson, et al, attempted to enhance the removal of middle molecular weight substances during hemodialysis with the use of intermittent hemodiafiltration.[55] A hemodiafilter consists of hollow fibers of Amicon Xm-50 membrane with approximately 12,000 bundles per coil. A diluting solution is added to the blood. Positive pressure is applied to the blood path resulting in movement of a greatly increased amount of fluid across the membrane into the dialysate. Ultrafiltration with this type of membrane enhances the clearances of the middle molecular weight substances by means of solvent drag. If too much fluid is ultrafiltrated across the membrane, this is measured and replaced by a comparable volume of fluid return to the patient. Clearances of inulin at 117 ml per minute approach that of the human kidney (150 ml per minute). This compares to a value of about 8 ml per minute in the standard artificial kidney membrane.

It is felt that because of their retention in the body, middle molecules may be responsible for some of the many metabolic abnormalities present in chronic renal failure, including carbohydrate intolerance, lipid abnormalities, vitamin D and calcium mishandling, coagulaton defects, impaired resistance to infection, altered immunologic reactivity, deposition of lipochromes in the skin, disturbed sexual function, and anemia.

Support of this theory was documented by Babb and his colleagues, who showed that, by using a so-called slow flow dialysis in which the blood flow rate was markedly diminished during dialysis, patients did not develop any deterioration of their motor nerve conduction velocities or any other evidence of neurological impairment during this study. However, the BUN and creatinine rose since the small molecules were removed less efficiently with slower flow rates. They demonstrated that by keeping the total time on dialysis and membrane surface area constant control of uremic neuropathy was maintained despite less efficient removal of the small molecular weight substances, thus supporting the theory of middle molecule-induced neuropathy. Nolph, et al, using an in vitro system to measure clearance and middle molecular weight substances such as BSP dye, showed that not only is surface area an important determinant of clearance of middle molecules, but ultrafiltration (the movement of excess fluid across the membrane) is equally important.[56] They demonstrated a direct linear relationship between the clearance of BSP dye and the ultrafiltration rate using coils in hollow fiber-type kidneys. They felt that ultrafiltration is a major determinant of the dialysance of middle molecules.

Further refinements had led to the development of more efficient membranes, such as Cuprophane™ and cellulose membranes. Ideally, a dialysis membrane should be one which allows for the most complete passage of toxic substances but holds back essential plasma components, such as albumin and antibodies. Further, ideally this is accomplished without a loss of membrane strength, because the membrane must be able to withstand the pressures generated by a dialyzer's pump and the outflow resistance without rupturing.

It is also true that a certain amount of surface area in the dialyzing membrane is necessary for hemodialysis to be efficient. Any increase in dialyzer membrane surface area results in an increased dialysance. Surface areas in the coil-type membranes vary from 0.7 to $1.9M^2$, in plate dialyzers from 0.5 to $2.0M^2$. The newest innovation in membranes for chronic dialysis is the use of minute hollow fibers made of polyelectrolytes. Many of these tiny hollow fibers are placed in a hollow tube through which dialysate circulates. Dialyzing membrane surface areas, comparable to those in coil and plate dialyzers, may thus be achieved in a device no more than 3 inches in diameter and 8 inches in length.

To maintain a steep concentration gradient from the patient's bloodstream to the dialysate bath used in the dialyzer, the bath must be changed as equilibration of substances approaches. In the older machines, the 100 L tank dialyzers, the bath must be changed every two hours. In newer models, where the dialysate is passed through a separate chamber containing a coiled membrane, the dialysate is discarded from the upper chamber. In this instance, enough dialysate can be mixed for an entire treatment and kept at room temperature (which retards bacterial growth) until it is all used. Some medical centers employ a twice-normal dialysis delivery rate and change the bath twice in order to maintain a greater concentration gradient.

An ideal dialyzer must not only remove toxic nitrogenous products of body metabolism, but must also remove water. Enhanced removal of excess body water (ultrafiltration) can be accomplished in hemodialysis by increasing the osmolality of the dialyzer bath through the addition of glucose, and by increasing the pressure gradient between blood and dialysate. The latter is accomplished by raising the outflow pressure in coil-type dialyzers and by exerting negative pressure in the Kiil parallel-plate devices.

DIALYSIS TECHNIQUES

The stable chronic patient can tolerate priming the dialyzer with his own blood volume. His arterial blood supply is connected to the inlet of the machine and unclamped. This should be done at a very slow flow (under 100 ml per minute). As blood reaches the bubble trap, it is observed for hemolysis; then the venous line is clamped and connected to the patient's venous access. When the clamps are released, the blood circuit is complete. This technique is usually utilized for the patient who is stable and fluid overloaded. If the patient is not fluid overloaded, he is given the priming saline from the dialyzer as both access routes are connected.

The patient should be dialyzed at a low blood flow initially. This should be gradually increased in order that sudden volume shifts do not occur. It has been demonstrated that blood flows of 200 to 300 ml per minute through the dialyzer provide for maximum dialysance and minimal damage to blood cells, though some centers consider blood flow rates below 300 ml per minute as minimum. This can depend on types of equipment used.

Dialysis of the chronic patient in center maintenance dialysis is conducted in a much different manner from that described for the acutely ill patient. Usually the patient is at home and hopefully is working at his usual daily occupation (job, housewife, student). One patient works 40 or more hours at his law practice after seven years on dialysis. He comes to the unit three times each week, weighs himself, and takes his vital signs in preparation for his dialysis. During the dialysis he reads and watches television. If he develops leg cramps or other symptoms of hypovolemia, he knows what he will need for fluid replacement. Very little, if any, physical nursing care is necessary for such a patient, but the nurse must offer support and encouragement to him.

When patients do not restrict their fluid intake, as directed, it is necessary to ultrafilter them during the dialysis. The amount of ultrafiltration needed is determined clinically by the estimated excess fluid weight of the patient prior to the dialysis. In the coil dialyzer, ultrafiltration is achieved by raising the pressure in the outflow line. It is generally not raised above 280 mm, a pressure which can bring about the removal of as much as eight pounds or more in six hours.

When this amount of fluid is removed in such a short period of time, the patient usually experiences symptoms of hypovolemia. Early in the procedure these symptoms are usually presented in the form of transient back pain, which is often related to increasing the blood flow to the dialyzer too rapidly. Later in the procedure the nurse may observe hyper- or hypotension, nausea, headache and leg cramps. Precordial pain is unusual but may be seen at the beginning of dialysis if there is a substantial volume shift to the dialyzer, or later in the run as large amounts of fluid are withdrawn. This may be related to a myocardial ischemia, secondary to rapid removal of circulating volume. These symptoms are alleviated by the administration of small amounts of normal saline or of solute such as mannitol (12.5 to 25 Gm) depending on the patient's fluid balance. As the patient's needs are established, these treatments are often given prophylactically.

Dialysis disequilibrium syndrome (see pp. 565-566) is seen less frequently with the use of the Kiil dialyzer. Ultrafiltration is achieved in this system by applying negative pressure to the dialysate outflow line. Though the same amounts of fluid are removed (often more), because it is done over a longer period of time, the patient tolerates the procedure better.

Patients are usually heparinized by means of intermittent systemic doses although some units use continuous systemic heparinization. Both methods are quite successful when used with care. In certain instances, regional heparinization is used, as described in the section on acute hemodialysis. Blood is transfused to these patients as indicated by clinical symptoms (i.e., fatigue and hematocrit values) in the form of washed or leukocyte-depleted packed cells. There is evidence that the use of washed or leukocyte-depleted red cells will decrease the exposure of the patient to foreign antigens. It has been observed recently that there is a decreased incidence of hepatitis in units using these blood preparations.

At the close of the dialysis, the blood within the dialyzer is reinfused into the patient by clamping the patient's arterial blood supply and pushing the blood through the dialyzer (Fig. 17-11). It is imperative that the maximal amount of blood is returned to the patient from the dialyzer as even minimal amounts (10 ml) will deplete the patient of a unit of blood (120 ml) in a month's time. This can be done using saline or air, but studies indicate that the membrane is best emptied with saline, and the hazard of air embolus is thus decreased. Vital signs and weight are again checked by the patient. The shunt is closed as described earlier. For patients with an A-V fistula, the needles are withdrawn and direct pressure is applied to the site until bleeding

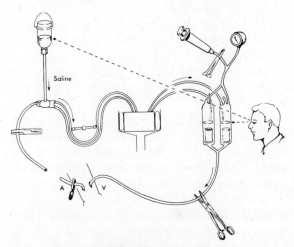

Saline

A   V

FIGURE 17-11.
Retransfusing blood back to the patient. Source: Nose, Y.: The Artificial kidney. St. Louis, C. V. Mosby, 1969, p. 53.

stops. A dressing or Band-Aid is applied. For both procedures the assistant to the patient must always wear gloves, to protect against contact with the patient's blood. The arm is wrapped, without occluding bruit, with an elastic bandage for a few hours, to prevent bleeding. (See Tables 17-4 and 17-5 on pages 560-561 for other pertinent patient teaching.)

Dialysis Disequilibrium Syndrome

One of the disturbing complications that can develop initially in a patient who is being dialyzed for the first time is the so-called dialysis disequilibrium syndrome which is manifested by altered cerebral activity with mental confusion and sometimes convulsions. These disturbances may last for several days. The etiology of this syndrome has escaped accurate definition. Some theories have held that the more rapid removal of urea from the body lowers the serum osmolality in comiarison to that of the brain in which urea may still be present. With the increased osmolality of the central nervous system, fluid is drawn into the central nervous system producing cerebral edema and the resultant neurologic picture.

More recently, Arieff, et al, have refuted the theory that urea causes cerebral edema.[57] They demonstrated this, by studying dogs, comparing so-called rapid hemodialysis with a blood flow of 12 ml per kg per minute, and so-called slow hemodialysis with a blood flow rate of 5 ml per kg per minute. Development of gross brain swelling, elevated cerebral spinal fluid pressure, and grand mal seizures only occurred in animals treated with rapid hemodialysis. The concentration of urea in the brain at the end of rapid hemodialysis was similar to that observed at the end of slow hemodialysis. However, the osmolality of the brain was significantly higher at the end of rapid hemodialysis, attributable perhaps to increased formation of organic acid since it was found that the hydrogen ion concentration rose.

It is for this reason that in some institutions the first hemodialysis in a patient with long-standing chronic uremia is done for a short period (2 to 4 hours) at a reduced blood flow rate. Some centers have utilized mannitol infusions intermittently in patients whose BUN is greater than 100 mg per 100 ml. In one case dialysis disequilibrium syndrome developed ten hours after the termination of the patient's 48-hour peritoneal dialysis which was carried out for edema, uremia, and severe hyponatremia. The question of an idiosyncratic reaction to prochlorperazine (Compazine) was raised, but intravenous diphenhydramine (Benadryl) had no effect. A dosage of 12.5 Gm of intravenous mannitol produced mental improvement within several hours, possibly by raising intravascular osmolality and decreasing the cerebral edema.

Pediatric Hemodialysis

Dialysis may be provided for the pediatric patient awaiting renal transplantation (see Part 3). Peritoneal dialysis may be successfully undertaken using small amounts of infused fluid in proportion to the body mass.

Extracorporeal hemodialysis may be used as an alternative therapy, though it will require greater technical expertise. Cannulation of the child's vessels requires special skill and modified equipment. Dialysis equipment must be adapted to safely expose the blood to dialysis surfaces without reducing the patient's circulating volume to dangerous levels. Special membranes with reduced capacity are available commercially. The care of the potential recipient on dialysis requires a much greater investment of time and ingenuity, and in most units suggests a one-to-one patient to staff ratio. Though the physical needs and treatments are similar, the psychological and sociological aspects of care are different; for the whole family must participate on a day-to-day basis in order for the patient to survive.

New Approaches to Hemodialysis

In an attempt to reduce the size of conventional dialysis equipment, a regenerative dialysis supply system has been described by Greenbaum and Gordon.[58] The system employs a sorbent to treat dialysate in an effort to reclaim and reuse it. In this technique developed by the Marquardt Corporation, a system is used in which a few liters of dialysate can be continually regenerated and reused through the course of a dialysis, thus eliminating the need for large volumes of dialysate and complicated plumbing. A combination of activated charcoal, urease, zirconium phosphate, and zirconium oxide is used in a disposable cartridge. This system will operate for an entire six hours of dialysis using 6 L or less of dialysate, compared to 120 L in a more conventional system.

Three basic types of hemodialyzers are used today: the coil dialyzer, the parallel-plate dialyzer, and the latest development, the hollow fiber cartridge dialyzer (often called HFAK for hollow fiber artificial kidney). In this last device, hollow capillary fibers made of cellulosic membranes are packed into a cartridge and connected to appropriate inlet and outlet blood lines (see Fig. 17-12). Dialysate circulates around the capillary fibers in the cartridge and is discarded. One of the principal advantages of the hollow fiber dialyzer is its compact size and small priming volume and its relatively infrequent rupture rate. Occasionally coils may have a disturbing problem with leakage, which causes blood loss to the patient, dialysis time lost, and exposes the dialysis personnel to hepatitis should the patient be infected.

SINGLE NEEDLE DIALYSIS

In 1972 Kopp, et al, introduced the concept of single needle dialysis.[59] With a special device blood is drawn from a cannula to the machine and blood is returned to the patient back through the same needle. This does not permit as high blood flow rates as with a double needle system but can be used quite well on a patient with a minimal venous system for blood access device. A great advantage of single needle dialysis is better acceptance by patients, who much prefer one "needle stick" to two. There is also some evidence that the life of the fistula is appreciably extended, especially with bovine grafts. Clearance rates may be reduced.

PORTABLE ARTIFICIAL KIDNEY

Looking toward the future, a wearable artificial kidney is being developed at the University of

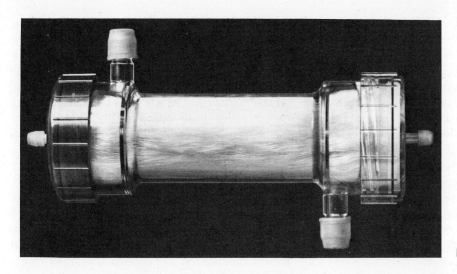

FIGURE 17-12.
Hollow fiber dialyzer.

Utah. This will permit the patient to perform daily dialyses of short duration (one to two hours), being self-administered when possible. The kidney will be wearable so that it can be carried about with ease and will use the single needle principle. Ultrafiltration will be needed to remove fluid with a recirculating dialysis bath utilizing sorbents.

In April 1975, a preliminary report was published in the Int. Med. News and Diagnosis newspaper which described a patient using a prototype seven paneled unit. This 20-year-old college student prefers this to conventional hemodialysis. Dialysis is carried out for three hours, five to six days a week, depending on residual function. However, it should be used in conjunction with a regular 20-liter dialysis bath for one to one and one-half hours each session. The additional dialysis bath is needed to remove urea, but it is felt that within the next year this problem should be under control, and a mass-produced unit is expected within two years.

The obvious advantage is that the patient is free to move about during treatment, which can be carried out any place, for example, at his desk if he works in an office. According to the report, the frequent daily dialysis allows freer protein and sodium intake. The only current disadvantage is that a new membrane, which costs between $15 and $25, must be used with each treatment. In the near future, this device may be a practical reality for many patients.

SHORTER DIALYSIS SCHEDULES

In an effort to shorten hemodialysis treatment time, the square meter per hour in the middle molecule hypothesis has been used to change clinical applications of various dialyzer schedules. Theoretically, hemodialysis for six hours using a 1 square meter coil could be duplicated by hemodialysis for four hours on a 1.5 square meter coil. Mirahmadi, et al, described 14 patients with chronic renal failure who were dialyzed for four hours three times per week, instead of the usual six hours three times per week schedule.[60] The patients all had a subjective improvement in well-being. Some had improvement in hematocrit and motor nerve conduction velocities. The decreased time on dialysis, cutting one third off the total dialysis time per week, was met with marked enthusiasm by the patients. Many centers have begun to evaluate larger membrane surface areas now that smaller volume coils and hollow fiber kidneys are available. Some patients, of course, are not able to tolerate the ultrafiltration rates with the larger coils, but this is an attempt to reduce total dialysis time without sacrificing dialysis efficiency. Personal experience has shown that many patients can tolerate shorter dialysis hours with larger coils; some patients cannot and experience deterioration of nerve conduction velocities. Patients must therefore be monitored closely for many months for evidences of inadequate dialysis.

Hepatitis

Sengar from the University of Ottawa described host immunity and antigen responses in a hemodialysis unit with hepatitis.[61] Eighty-six patients and 26 staff members took part in the study. Of the patients, 19.8 percent developed a positive hepatitis associated antibody as measured by counter electrophoresis method. Of these, 23 percent developed active hepatitis. This was in contrast to 23.4 percent of the staff members developing a positive hepatitis antigen in which 100 percent developed clinical hepatitis; whereas only 9 percent of the patients eventually developed antibodies, 38 percent of the staff members did so. The antigenemia persisted for longer than six months in 94 percent of the patients, whereas only 26.6 percent of the staff members had a positive antigenemia after six months' time. There was a definite association with HLA-8 antigen and it was felt the presence of HLA-8 in the blood probably predisposed to HAA (Hepatitis-Associated Antigen) infection in active hepatitis.

In February 1974, a point-prevalence study in 15 U.S. hemodialysis centers was published evaluating the hepatitis B infection problem.[62] Five-hundred eighty-three patients and 451 medical personnel were surveyed. Hepatitis B antigen was detected in 16.8 percent of the patients and in 2.4 percent of the medical staff. Specific antibody was detected in 34 percent and 31.3 percent respectively. The prevalence of hepatitis B infection was related to duration of dialysis treatment but not to blood transfusions. Of great interest was the finding that 61 percent of family contacts of dialysis patients with a history of hepatitis B infection were found to have hepatitis B antigen or antibody. It can be appreciated that hepatitis B infection is a major problem in dialysis centers since approximately one half of the patients and one third of the staff have evidence of exposure to the hepatitis B virus. The most severe outbreaks have caused a number of deaths among patients and staff following infection of almost an entire renal unit.[63]

The mechanism of hepatitis B virus transmission is not known. The parenteral route of infection with contaminated blood or blood products by means of transfusions, blood contaminated equipment or needle sticks, or other types of tissue penetration is well known. Hepatitis B antigen has been found in feces, nasopharyngeal washings, urine, and saliva. The possibilities of infection include contamination of mucous membranes, spilling of blood over intact skin, aerosol formation, and exposure to contaminated hands and limbs, although none of these have been officially documented as yet.

It appears, then, that nonparenteral routes of spread of infection must exist and that they probably greatly outweigh transfusions in relative importance. Another disturbing finding was the documentation of hepatitis B antigen recovered from such surfaces as gloved hands, door handles, needle clippers, furniture, and external parts of dialyzers, both with and without visible traces of blood.

Technical measures to protect patients and staff from hepatitis outbreaks have evolved, and renal units are subject to a number of precautions. Blood enzymes and HAA studies are frequently done on both patients (twice a month) and staff (at least once a month). Patients with elevated enzyme levels or antigen-positive results are isolated. Staff members with positive results are isolated. Staff members with positive results do not work without medical clearance until studies prove negative—a matter which often involves full financial compensation for two to three months or more. No new patient begins dialysis without these studies, and new staff members are likewise screened before employment. In terms of contamination via blood, a number of measures exist. All transfusions are given as washed, frozen, or leukocyte depleted cells. Gloves are worn for all blood contact by anyone—venipunctures, shunts, cleaning, handling dialysis membrane, excreta, clotting time, blood drawing, and so on. Patients are on blood and stool isolation, and blood or urine samples are kept in a separate refrigerator in an area isolated from anything edible. Dialysis machines are used by the same patient group, with a record being kept of each treatment. The machines are, of course, cleaned thoroughly after each patient use by staff who wear plastic aprons for this and for starting each dialysis. (Gowns and gloves are also worn by cleaning staff for bed-making and trash collection.) There are a number of precautions taken with respect to gastrointestinal cross-contamination; for example, if food is served to patients in the dialysis area, it is served on an isolation tray; no food is eaten in the unit by the staff, nor is any edible shared with patients. There must be no smoking, nail biting, and so on on the unit. Handwashing is strictly enforced, especially before entering the staff kitchen. Patient bathrooms are separated from those for the staff. Finally, all "positive" patients, should they require surgery, are placed last on the operating schedule for the day.

It is evident that, once an outbreak of hepatitis starts, it is very difficult to control. Therefore, measures noted above seem a reasonable way to prevent cross-infection from patient to staff and to isolate patients as much as possible from each other. It has proved helpful to provide each patient unit with enough equipment for each procedure so that staff members are not tempted to go with contaminated hands to another patient's area or to supply areas. Boxes for storage of these supplies are attached to each patient's bed. It is the nurse's responsibility to establish and maintain procedures which will protect the patient and the staff.

Air Embolism

Air embolism is a complication which is life-threatening to the patient. A number of sources within the blood circuit may allow for infusion of air to the patient. Small amounts of air may enter the circuit during the procedure from tubing leaks, cracks in syringes, or loose connections, which can result in a large cumulative amount of air being given to the patient. Large amounts have been given rapidly (200 cc per minute) when fluid replacements run dry, clamps fall off lines, or with poorly monitored air rinses at the close of the dialysis. The patient will experience symptoms which appear rapidly: deep respirations, coughing, cyanosis, gasping, followed by cessation of respirations. The patient's pulse will be weak and no blood pressure will be heard. Im-

mediate action must be taken to save the patient's life, and it is mandatory that all personnel caring for the patient, including the dialysis partner, must be familiar with the treatment. The blood circuit is immediately clamped off, while the patient is turned on his left side in Trendelenburg's position. The pathways of the air are seen in Fig. 17-13. This position is not changed until ordered by the physician. The arrest team should be alerted if necessary when this occurs in the hospital setting. It may be necessary to aspirate the air from the right heart. If the patient does not respond, it may be necessary to aspirate the air from the heart under direct visualization.

Preventive measures include visual monitoring of equipment and automatic monitoring of equipment when available, though there is no substitute for an alert and attentive staff. Plastic infusion bags are a definite improvement as they decrease the possibility of infusion of air when the container is emptied. The authors of this

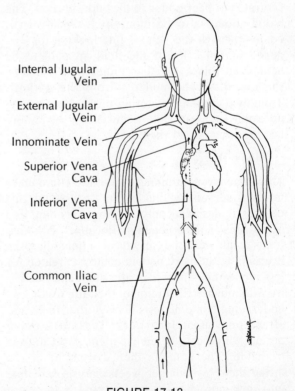

Internal Jugular Vein

External Jugular Vein

Innominate Vein

Superior Vena Cava

Inferior Vena Cava

Common Iliac Vein

FIGURE 17-13.
Circuit air embolism. Source: Adapted by Henderson, M. C.

chapter feel that fluid replacement should be given in amounts as necessary followed by clamping of the tubing, rather than by administering slow infusions through the day which could empty and be followed by air. Staff must attend the patient as blood is returned at the close of the procedure until the tubing is clamped. The membrane is rinsed with saline rather than air, as it is the safest method, as well as more efficient in returning blood.

Another life-threatening complication is hemolysis. This is associated with incorrectly prepared dialysis solutions and temperature changes and results in hemolysis of the patient's blood as it is exposed to the dialysate. With the prepared dialysis concentrates, this is seen less frequently. Before the bath solution is used, it should be checked by conductivity of sodium or by osmolarity. The membrane rinse saline is drained into the empty concentrate container as soon as possible, thus establishing that the concentrate has been added to the bath solution. The blood should also be monitored visually as it comes through the venous line looking for evidence of red cells. If the fluid appears to be hemolyzed (black or clear rather than cloudy), the circuit is clamped off from the patient. Treatment includes restoring the dialysis procedure as soon as possible, especially if the patient has received any of the blood.

Home Dialysis

The hemodialysis training unit at the community hospital served by one of the authors of this chapter is designed only for home training and acute renal failure patients. Because of limited funds available in the early days of hemodialysis, it was felt that more people could be treated for less money and enjoy a greater degree of flexibility with minimal disruption of their life routine by undergoing home dialysis. This author feels that after approximately a thirty session training period, 90 percent of their patient population is trainable. The patients then dialyze at home, fitting their 18 hour per week dialysis schedule into their normal routine. The goal is to return people to their previous level of life as quickly as possible. Only well-motivated patients are ac-

cepted into the program. It is emphasized to the patient and his family before the training program develops that it is his disease and his responsibility to set up and run the machine. In this way, the problem of over-zealous and dominant co-trainees and a passive-dependent patient is avoided. One patient is a 52-year-old, partially sighted man, who operates a food service at a local factory. It was his primary custom to rise at 4:30 A.M., start his work at 5:30, and conclude his day around 7:00 P.M. On those days in which he was involved in dialysis training program he would leave work at 6:30 A.M. and arrive at the Renal Unit at 7:00, finish his dialysis training between 3:00 and 4:00 P.M., and then return to work until 7:00 or 8:00 P.M. This he did, working his full work week.

The patient is seen alone for the first two to three weeks of the training session so that he learns to take primary responsibility for setting up his machine and choosing variations in flow rate, venous resistance, bath concentrate, and types of coil. Thus he is able to estimate fairly accurately his weight loss during a given dialysis period. In this way the patient masters the machine before the co-trainee arrives. The co-trainee's responsibility is primarily that of helping during emergencies.

Self-venipuncture is usually well accepted by patients and gives them increased independence. The authors have observed in one of their patient populations, that the major area of conflict arises when venipuncture is delegated to the dialysis partner; therefore, they do not train the partner in this technique. Patients repeatedly state that they experience less discomfort when they place their own needles. As stated before, local anesthesia is not used at the needle entry sites.

It has been the authors' experience that the teaching is best done by a nurse who can repeatedly teach techniques in a consistent way and can provide reassurance, while directing the patient in a way that makes him assume the responsibility for his own treatment. This is essential if the major advantage of home care (patient independence) is to be achieved. If this is not done, the dialysis partner, who initially is most eager to learn and to "help the patient," will become the expert. Later, the partner will begin to resent the responsibility which has been shifted from the dialysis staff to him, and he will eventually communicate this resentment to the patient both verbally and nonverbally. The partner is taught by the patient, which allows the staff to observe his knowledge. At this time emergency techniques are also reviewed. It is helpful to create problems for the patients to solve; such as power failures, blown fuses, and membrane leaks. The authors have utilized a room adjacent to the dialysis area for the purpose of gradually making the patient feel the responsibility prior to the start of dialysis at home.

At the conclusion of the course of instruction in home dialysis, the patient runs his own dialysis in the hospital without the assistance of the staff. When the staff and the patient are satisfied that he has a real understanding of the technique and that he has confidence in his knowledge, he is allowed to go home. During the training period, the home unit is equipped and set up. Before the patient conducts his first home dialysis, personnel from the dialysis unit inspect the home set-up. The dialysis personnel are on call for any problems encountered during dialysis. The patients are seen regularly at the hospital, or whenever necessary. Other units have felt it important to be with the patient for the first home run. An alternative method is the utilization of community nursing facilities to appraise the home situation on a regular basis. This is especially useful when the patient lives a considerable distance from the teaching unit. It is not mandatory that these nurses know the procedure completely, for they will be able to identify potential areas of concern either medically or psychologically and initiate care with the assistance of the teaching unit.

It is important at the onset of teaching to recognize that the patient at home has a much greater responsibility for his care than the patient in a medical facility and, therefore, must withstand many more psychological stresses. Hopefully, the patient selected for this method of therapy will possess these resources. It is necessary that the patient and his family realize that the teaching unit will continue to be available for

trouble shooting for technical problems, for medical care, and especially to assist them in the acceptance of this responsibility. The unit must always provide for back-up dialysis when necessary; this may need to be done simply to provide a break for the dialysis partner from time to time. It is often difficult for the patient to handle the absence of the continuous support and encouragement that he received in training, and it is difficult for the partner to provide this for the patient. Certainly it is a psychological advantage that the partner, especially in the case of the spouse, may now help the patient in a tangible way rather than being an observer. The community can also provide psychological support and motivation for the patient who returns to his former role as a responsible member.

The emotional impact of this program on the family is not to be underestimated. The burden of self-care is heavy, requiring many hours of maintenance of supplies and equipment. Frequently the roles of the family change (i.e., wife helping affected husband and thus supporting his life). The feasibility and success of the program is directly related to the general emotional stability of the participants.

It is essential for the psychological well-being of the patient that the family permit as much patient independence as is feasible for him. The dependence forced on him by his medical situation can be overwhelming—and psychologically crippling—as he views himself as having relinquished autonomy and at this time as being a burden to loved ones. This is particularly true of the male patient whose entire life style may be changed due to sexual impotence and inability to retain his role as family "bread-winner." The female patient may also feel that she is without purpose as she sees certain long-term goals as being unobtainable. However, the patient on home care has a more realistic hope of resolving these feelings and restoring order and purpose to his life than does the patient undergoing any other form of dialytic therapy.

The staff responsible for home care faces unique responsibilities and rewards as they instruct patients to conduct dialysis at home. As mentioned earlier, the nurse must provide a confident and competent approach to the patient continuously reassuring him that he will be capable of conducting the procedure and repeatedly reinforcing the advantages of assuming the responsibility of the techniques. She must be aware that, in most cases, the patient is being taught a technique that he does not want to learn and that he may try to tell her by repeated failures that he can not cope with this burden and would best be dialyzed in a limited-care facility.

It has been the authors' experience that a unit social worker is an integral part of the home-training program. In the patient's initial evaluation for chronic care, the social worker interviews the patient and his family to obtain information regarding the patient's preillness personality, his methods of coping with stress, past personal and family history of handling crisis, the reaction of the patient and his family to the present situation, and their understanding of the disease process and the prognosis. The social worker will also evaluate the feasibility of home dialysis in terms of the physical set-up of the home, the number of people living there, and other responsibilities of the family unit. This allows the health team to ascertain the practicality of placing a dialyzer in the home and expecting the family to make the necessary adaptations in their life patterns. Such information helps the nurse to see the patient as a "whole" person with a life pattern and responsibilities to which he is still obligated. This evaluation is especially helpful in planning the teaching program for each couple, utilizing information regarding each partner's past relationship to the other and to the family unit. In many cases, this has necessitated reorganizing the teaching format in order to adapt it to the couple who has developed an acceptable method of coping that does align with the instructional plan. For example, J. H., a woman who was a nurse, had great difficulty in assuming the responsibility for her dialysis treatment. When her dominant husband was included earlier than planned in her care and allowed to conduct the procedure entirely with her assistance, both were relieved and able to assume their usual roles and to assimilate the information with ease.

The patient on chronic maintenance hemodialysis may develop a multitude of physiological problems, but several potential problems must be evaluated and kept under control. His calcium and phosphorus metabolism must be carefully monitored with monthly blood tests, bone surveys and, hopefully, parathormone levels when they become commercially available. Keeping the inorganic phosphorus at a normal level is essential to prevent the development of uncontrolled secondary hyperparathyroidism.

Aluminum hydroxide and aluminum carbonate gels have been used extensively to lower the plasma phosphate by binding it in the gut with its subsequent passage into the stool. Several ounces are required per patient per day, and, because of the monotony of large volumes of fluid required, many patients fail to cooperate with the full dosage schedule. Studies have shown that the level of parathyroid hormone is directly correlated with the elevation of plasma phosphate so it is essential that phosphate levels be brought into the normal range. Because of the large size of the molecule and poor movement across the dialysis membrane, hemodialysis is, in itself, insufficient to lower the plasma phosphate to a normal range. In 1972, aluminum hydroxide capsules became available. These have been very helpful in enabling the patients to get their aluminum hydroxide dosage ingested. Patients take anywhere from 8 to 20 capsules per day and usually have none of the complaints they had when they were taking either Amphojel or Basaljel. In late 1973, an extra-strength Basaljel, aluminum carbonate liquid, was introduced, which is approximately three times more effective on a volume basis than the older aluminum hydroxide. This is also available in capsule form which should further reduce the volume of binding gel to be ingested. Aluminum hydroxide has also been incorporated in various cookie mixtures to make it more palatable.

Since most of the water soluble vitamins are lost in the dialysate it is essential that the patient take multivitamin preparation on a daily basis. Folic acid is not included in commercial vitamin preparations since it may completely mask the hematologic symptoms while allowing the neurologic symptoms of pernicious anemia to progress. All patients on maintenance hemodialysis should receive folic acid supplements. Some centers utilize as little as 1 mg orally after each dialysis and others give up to 5 mg per day. Still other centers add folic acid to the dialysis bath itself.

The hematocrit must be closely watched; this will usually stay at a precise level for any given patient. It is the authors' practice to perform bone marrow examinations on all patients before the start of dialysis, and, if iron deficiency exists, iron in the form of Imferon is given to replete the patient's iron stores. Because of the possibility of some small but significant blood loss during dialysis, most of the patients take oral iron on a daily basis.

Longnecker, et al, studied blood loss in patients on Kiil dialyzers and EXO#3 coils.[64] With losses during dialyzer rinse, ruptures of venipuncture sites, and diagnostic tests, he was able to show that up to 600 ml of blood could be lost per month. Most patients require no transfusions on chronic dialysis unless an acute bleeding episode should occur. An example is R. F., who started out with a hemoglobin of 5 and hematocrit of 15 percent. The patient's hemoglobin rose to approximately 10 over the next 18 months, at which time anabiolic steroids IM were added on a once every two weeks basis. Steroids were stopped when the patient had been on hemodialysis for 20 months and his hemoglobin was 16. Any sudden drop in the patient's hemoglobin should be thoroughly investigated since many patients on chronic hemodialysis may develop peptic ulcers which, more often than not, are asymptomatic.

R. P. Q., a patient with chronic glomerulonephritis, had maintained a hematocrit of 23 percent ever since starting dialysis. Two years later, because of this persistently low hematocrit, a bone marrow specimen was obtained and showed no stainable iron. Initially his bone marrow had shown rich iron stores. With a course of IM Imferon therapy, his hematocrit rose to 43 percent within three weeks. An upper GI series revealed an old ulcer. Stools were negative for occult blood. It was postulated that he had lost small amounts of blood during its active phase perhaps during periods of systemic heparinizations.

With adequate weight reduction, appropriate sodium concentration in the dialysate and avoidance of dietary sodium, most patients may be maintained at a normotensive level without resorting to oral antihypertensives such as methyldopa, propranolol, clonidine, minoxidil and hydralazine. Blood pressures should be taken not only during and after dialysis, but also on nondialysis days. Hypotension at the end of dialysis may be followed within several hours by return of blood pressure to normal or even hypertensive levels. In patients in whom volume depletion, ultrafiltration, and oral agents are ineffective in lowering blood pressure, bilateral nephrectomy may occasionally be necessary. Once bilateral nephrectomy has been carried out, blood pressure becomes much easier to treat and often the patient can be well maintained without any antihypertensives. Blood requirements will increase, probably due to lack of endogenously produced erythropoietin.

An example is W. B., a 33-year-old white female with a strong family history of hypertension who has been taking oral contraceptives for the past seven years. There was a six-month history of difficulty with vision. The patient recalls that approximately one year prior to admission she was told she had high blood pressure but did not seek follow-up care. On admission to a local emergency room, her diastolic blood pressure was 160 and her serum creatinine was 6. With vigorous treatment with antihypertensives, her creatinine rose to 10 mg per 100 ml, despite 100 mg of hydralazine, 80 mg of propranolol and 1 Gm of methyldopa every six hours. Her blood pressure was unresponsive to therapy. She required several peritoneal dialyses and eventually was placed on hemodialysis. Although there was a transient drop in blood pressure when the patient was managed as an outpatient, her diastolic blood pressure, despite all these medications, remained in the range of 150. She underwent bilateral nephrectomy and has been maintained without antihypertensives for 36 months.

Patients must also be admonished in not gaining too much weight between dialyses, since a 4 to 5 pound weight gain may result in significant hypertension.

The patient is instructed to keep his serum phosphate in the normal range at all times (see section on osteodystrophy). With these oral calcium supplements and a bath concentration of 7 mg per 100 ml it is usually possible to raise the patient's serum calcium to a normal range thus shutting off the stimulus for parathyroid hypersecretion. The calcium-phosphorus product should be kept at 50 or less. Values of greater than 60 or 70 are associated with metastatic calcification. Most patients on thrice weekly hemodialysis enjoy a relatively free food intake; the only thing being restricted is salt in patients who have a tendency toward hypertension, and foods containing excessive amounts of potassium. Occasional patients will require a tablespoon of kayexalate daily to keep their potassium within the normal range, and this is probably to be preferred rather than vigorously restricting potassium in the diet. The other alternative is lowering potassium concentration in the dialysate, although this may present problems in the digitalized patient. The patients are all told the consequences of hyperkalemia and are told in no uncertain terms that, if the serum potassium rises above 6, the danger of cardiac standstill is very real. One patient presented with syncopal episodes as a manifestation of his hyperkalemia. He had been enjoying the local peach crop and reported for dialysis one day with a history of fainting spells and dizzy spells every time he had tried to rise out of the chair for the last 24 hours. It was found on examination that he had a pulse of 40 and was unable to increase his pulse rate with any kind of exercise including sitting up. It was found that his serum potassium level was 9.0 and his P waves were no longer present and his QS complex had begun to widen.

Psychological/Sociological Aspects of Care for the Patient on Chronic Dialysis

"Mere preservation of life must not be the sole objective of the treatment."[65]

The patient on chronic dialysis needs and must have a great deal of support and encouragement from the dialysis team. The physician staff may change, but the the nurse remains the constant figure in the unit. As a result, the patient relies heavily upon her. She must provide sincere understanding and genuine concern for the many difficulties with which he is confronted.

The patient must be able to face reality and understand and accept his disease. Understandably, the patient with long-standing, slowly progressive renal disease is better able to accept his plight than the patient who is suddenly faced with a terminal disease process. No situation is as stressful to the patient and his family, and major adjustments in their thinking and living must be made. Though it is essential for the dialysis staff to encourage the patient and his family, it is important to realize that there is an overwhelming tendency for the patient to develop a closely dependent relationship with the staff. Studies reveal that the anxiety levels decrease as the patient develops confidence in the procedure; however, feelings of denial and isolation are usually present to some degree in all patients. The degree of success of the treatment is enhanced by pleasant surroundings in an environment which is soothing and promotes confidence. The role of the family members is critical to the patient's adjustment, since their understanding and strong support enable him to persevere in spite of the difficulties he experiences. The family experiences feelings of loss and frustration primarily related to the patient's psychological regression. It is particularly difficult for patients to deal with the problems of repeated cannulae failures, chronic fatigue and insomnia. Most patients demonstrate depression from time to time. However, even with all the difficulties, long-term dialysis restores to a reasonably productive life 90 percent of the patients who undergo it.

Difficulties of adjustment to a program of chronic long-term hemodialysis are well documented (see Bibliography at the end of this section). As with any major life change, many adaptations and compromises must be made, not only by the patient, but by the family as well. Often life in a new-found state of dependence and the need for undesirable life-style adaptations may be less acceptable to the patient than the alternative of death.

It has been observed by many that there are phases of adjustment to the care program that can be aligned to Kübler-Ross's process of adaptation to death and dying.[66] The patient with renal disease faces temporary, and often permanent, loss of his former life pattern. The patient must assume a role of dependence, relinquishing many hopes and long-term plans for himself and for his family. He must rely on them for tangible care and for support and encouragement. He must watch them make major changes in their lives as a result of his needs. With the resources of federal funds, the financial disasters which were once common are no longer a major concern; however, many patients are without funds for transportation to the treatment center and for the medications which are an essential part of their care. Although communities have provided resources to help, the large group in the urban areas still finds lack of funds a major concern.

With the advent of federal funding all patients requiring dialysis can now be accepted in chronic programs. This was a long-sought goal of all associated with this area of health care. The question has now been raised as to whether all patients must be dialyzed regardless of their "social worth." This would, of course, be a matter of individual interpretation. Selection committees are recommended to try to offer care to patients who can reasonably be expected to return to a responsible and meaningful quality of life in the judgments of the reviewing group. Others feel that all patients must be offered care, and no review group may make the above judgments. If the patient is to be returned to his former role in the family, he must be able to follow a complicated medical regime, work within the framework of a sophisticated medical setting, and make major adjustments in his life and of that of his family. For the middle-class patient, this can be done with the support of the family and of the medical facility, for this individual is accustomed to working within the framework of the institutional system. For the low socioeconomic group, this presents a major and, sometimes insur-

mountable, obstacle in the delivery of health care. The patient may feel that the medical staff are so far removed from his world to prohibit their understanding of his problems even if he were able to relate them. Communication and understanding of terms and information may be additional difficulties.

Limited-Care Facilities

As the number of patients on dialysis, and particularly the group awaiting transplantation, has grown (30,000 in 1977), it has become necessary to provide a variety of methods for providing dialytic therapy appropriate for the individual patient which will fully utilize his resources without stressing them to the extreme and which will provide safe medical care. Limited-care facilities have met the needs of the ever-increasing number of patients who, for a variety of reasons, cannot assume the responsibility of home care. In most cases, this is a result of the absence of a dialysis partner, as in the case of a single person, or the inability of the partner to participate in the patient's care. C. V., a male patient and minister, was unable to accept the care provided by his wife and his dependence on her, and she in turn could not accept the medical aspects (blood, needles, and the like) or his role reversal. He is now being cared for in a limited-care facility awaiting transplantation. In another situation, E. W.'s husband could not accept the burdens of providing home care, either in terms of responsibility or time; E. W. has been cared for in a limited-care unit for five years, returning to the hospital only for medical problems.

These units can provide care for large numbers (120) of patients with a low staff-patient ratio (5 to 20) in a low overhead area rather than in a hospital setting. The cost should be on a fee for service basis, as the hospital unit provides any special medical care (shunt declotting or surgery) and all back up facilities such as dietary instruction, social service and financial services. The responsibility for coordinating care for these patients cannot be undertaken lightly. The unit must provide the referring facility with continuous reports on patient care while demanding their continuing participation and responsibility for patient care.

These units provide decreased cost, facilities for gathering a large transplant recipient pool, removal of the patient from the "sick-setting" of the hospital and flexibility in scheduling which is difficult to obtain in the unit that must also provide emergency care. Disadvantages include the possible estrangement of the patient from the referring unit and the inherent problems of providing efficient communication methods for so many people. The risk of hepatitis is increased due to the large patient load, decreased staffing, and the mixing of patients from many referring sources.

Self-care facilities have been instituted in a number of areas and provide an alternative method for patient care (see Bibliography at the end of this section). In these units the patient does his own dialysis with minimal assistance from a small staff. This provides maximal patient independence without requiring the assistance of a family member. This facility is otherwise similar to the limited-care facility described above.

Projected Dialysis Needs in Future

In a recent study designed to project the dialysis and transplant needs for the state of Washington over the next ten years, Cooper and Blagg drew on their previous experience and a population of close to 2.7 million.[67] The yield of patients from their population went from a low of three new patients per million population in the early 1960s, when selection criteria were extremely strict and very few facilities were available, to 24.7 new patients per million in 1969, 39.7 new patients per million in 1972, with a figure of approximately 45 new patients per million population in 1973. Using a population figure of the United States of 210,000,000, it has been estimated that 50,500 people will be involved in the end stage renal disease program by 1981. Incidence rates may be as high as 100 new patients per million population per year.

Since 1969, the national dialysis registry has been compiling data. In the report as of January 1973, they had accumulated data on approxi-mately 11,000 patients being treated in more than 370 dialysis programs in the country.[68] The largest dialysis centers are in the northwest with the highest percentage of home patients. There are an average of 37.4 patients per million population ranging from a low of 23.8 in the south to 50.3 in the New England states. On the average, 36 percent of all patients are being treated at home. Almost twice as many men are on dialysis as women, with men comprising 64 percent and females 36 percent of the population. Ninety-eight percent of the patients are on hemodialysis with the remainder being on chronic peritoneal dialysis. The mean age for the men is now a little over 44, and for women slightly over 43 years. There has been significant increase in the male and female populations in the higher age groups, the geriatric population. Morbidity and mortality statistics show that heart disease is the primary cause of death in approximately 35 percent of all patient deaths, with infection being the next most important at 14 percent. Both male and female patients have roughly the same probability of survival. These survival statistics do not include patients who have been transplanted. On the patients that survived the first three months of dialysis, 12 month patient survivorship is 85 percent for the males, and an 18 month figure of 80 percent; 24 month figure of 75 percent; 30 month figure of approximately 71 percent. The figures for the females are almost identical. On the average, 88 percent of the population has survived one year of dialysis, 75 percent two years, and 65 percent three years. As of July 1, 1974 a total of 11,950 patients were on dialysis in a total of 452 Centers.[69] Of that total number, 11,509 were on hemodialysis with the remaining 296 on peritoneal dialysis. Social security administration which cares for approximately 94 percent of people with end stage renal disease was responsible for 30,186 people in the fall of 1976. This figure is broken down into 85 percent on dialysis and 15 percent alive with functioning transplants. Eight hundred sixty-six dialysis centers are operational.

In 1974, Linder, et al, analyzed data from the University of Washington and found an accelerated rate of atherosclerosis in patients on prolonged maintenance hemodialysis.[70] They examined the survival of 39 patients in the Seattle area being treated since 1960. The overall mortality rate was 56.4 percent at the end of the 13-year follow-up period, and 14 of the 23 deaths could be attributed to arteriosclerotic complications; 8 of the deaths were from myocardial infarction; 3 were from strokes; 3 were from refractory congestive heart failure.

In the early days of dialysis, technical problems, sepsis, and fluid overload were some of the major causes of mortality, but as these have been brought under control, it would appear that arteriosclerosis is the major unsolved problem. The coronary death rates were similar to those encountered in familial Type II hyperlipoproteinemia. The abnormal calcium metabolism and the abnormal triglyceride metabolism in patients on chronic hemodialysis may be contributing factors in these disturbing statistics.

Stenzel, et al, recently compared patient survival of hemodialysis and transplantation, analyzing 95 dialysis and 315 transplant patients.[71] The three-year predicted mortality was about 35 percent between 1963 and 1969, but fell to 8 percent during 1970 to 1973. During the latter period, the three-year mortality was 9 percent for related living and 7 percent for cadaver donor recipients. The mortality of chronic dialysis patients during this period was 11 percent. Most deaths occurred during the first 8 months of dialysis, and following this mortality fell to less than 4 percent.

Rehabilitation

In an attempt to assess rehabilitation capabilities in patients on chronic dialysis, patients and transplant patients were compared at the Northwest Kidney Center in Seattle in April 1973. One-hundred sixty-six patients (61 who had successful transplants and 105 treated by home dialysis) were included in the study.[72] The duration of treatment was at least six months and ranged up to six years in transplant patients and twelve years in patients on dialysis. The average age was 33.6 years for the dialysis patients and 32 years for the transplant patients. Twenty-nine

percent of dialysis patients and 30 percent of transplant patients were working full time. Of interest was the fact that 25 percent of the transplant patients had achieved greater responsibilities in their work following treatment compared to only 7 percent of the dialysis patients. Twenty-six percent of the dialysis patients had lesser work responsibilities. A significant difference was noted in the work effectiveness. One hundred percent of the working transplant patients rated their work effectiveness as good, compared to only 63 percent of the dialysis patients. The investigators felt that the greater well-being of successfully transplanted patients following treatment made him more aware of his previous limitations. The personal income had increased for 34 percent of working dialysis patients, and 71 percent of transplant patients. They concluded that good rehabilitation is possible with both home dialysis and transplantation in which patients can continue to contribute to society, family, and self in a similar way in both groups. The better rehabilitation of transplant patients was suggested by the fact that more of these had increased their responsibilities at work, while more of the dialysis patients had actually decreased their work responsibilities. In addition, the transplant patients rated their work effectiveness as good and more transplant patients who were working had an increase in their personal income.

References, Part 2

1. Kunkel, Henry G. and Dixon, Frank J.: Immunological aspects of renal disease: symposium. Kidney Int. 3.55, Feb. 1973.
2. Lerner, R. A., Glassock, R. J., and Dixon, F. J.: The role of anti-glomerular basement membrane antibody in the pathogenesis of human glomerulonephritis. J. Exper. Med. 6, 126:989, 1967.
3. Drummond, K. N.: Treatment with cyclophosphamide of resistant and relapsing nephrosis in childhood. Proc. 4th Int. Cong. Nephrology, Stockholm, 1969, Vol. 3 Karger, Basel/München/New York, 1970, p. 72.
4. Steinberg, A. D., et al: Cyclophosphamide in

lupus nephritis: a controlled trial. Annals Int. Med. 75:165, Aug. 1971.

5. Murray, T. and Goldberg, M.: Chronic interstitial nephritis: etiologic factors. Annals Int. Med. 82:453, 1975.

6. Myers, C. and Goldberg, M.: Personal communication.

7. Border, W. A., et al: Antitubular basement-membrane antibodies in methicillin nephritis. New Eng. J. Med. 291:381, Aug. 1974.

8. Symposium on Diabetic Nephropathy and End-stage Renal Disease. Kidney Int. 6, Supplement 1, 1974.

9. Gotch, F. C.: Symposium on Diabetic Nephropathy and Endstage Renal Disease. Kidney Int. 6, Supplement 1, 1974, pp. 5-32.

10. Simmonds, R. L.: Symposium on Diabetic Nephropathy and Endstage Renal Disease. Kidney Int. 6, Supplement 1, 1974, pp. 5-124.

11. Friedman, E. A., et al: Natural history of heroin-associated nephropathy. New Eng. J. Med. 290:19, 1974.

12. Fisher, J. W., et al: Erythropoietin production and inhibitors in serum in the anemia of uremia. Proc. Clin. Dialysis and Transplant Forum, 22, 1973.

13. Shepherd, A. M. M., et al: Peptic ulceration in chronic renal failure. Lancet, 1357, June 16, 1973.

14. Walzer, M.: Paper presented at the American Society of Nephrology, 1973.

15. DeLuca, H. F.: Parathyroid hormone as a tropic hormone for 1,25 dihydroxyvitamin D_3, the metabolically active form of vitamin D. New Eng. J. Med. 287:250, Aug. 1972; and The kidney as an endocrine organ involved in calcium homeostasis. Kidney Int. 4:80, 1973.

16. Rasmussen, H., et al: Hormonal control of skeletal and mineral homeostasis. Am. J. Med. 65:751, 1974.

17. Garabedian, M., Holick, M. F., DeLuca, H. F., et al: Control of 25-Hydroxycholecalciferol metabolism by the parathyroid glands. Proc. Nat. Acad. Sci. U.S.A. (in press).

18. Avioli, A.: American Soc. Nephrology Symposium, 1973.

19. Oettinger, G. W., et. al: Reduced calcium absorption after nephrectomy in uremic patients. New Eng. J. Med. 291:458, 1974.

20. Bricker, N. S.: On the pathogenesis of the uremic state: an exposition of the "trade-off" hypothesis. New Engl. J. Med. 286:1093, 1972.

21. Slatopolsky, E. and Bricker, N. S.: The role of phosphorus restriction in the prevention of secondary hyperparathyroidism in chronic renal disease. Kidney Int. 4:141, 1973.

22. Llach, F., et al: Skeletal resistance to endogenous parathyroid hormone in mild renal failure. Abstracts ASN:68, 1973.

23. Brickman, A. S., et al: Treatment of renal osteodystrophy with 1,25-dihydroxycholecalciferol. Abstracts ASN:15, 1973.

24. Fournier, A. E. and Johnson, W. J., et al: Etiology of hyperparathyroidism and bone disease during chronic hemodialysis. JCI 50:592, 1971.

25. Goldsmith, R. S. and Johnson, W. J.: Role of phosphate depletion and high dialysate calcium on controlling dialytic renal osteodystrophy. Kidney Int. 4:154, 1973.

26. Johnson, W. J., et al: Prevention and reversal of progressive secondary hyperparathyroidism in patients maintained by hemodialysis. Am. J. Med. 56:827, 1974.

27. Kaye, M., et al: Arrest of hyperparathyroid bone disease with dihydrotachysterol in patients undergoing chronic hemodialysis. Annals Int. Med. 73:225, Aug. 1970.

28. Hruska, K., et al: Parathyroid hormone metabolism in normal and uremic dogs. Abstracts ASN 50, 1973.

29. Stella, F. J., et al: Effect of acute uremia on vitamin D metabolism. Abstracts ASN 100, 1973.

30. Orrell, F. L., Butts, E. S., and Barbour, B. H.: Certain characteristics of dialysis in California. Dialysis and Transplantation 3:59, 1974.

31. Schwartz, A. B.: Treatment of malignant hypertension associated with renal insufficiency. *In* Hypertension: Mechanisms and Management, New York, Grune & Stratton, 1973, p. 783.

32. Woods, J. W. and Blythe, W. B.: Management of malignant hypertension complicated by renal insufficiency: further experience. Trans. Am. Clin. Climat. Assoc. 79:108, 1967.

33. Woods, J. W., Blythe, W. B., and Huffines, W. D.: Management of malignant hypertension complicated by renal insufficiency. New Eng. J. Med. 291:10, 1974.

34. Schwartz, *op. cit.*

35. Boen, S. T.: Kinetics of peritoneal dialysis: a comparison with the artificial kidney. Medicine, 40:243, 1961.

36. Henderson, L. W. and Nolph, K. D.: Altered permeability of the peritoneal membrane after using hypertonic peritoneal dialysis fluid. J. Clin. Invest. 48:992, 1969.

37. Gross, M. and MacDonald, H. P., Jr.: Effect of dialysate temperature and flow rate on peritoneal clearance. JAMA 202:263, 1967.

38. Hager, E. B. and Merrill, J. P.: Peritoneal dialysis and acute renal failure. Surg. Clin. North Am. 43:890, 1963.

39. Henderson, L. W., Merrill, J. P., and Craine, C.: Further experience with the inlying plastic conduit for chronic peritoneal dialysis. Trans. ASAIO 9:108, 1963.

40. Brewer, T. E., et al: Indwelling peritoneal (Tenckhoff) dialysis catheter. JAMA 219:1011, 1972; Rae, A. and Pendray, M.: Advantages of peritoneal dialysis in chronic renal failure. JAMA 225:937, Aug. 20, 1973; Tenckhoff, H. and Schechter, H.: A bacteriologically safe peritoneal access device. Trans. ASAIO 14:181, 1968.

41. O'Neill, M.: Peritoneal dialysis. Nurs. Clin. North Am. 1:18, 1969.

42. Abel, J. J., Rowntree, L. G., and Turner, B. B.: The removal of diffusible substances from the circulating blood by means of dialysis. Trans. ASAIO 28:51, 1913.

43. Inouye, W. Y. and Engelberg, J.: Simplified artificial dialyzer and ultrafilter. Surg. Forum, 4:438, 1953.

44. Teschan, P. E., et al: Prophylactic hemodialysis in the treatment of acute renal failure. Annals Int. Med. 53:992, 1960.

45. Quinton, W. E., Dillard, D., and Scribner, B. H.: Cannulation of blood vessels for prolonged hemodialysis. Trans. ASAIO 6:104, 1960.

46. Brescia, J. J., Cimino, J. E., Appel, K., and Hurwich, B. J.: Chronic hemodialysis using venipuncture and a surgically created arteriovenous fistula. New Eng. J. Med. 275:1089, 1966.

47. Thomas, G. I.: A large-vessel applique A-V shunt for hemodialysis. Trans. ASAIO 15:288, 1969.

48. Merrill, J. P., Schupak, E., Cameron, E. M., and Hampers, C. L.: Hemodialysis in the home. JAMA 190:468, 1964. Shaldon, S.: In *Proceedings of the Working Conference on Chronic Dialysis*. Seattle, Washington, 1964, p. 66. Curtis, K., Cole, J. J., Fellows, B. J., Tyler, L. J., and Scribner, B. H.: Hemodialysis in the home. Trans. ASAIO 11:7, 1965.

49. Pendras, J. P., Erikson, R. V.: Hemodialysis: a successful therapy for chronic uremia. Annals Int. Med. 64:293, Feb. 1966.

50. Retan, J. W. and Lewis, H. Y.: Repeated dialysis of indigent patients for chronic renal failure. Annals Int. Med. 64:284, Feb. 1966.

51. Lewis, E. J., et al: Survival data for patients undergoing chronic intermittent hemodialysis. Arch. Int. Med. 70:311, Feb. 1969.

52. Ginn, H. E.: Panel discussion, symposium on dialysis. Am. Soc. Neph., Third Annual Meeting. Washington, D.C., 1969.

53. Johnson, W. J., et al: Hemodialysis. Arch. Int. Med. 125:462, Mar. 1970.

54. Babb, A. L., et al: The genesis of the square meter-hour hypothesis. Trans. ASAIO, 27:81, 1971.

55. Henderson, L. W., et al: Hemodialfiltration. Trans. ASAIO 19:119, 1973.

56. Nolph, K. D., et al: Ultrafiltration: a mechanism for removal of intermediate molecular weight subtances in coil dialyzers. Kidney Int. 6:55, July 1974.

57. Arieff, A. I., Massry, S. G., Barientos, A., and Kleeman, C. A.: Brain water and electrolyte metabolism in uremia: effects of slow and rapid hemodialysis. Kidney Int. 4:197, Sept. 1973.

58. Greenbaum, M. A. and Gordon, A.: A regenerative dialysis supply system. Dialysis and Transplantation 1:19, 1972.

59. Kopp, K. F., et al: Single needle dialysis. Trans. ASAIO, 28:75, 1972.

60. Mirahmadi, K. S., et al: Clinical evaluation of patients dialyzed with 2 Gambro 4 hours, 3 times per week. Proc. Clin. Dialysis and Transplant Forum 3:247, 1973.

61. Sengar, H. A.: Trans. ASAIO, 1975. (In press).

62. Szmuness, W., et al: Hepatitis B infection: a point-prevalence study in 15 U.S. hemodialysis centers. JAMA 227:901, Feb. 1974.

63. Garibaldi, R. A., Forrest, J. N., Bryan, J. A., Hansen, B. F., and Dismukes, W. E.: Hemodialysis-associated hepatitis. JAMA 225:384-389, July 1973. Knight, A. H., Fox, R.

A., Baillord, R. A., Niazi, S. P., Sherlock, S., and Moorehead, J.: Hepatitis-associated antigen and antibody in hemodialysis patients and staff. Brit. J. Med. 603-606, Sept. 1970. London, W. T. D., Figlia, M., Sutnick, A. I., and Blumberg, B. P.: An epidemic of hepatitis in a chronic-hemodialysis unit. New Eng. J. Med. 281:571-578, Sept. 1969. Robsen, J. S.: The problem of hepatitis. Workshop of Dialysis and Transplant. Seattle, Washington, April 16, 1972, pp. 43-53.

64. Longnecker, R. E., et al: Blood loss during maintenance dialysis. Abstracts ASAIO 42, 1974.

65. Bull. N.W. Acad. of Med. 49:350, April 1973.

66. Kübler-Ross, E.: On Death and Dying. New York, Macmillan, 1969.

67. Cooper, K. and Blagg, C.: Modified Markov chain analysis in long-term planning of treatment programs for chronic renal failure. Proc. Clin. Dialysis and Transplant Forum 3:162, 1973.

68. National Dialysis Registry: Statistical analysis on reporting U.S. dialysis centers, Jan. 1, 1973.

69. Report of National Dyalysis and Transplant Registry, July 1974.

70. Linder, A., et al: Accelerated atherosclerosis in prolonged maintenance hemodialysis. New Eng. J. Med. 290:697, March 1974.

71. Stenzel, K. H., et al: Patient survival with hemodialysis and transplantation. Abstracts ASAIO, 69, 1974.

72. Blagg, C. R., et al: Rehabilitation of patients treated by dialysis or transplantation. Proc. Clin. Dialysis and Transplant Forum, 181, 1973.

Bibliography

Abram, H. S.: The psychiatrist, the treatment of chronic renal failure, and the prolongation of life. Am. J. Psychiat. 124:1351, 1968.

———: The psychiatrist, the treatment of chronic renal failure, and the prolongation of life, II, Am. J. Psychiat. 126:157-167, Aug. 2, 1969.

———: The psychiatrist, the treatment of chronic renal failure, and the prolongation of life, III. Am. J. Psychiat. 128:1534-1539, June 12, 1972.

Bailey, G. L., Mocelin, A. J., Hampers, C. L., and Merrill, J. P.: Adaptation of spouse pairs to home dialysis. Dial. & Transplant. 28-46, Oct.-Nov. 1972.

Beard, H.: Fear of death and fear of life. Arch. Gen. Psychiat. 21:373-380, Sept. 21, 1969.

Bilinsky, R. T., et al: Satellite dialysis: an economic approach to the delivery of hemodialysis care. JAMA 218:1809, 1971.

Blagg, R.: Home hemodialysis. Am. J. Med. Sci. 168-182, Sept. 1972.

Calland, C. H.: Iatrogenic problems in endstage renal failure. New. Eng. J. Med. 287:334-336, Aug. 17, 1972.

Cattran, D., et al: Hypertriglyceridemia in dialysis and triglyceride turnover studies to define pathogenesis. Abstracts ASAIO, 1974, p. 12.

Counts, S., Hickman, R., Garballio, A., and Tenckhoff, H.: Chronic home peritoneal dialysis in children. Trans. ASAIO 23, 1973.

Cutter, F.: Some psychological problems in hemodialysis. Omega 1:37-47, 1970.

DeNour, A. K.: Psychotherapy with patients on chronic hemodialysis. Am. J. Psychiat. 116:207-215, 1970.

DeNour, A. K. and Czaczkes, J. W.: Emotional problems and reactions of the medical team in a chronic hemodialysis unit. Lancet 2:987, 1968.

———: Personality factors in chronic hemodialysis patients causing noncompliance with the medical regimen. Psychosoma. Med. 34:333-344, July-Aug. 1972.

DeNour, A. K., Shaetiel, J., and Czaczkes, J. W.: Emotional reactions of patients on chronic hemodialysis. Psychosom. Med. 30:521, 1968.

Enelow, A. J. and Freed, G. O.: Psychosocial aspects of chronic hemodialysis. Arizona Med. 24:337, 1967.

Fine, R. N. and Schineider, C. J.: Renal homotransplantation in children. J. Pediatric 76:347-357, Mar. 1970.

Fishman, D. B., et al: Predicting emotional adjustment in home dialysis patients and their relatives. J. Chron. Disease 25:99-109, 1972.

Galton, R., Greenberg, S. M., and Shapiro, S.: Observations on the participation of nurses and physicians in chronic care. Bull. N.Y. Acad. Med. 49:112-119, Feb. 2, 1973.

Gelfman, M. and Wilson, E. J.: Emotional reactions in

a renal unit. Comprehen. Psych. 13:283-290, May 3, 1972.

Goldstein, A. M., and Reznikoff, M.: Suicide in chronic hemodialysis patients from an external locus of control framework. Am. J. Psychiat. 127:1204-1207, March 1971.

Gower, H. and Stubbs, R. K. T.: Some administrative problems in adaptation of houses for home dialysis. Brit. Med. J. 637-641, June 12, 1971; Gross, J. B., Keane, W. F., and McDonald, A. K.: Survival and rehabilitation of patients on home hemodialysis. Annals Int. Med. 78:341-346, Mar. 1973.

Hall, R. C. W.: Psychiatric complications of chronic hemodialysis and renal transplantation. New Physician 255-258, April 1971.

Halper, I. S.: Psychiatric observations in a chronic hemodialysis program. Med. Clin. North Am. 55:177-191, Jan. 1971.

Haviland, J. W.: Experience in establishing a community artificial kidney center. Am. Clin. Climat. Assoc. 77:125, 1965.

Henderson, L. W.: Rationale and evidence for the middle molecule in uremic man. Workshop on Dialysis and Transplantation, ASAIO, 1972, p. 69.

Hickey, K. M.: Impact of kidney disease on patient, family, and society. Soc. Casework 391-398, July 1972.

Kannel, W., Dawber, T., and Kagan, et al: Factors of risk in the development of coronary heart disease—six years follow-up experience: the Framingham Study. Annals Int. Med. 55:33, 1961.

Korsch, M., Fine, R. N., Grushkin, C. M., and Negrete, V. F.: Experiences with children and their families during extended hemodialysis and kidney transplantation. Pediatric Clin. North Am. 18:625-637, May 1971.

Kübler-Ross, E.: On Death and Dying. New York, Macmillan, 1969.

Lazarus, J. M., et al: Cardiovascular disease in uremic patients on hemodialysis. Kidney Int. (in press.)

Linder, A., et al: Accelerated atherosclerosis in prolonged maintenance hemodialysis. New Eng. J. Med. 290:697, Mar. 1974.

Massry, S. G., ed.: Divalent Ions in Renal Failure. Kidney Int. 4:71, Aug. 1973.

McKegney, F. P. and Laree, P.: The decision to no longer live on chronic hemodialysis. Am. J. Psychiat. 128-267-274, Sept. 1971.

Munitz, A., Wijzenbeek, H., Levi, J., Steiner, M., and Rosenbaum, M.: Psychological aspects of chronic hemodialysis. Psychiat. Neurol. Neurochir. 74:29-1223, 1971.

Nesbitt, L.: Nursing the patient on long-term hemodialysis. Canad. Nurse 40-41, Oct. 1967.

Norton, C. E.: Attitudes toward living and dying in patients on chronic hemodialysis. Annals N.Y. Acad. of Sci. 720-732, 1973.

Rae, A., Craig, P., and Miles, G.: Home dialysis: its costs and problems. Canad. Med. J. 106:1311-1315, June 1972.

Reichsman, F., and Levy, N. B., et al: Problems in adaptation to maintenance hemodialysis. Arch. Int. Med. 130:859-865, Dec. 1973.

Rosenheim, Lord, Chairman: Hepatitis and the treatment of chronic renal failure. Report of the advisory group 1970-1972. Published by the Department of Health and Social Security, Scottish Home and Health Department, Welsh Office, Cathays Park, Cardiff, Wales.

Sand, P., Livingston, G., and Wright, R. G.: Psychological assessment of candidates for a hemodialysis problem. Annals Int. Med. 64:602-609, April 1966.

Shambaugh, P. W., Hampers, C. L., and Merrill, J. P.: Hemodialysis in the home—emotional impact on the spouse. Trans. ASAIO 13:41, 1967.

Shea, E. J., Bogdon, D. F., Freeman, R. B., and Scheiner, G. E.: Hemodialysis for chronic renal failure: IV psychological considerations. Annals Int. Med. 62:558, 1965.

Siemsen, A. W., Ennis, J. A., McGowan, R., and Wong, E.: Limited care hemodialysis. Trans. ASAIO, April 1972.

Smith, E. K. M.: Hemodialysis in the home, problems and frustrations. Lancet 614, 1969.

Sorensen, T.: Group therapy in a community hospital dialysis unit. JAMA 221:899-901, Aug. 21, 1972.

Taylor, G., et al: Chronic renal failure, home dialysis and the liaison psychiatrist. Canad. Med. Assoc. J. 106:1318-1320, June 24, 1972.

Ward, M. K., Shadforth, M., Hill, A. V. L., and Kerr, D. N. S.: Air embolism during haemodialysis. Brit. Med. J. 74-78, July 10, 1971.

Weseley, S. A.: Air embolism during hemodialysis. Dial. & Transplant. 14-17, Aug.-Sept. 1972.

Wright, R. G., Sand, P., and Livingston, G.: Psychological stress during hemodialysis for chronic renal failure. Annals Int. Med. 64:611-620, April 1966.

PART THREE.
Renal Homotransplantation

HOWARD SILBERMAN and ELIZABETH M. CAMERON

Surgical Principles as Applied to Uremic Patients • Language of Transplantation • The History of Transplantation • The Biology of Transplantation • Selection of Recipients • Selection of Donors • The Recipient Operation • Rejection • Complications following Transplantation • Results • Outlook for the Future

Twenty years ago a laboratory phenomenon and only several years ago a clinical experiment, renal transplantation is now an acceptable, even preferable, therapeutic modality in endstage renal failure. Present-day knowledge allows salvage of many patients; yet, results are imperfect accounting for the intensive investigative work now in progress.

Renal transplantation is a truly multidisciplinary effort involving, among others, the immunologist, geneticist, nephrologist, surgeon, and nurse. It is with the latter that the patient develops a unique rapport, and even dependence, developed over the many years of illness, including dialysis, transplantation, and subsequent lifelong observation.

Surgical Principles as Applied to Uremic Patients

Although this section is devoted primarily to renal transplantation, the special considerations relevant to the management of uremic patients undergoing any surgical procedure (including transplantation) should be appreciated.

Patients with renal disease require surgical care with surprising frequency and under a variety of circumstances (Table 17-6). These pa-tients, of course, are subject to the same range of surgical illnesses as the general population, and, therefore, may require an operative procedure for coincidental diseases (e.g., appendicitis, cholecystitis, colon carcinoma). In addition, certain features of the uremic state may be amenable to surgical management. For instance, easy, repeated *access* to high flow vessels is required for hemodialysis. Consequently, all dialysis patients require the introduction of a Scribner-type shunt or a surgically created arteriovenous fistula. *Parathyroidectomy* is indicated in medically intractable secondary or tertiary hyperparathyroidism with bone pain, metastatic calcification, pathologic fractures, or pruritis (Wilson, 1971). *Bilateral nephrectomy* is advocated in severe hypertension (with encephalopathy, intractable congestive heart failure, papilledema)

TABLE 17-6
Operations in Uremic Patients

1. Arteriovenous fistulas
2. Parathyroidectomy
3. Nephrectomy
4. Renal biopsy
5. Splenectomy
6. Pericardiectomy
7. Renal transplantation
8. Operations for coincidental diseases

unresponsive to optimal dialysis and drug therapy (Lazarus, 1972). *Renal biopsy* may be indicated for diagnosis, for example, after prolonged oliguria in acute renal failure. *Splenectomy* has been reported to be of benefit in the small group of dialysis patients with hypersplenism, and *pericardiectomy* has been successful employed in the management of uremic pericarditis with cardiac tamponade. Finally, *renal transplantation* may be indicated in terminal renal failure.

The conduct of surgical operations in uremic patients is an extraordinary challenge to the physician. *Preoperative considerations* include evaluation and correction of fluid and electrolyte abnormalities, control of hypertension, management of anemia and nutritional depletion, modification of drug regimens, and dialysis.

Fluid and electrolyte balance is frequently abnormal. Hypervolemia and increased total body sodium (manifest by edema, hypertension, and congestive heart failure) and hyperkalemia are derangements best managed by adequate preoperative dialysis often within the 24 hours preceding operation.

These nutritionally depleted, catabolic patients are clearly less than ideal surgical candidates; unfortunately, this state is difficult to reverse. In a few reported series to date, intravenous hyperalimentation utilizing essential amino acids and 50 to 70 percent glucose has resulted in positive nitrogen balance, reversal of hyperkalemia and acidosis, and reduction in azotemia (Abel, 1972; Dudrick, 1970).

Uremic patients invariably have a marked normochromic, normovolemic anemia which, however, is generally well-tolerated. Transfusions to raise hemoglobin levels above 7 to 8 Gm are unnecessary and even inadvisable since transfusions subject the patients to the risk of potassium administration, congestive failure, and hepatitis. When required, transfusions of washed or frozen red cells minimize these hazards.

Drug regimens have to be modified in consideration of their altered metabolism in renal disease (Table 17-7). Digitalis, largely renally excreted and nondialyzable, is infrequently required in the parasurgical period. Its use may precipitate toxicity associated with fluctuations in potassium and calcium levels related to uremia, dialysis, and operative trauma. Dosage schedules of kanamycin and gentamicin must be modified in view of the renal excretion of these antibiotics. In contrast, the commonly prescribed narcotic analgesics and anticoagulants can be given in the usual manner when indicated.

Intraoperative considerations include anesthetic management as well as the technical aspects of the operation. Spinal anesthesia may well be the anesthetic technique of choice when applicable. However, thiopental, nitrous oxide, halothane, ether, and cyclopropane have all been used successfully in uremic patients, although

TABLE 17-7
Medications in Renal Disease

		Maintenance Dose Interval				
Drug	Normal	Mild C_{Cr} 50-80	Renal Failure Moderate C_{Cr} 10-50	Severe C_{Cr} <10	Significant Dialysis of Drug	Major Route of Excretion
Cephalothin	Q6H	Q6H	Q6H	Q8-12H	Yes	Renal, Hepatic
Chloramphenicol	Q6H	Q6H	Q6H	Q6H	No	Hepatic
Gentamicin	Q8H	Q8-12H	Q12-24H	Q48H	Yes	Renal
Kanamycin	Q8H	Q24H	Q24-72H	Q72-96H	Yes	Renal
Penicillin G	Q8H	Q8H	Q8H	Q12H	No	Renal, Hepatic
Meperidine	Q4H	Q4H	Q4H	Q4H	?	Hepatic
Morphine	Q4H	Q4H	Q4H	Q4H	?	Hepatic
Heparin	Q4H	Q4H	Q4H	Q4H	?	Nonrenal
Warfarin	Q24H	Q24H	Q24H	Q24H	?	Hepatic

Modified from Bennett W., et al. A practical guide to drug usage in adult patients with impaired renal function. JAMA 214:1468, 1970.

there seems to be an increased incidence of arrhythmias with cyclopropane and ether. Methoxyflurane has renal toxicity and is best avoided if there is any residual renal function, when the uremic state is potentially reversible, or in transplant operations.

Succinylcholine is a frequently employed muscle relaxant but is known to cause slight increments in serum potassium, up to 0.5 mEq per L, and should, therefore, be used cautiously in hyperkalemic patients (Aldrete, 1970; Koide, 1972). Curare though renally excreted is also detoxified by internal redistribution and, consequently, can be safely administered. The margin of safety is reduced in patients receiving potentiating antibiotics (e.g., colistin, kanamycin, streptomycin). Gallamine is exclusively excreted in the urine and is contraindicated.

The anesthesiologist should hyperventilate the uremic patient intraoperatively to sustain the normal compensatory mechanism for the metabolic acidosis of renal failure and to avoid respiratory acidosis which aggravates hyperkalemia. Anemia, though well tolerated under ordinary circumstances, requires some special attention during operation. Anemia of the magnitude seen in these patients reduces oxygen-carrying capacity to less than 50 percent of normal, posing the threat of anemic hypoxia in the face of normal arterial blood gases. Increased inspired oxygen concentrations are administered but cannot make up the deficiency. Increased cardiac output is the important compensatory mechanism for anemia; it is critical, therefore, to minimize myocardial depression during operation.

Surgical technique emphasizing compulsive attention to hemostasis is essential in uremic patients because of a bleeding tendency characterized by a qualitative defect in platelet function. Adequate dialysis tends to normalize this defect.

There is some reason to believe that wound healing is impaired in these patients on the basis of azotemia, anemia, and nutritional depletion. For this reason, it may be advisable to use monofilament, nonabsorbable suture material in securing wounds. In addition, adequate dialysis appears to reduce wound problems.

Fluid balance, dialysis, and management of any complications are among the *postoperative considerations*. (The specific features in the management of patients receiving renal transplants which function immediately are discussed on page 594.) Orders for fluid administration are calculated to cover insensible losses (i.e., 400 to 800 ml per 24 hour) and measured losses (urine, gastrointestinal secretions, drainage).

Operative trauma tends to aggravate azotemia and hyperkalemia so that dialysis is generally undertaken within the first few postoperative days. Hemodialysis in the early postoperative period is best carried out utilizing minimal anticoagulation or regional heparinization. This latter technique is not without hazard, however, since the more rapid degradation of protamine may produce a relative heparin excess resulting in rebound heparinization and therefore the hazards of systemic anticoagulation in the fresh postoperative patient. Peritoneal dialysis in the immediate postoperative period has been described but in a less efficient method.

Uremic patients are subject to a wide range of postoperative morbidity (Table 17-8). These patients have an increased susceptibility to infection attributable in part to impaired cellular immunity (Mannick, 1961) and leukocyte function (Montgomerie, 1972) and possibly some impaired antibody responses as well (Wilson, 1965). In addition, there is a high incidence of shunt thrombosis which may reflect awkward positioning during operation or a period of increased coagulability immediately postoperatively.

ILLUSTRATIVE CASE REPORT. A 34-year-old woman on chronic hemodialysis underwent cholecystectomy and bilateral nephrectomy. On the first postoperative night, oozing from the

TABLE 17-8
Postoperative Morbidity

1. Infections
2. Shunt thrombosis
3. Hemorrhage
4. Pancreatitis
5. Pericarditis
6. Ileus
7. Hiccups
8. Hyperkalemia
9. Cardiac arrhythmias

wound developed which required suture ligation. Thrombosis of the arteriovenous fistula was noted on the evening of the operation requiring operative revision. The patient was hemodialyzed on the third postoperative day following which the shunt again required revision because of thrombosis. Thereafter, the wound healed without complication, the fistula remained patent, and the patient was discharged on the fourteenth postoperative day.

In summary, operations upon uremic patients can be carried out successfully but are challenging. Preoperative and postoperative dialysis is a critical feature in the perioperative management of these patients since dialysis tends to normalize the metabolic derangements, to improve coagulation, and to reduce wound complication.

The Language of Transplantation

The tissue to be transplanted is designated the *transplant*, or *graft*. The biological relationship between the donor and the recipient (host) is denoted by the terms *autograft, isograft, homograft (allograft),* or *heterograft (xenograft)*. Tissues grafted to a different site in the same individual are *autografts*. *Isografts* are transplants derived from donors genetically identical to the recipient (for example, grafts between monozygotic twins). *Homografts* and *heterografts* are obtained from genetically dissimilar individuals of the same species and individuals of different species, respectively. Grafts are *orthotopic* if they are placed in the normal anatomic position in the recipient. In contrast, *heterotopic* grafts are located in ectopic positions. Kidney transplants are generally placed in the recipient's pelvis and are, therefore, properly termed heterotopic grafts.

The History of Transplantation

Although renal transplantation was attempted as early as 1902, concerted efforts to achieve renal graft survival in humans were first made in the early 1950s. In these early days, human kidneys transplanted to unrelated human hosts often produced urine for variable periods, but graft survival was consistently short-lived. Nevertheless, these instances of sporadic graft function confirmed the feasibility of the surgical operation.

In 1954, a unique opportunity was afforded Drs. John Merrill, Hartwell Harrison, and Joseph Murray when a chronically uremic patient with an identical twin brother was referred to them at the Peter Bent Brigham Hospital in Boston. These physicians had derived considerable technical experience from their earlier series of unmodified renal transplants between unrelated individuals. In addition, it had long been thought that identical twins were so similar that their tissues could be freely exchanged. With this background, the Boston group undertook the first transplant between monozygotic twins in December 1954. The patient survived eight years on his new kidney.

The likelihood of a renal failure patient having an identical twin is distinctly remote. It became evident, therefore, that the practical application of transplantation to clinical medicine would require the use of genetically disparate donor kidneys. Moreover, the inevitable biological attack upon such foreign tissue would have to be overcome.

In 1943, Gibson and Medawar discovered that this phenomenon of graft rejection was an immunological event in which the recipient became immunized against the foreign tissue.[1] Subsequent research, therefore, was directed toward circumventing or modifying this acquired immune response which results in graft destruction.

In 1952, Dixon demonstrated immunosuppression in rabbits by total body irradiation, a discovery applied to humans in 1958.[2] The following year, the first successes using this immunosuppressive modality in humans were reported. Merrill, in Boston, and, shortly thereafter, Hamburger, in Paris, each reported a case of kidney transplantation in which the irradiated recipient received a graft from a fraternal twin. Both of these patients survive today and represent the longest surviving individuals bearing functioning, life-sustaining, renal homografts.[3] Despite these successes, the general experience with total body irradiation was unsatisfactory.

The doses of irradiation required to suppress the immunologic attack against the kidney produced impairment of all body defenses, subjecting recipients to unacceptable toxicity including overwhelming infection. Gentler immunosuppression had to be found.

In 1960, Schwartz and Damashek demonstrated extended survival of skin homografts in rabbits receiving the antimetabolite, 6-mercaptopurine.[4] The less toxic analog of 6-mercaptopurine, azathioprine, has become a standard in present immunosuppressive regimens. In 1961, Murray and associates transplanted the first patient to enjoy prolonged kidney graft survival using azathioprine immunosuppression.[5]

In 1963, Starzl reported a high rate of success using a combination of azathioprine and the corticosteroid prednisone.[6] This latter agent potentiates the efficacy of azathioprine. Three years later, in 1966, Starzl added antilymphocyte serum to his immunosuppressive regimen and reported an improved early course following transplantation and a reduction in the required doses of other immunosuppressive agents.[7]

The Biology of Transplantation

Antigens present on cellular membranes which characterize a given individual and provoke the homograft reaction are known as histocompatibility antigens. These antigens are determined by histocompatibility genes located on chromosomes at histocompatibility loci. Transplanted tissues bearing antigens absent in host tissues stimulate specific immunity against the foreign antigens. (See Chapter 22 *The Immune Process* for further discussion of immunity.)

Homografts exchanged between healthy individuals thrive for a variable but limited period of time then become subject to an immunologic destructive process, the *first set homograft reaction*. The vigor of this process of graft rejection is related to the degree of antigenic disparity between donor and recipient.

A renewed exposure to an antigen against which an individual has been previously immunized provokes a more rapid, more vigorous immune response, the *second set (anamnestic)* *reaction*. Thus, alien tissue transplanted to a host previously having rejected a graft bearing the same histocompatibility antigens may undergo accelerated, even violent, destruction.

The mode of host recognition of and reaction to alien histocompatibility antigens is complex and, in part, incompletely defined. In general, foreign antigenic material interacts with immunocompetent host cells setting forth a series of events culminating in the elaboration of specific antibody (humoral immunity) or in a population of specifically sensitized lymphocytes (cellular immunity) or both (Fig. 17-14).

Antigenic material from the graft may reach lymph nodes via afferent lymphatics or veins draining the graft thereby engaging host immunocompetent cells. The afferent lymphatic vessels are critical for sensitization of skin homografts. Such skin grafts placed in pedicled skin flaps devoid of lymphatic drainage enjoy prolonged survival; however, reestablishment of lymphatic drainage results in prompt rejection (Barker, 1968).

In contrast, organ homografts whose circulation is re-established by surgical anastomosis (unlike free skin homografts) provoke the homograft reaction even in the absence of lymphatic drainage. According to the theory of *peripheral sensitization*, circulating host immunocompetent lymphocytes pass through the newly vascularized graft contacting donor cells whose surfaces bear alien antigens. These circulating host cells return to regional lymph nodes and undergo a proliferative phase producing a population of sensitized cells which, when circulating through the graft, effect their destructive function. (Strober, 1965).

Selection of Recipients

Patients with irreversible renal dysfunction so severe as to endanger life or require hemodialysis to maintain homeostasis come under consideration for renal transplantation.

Factors to be considered in determining the suitability of a patient with endstage renal failure for transplantation include the specific renal diagnosis, the general medical and immunologic

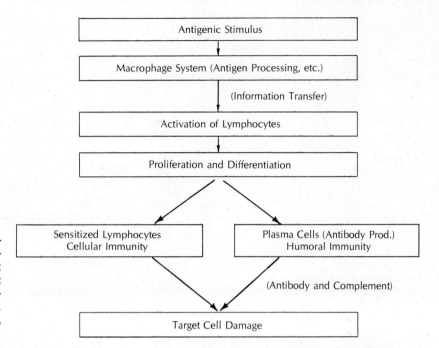

FIGURE 17-14.
Schematic view of mechanisms operating in the immune response. Source: Adapted from Santos, G. W.: The pharmacology of immunosuppressive drugs. Pharmacol. Physicians 2, 8, 1968.

status of the candidate, and the availability of an acceptable donor.

An ever-expanding range of renal pathology is being managed successfully by transplantation (Table 17-9). Glomerulonephritis continues to be the commonest diagnosis among patients receiving kidney grafts. Pyelonephritis follows in frequency; and these two diseases underlie the renal failure in 75 percent of transplant patients.[8]

Factors which enhance the risk of every major operative procedure naturally increase the hazards of transplantation as well. Advanced age, arteriosclerotic cardiovascular disease, diabetes mellitus, and obesity are among such risk factors. The immunosuppressive drugs required following transplantation subject all patients to potential complications but create additional hazards for some patients. For example, the drug regimen, including corticosteroids, is apt to aggravate diabetes, chronic infections, peptic ulcer diathesis, and neoplastic diseases.

"Ideal-risk" patients have generally included those 17 to 45 years of age with normal lower urinary tracts and without infection or malignancy.[9] Recent studies, however, indicate that transplantation can be carried out in certain high-risk patients with rates of success equal to those in ideal-risk patients. Such favorable outcomes have been reported in children, diabetics, and persons over age 45 receiving related kidneys, and patients with peptic ulcer disease, coronary artery disease, and abnormal bladder function.[10]

Disseminated malignancy is an absolute contraindication to transplantation. Transplantation may be feasible in patients with malignancy previously treated for cure.

Recipients of cadaveric kidneys who are over age 45 or are diabetic are at significant risk compared to other transplant candidates. Hypertensive encephalopathy, polyarteritis, inactive tuberculosis, and a history of gastrointestinal hemorrhage may increase risk of failure or death. Infants appear to be poorer candidates than children over one year of age.

It is well established that transplantation is doomed to failure if the recipient has circulating antibodies against donor histocompatibility antigens. Under these circumstances another donor has generally been sought. However, some evidence suggests that recipients with antibodies against *any* histocompatibility antigens (i.e., even in the absence of antibodies against donor-specific antigens) have low rates of satisfactory

TABLE 17-9
Diagnoses Submitted to Registry

DISEASE	NUMBER REPORTED	% OF TOTAL
Glomerulonephritis	3,403	59.8
Pyelonephritis	892	15.7
More than one primary disease	301	5.3
Polycystic kidneys	259	4.6
Malignant hypertension	160	2.8
Renal disease, unspecified	137	2.4
Glomerulonephritis and pyelonephritis	100	1.8
Familial nephropathy	83	1.5
Congenital, nonobstructive	79	1.4
Nephritis secondary to drugs	39	0.7
Medullary cystic disease	31	0.5
Obstructive uropathy	24	0.4
Diabetic glomerulosclerosis	19	0.3
Cortical necrosis	19	0.3
Lupus nephritis	16	0.3
Traumatic loss or removal	16	0.3
Cancer of kidney	13	0.2
Goodpasture's syndrome	11	0.2
Congenital, obstructive	10	0.2
Gout	10	0.2
Tuberculosis	9	0.2
Amyloidosis	8	0.1
Cystinosis	8	0.1
Nephrocalcinosis	8	0.1
Oxalosis-oxaluria	8	0.1
Tubular necrosis	8	0.1
Calculus disease	4	0.1
Radiation nephritis	4	0.1
Hyperparathyroid	2	0
Angiokeratoma corporis diffusum (Fabry's)	2	0
Periarteritis nodosa	1	0
Subacute bacterial endocarditis	1	0
Collagen disease	1	0
Nail-patella syndrome	1	0
Endocarditis	1	0

From Ninth Report of the Human Renal Transplant Registry. JAMA 220:253, 1972.

graft function (Patel, 1971). These recipient candidates may, therefore, represent another true high-risk group.

Selection of Donors

Kidneys for transplantation can be derived from living blood relatives or from unrelated individuals (cadavers).

It is clear from the experimental laboratory that the probability of successful tissue transplantation correlates with minimal genetic disparity between donor and host. How to determine who among a panel of otherwise suitable donors is most compatible with the recipient is one of the major problems facing clinical transplantation today. In general, a monozygotic twin, a sibling, a parent, another related, or an unrelated individual (cadaver) are satisfactory donors in descending order of preference.

In addition to these genetic considerations, other factors in donor selection include the general health of prospective living donors, the pathologic status including renal function of cadaveric donors, and the renovascular anatomy in either case.

TISSUE TYPING

At least three genetic systems are responsible for histocompatibility in humans: The ABO system of erythrocyte antigens, the HLA system, and mixed lymphocyte culture reactivity.

The major blood group antigens (ABO) are strong histocompatibility antigens. It is unwise to perform transplants into patients with known preformed isohemagglutinins against the donor blood type. Thus, an individual must be a compatible blood donor in order to be an acceptable kidney donor. Transplantation carried out across an ABO incompatibility may result in *hyperacute rejection*. There is no convincing evidence that minor blood group factors (Rh, Duffy, Kell) act as histocompatibility antigens.[11]

A series of strong histocompatibility antigens is genetically determined by the HLA locus. The HLA locus, the major histocompatibility locus in humans, is located on an autosomal chromosome and consists of at least two closely approximated subloci, HLA-A and HLA-B (Bach, 1976). Each individual inherits two such chromosomes (one from each parent) and, therefore, four HLA genes (two from the A series and two from the B series) which determine four HLA antigens on his tissue cells. An individual may have as few as two *different* HLA antigens since he may be homozygous for one or both pairs of allelic genes at the two subloci.

About 35 different HLA antigens have been identified in human populations. The HLA antigens of donors and recipients can be determined by the lymphocytotoxicity method of Terasaki.[12] The test is performed by incubating lymphocytes (which bear HLA antigens) with antisera of known specificity. Destruction of the lymphocytes by a specific antiserum implies the presence of the antigen. In addition, the presence in the recipient of circulating cytotoxic antibodies directed against donor histocompatibility antigens may be determined by the cross-match test. Here, donor lymphocytes are incubated with recipient serum; destruction of the donor lymphocytes constitutes a positive test.

Based on the results of these tests, a histocompatibility grade between donor and recipient can be designated. In one grading system, an *A match* (identity) indicates that the donor and the recipient have identical HLA antigens. In *B matches* (compatible) all donor antigens are present in the recipient, but the recipient has an antigen not identified in the donor. Here, no donor antigens are foreign to the recipient. When the donor has one antigen not identified in the recipient, the match is rated *C*. When two or more donor antigens are lacking in the recipient a *D match* exists. An *F match* indicates a positive cross-match; that is, the recipient has circulating antibodies against donor antigens (Fig. 17-15).

The utility of HLA tissue typing in predicting homograft success is uncertain at the present time. Two principles are clear, however. An *A match* between siblings is highly predictive of homograft success; some groups report over 95 percent success rate in such cases.[13] At the other end of the spectrum, grafting in the face of an *F match* is contraindicated. Although a donor with the "best" match is generally chosen, there appears to be little correlation between HLA tissue typing and homograft success beyond the principles alluded to above. Thus, recipients of poorly matched kidneys are not considered high risk-patients.

Mixed lymphocyte culture (MLC) reactivity is another genetic system influencing histocompatibility. In this *in vitro* test, donor and recipient lymphocytes are incubated in a nutrient medium containing tritium-labeled thymidine. Antigenic differences between donor and recipient stimulate protein synthesis by these immunocompetent cells. The extent of stimulation is quantitated by measuring thymidine uptake. The MLC reactivity is governed by a locus, HLA-D, which lies on the same chromosome as the A and B loci but is separate from them. It appears that minimal MLC reactivity correlates with transplant success.

The inability to consistently predict homograft outcome by tissue typing is at present the subject of intensive investigation. It is likely that additional genetic loci controlling important histocompatibility antigens are as yet unidentified.[14]

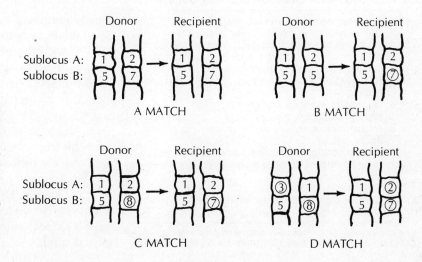

FIGURE 17-15. Schematic representation of the HLA locus consisting of two closely approximated subloci (A and B). The various HLA tissue types are shown as defined in the text. Source: Modified after Turcotte J. G., et al: Histocompatibility and the success of intrafamilial renal transplantation. Surg. Gynecol. Obstet. *135*:193, 1972.

LIVING DONORS

Results to date indicate that relatives of prospective homograft recipients provide the best tissues for transplantation. Living persons unrelated to recipients are no longer acceptable donor candidates since cadaveric tissues produce equally good results.

Individuals offering a kidney should be true volunteers; their motivation should be altruistic rather than deriving from a sense of obligation or guilt.

Despite the limitations alluded to above, tissue typing is generally carried out among prospective donors, and the donor with the best match is selected for an intensive general medical evaluation. When his excellent general health is confirmed, the individual's renal function is assessed including urinalysis, urine culture, urogram, urea, creatinine, and creatinine clearance (Table 17-10). If all these parameters are normal, the renovascular anatomy is determined arteriographically. Multiple renal arteries increase the technical difficulty of transplantation since all arterial branches (each an end-artery) must be revascularized. The presence of multiple vessels may make the opposite kidney preferable.

The recipient and donor are operated upon simultaneously in adjacent operating rooms. The operations are coordinated so that the donor kidney is removed just as the recipient is prepared to receive it. The donor nephrectomy is carried out with special effort to preserve long segments of artery, vein, and ureter.

The renal *ischemia time* is that time between vascular occlusion of the kidney in the donor and re-establishment of blood flow in the recipient. The ischemic damage to which the kidney is subject during this period may be minimized by rapid cooling of the organ. This is accomplished immediately on removal by emersion in ice saline slush and by perfusion through the renal artery with a cold solution similar in composition to intracellular fluid (Collins, 1976).

The risks to the donor of nephrectomy are small but finite. Among nearly 4,000 donors studied, nephrectomy resulted in three deaths, a mortality rate of less than 0.1 percent.[15] Significant complications are uncommon, but nearly half of a group of donors studied at the University of Colorado experienced some morbidity. Atelectasis, pneumonitis, pneumothorax, and urinary infection were the commonest postoperative problems. No instances of renal insufficiency were reported.[16]

Nursing Implications

The medical evaluation is a difficult time for the donor. Throughout the routine studies it is the nurse's responsibility to explain the purpose and techniques of the procedures. She should encourage him to discuss the proposed operation and to ask questions. If she feels that the donor needs additional support or explanation, or if she is in doubt regarding his motivation, she should confer with the physician. After close study, if the motivation of the proposed donor seems questionable, he may be told that the tissue match is incompatible or that his kidney is unsatisfactory for some reason. This provides an excuse which allows the potential donor to live with his conscience and his family. It is important that the nurse be sure the rejected donor and his family understand and accept his inability to give his kidney. On the other hand if the donor is emotionally stable and secure in his decision to give a kidney, and if he is physically fit, the proposed surgery is discussed with him.

TABLE 17-10
Criteria for Selection of Living Donors

1. Voluntary donation without coercion.
2. Stable social and psychological history.
3. Complete history and physical examination normal.
4. Absence of renal disease, hypertension, significant diabetes, or transmittable neoplasm.
5. Normal CBC, ECG, chest x-ray, SMA-12, coagulation profile, STS.
6. Normal intravenous urogram.
7. Normal creatinine clearance.
8. Negative urine culture on two occasions; normal urinalysis.
9. Normal aortogram and renal arteriograms (major renal anomalies or more than two renal arteries may exclude donor).
10. Compatible ABO typing.
11. Compatible HLA tissue typing (D match or better).
12. Negative cross-match with recipient.

From Colberg, J. E.: Selection and management of patients for renal transplantation. Surg. Clin. North Am. 53:685, 1973.

The donor is admitted to the hospital several days preceding surgery. He is permitted unrestricted activity and diet. The nurse describes what he may expect in the postoperative course. He receives instruction in coughing and deep-breathing exercises. Because this is a stressful time for him, he should be given every opportunity to discuss his fears and concerns. Skin preparation is the same as for routine nephrectomy.

Postoperatively, the donor goes from the recovery room to the ward where he is given the usual postnephrectomy care. Coughing and deep breathing are stressed, and progressive ambulation is started.

It is important that the nurse continue to support the donor, as he may be inadvertently neglected due to the enthusiasm surrounding the recipient's progress. He is generally discharged within 7 to 14 days and is followed as an outpatient. In the event that the graft is rejected, the donor deserves consideration and support lest guilt and depression supervene. It has been observed, however, that even when the graft fails, the donor's sense of satisfaction in contributing to the recipient can be a source of comfort to him.

CADAVERIC DONORS

Kidneys for transplantation have been increasingly obtained from cadaveric donors. Such donors have often been pronounced dead according to "brain death" criteria rather than by the traditional diagnostic signs of cessation of spontaneous heartbeat and respiration which are obscured by resuscitative machinery. Persons whose kidneys are suitable for transplantation under these circumstances are in a state of irreversible coma, yet have a heartbeat and blood pressure sufficient to maintain near-normal perfusion and oxygenation of their kidneys so that renal function and urinary output are essentially normal. *Irreversible coma* is defined as complete unreceptivity and unresponsitivity to even the most intensely painful stimuli; there are no spontaneous muscular movements, spontaneous respirations, or reflexes. Furthermore, the electroencephalogram is flat. The patient is pronounced dead when there are no changes in these tests 24 hours after the initial examination. The process underlying irreversible coma may be cardiac arrest, asphyxia with respiratory arrest, or massive brain damage (e.g., due to trauma or vascular accident). Suitable donors are free from malignancy (except central nervous system), sepsis, or other transmissible diseases (e.g., hepatitis). The donor and recipient must be ABO compatible and the cross-match must be negative.

The donor kidney may be removed and placed in the recipient immediately, as with living donors. Alternatively, the harvested kidney may be preserved by a variety of techniques for variable periods before grafting. *In vitro* tissue preservation is advantageous because it allows evaluation and examination of the kidney before committing the recipient to operation. In addition, tissue typing, including cross-matching, may be carried out more leisurely, and the recipient operation can be scheduled electively. Perhaps most important is that adequate preservation allows transportation of a kidney to a distant hospital.

Simple hypothermia utilizing ice slush and a cold intracellular-like perfusate allows preservation of renal function up to 24 to 48 hours. (Collins, 1976). Preservation without renal functional impairment up to 24 hours (and perhaps longer) may be achieved with an apparatus incorporating hypothermia, pulsatile perfusion, and static membrane oxygenation (Fig. 17-16). (Toledo-Pereyra, 1976).

Procurement of cadaveric donor organs has been hampered in the past by medico-legal obstacles. These problems have been obviated to some extent by the recent adoption by nearly all the States of laws based on the *Uniform Anatomical Gift Act.* This act provides that any individual of sound mind may give all or any part of his body for medical purposes, the gift to take effect upon death. Such a gift may be made by will or other written document such as a card designed to be carried on the person (Fig. 17-17). Moreover, if the individual has made no directive the next of kin may give all or any part of the decedent's body for medical purposes. (Sadler, 1971).

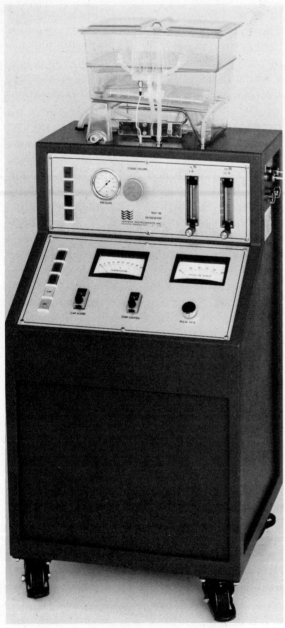

FIGURE 17-16.
Transport module of Minnesota organ Perfusion System. Source: Moberg, A. W., et al: Transportable organ perfusion system for kidney preservation. Lancet 2:1403, 1971.

Despite these medico-legal advances, the problem of donor tissue procurement is acute since demand far exceeds supply.

The Recipient Operation

PREOPERATIVE CONSIDERATIONS

Operations upon uremic patients present special problems as discussed previously.

Although there is little indication to transfuse these patients beyond 7 to 8 Gm of hemoglobin, in the weeks, months, or years preceding transplantation, these patients often have received multiple transfusions. Such transfusions have generally been regarded as detrimental to transplant outcome because the leukocytes (which bear HLA antigens) tend to presensitize prospective graft recipients to HLA antigens. Studies challenging this view have shown that, whereas transfusions are capable of producing sensitization in 25 to 40 percent of potential recipients, in the remainder such transfusions actually may have a salutary effect by inducing a state of immunologic unresponsiveness.[17] When transfusion is indicated, leukocyte-poor blood (frozen or washed red cells) rather than whole blood has usually been recommended. The view that such preparations decrease the sensitizing potential of blood transfusions has been confirmed by recent experimental work.[18] Nevertheless, it appears that such leukocyte-poor preparations have the same potential to induce protective blocking or enhancing antibodies as transfusions of whole blood (Strom, 1977).

Under certain circumstances pretransplant nephrectomy or splenectomy are indicated. Bilateral nephrectomy is indicated for intractable severe hypertension, documented urinary tract infection, and Goodpasture's syndrome. It may also be indicated in patients with polycystic kidney disease, vesico-ureteral reflux, and massive proteinuria. In the absence of specific indication for preoperative nephrectomy, many groups remove the kidneys at the time of transplantation.

Pretransplant splenectomy appears to benefit patients with hypersplenism by improving the hematologic derangements. The benefit of routine splenectomy before or at the time of transplantation is less clear. Recent reports indicate that splenectomy increases tolerance to azathioprine and reduces the incidence of leukopenia associated with moderate doses of the drug.[19] Dialysis is generally carried out on

UNIFORM DONOR CARD

OF_____

<small>Print or type name of donor</small>

In the hope that I may help others, I hereby make this anatomical gift, if medically acceptable, to take effect upon my death. The words and marks below indicate my desires.

I give: (a) _____ any needed organs or parts

       (b) _____ only the following organs or parts

_____

<small>Specify the organ(s) or part(s)</small>

for the purposes of transplantation, therapy, medical research or education;

       (c) _____ my body for anatomical study if needed.

Limitations or
special wishes, if any :_____

Signed by the donor and the following two witnesses in the presence of each other:

_____   _____
<small>Signature of Donor   Date of Birth of Donor</small>

_____   _____
<small>Date Signed   City & State</small>

_____   _____
<small>Witness   Witness</small>

This is a legal document under the Uniform Anatomical Gift Act or similar laws.

For further information consult your physician or

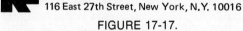 National Kidney Foundation
116 East 27th Street, New York, N.Y. 10016

FIGURE 17-17.
Uniform donor card.

the day preceding transplantation in order to minimize fluid, electrolyte, and acid-base derangements, and to reduce azotemia and hypertension.

Nursing Care

The care of patients receiving renal transplants is one of the most challenging areas of nursing. It is unique, for every area of nursing expertise is utilized, especially that required to promote the psychological well-being of the patient and his family. The nurse should be acquainted with the experiences which the patient has had prior to coming to the transplant center for evaluation. The majority of these patients come with a long history of renal disease and all the accompanying implications of a prolonged illness. Transplantation is reserved for those who have reached a terminal phase of their illness. Yet, the prospective recipient often is unaware of the advanced stage of his disease, and generally he is uncertain of the exact time of surgery until the donor has been selected. All these factors contribute to the patient's anxiety which may be allayed by tactful and thoughtful explanation and support.

The preoperative care of the recipient includes maintenance of fluid and electrolyte balance at an optimal level. The patient is dialyzed as needed, usually within 24 to 36 hours preceding surgery. Extracorporeal hemodialysis is usually the procedure of choice because it avoids the chance of infecting the surgical field. However, some groups have used peritoneal dialysis safely in controlled circumstances.[20] Hemodialysis is carried out in routine fashion using systemic heparinization. During the last several dialyses prior to surgery, the patient receives washed or frozen cells bringing his hemoglobin to 7 to 8 Gm.

Preoperatively, every effort is made to discuss the various aspects of the operative and postoperative course with the patient. The hours of hemodialysis prior to surgery afford the nurse many opportunities to review the patient's understanding of the situation in an attempt to alleviate his fears. A brief description of the surgery is given, including the time required and the location of the new organ. The frequent posttransplant diuresis and the method for fluid replacement are described. The patient is reminded that a rejection episode is expected to occur at some time and can be treated successfully. He is told that he may see much that could confuse or concern him and that he should always ask questions. The authors of this chapter also discuss the possible need for hemodialysis postoperatively. It is stressed that this is, hopefully, only for the short period until his new kidney functions adequately.

The patient is instructed in coughing and deep breathing postoperatively, and the importance of these measures is explained. He is taught to splint his incision during the exercises in order to lessen the discomfort.

The preoperative skin preparation is carried out according to standard methods; it includes cleaning and shaving from nipples to knees including pubis. Any area which appears to be infected is reported to the surgeon.

OPERATIVE TECHNIQUE

Following the induction of general endotracheal anesthesia, a Foley catheter is introduced which allows careful monitoring of urine output and protects any bladder suture lines postoperatively.

Following appropriate skin preparation and draping, the iliac vessels are exposed retroperitoneally through an anterolateral incision which is made several centimeters above and parallel to the inguinal ligament.

The internal iliac (hypogastric) artery is dissected free and divided distally preserving sufficient length to allow end-to-end anastomosis with the donor renal artery. The external iliac vein is likewise exposed following which a longitudinal incision is made in its anterior wall. An anastomosis is then created between the end of the donor renal vein and the side of the external iliac vein. The kidney, placed in the iliac fossa, is thus revascularized. Next, urinary outflow continuity is reestablished by implanting the donor ureter into a new opening in the bladder (ureteronecystostomy). Alternatively, the donor renal pelvis may be anastomosed to the recipient ureter (ureteropyeloplasty) (Fig. 17-18).

In young children where vessels are small and the kidney too large to fit comfortably in the iliac fossa, the graft is placed intraperitoneally with anastomoses to the inferior vena cava and aorta.

Following closure of the operative wound and arousal from anesthesia, the patient is admitted to the transplant unit or to an intensive care facility.

POSTOPERATIVE COURSE

Under the most favorable circumstances, urine production follows within minutes of graft revascularization. In Starzl's experience patients receiving kidneys from living, related donors produce an average of 444 ml of urine per hour for the first 12 hours. The diuresis usually begins to subside after 8 to 24 hours.[21] This early post-transplant diuresis appears to be caused by a

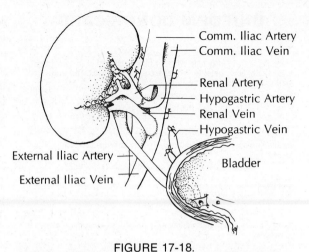

FIGURE 17-18.
Vascular anastomoses in renal transplantation. Source: Adapted from Hume, D. M.: Transplantation. *In* Schwartz, S. I. (ed.): Principles of Surgery. New York, McGraw-Hill, 1969, p. 279.

self-limited defect in the proximal tubular transport system for sodium and glucose. Such a massive obligatory diuresis may result in rapid changes in fluid and electrolyte balance. Consequently, careful, frequent analysis of serum and sometimes urine electrolyte composition is required. Intravenous fluid orders generally call for the administration of solutions similar in volume and composition to the previous hour's urinary output. These orders are naturally modified by other parameters including pre-existing deficits, central venous pressure, other external losses (emesis, drainage), and insensible losses. The uremic state is rapidly relieved by immediately functioning grafts. In contrast, early postoperative hemodialysis may be required for recipients whose initial graft function is delayed.

Following surgery, the vital signs are monitored closely as the patient awakens from anesthesia. Vigorous chest physical therapy is started using the techniques taught preoperatively. The patient should be offered medication for pain prior to these treatments in order to obtain his full cooperation. He should be shown how to splint his incisions and reassured that they are intact even though he may fear that they are splitting apart. The patient is turned frequently.

The head of his bed may be elevated; ambulation usually is initiated on the first postoperative day.

Dressings should remain sterile and dry. They may be changed with the surgeon's permission, utilizing sterile technique. Wet dressings overlying significantly draining wounds should be weighed in order to accurately assess losses.

Oral hygiene is an important aspect of nursing care because so many of these patients develop annoying bacterial and fungal infections; a high incidence of herpes stomatitis has also been observed. In addition to routine mouth care, antifungal mouth washes are frequently prescribed.

Shunt dressings are changed by the dialysis team. A special loop is incorporated into the shunt so that it can be used for drawing the frequent blood samples. There is a marked increase in clotting of shunts and fistulas in the postoperative period, and, therefore, they should be observed frequently and declotted as necessary.

Diet is advanced in accordance with the patient's progress, and the patient is weighed daily. Dietary restrictions, so important in the preoperative uremic state, are now often unnecessary if graft function is adequate.

Although rigid reverse isolation techniques are infrequently recommended today, recipients should be protected from potential sources of infection in the hospital environment. When patients must leave the transplant unit for care in other areas of the hospital (e.g., radiology department) they are generally attired in gown and mask. Visitors should be free of even minor infectious diseases and are usually restricted to spouse or parents.

Nurses should remember that patients in intensive care units are subject to peculiar "ICU syndromes" related to alterations in sensory stimuli. Day becomes indistinguishable from night and track of time is lost. The stress and apprehension inherent in being in an intensive care area can be relieved to a great extent by the nurse's approach and attitude. She should help the patient retain contact with the environment beyond his room by orienting him to time, weather, news, sports and the like. (Other helpful measures are discussed in detail in Chapter 18, concerning sensory deprivation.)

Rejection

Rejection is the clinical counterpart of the homograft reaction; it is the immune attack against the donor organ stimulated by foreign histocompatibility antigens. Three varieties of clinical rejection can be recognized: 1) hyperacute rejection, 2) acute rejection, 3) chronic rejection.

Hyperacute rejection occurs in presensitized recipients; circulating cytotoxic antibodies promptly destroy the graft, often within minutes of revascularization. The kidney fails to regain its normal tissue turgor and pink color. There is a sequestration of antibodies, platelets, white cells, and clotting factors within the graft leading to intrarenal vascular thrombosis. Nephrectomy is indicated following diagnosis.

Acute rejection is a primarily cell-mediated, usually reversible, process, episodes of which occur in the majority of patients sometime in their course. The first episode generally occurs within the first six weeks and most commonly about two weeks after grafting. Pathologically, acute rejection is characterized by marked interstitial edema of the kidney with mononuclear cell infiltration and a vasculitis with intramural edema and deposition of fibrinoid material.

Clinical features of acute rejection include fever, leukocytosis, acute hypertension, and diminished renal function manifest by increasing blood urea and creatinine and diminished creatinine clearance, urinary output, and urinary sodium.

Anuria or oliguria in the early postoperative period may signify a rejection crisis, arterial or venous thrombosis, ureteral obstruction, or other technical problems but usually are manifestations of ischemic renal failure, often reversible. Urography, renograms, and infrequently arteriography, and renal biopsy may be indicated to assist in distinguishing between these entities. Later, instances of rejection must be distinguished most importantly from infection. This critical distinction is often difficult since the fever and leukocytosis (seen in both infection and rejection) in rejection may precede the usual renal functional deterioraton. Increments in corticosteroids indicated for rejection tend to aggravate infectious processes. To compound the problem, it appears that mild infection may trigger graft rejection.

Unfortunately, no pathognomonic clinical or laboratory tests for rejection are known. The diagnosis is based on clinical and laboratory examination and the exclusion of other entities in the differential.

In contrast to the acute process, *chronic rejection* is manifest by slow, indolent deterioration of renal function usually with few systemic signs or symptoms. It appears to be, at least in part, antibody mediated. Chronic rejection may occur weeks or months following transplantation and is often resistant to therapy.

IMMUNOSUPPRESSIVE AGENTS

Azathioprine and corticosteroids are basic constituents of nearly every immunosuppressive regime. Azathioprine, a less toxic analog of 6-mercaptopurine, appears to impede the proliferation of immunocompetent cells and, in addition, has some anti-inflammatory effect.

The salutary effect of corticosteroids is poorly understood, but their anti-inflammatory and lympholytic properties appear to play an important role. Steroids are of little value as immunosuppressive agents when used alone; graft prolongation is minimal. They are most effective in association with other immunosuppressive agents whose actions they potentiate.

Antilymphocyte serum (ALS) is a heterologous serum containing antibodies against lymphocytes. A suspension of human lymphocytes, derived from thymus, spleen or cultured lymphoblasts, is injected into animals of another species (e.g., horses, rabbits, goats) according to various protocols. Serum from the immunized animal is drawn and the antibody-containing fraction isolated, sterilized, and frozen until used. ALS is an extremely potent immunosuppressive agent in laboratory animals. It evidently acts by selectively depleting lymphocytes responsible for cell-mediated immunity; cells coated with antibody are lysed or phagocytized. The efficacy of present preparations in human renal transplantation is less clear. Prolongation

of cadaveric graft survival when ALS is added to azathioprine and steroids has been reported by Najarian and Sheil.[22,23] In contrast, Turcotte could not confirm these findings with cadaveric grafts, although enhanced survival was achieved with ALS in patients receiving an incompatible intrafamilial graft.[24] Some groups do not use this material at all.

The optimal protocols for preparation, assay and administration of ALS remain inadequately defined. Discrepancies in apparent efficacy are probably in part related to nonstandardized preparation and administration, making comparisons of results reported from different medical centers difficult.

Immunosuppressive drugs are administered to patients undergoing transplantation prophylactically in the hope of delaying or even preventing entirely rejection crises (Table 17-11). At one hospital, patients receive antilymphocyte globulin (ALG, the globulin fraction of ALS) for five days preoperatively. In addition azathioprine is started the evening preceding operation. Two to three Gm of methylprednisolone are administered intravenously over 24 hours starting at operation.[25] Azathioprine and corticosteroids (prednisone) are continued for life. Generally, the highest dose of azathioprine consistent with a normal leukocyte count is prescribed postoperatively (usually 2 to 3 mg per kg). In contrast, the lowest doses of prednisone consistent with normal renal function are administered. Transplant groups using antilymphocyte serum or its derivatives prescribe this material for varying periods postoperatively, usually two weeks to four months. Discontinuation of all immunosuppressive drugs ultimately results in graft destruction.

Once rejection occurs, additional therapy is required (Table 17-12). Increased doses of steroids are prescribed. Massive, intermittent, intravenous doses of methylprednisolone appear to be especially effective. In addition, local graft irradiation may be of value in reversing the rejection process.

Nursing Aspects

Nurses should exercise unusual caution in calculating and administering immunosuppresive

TABLE 17-11
Prophylactic Immunosuppression for Renal
Transplantation at University of Minnesota

ANTILYMPHOBLAST GLOBULIN (ALG)

30 mg/kg IV daily for cadaver recipients for two weeks

20 mg/kg IV daily for related recipients for two weeks

AZATHIOPRINE (EVENING DOSE AFTER CHECKING LEUKOCYTE COUNT)

Preop dosage—5 mg/kg/day for two days

First and second postop days—5 mg/kg

Third through sixth postop days—4 mg/kg

Seventh postop day—3 mg/kg; maintain at 2-3 mg/kg

Adjust at all times with respect to WBC, platelet count, and renal function.

Caution: Reduce dosage to 1½ mg/kg for severe renal functional impairment

PREDNISONE

Related kidney:

0.25 mg/kg every six hours beginning 36 hours prior to transplant

First and second postop days—1 mg/kg/day

Third through sixth postop days—0.75 mg/kg/day

Seventh through ninth postop days—0.5 mg/kg/day

Reduce level slowly to achieve a maintenance dose of 0.15-0.25 mg/kg/day

Cadaver kidney:

0.5 mg/kg every six hours on first three postop days (total dose 2.0 mg/kg/day)

1.5 mg/kg/day for the next three days

1.0 mg/kg/day for three days

0.75 mg/kg/day for three days

0.5 mg/kg/day until discharge

Reduce dose slowly to achieve a maintenance dose of 0.3-0.4 mg/kg/day

METHYLPREDNISONE

20 mg/kg/day IV on evening of transplantation and on first two postop days

From Simmons, R. L. and Kjellstrand, C. M.: Kidney: technique, complications and results. In Najarian, J. S. and Simmons, R. L. (eds.): Transplantation. Philadelphia, Lea & Febiger, 1972, p. 460.

TABLE 17-12
Standard Antirejection Therapy at the University of Minnesota

THERAPY

Solu-Medrol—20 mg/kg/day IV × 3

Prednisone—2 mg/kg × 3 days

Then 1.5 mg/kg × 3 days

Then 1.0 mg/kg × 3 days

Thereafter reduce prednisone slowly to a maintenance dosage.

Azathioprine—Regulate dose to prevent leukopenia; do not increase

Irradiate kidney transplant—150 R every other day for three doses

From Simmons, R. L., and Kjellstrand, C. M.: Kidney: technique, complications, and results. In Najarian, J. S. and Simmons, P. L. (eds.): Transplantation. Philadelphia, Lea & Febiger, 1972, p. 470.

drugs. Special immunosuppressive order sheets are frequently printed (Fig. 17-19). In addition, patients are familiarized with medications including their appearance and doses, so that patients become responsible early in their course for recognizing and questioning alterations in medications and dosages. Cushingoid facies, acne, and hirsuitism in women are side effects of steroids distressing to all patients but especially to teenagers. Patients appreciate it when nurses and physicians take these problems seriously. (See Chapter 18, regarding the effects of Corticosteroid therapy.)

Patients are discharged from the hospital when optimal renal function has been achieved and operative wounds are satisfactorily healed, generally three to five weeks after operation. Following discharge, the patient assumes substantial responsibility for his own care (Table 17-13). The patient is seen frequently initially (even daily), then at increasing intervals as his drug dosages and renal function stabilize and he develops a sense of security and confidence at home. During outpatient visits blood is drawn for creatinine and leukocyte count, creatinine clearance is calculated, and the patient's progress is assessed by the transplant team. Later the same day, when laboratory values are available, the patient telephones the transplant clinic and drug doses are prescribed.

Complications Following Transplantation

A wide spectrum of morbidity has been reported in transplant patients. The increased susceptibility of these patients to complications is generally attributed to one or more of the immunosuppressive drugs, but severe preoperative debility and technical problems also contribute to morbidity.

Infectious processes are common, and unusual pathogens are frequently implicated. Pulmonary sepsis contributes significantly to mortality; its onset appears related to periods of increased immunosuppression with prednisone associated with rejection episodes. Opportunistic organisms underlying severe pneumonias have included Nocardia asteroides, Pneumocystis carinii, and Aspergillus fumigatus.

NAME _____

HUP No. _____ TELE. _____

DATE OF SURGERY _____

DATE	BLOOD		HEMATOLOGY			URINE		PROCEDURES				DRUG DOSAGE			ORDER BY
	BUN	Creat.	Hgb	Hct	WBC	Creat.	Cr. Cl.	BP	Wt.	In	Out	ALG	Imur.	Pred.	

FIGURE 17-19.
Immunosuppressive order sheet used at the Hospital of the University of Pennsylvania.

TABLE 17-13

General Home Instructions to Patient with Kidney Transplant (Hospital of University of Pennsylvania)

I. Hospital visits
 a. Daily at 9 A.M. until changed by your physician. You will be seen in the dialysis unit, 631 Maloney Building. Call 662-2646 if you anticipate being late.
 b. Weekly, on Tuesdays, come to 6 West Gates Building, no later than 8:30 A.M.
II. Bring to each Hospital visit:
 a. 24-hour urine collection
 b. Record of intake and output
 c. Record of weight
 d. Record of temperatures if required
 e. List of questions, problems and drugs needed.
III. Clinic
 a. Obtain a spot urine and label
 b. Measure 24-hour urine and label
 c. Call at 4 P.M. for drug order—662-2646.
IV. Home
 a. Avoid contact with all persons with colds, infections, and other illness
 b. Record daily intake and output
 c. Collect 24-hour urine
 d. Record weight, temperature, and blood pressure p.r.n.
 e. Keep a record of drugs:
  1. what drug
  2. when used
  3. how much used

Do not take any other drugs without consulting physician.

TAKE ALL DRUGS ONLY AS PRESCRIBED!!!

SERIOUS ILLNESS CAN RESULT FROM MISSING *ONE* DRUG DOSAGE!!
Call the dialysis unit, 662-2646 on weekdays if you have any problems or questions. Call the Hospital operator, 662-4000 at any time or when there is no answer in the unit and ask for the "transplant fellow on call." Never hesitate to call. Reasons for calling might be feeling generally poor, presence of an elevated temperature, decreased output, or discomfort in the area of your surgery.

The appearance of malignant neoplasms following transplantation occurs at a considerably greater rate than in the general population. The risk of developing lymphoma is about 35 times higher than normal and is derived almost entirely from a risk of reticulum cell sarcoma. The incidence of skin cancer is four times normal, and other cancers appear in men more than twice as often as expected. Women may not be at increased risk of these other cancers. Superficial carcinomas (e.g., skin, lip, cervix) respond to conventional surgical treatment. On the other hand, deep carcinomas in the body cavities as well as lymphomas have a poor prognosis. In these cases immunosuppression is drastically reduced or stopped even at the expense of the kidney in order to salvage the patient (Penn, 1971; Hoover, 1973). (See Chapter 22 *The Immune Process* for further discussion of tumors and altered immunity.)

Urologic morbidity has included bladder neck contracture, ureteral necrosis, ureteropelvic junction obstruction, ureterocutaneous fistula, and orchitis and epididymitis.

Aseptic necrosis, usually of the femoral head, is generally attributed to corticosteroid therapy. Cruess reported the occurrence of aseptic necrosis in ten of 27 patients who survived over six years.[26]

In an analysis of transplant recipients at the University of Cambridge, nearly 25 percent of patients suffered some gastrointestinal complication.[27] Immunosuppressed patients are at increased risk of acid-peptic disease, including hemorrhage and perforation. Colonic diseases reported in association with homografting include perforated sigmoid diverticulitis, pseudomembranous enterocolitis, ischemic colitis, fecal impaction, gangrenous appendicitis, and Candidiasis. Pancreatitis occurs in nearly 2 percent of recipients half of whom succumb to the disease.[28]

Ocular complications following transplantation include posterior subcapsular cataracts, acute cytomegalic retinitis, and steroid-induced glaucoma.

Results

One of several outcomes ensues following renal transplantation. Patients surviving may have grafts sustaining life with normal or somewhat impaired function. Other surviving patients may lose graft function and return to dialysis or be retransplanted. The remaining patients die.

In a recent report, the Human Renal Transplant Registry analyzed the results of 12,389 transplants carried out between 1951 and 1972.[29] Among 10,357 patients for which follow-up information is complete, 4,934 (47.6 percent) are alive with graft function; 1,880 (18.2 percent) are alive without graft function; and the remaining 3,543 (34.2 percent) are deceased. Among patients receiving transplants in 1972 from sibling, parent, or cadaver donors, patient survival at one year was 87.4 percent, 91.7 percent, and 71.8 percent, respectively. The corresponding figures for graft survival were 74.0 percent, 76.4 percent, and 45.4 percent (Table 17-14).

In an analysis of results following transplantation or dialysis at the Peter Bent Brigham Hospital, Lowrie and associates found that in comparing patient mortality rates, parental and sibling recipients did significantly better than cadaver recipients.[30] There was no significant

TABLE 17-14
Patient Survival and Transplant Function of First Transplant

YEAR OF TRANSPLANT	SAMPLE SIZE	ONE YEAR		TWO YEARS		THREE YEARS		FOUR YEARS		FIVE YEARS	
		% ALIVE	% FUNC-TIONAL	% ALIVE	% FUNC-TIONAL	% ALIVE	% FUNC-TIONAL	% ALIVE	% FUNC-TIONAL	% ALIVE	% FUNC-TIONAL
SIBLING											
1951-1966	243	68.5	64.1	62.2	57.3	58.5	53.1	56.1	49.3	54.1	46.2
1967	144	84.6	78.4	77.7	71.3	72.9	66.2	66.3	59.5	63.0	55.6
1968	193	89.0	81.3	83.8	75.5	81.4	72.3	77.6	66.2	71.4	59.4
1969	210	82.5	76.2	78.2	71.3	76.9	68.4	73.7	65.6	...	...
1970	259	87.1	82.5	85.0	79.1	82.5	73.3	...	...	...	...
1971	364	85.8	73.8	81.7	69.6	...	...	...	...	...	...
1972	202	87.4	74.0	...	...	...	...	...	...	...	...
PARENT											
1951-1966	403	61.2	56.4	56.6	50.2	52.9	45.4	51.0	42.7	50.4	40.7
1967	148	74.9	72.2	69.1	63.9	64.6	58.4	63.0	55.5	60.8	51.7
1968	201	79.2	72.5	75.2	67.3	71.0	61.0	66.5	52.8	66.5	51.4
1969	213	80.8	71.7	75.3	65.0	70.6	59.3	67.4	55.3	...	...
1970	246	84.9	74.2	80.5	68.6	79.2	63.2	...	...	...	...
1971	292	86.6	72.9	82.4	67.7	...	...	...	...	...	...
1972	155	91.7	76.4	...	...	...	...	...	...	...	...
CADAVER											
1951-1966	683	42.0	35.6	34.0	27.8	28.7	22.3	25.9	19.5	23.2	16.3
1967	395	56.0	45.3	49.1	38.7	44.7	33.9	40.3	29.1	39.3	26.6
1968	641	58.3	47.5	51.3	40.3	46.1	34.9	44.1	32.2	42.6	29.4
1969	839	66.2	54.9	59.9	47.7	55.2	42.0	53.6	39.7	...	...
1970	1,083	70.2	56.1	64.1	47.2	60.6	42.3	...	...	...	...
1971	1,390	69.6	52.8	64.7	46.6	...	...	...	...	...	...
1972	669	71.8	45.4	...	...	...	...	...	...	...	...

Source: JAMA 226:1197, 1973.

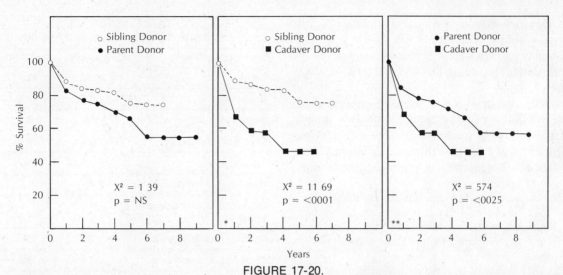

FIGURE 17-20.
Comparative Patient Survival Curves for Recipients of Cadaver, Parental and Sibling Allografts. X^2 indicates the significance of the difference between the total curves. *Yearly decrement significantly different (p<0.005); **yearly decrement significantly different (p<0.05). Source: Lowrie, E. G., et al: Survival of patients undergoing chronic hemodialysis and renal transplantation. New Eng. J. Med. *288*:863, 1973.

difference in survival among patients receiving grafts from parents or siblings (Fig. 17-20).

In addition, no significant difference between home dialysis patients and recipients of either sibling or parental grafts could be demonstrated in survival curves. Moreover, survival was statistically better in home dialysis patients than in recipients of cadaver transplants (Fig. 17-21).

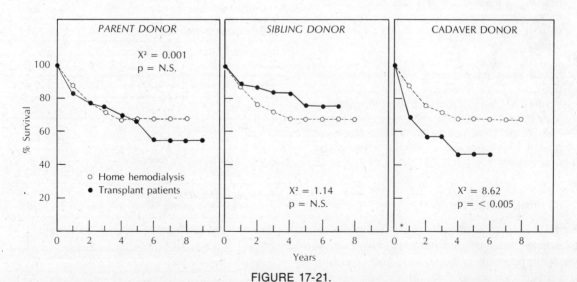

FIGURE 17-21.
Survival Curves Comparing Home-Dialysis Patients with Recipients of Cadaver, Parental and Sibling Transplants. X^2 indicates the significance of the difference between the total curves. *Yearly decrement significantly different (p<0.001). Source: Lowrie, E. G., et al.: Survival of patients undergoing chronic hemodialysis and renal transplantation. New Eng. J. Med. *288*:863, 1973.

Death following homografting may result from a variety of causes (Table 17-15) but infection plays a major role. Sepsis accounted for, or contributed to, death in 45.8 percent of cases analyzed.

Whereas survival is of supreme importance in the evaluation of a therapeutic modality, quality of life following treatment is also a critical parameter. It is here that transplantation has great potential. Statements by graft recipients illustrate this point:

> I now wake up each morning feeling that I can move mountains. I can now run instead of walking slowly; when my hematocrit was as low as ten to twelve (during dialysis) that was not possible. . . .
> My body has become normal in all respects again. My color is clear and rosy instead of muddy and grey. . . .[31]

> In chronic dialysis, the problem of the shunt, the twice or thrice-weekly dialyses and the time spent on it, the anxiety, and the cost, are problems which can be wiped off by a successful transplant.[32]

> Hemodialysis is a wonderful thing. . . . The machine makes life both possible and miserable. . . . All activities are scheduled around those eighteen hours of dialysis in the week. The salt-free diet limits what you can eat and drink. . . .[33]

> Seven years have passed since (transplantation). . . . Those years can be summarized by saying that I have indeed lived that normal life. I have been able to fulfill some dreams that I once had; I have returned to work, and have not missed a day because of illness in those last seven years.[34]

Outlook for the Future

Renal transplantation in its present state restores health to many uremic patients. However, immunosuppression is imperfect, and rejection is frequently unmanageable. Moreover, available immunosuppressants are nonspecific in the sense that they produce a generalized impairment of all immune defense mechanisms thereby subjecting recipients to a wide spectrum of morbidity.

TABLE 17-15
Causes of Death in Renal Transplant Recipients

Cause of Death	Frequency	% of Total
Sepsis	792	31.1
Unknown	325	12.8
Rejection	235	9.2
Rejection and sepsis	221	8.7
Technical	145	5.7
Unrelated to transplant	141	5.5
Gastrointestinal hemorrhage and ulceration	96	3.8
Myocardial infarction	96	3.8
Technical and sepsis	74	2.9
Cardiac arrest	58	2.3
Cerebrovascular accident	54	2.1
Immunosuppression	49	1.9
Pulmonary embolus	34	1.3
Cancer	32	1.3
Immunosuppression and sepsis	29	1.1
Pancreatitis	27	1.0
Rejection, technical and sepsis	23	0.9
Tubular necrosis	21	0.8
Rejection and technical	16	0.6
Rejection, immunosuppression and sepsis	16	0.6
Diffuse vasculitis	14	0.5
Hepatitis	13	0.5
Immunosuppression and technical	8	0.3
Immunosuppression, technical and sepsis	8	0.3
Rejection, immunosuppression, technical and sepsis	5	0.2
Rejection and immunosuppression	5	0.2
Subdural hematoma	3	0.1
Rejection, immunosuppression and technical	2	0.1
Liver failure	1	0.1

Source: JAMA 221:1496, 1972.

Production of host nonreactivity specific for donor histocompatibility antigens is a goal which holds promise for the future.

Procurement of donor organs is a present-day problem since demand outstrips the supply of donated tissue. Public education to encourage donation of organs is a reasonable approach. More exciting, however, is the prospect that elucidation of the immunobiology of heterografting will allow use of organs from other species for human benefit.

References for Part 3

1. Gibson, T. and Medawar, P. B.: The fate of skin homografts in man. J. Anat. 77:299, 1942-43.
2. Dixon, F. J., Talmage, D. W., and Maurer, P. H.: Radiosensitive and radioresistant phase in antibody response. J. Immunol. 68:693, 1952.
3. Moore, F. D.: Transplant: The Give and Take of Tissue Transplantation. New York, Simon & Schuster, 1972.
4. Schwartz, R. and Dameshek, W.: Effects of 6-mercaptopurine on homograft reactions. J. Clin. Invest. 39:952, 1960.
5. Groth, C. G.: Landmarks in clinical renal transplantation. Surg. Ob-Gyn. 134:323, 1972.
6. Starzl, T. E., Marchioro, T. L., and Waddell, W. R.: The reversal of rejection in human renal homografts with subsequent development of homograft tolerance. Surg. Ob-Gyn. 117:385, 1963.
7. Starzl, T. E., Porter, K. A., Iwasaki, Y., Marchioro, T. L., and Kashiwagi, N.: The use of heterologous antilymphocyte globulin in human renal homograft transplantation. In Wolstenholme, G. E. W. (ed.): Antilymphocyte Serum. Boston, Little, Brown, 1968.
8. Ninth Report of the Human Renal Transplant Registry. JAMA 220:253, 1972.
9. Simmons, R. L., Kjellstrand, C. M., Buselmeier, T. J., and Najarian, J. S.: Renal transplantation in high risk patients. Arch. Surg. 103:290, 1971.
10. Najarian, J. S., Simmons, R. L., Tallent, M. B., Kjellstrand, C. M., Buselmeier, T. J., Vernier, R. L., and Michael, A. F.: Renal transplantation in infants and children. Annals Surg. 174:538, 1971. Fine, R. N., Edelbreck, H. H., Brennan, L. P., Gruskin, C. M., Korsch, B. M., Riddell, H., Stiles, Q., and Lieberman, E.: Cadaveric renal transplantation in children. Lancet 1:1087, 1971. Woods, J. E., Anderson, C. F., Johnson, W. J., Donadio, J. V., Frohnert, P. P., Leary, F. J., DeWeerd, J. H., and Taswell, H. F.: Experiences with renal transplantation in high risk patients Surg. Ob-Gyn. 137:393, 1973.
11. Simmons, R. L., Kjellstrand, C. M.: Kidney: technique, complications, and results. In Najarian, J. S. and Simmons, R. L. (eds.): Transplantation. Philadelphia, Lea & Febiger, 1972.
12. Terasaki, P. I. and McClelland, J. D.: Microdrop assay of human serum cytotoxins. Nature 204:998, 1964.
13. Williams, G. M.: Transplantation. Surg. Ob-Gyn. 136:212, 1973.
14. *Ibid.*
15. Leary, F. J., and DeWeerd, J. H.: Living donor nephrectomy. J. Urol. 109:947, 1973.
16. Penn, I., Halgrimson, C. G., Ogden, D., and Starzl, T. E.: Use of living donors in kidney transplantation in man. Arch Surg. 101:226, 1970.
17. Opelz, G., Mickey, M. R., and Terasaki, P. I.: Identification of unresponsive kidney-transplant recipients. Lancet 1:868, 1972.
18. Currier, C. B., Pierce, J. C., and Hume, D. M.: Canine renal allograft rejection and antibody formation following blood transfusions. Surg. Forum 24:279, 1973.
19. Woods, J. E., DeWeerd, J. H., Johnson, W. J., Anderson, C. F.: Splenectomy in renal transplantation: influence on azathioprine sensitivity. JAMA 218:1430, 1971.
20. Robinson, Y.: Peritoneal dialysis for long-term maintenance. In Dialysis Symposium for Nurses, Philadelphia, 1969.
21. Starzl, T. E.: Experience in Renal Transplantation. Philadelphia, W. B. Saunders, 1964.
22. Najarian, J. S. and Simmons, R. L.: Clinical use of antilymphocyte globulin. New Eng. J. Med. 285:158, 1971.
23. Sheil, A. G. R., Mears, D., Johnson, J. R., Kelly, G. E., May, J., Ibels, L. S., and Stewart, J. H.: Antilymphocyte globulin in patients with renal allografts from cadaveric donors: late results of a controlled trial. Lancet 2:227, 1973.

24. Turcotte, J. G., Feduska, N. J., Haines, R. F., Frier, M. D., Gikas, P. W., MacDonald, F. D., Johnson, A. G., Morrell, R. M., and Thompson, N. W.: Antithymocyte globulin in renal transplant recipients: a clinical trial. Arch. Surg. 106:484, 1973.

25. Silberman, H., Barker, C. F., Henderson, L. W., Gardner, L., Murphy, J. J.: Functional ureteral obstruction and massive diuresis following renal homotransplantation. J. Urol. 108:858, 1972.

26. Cruess, R. L., Blennerhassett, J., MacDonald, F. R., MacLean, L. D., and Dossetor, J.: Aseptic necrosis following renal transplantation. J. Bone Joint Surg. 50A:1577, 1968.

27. Hadjiyannakis, E. J., Smellie, W. A. B., Evans, D. B., and Calne, R. Y.: Gastrointestinal complications after renal transplantation. Lancet 2:781, 1971.

28. Johnson, W. C. and Nabseth, D. C.: Pancreatitis in renal transplantation. Annals Surg. 171:309, 1970.

29. Eleventh report of the Human Renal Transplant Registry. JAMA 226:1197, 1973.

30. Lowrie, E. G., Lazarus, J. M., Mocelin, A. J., Bailey, G. L., Hampers, C. L., Wilson, R. E., and Merrill, J. P.: Survival of patients undergoing chronic hemodialysis and renal transplantation. New Eng. J. Med. 288:863, 1973.

31. West, D.: The world is a beautiful place. Transplant. Proc. 5:1077, 1973.

32. Lobo, L. H.: Experience of a physician-patient after renal transplantation. Transplant. Proc. 5:1081, 1973.

33. Rose, C. A., Jr.: Kidney transplant: a personal case history. Transplant. Proc. 5:1091, 1973.

34. Blackburn, W. W.: Survival with a living-related donor transplant. Transplant. Proc. 5:1093, 1973.

Further Reading

Abel, R. M., Abbott, W. M., and Fischer, J. E.: Intravenous essential L-amino acids and hypertonic dextrose in patients with acute renal failure. Effects on serum potassium, phosphate and magnesium. Am. J. Surg. 123:632, 1972.

Aldrete, J. A., O'Higgins, J. W., and Starzl, T. E.: Changes of serum potassium during renal homotransplantation. Arch. Surg. 101:82, 1970.

Bach, F. H. and van Rood, J. J.: The major histocompatibility complex—genetics and biology. New Eng. J. Med. 295:806, 1976.

Barker, C. F. and Billingham, R. E.: The role of afferent lymphatics in the rejection of skin homografts. J. Exptl. Med. 128:197, 1968.

Collins, G. M. and Halasz, N. A.: Forty-eight hour ice storage of kidneys: importance of cation content. Surgery 79:432, 1976.

Dudrick, S. J., Steiger, E., and Long, J. M.: Renal failure in surgical patients. Treatment with intravenous essential amino acids and hypertonic glucose. Surgery 68:180, 1970.

Hoover, R. and Fraumeni, J. F. Jr.: Risk of cancer in renal transplant recipients. Lancet 2:55, 1973.

Koidc, M. and Waud, B. E.: Serum potassium concentrations after succinylcholine in patients with renal failure. Anesthesiology 36:142, 1972.

Lazarus, J. M., Hampers, C. L., Bennett, A. H., Vandam, L. D., and Merrill, J. P.: Urgent bilateral nephrectomy for severe hypertension. Annals Int. Med. 76:733, 1972.

Mannick, J. A., Powers, J. H., Mithoefer, J., and Ferrebee, J. W.: Renal transplantation in uremic dogs. Surgery 47:34, 1961.

Montgomerie, J. Z., Kalmanson, G. M., and Guze, L. B.: Leukocyte phagocytosis and serum bactericidal activity in chronic renal failure. Am. J. Med. Sci. 264:385, 1972.

Patel, R., Merrill, J. P. and Briggs, W. A.: Analysis of results of kidney transplantation: Comparison in recipients with and without performed antileukocyte antibodies. New Eng. J. Med. 285:274, 1971.

Penn, I., Halgrimson, C. G., and Starzl, T. E.: De novo malignant tumors in organ transplant recipients. Transplant. Proc. 3:733, 1971.

Sadler, A. M. Jr. and Sadler, B. L.: Recent developments in the legal aspects of transplantation in the United States. Transplant. Proc. 3:293, 1971.

Strober, S. and Gowan, J. L.: The role of lymphocytes in the sensitization of rats to renal homografts. J. Exptl. Med. 122:347, 1965.

Strom, T. B. and Merrill, J. P.: Hepatitis B, transfusions and renal transplantation. New Eng. J. Med. 296:225, 1977.

Toledo-Pereyra, L. H., Simmons, R. L., Olson, L. C., and Najarian, J. S.: Perfusion time and the survival of cadaver transplants. Surgery 79:377, 1976.

Wilson, R. E., Hampers, C. L., Bernstein, D. S.,

Johnson, J. W., and Merrill, J. P.: Subtotal parathyroidectomy in chronic renal failure: a seven year experience in a dialysis and transplant program. Ann. Surg. 174:640, 1971.

Wilson, W. E. C., Kirkpatrick, C. H., and Talmage, D. W.: Suppression of immunologic responsiveness in uremia. Annals Int. Med. 62:1, 1965.

18

Nursing Intervention for Patients Receiving Corticosteroid Therapy

MARY EVANS MELICK

Effects and Uses of Corticosteroids ● Administration, Dosage and Choice of Agent ● Complications

There are so many preparations of corticosteroids being used in the treatment of so many maladies that one is reminded of the old-time patent medicine salesman's pitch: "It's good for what ails ya." For many individuals receiving corticosteroid therapy, this statement is true; however, these drugs are not without adverse effects which range from mild metabolic disturbances to death. The nurse is in continual contact with people receiving corticosteroid therapy, both inside and outside the hospital. She can assist them to maximize the therapeutic effects and to minimize the toxic effects of their drug therapy, if she is sufficiently knowledgeable about this group of drugs.

Approximately 30 steroid hormones have been isolated from the adrenal cortex. They are classified by their major metabolic effects on the body as: mineralocorticoids, glucocorticoids, and sex hormones. The mineralocorticoids, produced by the zona glomerulosa, are concerned with sodium and water retention and potassium excretion. Examples of mineralocorticoids are aldosterone and 11-desoxycorticosterone. The glucocorticoids, produced by the zona fasciculata, have many metabolic effects including those on carbohydrate metabolism. Examples of this group of hormones are cortisol and corticosterone. The sex hormones, produced by the zona reticularis, include androgens such as dehydroepiandrosterone and testosterone, estrogens such as estradiol, and progestins such as progesterone. The adrenal sex hormones are of importance when they are secreted in excess amounts or when they stimulate the growth of hormone-sensitive cancers.

Classification of hormones into the categories of mineralocorticoids and glucocorticoids is largely for the sake of convenience, because many hormones possess characteristics of both groups. For this reason, the majority of commonly used adrenal hormones can be thought of as existing on a continuum ranging from pure mineralocorticoids at one end to pure glucocorticoids at the other. Using this type of model, aldosterone would be an example of a mineralocorticoid; cortisone would occupy a position with both mineralocorticoid and glucocorticoid activity; dexamethasone would be an example of a glucocorticoid. The glucocorticoids, which are the subject here, are frequently called corticosteroids, anti-inflammatory steroids, and steroids.

The therapeutic use of the glucocorticioids is of relatively recent origin. In the early 1940s, they were used in the treatment of Addison's disease. In 1949, Hensch and his associates first used them for their pharmacological effects in the treatment of rheumatoid arthritis. Initially cortisone and cortisol, also known as hydrocortisone, were the preparations available. Because of their salt- and water-retaining effects, in addition to their glucocorticoid effects, these naturally occurring steroids were found to produce signs and symptoms of Cushing's syndrome. Since that time, many synthetic preparations of steroids have been introduced to increase the anti-inflammatory effect while decreasing the fluid-retaining potential. Other serious side effects of the steroids, once believed innocuous, have become apparent. In 1952, the first postoperative death due to steroid-induced adrenal suppression was reported. With the recognition of the relationship between steroid treatment and complications, such as peptic ulcer, there has been an increasing need for careful monitoring of the patient receiving steroid therapy.

Effects and Uses of Corticosteroids

Although the major effect of the glucocorticoids is on carbohydrate metabolism, there are many other effects which form the basis for the therapeutic use of the steroids. In general, this group of hormones:

1. Influences carbohydrate metabolism by antagonizing the action of insulin and by promoting gluconeogenesis. These actions increase the body's glucose pool.
2. Enhances protein breakdown and inhibits protein synthesis.
3. Increases the breakdown of fatty acids.
4. Influences defense mechanisms by suppressing inflammation, inhibiting scar tissue formation, blocking allergic responses, decreasing the number of circulating eosinophils and leukocytes, and decreasing the size of lymphatic tissue.
5. Exerts a permissive action on all effects caused by the catecholamines. Permissive action means

that the glucocorticoids allow the full expression of the effects of another hormone or system.
6. Exerts a permissive action on the functioning of the central nervous system. In this way they influence emotional functioning.
7. Inhibits the release of adrenocorticotropin-releasing factor by the hypothalamus and adrenocorticotropin by the anterior pituitary.

In general, when the glucocorticoids are present in physiological amounts, they give an organism the capacity to resist all types of noxious stimuli and environmental change. Selye proposed that when an organism encounters stress, the initial response is an alarm reaction in which the sympathetic nervous system is activated and the adrenal cortex discharges hormones. This stage is followed by a stage of resistance, during which the adrenal cortex accumulates a reserve supply of hormones. If the organism continues to be exposed to the stressor, the acquired adaptation is lost, and a stage of exhaustion follows.[1] Therefore, although the corticosteroids are essential for life and confer a capacity to resist stress, this capacity is not boundless.

In clinical medicine, the steroids are used in one of three ways:

1. In a *physiological* sense to correct deficiency, underfunction, or malfunction of a particular endocrine organ or system. An example is the administration of cortisone and fludrocortisone acetate in the management of Addison's disease.
2. As *diagnostic* aids to determine the adequacy of function of the endocrine system. For example, steroids such as dexamethasone can be used in the assessment of adrenal function.
3. In a *pharmacological* sense as a drug exerting effects upon the body which may be an exaggeration of its physiological effect or entirely new effects, not observed when only physiological amounts are used.[2]

Steroids are widely and most commonly used for their pharmacological effect. They have been used in the treatment of conditions with widely different etiologies, and in some conditions of unknown etiology. A partial list of their uses includes:

1. The prevention and treatment of cerebral edema.

2. The treatment of rheumatoid arthritis.
3. The treatment of acute rheumatic fever.
4. Treatment in connection with tuberculosis. Although the presence of tuberculosis generally constitutes a contraindication to glucocorticoid therapy, physicians have reported beneficial effects with the concurrent administration of corticosteroids and antituberculosis treatment. This is not a routine method of treatment, however, and corticosteroids are more frequently used in the treatment of complications such as tuberculosis meningitis.
5. The treatment of hematological disorders such as idiopathic thrombocytopenic purpura and leukemia.
6. The treatment of allergic diseases such as bronchial asthma, allergic rhinitis, and angioneurotic edema.
7. The treatment of dermatological disorders, especially when inflammation is prominent or allergy is an important factor. For example, steroids are useful in the treatment of neurodermatitis, discoid lupus erythematosus, and atopic dermatitis.
8. The treatment of ocular diseases such as conjunctivitis, uveitis, and choroiditis.
9. The treatment of collagen diseases, such as systemic lupus erythematosus, periarteritis nodosa, pemphigus, and dermatomyositis.
10. The treatment of the nephrotic syndrome.
11. The treatment of ulcerative colitis.
12. Use as an immunosuppressive agent in patients who are organ-transplant recipients.
13. Use in miscellaneous conditions such as shock, gout, multiple sclerosis, and ascites. In the latter condition it is used for its value as a diuretic, based on the ability of corticosteroids to increase the glomerular filtration rate.

Before treatment is instituted in patients who will be receiving long-term therapy, a number of diagnostic studies should be performed. These studies include a thorough medical history and physical examination, a glucose tolerance test, a tuberculin sensitivity study, and an upper gastrointestinal radiographic study. These studies help to determine such factors as the presence of peptic ulcers and diabetes mellitus, which may complicate or contraindicate drug therapy. It is important that the tuberculin sensitivity test be completed before therapy is begun because, following the administration of steroids, the patient's hypersensitivity to tuberculin may be suppressed. Further, if the sensitivity test is positive, the patient should receive antituberculous therapy (isoniazid) concomitantly with steroids. Thorn recommends that all patients who will be on long-term, high dosage therapy have an evaluation of their level of steroid secretion before treatment. The reasons for this suggestion are to: discover pituitary-adrenal hypofunction which will require life-long physiological doses of hormones, alert the physician to the need for high doses in patients with high levels of steroids, and help the physician determine to what extent pituitary-adrenal inactivation may be due to therapy.[3]

The patient should have an explanation of the procedures of the various tests and why he is receiving them. This responsibility may be assumed by the physician, delegated to the nurse, or be shared by both. The explanation must be geared to the individual patient's level of understanding and interest, but should communicate the feeling that the health team members are interested in the patient and wish to be certain that there is no reason why he cannot or should not receive steroid medication.

Administration, Dosage and Choice of Agent

Not all steroids are equally suited for administration to all patients. The choice of a medication will depend on whether mineralocorticoid effects are desired, such as in the treatment of Addison's disease, or not desired, such as in the treatment of a hypertensive asthmatic patient. The cost of the medication influences its usability. Cortisone, cortisol, and prednisone are less expensive for long-term use than the newer analogues such as dexamethasone. The route of administration will influence the choice, because not all preparations are equally well absorbed by all routes. The physician's experience with a drug also influences his choice.

Table 18-1 lists the commonly used corticosteroids and their usual dosages.

There is no set dosage of steroids which is

TABLE 18-1
Corticosteroid Drugs[*4]

NONPROPRIETARY OR OFFICIAL NAME	SYNONYM OR PROPRIETARY NAME	USUAL DOSAGE† AND DOSAGE RANGES
Betamethasone N.F.	Celestone	600 mcg to 4.8 mg daily, oral
Cortisone acetate N.F.	Cortogen; Cortone	Oral 25 mg 4 times daily; IM 100 mg daily
Dexamethasone N.F.	Decadron; Deronil; Decameth; Gammacorten; Hexadrol	500 mcg to 6 mg daily; 750 mcg 2 to 4 times daily
Dexamethasone sodium phosphate N.F.	Decadron phosphate	0.4 to 6 mg per local injection
Hydrocortisone U.S.P.	Cortisol; Cortef; Crotifoam; Cortril; Hydrocortisone, etc.	10 to 300 mg daily; oral 10 mg up to 4 times daily
Hydrocortisone acetate U.S.P.	Cortef acetate, etc.	10 to 50 mg intra-articular
Hydrocortisone cypionate	Cortef fluid	Initially 20 to 500 mg; maintenance 10 to 260 mg
Hydrocortisone sodium succinate U.S.P.	Solu-Cortef	50 to 300 mg daily IV or IM
Methylprednisolone sodium succinate N.F.	Solu-Medrol	10 to 40 mg daily IV or IM
Methylprednisolone N.F.	Medrol	Oral 4 mg 4 times daily or 2 to 60 mg daily
Paramethasone acetate	Haldrone	Oral 6 to 12 mg initially; 1 to 8 mg maintenance
Prednisolone U.S.P.	Delta-Cortef; Hydeltra; Meticortelone; Meti-Derm; Paracortol; Sterane; Sterolone	Oral 5 mg 1 to 4 times daily for 2 to 7 days; then 5 mg one or more times a day. Range: 5 to 80 mg daily
Prednisolone acetate U.S.P.	Sterane	5 to 50 mg intra-articular; 5 to 80 mg daily IM
Prednisolone sodium phosphate U.S.P.	Hydeltrasol	10 to 100 mg IM or IV
Prednisone U.S.P.	Deltasone; Deltra; Meticorten; Paracort	Initially 5 mg 2 to 4 times a day for 2 to 7 days; maintenance, up to 5 mg one or more times a day. Range: 5 to 80 mg daily
Triamcinolone	Aristocort; Kenacort	Initially 8 to 30 mg daily orally for adults; 4 to 16 mg daily for children; reduce for maintenance

*These drugs are administered orally or parenterally for systemic or intra-articular actions of an anti-inflammatory or anti-stress type. Other steroids and dosage forms are available for topical application and for mineralocorticoid activity.
†Dosages vary widely, depending on the nature and severity of the condition that is being treated.

suitable for all patients or for all patients with a similar condition. A recommended dosage for a postmenopausal woman with rheumatoid arthritis may be prescribed, but in reality a clinical bio-assay is conducted in each patient because of variations in response to corticosteroids. The nurse assists the physician in determining the proper dosage for each patient by observing and reporting therapeutic effects and side effects—for example, that it becomes easier for an arthritic patient to button a blouse. This professional function of the nurse is a form of monitoring.

The physician will determine the route of administration. However, the nurse should know the routes by which corticosteroids may be administered, the advantages and disadvantages of each, and the reason why a given route was chosen. Corticosteroids may be given for either local or systemic effects. They can be administered orally, parenterally, by inhalation, sublingually, rectally, or applied directly to the skin or mucous membranes. The local methods of administration are used to prevent systemic absorption and minimize complications, while enhancing the effectiveness of the medication at the site of administration. Examples of situations in which local methods of administration are of value are the treatment of circumscribed skin lesions, the treatment of inflammatory conditions of the anterior capsule of the eye, and injection into arthritic joints when only one or a few joints are affected.

Local administration is not without side effects. It has been noted that application of steroids to the skin in combination with occlusive dressings may, when applied for long periods to large areas, cause a decrease in plasma cortisol such as that noted with suppression of the hypothalamic-pituitary-adrenal system. Several studies of patients with chronic skin diseases who have used potent glucocorticoids for prolonged periods of time have shown little evidence of adrenal suppression.[5,6] However, it is well to bear in mind that some systemic absorption is increased when the integrity of the epidermis is disrupted, and the use of occlusive dressings may increase absorption because of in-

creased penetration of the medication due to increased temperature and humidity of the skin.[7] Systemic absorption with hypothalamic-pituitary-adrenal suppression may be more likely to occur in infants and small children, especially those in whom treatment involves a large proportion of the total body surface. The local administration of corticosteroids to the eye has been associated with complications such as corneal ulceration, an increase in intra-ocular pressure and herpetic infection of the eye. Recently introduced medrysone seldom produces a significant increase in intra-ocular pressure, although marked pressure increases can occur in some individuals.[8]

When a physician prescribes steroids for a patient, he may or may not indicate precisely the hour he wishes the medication given. The nurse should ask the physician about the desired effect of the medication and how this can be maximized. It may be desirable or necessary to maintain a blood level of a corticosteroid. In this instance, the dosage would be divided equally over a given period of time. In many cases it is desirable to simulate the normal circadian rhythm with the highest dosage in the early morning, tapering to lower doses in the evening. Many patients experience restlessness or insomnia if the last daily does is large or given late in the evening. Sleeplessness may be prevented by giving the last dose for the day no later than 6 P.M. If therapy is directed toward adrenocortical suppression to avoid excessive androgenicity, the last dose of steroids should be given as close to midnight as possible, inhibiting the increase in the activity of the pituitary-adrenal system, which normally occurs about 2 A.M.[9]

In 1963, Harter, Reddy, and Thorn published their studies on intermittent corticosteroid therapy. Based on the knowledge that the therapeutic effects of steroids last longer than the metabolic effects, they administered one dose of the medication every other day. The stated advantages of every-other-day therapy are a lower incidence of side effects, better maintenance of hypothalamic-pituitary-adrenal reserve function, and facilitation of transition to the withdrawal of corticosteroids.[10] Thorn noted that the escape of the body from elevated plasma steroid levels, for even brief periods, may help protect the hypothalamic-pituitary-adrenal system from structural deterioration. Thorn also believes that intermittent therapy, because of the periodic awareness of symptoms, increases the patient's understanding of his condition and the palliative, but not curative effects of his drug therapy.[11]

Patients on intermittent therapy frequently require explanations about the reason they will not be taking the medication every day. This is especially true in patients who experience an increase in discomfort or symptomatology shortly before the administration of the next dose of steroids. The patient will want to know why, if the medication is so effective in controlling the symptoms of his disease, he must be limited to taking it every other day. The nurse is frequently the person to whom this question is directed. She may wish to tell the patient about the lower incidence of side effects and encourage him to further discuss his feelings with the physician. She may need to reinforce the physician's instructions about taking the medication every other day, because the temptation to take an extra pill may be great.

The nurse will encounter several other situations in which she may be helpful to the patient receiving corticosteroids. The first situation concerns the patient who is being withdrawn from steroids or whose dosage is being reduced. The activity of the hypothalamic-pituitary-adrenal system can be restored in nearly everyone, even after years of continuous steroid treatment. The feedback responsiveness (that is, the ability to respond to low levels of corticosteroids by increasing the stimulation to the adrenal cortex) returns before the ability to respond to a stress situation with a sufficient increase in corticosteroids. The feedback responsiveness may take several months to return to normal, while the responsiveness to stress may require a year or longer. During the time the patient is being withdrawn from steroids, he is instructed to report to his physician any stress situation, physical or mental, which may require temporary coverage with steroids. Such situations include surgical procedures, death of a family member, or pregnancy. During the withdrawal period the patient's intrinsic level of steroid production may be monitored by determinations of the 11-hydroxycorticosteroid level in the urine. The patient should be instructed to save all his urine for 24 hours and should be told why this study will need to be done repeatedly.

Even though the period of withdrawal is gradual, a patient may experience symptoms such as muscular weakness, lethargy, and possibly exhaustion. These symptoms abate when the patient's adrenal cortex begins to produce higher levels of corticosteroids. The nurse observes and reports the patient's symptoms, while reassuring him that his symptoms are temporary.

When a patient's dosage of corticosteroids is reduced so that he experiences symptoms of his disease, the nurse may help him adjust to the new medication dosage by showing an understanding of his concern. She may also help by reinforcing the physician's explanation for the decrease in dosage. To facilitate patient understanding and compliance, the nurse may wish to do the same for the patient's family.

The second situation, involving the nurse as the dispenser of medications, concerns patients receiving continuous intravenous therapy. These patients may be pre- or postoperative, be in life-threatening situations, or have adrenal crisis. It is imperative that the physician's schedule for the administration of the medication be followed precisely. This may involve determining the rate of flow necessary to administer a given amount of medication and fluid within a given time. It involves careful monitoring of the flow of the solution. Any abnormality of flow must be promptly remedied.

Monitoring the administration of intravenous fluids was very important in the care of Mr. M., a patient with a long history of ulcerative colitis. He was admitted to the hospital with frequent episodes of diarrhea, weakness, and dehydration. For several weeks he received intravenous infusions containing vitamins and hydrocortisone as part of his therapy. Although he was better hydrated at the end of this time, he continued to be anorexic, to lose weight, and to have frequent episodes of diarrhea. A colectomy was planned, and the physician ordered several days of intravenous fluids, to which varying amounts of hydrocortisone were to be added, in order to prepare Mr. M. to withstand the stress of surgery. The intravenous fluids seldom ran properly, due to clogging or dislodging of the needle or catheter and to the patient's restlessness. Consequently, the patient was not receiving the scheduled amounts of hydrocortisone at the proper times. Some intramuscular doses of corticosteroids were given to try to maintain the schedule. Mr. M. underwent surgery on the day planned. About 12 hours after surgery, while in the intensive care unit, Mr. M. became very restless and hypotensive. He responded poorly to vasopressor and corticosteroid therapy and died on the second postoperative day. The cause of death was adrenal crisis. Although this is an extreme example, it illustrates the importance of the nurse as a monitor of intravenous corticosteroid therapy. The nurse could have increased the efficiency of monitoring the administration of steroids simply by removing Mr. M. closer to the nurses' station where the intravenous flow could be checked more easily and quickly. It also illustrates the importance of continued communication between nurse and physician concerning the progress of medication administration.

Patients with known adrenal hypofunction due to Addison's disease, adrenalectomy, or iatrogenic suppression must be carefully observed for signs and symptoms of adrenal crisis. The nurse is alert for: hypotension, restlessness, severe weakness, lethargy, headache, dehydration, nausea, vomiting, or diarrhea.

Complications

It is the pharmacological, not the physiological, dose which results in side effects. Approximately 20 mg. of cortisol are secreted by the adrenal cortex daily. Doses of steroids larger than the equivalent of this amount of cortisol are considered pharmacological doses. (See Table 18-2 for common dose equivalents.) These side effects represent an exaggeration of the physiological functions of the steroids. For example, insulin antagonism and gluconeogenesis may eventually result in steroid diabetes. Indeed, the side effects of corticosteroid therapy may be more of an inconvenience and hazard to the patient than his initial pathology.

The side effects may be divided into those resulting from mineralocorticoid and those resulting from glucocorticoid activity. Side effects resulting from mineralocorticoid activity are weight gain, edema, hypertension resulting from sodium and water retention, weakness, fatigue, and alkalosis resulting from potassium depletion. Examples of side effects resulting from glucocorticoid activity are osteoporosis, steroid diabetes, exacerbation of tuberculosis, and masking of infections. The side effects resulting from mineralocorticoid activity have been virtually eliminated by the use of the newer synthetic steroids, such as triamcinolone. It has been impossible to separate the desired therapeutic effects of the steroids from the side effects resulting from glucocorticoid activity. For information on the relative anti-inflammatory and sodium retaining potencies of commonly used corticosteroids, see Table 18-3. In this table hydrocortisone (cortisol) has arbitrarily been assigned a value of 1; the other preparations receive relative values as a result of comparison with cortisol. This table is a valid measure of comparison only when oral or intravenous routes are used.

The nurse can play a major role in the detection and prevention of complications. In assessing the effects of treatment with steroids, there are no sensitive machines, such as cardiac monitors, to supply constant information. This

TABLE 18-2
Common Equivalents of Selected Corticosteroids[12]

Steroid	Dosage in Mg
Cortisone	25
Hydrocortisone	20
Prednisolone	5
Prednisone	5
Methylprednisolone	4
Triamcinolone	4
Paramethasone	2
Betamethasone	0.75
Dexamethasone	0.75

TABLE 18-3
Relative Anti-inflammatory and Sodium Retaining
Potencies of Some Corticosteroids[13]

COMPOUND	RELATIVE ANTI-INFLAMMATORY POTENCY	RELATIVE SODIUM RETAINING POTENCY
Cortisol	1	1
Cortisone	0.8	0.8
Prednisone	3.5	0.8
Prednisolone	4	0.8
6 α-Methylprednisolone	5	0
Triamcinolone	5	0
Paramethasone	10	0
Betamethasone	25	0
Dexamethasone	25	0
9 α-Flurocortisol	15	125

lack increases the importance of the human monitor. The nurse who is in continual contact with the patient in the hospital, and who may see him as an outpatient in a clinic or in his home, is in a good position to monitor the patient's progress. The nurse assesses, records, and reports the effects of treatment to the physician. To do this she must be familiar with the common problems encountered in corticosteroid therapy and the appropriate measures for preventing these problems.

The undesirable effects of steroid therapy can easily be recalled if they are categorized according to systems. The glucose pool of the body is increased by gluconeogenesis and insulin antagonism. This results in hyperglycemia, glucosuria, and decreased carbohydrate tolerance. In some patients steroid diabetes results. This type of diabetes is characterized by a marked decrease in the sensitivity to insulin and by reversibility when steroid treatment is discontinued. The nurse remains alert for symptoms of diabetes. If visiting a patient in his home, especially if he neglects regular checkups by a physician, the nurse may wish to test his urine for glucose. (See Chapter 15.)

Corticosteroids affect protein metabolism producing a negative nitrogen balance. This is responsible, in part, for the catabolic effects of therapy. Preventing or decreasing negative nitrogen balance may be accomplished by a high protein, high carbohydrate diet.

An unknown mechanism is responsible for the characteristic adiposity of Cushing's syndrome, which occurs in some patients treated with steroids. Patients may develop moon facies, trunchal obesity, and a buffalo hump.

Patients receiving corticosteroids which possess mineralocorticoid effects may experience sodium retention and potassium depletion with edema, weight gain, and metabolic alkalosis. The physician may prescribe a diet restricted in sodium. The nurse can help the patient in planning menus. The patient can be encouraged to increase his potassium intake by selecting foods high in potassium such as fruit and fruit juices. Lemon juice, for example, has the double advantage of being high in potassium and low in sodium. The nurse should routinely check the patient's blood pressure and weight, and note any evidences of edema in patients receiving corticosteroids with mineralocorticoid effects. When sodium and water retention are a problem, the nurse avoids the use of saline as a diluent when preparing injectable medications.

Corticosteroid therapy causes atrophy of the zona reticularis and zona fasciculata of the adrenal cortex. The hypothalamic-pituitary-adrenal system becomes unable to respond to stress. Therefore, all patients on long-term steroid therapy, whether on physiological doses or pharmacological doses, should carry an identification card stating their physician's name, the medication they are taking, and instructions for emergency treatment. Since the patient will no longer be able to respond appropriately to stress, the physician instructs him on the adjustment of dosage in stress situations. The nurse reinforces the physician's explanation. She can also assist the patient to identify stressors and discuss ways of modifying or avoiding stress. Many individuals do not think of extremes in temperature or minor infections as stressors, and the nurse can help the patient become more aware of the multitude of stressors which affect him daily.

The musculoskeletal system is affected by steroid therapy, and muscular weakness, partly a result of potassium depletion, may be a prominent symptom. Also, the increased output of calcium and phosphorus may cause osteoporosis, or may intensify already existing osteoporosis. Pathologic fractures may occur. The occurrence of osteoporosis depends on the age, sex, and physical disability of the patient. Post-menopausal women are most prone to osteoporosis. A diet high in calcium and protein may help to prevent or alleviate osteoporosis. Since calcium leaves the bones more readily in an inactive than in an active individual, the nurse will encourage activity. Range-of-motion exercises are helpful in bedfast patients. The nurse and the patient discuss safety measures for use at home and in the hospital to decrease the possibility of fracturing a bone.

In patients taking corticosteroids there is an altered response to injury, regardless of the inciting cause. Steroids interfere with the function of fibroblasts, granulation tissue, and ground substance.[14] They impair the growth of blood vessels into new tissue. If the patient is postoperative or injures himself, wound healing is delayed. An example of this is Mrs. G., a patient who had an abdominal hysterectomy. She had received large doses of hydrocortisone both before and after surgery because of an isolated adrenocorticotropin deficiency. In addition, she was obese and had been placed on a diet restricted in calories. She appeared to be doing well postoperatively and ambulated on the first postoperative day without difficulty. On the fifth postoperative day, as she lay in bed, she experienced a strange sensation, and looking down, noticed a wound dehiscence. She was returned to the operating room for closure. This case illustrates the importance of regular examinations by physician or nurse to determine the progress of healing in surgical or traumatic wounds. A word of caution to the patient about the prevention of trauma may be very beneficial.

Some patients receiving steroid therapy develop or aggravate an existing peptic ulcer. In one study of terminal cancer patients, 2 percent of those not receiving steroids and 10 percent of those receiving steroids developed peptic ulcers. In 11 of the 18 persons who developed ulceration while taking steroids, the ulcer was the major cause of death.[15] Corticosteroids cause an increase in hydrochloric acid secretion. They also

appear to have an inhibitory effect on the secretion of mucus by the gastric antrum.[16] These ulcers heal very slowly because of the anti-inflammatory and catabolic effects of steroids. As a preventive measure, the physician may order the steroid to be taken with an antacid or the patient may be placed on an ulcer diet prophylactically and may receive anticholinergic drugs. The nurse may suggest taking the steroid with food or milk. The nurse assesses the patient's food tolerance and habits, and is alert for epigastric pain. Blood in the feces or emesis may be the first sign of ulceration. A specimen should be retained, and the physician notified promptly. Periodic radiological examination of the upper gastrointestinal tract and stool examination for occult blood may be beneficial in identifying early ulceration. Any patient with a history of peptic ulceration must be observed closely for recurrence and perforation.

Some patients experience an increase in appetite which may contribute to weight gain. In some this is a desirable side effect, while in others it is not. The nurse may need to guide the patient in choosing low calorie menus if weight gain is undesirable. Such guidance was necessary in the case of the S. family. Scott, age three and one-half, was recently diagnosed as having acute lymphocytic leukemia. He was sent home from the hospital with a bewildering array of medications including prednisone. The high doses of the steroid resulted in a greatly increased appetite, and Scott consumed so much food, especially snack food, that he became obese, and walking became difficult for him. Still he managed to steal food from the refrigerator and went from door to door begging cookies which were freely given since the neighbors felt sorry for him. Noting this situation, a nurse neighbor visited Mrs. S. and helped her to plan a schedule of medication administration to decrease gastric discomfort and insomnia. Medication was given with meals whenever possible or with applesauce or milk as a snack. The pills mixed with applesauce were easily swallowed and provided a midafternoon snack. Menus and substitute low calorie snack foods such as celery and cheese were suggested. Skim milk was alternated with whole milk. The importance of exercise was stressed, and nearby neighbors were advised about substitute snack food. The plan worked very well and is implemented prophylactically by Mrs. S. whenever Scott is placed on a periodic course of prednisone.

Corticosteroids may cause thinning of skin, the appearance of purple-red striae, acne, and hirsutism. The patient beginning therapy should be encouraged to report any unusual changes in his skin to his physician.

Corticosteroids increase the excitability of the central nervous system, and convulsive seizures, especially in children, may occur. Patients may experience alterations in their moods. Some patients are euphoric, others become depressed, restless, or psychotic. Weird dreams and withdrawal from social contact are symptoms for which the nurse is alert. These should be reported to the physician as should all references to suicide. The nurse should protect the patient from individuals and situations which are upsetting and act as a buffer between the patient and his environment.

The patient taking corticosteroids has an altered blood count. The eosinophils and reticulocytes are decreased while the number of red blood cells is increased, especially in anemic persons. Some patients experience an increased incidence of thrombophlebitis. Nursing measures such as the prevention of stasis by proper positioning and exercises should be employed. Because of the decrease in lymphocytes, the patient is more susceptible to infections. Signs and symptoms of infection, such as fever, heat, redness, pain, and swelling, may be masked by steroids. The nurse takes precautions to limit the patient's contact with infectious agents. This includes encouraging the patient to avoid contact with crowds and persons known to have infections, and using meticulous sterile technique when performing procedures as well as faithfully practicing handwashing between patients. Some patients, such as those receiving cancer chemotherapy and those with organ transplants (see Chapter 17) receiving immunosuppressive therapy are especially prone to infections. If placed on corticosteroid therapy, reverse isolation may be required to prevent life-threatening infections.

Some patients receiving corticosteroids, experience alterations in the function of their cardiovascular system. Hypertension and ecchymoses are the most common problems. Coronary occlusion may occur with the cessation of steroid therapy.

With the introduction of more potent anti-inflammatory steroids, new side effects have become apparent. Some of the complications in which these new drugs play a role are: avascular necrosis of bone, cataracts, acute pancreatitis, the development of subcutaneous fatty tumors, arthropathy of the hip, and fat embolism.[17]

Several roles of the nurse have been stressed: dispenser of medications, monitor, and preventor of complications. Another important role is that of assessor and planner of nursing care. Assessment of the patient begins on the first contact between nurse and patient. Using observation and interview, the nurse gathers information from the patient, from the medical records and from others such as members of the health team, the patient's family and friends. The goal is to formulate a pertinent nursing care plan. It is essential that the nurse know which of her patients have received or are receiving corticosteroids. This alerts her to possible complications. When the nurse requests information about medicines which have been taken, it may be necessary to review all the brand names of the commonly used corticosteroids. The patient may not know that the question, "Have you ever taken cortisone?" may also refer to dexamethasone, prednisone, and others. If the patient has taken a corticosteroid within one year, this fact should be prominently displayed on the care plan and in the patient's chart. Before the patient undergoes any surgical procedure, the nurse must be certain that the physician knows about past steroid therapy. Preoperative preparation with steroids may prevent fatalities.

The nurse will want to know why the patient is receiving a corticosteroid, and the dosage and route of administration of the drug. These are factors which will influence the plan of care and alert the nurse to specific problems which may arise. She may wish to systematically assess the patient using a tool, such as McCain's *Guide to the Functional Ability of a Patient,*[18] or to devise a personal guide using the major areas discussed under complications. Periodic reassessment would then indicate the changes which have taken place which require a change in the plan of medical and/or nursing care.

Finally, we come to the role of the nurse as a teacher. This is quite possibly the most important role. It is essential that the patient and his family understand what medication he is receiving, why he is receiving it and what effects are desired. They must know what complications could occur, what to do if a complication does occur, and how to prevent complications. They must understand the relationship between stress and the amount of steroid required by the body. The patient must be instructed never to let anyone else take his medication. He must know that, in his contact with a physician or nurse unfamiliar with his care, he should report that he has been receiving corticosteroids.

This information is complex and unfamiliar to the patient, and yet his well-being depends on his understanding of it. The information given to the patient must be given when he is ready to receive it. The day the patient receives confirmation that he has lupus erythematosus, or the day of discharge, are poor choices for teaching. Teaching should be spread over several days, if possible, and should include review and time for questions. The patient should play an active role in his learning. When possible, someone close to the patient should also be instructed, in case the patient becomes unable to care for himself. In all contacts with the patient the nurse should repeatedly stress the importance of regular care by a physician.

In summary, there are many preparations of corticosteroids available for use. These drugs are beneficial in the treatment of a wide variety of clinical problems. They are, however, capable of producing side effects as dangerous, or more so, as the patient's disease. The nurse, through the performance of roles as dispenser of medication, monitor, preventer of complications, assessor and planner of nursing care, and teacher, can assist in maximizing the therapeutic effects while minimizing the untoward effects of corticosteroid therapy.

References

1. Selye, H.: The Stress of Life. New York, McGraw-Hill, 1956, pp. 31-33.
2. Rasmussan, H.: Organization and control of the endocrine system. *In* R. H. Williams (ed.): Textbook of Endocrinology, ed. 5. Philadelphia, W. B. Saunders, 1974, p. 30.
3. Thorn, G. W. : Clinical considerations in the use of corticosteroids. New Eng. J. Med. 274:777, Apr. 7, 1966.
4. Rodman, M. J. and Smith, D. W.: Pharmacology and Drug Therapy in Nursing. Philadelphia, J. B. Lippincott, 1968.
5. Munro, D. D. and Clift, D. C.: Pituitary-adrenal function after prolonged use of topical corticosteroids. Brit. J. Derm. 88:381-385, Apr. 1973.
6. Wilson, L., Williams, D. I. and Marsh, S. D.: Plasma corticosteroid levels in out-patients treated with topical steroids. Brit. J. Derm. 88:373-380, Apr. 1973.
7. Munro and Clift, *op cit.*
8. Medrysone: a review. Drugs 2:5-19, 1971.
9. Forsham, P.: The adrenal cortex. *In* R. H. Williams (ed.): Textbook of Endocrinology, ed. 3. Philadelphia, W. B. Saunders, 1968, p. 374.
10. Harter, J. G., Reddy, W. J. and Thorn, G. W.: Studies on intermittent corticosteroid dosage regimen. New Eng. J. Med. 269:591-596, Sept. 19, 1963.
11. Thorn, G. W.: The adrenal cortex. Johns Hopkins Med. J., 123:73, July 1968.
12. Hayes, R. C., Jr., and Larner, J.: Adrenocorticotropic hormone; adrenocortical steroids and their synthetic analogs; inhibitors of adrenocortical steroid biosynthesis. *In* L. S. Goodman and A. Gilman (eds.): The Pharmacological Basis of Therapeutics, ed. 5. New York, Macmillan, 1975, p. 1499.
13. *Ibid.,* p. 1491.
14. Frohman, I. P.: The adrenocorticoids. Am. J. Nurs., 64:121, Nov. 1964.
15. Schell, H. W.: Adrenal corticosteroid therapy in far advanced cancer. Geriatrics 27:131-141, Jan. 1972.

16. Glenn, F. and Grafe, W. R.: Surgical complications of adrenal steroid therapy. Ann. Surg., 165:1030, June 1967.
17. Beckman, H. (ed.): Yearbook of Drug Therapy—1969. Chicago, Year Book Medical Publishers, Inc., 1969, p. 221.
18. McCain, R. F.: Nursing by assessment—not intuition. Am. J. Nurs. 65:82-84, Apr. 1965.

Bibliography

Arman, E., et al: Calcium retention and skeletal calcium uptake in asthmatic subjects. Acta Allerg. 25:456-474, Dec. 1970.

Criep, L. H. : Corticoid therapy in chronic obstructive pulmonary disease. Geriatrics 28:111-115, Jan. 1973.

Danowski, T. S.: Answers to questions on adrenocorticoids. Hosp. Med. 4:33-37, Apr. 1968.

Eisen, A. A. and Norris, J. W.: Adrenal steroid therapy in neurologic disease. Canad. Med. Assoc. J., 100, Part I:27-30 Jan. 4, 1969, and Part II:66-70 Jan. 11, 1969.

Goodman, D. H.: Systemic fungal infection complications in asthmatic patients treated with steroids. Ann. Allerg. 31:205-208, Apr. 1973.

Goodman, L. S. and Gilman, A. (eds.): The Pharmacologic Basis of Therapeutics, ed. 5. New York, Macmillan, 1975.

Kehlet, H. and Binder, C.: Value of an ACTH test in assessing hypothalamic-pituitary-adrenocortical function in glucocorticoid treated patients. Brit. J. Med. 2:147-149, Apr. 21, 1973.

Kenny, F. M.: Clinical observations on the use of adrenal steroids. Clin. Ped. 11:395-402, July 1972.

Klevit, H.: Corticosteroid therapy in the neonatal period. Ped. Clin. North Am. 17:1003-1013, Nov. 1970.

Medansky, R. S. and Handler, R. M.: New steroid aerosol in dermatoses: a double-blind multicentric analysis. Southern Med. J. 65:855-858, July, 1972.

Quintero, J. M., Wymer, B. and Glass, D. D.: A more rapid route of administration of corticosteroids in bronchial asthma. Ann. Allerg. 26:501, Sept. 1968.

Rodman, M. J. and Smith, D. W.: Pharmacology and Drug Therapy in Nursing. Philadelphia, J. B. Lippincott, 1968.

Smith, R. A. and W. A.: Steroid therapy of cerebral edema. J. Med. Ass. Ga. 56:324-328, Aug. 1967.

Soika, C. V.: Combating Osteoporosis. Am. J. Nurs. 73:1193-1197, July 1973.

Statement by the Committee on Therapy of the American Thoracic Society. Adrenal corticosteroids and tuberculosis. Am. Rev. Resp. Dis. 97:484-485, Mar. 1968.

Vetten, K. B.: Steroids, antibiotics, sulphonamides and the anaesthetist. South African J. Surg. 8:41-51, Apr.-June 1970.

Wheeler, C. E., Jr., Briggaman, R. A. and Puritz, E. M.: Corticosteroids in the treatment of skin disorders. Am. Fam. Physician 7:130-140, Jan. 1973.

19

Nursing Implications in the Care of the Patient Experiencing Sensory Deprivation

JUDITH DEIGNAN WORRELL

Sensory and Cognitive Effects of Sensory Deprivation ● Sensory Deprivation Research ● Clinical Sensory Deprivation ● Nursing Implications ● Summary

Man exists in a state of tension. He is seeking a balance between the stimulation of continuous sensory input from an ever-changing environment and his responses which continuously modify his relationship with this environment.

Man is unique in his capacity to adapt to the multi stimuli from his internal and external environment. In fact, he appears to be dependent upon a certain amount of stimuli for his sense of well-being. The continuous stimulation and his subsequent responses provide him with the assurance that he can exert control over himself and that his basic needs will be met.

This adaptive capacity, which is usually taken for granted, varies from individual to individual, and, at times, in the same individual depending upon his physiological and psychological needs. In addition, continuous bombardment of stimuli as well as continued deprivation of stimuli may threaten the survival of even the most "fit" individual. Not only is man unable to tolerate extensive periods of inactivity, he also experiences hunger for stimulation and change.[1] It is becoming apparent that monotony is objectionable not only because of the boredom it brings about, but because it can become an etiological agent for various types of mental disorders. This reduction of incoming stimuli has been termed sensory deprivation.

There is increasing evidence to support the theory that reduced stimulation has deleterious effects on human beings.[2] Various types of mental aberrations commonly occur among prisoners in solitary confinement or among otherwise normal people isolated during arctic and space explorations, within fallout shelter confines, and even among pilots in the course of prolonged, monotonous air travel. In addition, physiological and mental disturbances have been associated with the monotony of automated work and dial-watching tasks such as observing radar screens. Although the responses to reduced sensory input differ from one individual to another, certain manifestations of this reduced input are common enough to invite generalization. These include abnormalities in feeling states, deterioration of the ability to think, perceptual distortions, vivid imagery, illusions, and hallucinations.

The syndrome of sensory deprivation is a relatively new concept for nurses; yet over a century ago Florence Nightingale included a chapter in her book *Notes on Nursing* titled "Variety."

> Little as we know about the way in which we are affected by form, by colour, and light, we do know this, that they have an actual physical effect. . . . It is an ever recurring wonder to see educated people, who call themselves nurses, acting thus. They vary their own objects . . . and while nursing(!) some bed-ridden sufferer, they let him lie there staring at a dead wall, without any change of object to . . . vary his thoughts. . . .[3]

Upon reflection it seems obvious, as it did to Florence Nightingale, that persons who are clinically ill are more susceptible than the average human being to changes in sensory input. In many cases, the illness itself may reduce the efficiency of the sense organs. In other cases, the therapeutic routine may bring about reduced or intensified sensory stimulation to which the individual may or may not be able to adapt.

Much of the aberrant behavior characteristic of persons who are sensorily deprived can and should be anticipated. If these contributing factors can be identified and modified, such behavior might be minimized. This chapter will highlight some of the research investigations in the field of sensory deprivation, discuss the sensory and cognitive effects of sensory deprivation and the terminology employed by the investigators, and emphasize the application of research findings to the clinical situation. However, identification of nursing implications which may alter sensory input or reduce sensory deprivation is the primary goal of this chapter.

Sensory and Cognitive Effects of Sensory Deprivation

TERMINOLOGY

An understanding of research in sensory deprivation is hampered by the absence of a standard terminology. The many ambiguous terms coined by different investigators cloud the significance of findings and make comparison of data difficult. Although the term "sensory deprivation" is often used, there is, in fact, no unequivocal term to describe this field of research. Thus, clarification of the more common terms is necessary. Basically, there are five main avenues of scientific investigation at present, each of which has its own terminology.[4]

1. REDUCTION OF STIMULUS INPUT VARIABLES. The term "sensory deprivation" is most frequently employed with reference to this avenue of investigation. As noted previously, sensory deprivation is defined as an absolute reduction in variety and intensity of sensory input, with or without a change in pattern. Thus, an environment of silence and darkness would be an example of sensory deprivation.

2. REDUCTION OF STIMULUS VARIABILITY. Absence or reduction of stimulus variability is called "perceptual deprivation" or "perceptual isolation." This occurs when the quantity of stimuli from the environment remains constant but there is reduced patterning, imposed structuring, and homogeneous stimulation. An environment in which sound is muffled (white noise), light is diffused, and bodily sensations are nondistinct is one of perceptual deprivation.

Sensory deprivation and perceptual deprivation have been compared to determine which is more stressful to the individual. Marvin Zuckerman reported that while neither sensory deprivation nor perceptual deprivation seems more stressful, as measured by endurance or verbal reports, perceptual deprivation seems to produce a more extensive cognitive and perceptual impairment than does sensory deprivation.

Body confinement, resulting in perceptual deprivation, was found to be quite stressful, producing bodily discomfort and thinking difficulties. The major source of subjective stress produced by sensory or perceptual deprivation appears to stem from the loss of contact with reality. The individual experiences a confusion of internal and external sensations, an increase in primary process thinking, and disorientation in space and mind.[5]

3. SOCIAL ISOLATION. Social isolation refers to isolation from people and from a familiar environment. An environment of social isolation includes some perceptual deprivation because of the reduced or nonstructured auditory stimuli as-

sociated with the isolated conditions. In an experimental setting, subjects are not entirely socially isolated. They know that they can be heard through the intercom system and can terminate the experiment at will. Consequently, the true effects of social isolation in the clinical situation have yet to be determined.

4. CONFINEMENT. Confinement refers to motor restriction and is often called "immobility." It is difficult to discuss the effects of confinement exclusively, because studies involving sensory input reduction, variability reduction, and isolation have also involved some degree of confinement and vice versa.

The effects of confinement in the laboratory have been compared with those of sensory and perceptual deprivation. Zuckerman and Persky concluded that: 1) most of the stress of sensory deprivation, including adrenal-medullary responses and verbally reported stress, is produced by confinement alone, without sensory or social isolation; 2) social isolation, even without sensory deprivation, produces more contemplative responses, dreams, memories, and reports of inefficiencies of directed thinking than confinement with social stimulation; and 3) sensory deprivation produces more reports of visual and auditory sensations or imagery, dreams, and feelings of unreality than social isolation.[6] Therefore, confinement to a bed in a small cubicle for about eight hours produces generalized stress relative to a normal environment. Social isolation would add to this stress an increase in unstructured cognitive activity, and the addition of sensory deprivation would yield the feeling of a loss of touch with reality and the emergence into consciousness of hallucinations and fantasies (primary process-thinking).

5. INCREASED SENSORY INPUT. "Sensory stimulation," "sensory bombardment," or "sensory overload" are the terms most frequently used in discussing this avenue of research. Sensory overload refers to the presence of multisensory experiences which act simultaneously and at levels of intensity greater than normal. It can be readily deduced that the individual experiencing sensory overload is also experiencing a type of sensory deprivation, as certain stimuli are reduced or absent in the presence of greater intensity of others (see Chapter 10.)

The findings of Davis, McCourt, and Solomon, who investigated the role of sensory stimulation, appear to be applicable to clinical sensory deprivation situations. These authors first produced an environment of sensory deprivation and then introduced a variety of visual stimuli. Essentially the same mental aberrations occurred in the latter environment as occurred in the deprivation states. They hypothesized that it is not the absence of sensory stimulation per se; but the absence of *meaningful* stimulation which produces the effects of sensory deprivation. It appears that it may not be the quantity or change in sensation that the brain requires for normal functioning, but a continuous, meaningful contact with the outside world.[7] It may well be this lack of meaningful stimuli that contributes to the behavioral manifestations which occur in situations of sensory overload.

Sensory Deprivation Research

During the past several years, many investigators have reproduced the effects of altered sensory input using volunteers in the laboratory. The general technique consists of placing healthy individuals in environments in which they are isolated from sensory stimuli or from patterned visual or auditory perceptions. In this context, the term "patterned stimuli" refers to the rhythm, intensity, and frequency of the stimuli which facilitate its differentiation.

A few of the more classical research studies are presented here to provide the reader with necessary background information and a glimpse at the exciting findings which have evoked so much interest in this field over the last several years. D. O. Hebb at McGill University published the first reports describing the experimental results of sensory deprivation on human behavior. The chief impetus for this work was the effectiveness of the Chinese communist technique of "brainwashing" prisoners of war. Hebb and his associates designed an environment of homogeneous light and sound as their experimental medium. Volunteer college students were placed in soundproof chambers for up to five days. The subjects wore translucent goggles which permitted some light; hearing was reduced by pillows and the unpatterned noise of an air-conditioner. Kinesthetic and tactile stimuli were partially reduced by the use of cardboard cuffs and gloves. The experimental results indicated that it was possible to produce a wide variety of behavioral changes on the basis of reduced sensory and perceptual input.[8]

Another important study was that of Lilly and his associates who invented the water immersion technique of sensory and perceptual deprivation. They immersed subjects, except for face masks and breathing apparatuses, into tanks of water. Sound and light were eliminated; touch and pressure were minimal. Under these conditions, hunger for stimulus developed rapidly, vivid imagery appeared after one to three hours, and vivid fantasies occurred. Lilly concluded that persons in perceptual and sensory isolation experience many, if not all, of the symptoms of the mentally ill.[9]

A series of studies using tank respirator confinement, as well as the conventional techniques, to structure the environment with nonvarying, nonrepetitive stimuli has been undertaken. Solomon and Leiderman placed volunteers in respirators for ten hours or more. The subjects could breathe for themselves, vision was reduced to a patch on the ceiling, and the respirator produced dull, continuous sounds. Kinesthetic and tactile senses were reduced by having the subjects' arms encased in cylinders within the tanks. Notable here is the fact that positioning each subject in such fashion meant that he could never see any part of his own body. All subjects reported difficulty in concentration, periodic feelings of anxiety, and loss of the ability to judge time. Some subjects also reported reality distortion, panic, and pronounced anxiety.[10]

Social isolation has been shown to produce some of the effects found in sensory deprivation experiments. Davis and McCourt made several investigations to determine whether reduced sensory input, social isolation, or reduction in kinesthetic cues due to immobility was the primary factor. Samples of their studies to assess

the importance of social contact in reducing the effects of sensory deprivation are presented below.

In one study, ten males were placed in isolation in pairs and allowed to converse. Although there was not a great deal of communication between the strangers, 90 percent were able to remain in the isolated environment for ten hours as compared with 30 percent of singly isolated male volunteers in a previous experiment.

In another study in which eleven married couples were isolated, placed in respirators, and allowed to converse, only one of the eleven couples remained ten hours. The male strangers seemed to perceive the situation as a competitive one, whereas the married couples discussed their discomfort and supported each others' decision to terminate the experiment. The social stimulation in the experiment with married couples resulted in fewer hallucinations, somatic complaints, and mental cloudiness. The male strangers' reactions were more comparable to those of the single males in sensory deprivation. On the basis of these results, the authors concluded that social contact ameliorated, but did not eliminate, the effects of sensory deprivation.[11]

Such studies reveal that unusual mental and physical manifestations of sensory deprivation are common. Subjects report all or some of the following experiences in the laboratory: vivid and elaborate visual hallucinations; inability to think and reason (secondary process thinking); distortion of time sense; feelings of unreality; disturbances in feeling states and primary process thinking. In addition, subjects who experience prolonged perceptual isolation report typical experiences of body illusions or delusions, somatic discomforts, and feelings of paranoia, anxiety, and apprehension.

Several theoretical models have been suggested by investigators, but none seems to be conclusive. One explanation offered by psychoanalytic theory focuses upon ego autonomy and reality testing. It has been stated that "the ego when deprived of a normal amount of external stimuli turns inward in an attempt to find meaning and order in all available stimuli.

The ego's process of turning inward results in a deterioration of its function of reality testing."[12] The process of seeking order where there is none and attempting to incorporate nonorder into previously existing schemata accounts for the perceptual changes, instabilities, and inconsistencies. Thus, when an individual must turn inward to find meaningful organization of stimuli which are bombarding him, he may misinterpret stimuli, lose accurate time awareness, experience abnormalities in feeling states, deteriorate in his ability to think, and experience vivid imagery illusions and hallucinations.

On the other hand, the neurophysiologist states that these changes stem from the reticular formation. The reticular activating system is that diffuse neural tract system responsible for integrating and conveying a variety of impulses associated with poorly localized pain, the sleep arousal cycle, and affect expressions. It is believed that sensory stimulation ultimately may control cortical activation or alertness through its regulation of activation of the reticular activation system. The brain depends upon a continuing arousal reaction generated in the reticular formation, which in turn depends on constant sensory stimulation. If stimuli are restricted to the monotonously repeated stimuli of an unchanging environment, they are unable to produce the arousal reaction and mental disorganization results.

In summary, theories of sensory deprivation represent broad areas of investigation: 1) *physiological,* which emphasizes the reciprocal relationships among the receptors, reticular formation, and cerebral cortex. In this area sensory deprivation is seen by some as one of a class of stress situations (the effects of deprivation of long duration and the effects of sensory deprivation on the person who is ill; 2) *personality,* particularly psychoanalytic, body-field orientation, introversion-extroversion, and optimal stimulation level approaches; 3) *drive or need,* which postulates a specific drive for varied stimulation or information; 4) *social influence,* which emphasizes set expectation and demand characteristics of the sensory deprivation situation and 5) *cognitive or perceptual theories.*[13,14]

Many of the early research studies have been criticized because of the absence of control groups and the limiting of age of the volunteers. In the late 1960s, studies became more sophisticated, partly because of more exacting tools of measurement and partly because of the collaboration of various investigators in adapting a standard terminology within the field.

Any number of variables can affect the individual's response to a sensory-deprivation experience. Psychological testing, evaluation of arousal levels by electroencephalogram (EEG) recordings, and biochemical assays to measure psychological respone to stress are examples of the techniques used to identify these variables. No single factor accounts for the major portion of individual differences in response to sensory deprivation.[15]

The importance of personality factors as possible determinants of subject's toleration to stress has been suggested. No clear-cut relationships have been established to date. However, it appears that the more outgoing the individual and the better his social orientation, the better he is able to adapt to sensory deprivation. In addition, subjects who are less able to generate internal mental stimulation or guidelines experience the effects of deprivation more strongly, and subjects of higher intelligence or complexity appear to exhibit more resistance to the effects of sensory deprivation.[16]

Changes in brain wave activity during sensory deprivation have been studied extensively. Definite changes have been noted in the EEG activity following prolonged periods of isolation. A progressive slowing of frequencies in the alpha range occurs. This change is greater during perceptual deprivation than during sensory deprivation, and it may indicate that the crucial factor is the variation in sensory input, rather than a reduction in the level of sensory stimulation.[17] Zubek's studies reveal that the introduction of physical exercises during isolation can counteract or minimize both EEG and behavioral disturbances.[18]

Biochemical changes have only recently received attention. Results to date indicate that the activity of the sympatho-adrenal system is affected little, if at all, by perceptual deprivation or by confinement in groups. However, catecholamine levels have increased in some of the people who have terminated the experiment early. In several experiments, this increase in catecholamine level was effectively counteracted by a program of mental exercises.[19]

Sex difference has been studied as a factor affecting toleration of a deprivation environment. Male versus female differences in toleration have been measured in terms of the subject terminating the experience and the kind of sensations reported. No significant difference was found. In general, females seemed more ready to admit their discomfort than males and were less likely to view the situation as a test of their adequacy as individuals.[20]

Clinical Sensory Deprivation

Applications of the controlled laboratory experimental findings to the clinically ill individual are suggested in the literature. However, specific scientific studies to confirm the presence of a sensory deprivation experience in the clinical setting are only beginning to emerge. One obvious stumbling block is the recognition of the point at which sensory alteration becomes sensory deprivation or overload. Until baselines of "normal" behavioral response to sensory stimuli are established, this difficulty will remain.

The problem of determining a baseline of behavioral response becomes more complex when one considers all of the sense modalities—visual, auditory, tactile, olfactory, kinesthetic, gustatory, and proprioceptive.

Characteristically, these senses function in the manner of intersensory perception. Although not all sensory avenues in man are stimulated simultaneously, a specific sensory experience is interpreted on the basis of what has been learned from all sensory experience. For example, when a sensory input is lacking (deafness), the experience gained from remaining senses is structured differently. There is reduced perceptual reciprocation. To further clarify, consider organizing the five senses into close (olfactory, gustatory,

and tactile) and distant (auditory and visual) senses. Distant senses serve as lead senses for the purposes of exploring and acquiring experience. Again using deafness as an example, as auditory sensation is reduced, alteration in the use of the other senses and altered perceptual organization is necessary for the person to maintain an adequate balance between inner needs and external circumstances.[21]

Fundamentally, when the individual is deprived of a distant sense he is forced into greater dependence on the close senses. Severe emotional disturbances in both children and adults may result in their relinquishing the use of the distant senses. An example would be the schizophrenic child who uses olfaction as a lead sense, or as a basic exploratory sense.

In the clinical setting, a patient concurrently experiences highly varied stimuli from several sense modalities. He may be reacting to reduced intensity of some stimuli, to reduced patterning of stimuli, to increased intensity of other stimuli, to the addition of new stimuli, and to change in the meaning of stimuli. Therefore, patient behavior should not be categorized as exemplifying a particular type of deprivation (sensory, perceptual, and so on) but rather as a manifestation of the total phenomenon of sensory deprivation.

Characteristic behavioral manifestations may differ for people within a single group and will certainly change for different groups of people in different situations. Therefore, one cannot meaningfully discuss the effects of clinical sensory deprivation until one examines the type of sensory input for a particular group of people in a specific situation. Sensory deprivation studies in the laboratory strongly suggest that certain medical and surgical patients develop psychoticlike manifestations from silence, darkness, and loneliness rather than from organic and toxic causes. Three such groups of clinically ill patients are described below.

1. There are patients who have experienced trauma to the sense organs themselves, resulting in reduced sensory functioning. Examples are patients with temporary or permanent eye disorders, the deaf, those with loss of sensation to a body part, the elderly, amputees, and individuals

who have lost the sense of taste or smell, perhaps as a result of radiotherapy.

Those most frequently identified with clinical sensory deprivation are patients hospitalized for eye surgery. Such patients, particularly those with cataracts or detached retinas, frequently experience sensory and behavioral disturbances when their vision is suddenly lost. These disturbances are similar to those reported by normal subjects during laboratory studies of sensory deprivation. As early as 1900, reports of disturbances following eye surgery appeared in the literature. Later summaries and studies include those by Linn, Ziskind, Dayton, and Jackson (see Bibliography).

Research reports indicate a typical sequence of events. Following surgery for either a cataract or a detached retina, one or both eyes are patched for the duration of the hospitalization. Both groups of patients receive medications and must remain in a recumbent position for at least the early postoperative stage. Most of the unusual behavioral experiences begin by the second postoperative day, occur during the day and night, are experienced by both men and women, and may last from several days to weeks. Most of the patients improve radically when the eye patch is removed from the good eye, allowing them at least partial vision. The frequency of the reported behavioral experiences ranges from 30 percent to 90 percent.[22]

The theory that these patients are experiencing sensory deprivation has relevance. There is reduction in visual stimulation because of the basic eye pathology and because of the eye patching. Most of these candidates are elderly and may also be experiencing decreased hearing acuity. Prolonged recumbent position and drug ingestion may further decrease sensory input. In addition, the unfamiliarity of the hospital and the inability to perform usual activities add to the complex of sensory deprivation variables affecting these patients.

As a group, the deaf have received little attention from a nursing practice geared to a hearing world. Although psychiatric research programs have been operating for the deaf, the understanding of the psychology of deafness was blocked by obstacles to communication. Many people unconsciously equate the soundless world of the deaf with lifelessness, with impenetrability, and with hopelessness regarding vital human contacts.

Rainer and Altshuler reported certain personality maladjustments for subjects who were congenitally deaf or deaf since early childhood. Some of the maladjustments identified in this group were diminished understanding for the feelings of others and a tendency toward impulsive behavior with little constraint.[23] Here was a group of people who were making slow progress toward educational and vocational opportunity and who had generally poor preparation for family living. One wonders whether these character traits are related to the general lack of verbal interchange or to the lack of parent-child communication in the early years. Many investigators have noted similarities in character traits between the deaf child and the culturally deprived child.

A three-year project funded by the department of HEW and conducted at Catholic University studied nurse attitudes toward deaf and blind patients. One hundred seventy-nine nurses were surveyed regarding their knowledge of physical, psychological, and social aspects of deafness and blindness, and their personal experience in dealing with deaf patients. In general, the nurses felt that the physical needs of these patients were met. The nurses indicated that they explained procedures to the deaf patient either verbally or in writing. They indicated a belief that deaf patients read lips well. Only in exceptional cases was an interpreter used.[24]

Contrary to opinion, few deaf persons are competent lip readers. In the Journal of Speech and Hearing Research, McCoy states that most deaf persons have extreme difficulty with oral communication and the speech reader does well to discern 20 to 30 percent of spoken words under ideal conditions. In addition, many of these persons have not mastered a reading level beyond the fourth grade. How realistic are we then in evaluating the effectiveness of nursing care to these patients?[25]

2. There are patients who are immobilized

either as an enforced therapeutic approach to an illness or because of loss of mobility. Examples are the patient whose movements are severely restricted by bedrest, body casts, or traction; the person with spinal cord injuries; the patient with a cerebrovascular accident; the patient on a respirator; the patient recovering from a myocardial infarction and the postoperative patient who is confined by pain and equipment.

Immobility or confinement reduces the quantity and quality of sensory input available to the patient. His ability to react and interact with his environment is reduced. Olson reported that studies of isolated or immobilized subjects have demonstrated the subject's decreased motivation to learn, decreased retention, and decreased ability to discriminate. She noted that the accompanying psychological reaction to isolation and immobility may be related to changes in body image.[26]

Immobility often connotes chronic illness. To understand the effects of chronic illness on body image, one must consider the emotional reactions these disabilities elicit. Leonard suggests that people invest emotions in their body and its well-being and that they feel anxious if change occurs.[27] Any bodily alteration is a disturbance of one's integrity, a threat to one's self. Some of the disabled patients interviewed expressed fears of abandonment, incapacitation, pain, loss of self-esteem, and disturbance of interpersonal relationships.[28] These fears are reality-oriented; they are not delusions.

The person with a cerebrovascular accident is a prime example of an immobilized, chronically ill individual. He may be confined to a wheelchair and, in addition, lose control of bowel and bladder function and speech. Arnhoff notes in his study on body boundaries, that chronically ill patients confined to wheelchairs often develop personality disruption. The body no longer serves its normal function of contact with the environment since the wheelchair is now interposed between the body and the external world. The patient does not receive the feedback necessary for adequate and current evaluation of the body's status.[29] As previously mentioned, numerous sensory experiences contribute to integrating one's body image into a highly organized arrangement. As the number of environmental and body organ influences are decreased due to organic brain damage (e.g., stroke), the person loses his orientation to his body sphere. "He feels as though he's in a maze and can't get out; he is confused, and feels trapped within the limits of his own body."

The patient who has had cardiac surgery is an example of a postoperative patient who is immobilized and exposed to altered patterns of stimuli. During the past decade, there has been major interest in the incidence of psychiatric symptoms following open-heart surgery.[30] Although primarily associated with cardiac surgery, the incidence of psychiatric complications has become notable in other patients experiencing catastrophic stress and treated in the intensive care unit: the patient having an organ transplant and the patient on dialysis. Psychiatric complications rarely occur following general surgical procedures.

The clinical picture of these complications varies and may include visual and auditory hallucinations, perceptual distortion, delusions, confusion, excitement, depression, and disorientation to one or more spheres. Characteristically, the onset of these symptoms follows a three- or four-day lucid interval. The symptoms often disappear within 48 hours.[31] There exists a wide divergence of opinion regarding the cause of these symptoms. Many theories have suggested a range of organic and psychological origins which include increased dependency needs, preoperative anxiety, sleep deprivation, cerebral injury, emboli, chemical changes secondary to oxygen want, metabolism of neurohormones, and the effects of cardiopulmonary bypass.

Several investigators have studied the intensive care and have suggested that mental aberrations result from both the overstimulation and the sensory deprivation of this environment. Authorities agree that the postoperative cardiac surgery patient experiences some degree of confinement or immobilization, deprivation of sleep, overstimulation of some sense modalities, and understimulation of others.

Among the most frequently cited studies

demonstrating these findings are those by Kornfeld et al. and by Abrams, Kornfeld, Zimberg, and Malm reviewed the charts of 119 patients who had heart surgery to determine the incidence of these disturbances. They also identified certain factors which might contribute to the postoperative psychiatric disturbances. Data analysis revealed that such factors as age, sex, marital status, and evidence of rheumatic heart disease were not significant. A positive relationship appeared to exist between the severity of operative risk and the incidence of delirium as well as between the increased time on the cardiopulmonary bypass machine and the incidence of delirium. However, after further analysis, the investigators concluded that the environment of the intensive care unit was a major contributing factor. Here the necessities of specialized care produced an atmosphere of sensory and sleep deprivation[32] (see Chapter 10).

In 1965, Abrams published a study emphasizing the individual patient's reaction to the stress of open-heart surgery. He interviewed 23 patients preoperatively and followed them postoperatively in the role of a psychiatric consultant. Postoperatively, 16 percent of the patients who survived the surgery developed severe psychotic episodes; one patient became severely depressed and another became very anxious.

Abrams concluded that both sensory deprivation and sensory stimulation were significant factors in the formation of these psychotic symptoms. The deprivation resulted from the imposed immobility and from the patient's estrangement from a familiar environment. The increased sensory stimulation was attributed to the foreign and incongruous stimuli which the patient received from the activity and equipment in the intensive care unit.[33]

Lazarus and Hagens published one of the first experimental studies designed to evaluate the intensive care unit environment as a significant variable. This study, published in 1968, included a control group of 33 patients at hospital A and an experimental group of 21 patients at hospital B. The same surgical team performed surgery in both settings, and the postoperative routine was the same.

A psychiatrist assisted in planning the post-operative management for the experimental group. He held a therapeutic interview with each patient preoperatively and made specific recommendations for postoperative nursing care to try to lessen the effects of sensory and sleep deprivation. He alerted nurses to the psychological needs of these patients and suggested that such considerations as the establishment of a positive, supportive, and reality-oriented relationship with the patient and provision of rest periods become a part of the postoperative routine.

Results indicated that 33 percent of the control group and 14 percent of the experimental group experienced psychiatric complications. No increase in the incidence of psychoses with increased operative procedure time or cardiopulmonary bypass time was detected. The authors concluded that adequate attention to anxiety before surgery and a personal relationship between the patient and the nurse appeared to be the most crucial factors in reducing psychological stress in the postoperative period.[34]

If a significant part of this psychosis reflects unsuccessful interpersonal relationships, non-English-speaking patients having operations in the United States would theoretically be more prone to develop an acute psychosis postoperatively. This thesis was explored by Danilowicz and Gabriel who compared results from two groups of patients undergoing heart surgery at the National Heart Institute. Results proved the incidence of psychosis to be significantly higher in the non-English-speaking patients (29.4 percent) than in the U.S. patients (3.9 percent).[35] Correlation of psychosis with the degree of medical complication did not reach statistical significance. The majority of psychoses in the foreign patients occurred in men.

The role of language and cultural factors has received little attention by other investigators. Although these factors may not be direct etiologic agents in postcardiotomy delerium, the unusually high incidence of delerium among these foreign patients indicates that the ability to communicate and become familiar with surroundings may help to prevent psychological disintegration.

Danilowicz and Gabriel suggest that the intensive care unit is a distinct subculture with its own rules of behavior. Lack of familiarity and the inability to communicate add to sensory deprivation. Routine medical procedures as well as the unusual array of sounds and machinery would represent panic-provoking behavior for the non-English-speaking patients since these patients would not have the added support of meaningful explanation and psychological comfort available to English-speaking patients.

Certainly non-English-speaking patients should be prepared preoperatively and should be provided with someone who can communicate with them in the postoperative period. If staff with the necessary linguistic skills are unavailable, it is reasonable to expect that rules governing intensive care units be made more flexible to allow a family member or friend to be in constant attendance.

With increasing knowledge about man's reactions to his environment, nurses must examine the physical as well as the psychosocial environment in which patients are confined. The highly technical and efficiency-oriented intensive care unit is one area which must be examined objectively. Wilson and Larkin studied the physical environment of the intensive care unit. They compared the incidence of postoperative delerium in two units which resembled each other in all respects except for the total absence of windows in one unit. Fifty consecutive surgical patients treated for at least 72 hours in each intensive care unit were observed. Results indicated that 40 percent of the patients experienced delerium in the unit without windows compared with only 9 percent of the patients in the unit with windows.[36] Other variables such as age, type of procedure, complications, and differences in medical management were not statistically significant.

The study of noise and its relationship to patient discomfort by Minckley also focuses upon the patient's environment. Minckley hypothesized that the postoperative patient was made more uncomfortable as noise over which he had no control increased. The amount of pain medication requested during high and low noise levels was the criterion of measurement. Patients did not respond to sounds of snoring and telephones,

seemingly because they did not connote human distress. They were distressed by cries of other patients, sounds of equipment, vomiting, and laughter and banter by the staff. Their requests for pain medication reflected this distress.[37]

As previously mentioned, patients are cognizant of unusual sensory experiences while undergoing them. An unpublished masters study carried out in 1971 found that patients were not only willing to reveal these experiences, but indicated a need to talk about them.[38] This study focused upon two questions: 1) Are the sensory and cognitive experiences reported by cardiac surgery patients similar to the kinds of experiences elicited in laboratory experiments of sensory deprivation? 2) Do patients who experience greater alteration in sensory input (sensory bombardment or sensory deprivation) report a greater incidence of these experiences than patients who experience less alteration in sensory input?

Fourteen patients were interviewed on the seventh to tenth postoperative day to ascertain the presence of unusual sensory and cognitive experiences. Responses were organized into reactant and nonreactant groups. The reactant group (those who admitted to unusual sensory experiences) was separated into two groups according to the degree of complications and complexity of postoperative management required. These patients were further categorized according to the quality of experience revealed. Comparisons were made to discern whether patients who experienced a greater alteration in sensory input reported more complex experiences.

Thirteen of the 14 patients interviewed reported one or more unusual sensory or cognitive experience postoperatively. The reported experiences were similar to those reported in sensory deprivation experiments. Patients with greater alteration in sensory input (patients subjected to longer time in the intensive care unit, to pain, and to complex medical procedures) reported a greater frequency of and more complex sensory and cognitive experiences than did patients with less alteration in sensory input.

Responses ranged from: "I can't concentrate, I forget everything"; "I'm always floating"; "I saw things on the wall; there were strange noises with them'' to: ''My husband, friends, the doctors, and nurses are planning to do away with everyone. I heard their voices. I knew it was true when I saw blood on the nurse's uniform.'' And another patient replied, ''Someone asked me if I would choose between having all my blood removed or dying like most people do. I remember getting colder. I must have been making up my mind.'' The more complex responses such as the last two examples seemed to be related to advanced age, need for sleep, presence of physical limitations prior to surgery, and to the presence of complications following surgery.

3. There are the group of patients who are physically isolated from people and from familiar surroundings. Examples of these include people with communicable disease who are isolated for the protection of others; persons who are susceptible to infection and are isolated for their own protection (the patient who has been burned, the patient with a low white blood cell count, the patient receiving immunosuppressive drugs). In addition, there is the patient subjected to long-term hospitalization, the patient isolated because of a language barrier, the patient who cannot speak following a tracheostomy, or a laryngectomy, the dying patient and the elderly patient.

The dying patient is often the recipient of imposed social isolation by the medical and nursing staff. Illness itself isolates one from a segment of humanity, so much more so when one is dying. It is a commonplace observation that, when death approaches, others literally depart. Death is perceived as a failure, or, at best, an accident in what has become our ''death denying'' culture. This attitude is readily recognized in medicine by the reluctance to talk about death or to tell the patient that he is dying. Minimizing contact with the dying patient has also served as a convenient means for physicians and nurses to protect themselves from emotional involvement and from being asked unanswerable questions. This imposed social isolation is subtle, taking the form of rotation of staff assignments, reluctance to answer call bells, and avoidance of the family. Our concern has centered upon the technical aspects of death, rather than upon ways to help the pa-

tient resolve the death crisis in a manner that would enhance his self-esteem and dignity. Consequently, the patient feels abandoned and has little opportunity to establish a therapeutic relationship with any one person. He may die socially before he dies biologically.

Dying is a social experience as well as a biological one. Dying is a process; therefore, patients who are dying are also living a human experience that culminates in death. To focus solely upon whether or not to tell the patient that he is dying is to miss the point. What the dying patient seems to fear most is the process that brings about the progressive dissolution of the things that he has considered to be the act of living.[39]

How one experiences death is determined to a great extent by where in the life cycle death occurs. Each stage of life affords a particular view of one's own life and one's relation to others. For the child, death is primarily an experience of separation, fear of pain, and punishment. For the adult, dying poses a problem of loss—loss of one's healthy body, of self-image, of involvement with mate, children, work, or play. For the elderly, dying means being faced with the consequences and meaning of one's life.[40]

Dying is a crisis. The person is faced with an insoluble event with which he may not have the resources to deal. Impending death carries with it social and psychological consequences, which may be as important to the dying patient as the physical consequences. Admittedly there exists great divergence among people in their attitudes and reactions to impending death. Yet researchers such as Kübler-Ross who interviewed dying patients found that when it comes to actually being faced with death there are certain common feelings that transcend culture, beliefs, and experience.

Kübler-Ross found that dying patients wanted to avoid loneliness and to maintain hope and their dignity as human beings. She suggested that failure to communicate with the dying patient stems partly from lack of awareness of the emotional response the patient is having to the reality of his dying. She describes five stages of coping mechanisms which the individual passes through in the process of dying:

1. Denial and isolation in which the patient does not believe death could be real for him.
2. Anger in which the patient is resentful and hostile about the unfairness of events.
3. Bargaining in which the patient is trying to make a deal, usually with God, to change his situation.
4. Depression in which the patient can no longer deny his illness and is grieving over his loss.
5. Acceptance—not resignation, but a feeling that life is finished.[41]

The death process cannot be reversed, yet nursing can help the patient live this experience to the fullest. The nurse must be available for a meaningful relationship with the patient. The patient may learn to endure the inevitable degree of separation that occurs if he is not deprived of human contact. He can be helped to face the loss of family, friends, and activity, and actively mourn their loss if he is helped to define and accept his grief. He may be able to tolerate loss of self-control if it is not perceived by him and by staff as a shameful experience. He may be able to retain dignity and self-respect when he is encouraged to maintain power over himself to the degree that he is able.

Nursing this patient successfully demands the formulation of a relationship that has continuity and that is nonthreatening. It implies clarifying the realities of the day-to-day existence which can be dealt with by the patient. It demands that human contact be available and rewarding to the patient.

The elderly patient is another example of an individual often isolated from social interaction. The effects of isolation upon the aged ego have yet to be studied. Yet we have all observed the geriatric patient who, when removed from normal surroundings and placed in an unfamiliar environment, for example, a hospital, displays disoriented or senile behavior not directly related to his illness. Clinical experience leads one to the thesis that isolated living without the input of meaningful interactions results in psychologically degenerative processes. The elderly person appears to be especially vulnerable.

There are several theories about the elderly person's apparent disassociation with the world about him. Cumming and Henry's theory of disengagement postulates that aging is an inevitable mutual withdrawal resulting in decreased interaction between the aging person and others.[42] In this normal aging process, disengagement is an adjustment mechanism employed by the elderly to cope with internal and external pressures. It is a mechanism of withdrawal by which a person limits his sensory input and reduces his social involvement.

Other authors disagree that old age produces disengagement. Rather they state that the impact of physical and social stress increases with age causing some elderly persons to disengage from the world around them. Regardless of which theoretical framework one choses, it would seem appropriate to question whether the environment encourages the elderly patient to engage, or whether it forces him to disengage in self-defense. Current hospital routines lend themselves to scrutiny. The limitation of visitors, discouragement of having personal belongings at the bedside, segregation by age, the highly regimented routines, and the limited opportunity for the patient to make even minor decisions (e.g., when to go to sleep) hardly encourages engagement. Senility and aging are not synonymous. Removing the patient's right to make decisions is a form of intellectual deprivation.

In some instances, the elderly patient who becomes disoriented at night is isolated from other patients and is often forcibly secured to the bed. Such treatment only intensifies the deprivation and often increases the disorientation. Such seclusion as a treatment is frequently initiated, implemented, and terminated at will by the nursing staff. Yet there exists little criteria available on which to base such decisions. A better alternative would be getting to know the patient and discovering the patient's interpretation of impending events. Such an alternative involves human contact and meaningful interpretation to the patient of the realities of his situation.

Sylvia Carlson's study of the effects of increasing sensory input for elderly female patients is one example of helping patients to engage.[43] Within a hospital setting two six-bed units were used; one, very plain, white-walled room was designated the control room, the second, a circular room with many windows, TV, and books was designated the study room. The investigator remained with study patients for seven days from 4 to 8 P.M. and attempted to increase the input through conversation, music, flowers, and pictures, back rubs to stimulate touch sensation, and craft lessons. Even patients previously withdrawn became involved. At the end of five days both groups of patients were given psychological testing (Neugarten Life Satisfaction test). Results supported the belief that this program of sensory stimulation contributed to greater life satisfaction in the study group.

Nursing Implications

Disorganized or aberrant behavior is frequently duc to a combination of physiological, psychological, and environmental factors, all of which must be evaluated. The formulation of a nursing diagnosis followed by the implementation of carefully planned nursing intervention is only the beginning. For the nursing diagnosis to be dynamic, it must change with the alterations in the patient's condition. Thus, it necessitates constant reevaluation throughout the patient's illness experience. The following discussion of nursing intervention for patients susceptible to sensory deprivation is directed toward three major goals:

1. To identify measures which can effectively prevent the occurrence of a sensory deprivation experience or situation;
2. To identify the presence of a sensory deprivation experience;
3. To assist the patient to cope with this experience.

PREVENTING THE OCCURRENCE OF A SENSORY DEPRIVATION EXPERIENCE

Concern with preventing a sensory deprivation situation must extend to the entirety of events and forces that the patient encounters during his illness experience. The nurse who is aware of the inherent dangers from the physical and social environment mobilizes her resources toward making sensory input meaningful to the patient. Suggestions for preventing the occurrence of a

sensory deprivation experience focus upon seven major points: 1) creating an environment with a minimum of sensory monotony or overload; 2) familiarizing the environment for the patient; 3) assisting the patient to interpret incoming stimuli; 4) orienting him to the reality of the moment; 5) providing him with an active role in his care; 6) encouraging him to use the highest form of cognitive functioning possible; and 7) providing him with uninterrupted rest periods.

Creating an environment with a minimum of sensory monotony or overload to prevent neurological, intellectual, or physical degeneration is not an easy task. The use of the telephone, radio, and television, so often accepted as the panaceas of diversion, are of great help if used selectively. Selective use of these devices provides opportunities for the patient to make some decisions. Any decision-making activity improves the patient's self-esteem by creating a more active role for him.

Many innovations on the part of the nurse reduce the monotony of a long hospitalization. Positioning the patient within view of a window or where he can observe activity provides a constant diversion. The nurse can extend the patient's environment beyond his room by moving his bed into the patient lounge for part of the day. Transporting him to other areas of the hospital or to the bedside of another patient increases his social contacts. Proper lighting, a clock, a colorful poster, calendar, greeting cards, and pictures add visual stimulus by providing a focus of interest.

The nurse can help the patient establish positive self-identity by encouraging some personal possessions at the bedside and providing cues within the immediate environment that would keep him oriented to reality and bridge the gap between past and present. Visiting hours can be altered to allow the family to be of more comfort to the patient. It may be advisable to encourage a family member to participate in the therapeutic program.

In the case of the elderly patient, the nurse would attempt to provide meaningful diversional activity that would help the patient establish a sense of belonging and usefulness. Diversional activity is successful only when purposeful. Too much emphasis upon fun and games (e.g., old timer sing-a-longs) presents an artificial world accentuating the sense of powerlessness felt by the elderly. Goals should exist. Activities can be designed to replace the void resulting from lack of employment and loss of family identity. Contact with the opposite sex should be encouraged as should contact with different age groups. Elderly patients who are capable would probably enjoy reading to hospitalized children or to other adults.

Assisting the blind or deaf patient to become more familiar with his environment taxes the imagination. Certainly two objectives would be to restore the patient's sense of physical integrity and restore his confidence in his remaining senses. The nurse is cautioned to avoid reliance upon children's guessing games of identifying sounds, smell, and touch. A more appropriate rehabilitative program could be planned to include cautious mobility, typing, and learning braille.

Because the patient may be reacting to many stimuli at any one time, he often requires assistance in interpreting these incoming stimuli. Application of the theory of cybernetics to human communication helps the nurse to understand how the patient reacts to sensory input. This theory suggests that stimuli impinging on external sense organs must be such that the subject can understand the existing circumstances in the environment. These stimuli must also be such that the subject can make decisions about them based upon his past performance. "Stimuli fed into the organism go through the cybernetic loop; the stimuli impinging on the sense organs are carried by sensory pathways to the central mechanism. Here a scanner identifies the appropriate data stored in the memory, including past experiences and past decisions. Based on the retrieved data, decisions for action are made at the synapses and are carried along efferent pathways to produce results in the environment."[44] Therefore, since reality is constantly changing, the individual requires constant information about the reality of the moment so that he can react to these changes.

A therapeutic nursing approach should, then, be geared toward helping the patient understand the incoming stimuli. Such an approach is of particular importance to the patient who may be experiencing sensory overload.

In the intensive care unit, Mr. B. was essentially immobilized. The electrocardiograph monitor leads, a urinary catheter, intravenous infusions, a central venous pressure catheter in the subclavian vein, a tracheotomy tube attached to a volume respirator, and the pain of a transthoracic incision limited any activity. Constant unpatterned sounds, a combination of the public address system, the respirator, the monitoring equipment, and the excited voices of the intensive care unit staff, added more stimuli to the already stressful situation.

Mr. B. was experiencing marked sleep deprivation as a result of endless nursing and medical procedures, several of which were performed every 15 minutes. The nurse attempted to provide Mr. B. with uninterrupted rest periods. Activities were organized into those which could be accomplished while he rested and those which would necessitate disturbing him. Although this plan was not always successful, even a little rest was a welcome relief for Mr. B.

During the postoperative phase, the nurse used the various pieces of equipment, attachments, and sounds as foci for reality orientation. The equipment also served as a means of stimulating secondary process thinking. The nurse explained what she was about to do and identified the equipment used. She also explained the source of certain noises and activities taking place in the unit.

Reducing the environmental sounds was difficult on a busy unit. The staff attempted to evaluate the necessity of the diverse auditory stimuli. They helped to reduce this stimuli by lowering their voices and confining conversation to the nurses' station. The monitor "beep" was also eliminated. No danger to the patient was involved since the electrocardiograph pattern remained continuously observable.

During conversation, attempts were made to associate the postoperative routine with what had been taught to Mr. B. preoperatively. Because he had a tracheostomy, a signal system was established to facilitate communication. Because he was too weak to write, he would move his index finger to demonstrate understanding.

Mr. B.'s postoperative course was not entirely without incident. About five days following surgery he awakened confused and mumbling. He responded to conversation but blurted that "strange things were going on in this hole of Calcutta." He announced that he was leaving, and then was suddenly startled by the confining monitor leads. The nurse talked with him and emphasized that these periods of confusion were normal. She urged him to talk about his feelings. A review of events from surgery to the present seemed to help him regain his orientation. He had no further difficulty.

As the days progressed, the nurse encouraged the highest form of cognitive functioning by helping Mr. B. recall events and people, by engaging in activities such as reading the newspaper, and by seeking his opinion where possible. He responded to this approach and seized every opportunity to talk about the events of the past week. He recognized when he had the "blues" and talked easily about any mood swings he experienced. During a later conversation about his postoperative experience, he stated, "Boy, you really straightened me out. I thought I was losing my grip."

Some social isolation in addition to sensory bombardment can be anticipated with a patient like Mr. B. This can occur in spite of or even because of the large number of persons who attend the bedside of the cardiac patient. This constant attention of many impersonal beings can result in the absence of meaningful interaction with any one person. The nursing personnel in the intensive care unit must be aware that this lack of identification with any one person contributes to the stress of the postoperative experience. Therefore, the protocol for patients having heart surgery in one particular hospital afforded the patient the opportunity of meeting his nurse before surgery and having her care for him for several consecutive days postoperatively. This goal of providing some continuity of care has been beneficial to patients. Continuity of care

also enables the nursing staff to evaluate the results of their efforts.

Periods of uninterrupted rest or sleep are essential in helping the patient to fortify his resistance to the effects of sensory deprivation. Research into the phenomena of sleep has demonstrated that sleep deprivation can produce personality and task performance changes.[45] Withdrawal, depression, and apathy as well as periods of irritability and aggression, confusion and hallucination are found with even moderate sleep deprivation. Quiet conversation, a back rub, and perhaps instructing the patient in some of the isometric relaxation exercises will provide the period of quiescence necessary for physical and mental rest.

Relaxation exercises serve dual purposes. They result in tension release and subsequent sleep, and they provide the patient with another opportunity to participate in his therapeutic progam. Isometric exercises provide muscle relaxation and are simple to perform. Essentially these contract muscles without producing movement or demanding appreciable amounts of oxygen. One set of muscles is tensed against another set of muscles or against an immovable object. The patient can learn to relax these muscle groups. A simple exercise is to hold the hands in front of oneself, tighten the forearm muscles so that the hands and fingers are straight. Abruptly relax them so that the hands fall limply. Try this with other muscles; tighten, then relax. Urge the patient to start with muscle groups in his feet and progress to include all voluntary muscle groups.

IDENTIFYING THE SENSORY DEPRIVATION EXPERIENCE

This discussion emphasizes methods of assessing the patient situation to identify his experience. Foremost, the nurse must be alert to the possibility that the patient may want to conceal any information about unusual sensations, feelings, or visions. He may fear that these manifestations indicate a mental disorder. He may be frightened by a feeling of powerlessness, a perceived loss of internal control over events or situations affecting him. Engaging the patient in conversation about unusual sensory experiences may be the bridge to confidence needed for the patient to unleash his feelings of apprehension. The nurse should emphasize that such experiences are normal for people in these situations.

However, the patient may remain reluctant to disclose these feelings. In that case, the nurse must rely on her observations. Does the patient seem indifferent to people and events affecting him? Does the nurse encounter difficulty in getting the patient's attention? The nurse's evaluation of the patient's sleeping patterns, appetite, reactions to visitors, conversation, and attention to personal hygiene reveal valuable information. Ellis suggests several assessments which the nurse can make to determine whether the patient's sensations or unusual behavior follow any particular pattern.[46] Do they go away when he sleeps? Do they keep him awake? Are they always present? Does the patient do something which seems to set off the experience? Once a pattern is recognized, concrete plans can be made either to modify the contributing factors or to help the patient in adjusting to them.

Mr. H. was a prime candidate for sensory deprivation. He had been in Room 300 for five months. He had been burned severely and was now in the process of having skin grafts and healing decubitus ulcers. He was confined to a circ-Olectric bed and was alone in the room. A television played most of the day; it was his main diversion.

A review of Mr. H.'s chart and discussion with the nurses revealed that he ate poorly and had no interest in himself or his surroundings. He had many decubitus ulcers which were not healing because of his poor nutritional state. He refused personal grooming and would not perform his exercises. He was becoming progressively weaker. Further evaluation revealed that he was receiving only weekly visits from his family. There were no other visitors. His care was rotated between members of the nursing staff, as they found him a "difficult" patient. "He's just been here too long." Conversational exchange with the patient was almost nonexistent. He responded in a hardly audible voice with comments such as "Do whatever you want, just don't hurt me"; "What does it matter? They all do what they want anyway."

After several days of administering his care, some rapport was established between one nurse and Mr. H. She felt that to gain his confidence she must be available to him and display an interest in him. Eventually their conversation acquired meaning. Mr. H. revealed a fear that he would never leave his room. He told of dreaming about escaping but of being "chained to the bed." He admitted having periods of confusion, losing all track of time and seeing "strange things." He had been afraid to talk of these experiences.

A nursing approach was designed to give Mr. H. reassurance and to provide him with meaningful stimulation. He became involved in some decision making and displayed some interest in his surroundings. Simply giving him a roommate and another room effected a remarkable change. The creation of a meaningful relationship with another individual seemed to reduce his sense of social isolation.

Clues to the presence of these experiences are often present in the form of dreams, fantasies, confusion, or nightmares. Some patients have admitted being fearful of sleep because of disturbing dreams. Many patients relate these experiences within the framework of what they consider to be normal experiences. It is then up to the nurse to delve into what the patient has said in order that they both understand its meaning.

Orientation of the patient to time, place, and person is a familiar index for the evaluation of the patient's state of wellness. Consider, however, the potentialities of the patient's orientation to time. The ability of the patient to estimate time intervals between events, the relationship of the past to the present and to the future, and his ability to relate the sequence of events are additional parameters to be assessed. It is often within these more subtle areas that distortion of reality is most apparent.

Very often therapeutic procedures themselves result in a change or reduction of sensory input from the environment. Hypnotic and tranquilizing drugs used to reduce anxiety effect a sensory alteration in some patients. Linton reports that marked symptoms of anxiety, rather than tranquility, have been observed in some patients receiving the psychoactive drugs. This reaction was observed most frequently in the early stages of treatment with the phenothiazine compounds.[47] These patients complained of feeling "strange." They reported symptoms of tension, restlessness and somatic complaints. They appeared to be more vulnerable than the usual individual to separation from familiar surroundings and to a change in the environment.[48]

The respirator, the Stryker frame, and the water bed are additional examples of therapeutic measures which alter the sensory input to the patient. One patient treated with the water bed to relieve the pressure of sacral and hip decubitus ulcers said, "When they put me into this bed I feel like I'm being lowered into a casket. I'm waiting for the top to close so they can bury me." The woman became so anxious that this method of treatment had to be abandoned.

ASSISTING THE PATIENT TO COPE

The goal of assisting the patient to cope with the sensory deprivation experience is no less challenging than the previous two. Suggestions for accomplishing this goal will emphasize: 1) helping the patient to explore his feelings, 2) providing reassurance, 3) improving the patient's self-esteem, 4) stimulating as many senses as possible, 5) using available sounds and unfamiliar equipment as foci for reality orientation, and 6) helping the patient to develop coping mechanisms.

Researchers have depended upon the subject's memory and verbal report of unusual experiences occurring during deprivation states. One can assume, therefore, that the subject is not out of contact with reality or necessarily confused. On the contrary, he may be able to talk logically about the experience, either following it or while going through it. One should encourage the patient to relate these experiences. Talking with the patient about his perceptions of these experiences may reduce the stress. In addition, helping him to explore his distress and the meaning it has for him gives the nurse direction in rendering care.

Reassuring the patient also enables him to cope. Dorothy Gregg writes, "Reassurance is the restoration of confidence . . so that one can discard the non-rational solutions made in panic and begin to work toward a realistic outcome."[49] The patient is reassured by trust, by competence, by authentic information given by one whom he trusts, and by having appropriate limits set for him. Gregg suggests that the patient is reassured when he finds that he is respected and understood by the nurse who cares for him. It is the development of the patient's own resources that restores the necessary confidence in himself and improves his self-esteem.

For the patient receiving reduced sensory input, careful planning to stimulate as many senses as possible is beneficial. Taste, smell, hearing, and tactile sensations can be stimulated during the daily administration of care by an imaginative nurse. The elderly patient in particular responds to this kind of approach.

Patients receiving reduced or increased sensory input must be oriented to events occurring to and around them. Various sounds and equipment in the patient's immediate environment provide foci for reality orientation. This approach was of great value in helping Mr. B. regain his orientation. Interviews with patients such as Mr. B. reveal that unfamiliar equipment, sounds and the distorted vision from within an oxygen tent may be percieved as hostile agents.[50] Often the patient's hallucinations are associated with these agents. One patient who was interviewed stated that the alarm buzz which periodically indicated an altered electrocardiogram pattern was a fire alarm. She was convinced that the room was on fire. Another patient who was interviewed stated that all her blood was "being drained away through the tubes in her chest and the hanging bottle of blood." And another patient revealed a fear of going to sleep because "the respirator would suck the air out of my lungs."

The elderly patient is a prime example of one who needs frequent orientation. So often the aged patient who becomes disoriented during the night is restrained or isolated to avoid disturbing other patients. These measures intensify any sensory deprivation which may already be present. An evaluation of the patient's sleeping patterns and the kinds of medication taken may yield useful information for planning the care of this kind of patient. Keeping a night light on and having the patient touch the side rail of the bed for orientation are often quite helpful.

The case of Mrs. M. is an example of a patient who profited from an approach of reality orientation. She had been burned over approximately 75 percent of her body and was positioned on a circOlectric bed. Burned areas included both of her legs, anterior and posterior trunk, forearms, hands, and some areas about the face.

Approximately three weeks following her admission, Mrs. M. displayed marked disorientation of thought, restlessness, hallucinations, and panic. Disorientation was so severe that she managed to get out of the circOlectric bed and attempt to flee. During this period her fluid and electrolyte balance remained stable, ruling out a physiological basis for her disorientation. Restraints had been attempted but discarded, because of the limited area of unburned skin and the fear of intensifying her apparent panic reaction. Mrs. M. had intermittent lucid periods but soon drifted off into a state of mumbling and continuous movement of extremities.

The observation was made that when one conversed directly with Mrs. M., her attention was maintained. Nursing staff evaluation of the situation further revealed that Mrs. M's vision was limited to the ceiling and floor because of the position of the bed. Sound within the room was of an unpatterned nature—a combination of the muffled public address system, voices from the ward activity and from persons out of Mrs. M.'s range of vision. In addition to the altered auditory stimuli, most physical contact was associated with discomfort, if not with pain.

A regimen of reorienting Mrs. M. was attempted; the approach decided upon was conveyed to each person participating in her care. All persons who conversed with the patient were to place themselves in her range of vision and attract her attention before progressing. Conversations were directed toward familiar items, her

family, her home, and her interests. Mrs. M. was urged to participate and offer her opinions.

A platform was placed beneath the bed which held items such as a clock and pictures of her family. The clock was a source of orientation and the pictures provided visual stimulus. Pictures were placed on the ceiling as well.

Within two weeks, positive results were realized. Mr. M. engaged in her first conversational exchange. She asked about her family and was noted to lie quietly at intervals. The mumbling, restlessness, and crying out had markedly decreased.

The nurse can help the patient to develop coping mechanisms. Laboratory studies of cognitive functioning indicate that the mere assignment of tasks increases the subject's vigilance and helps him to utilize his inner resources during sensory deprivation.[51] The occupational therapist is of great help to the nurse in suggesting tasks in which the patient can participate unaided. In addition the patient can participate in his own health care. Selecting his own menu, keeping a record of his fluid intake and tasks such as sorting mail provide him with daily activities he can anticipate.

Spontaneous verbalization allows the patient to provide himself with self-stimulation techniques. Self-stimulating techniques such as humming aloud, recitation and memory review provide resource when the patient is alone. In addition, talking, problem solving and planning for the future help the patient to engage in secondary process thinking and retain a hold on his mental orientation.

Summary

The purpose of this chapter was to survey selected research studies of sensory deprivation, to discuss application to the clinical situation, and to suggest methods of nursing intervention which benefit the patient experiencing sensory deprivation. In laboratory sensory deprivation studies, well-documented symptoms of abnormalities in feeling state, deterioration in the ability to think, perceptual distortion, vivid imagery, illusions, and hallucinations have been described.

Clinically ill persons are more susceptible than the average laboratory volunteer to changes in sensory input. In the hospital setting, additional influential variables are present—psychological stress drugs and a confining therapeutic regime. A deliberative nursing approach prevents or modifies the sensory deprivation experience for the patient. Some patients are helped to cope with sensory disturbances while they are experiencing them. Examples of patient situations were included in this chapter to illustrate selected nursing approaches. Mr. B. experienced sensory overload. Mrs. M. and Mr. H. suffered from sensory monotony. All three patients improved markedly with a deliberative nursing approach.

Nursing research is needed to examine the kinds of sensory disturbances experienced by a common group of patients in the clinical setting. Additional research also should evaluate the effectiveness of a particular approach in nursing these groups of patients. Such research builds nursing theories.

References

1. Hebb, D. O.: The mammal and his environment. Am. J. Psychiat. 111:286, 1955.
2. Kubanski, P. E.: The effects of reduced environmental stimulation on human behavior: a review. *In* A. D. Biderman and H. Zimmerman (eds.): The Manipulation of Human Behavior. New York, John Wiley & Sons, 1961, pp. 10-14.
3. Nightingale, F.: Notes on Nursing. London, Harrison, 1860. (Reprint, University of Pennsylvania Press, 1965.)
4. Goldberger, L.: Experimental isolation, an overview. Am. J. Psychiat. 122:774-782, Jan. 1966.
5. Zuckerman, Marvin,: Variables affecting deprivation results. *In* J. Zubek (ed.): Sensory Deprivation: Fifteen Years of Research. New York, Appleton-Century Crofts, 1969, 51-57.
6. *Ibid.*
7. Davis, J., et al.: The effects of visual stimulation on hallucinations and other mental experiences during sensory deprivation. Am. J. Psychiat. 116:889, Apr. 1960.
8. Kubanski, *op. cit.*, pp. 10-14.
9. Ruff, G.: Isolation and sensory deprivation. *In* S. Arietic (ed.): American Handbook of Psychiatry. New York, Basic Books, 1966, pp. 362-72.
10. Leiderman, P. H., et al.: Sensory deprivation—clinical aspects. Arch. Int. Med. 101:389-96, Feb. 1958.
11. Davis, J., et al.: Sensory deprivation: the role of social isolation. Arch. Gen. Psychiat. 5:84-90, July 1961.
12. Zubek, J. (ed.): Sensory Deprivation: Fifteen Years of Research. New York, Appleton-Century Crofts, 1969.
13. Zuckerman, M.: Theoretical formulations I. *In* J. Zubek (ed.): Sensory Deprivation: Fifteen Years of Research. New York, Appleton-Century Crofts, 1969, p. 407.
14. *Ibid.,* p. 407.
15. Suedfeld, P.: Changes in intellectual performance and susceptibility to influence. *In* J. Zubek (ed.): Sensory Deprivation: Fifteen Years of Research. New York, Appleton-Century Crofts, 1969, pp. 126-166.
16. *Ibid.*
17. Zubek, J.: Physiological and biochemical effects. *In* J. Zubek (ed.): Sensory Deprivation: Fifteen Years of Research. New York, Appleton-Century Crofts, 1969, pp. 255-288.
18. *Ibid.,* p. 286.
19. *Ibid.*
20. *Ibid.*
21. Myklebust, H.: Sensory deprivation and behavior. *In* H. Myklebust (ed.): The Psychology of Deafness. New York, Grune & Stratton, 1964, pp. 45-55.
22. Jackson, C. W.: Clinical sensory deprivation: a review of hospitalized eye-surgery patients. *In* J. Zubeck (ed.): Sensory Deprivation: Fifteen Years of Research. New York, Appleton-Century Crofts, 1969, pp. 332-73.
23. Rainer, J. D. and Altshuler, K.: A psychiatric program for the deaf: experiences and implications. Am. J. Psychiat., 137:103-108, May 1971.
24. Carty, R.: Patients who cannot hear. Nurs. Forum II, 3:290-299, 1972.
25. McCay, B., et al.: Psychological adjustments of profound hearing loss. J. Speech and Hearing Research 12, 3:546-555, Sept. 1969.
26. Olson, E.: Effects of immobility on psychosocial equilibrium. Am. J. Nurs. 67:194-97, Apr. 1967.

27. Leonard, B. J.: Body image change in chronic illness, Nurs. Clin. N. Am. 7,: 687-695, Dec. 1972.

28. *Ibid.*

29. Arnhoff, F.: Body image deterioration in paraplegia. J. Nervous and Mental Diseases: 137: 88-92, 1963.

30. Hazan, S. J.: Psychiatric complications following cardiac surgery: a review. J. Thorac. Cardiovas. Surg. 51:307-18, Nov. 1966.

31. Abram, H. S.: Adaptation to open-heart surgery: a psychiatric study of response to the threat of death. Am. J. Psychiat. 122:662, Dec. 1965.

32. Kornfeld, D., Zimberg, S. and Malm, J.: Psychiatric complications of open-heart surgery. New Eng. J. Med. 273:287-92, Aug. 5, 1965.

33. Abram, *op. cit.*

34. Lazarus, H. and Hagens, J.: Prevention of psychosis following open-heart surgery. Am. J. Psychiat. 124:76-81, Mar. 1968.

35. Danilowicz, D. and Gabriel, P.: Postcardiotomy psychosis in non-English-speaking patients. Psychiat. Med., 2:314-319, 1971.

36. Wilson, L.: Effect of outside deprivation in a windowless unit. Arch. Int. Med., 130:225-6, Aug. 1972.

37. Minckley, N.: Study of noise and its relationship to patient discomfort in recovery room. Nurs. Research 27, May-June 1968.

38. Worrell, J.: A Comparison of the Sensory and Cognitive Experiences Reported by Cardiac Surgery Patients with those Experiences Elicited in Sensory Deprivation Experiments. Unpublished Masters project, University of Pennsylvania, 1971.

39. Pattison, E. M.: The experience of dying. Am. J. Psychotherapy, 21:32-43, Jan. 1967.

40. *Ibid,* 34.

41. Kübler-Ross, E.: On Death and Dying. New York, Macmillan, 1969.

42. Cumming, E., et al.,: Growing Old: The Process of Disengagement. New York, Basic Books, 1961.

43. Carlson, S.: Communication and social interaction in the aged. Nurs. Clin. N. Am., 7: 269-279, June 1972.

44. Price, L. F. : An adrenal stress index as a criterion measure for nursing. Nurs. Research, 294, July-Aug. 1968.

45. Long, B.: Sleep. Am. J. Nurs., 69, Sept. 1969.

46. Ellis, R.: Suggestions for the care of eye surgery patients who experience reduced sensory input. American Nurses Association, Regional Clinical Conferences, 1967, pp. 131-136.

47. Linton, P.: Sensory deprivation in hospitalized patients, Alabama J. Med. Sci., 2:256-258, July 1965.

48. *Ibid.*

49. Gregg, D.: Reassurance. *In* C. Skipper and B. J. Leonard (eds.): Social Interaction and Patient Care. Philadelphia, J. B. Lippincott, 1965, pp. 133-135.

50. Worrell, J.: A Comparison of the Sensory and Cognitive Experiences Reported by Cardiac Surgery Patients with those Experiences Elicited in Sensory Deprivation Experiments. Unpublished Masters project, University of Pennsylvania, 1970.

51. Rossi, A. M.: General methodical consideration. *In* J. Zubek (ed.): Sensory Deprivation: Fifteen Years of Research. New York, Appleton-Century Crofts, 1969.

Bibliography

Abram, H. S.: Psychological reactions to cardiac operations: an historical perspective. Psychiat. Med., 277-293,

Black, Sr., Kathleen: Social isolation and the nursing process. Nurs. Clin. N. Am., 8: 575-586, Dec. 1973.

Carlson, S.: Selected sensory input and life satisfactions of immobilized geriatric female patients. Am. Nurs. Assoc. Clinical Sessions. Dallas, Appleton-Century Crofts, 1968, pp. 117-123.

Chambers, C.: Senility of deprivation, Am. Nurs. Assoc. Clinical Sessions. San Francisco, Appleton-Century Crofts, 1966, pp. 6-12.

Comer, N.: Observations of sensory deprivation in a life thinking situation. Am. J. Psychiat., 124:164-169, Aug. 1967.

Cooper, G. D., et al.: Personality changes after sensory deprivation. J. Nervous and Mental Diseases, 125:103-118, Feb. 1965.

Dayton, G. O., et al.: Overt behavior manifested in bilaterally patched patients. Am. J. Ophthalmol. 16, 1965.

Downs, F.: Bedrest and sensory disturbances. Am. J. Nurs., 75:434-438, Mar. 1974.

Elsberry, N. L.: Psychological Responses to open heart surgery—a review. Nurs. Research, 220-227, May-June 1972.

Fitzgerald, R. G.: Visual phenomenology in recently blind adults. Am. J. Psychiat., 127: 1533-1539, May 1971.

Jackson, C. W. J. and O'Neil, M.: Experiences associated with sensory deprivation reported for patients having eye surgery, *In* J. E. Jeffries (ed.): Disturbances in Sensory Input in Nursing Practice and Research, Ross Roundtable on Maternal and Child Nursing, Columbus, Ohio, 1966.

Kornfeld, M.: Psychological hazards of the intensive care unit. Nurs. Clin. N. Am, 3: 41-51, Mar. 1968.

Linn, L.: Psychiatric reactions complicating cataract surgery. Internat. Ophthalmology Clin., 5, 1965.

Rock, I. and Harris, C.: Vision and touch. Sci-Am. 96-104, May 1967.

Seeman, M., et al: Alienation and learning in a hospital setting. Am. Sociol. Review, 27: 772-782, Dec. 1962.

Soloman, P.: Sensory Deprivation. Cambridge, Harvard Press, 1965.

Thompson, L. R.: Sensory deprivation: a personal experience. Am. J. Nurs., 73:266-268, Feb. 1973.

Ujhely, G. G.: The environment of the elderly. Nurs. Clin. N. Am., 7: 281-289, June 1972.

Woodburn, H.: Pathology of boredom. Sci-Am., 56,67, Jan. 1957.

Ziskind, E., et al.: Observations on mental symptoms in eye patched patients: hypnagogic symptoms in sensory deprivation. Am. J. Psychiat., 116, 196.

———: Isolation stress in medical and mental illness. JAMA, 1427-1430, Nov. 15, 1958.

20

Nursing Assessment and Intervention for the Patient with Central Nervous System Dysfunction

MARIANNE COSTOPOULOS SLATER

Nursing Assessment, Diagnosis, and Care Planning • Neurologic Examination • Nursing Intervention for the Comatose Patient • Nursing Observation and Intervention in Increased Intracranial Pressure • Neurologic Problems and Dysfunction

One of the greatest health problems existing today concerns the vast number of persons with neurologic disorders. Neurologic diseases not only claim countless lives each year, but also cause varied and disturbing disabilities which affect the individual, the family, society, and the nation as a whole. The National Committee for Research in Neurological Disorders has estimated the following prevalence of neurologic disorders:

1. One in every 16 babies born in the United States suffers from some form of neurologic disability.
2. Several hundred thousand deaths occur each year from neurologic and sensory disorders—almost 190,000 from strokes alone.
3. Cerebrovascular accidents rank third as the major cause of death.
4. More than 8 million persons are disabled by diseases affecting the brain or spinal cord.
5. Nearly 6 million Americans have hearing problems.
6. Over one-half million cases of Parkinson's disease are estimated.
7. More than one million Americans are disabled by strokes; another half million suffer from cerebral palsy.

It is apparent from these statistics that all members of the health team have a tremendous task and challenge in providing health care for the great number of patients with neurologic disorders.

In recent years, the nurse's role has expanded to include greater responsibility and specialized functions in nursing assessment and intervention, diagnosis and treatment, prevention of illness, case finding, and health management. It becomes necessary for the nurse to have greater knowledge to deal effectively with these newer areas of responsibility.

Nursing Assessment, Diagnosis, and Care Planning

The degenerative and debilitative nature of most neurologic conditions creates a tremendous need for personalized and individualized care. The patient may be faced with a chronic problem, such as seizures or neurologic deficits following cerebral or spinal injury, or be confronted with a chronic crippling disease. For many, there are no cures as yet. The majority of patients must cope with changes in their life styles, goals, and activities of daily living. Not only is the patient's life affected, but that of his family as well. In addition, neurologic diseases manifest themselves in different ways, and patients demonstrate complex and varying symptomatology. Therefore, it is essential that *all* patients receive individualized care. The nurse must be aware of the patient's physiological, psychological, and social needs and problems. This is most readily accomplished through use of a nursing assessment tool.

Neurologic patients require a comprehensive team approach in order to make the most of their abilities and the best possible adjustments to life. Components of this team approach include the physician's diagnosis and treatment, nursing assessment and intervention, teaching, coordination of health team members, rehabilitation and follow-up services, and, in many instances, provision for care after discharge. The nurse is a major part of this team and is with the patient more than any other health team member. It is imperative, then, that the nurse face her responsibilities in the care of neurologic patients through a rational, systematic nursing process.

To discuss the nursing assessment and process of the neurologic patient, one must begin with a definition of nursing. Virginia Henderson has defined nursing to be:

> primarily assisting the individual (sick or well) in the performance of those activities contributing to health, or its recovery (or to a peaceful death) that he would perform unaided if he had the necessary strength, will or knowledge. It is likewise the unique contribution of nursing to help the individual to be independent of such assistance as soon as possible.[1]

The above definition requires that the nurse assist the *individual,* individual meaning "unique, or existing as a distinct entity." The nurse must understand the patient's background, strengths, weaknesses, habits, perceptions of illness, coping mechanisms, idiosyncrasies, and so on, if she is to assist him to function at full capacity. Upon arrival at the hospital, the patient is stripped of his personal possessions and placed in a seemingly endless assembly line of red tape and procedures. He is soon divested of much of his personal identity. All too often he is labeled descriptively by diagnosis or by some personal judgment. Nursing care must not be intuitive, accidental, and haphazard, but must be conscientiously planned if the nurse is to assist the individual and contribute to health, recovery, or peaceful death. This can be accomplished by acquiring and organizing data from various sources (e.g., patient, family, significant other, hospital records, medical history, past records) which aid in the assessment of the patient's needs, identification of his nursing problems, and the formulation of nursing goals. The Nursing History form developed at the University of Florida College of Nursing is one method of organizing data relevant to the care of the neurologic patient. It should be noted that the tool is used in the assessment and nursing care of *all* patients, not only of patients with nervous system dysfunction.

The above nursing goals and orders were specific and routinized for this particular patient. It was most important that Mr. R. have continuity of care and order in his activities of daily living. To have someone care for him who was new and did not know his routine and habits upset and frustrated him. This attitude is true of many patients with central nervous system dysfunction, especially those with a degenerative process. Having a daily routine he can look forward to provides the patient with security. He should be allowed to participate in planning his care as much as possible. In the case of Mr. R., he had difficulty asking for help and liked things done his own way. Allowing him to participate in his care increased his self-worth, and independence and lessened his frustration.

Nursing History[2]

I. Vital statistics.
1. Name:
2. Hospital number:
3. Number of _____ hospital admissions:
4. Age:
5. Sex:
6. Race:
7. Marital status:
8. City of residence:
9. Medical diagnosis:
10. Admitting vital signs:

Temperature   *Pulse*   *Respiration*   *Blood Pressure*   *Pupils*

II. Appearance on first sight. Might include the following:
1. Build—Tall, slim, obese, emaciated, average.
2. Appearance—Tidy, makeup, neat, clean, shaven, unwashed. Noticeable abnormalities—lid ptosis (drooping of the eyelid), facial paralysis, muscle atrophy or rigidity, contractures, absence of extremities, prosthesis, paralysis.
3. Presence—Eager, relaxed, strained, attempting to relieve pain, shutting out interviewer.
4. Speech flow—Articulate, slurred, staccatolike, hoarse, stammering, stuttering, monotonous, tremulous, whispering, jerky, scanning, lisping, expressive aphasia, dysphonia—difficulty in speaking, dysarthria—difficulty in articulation, loud or soft voice, memory failure.
5. Distinguishing marks or scars.
6. Clothing—Warm enough robe, pajamas, slippers, shoes.
7. Activity—How the patient was engaged when interviewed.
8. Other observations—Visitors, personal equipment—wheelchair, walker, cane, crutches, hearing aid.

III. Patient's understanding of illness.
1. Does he know what led up to his illness?
2. What does he know about his illness?
3. What was he doing and who was he with when his symptoms first appeared?
4. How has it altered his pattern of living, if at all?
5. What drugs was he taking and for what reason?

IV. Indications of the patient's expectations.
1. What does he expect will be the result of his hospital care?
2. What does he think his abilities will be after discharge?
3. What does hospitalization mean to him?
4. What does he expect from the nursing staff?

V. Brief social and cultural history.
1. Occupation.
2. Educational level achieved.
3. Family members. What effect does the patient's hospitalization have on them? Does he have any concerns about them?
4. What or who is significant to the patient? Church, clubs, hobbies?
5. How does the patient cope with new situations?

VI. Significant data.
1. Rest and sleep patterns—Amount of sleep required; naps; sleep medications; other methods used to achieve sleep; any rituals upon retiring or awaking.
2. Elimination—Time and frequency of voiding and defecation; void during the night; any difficulty; medication or mechanical aids such as coffee, prune juice.
3. Breathing—Shortness of breath, dyspnea, other difficulties; what influences or worsens difficulties; how the patient counteracts difficulties; allergic conditions such as asthma or hay fever; paralysis or paresis of muscles needed for proper ventilation; tracheostomy; requires oxygen (e.g., IPPB, hand nebulizer, nasal catheter), any particular position for sleeping—extra pillows, elevated bed.

4. Eating—Patient feeds himself; difficulty chewing or swallowing; particular eating pattern such as large lunch or breakfast; likes and dislikes in food; special diet; allergies; appetite stimulants or depressants; dentures; eats more or less when upset.
5. Skin integrity—Edema, bruises, decubitus ulcers, reddened areas, eruptions, rashes, turgor, texture, color, oiliness, moistness, special soaps or other cleansing agents.
6. Mobility—Any limitation in movement, balance, safe ambulation; walking pattern—leaning to one side, shuffling gait; able to manage most activities, or needs help; coordination, paresis, spasticity, rigidity, contractures; abnormal movements—hemiballismus (involuntary, violent, wild choreiform, usually present in one limb or one side of body), athetosis (involuntary slow, wormlike, sinuous, writhing of the extremities, particularly fingers and wrists), dystonic (resembles athetoid movements but involves larger areas of body, particularly muscles of trunk and girdle); strength.
7. Activity—Hobbies and interests; how the patient spends his spare time.
8. Interpersonal and communicative patterns—Volunteers and gives information readily; evades questions, changes subject, reluctant to talk; literate, ability to communicate; nervous habits—shifting positions, tapping fingers, biting nails.
9. Temperament—Angry, argumentative, docile, good-natured, shy, quick-tempered, withdrawn, verbalizes and demonstrates anger in upsetting situations.
10. Dependency and independency—Patient gets what he wants; allows others to care for him; wishes to do for himself; asks for help; usually depends upon others to meet his needs or demands.
11. Senses—Level of consciousness, oriented to time, place and person; right- or left-handed; any impairment in sensation, vision, hearing and other senses.

VII. **What is important to this patient? What will tend to help him feel secure, comfortable, protected, cared for?**

VIII. **Nursing Diagnosis.**
The nursing diagnosis is a list of the patient's problems as identified by the nurse and/or nursing staff. Mayers defines a problem as an "actual or potential difficulty or concern with which a patient is not coping satisfactorily."[3] During the interview, the nurse should strive to identify the patient's difficulties from the data obtained. Nursing diagnosis should also include a list of the patient's strengths, resources, and so on. This knowledge is helpful in planning nursing care and assisting the patient to cope with his problems.

IX. **Nursing care objectives.**
This is a statement describing an activity, behavior, appearance, physical condition, and so on, the nurse expects the patient to demonstrate by a specific time. The objectives are written in positive terms, should be concise, and include limits or deadlines. These criteria are necessary to be able to evaluate the effectiveness of nursing actions. Examples of nursing care objectives might be:
1. The patient will take in 2,500 cc's daily.
2. The patient will have a decreased area of decubitus ulcer by (date).
3. The patient will be knowledgeable in a diabetic diet by (date).
4. The patient will show less anxiety over hospitalization (daily).
5. The patient will take his IPPB b.i.d.

X. **Achievement of objectives.**
Factors which inhibit or enhance.

XI. **Nursing Orders** most likely to achieve the objectives. The nursing orders (also called actions) are those specific nursing activities or methods which will achieve the nursing care objective. For example, if the nursing care objective is that the patient will eat three nutritional meals each day, the nursing orders might include the following:
1. Clean patient's dentures before feeding.
2. Feed patient on the left (unaffected) side of the mouth.
3. Use straws when giving all fluids and place on left side of mouth.
4. Allow at least 30 minutes for each feeding.
5. Reheat food, particularly coffee, if it is cold.

XII. **Evaluation** of nursing care through the use of objective-related progress notes.

XIII. **Modification** addition, and/or deletion of the objectives and nursing orders in light of the patient's progress.

XIV. **Nursing Discharge Summary.**
At the conclusion of the patient's hospitalization, a summary of the nursing care is placed in the chart. This includes a resume of nursing orders, their successes and failures, the patient's condition upon discharge (from a nursing standpoint), and future plans of the patient such as returning home or transferring to a rehabilitation center, nursing home, or the like.

The following Nursing History illustrates data collection and formulation of nursing goals and orders based on the information acquired. The interview was conducted with both the patient and his wife present. The patient could not articulate due to severe dysarthria and could not write extensive answers to questions due to the weakness and contractures of his fingers and hands. Thus, it was helpful to question his wife during various aspects of the interview to obtain the necessary data.

Nursing History

I. Vital statistics.

Name: Mr. R.
Number of _____ Teaching Hospital admissions: None
Age: 54
Sex: Male
Race: Caucasian
Marital Status: Married
City of residence:
Medical diagnosis: Amyotrophic Lateral Sclerosis
Admitting vital signs:

Temperature	Pulse	Respiration	Blood Pressure	Pupils
37.1°C.	84	20	130/80	Equal and reactive to light

II. Appearance on first sight.

When first observed, patient was lying in bed with head of bed elevated about 45°. Lay very still and rigid with his hands holding tissue box. Thin, gaunt, and wasted, but neat and meticulously groomed. Considerable drooling from mouth. Was wearing his own pajamas and a bib was placed around his collar to prevent soiling. Attempted a slight smile when the interviewer introduced herself. Unable to speak and could only make an ah-like groan. Communicated with interviewer by using a Magic Slate and wrote answers to questions on it. Marked contractures and atrophy of fingers of both hands; legs thin and wasted. The patient's wife was at his bedside. The patient brought his own walker and wheelchair.

III. Patient's understanding of illness.

He is aware that he has a degenerative disease. Wrote, "I have amyotrophic lateral sclerosis. There's no cure yet." Approximately a year ago he developed weakness of his lower extremities and hands. Patient wrote, "I couldn't open or lift things very well." He went to his local physician who referred him to a neurologist. The diagnosis of ALS was established. The patient has gotten progressively worse and more disabled. He now is unable to speak and has dysphagia (difficulty swallowing) and difficulty with most activities. Patient also has muscular aches and pains as well as weakness of all extremities and trunk.

IV. Indications of expectations.

Hopes to be helped and has come to the hospital specifically for experimental therapy and drugs. He wrote, "I hope Dr. _____ can help me. He's why I'm here." The patient's wife stated, "We are prepared to stay as long as is necessary while tests and drugs are tried." They both appear hopeful that his hospital stay will be productive and that good results will be obtained.

V. Social and cultural history.

Mr. R. has been married for 30 years, has three children (none at home), graduated from college with degree in business administration, worked as accountant all his life, retired six months ago due to illness. The most significant person to him is his wife who is employed as an elementary schoolteacher. A hired woman cares for Mr. R. during the day; Mrs. R. assumes care during evening and nights. Both husband and wife attend the Episcopal church.

VI. Significant data.

1. Rest and sleep patterns—Has difficulty sleeping, due to muscular aches and pains of both upper and lower extremities, and because of choking and coughing spells which awaken him. Has not been taking any sleep medications, prefers to sleep with a light on and without any covers. Difficult to find comfortable position and cannot turn easily with covers over him. Has always followed a routine of going to bed around 10 P.M. and waking up at 6 A.M. Due to weakness, naps frequently during the day, usually after his morning care, after lunch, and after supper. Changing positions usually helps him to fall asleep once awakened; prefers to sleep on his side with two or three pillows under head.

2. Elimination—Has one bowel movement a day, almost always after breakfast, is assisted to bathroom with walker after breakfast, uses no particular mechanical aid. If constipation occurs, patient benefits by using Milk of Magnesia, has to be in a standing position to void, cannot void in sitting position, or sitting on side of bed.

3. Breathing—The patient wrote, "I get choking spells a lot." Choking occurs particularly when eating, and on his own secretions. Prefers to have his head elevated 45° or more both when awake and asleep, no known allergies, never smoked.

4. Eating—Has great difficulty swallowing. Coughs and chokes when eating and regurgitation of food and fluid occurs through nose, has been eating soft foods while at home, has great difficulty swallowing liquids, especially water. He wrote, "Tongue nearly paralyzed, making chewing impossible." Prefers eating with a soup spoon and takes liquids from a large cup, dentulous.

5. Skin integrity—No observable signs of skin breakdown or decubitus ulcers, no blanching or redness; skin is dry and many bony prominences, prefers no special soap and uses favorite aftershave lotion each day. Mrs. R. applies baby lotion and powder after his bath.

6. Mobility—Marked weakness and atrophy of both upper and lower extremities, severe contractures of fingers of each hand, great difficulty manipulating anything with hands; unable to feed himself or perform any activities of daily living without assistance; ambulates a short distance using walker but requires assistance getting to walker and into proper position for using it.

7. Activity—Enjoys reading, working crossword puzzles, and playing chess; prefers indoor activities in general; likes nonfiction literature; reads newspaper each day.

8. Interpersonal and communicative patterns—Considering extreme difficulty in communication and the weakness, he volunteered information willingly; attempted to write answers on Magic Slate; very friendly and cooperative; not capable of uttering intelligible speech; groans but hard to tell what this means; face is not expressive (due to illness); shakes head and nods to Yes and No questions; when unable to write, forms letters on top of left hand with right index finger.

9. Temperament—In response to questioning, wrote: "I'm easy to get along with. I don't get upset very easily." Wife agreed and stated, "My husband isn't the screaming type. He usually goes off by himself if he gets mad about something." Lately, according to wife, patient very depressed and frustrated, due to inability to do things for himself and increasing weakness.

10. Dependency and independency—The patient wrote, "I like doing most things myself and to my specifications." Also mentioned, "I hate waiting for others to do things." Wife stated "He has always been the boss and organized everything." Patient has always managed own affairs and lived by routine.

11. Senses—Quite alert, oriented in all spheres. Even though he is unable to speak, understands everything spoken to him. Wears glasses to read and has slight difficulty with hearing at times; sensation is intact (has just motor involvement); righthanded.

VII. What is important to this patient?

"To have someone come when I need him and to have the same person take care of me. I hate to train somebody new all the time." The patient also wrote, "I like to have my routine followed as much as possible."

VIII. Nursing Diagnosis.

The patient's particular problems were identified from the nursing history, past medical history, and family. These included:

1. Difficulty sleeping due to anxiety and discomfort.
2. Difficulty communicating with others and making his needs known due to degeneration of bulbar nerves (*severe* dysarthria).
3. Severe difficulty in swallowing and eating due to bulbar involvement.
4. Possible complications due to immobility and weakness.
5. Inability to perform most activities of daily living without assistance due to atrophy and weakness of muscles.
6. Anxiety and fear over hospitalization and increased dependency on others.

Some of Mr. R's strengths include: He seems cooperative and pleasant and communicates willingly with the nursing staff, even in light of his severe debilitation. He appears to like to do things himself and his need for independence can be readily integrated into the plan of care.

IX. The following objectives and orders were formulated from the data. The orders in italics were added to the care plan by other staff nurses during the course of his stay.

Objectives

1. The patient will sleep comfortably six to eight hours during the night.

2. The patient will maintain communication and interpersonal relationships with the staff.

3. With assistance, the patient will eat three meals and drink 1,500 ml a day.

4. The patient will remain free of complications during hospitalization.

Nursing Orders

1. Position patient on his side with two to three pillows under his head.
2. Help him to change positions if he awakens.
3. Tie light cord to right side rail and keep right side rail up.
4. Keep on light in alcove at night.
5. Do not cover patient with sheet unless he so requests.
6. Do not rush patient and let him do as much as he can for himself.
7. Handle patient and extremities gently, for he has muscular aches and pains.
8. *Check patient every half hour at night.*

1. Provide Magic Slate and pencil.
2. Ask questions that can be answered in short sentences or "yes" and "no."
3. Observe patient's left hand if he is unable to write on Magic Slate (forms letters on top of left hand with right index finger).
4. *Don't become alarmed if patient has explosive, uncontrollable outbursts of laughing and crying (it is part of his illness and quite characteristic of pseudobulbar palsy).*
5. *Make sure patient has his glasses on when trying to write or read.*

1. Allow 45 minutes to an hour for feeding.
2. Feed patient with soup spoon.
3. Feed patient sitting on side of bed or in chair with towel over lap.
4. Offer all liquids in a cup.
5. Remain with patient while eating and drinking.
6. Maintain suction-machine setup at bedside at all times.
7. *Mash medications and give with meals.*
8. *Stop frequently. Let patient burp, since he swallows a lot of air.*
9. *Allow patient to determine when he is ready to eat.*
10. *Break toast into small pieces and pour milk over it. Feed this to patient last.*

1. Use footboard to prevent footdrop. Make sure patient's feet are supported by it.
2. Extend and exercise fingers three times a day.
3. Place extremities through passive range of motion three times a day.
4. Keep sheepskin under patient.
5. Keep head of bed elevated around 45°, to prevent choking aspiration, and to maintain patent airway.
6. Turn patient every two hours and massage back, particularly over bony prominences. At night, do back care only when patient is awake.
7. *Assist patient to walk frequently during the day (as much as he desires).*

Objectives	*Nursing Orders*
5. The patient will perform activities of daily living with assistance.	1. Stand patient to void, balancing himself with walker. 2. After breakfast, have patient walk to bathroom (use walker) for bowel movement.
	1. Assist the patient with bath care and morning care. 2. *Sit patient on edge of bed while face, chest, and arms are washed.* 3. *Have patient lie back in bed and finish bath.* 4. *Shave patient every other day, while he is in a sitting position.* 5. *Apply lotion over body.* 6. *Put your right arm under his shoulders and pull to sitting position (less painful this way).* 7. *Assist patient to brush his teeth while in bathroom, after bowel movement.*
	1. Assist the patient to ambulate by using his walker. 2. *Pull legs to side of bed and put on his shoes.* 3. *Pull patient to a sitting position.* 4. *Put walker in front of patient.* 5. *Help patient to stand; grasp only under armpits, since arms are sore.* 6. *Place patient's hands on the walker. Make sure he has good grip.* 7. *When patient is balanced, let him walk alone to chair.* 8. *Help him sit down in chair by placing arms around his waist.*
6. The patient will show less anxiety and fear by (date).	1. Maintain one-to-one relationship on each shift, if possible, having same personnel care for patient each day. 2. Follow routine that has been set up (see above). 3. *Explain all tests, procedures and inform patient of the schedule.* 4. *Encourage patient to participate and make decisions concerning his care.*

Mr. R. remained relatively "status quo" while he was hospitalized. His condition changed very little and he had no response to therapy. The decision was made by his family to have him transferred to a nursing home. Upon discharge, a copy of his nursing history and "routine" was sent with him to the nursing home, in order to maintain continuity of care and to make this transition as smooth as possible for him. A nursing discharge summary was placed on his chart; it was a résumé of the nursing care he had received and its effectiveness.

There will be many instances in which a complete nursing history and physician's examination cannot be obtained, due to the patient's unresponsiveness or extreme distress. If complete information cannot be obtained from the patient and family, the nurse must rely more upon her observations, the physician's workup, and past medical records (if available). The following partial interview illustrates how even a short, structured interview can elicit data needed for arriving at a nursing assessment and for planning intervention. More inclusive data concerning the patient's family, socioeconomic status, activities of daily living, and expectations were obtained when the patient improved and was not in acute distress. It is not necessarily the quantity of data which is important in planning patient care but rather the quality.

Mrs. R. is a 42-year-old housewife whose admitting diagnosis is myasthenia gravis. She has been hospitalized twice previously at the Myasthenia Gravis Clinic in New York and appears to have much insight into and knowledge about her illness. The following is a clinical nursing observation and partial interview:

Patient was lying in bed with the head of the bed elevated to almost 90°. Lid ptosis was extremely visible. She was unable to raise her left lid and it remained closed during the entire observation. Right lid was halfway closed. Speech was breathy and nasal, paused to catch breath frequently during brief interview. Respirations shallow and rapid (28 a minute). Pleasant, cooperative, and talked willingly about illness. She stated, "I'm unable to walk any more and fell four days ago. I've been taking Prostigmin every three or four hours, but it isn't helping any more. I'm unable to do anything but stay in bed."

Patient's jaw dropped and mouth hung open, with drooling apparent. Could barely force a smile; stated, "Sometimes I get so tired that I am unable to move my upper lip or tongue and then I can hardly talk." Dysphagic and could not swallow meat or even soft foods. Liquids and milk increased salivation and frequently came back through nose. She stated, "I have difficulty getting anything down anymore."

Has difficulty with double vision and focusing left eye, due to rapid movements of it. Generalized weakness and could raise hands only about 9 inches from bed. She said, "I'm so weak that I can't even push myself up in bed." Gets weaker as day progresses.

Patient also had extreme difficulty with diarrhea over last week prior to admission, buttocks chafed. Attributed diarrhea to Prostigmin she was taking at frequent intervals. Found herself taking injections almost on "whenever necessary" basis.

Interview terminated due to patient's distress.

From the brief nursing history, interview, and physical assessment, many areas of concern were identified. These were the patient's:

1. Difficulty in breathing.
2. Extreme weakness.
3. Inability to carry out most activities.
4. Dysphagia.
5. Double vision.
6. Chafed buttocks.
7. Dysarthria.
8. Drooling and increased salivation.
9. Danger of aspiration.

It was also established that although this patient had knowledge of her illness, she had been taking medications as she felt necessary. The nursing staff also anticipated that the physician might perform a tracheotomy on the patient, should her condition worsen. From this assessment, it was decided that nursing intervention should involve the following goals for the patient:

1. Observe closely for signs of respiratory failure.
2. Assist with all activities of daily living.
3. Maintain skin integrity and prevent possible development of decubitus ulcers.
4. Help provide adequate nourishment.
5. Maintain communication.
6. Observe for complications of myasthenic and cholinergic crises.

Specific nursing orders were then formulated and placed on the Kardex, a step which would lead to the realization of the nursing goals. As the patient's condition improved, the goals and orders were modified and/or new ones were formulated, as was necessary. Nursing intervention is neither a static nor a "one-shot" process. Nursing care consists of continual evaluation, modifications, additions, and revisions, if it is to be as effective and therapeutic as possible.

After the patient improved sufficiently, a more complete nursing history was obtained concerning her social and cultural history, her role in the family and routine at home, coping mechanisms, and so on. New nursing goals were formulated which included teaching the patient aspects of self-care and about her illness, particularly the medications she would be taking. Provision for a community health consultant was made in order to assist in the attainment of long-range rehabilitative goals at home.

Neurologic Examination

In addition to obtaining a nursing history, nursing assessment involves a physical examination of the patient. Assessment of the person's neurologic status is essential in planning patient care and provides helpful baseline data by which to judge improvement or deterioration. Even though a complete neurologic examination is done by the physician upon the patient's admission, the nurse remains responsible for observing changes in neurologic status and testing for neurologic function.

The neurologic examination is utilized to determine the existence of nervous system dysfunction, the location and nature of the dysfunction, improvement or worsening of nervous system function, and prognosis. It involves assessing the function of the following areas of the nervous system: the cerebral cortex, cranial nerves, cerebellum, motor and sensory systems, reflexes, and cerebrovascular system.

It is beyond the scope of this chapter to include every aspect of the neurologic examination; therefore, only the most basic and relevant procedures will be discussed. Individual nurses desiring more comprehensive knowledge should consult the bibliography at the end of this chapter.

ASSESSMENT OF CEREBRAL FUNCTION

Evaluation of cerebral function aids in obtaining differential diagnosis (various neurologic conditions affect cerebral function) and helps to differentiate organic from functional neurologic illness. The mental examination also gathers data concerning the patient's ability to communicate with and relate to others which is of primary importance when planning therapeutic intervention.

LEVEL OF CONSCIOUSNESS. An assessment of the patient's awareness of his environment, and psychological and sensory stimuli is made.

GENERAL BEHAVIOR. The nurse should observe for general appearance, interpersonal interaction, manner, expressions, attitude, reactions to the interviewing and to the nurse, and speech patterns.

EMOTIONAL STATUS. The nurse observes for such parameters of emotionality as depression, bizarre behavior, euphoria, indifference, tenseness, anger, hostility, silliness or inappropriate responses, suspiciousness, emotional lability, manic behavior, anxiety, withdrawal, worried state, calmness, and the like.

TRAIN OF THOUGHT. The nurse observes for alterations in thought content such as paranoia, hallucinations, delusions, obsessions, phobias, depersonalization, suicidal thoughts, feelings of grandeur, flight of ideas, or excessive preoccupations.

INTELLECTUAL FUNCTION. To test for orientation to time, place, and person, the nurse asks the patient his name, age, date and day of the week, year, residence, personal history such as marriage, job, and the name of the hospital or institution in which the interview is taking place. She tests for remote memory by asking questions related to early events such as the patient's birthday, date of marriage, place of birth, and so on. Recent memory can be assessed by asking questions about what has transpired within the last week or the last few days. Other intellectual function tests include attention span, calculations (patient multiplies or adds by two digits, counts forward or backward) and abstract judgment. The most common test for abstract reasoning is interpretation of proverbs. The patient's general knowledge, and his ability to read and write are also assessed.

LANGUAGE FUNCTION. (For assessment of language function, see aphasia, pp. 692-696.)

CORTICAL SENSORY FUNCTION. The cerebral cortex is composed of cortical areas where recognition and interpretation of objects and stimuli occur. *Agnosia* is the inability to recognize or interpret objects through a particular sensory modality, at the cortical level. *Visual agnosia* is an inability to identify objects through visual means. *Tactile agnosia* (astereognosis) is an inability to recognize the shape and texture of objects by touching. *Auditory agnosia* is a lack of ability to interpret and identify sounds. *Autotopagnosia* occurs when an individual has difficulty identifying his body parts, or the orientation of his body parts (recognizing right from left, unawareness of a particular part or even one-half of the body).

ASSESSMENT TECHNIQUES

Visual agnosia—occipital lobe is affected	The patient is asked to identify objects or pictures of objects which are placed in front of him and colors. Identification of letters and words is not necessary as this tests for aphasia.

Auditory agnosia—temporal lobe is affected	The patient is asked to identify various sounds with his eyes closed, such as a ringing bell, whistling, water being poured, rattling paper, and so on.
Tactile agnosia—parietal lobe is affected	With the eyes closed, the patient is asked to identify familiar objects such as keys, a comb, coins, a paper cup, pencil, and so on.
Autotopagnosia—usually nondominant parietal lobe is affected	The patient is asked to identify his body parts and also his right from left (e.g., extending his left hand; touching his left ear; lifting his right leg).

CORTICAL MOTOR FUNCTION. Apraxia is the loss of ability to perform a skilled act in the absence of paralysis, rigidity, bradykinesia, difficulty with coordination or other motor involvement. *Motor* apraxia usually occurs in one extremity such as the arm. There is loss of ability to perform skilled movements with the fingers, even though there is no motor weakness present. This type of apraxia is almost always contralateral to a lesion in the precentral or premotor cortex. *Idiokinetic apraxia* results from a discontinuity between association areas where ideational planning occurs and the motor center which controls voluntary movement. Consequently, a person may know what he wishes to do, but be unable to perform the act. An example of this occurred in a woman who had suffered a left middle cerebral artery stroke. When she returned home from the hospital, she noted she could not make a bed. She knew what she wanted to do, but when she attempted to make the bed, she could not. *Ideational* apraxia is difficulty formulating or planning the necessary steps needed to perform skilled acts. Movements in a given act may be out of sequence, omitted, or incorrect. The nurse often sees this in a patient who has an apraxia for dressing. The patient may begin to dress himself, but omits necessary steps, and does it incorrectly. He may neglect to put an arm through a sleeve or may button only one buttonhole. Ideational and idiokinetic apraxia are often difficult to differentiate since they overlap to a great degree.

ASSESSMENT OF APRAXIA

Motor apraxia	The patient is tested for fine hand movements by being asked to open and close a safety pin, pick up small coins, handle a comb, tie a bow, open a cup with a lid, and so on.
Idiokinetic (apraxia ideomotor)	Various tests can include having the patient pretend to hammer a nail or to open a lock, cut something out with scissors, put on a robe, comb the hair, drink from a cup.
Ideational apraxia	The patient is asked to perform some of the same tests used for the assessment of idiokinetic apraxia. He is observed for forgetfulness, absent-mindedness, incorrect movements, sudden stopping of movements before the act is completed.

ASSESSMENT OF CRANIAL NERVE FUNCTION

CRANIAL NERVE I (OLFACTORY). The olfactory nerve is a visceral afferent nerve which conducts sensory impulses from the nasal mucosa to the central nervous system, thereby transmitting the sense of smell. Testing of olfactory nerve function is important as lesions (particularly tumors) may compress the olfactory groove and cause anosmia (loss of smell). In testing, the examiner asks the patient to identify familiar odors, such as coffee, cloves, tobacco, cinnamon, with his eyes closed. Each nostril is tested separately.

CRANIAL NERVE II (OPTIC). Optic nerve fibers arise from each retina and constitute the visual pathway to the brain. The fibers which arise from the nasal halves of each retina cross while passing through the optic chiasm, whereas the fibers from the temporal halves do not. The optic nerve proper consists of optic fibers which extend from the retina to the optic chiasm. Fibers behind the chiasm are called optic tracts.

Loss of the temporal portion of vision in each eye is *bitemporal hemianopia*. Loss of vision in the left field of vision in both eyes is *left homonymous hemianopia*. *Right homonymous hemianopia* occurs with loss of right field of vision in both eyes. Quadrant field cuts occur due to damage of the fibers which arise from the lateral geniculate bodies and extend to the occipital cortex.

Assessment of optic nerve function includes tests for visual acuity for distant and near vision and visual fields, and an ophthalmoscopic examination.

Visual Acuity. Visual acuity for distant vision is tested by the standard Snellen eye chart as described in Chapter 4, p. 60. Visual acuity for near vision is tested by the Jaeger reading chart. If the patient wears glasses, he is instructed to keep them on while being tested for acuity.

Visual Fields. The confrontation method is used most often to detect obvious defects in the visual field. The examiner moves his index finger, a cotton-tipped applicator or a large white-tipped hat pin into the patient's visual field from various meridians starting from the periphery and moving into the center of vision. The examiner and the patient should be facing each other approximately two feet apart. Each eye is tested separately while the other eye remains closed. With the confrontation method, the patient's visual fields are compared with the examiner's. To test the patient's right eye, the examiner asks the patient to close his left eye while the examiner closes his right eye. The patient is asked to respond when he detects any movement of the finger (or whatever object is being used), when he first sees the object, and when he can identify the object. Some examiners have the patient count fingers, suggesting this produces more sensitive results. There are other more precise methods available to test visual fields such as the perimeter and tangent screen. These tests are usually conducted by a neurologist or a neuro-ophthalmologist.

Ophthalmoscopic Examination. The eyes are examined with an ophthalmoscope to visualize the fundus (eyeground). (See Chapter 4, pp. 62-63.)

The ophthalmoscopic examination is extremely important because various neurologic conditions are manifested by changes in the optic disc or vessels. Papilledema (swelling or choking of the optic disc) indicates increased intracranial pressure. When papilledema occurs, the margins of the disc become blurred, the retinal veins dilate, and hemorrhages occur around the disc. Other conditions producing changes in the fundus include optic neuritis, retinal arteriosclerosis, hypertension, diabetes, retinitis pigmentosa, and retrobulbar neuritis.

OCULAR NERVES: CRANIAL NERVE III (OCULOMOTOR), CRANIAL NERVE IV (TROCHLEAR), AND CRANIAL NERVE VI (ABDUCENS). Oculomotor, trochlear, and abducens nerve function is determined by testing extraocular movements and pupillary reflexes of the eye. Since these three nerves supply muscles of the eye necessary for movement, they are viewed as a specific unit and are tested at the same time.

Assessment of Extraocular Movements. Initial observation for any ptosis, exophthalmos, deviation of the eyes, position of the eyeballs is made. To test extraocular movements, the examiner asks the patient to look in the following directions: up, down, laterally, medially, upward and medially (upward and inward), upward and laterally (upward and outward), downward and medially, downward and laterally. Observation for conjugate gaze (eyes moving in the same direction) is made. Any difficulty in gaze, paresis or paralysis of movement, or diplopia is noted. The eyes are also tested for convergence (the coordinated movement toward fixation at a near point). The patient watches the examiner's finger as it moves from a distance to a point between the eyes. Normally, the eyes converge.

Testing Pupillary Reflexes. Pupillary reflexes are tested to determine the function of the retina, optic nerve, optic chiasm, optic tract, brain stem, and oculomotor nerve. Testing pupillary reflexes is one of the most important areas of the neurologic examination.

Pupillary Light Reflex. Normally, the pupil constricts when light is shone into the eye and dilates when the light is removed. This is the *direct light reflex.* The light stimulus is transmitted from the retina via optic nerve fibers through the optic chiasm to the dorsal portion of the midbrain. Internuncial neurons in this area then carry the impulse to the Edinger-Westphal nucleus. The Edinger-Westphal nucleus is part of the parasympathetic division of the autonomic nervous system and is located rostrally to the oculomotor nucleus. The axons of the Edinger-Westphal nucleus become part of the

NERVE	INNERVATION AND FUNCTION	OCULAR DISTURBANCE
Oculomotor	Supplies parasympathetic innervation to the pupil. Supplies the following ocular muscles: *Superior rectus* which turns eye upward and inward; *Medial rectus* which adducts eye; *Inferior oblique* which moves eye upward and outward; *Inferior rectus* which turns eye downward and inward; *Levator palpebrae superioris* which elevates the eyelid.	Isolated third nerve palsy occurs frequently due to location of nerve. Paralysis produces 1. Ptosis of the eyelid due to involved levator palpebrae superioris muscle. 2. Inability to move the eye inward, downward or upward. Lateral eye deviation occurs due to pulling by the lateral rectus muscle. Deviation of the eye downward occurs due to the pull of the superior oblique muscle. Diplopia (double vision) results. 3. Dilated pupil which is nonreactive to light and accomodation.
Trochlear	Supplies the superior oblique muscle which depresses the eye and turns it outward.	Isolated fourth nerve palsy is less common. Paralysis or weakness causes difficulty on downward and outward gaze. With an isolated fourth nerve palsy, binocular vision can be maintained by tilting the head to the opposite shoulder.[4]
Abducens	Supplies the lateral rectus muscle which controls lateral movement of the eye.	Due to its location and length, the abducens nerve becomes affected in many neurologic conditions. Paralysis produces loss of ability to turn eye laterally. Eye is turned inward due to pull of other ocular muscles. Diplopia occurs.

oculomotor nerve upon leaving the midbrain and constitute the efferent pathway to the ciliary ganglion which controls the sphincter of the pupil. It should be noted that internuncial neurons conduct impulses to the Edinger-Westphal nucleus on both sides. Therefore, the opposite pupil from the one being tested will also constrict, although less vigorously. The response to light by the contralateral pupil is the *consensual light reflex*. A lesion or damage to the oculomotor nerve will result in a loss of the direct and consensual light reflex on the affected side. The direct light reflex is absent in a blind eye due to the involvement of the optic nerve and the afferent pathway to the midbrain.

Pupillary reaction tests should be performed

diligently and with utmost accuracy. The nurse should first observe the size, shape, and equality of the pupils. Since some patients may have unequal pupils, nonreactive pupil,[5] or eccentric location, information should be obtained concerning the status prior to admission. Next, reaction to light should be tested in a darkened room with the use of a small bright flashlight. All too often inadequate equipment and techniques are used, resulting in inaccurate responses. The patient should look at a distant point when testing the light reflex, since the pupils constrict on accommodation. The light should be shone into the eye and the direct and consensual responses noted.

A normal pupil constricts briskly when exposed to light. Both pupils should be tested for reaction and any difference noted. (Often in the presence of increasing intracranial pressure, the affected pupil reacts more slowly than the other, or is slightly constricted before dilatation and fixation ensues.) If both pupils are equal and react to light, the following abbreviation is often used: PEARL (pupils equal and react to light). When pupil reactions are recorded separately, RB (reacting briskly) and RS (reacting sluggishly or slowly) are used to denote the response. As the pupil becomes dilated and fixed, it may be recorded as DNR (dilated and nonreactive). Abbreviations vary with recording tools used and with the institution.

It is extremely important that the nurse carry out the procedure as ordered. Acute observations can often aid the physician in localizing a lesion or changes in the condition of the patient. Understanding the physiological and scientific principles underlying increased intracranial pressure and pupillary changes impresses one with the fact that "routine" pupil checks can be vital and lifesaving.

Testing for accommodation is done during the pupillary examination. The patient after looking into the distance is asked to direct his gaze to a near object. The following responses normally occur:

1. Convergence of the eyes due to the action of the medial recti muscles to maintain visual focus.
2. Thickening of the lens.
3. The pupils constrict.

Assessing Abnormal Eye Movements. Nystagmus (talantropia) is a condition of involuntary, coordinated, rapid movement or oscillation of the eyeball. It is most often acquired, but may be congenital and is frequently seen in neurologic disease as well as disease of the inner ear. Nystagmus may occur in any direction: horizontally, vertically, obliquely, or rotatory. The eyeball movements can be fine (scarcely visible) or very coarse. Rate of movement is recorded as slow, medium, or rapid. If the movement is horizontal and equal without a quick and slow component, it is *pendular nystagmus*. Nystagmus which is jerky in nature and has both slow and quick components (unequal oscillation) is *rhythmical nystagmus*. The direction of the quick component is used to determine the direction of nystagmus. The intensity of nystagmus refers to the degree to which it is present in various directions. First-degree nystagmus is the presence of nystagmus only when the eyes are turned in the direction of the quick component. Second-degree nystagmus is the presence of nystagmus when the eyes are looking in the neutral direction and when the eyes are looking in the direction of the quick component. Third-degree nystagmus is the presence of nystagmus even when the eyes are moved in the direction of the slow component.

The vestibular nerve, vestibular-ocular reflex, cerebellum, basal ganglion, ocular nuclei, and medial longitudinal fasciculus pathways all influence eye movements. Involvement of the vestibular circuits and their pathways can produce nystagmus. Forms of nystagmus frequently seen in neurologic disease include vestibular nystagmus, cerebellar nystagmus, and nystagmus due to involvement of the medial longitudinal fasciculus.

Testing for nystagmus is done while testing extraocular movements. Observation is made for the type, direction, amplitude, rate and degree of nystagmus. If present, the examiner should determine if changes in position or movement of the eyes and head affect the nystagmus.

CRANIAL NERVE V (TRIGEMINAL). The trigeminal nerve is both a motor and sensory (mixed) nerve and has three branches: the ophthalmic, maxillary, and mandibular. Motor fibers which enter the mandibular branch supply the muscles of mastication which include the masseter, temporalis, and pterygoid (internal and external) muscles of the face. These muscles help to elevate and depress the mandible and move the jaw from side to side.

Testing the Motor Portion of the Trigeminal Nerve. The muscles of mastication are tested for power, strength, and movement.

1. The patient clenches his jaw which will contract the temporalis and masseter muscles. The examiner palpates the contraction of these muscles by placing the fingers over the patient's cheeks and temples, and feels for any difference in contractions or loss of contraction which indicates paresis or paralysis on one side.

2. The examiner asks the patient to open his mouth and notes any deviation of the jaw. Since the pterygoid muscles draw the jaw forward and toward the middle of the mouth, deviation will be toward the side of the paralyzed muscles.

3. To test for action of the pterygoid muscles which produce jaw movement side to side, the examiner asks the patient to move his jaw side to side against resistance of the examiner's hand. When paralysis occurs, the patient is unable to move the jaw toward the nonparalyzed side.

4. The examiner notes any atrophy, fasciculations, tremors of the muscles.

5. To test the jaw reflex (masseter reflex), the examiner taps the middle of the chin with a reflex hammer while the mouth is partially opened and relaxed. Normally, the jaw contracts and the mouth closes. In supranuclear (upper motor neuron lesions) the jaw reflex is exaggerated, whereas in a nuclear or lower motor neuron lesion of the trigeminal nerve it is absent or diminished.

In assessing motor function of the trigeminal nerve, the nurse should be aware that the motor nuclei of the fifth nerve receive upper motor neuron connections from both the right and left cortex. Therefore, a supranuclear (upper motor neuron) lesion does not usually produce any marked paresis or symptoms. Paralysis of the masticator muscles is most apparent following a nuclear or lower motor neuron lesion such as occurs in bulbar palsy, multiple sclerosis, and poliomyelitis. Bilateral trigeminal involvement is frequently seen in infranuclear processes such as myasthenia gravis which affects the myoneural junction. Bilateral involvement is characterized by drooping of the jaw, and bilateral weakness of the muscles with resulting loss of movements of mastication.

Testing the Sensory Portion of the Trigeminal Nerve. Each of the individual branches of the trigeminal nerve supplies sensation from various areas of the face. The ophthalmic division transmits sensations from the forehead, eyes, anterior temples, scalp, anterior and lateral surfaces of the nose, cornea, upper nasal mucosa, and paranasal sinuses. The maxillary branch carries sensations from the lower nose, cheeks, lower eyelid, upper jaw, upper lip, upper teeth, hard palate, nasal mucosa, and maxillary sinuses. The mandibular branch transmits sensation from the lower jaw, lower lip and chin, tongue, lower teeth, buccal mucosa, posterior cheek and temple, and portions of the external auditory canal.

To determine sensory function of the trigeminal nerve, the examiner tests both sides of the face, and the oral and nasal cavities for sensations of light touch, pain, and temperature. A wisp of cotton is used to test for light touch of the face, and a wooden applicator is used to test the mucous membranes. A pin is used to test for pain sensation and tubes of hot and cold water are applied to assess temperature sensation.

The *corneal reflex* is regulated partly by the ophthalmic division of the trigeminal nerve and is considered an important diagnostic test for lesions of the trigeminal nerve. The corneal reflex is present if the eye blinks when the cornea is touched lightly with a piece of cotton. When testing, the examiner stands at the side of the patient and strokes the cornea gently while the patient looks in the opposite direction. The eye tested should blink (direct corneal reflex). The opposite eye will also blink (*consensual* corneal reflex). A lesion of the trigeminal nerve will abolish both the direct and consensual corneal reflex. The corneal reflex is often used in assessing the level of coma.

The most common neurologic disorder which

affects the trigeminal nerve is trigeminal neuralgia (tic douloureux).

CRANIAL NERVE VII (FACIAL). The facial nerve is primarily a motor nerve and supplies the muscles of facial expression and the orbicularis oculi which closes the eye. The part of the facial nerve which carries the parasympathetic and sensory portions is called the nervus intermedius. It supplies parasympathetic secretory fibers to the oral and nasal cavities, the salivary and lacrimal glands. It conveys sensation from the anterior part of the tongue, the eardrum, salivary glands, nasal and pharyngeal mucosa, and conveys deep proprioceptive sensation from the facial muscles.

Assessing Motor Function of the Facial Nerve. Initially, the nurse should observe for any asymmetry of the face or abnormality of the facial muscles. She observes for drooping of the mouth, flattening of the nasolabial fold, absence of facial expression, a widening palpebral fissure, absence of blinking, lack of mobility of muscles, drooling of the mouth, or tearing of the eye.

The patient is asked to perform the following movements which utilize the various facial muscles: raising the eyebrows, frowning, wrinkling the forehead, lifting the forehead, closing the eyes against resistance, smiling, whistling, puckering the lips, blowing out the cheeks, retracting the angles of the mouth and "making a face." Any abnormality, immobility, atrophy, or contracture is noted.

The orbicularis oculi reflex is elicited by percussing the supraorbital ridge. Normally, the eye should close following percussion.

Assessing Sensory Function of Facial Nerves: The sense of taste is determined by having the patient identify sugar, acid, and salt when they are each placed on the anterior part of the tongue. Both sides of the tongue should be tested separately. The patient should not speak and should keep the tongue protruded to avoid the substance spreading to other parts of the tongue.

Peripheral lesions of the facial nerves, such as Bell's palsy, result in drooping or sagging of the face on the affected side, inability to close the eye, inability to raise the eyebrow, frown, or smile, sagging of the lower lid, and tearing of the

affected eye. The person is unable to whistle, purse his lips, or show his teeth on the affected side. Due to paralysis of the facial muscles surrounding the lips, there is difficulty in pronouncing words and speaking articulately. Drooling from the mouth on the affected side often occurs. Particles of food lodge in the mouth due to lack of movement of the cheek and can cause irritation and difficulty maintaining oral hygiene.

CRANIAL NERVE VIII. (ACOUSTIC). The acoustic nerve has two branches, the cochlear and the vestibular, both of which have different peripheral receptors and central connections. The cochlear branch is the nerve for hearing. The vestibular nerve conveys messages which are necessary for controlling balance, equilibrium, and orientation in space.

Cochlear Nerve Function. The following tests are routinely done to determine hearing function.

1. Hearing acuity is determined by covering one ear and testing the other with either a ticking watch or the whispered voice. The furthest distance the sound is heard is noted. Both ears are tested. The patient should close his eyes to avoid seeing the examiner's movements.

2. Lateralization (Weber Test). A vibrating tuning fork is placed over the forehead or vertex of the skull. Normally it should be heard in both ears and not to one side (lateralized).

3. Air and Bone Conduction (Rinné Test). In this test, air and bone conduction are compared. First bone conduction (BC) is tested by placing the tuning fork on the mastoid process. The examiner notes how long the patient hears it. Then air conduction is determined by placing the tuning fork in front of the ear. Normally, air conduction (AC) is greater and heard much longer than bone conduction. The Rinné test is useful in determining the type of deafness. In conductive deafness, air conduction is decreased and bone conduction maintained. In perceptive or nerve deafness both air and bone conduction are reduced.

Audiometry is a more accurate means of testing hearing function. Symptoms of cochlear nerve involvement include tinnitus (ringing, roaring, buzzing noises in the ear), loss of hearing, and deafness. The patient's ability to hear is important not only from a neurologic diagnostic standpoint, but also from a psychosocial one.

Vestibular Nerve Function. Assessment of vestibular function is obtained by the cold caloric test and is not a routine part of the neurologic examination.

CRANIAL NERVE IX (GLOSSOPHARYNGEAL). The glossopharyngeal nerve and the vagus nerve are usually tested together due to their similarities in function and overlapping innervation to the pharynx. However, for purposes of clarity, they will be discussed separately.

The glossopharyngeal nerve supplies motor fibers to the stylopharyngeus muscle of the pharynx which elevates the pharynx, and parasympathetic fibers to the parotid gland which stimulates salivation and supplies sensation to the pharynx and posterior third of the tongue. Through its carotid branch, it supplies receptors in the carotid body and carotid sinus which provide for reflex control of heart rate, blood pressure, and respiration.

Tests used to evaluate glossopharyngeal function include sensory testing of the posterior pharynx and the pharyngeal (gag) reflex. Sensation to the pharynx and posterior third of the tongue is tested with a long wooden applicator.

The gag reflex is elicited by stimulating each side of the posterior pharynx with a tongue blade. Stimulation normally produces elevation and constriction of the pharynx and retraction of the tongue (gagging). The gag reflex is important because it initiates the act of swallowing. Its reflex arc consists of afferent (sensory) impulses which are conducted to the medulla via the glossopharyngeal nerve and the efferent (motor) pathway which is carried by the vagus nerve. Consequently, the pharyngeal (gag) reflex tests for both glossopharyngeal and vagal nerve function.

Isolated lesions of the glossopharyngeal nerve are rare and produce only slight dysphagia (difficulty swallowing). More often, lesions occur in association with the other bulbar nerves, such as in bulbar palsy, multiple sclerosis, botulism, and poliomyelitis.

CRANIAL NERVE X (VAGUS). The vagus nerve has many branches and the greatest distri-bution of all the cranial nerves. The motor portion of the vagus nerve supplies the muscles of the pharynx, soft palate, and larynx. The parasympathetic pathways of the vagus nerve supply thoracic and abdominal viscera, which inhibit and slow the heart rate, increase and stimulate gastrointestinal peristalsis, and gastric and pancreatic secretion, and stimulate gallbladder, hepatic, and splenic activity. The sensory fibers of the vagus nerve originate in the jugular ganglion and the ganglion nodosum and supply sensation to the lower pharynx, larynx, thoracic and abdominal viscera.

Examination of vagus nerve function consists of testing the motor functions of the soft palate, pharynx, and larynx and assessing the autonomic carotid sinus reflex.

Observation of the Soft Palate. The palate is observed while the mouth is open and at rest. (Fig. 20-1, A). The examiner observes for symmetry and position of the uvula, median raphe, and palatal arches. Elevation of the palate is tested by having the patient say "ah." The palate should elevate equally and not to one side, and the uvula should rise in the midline. In unilateral vagus paralysis, there is weakness of the soft palate on the affected side and lowering of the palatal arch. (Fig. 20-1, B). On phonation, the affected side elevates toward the normal side, and the uvula is deviated toward the normal side (Fig. 20-1, C). The palate does not rise on phonation in bilateral vagus paralysis.

Palatal Reflex. The palatal reflex is obtained by stroking each side of the uvula with a cotton-tipped applicator. Stimulation produces elevation of the soft palate on the side tested. In unilateral vagus paralysis, the palatal reflex is lost on the affected side. Bilateral involvement produces loss of palatal reflexes bilaterally.

Observation of the Pharynx. The gag (pharyngeal) reflex is also a test for vagus nerve function as the efferent pathway of the pharyngeal reflex is transmitted by the vagus nerve.

The ability to swallow liquids and solids should also be assessed, since the pharyngeal musculature is essential in deglutition. The pharyngeal muscles not only block off the nasal

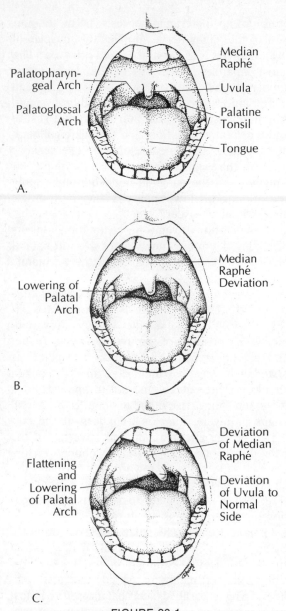

FIGURE 20-1.
Observing the palate. (A) Normal palate with mouth open and at rest. (B) Right unilateral vagus paralysis, mouth at rest. (C) Right unilaterial vagus paralysis on pronation.

passages in the act of swallowing, but help to force food into the esophagus. Unilateral vagus paralysis produces difficulty swallowing liquids and solids and causes regurgitation of liquids through the nose. Bilateral involvement causes marked dysphagia with severe choking, coughing, and regurgitation, and is frequently seen in bulbar palsy. Assessment of the gag reflex and swallowing functions is necessary to determine nursing methods for promoting nutritional intake.

Observation of the Larynx. The superior laryngeal branch of the vagus innervates the cricothyroid muscle and supplies the mucous membrane of the larynx above the vocal cord. The recurrent laryngeal branch supplies all the intrinsic muscles of the larynx. In evaluating laryngeal function, the examiner observes the patient's voice for hoarseness, dysphonia, and for pitch. Unilateral vagus paralysis produces hoarseness, dyspnea, coughing, and often the speech will become nasal in sound. The examiner observes for respiratory stridor. During inspiration, the cords are normally abducted by the action of the posterior cricoarytenoids (abductor muscles of the larynx). When paralysis of the abductor muscle occurs, the vocal cords cannot be separated fully and inspiratory stridor is heard. In bilateral abductor palsies (seen in bilateral vagus paralysis), inspiratory stridor is marked with severe dyspnea.

Carotid Sinus Reflex. Applying pressure over the carotid sinus produces reflex stimulation of the vagus which results in cardiac slowing. Testing should be carried out with extreme caution in patients with suspected or known vascular disease.

CRANIAL NERVE XI (ACCESSORY). The accessory nerve is a motor nerve which innervates the sternocleidomastoid muscle and also the upper part of the trapezius muscle. The sternocleidomastoid muscle assists in turning the head from side to side. The trapezius raises, depresses, and rotates the scapula.

Assessment of accessory nerve function involves testing both the trapezius and the sternocleidomastoid muscles for strength. Initial observation is made for atrophy, hypertrophy of the muscles, position of the head, and shoulder droop. To test the strength of the trapezius muscle, the examiner asks the patient to shrug his shoulders against resistance and palpates the contraction. Strength and contraction of the sternocleidomastoid muscle is ascertained by having the patient rotate his head toward the opposite shoulder against resistance.

The most common disorder affecting the sternocleidomastoid muscle is spasmodic torticollis, a spasmodic turning or deviation of the head and neck toward the opposite side. Paralysis of the sternocleidomastoid and trapezius muscles is most often the result of peripheral lesion of the accessory nerve from injury, trauma, neoplasms, and intracranial hemorrhages. Muscular disorders also cause paralysis and atrophy such as myopathies, myositis, amotrophic lateral sclerosis, and myasthenia gravis. If a person has difficulty turning his head toward a particular side, personal items, bedside tables, and so on should be placed on the opposite side.

CRANIAL NERVE XII (HYPOGLOSSAL). The hypoglossal nerve supplies the muscles of the tongue and is a pure motor nerve. Observation of the tongue for atrophy and deviation is made while the tongue is protruded. To test for strength, the examiner asks the patient to protrude the tongue and move it from side to side against resistance. Intelligible speech should be noted to detect difficulty pronouncing the linguals. In unilateral paralysis, speech and swallowing are only slightly affected. Bilateral paralysis of the tongue produces marked speech and swallowing difficulties. Respiration may be affected as the tongue falls back in the throat.

ASSESSMENT OF CEREBELLAR FUNCTION

The cerebellum with its cerebral and vestibular connections helps to control balance, coordination, and posture. The following tests are used to determine cerebellar function.

TESTING FOR RAPID ALTERNATING MOVEMENT. The patient is asked to alternate the palmar and back side of his hands on his knees rapidly. Other tests used include tapping the foot on the floor, pronating and supinating the extended forearm, tapping the fingers up and down, touching each finger to the thumb in quick succession. The patient is observed for speed, accuracy, and skill of movements. Difficulty in performing rapid alternating movements is *dysdiadochokinesia*.

FINGER TO NOSE TEST. With the eyes open, the patient is asked to extend his arm and touch the tip of his nose with his index finger. The finger-to-nose test is done slowly at first and then with increasing rapidity, with the arm outstretched in different positions. During testing, the examiner observes for tremor, inaccuracy, jerkiness, past-pointing, and *dysmetria* (the inability to direct or stop movements at the proper point). Both hands should be tested.

HEEL-TO KNEE-TO TOE TEST. In a lying position, the patient brings the heel of one foot dorsiflexed to the opposite knee and then slides the heel down on the shin in a straight line to the great toe. The examiner observes for dysmetria, action tremor, jerky movements, and inaccuracy. Both feet are tested. Other tests used to assess coordination in the lower extremities include making figure 8's in the air with each foot and pointing to some fixed object (examiner's index finger or chair) with each great toe.

TREMOR. During testing, the examiner observes for intention tremor. This tremor occurs upon movement, is coarse and irregular, and is a symptom of cerebellar dysfunction.

ARM DRIFT. With the arms held in a forward position, the affected arm tends to deviate or drift outward in cerebellar disease.

DYSARTHRIA. Inability to articulate is observed. In cerebellar disease speech may be slurred or scanning in nature, due to inability to coordinate movements necessary for articulation.

POSTURE AND GAIT. The examiner observes the patient's posture, first while he is sitting and then while he is standing. She notes the position of the arms, body, and legs to maintain the upright position, and observes for any unsteadiness, wobbling, or swaying. She ascertains whether balance can be maintained with the feet placed close together. To test for gait, the examiner has the patient walk forward and observes for ataxia (difficulty in gait). She notes any falling, staggering, or swaying and in what direction; position of arms, trunk, and lower extremities while walking; difficulty in maintaining posture and wobbly balance. Other tests to assess gait include walking backwards, sideways, turning quickly, running, rising from a sitting position, walking in a circle, and tandem walking (placing one foot directly in front of the other on a straight course). In cerebellar disease, ataxia tends to be toward the side of the lesion, and the ataxia is present with the eyes open or closed.

ASSESSMENT OF MOTOR FUNCTION

EXAMINATION OF MUSCLE SIZE. The muscles are inspected for wasting, atrophy, contractures, changes in contour, loss of bulk, and fasciculations. Differences of muscle size in the upper and lower extremities should be accurately recorded with a tape measure. Muscle movement is determined by having the person perform movements and activities which utilize various muscle groups such as rotation of the neck, movement of the arms, movement of thorax, movement of the legs, and the like.

GAIT. Observing a person walk is a useful test for assessing the function of various muscles and for determining a neurologic diagnosis. The following gait disturbances are seen in neurologic illness.

The *cerebellar ataxic gait* is characterized by wide-based, staggering, drunkenlike movements. The person is unsteady and may sway to a particular side. Ataxia is present with the eyes open or closed. It is present in such cerebellar diseases as cerebellar tumors, Freidreich's ataxia, and multiple sclerosis.

The *tabetic ataxic gait* ("slapping gait") is caused by degeneration of the posterior columns which produces a loss of position sense in the lower extremities. Consequently, the person is not sure of the position of his legs and, in order to walk, must watch them closely to make the necessary adjustments and compensations. Movements of the lower extremities are jerky and often flail-like. The gait is wide-based, the feet are lifted high and brought down heels first followed by slapping of the toes. Ataxia is more marked with the eyes closed.

The *hemiplegic gait* is most often caused by a cerebrovascular accident with corticospinal tract involvement and hemiplegia. The gait is unilateral. The affected upper extremity is semiflexed at the elbow and held close to the abdomen, and adducted at the shoulder. The fingers and the wrist are flexed so that wristdrop occurs. The affected leg is extended at the hip, stiff at the knee, extended at the ankle (footdrop), and the ankle turns inward. When walking, the person leans toward the affected side and swings the affected leg in a semicircle to enable the foot to clear the floor. Sometimes the person will slide or drag the leg around rather than lift it.

The *scissors gait* results from spasticity of the adductor muscles of the thigh due to spastic paraplegia such as cerebral palsy. Due to spasticity of the adductor muscles, the knees are brought together inward (knock-kneed). The gait consists of alternating crossing of the legs in short steps with concomitant swinging of the hips. Since the leg is brought over the opposite knee, it resembles the movement of scissors; hence, the name scissors gait. In this gait, the person walks on his toes and the heels often do not touch the floor.

The *Parkinsonian or festinating gait* is seen in Parkinson's disease. The person walks with his head and body hunched rigidly forward. The gait is characterized by rigid posturing of the body, lack of arm-swinging, and short, rigid shuffling steps. There is difficulty initiating movement, but, once walking, the person tends to be propelled forward faster and faster in a rapidly accelerating (festinant) manner.

The *athetoid gait* results from damage and/or involvement of the basal ganglia. The gait is staggering, often in a sidewards direction, accompanied by wormlike writhing movements of the arms, head, and legs.

The *shuffling gait* is also called the "flat-footed" gait because the heel and toe touch the floor simultaneously as there is inability to raise the heel off the floor. This gait is caused by polio or other toxic disorders which produce weakness of the gastrocnemius, soleus, tibialis anticus, peroneus brevis, and extensor digitorum longus muscles.

The *steppage gait* ("footdrop" gait) is characterized by inability to dorsiflex the foot with resulting footdrop. Since there is weakness of the muscles which dorsiflex the foot, the toes drag and the person compensates for this with very high steps in order for the toes to clear the floor. The gait consists of flopping or slapping of the feet with high steps and may be unilateral or bilateral. It occurs in peroneal atrophy (Charcot-Marie-Tooth), peroneal nerve injury, and other conditions, such as poliomyelitis, which cause weakness of the muscles which dorsiflex the foot.

The *waddling gait* is seen in muscular dystrophy and in other conditions which cause weakness of the psoas muscles of the hip and quadriceps muscles of the thigh. Due to weakness of the hip girdle, pelvis, gluteal, and thigh muscles the person develops severe lordosis. The gait is broad-based, and the hips and trunk are jerked and rotated to the opposite side with each step.

MUSCLE TONUS. The stretch reflex (myotatic reflex) is responsible for maintaining muscle tonus or tension of the muscles and occurs whenever a muscle is stretched. The stretch reflex is a simple reflex requiring only one sensory and one motor neuron and, unlike most reflex arcs, does not require any other connecting neurons. When a muscle is stretched, the muscle spindle is also stretched and sensory endings of the neuromuscular spindle become stimulated. Afferent sensory impulses from the neuromuscular spindles reach the spinal cord via the dorsal root, and travel ventrally to the anterior horn and synapse with anterior motoneurons. Axons of these anterior motor neurons transmit impulses from the spinal cord to the motor end-plates in skeletal muscle fiber and excite the muscle fibers to produce greater tension and oppose the stretch (Fig. 20-2).

Changes in muscle tone accompany a variety of neurologic disorders. Abnormalities of tone can be due to lesions affecting the spinomuscular level (anterior horn cell), peripheral nerve, myoneural junction, or even the muscle itself. Tone can be affected by involvement of higher cerebral centers such as pyramidal and extrapyramidal systems and midbrain centers. Disturbances in proprioceptive pathways can also produce changes in muscle tone.

Reduced muscle tone (hypotonicity, flaccidity) occurs when there is decreased resistance to

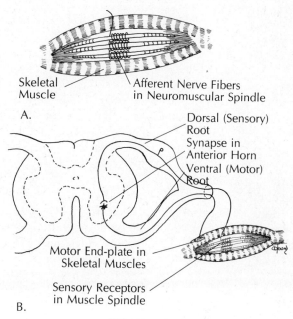

FIGURE. 20-2.
(A) Neuromuscular spindle. (B) Stretch reflex.

passive movement of the limbs and other areas of the body. Increased muscle tone (hypertonicity) is evident when there is increased resistance to passive manipulation of limbs.

The degree of muscle tone present is often difficult to assess. The patient should be as relaxed as possible to insure accurate evaluation. The resistance to passive movement is noted. The extremities should be taken through complete range of motion. Examination is made for resistance to movement and the ability to maintain position. Both slow and rapid movement should be tested. Observation is made for spasticity, rigidity, or flaccidity.

It is important to assess muscle tone because abnormalities in muscle tone are present in various neurologic diseases. *Flaccidity* results from damage to the spinal-neural-muscular pathways which interfere with or interrupt the efferent side of the reflex arc. These pathways include the anterior horn cells, ventral nerve roots, motor fibers of peripheral nerves, the myoneural junction, and muscle fiber. Flaccidity is characterized by decrease in tone of the affected muscles, decreased resistance of the muscles to passive manipulation, decrease in or loss of tendon reflexes, and, eventually, atrophy in the muscles affected.

Lesions of the dorsal root ganglia and/or posterior columns, as seen in tabes dorsalis, disrupt afferent proprioceptive pathways of the stretch reflex and produce hypotonicity in muscles. Cerebellar disease produces hypotonicity but not to the extent seen in lower motor neuron lesions.

Hypertonicity is usually caused by damage to the pyramidal tract and extrapyramidal areas central to the anterior horn cell. The two major forms of hypertonicity are spasticity present in pyramidal tract involvement and rigidity (extrapyramidal rigidity) occurring in lesions of the basal ganglion and/or extrapyramidal areas.

Spasticity is a state of increased tonus or tension in muscle due to overactivity of the stretch reflex. The exact cause is unknown. The pyramidal cortex has been considered to exert an inhibiting influence on the anterior horn cells and consequently the stretch reflex. Damage of the pyramidal areas removes this inhibiting influence allowing for unrestricted activity of the stretch reflex, producing spasticity.

The nurse most frequently observes spasticity in the cerebral hemiplegic patient. It is most apparent in the flexor muscles of the upper extremity. The forearm is flexed at the elbow and the arm is adducted at the shoulder. The wrist and fingers are also flexed tightly. On attempting to move the arm, one encounters increased resistance to passive manipulation followed by relaxation of the limb which gives dramatically away in a clasp-knife manner. At times, an extremity cannot be moved passively due to marked spasticity. Spasticity is accompanied by hyperactive tendon reflexes and clonus may also be present.

Rigidity (extrapyramidal hypertonicity) is present in diseases of the basal ganglion or of the extrapyramidal system. It is most commonly seen in Parkinson's disease. The rigidity affects both flexor and extensor muscles so that there is a steady muscular tension in both muscle groups. Resistance remains constant in all directions through the entire range of motion and does not give way like that seen in "clasp-knife" spasticity. When the extremity or part is moved to a new position, the extremity will assume a fixed posture. Occasionally, *cog-wheel rigidity* is present whereby upon passive movement of the part, resistance gives away in degrees or intervals rather than all at once producing a jerking motion of the muscles.

The extrapyramidal system is considered to contain facilitory (excitatory) and inhibitory (suppressor) fibers which regulate the stretch reflex. In lesions of the basal ganglion or other disturbances on the extrapyramidal level, interruption of these inhibitory fibers to lower reflex arcs are felt to contribute to the rigidity.

INVOLUNTARY MOVEMENTS. A tremor is an involuntary rhythmical movement of a part of the body in which there are alternate contractions of opposing muscle groups, for example, agonists and antagonists. Tremors are most often seen in the extremities but are located in other parts of the body and may be unilateral or bilateral in nature. Slow tremors are present when oscillations of three to five per second occur, whereas rapid tremors have oscillations of ten to twenty per second. Amplitude of a tremor refers to whether it is fine (movements are barely visible and usually rapid), medium, or coarse (movements are forceful and slower so that the entire limb or body part shakes and is easily detected). Tremors are affected and often worsened by emotional upset, overexertion, heat and cold, lack of sleep, and medication. They usually disappear during sleep.

Intention tremor occurs upon initiation of movement, worsens with voluntary movement, and is not present at rest. It is sometimes called action tremor, or kinetic tremor. It is medium to coarse in amplitude causing the body part to shake upon movement. The extremities, head, and body can be affected. Intention tremor is seen most often in multiple sclerosis and other cerebellar syndromes.

Toxic tremor is present in toxic conditions such as chronic alcoholism, hyperthyroidism, and drug toxicity (e.g., nicotine, caffeine, cocaine, amphetamines). The tremor is fine and rapid and involves primarily the fingers, hands, lips, and tongue.

Resting tremor (static tremor) is a coarse, alternating tremor seen most frequently in Parkinson's disease and involvement of the basal ganglion. The slow coarse tremor is present at rest and lessens or disappears with action. The thumb moves in a repetitive fashion over the first two fingers while the wrist moves alternately back and forth, and resembles the action used by early apothecaries to roll pills. Resting tremors may involve the head, tongue, and lips, as well as the extremities, and are particularly affected by emotional stimuli.

Flapping tremor is seen in advanced liver disease such as hepatic coma. The hands flap like bird wings when the arms are held outstretched.

Fasciculations are sudden fine twitching movements of muscle fasciculus. They are difficult to see or feel, but when observed the skin can be seen to slightly twitch or ripple. Unlike tremors, fasciculations are not affected by emotional or psychological stimuli and are present during sleep. Fasciculations are present most frequently in conditions which affect the anterior horn cells, in lesions of the spinal cord and motor nuclei of the cranial nerves.

Choreatic movements consist of rapid, jerky irregular involuntary movements which may affect the entire body and extremities. The distal muscles are more often affected. The abnormal movements are asymmetric and unpredictable. There may be grimacing of the face and difficulty in chewing, speaking, and swallowing due to rapid jerky movements. Jerking movements increase with purposeful movement, making activities of living most difficult to perform. Choreatic movements usually disappear during sleep. They are present in Sydenham's chorea and in Huntington's chorea.

Athetoid movements are slower, more continuous involuntary movements than choreatic movements, and also involve primarily the distal muscle groups. The movements resemble that of wormlike writhing and may be unilateral or bilateral. They also disappear during sleep. Due to the continuous movements, purposeful coordinated actions are very difficult to perform. Athetoid movements are due to lesions of the basal ganglion (caudate and putamen).

Dystonic movements resemble athetosis, except that they involve larger segments of muscle causing larger portions of the body to be affected. The involuntary movements are slow, undulating, and very distorted. Writhing and twisting movements of the trunk and spine may be present. Hypertonicity of the musculature is usually present which can lead to development of contractures and/or deformities. Voluntary activity and emotional tension accentuate and increase dystonic movements. Dystonic movements are present in dystonia musculorum deformans, a heredofamilial disease which affects the basal ganglion.

Hemiballismus movements are caused by a lesion in the subthalamic nucleus. The side of the body contralateral to the lesion is affected. Movements are usually in the extremities but may involve the face and trunk, and are unilateral. Involuntary movement consists of continuous wild flinging flailing movements of the area involved which disappear only during sleep, and which can lead to exhaustion. Chafing, sheet burns, and other skin irritations occur easily if the person is bedridden, due to the continuous movement. The elbows, buttocks, and heels are particularly prone to skin irritation.

Spasms. Involuntary contractions of a single muscle or a group of muscles produce spasms. Spasms may occur in any of the body musculature. Spasm may be due to irritation of the cortex or its descending motor pathways, irritation or lesions of the motor nuclei on the brain stem and spinal cord, injury or irritation to the peripheral nerves, vascular insufficiency to the muscle, metabolic imbalance affecting the muscle, and in diseases of muscles. Habit spasms (tics) are considered to be nervous spasms of psychogenic origin. Tics are seen most commonly in children. They can involve repetitious blinking of the eyes, facial grimacing, throat clearing, shrugging of the shoulders, snorting noises, and a variety of movements.

Convulsions are a major form of involuntary movement (see Neurologic Problems and Dysfunction, pp. 682-698).

MUSCLE STRENGTH. In examining muscle strength, the patient first moves the extremities to ascertain the presence of voluntary movement. Paresis (muscle weakness) or paralysis (loss of power) is noted. Strength of various muscle groups is then tested by having the patient perform movements while the examiner offers resistance or, the patient offers resistance while the examiner flexes or extends the elbows, wrists, shoulders, thighs, knees, and ankles. Corresponding muscles on each side should be compared for strength. Grip is tested by having the patient grasp the examiner's index finger tightly to prevent the examiner from withdrawing his finger. Individual muscle testing is very detailed and beyond the scope of this chapter. The patient's handed-ness should be ascertained to account for differences in strength on a particular side.

In assessing motor function for paralysis, tone, muscle wasting, and movement, the nurse should know the principal signs and symptoms which occur in diseases of the motor pathway. The motor pathway has been divided into two main divisions or components. They include upper motor neurons (pyramidal fibers), and lower motor neurons (peripheral nerve fibers), and are the spinomuscular component of man's nervous system. Therefore, disturbances in motor power are classified as upper motor neuron lesions or lower motor neuron lesions.

Upper motor neurons (pyramidal fibers) originate in the nerve cells (Betz cells) of the motor cortex and are essential in providing *voluntary* muscular activity. The nerve fibers originating in the Betz cell travel downward and cross to the opposite side, terminating in the voluntary motor nuclei of cranial nerves and in the anterior motor cells of the spinal cord. Upper motor neuron fibers consist of the corticospinal tract (pyramidal tract) which is the main motor pathway that descends from the cerebral cortex to the spinal cord. Other upper motor neuron fibers include the corticobulbar tract and the corticomesencephalic tract. Corticobulbar fibers descend from the cerebral cortex to the brain stem and terminate in the voluntary motor nuclei of the trigeminal, facial, glossopharyngeal, vagus, spinal accessory, and hypoglossal nerves. Corticomesencephalic fibers descend from the cortex to the nuclei of the oculomotor, trochlear, and abducen nerves. Upper motor lesions may be located in the cerebral cortex, the internal capsule, cerebral peduncles (pair of bands which join the pons and medulla with the cerebrum), brain stem, and the spinal cord. Since the majority of upper motor neuron fibers cross to the opposite side, an upper motor neuron lesion causes contralateral hemiparesis. An example of upper motor neuron lesion commonly seen is a cerebrovascular accident resulting in hemiplegia.

Lower motor neurons consist of large cell bodies located in the anterior gray column (anterior horn cell) of the spinal cord and also in the motor nuclei of cranial nerves located in the brain stem. Lower motor neuron fibers leave the spinal cord and emerge with the dorsal root fibers to form peripheral nerves which terminate in the motor end-plates of muscle. As many as 300 separate muscle fibers may be supplied by one lower motor neuron. In short, the lower motor neuron is the motor cell concerned with skeletal activity. It is often called the "final common pathway," since it is acted upon by many descending tracts, such as the corticospinal, vestibulospinal, reticulospinal, rubrospinal, olivospinal, and tectospinal. Lower motor neuron lesions may be located in the anterior gray column of the spinal cord, or brain stem, or in their axons (spinal or cranial nerves). The lower motor neuron lesion would involve those specific muscle groups supplied by the lower motor neuron (Fig. 20-3).

ASSESSMENT OF THE REFLEXES

There are three types of reflexes: deep tendon reflexes, superficial reflexes, and pathological reflexes.

DEEP TENDON REFLEXES (DTR'S). In a sense, this term is a misnomer because the deep reflexes are actually muscle stretch reflexes. Since these reflexes are elicited by percussion of the tendons which initiate stretching of the muscle followed by reflex contraction, they are called tendon reflexes.

Testing for deep reflexes is performed with a reflex hammer, although highly skilled practitioners can often use the tip of the middle

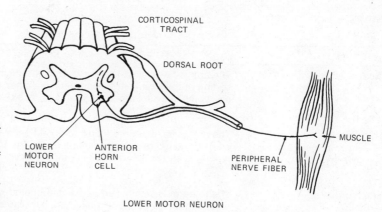

CORTICOSPINAL
TRACT

DORSAL ROOT

MUSCLE

LOWER
MOTOR
NEURON

ANTERIOR
HORN
CELL

PERIPHERAL
NERVE FIBER

LOWER MOTOR NEURON

FIGURE 20-3.
Upper motor neuron and lower motor neuron lesions. Source: Gatz, A. J.: Manter's Essentials of Clinical Neuroanatomy and Neurophysiology, ed. 3. Philadelphia, F. A. Davis, 1966, p. 9. Used with permission.

finger. Prior to testing, the muscle should be slightly stretched and the limb relaxed.

Reflex responses are usually graded in various ways. Descriptive words such as absent, dull, or brisk are sometimes used, or a number system can be employed from a scale of 0-5:

0. Not elicited or absent reflex
1. Sluggish or trace or diminished
2. Active or normal
3. Very active or brisk
4. Transient or unsustained clonus
5. Permanent or sustained clonus

Deep reflex responses can be diagnostic indicators of pyramidal tract disease, lower motor neuron involvement, and other neurologic conditions.

Testing of the reflexes is an essential part of the neurologic examination. Five of the most important deep tendon reflexes are listed in Table 20-1.

SUPERFICIAL REFLEXES are obtained by stroking or stimulating a sensory zone such as skin or mucous membrane. They differ from deep tendon reflexes since they are elicited by stimulating a sensory zone rather than by muscle stretching. Therefore, they are not considered muscle stretch reflexes but rather superficial reflexes.

Corneal, pharyngeal and palatal reflexes are superficial reflexes and are discussed under cranial nerves V, IX, and X.

Abdominal reflexes include upper and lower abdominal reflexes. The upper abdominal reflex is elicited by stroking the skin of the upper abdominal quadrants; the lower abdominal reflex is evoked by stimulating the lower abdominal quadrants. In either reflex, contraction of the abdominal musculature is toward the site of the stimulus.

The *cremasteric reflex* is a superficial reflex present only in men. The inner side of the thigh is stroked producing contraction of the cremasteric muscle and ipsilateral elevation of the testicle.

The *plantar* reflex is produced by stimulating the outer sole of the foot beginning from the heels and moving toward the toes. Normally, flexion of the toes occurs.

PATHOLOGICAL REFLEXES. Various reflex responses can be pathognomonic of neurologic disease and can also aid in localizing the disease process. Some of the most common pathological responses are listed in Table 20-2.

ASSESSMENT OF SENSORY FUNCTION

The sensory examination involves testing for pain, touch, temperature, position, vibratory sensations, and cortical sensory function. The special senses such as vision, hearing, smell, and taste are tested during the cranial nerve examination.

The patient must be alert and able to respond reliably during sensory testing. Testing for sensory function is conducted with the *patient's eyes closed*.

Knowledge of peripheral nerve distribution and segmental distribution (dermatomes inner-

TABLE 20-1
Deep Tendon Reflexes

Reflexes	Elicitation of Reflex	Normal Response
Biceps reflex	The arm is half-flexed at the elbow with the elbow resting in the examiner's hand. The examiner places his thumb over the biceps tendon and taps the tendon with a reflex hammer.	Flexion of the forearm and contraction of the biceps muscle.
Triceps reflex	The arm is flexed at the elbow and held across the chest or rested on the examiner's hand. The triceps tendon is struck above the olecranon process.	Contraction of the triceps muscle with extension of the forearm.
Brachiordialis reflex	The forearm is semiflexed and semipronated with the hand supported by the examiner's hand. The styloid process of the radius is tapped.	Flexion of the forearm and supination of the forearm.
Patellar reflex (quadriceps reflex, "knee jerk")	*Sitting position*: The legs hang freely over the bed or an examining table. The patellar tendon is struck just below the knee. The examiner should place one hand over the quadriceps femoris muscle as he strikes the patellar tendon with the other in order to feel the contraction of the muscle. *Lying position*: The person's knee is flexed slightly by placing the hand under the knee and raising the knee off the bed. The patellar tendon is tapped.	Extension of the leg at the knee and contraction of the quadriceps femoris muscle.
Achilles reflex ("ankle jerk" or triceps surae reflex)	*Sitting position*: The legs should dangle freely over the bed or table. The patient's foot is grasped and pressure exerted upward on the ball of the foot to a position of moderate dorsiflexion. The Achilles tendon is tapped on the posterior surface of the calcaneous. *Lying position*: The thigh and leg are rotated slightly outward and the knee is flexed. The examiner places his hand under the foot and exerts pressure upward to produce dorsiflexion. The Achilles tendon is tapped.	Contraction of the gastrocnemius, soleus, and plantaris muscles which produce plantar flexion of the foot.

vated by specific spinal cord segments) is essential in testing and recording changes in sensation.

PAIN SENSATION. Superficial pain is tested by pricking various parts of the body with a pin (hat or tailor's pin) and noting the patient's response. To test for accuracy, the examiner sometimes uses the head of the pin to see if the patient can differentiate between sharp and dull pain. The ability to sense pain is *algesia*. Decreased or reduced pain sensibility is *hypalgesia*. Increased sensitivity to pain is *hyperalgesia*. Loss or absence of pain sensation is *analgesia*.

TOUCH is tested by touching the skin lightly with a wisp of cotton or a camel's hair brush. Reduced or decreased sensation to touch is *hypesthesia*. Loss or absence of touch is *anesthesia*. *Hyperesthesia* is increased sensitivity to touch.

TEMPERATURE SENSE (THERMESTHESIA). Two test tubes, one containing hot water and the other cracked ice, are used in testing. The patient is asked to identify which tube is being placed over various body sites.

POSITION AND MOTION SENSE is the person's

TABLE 20-2
Pathological Reflexes

Pathological Reflex	Site of Stimulus	Response to Stimulus
Babinski—One of the most important tests for neurologic disease. Indicative of pyramidal tract involvement and occurs most frequently in pyramidal tract disease.	The lateral (outer) aspect of the sole of the foot is stroked with a blunt point from the midpoint of the heel up to the ball of the foot and then across the ball of the foot.	Dorsiflexion of the great toe and fanning of the small toes. Dorsiflexion of the foot and flexion of the knee occur concomitantly.
Chaddock's sign—Appears in pyramidal tract disease.	The lateral aspect of the foot under the external malleolus is stimulated.	Dorsiflexion of the great toe.
Gordon's sign—Pyramidal tract response.	Deep pressure is applied to the calf muscles by squeezing or pressing firmly.	Dorsiflexion of the great toe.
Oppenheim's sign—Pyramidal tract response.	The examiner strokes downward on the anteromedial tibial surface toward the ankles with the thumb and index finger or with the knuckles of the fingers.	Dorsiflexion of the great toe.
Hoffman's sign—Pathological hand reflex seen in pyramidal tract involvement.	Flicking or snapping the nail of the middle finger.	Flexion of the index finger. Flexion and adduction of the thumb.
Clonus—A continuous contraction of muscle which has been stimulated through stretch. Present in pyramidal tract disease.	*Finger clonus*—The patient's fingers are held and the hand is quickly dorsiflexed at the wrist.	Alternating flexion and extension at the wrist.
	Quadriceps (patellar) clonus—With the leg in extension and lying flat, the knee is held with the thumb and index finger and pushed down toward the feet.	Rhythmical movements of the patella.
	Ankle clonus—With the knee flexed, relaxed and supported, the foot is held with the free hand and quickly dorsiflexed.	Alternate flexion and extension of the foot due to repeated contractions of triceps surae muscle.

ability to sense or recognize the position and movement of parts of the body in space. Position sense is examined by moving the fingers, toes, and limbs passively to a particular position and asking the patient to identify the position or to imitate the position with a comparable body part. The digits are held lightly with the examiner's thumb and index finger. The digits must be relaxed for testing to be effective.

VIBRATORY SENSE is the ability to feel vibration from a vibrating tuning fork placed over the bony prominences. Bony prominences usually tested include the finger joints, styloid processes of the radius and ulna, elbows, ankles, shins (tibia), knees, clavicles, sternum, anterior iliac and vertebral spinous processes. The vibrating tuning fork is placed over the bony prominence. The examiner notes the patient's ability to perceive the vibration (buzzing) and its duration. Testing is done with the patient's eyes closed. Both sides should be compared. Vibratory sense is *pallesthesia*. *Pallanesthesia* is decreased vibratory sense.

CORTICAL SENSORY TESTING. The sensations

described below are more complex sensations which necessitate interpretation by the cerebral cortex (parietal lobe). These sensations require two- or three-dimensional discrimination such as size, shape, form, identification of objects, and so on.

Sterognosis is the ability to recognize objects by touching and feeling them with the eyes closed. Such objects as a key, pencil, safety pin, comb, coin, ball, are put in the patient's hand. Inability to recognize the object in the above manner is *astereognosis*.

Two-Point Discrimination involves the recognition of two points applied simultaneously to the skin. A compass or two pins are applied to various parts of the body and the patient states whether one or two points is touching him. The distance between the two points, which is necessary to differentiate two-point discrimination, varies for different parts of the body. The distance is small on the tongue and fingertips, larger on the trunk (chest and back) and proximal extremities.

Texture Discrimination is tested by having the patient differentiate between objects of metal, wood, cotton, glass, and various cloth textures, for example, silk, cotton, wool.

Graphesthesia refers to recognizing and identifying letters or numbers written on the skin (backs of the palms, trunk) with a blunt point. To avoid confusion, the patient should be told whether numbers or letters are being written.

Test for Extinction is conducted by touching identical areas in opposite parts of the body (the backs of both hands) simultaneously with a pin or the fingertips. Normally, both sides should be perceived. Extinction or inattention occurs when the patient is unable to perceive the stimulus on one side when both sides have been touched simultaneously, and is seen in parietal lobe disease.

ASSESSMENT OF CEREBROVASCULAR FUNCTION

Components of the cerebrovascular examination include the ophthalmoscopic examination, blood pressure, palpation of arteries, and auscultation.

The *ophthalmoscopic examination* is done to observe for vascular changes in the retina such as hemorrhages, exudates and atherosclerosis of the arterioles, infarction and retinal ischemia.

Blood pressures in each arm are compared in both a lying and standing position. The examiner observes for unequal blood pressures (systolics differ by 20 mm Hg) in the arms which may indicate vascular disease. Blood pressure is also taken during and after Valsalva's maneuver in which the examiner observes for postural hypotension, decreased cardiac output, and cardiac insufficiency.

Palpation of the corresponding arteries on each side is done simultaneously. These include the superficial arteries of the head (temporal, occipital), the carotids at the region of the bifurcation, subclavian arteries, the ulnar and radial arteries, abdominal aorta, iliac arteries, femoral arteries, and pedal pulses. Observation is made for absence of pulsations, diminished pulsation, increased pulsation, or delays in the pulse on a particular side, all of which may be indicative of vascular disease.

Auscultation for bruits (murmurs) is done along the vertebral and carotid arteries and the orbits of the eye. Bruits often indicate atherosclerotic vessel disease.

Nursing Intervention for the Comatose Patient

The unconscious patient presents one of the most difficult challenges in nursing. Being totally dependent, the comatose patient cannot survive for long without diligent medical and nursing intervention. Since many neurologic conditions manifest some degree of coma, the nurse must know the principles and nursing methods underlying the care of the comatose patient. In addition, coma and decreased consciousness signify brain dysfunction. It is an acute and life-threatening problem and demands attention and intervention from all members of the health team.

There are many diseases and conditions which lead to coma, not all neurologic in origin, including vascular lesions, trauma, meningitis, encephalitis, brain tumors, brain abscesses, alcoholism, poisoning, drug intoxication, diabetes, uremia, hepatitis, hypoglycemia, pneumonia, congestive heart failure, epilepsy, and many more. Regardless of the cause, the nurse has a two-fold responsibility: to carry out the ordered medical and/or surgical treatment and to formulate nursing intervention. Nursing intervention for the patient should be to:

1. Maintain a patent airway and adequate oxygenation.
2. Help preserve the patient's normal physiological functioning.
3. Observe the patient for both general and neurologic changes.
4. Prevent complications of immobility and the comatose state.
5. Help provide rehabilitation in order to assist the patient to maximum recovery as quickly as possible.

Although maintaining a patent airway is an immediate priority, all areas of care are vitally important if the patient is to make as full a recovery as possible. If maintaining a patent airway is accomplished, but the patient's eyes are neglected, resulting in blindness, the purpose of intervention has been defeated.

PHILOSOPHICAL CONSIDERATIONS

The maintenance of dignity and worth should be of primary concern in caring for the comatose patient. Since he is unresponsive and noninteracting, he is often approached as a mystical object on whom a series of procedures and tasks must be carried out day after day and sometimes month after month. He has been talked around and over, but rarely talked to by those caring for him. He is more often screamed at to "Squeeze my hand"; or "Stick out your tongue." While these techniques are needed to assess the neurologic status, they do little to promote treatment of the patient as an individual. Some feel that since the patient cannot respond or hear, there is no sense in carrying on a conversation with him or explaining what one is about to do. Scientifically and philosophically, this is far from being true. Electoencephalographs show response to auditory stimulation even in moderately deep coma. There is, however, no way of knowing whether this auditory stimulation is meaningful for the patient or not. Nevertheless,

hearing is usually the first sense to return upon gaining consciousness. Talking to the patient may help orient and bring him to a state of consciousness sooner. Often a patient is aware of voices and words, but is unable to respond.

The nurse should treat the comatose patient with all the respect, dignity, gentleness, and compassion she would any conscious well person, even though he gives back nothing. Virginia Henderson said, "The nurse is temporarily the consciousness of the unconscious." In all aspects of care, she should explain what she is about to do to the patient and talk to him. Modesty, privacy, and individual worth should be preserved. Because the patient is unconscious is no excuse for being careless about keeping him adequately clothed or drawing curtains when procedures are being carried out.

Family members also need individual attention and support. It is frightening to see a loved one in continual sleep and many fear that he will never awaken. They are afraid to be alone with him and feel inadequate. The example set by the nurse, through her confidence, gentleness, and purposeful care, can do much to allay the anxieties and fears of the family. The family should be informed of explanations and procedures concerning the care of the patient. Since family members often become upset when neurologic testing for level of consciousness and motor and sensory function is done, it is often better that they are not present at this time. Relationships with the patient's family can best be promoted by treating the patient with dignity.

ASSESSMENT OF THE LEVEL OF CONSCIOUSNESS

Consciousness is a state in which the individual is aware of his environment and himself and is responsive to psychological and sensory stimuli. It is difficult to define consciousness and all the stages which exist between the conscious and unconscious states. To compound matters, such terms as stupor, confusion, coma, and semicomatose all have been given many meanings. The nurse needs to know more specifically the observations, actions, and behavior which denote a lowering of consciousness rather than to use ambiguous and nonspecific descriptions. The following are descriptions of the state of consciousness in relative order of decreasing awareness. A patient may or may not pass through each phase and further, he may exhibit a combination of phases.

1. The patient is aware of himself and his environment, follows commands well, is cooperative, and is oriented to time, place, and person. Many patients quickly lose track of time or date while hospitalized, but otherwise remain alert.

2. The patient may be very sleepy and/or irritable or restless. Increased restlessness is often an indication that cerebral function may worsen and the patient become unresponsive. The patient may be quite excitable when aroused and generally uncooperative.

3. The patient is lethargic and sleepy, can be aroused with verbal stimulation, and is able to carry out simple commands well. However, following stimulation he usually falls asleep again.

4. The patient can still be aroused with verbal stimulation, but is unable to follow simple commands well (such as squeezing the examiner's hand, protruding the tongue, blinking the eyes).

5. The patient arouses to deep pain rather than verbal stimulation. Deep pain may include pinching of the skin, shaking, pricking with a pin. The patient once aroused is able to carry out some simple commands.

6. The patient can still be aroused with painful rather than verbal stimulation. However, he does not follow simple commands. His response is usually that of pushing the examiner away, wincing, withdrawing the part of the body stimulated.

7. The patient is unresponsive. He responds to deep pain upon stimulation by withdrawal only (there is an attempt to withdraw the portion of the body stimulated).

8. The patient responds to deep pain by extension only. He may have extensor rigidity of the limbs, which indicates decerebration.

9. In profound coma, there is no response to deep pain. Corneal, pupillary, and pharyngeal reflexes are not present. Swallowing and cough reflexes are abolished. The patient is incontinent of urine and feces.

In addition, there are subtle changes in the patient's behavior which often indicate a lowering of consciousness. For instance, a patient who is unable to feed himself or lacks the interest to eat may deteriorate slowly. Of all health team members, the nurse is in the best position to pick up these clues. She should observe and report such things as incontinence, irritability with staff and family, and lack of interest or activity. Observable pupillary changes should be noted since the pupils may be contracted or dilated in various degrees of unresponsiveness and coma.

OBSERVATIONS OF CHANGES IN MOTOR AND SENSORY FUNCTION

Observation for changes in motor and sensory function is another responsibility of the nurse caring for the patient with cerebral dysfunction. Usually, this does not present a problem with the conscious or alert patient, since the nurse is able to observe and question him. However, in the less conscious patient, responses to questioning cannot be obtained, and so the nurse must rely on observation and neurologic testing. To test for sensory function, she should apply painful stimulation on some part of the body—pinching the skin, squeezing the muscles or tendons, pricking with a pin, pressing on the knuckles, or applying pressure over the eyes or supraorbital notches. (Care should be taken not to bruise the patient.) If sensory function is intact (and coma not profound), the patient winces or shows expression on the face. In addition, he withdraws the portion of the body which was stimulated. (If paralysis is present, the patient may grimace or wince but not withdraw the portion stimulated.)

In testing for motor function, the nurse should first observe the patient for positioning of extremities, flaccidity, loss of tone, spasticity, contractures, and movements such as decerebrate or decorticate rigidity. If the patient is responsive to questioning, he should be asked to move his extremities, smile, and squeeze the examiner's hand. *Both* arms and extremities should be tested, because often unilateral paresis or paralysis is present and comparisons should be made. If the patient is unresponsive, noxious and painful stimuli should be applied to determine motor function. The patient should withdraw the extremity or part of the body stimulated. If no move is elicited, additional testing should be carried out. Paralysis of the arms can be ascertained by lifting them simultaneously and then releasing them. The paralyzed arm falls more quickly and in a flail-like manner. Delong states that another way to test the arms is to place the elbows on the bed at right angles to the forearm. the affected extremity falls faster and often strikes the face. The legs may be tested by flexing them with the heels on the bed. When released, the paretic limb falls to an extended position with the hip in outward rotation, whereas the unaffected limb maintains the posture for a few moments and gradually returns to its original position.[6]

The nurse should also observe and test for facial paralysis. With facial paralysis, there may be noticeable asymmetry of the face, drooping of the mouth, and drooling. To examine facial nerve function, firm pressure over the eyeball or supraorbital notch should be applied. Retraction and movement of muscles or a grimace should be noted if there is normal functioning, whereas the paralyzed side would demonstrate no movement. Facial paralysis may also be tested by attempting to open the eyes when closed firmly. No resistance would be present on the paralyzed side.

Motor response to painful stimulation may be one of decerebrate or decorticate rigidity. In addition, decerebrate or decorticate posturing may be present in the patient without stimulation due to cerebral dysfunction. The nurse should be able to recognize and observe these changes, since they are indicative of cerebral damage at various levels and produce changes in muscular tonus.

Decorticate rigidity is characterized by flexion of the wrist, arms, and fingers. The upper extremity is adducted and flexed at the shoulder; the lower extremity is extended and internally rotated with plantar flexion of the foot. This pattern is most commonly seen in spastic hemiplegia and with lesions of the internal capsule which interrupt the corticospinal pathways.

Increased tonus occurs with resulting firmness and stiffness of muscles and increased resistance to manipulation. When attempts are made to move the affected extremity, resistance is very strong at first, but gives way as more

force is applied. Also spasticity is greater in the extensors in the leg, while in the arm, the flexors are most affected (see Assessment of Muscle Tonus).

Decerebrate rigidity usually occurs as a result of upper brain stem damage and is characterized by rigidity and contraction of all the extensor muscles. The legs are stiffly extended with the feet plantar flexed. The arms are extended and hyperpronated, the back arched and in opisthotonous. The patient's jaws are closed, teeth clenched, and head erect. It is believed that it follows transection of the brain stem which releases vestibular nuclei from extrapyramidal control. The loss of inhibitory effects on the vestibular portion of the reticular formation is possibly responsible for the increased activity of the stretch reflexes of extensor muscles. Guyton points out that transection of the brain stem beneath the superior colliculus, which is located in the dorsal portion of the midbrain (tectum), causes marked increase in muscular tone throughout the body.[7] This results from removal of inhibitory influences normally transmitted from above. Since the greater portion of the reticular formation is facilitory rather than inhibitory, the normal effect is to facilitate all muscles throughout the body, causing a general increase in muscular tone.

The nurse should be aware of signs of decorticate and decerebrate rigidity and should report them at once, since they indicate areas of cerebral involvement as well as a change in the patient's condition.

Observation for Pupillary Reaction

One of the most important functions in caring for the patient with central nervous system dysfunction is testing for pupillary reaction. Pupillary changes may be indicative of increasing intracranial pressure or localizing signs of cerebral dysfunction. In pontine lesions, pupils are bilaterally small and nonreactive to light, due to interruption of sympathetic pathways. Midbrain damage produces dilatation and abolition of the light reflex. Small pupils may be seen with metabolic brain disease, but pupillary light reflex is usually maintained until the terminal stages of coma. Bilaterally dilated and fixed pupils occur with anoxic states such as cardiac arrest. Unilateral dilatation of the pupil is usually indicative of increased intracranial pressure.

There are various drugs which do have pharmacological effects on pupils, and which may confuse interpretation or mask changes in the clinical picture of the patient. It is the responsibility of the physician to order drugs, but the nurse should be aware of side effects and various contraindications. The following drugs are apt to cause pupillary changes: mydriatics, by sympathetic stimulation or paralysis of the parasympathetic division; miotics, through paralysis of the sympathetic division or through stimulation of the parasympathetic division. Drugs causing dilatation of the pupil include scopolamine, atropine, homatropine, amphetamine, cocaine, ephedrine, epinephrine, and glutethimide. Constrictors include ergot derivatives, histamine, pilocarpine, mecholyl, muscarine, neostigmin, and physostigmine. Heroin and morphine produce pinpoint pupils like that seen in damage to the pons.

The *ciliospinal reflex* (ipsilateral dilatation of the pupil upon pinching the side of the neck) is often tested in the comatose patient to evaluate the depth of coma. This reflex disappears in pontine and medullary deterioration (deep coma).

Observation of Ocular Movements

Eye movements in the comatose patient remain motionless (prolonged stare) or can oscillate from side to side very slowly (which sometimes gives the impression that the patient is watching objects around him).

The *oculocephalic reflex* (doll's head phenomenon) is a reflex ocular movement which is present in unconscious states, and cannot be elicited in the conscious person. The doll's head phenomenon is tested in the unconscious patient by holding the eyelids open and passively and quickly turning the head first to one side and then the other. The oculocephalic reflex is present when the eyes move in an opposite direction from the side to which the head is turned, that is, the eyes will turn to the left when the head is turned to the right. This reflex response disappears and cannot be elicited in severe lower pontine and brain stem involvement. For this reason, it is a useful test for evaluating the depth of coma.

Respiration

One of the primary concerns in the care of the comatose patient (and of all patients) is the maintenance of a patent airway. The unconscious patient is deprived of his cough reflex and is completely immobile. No better conditions exist for the development of respiratory complications. Therefore, the patient should lie in a lateral (side-lying) position, permitting drainage from the mouth, promoting better drainage of mucus from the lungs, and preventing the tongue from falling back and asphyxiating the patient. Both the mouth and the nose should be unobstructed. The nose can be cleansed and removed of exudate by sterile cotton swabs or by suctioning. Suctioning is also used to remove secretions from the oropharynx and mouth. During suctioning, a proper suction catheter should be used gently to avoid trauma and tearing of the mucous membranes. Adequate suction equipment should be at the bedside at all times, since there is a danger of aspiration. New suction catheters should be used each time, since there is a tendency toward the growth of microorganisms, particularly Pseudomonas, when suction catheters are allowed to soak.

In many instances, a clear airway can be established only through a tracheostomy, using a cuff-type tracheostomy tube. Sterile precautions, disposable catheters, and gloves should also be used to avoid infection. The inner cannula should be removed whenever necessary and kept as clean and patent as possible. Pipe cleaners and gauze can be used to clean the inner cannula after soaking in hydrogen peroxide solution. The skin around the tracheostomy should be kept clean and free from mucus. Humidifiers may be used to moisten secretions and prevent drying of mucosa. If a cuff-type tracheostomy tube is used, the cuff should be inflated prior to tube feeding to prevent aspiration. With an inflatable cuff, intermittent positive pressure can be used to assist breathing.

The nurse should observe the rate, depth, type, and rhythm of respiration. Respiratory signs are useful in diagnosing diseases which produce coma. Changes in respiration also indicate a deterioration of condition, or cerebral involvement at various levels. Plum and Posner describe various abnormal respiratory patterns associated with pathologic lesions at various levels of the brain and seen in coma (Fig. 20-4).

According to Plum and Posner, Cheyne-Stokes respiration (CSR) is the most common type of periodic breathing whereby hyperpnea regularly alternates with apnea.[8] The breathing is characterized by slow waxing and waning of respirations. The hyperpneic phase usually lasts longer than the apneic stage, with the cycle occurring over again every 45 seconds to 3 minutes. The pathogenesis of CSR is a combination of an abnormally increased ventilatory response to cardon dioxide stimulation causing hyperpnea and an abnormal forebrain ventilatory stimulus, subsequently permitting postventilation apnea. Cheyne-Stokes respiration in patients with neurologic disease implies bilateral dysfunction of neurologic structures, usually of those deep in the hemispheres or diencephalon.

Central neurogenic hyperventilation is described by Plum and Posner as sustained, regular, rapid, and fairly deep hyperpnea, occurring in certain patients with dysfunction of the brain stem tegmentum.[9] Central hyperventilation occurs with midbrain pontine infarcts and with anoxia affecting the same area. The breathing pattern is frequent in patients with midbrain compression secondary to transtentorial herniation, particularly when cerebral hemorrhage is the cause.

Another pattern of breathing found in the patient with central nervous dysfunction is apneustic breathing. Plum and Posner state that apneusis is a prolonged inspiratory cramp—a pause at full inspiration.[10] Quite common are brief end-respiratory pauses lasting two or three seconds. Apneustic breathing results from damage to the respiratory control mechanisms located at the mid- or caudal-pontine level and usually denotes pontine infarction.

Lesions in the dorsomedial part of the medulla and extending down or just below the obex (the portion near the fourth ventricle) cause respiratory ataxia. Ataxic breathing, according to Plum and Posner, has a completely irregular pattern in which both deep and shallow breaths occur randomly.[11] Irregular pauses appear haphazardly, and there is no predicting the future respiratory rhythm from the pattern of past breaths. The respiratory rate tends to be slow and may progressively decelerate to apnea. Its

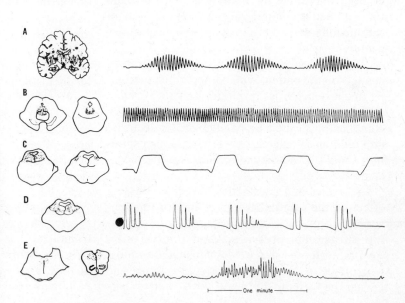

FIGURE 20-4.
Abnormal respiratory patterns associated with pathological lesions (shaded areas) at various levels of the brain. Tracings by chest-abdomen pneumograph, inspiration reads up. (A) Cheyne-Stokes respiration. (B) Central neurogenic hyperventilation. (C) Apneusis. (D) Cluster breathing. (E) Ataxic breathing. Source: Plum, F. and Posner, J. B.: Diagnosis of Stupor and Coma. Contemporary Neurology Series. Philadelphia, F. A. Davis, 1966, p. 16. Used with permission.

irregularity differentiates it from the regular waxing and waning of Cheyne-Stokes respiration and is the respiratory abnormality that Biot described.[12] Therefore, this type of periodic breathing is sometimes called Biot's breathing.

Cluster breathing occurs when the lesion is high in the medulla. Plum and Posner elucidate that clusters of breath may follow each other in disorderly sequence with irregular pauses in between.[13] These merge with various patterns of gasping respirations in which deep "all or none" breaths occur, usually at a slow rate.

In assessing respiration, it is extremely important that the nurse be as descriptive as possible. To simply give the rate without indicating the quality or rhythm, denotes poor observation. In addition, any cyanosis, pallor, or other signs of respiratory difficulty should be noted. The nurse must learn to observe with ears and hands as well as with eyes. Respiratory changes, particularly depression, in the patient with central nervous system dysfunction are usually indicative of increasing intracranial pressure, brain edema, or pressure conus. Brain edema results in swelling of brain tissue compressing cerebral arteries and causing blockage of cerebral blood supply. Depression or inactivation of the respiratory center occurs because of inadequate blood supply. With a pressure conus, pressure in the cranium may force the brain downward through the foramen magnum, causing compression of the medulla and, consequently, the respiratory center.

Many other conditions produce respiratory changes in the patient with cerebral dysfunction, particularly acidosis, respiratory alkalosis, electrolyte disturbances, and frequently respiratory complications, such as pneumonia, atelectasis, and pulmonary edema. Any changes in respiration should be noted and reported to the physician.

Narcotics and anesthetics have a depressing effect on the respiratory center and for this reason are contraindicated in patients with increasing intracranial pressure, head injury, brain tumors, in those who are comatose and in most neurologic patients. In particular, morphine causes depression of respirations and masks other clinical signs, such as pupillary changes, and is contraindicated in the patient with central nervous system dysfunction.

Thus, the nurse has a dual role in the care of the comatose patient—to maintain a patent airway, thus helping to provide adequate oxygenation in the patient, and to observe any changes in respirations. The importance of both roles cannot be overemphasized.

Blood Pressure, Pulse, and Temperature

Observation for changes in vital signs is important in the comatose and neurologic patient. In the comatose patient, they may be ordered as often as every 15 minutes in the acute stage. As the patient's condition becomes stable, they are usually ordered hourly or at longer intervals. Changes in vital signs may be indicative of increased intracranial pressure (see pp. 677-682), or may denote shock, hemorrhage, electrolyte imbalance and other disturbances. It is best if recordings of vital signs are left in close proximity to the patient so that quick comparisons can be made.

In checking the pulse, the volume, rate, and rhythm should be noted. The nurse should be aware if the patient is receiving drugs, such as digitalis, which may affect the readings.

The temperature is taken rectally in the comatose patient as well as in all seizure patients, those with tracheostomies, or those who are restless or confused, or postoperative. The patient should not be left unattended with a thermometer in place. In cases of hyperthermia, alcohol sponging *with massage* (for maximum cooling) and aspirin suppositories may be ordered. In caring for the patient receiving hypothermia, the nurse's responsibility is increased even more, due to the danger of burns, skin breakdown, and the masking of signs of infection and changes in vital signs.

PREVENTION OF COMPLICATIONS AND PRESERVATION OF NORMAL BODY FUNCTIONS

Comatose and neurologic patients are particularly prone to complications, due to a number of factors. First, many patients are completely immobilized, or have varying degrees of immobility. They may have paralysis or paresis of muscles which affect their activity, loss of sensation, rigidity of movement, overactive movements such as hemiballismus or dystonia, confusional episodes, mental deterioration, and so on. It is not unusual to have over half the patients admitted to a neurological unit bedridden and in need of assistance with activities.

Prevention of Skin Breakdown

The most frequent complication is skin breakdown resulting in pressure sores (decubitus ulcers). Regardless of how sick a patient may be, skin breakdown can be prevented to a large extent. It is primarily a nursing responsibility to see that the patient receives proper skin care. No physician should have to order back care, turning, and so on. In the case of decubitus ulcers, blanching of the skin occurs prior to any reddening and is indicative of ischemia in the area. At any sign of blanching, extreme measures should be instituted to prevent a decubitus ulcer from forming. The area should be massaged and the patient kept off the site as much as possible. Comatose patients should be turned every two hours. Many patients, particularly those on hypothermia blankets, should be turned more often.

Alternating pressure mattresses, sheepskins, and the newer water beds are also effective methods which can be utilized to prevent skin breakdown. Sheepskin is particularly helpful in preventing decubitus ulcers in patients with hemiballismus or other hyperkinetic disorders. These patients are prone to chafing of the extremities, skin burns, and consequent skin breakdown. Good results have been obtained by using sheepskin.

The best remedy for decubitus ulcers is simply prevention. With the neurologic patient, turning, massaging the body surfaces, positioning properly, and distributing weight over as wide an area as possible are essential for maintaining skin integrity. In addition, the bed should be free of wrinkles and soilage. Many patients are incontinent of both urine and feces, increasing the likelihood of skin breakdown. Cleanliness of the patient cannot be overemphasized.

Although the sacrum, ischial tuberosities, femoral trochanters, and scapulae are the usual sites of decubitus ulcer formation, the ears, elbows, heels, and iliac crests are more often affected in the comatose patient, due to the side-lying position. Particular attention should be given to ears, elbows, heels, and iliac crests. As soon as the patient's condition permits, he should be turned on his back as well as his side. When lying on his back, a small flat pillow under the ankles can be used to prevent pressure on the heels. (Doughnuts should not be used, since they simply apply an increased pressure around the surrounding area.) When turning the patient on his side, care should be taken to make sure the ear is in proper position under him and that the area under the ear is dry and clean. Often mucus and oral secretions accumulate on the pillow, irritating the ear and face.

Prevention of Injury

Hot water bags and other heating applications should not be used on the comatose patient, or on those having loss of sensation or paralysis, unless ordered by the physician. Ice caps and ice bags also can cause burns, as can hypothermia blankets, and their use is discouraged unless the patient is febrile. The nurse must observe the patient carefully for any signs of irritation, burns, ischemia, cyanosis, and skin breakdown.

There are other salient points of safety which should be emphasized for the comatose and/or neurologic patient. For instance, in transporting patients, extremities should not hang over or outward from stretchers and wheelchairs, for injury can occur. Support should be provided in order to prevent subluxation of the shoulder, bruised feet from wheelchairs, and other injuries. One extreme example of injury occurred when a patient on a CircOlectric bed caught his foot in it and was cut as he was being turned. Though he was paralyzed, his sensation was intact. He was unable to communicate fast enough, due to tracheostomy, bulbar palsy, and generalized weakness, although he was aware that his foot had slipped and was caught. It should be emphasized that although a patient's sensation may be intact, he may not have the strength or ability to help himself when such a situation occurs.

For patients who are unconscious, restless, or confused bedside rails should be raised and padded. Restlessness may be a sign of a variety of problems, including increasing intracranial pressure, full bladder, fecal impaction, and fracture. Therefore, signs of restlessness should be reported to the physician for his appraisal. Restraints are usually not indicated, since they merely serve to increase the agitation of the patient. If the patient is pulling at nasogastric or other tubes, gauze mittens (resembling boxer's gloves) can be used and secured with tape. However, some resourceful patients manage to pull out tubes even with the mittens on their hands. In extreme cases, medications such as chlorpromazine, codeine, or paraldehyde may have to be ordered to keep the patient quiet and resting. If the patient is conscious, the presence of staff or a family member is often calming to him. The point is that the patient must be protected from harming himself (and others) while he is in an irresponsible state. He must have intensive and close observation. Restlessness also increases the intracranial pressure, a condition which can be deleterious in the neurologic patient.

Prevention of Eye Complications

Corneal ulcerations and other eye complications need to be prevented in the comatose patient and in neurologic patients who have loss of the corneal reflex. If the eyes are allowed to remain open, the cornea dries and ulceration occurs. With comatose patients, the eyes should be kept closed with gauze butterfly dressings or with eye shields. Drops of ophthalmic solution and/or antibiotic drops may be ordered given every two hours. Inspection of each eye should be made for signs of inflammation, irritation, and exudate whenever eye care and pupillary checks are made. In some cases, eyelids may be temporarily sutured closed by the physician. Upon admission, patients wearing contact lenses should have them removed immediately. In the absence of moisture they are irritating to the eyes and can quickly cause corneal ulcerations, particularly if the patient has worn them eight to ten hours prior to injury.

Prevention of Deformities

The prevention of deformities is of utmost importance in the patient who has had central nervous system involvement. Two of the most important nursing goals in the prevention of deformities are 1) to maintain correct body positioning, and 2) to provide range of motion to all joints as soon as possible.

At first, the unconscious patient is placed in the lateral position. It is very important that both the upper arm and leg be supported properly with pillows so that they are in a plane with proper trunk alignment. The forearm and wrist should be supported on the same level as the arm, or slightly higher. The wrist should be in a neutral position, or in slight extension. Splints can be used to prevent wristdrop and to maintain this position. Hand rolls should be used to prevent flexion contractures of the fingers. A properly constructed hand roll keeps the fingers and thumb opposed to each other. The upper leg should be flexed at the knee at an approximate right angle to the hip. The leg should be placed in such a way that it does not twist or rotate the pelvis forward. Legs should be supported so that the weight on one does not fall on the other. The back should be straight. A small pillow or pad placed under the head keeps the cervical vertebrae in alignment with the spinal column. The feet should be maintained in a position of dorsiflexion, by using footboards, splints, or sandbags. The best prevention for footdrop is passive range of motion, which should be instituted as soon as possible. Weight should be taken off the limbs by use of either bed cradles or a footboard.

Paralyzed muscles need more support than do normal muscles. Consequently, sandbags, pillows, splints and other devices are necessary to maintain proper positioning. An affected arm in the side-lying position should be placed in a position which discourages adduction. Adduction should be prevented, since shoulder tightness and fibrosis may develop, causing deformity and difficulty with range of motion and rehabilitation.

Positions of abduction and extension of the arm are necessary to prevent shoulder tightness. An affected leg should be positioned to prevent external rotation, since extensor muscles of the leg are stronger than flexors. It is best to place the leg in slight internal rotation to achieve a neutral position.

As soon as back-lying and the supine position are allowed, the patient should be encouraged to assume this position as well. If his head is elevated, care should be taken not to roll the shoulder forward, further tightening the shoulder girdle. He should be encouraged to lie flat at frequent intervals, since elevation of the head of the bed causes hip flexion. Flexion contractures occur easily in the hip and knees and should be avoided. Pillows should not be placed beneath the knees, since this increases knee flexion deformity. Also with knee flexion, there is plantar flexion of the feet and a shortening of the Achilles tendon. If a small pad is used under the knees to relax the muscles of the leg, the feet must be supported firmly in dorsiflexion. A small pad can be placed under the lower leg and ankles to prevent pressure on the heels and decubitus ulcers from occurring. A paralyzed leg should be supported by sandbags and trochanter rolls to prevent external rotation in the supine position. Also the affected arm should be supported on a pillow to prevent adduction. Alternate positions of abduction and extension are also necessary to prevent shoulder tightness and shortening of the pectoral muscles. Hand rolls and splints should be used to prevent wristdrop and flexion contractures of the fingers.

In positions of sitting and walking, support should be given to the affected arm. A paralyzed arm should be placed in a sling to prevent dislocation of the shoulder and possible injury to the arm. Since the patient is prone to losing his balance easily, he should be secured in a wheelchair or chair with a sheet. In the case of hemiplegia, support and assistance with walking should be given on the unaffected side.

Provision for passive range of motion exercises is necessary as soon as the physician permits. It is a nursing responsibility to check with the physician and obtain permission to begin passive exercises. In most cases, if hemorrhage is not apparent, these activities can be initiated as early as 48 hours after injury, otherwise stiffening of the shoulder of the involved arm can occur. Deformities and pain from abnormal muscle tensions develop very rapidly! Passive range of motion should be done as often as three times a day. Unnecessary delay does the patient more harm than good. It does not matter whether he is hemiplegic, monoplegic, or paraplegic, exercises are necessary if rehabilitation is to be effectively initiated. The principles of good body positioning and range of motion exercises are important for all these patients. Once deformities and contractures occur, retraining of activities of daily living, fittings for braces, and other rehabilitative processes are delayed, posing an even greater setback.

ELIMINATION. The comatose patient is incontinent of both urine and feces. Therefore, an indwelling catheter is inserted to prevent bladder distention. The catheter should be taped to the inner part of the thigh to prevent pulling and subsequent irritation to the wall of the bladder and internal sphincter. Care of the catheter and drainage system should involve the strictest aseptic technique, even though the patient is on prophylactic antibiotics. Irrigations of the catheter are usually ordered to insure its patency. Since bacteria thrive in an alkaline medium, measures to maintain the acidity of the urine may be a part of the program to prevent infection and may include medication such as mandelic acid (Mandelamine) and fruit juices, particularly cranberry and prune. Fluids (unless the patient's status prohibits) should be forced to prevent infection and to help maintain the patency of the system. Also, antibiotics may be given prophylactically to help ward off infection.

Bowels should be evacuated, if possible, once a day. Suppositories or mild laxatives may be ordered. The nurse should observe carefully for fecal impaction, which is characterized by frequent small seepage of loose stools. The patient may also show signs of restlessness and discomfort. It was discovered that one unconscious patient who grimaced and writhed in apparent discomfort hadn't had a bowel movement for four days. Digital manipulation was necessary. After a sizable evacuation, the patient manifested no more restlessness or discomfort. Fecal impaction should be avoided as well as straining at bowel movement, since they increase intracranial pressure and the possibility of cerebral hemorrhage. A regular bowel movement regime is important not only with the unconscious patient but with all neurologic patients, particularly the paralyzed. Any effective bowel training program depends upon regularity and consistency of effort both on the part of the nurse and on the patient.

FOOD AND FLUIDS. The comatose patient must be maintained on intravenous feedings. As soon as bowel sounds return and conditions permit, feedings by nasogastric tube are in order. The nurse should ascertain whether the tube is in the stomach and aspirate before each feeding to determine if there is gastric retention. The tube should be brought down laterally from the nose and taped in this position to prevent pressure and ulcerations of the nasal mucosa. Fluids should be warmed to room temperature and never given directly from the refrigerator. They should not be forced but allowed to flow into the stomach by gravity. After the feeding, the tube should be irrigated with warm water and then clamped. Any contents aspirated from the stomach should be included when recording output.

An *accurate* record of intake and output is essential, since both dehydration and overhydration produce symptoms similar to head injury or trauma. Intake should include intravenous infusion, tube feeding, blood transfusion, clysis, rectal instillations. All output including that from voided, vomited, and gastric drainage, diaphoresis, cerebrospinal fluid drainage, hemorrhage, diarrhea, and wound or cavity drainage and excessive mucus should be recorded. Since adequate fluid balance is vital, the patient is placed on daily weights. He should be weighed on the same scale using the same procedure at the same time daily.

Daily dietary requirements are determined by the patient's status. During the early stages following injury or cerebral insult, negative nitrogen balance may occur (particularly after head injury). During this phase, catabolism is greater than anabolism and losses of up to 10 Gm of protein a day may occur. These losses are not influenced by caloric intake, and very little affected by increasing the protein intake.[14] After the catabolic phase has passed, both protein and caloric intake are usually increased to counteract the losses incurred.

After the patient has regained consciousness, oral intake can be resumed, providing the gag reflex is present and the patient is able to swallow. If he is recovering from a cerebral vascular accident, he may have unilateral facial paralysis and difficulty in eating, chewing, drinking, and even swallowing to some extent. The patient should be fed and encouraged to chew on the unaffected side. Sufficient time should be allowed for feeding. Often the patient has little appetite or enthusiasm. Feeding the patient with neurologic dysfunction is above all an act of perseverance. If the patient is being fed by ancillary personnel, specific instructions should be communicated to them concerning how they should feed the patient. However, it is believed that the feeding of the patient with neurologic dysfunction should be a nursing function. All too often he has little oral intake simply because no one takes the time to really assist him and teach him how he can eat more easily.

REHABILITATION

As discussed previously, provision for rehabilitation of the neurologic patient should be initiated by the nurse on the day of admission, through careful assessment and deliberate nursing intervention. Unless the philosophy of helping the patient to recover maximum functioning is held, the patient may inevitably be condemned to a bedridden existence. One of the primary goals, although it may be a long-term one, is to mobilize the patient as quickly as possible by having him participate in his care and help himself as much as possible.

The nursing role in assisting the patient to cope with his disabilities should be done in conjunction with the physician, patient, family, and other members of the health team such as physical, occupational and speech therapists, vocational counselors, and so on. The nurse must coordinate and incorporate into the nursing care what others are teaching the patient and the patient's daily activities. This necessitates having conferences with the health team members at frequent intervals for collaboration and planning, and when necessary to provide for continuity of care.

Due to the disabling effects of many neurologic disorders, planning for discharge necessitates follow-up care and extension of nursing or various services in the home. The patient and his family should be assisted in obtaining help and information from appropriate agencies which can facilitate rehabilitation assistance and care after discharge.

Nursing Observation and Intervention in Increased Intracranial Pressure

Intelligent observation, combined with appropriate recording and reporting of the signs and symptoms of increasing intracranial pressure, is one of the great responsibilities of the nurse caring for the patient with central nervous system dysfunction. Astute and accurate observations may assist the physician in obtaining a diagnosis and therefore effect treatment. Indeed, they may render him lifesaving intervention. To make intelligent observations and interpretations and to act effectively, the nurse must understand the scientific basis and physiological signs and symptoms of increased intracranial pressure. Understanding the mechanisms involved and the necessity for acute observation enables her to see more subtle changes in the patient's condition before the situation becomes irreversible, due to severe brain damage.

In the adult, the brain is encased in a rigid, bony structure and literally has no room for "excess baggage." Since the cranium is a compact and tight compartment offering no room for expansion, any increase in one of its elements (blood, cerebrospinal fluid, nervous tissue) can do so only at the expense of other elements.[15] The volume of brain tissue simply cannot expand without having deleterious effects on the flow

and amount of cerebrospinal fluid and cerebral circulation. Anything which obstructs the normal passage of cerebrospinal fluid consequently leads to an increase of intracranial pressure.

Increased intracranial pressure may be caused by various space-occupying masses such as neoplasms, abscesses, and hematomas, or processes such as trauma, hemorrhage, inflammation, hydrocephalus, and the like which cause compression, interfere with normal circulation of cerebrospinal fluid, or produce edema in surrounding brain tissue. A space-occupying mass develops at the expense of other elements. As the subarachnoid and ventricular space is reduced, cerebrospinal fluid becomes compressed and there is a rise in intracranial pressure. Initially, partial temporary relief is permitted by displacement of fluid into the spinal and perioptic subarachnoid spaces. Further increase in pressure soon leads to venous compression, resulting in impaired cerebral circulation and stasis of blood. The following signs, symptoms, alterations, and complications occur as a result of the increasing intracranial pressure and should be critically observed by the nurse.

BLOOD PRESSURE AND PULSE. As the elevation of venous pressure occurs and intracranial pressure rises, blood stasis results and cerebral blood flow diminishes. Compensatory vasodilatation of arteries and arterioles attempts to improve cerebral circulation. But if the rise in pressure is rapid and to high levels approaching diastolic, the blood pressure must rise in order to maintain blood flow.[16] Usually there is a greater rise in the systolic blood pressure than in the diastolic pressure, resulting in an increase in pulse pressure. The rising of the blood pressure is accompanied by a slow, bounding pulse. It is thought that the changes in blood pressure and pulse are due to venous stasis and the accumulation of carbon dioxide in the vasomotor center of the medulla. In short, the more crowded and compressed the brain becomes, the less blood and oxygen are available to maintain optimal cerebral functioning and life. (One analogy is that of a woman who gains 15 pounds, in her abdomen, and does not bother to buy a larger girdle.)

Accurate and accessible recordings of blood

pressure and pulse are extremely important indicators of increasing intracranial pressure. Comparisons should be made with other readings to delineate subtle, gradual, or rapid changes. A graphic sheet on which readings can be plotted as often as necessary is a successful tool for noting any changes. Many patients other than the acutely ill can develop increasing intracranial pressure. Patients who are admitted to the ward for a "tumor workup," for instance, may not have vital signs ordered as frequently as does the patient receiving intensive care. The nurse, in this instance, must be extremely alert for any clues which might indiciate a worsening in the patient's condition. *Changes in blood pressure or pulse may be one of the first noticeable signs of increasing intracranial pressure* (although changes in level of consciousness usually precede changes in vital signs).

CHANGES IN THE LEVEL OF CONSCIOUSNESS. The most reliable index of cerebral status is the state of consciousness. Increased intracranial pressure produces changes in the level of consciousness and cerebral function. Although the exact mechanisms are not known, lowering of the level of consciousness is probably due to compression and ischemia of brain cells. Electroencephalographic studies demonstrate diffuse slowing of electrical activity of the cortex. The higher centers are usually affected first, with the patient showing dullness of thought and perception. He may appear lethargic, forgetful, confused, disoriented, and restless. Eventually, he may lapse into coma as the midbrain and ascending reticular system are involved. If the condition is not alleviated, midbrain ischemia soon occurs and deterioration proceeds rapidly. The nurse should observe any changes in the level of consciousness, as described previously, and report them at once to the physician. *A lowering in the level of consciousness should be reported, even though there is no change in vital signs.* In some instances, vital signs may not show characteristic changes; one may be altered without the other, or changes may occur late in the process.

RESPIRATION. The respiratory changes which occur are due to pressure and anoxia in the respiratory center in the medulla. Increased intracra-

nial pressure usually causes irregularities and alterations in respiration. There may be a slight initial increase followed soon by *slowing* of respiration. As the condition worsens, Cheyne-Stokes respiration occurs. This is a serious situation and if not corrected, leads to death. Any changes in respiration should be reported immediately.

TEMPERATURE. The temperature is not necessarily a reliable indicator of increasing intracranial pressure. Rises may occur with compression of the hypothalamus, but may also indicate an infection, particularly respiratory, urinary, skin, wound, or decubitus ulcer. Dehydration may also contribute to a rise in temperature. But an elevation in temperature should be reported. Each degree of temperature elevation increases metabolism in the brain and is detrimental to an ischemic and insulted brain. Temperature should be taken rectally as ordered.

PUPILLARY CHANGES. Pupillary changes and signs are among the most important neurologic signs and should be reported at once. One of the most consistent signs of increased intracranial pressure is a unilateral dilatation of the pupil which results from uncal herniation and lateral brainstem compression. The uncus is the anterior hooklike protrusion of the hippocampal gyrus which extends along the inferomedian aspect portion of the temporal lobe. Uncal herniation occurs when supratentorial pressure (usually due to lesions of the temporal lobe) causes the uncus and the hippocampal gyrus to shift toward the midline and the lateral edge of the tentorium, a transverse fold of dura stretching over the cerebellum and separating it from the cerebrum. Since the oculomotor nerve crosses the anterior portion of the tentorial opening, it is frequently displaced downward and stretched by herniating tissue against the incisura or tentorial notch (Kernohan's notching), which is a large semioval opening extending down into the center of the tentorium. Compression and stretching of the oculomotor nerve in this manner causes ipsilateral dilatation of the pupil. In bilateral dilatation both hemispheres are involved. Ipsilateral dilatation of the pupil is a serious sign, for deterioration may proceed at a very rapid rate. If treatment is not carried out and the pressure or lesion removed, irreversible brainstem damage occurs and death results (Fig. 20-5).

MOTOR ABNORMALITIES. Motor abnormalities occur when pressure is exerted on the pyramidal tract in the cerebral peduncle. The cerebral peduncle (crus cerebri) which contains motor fibers (corticospinal and corticopontile) to the cord below, is the basal portion of the midbrain. As compression or displacement of the midbrain occurs, the ipsilateral cerebral peduncle may be compressed, leading to contralateral hemiparesis or hemiplegia. Frequently the opposite peduncle is wedged against the edge of the tentorium, producing ipsilateral hemiparesis or hemiplegia. Ipsilateral or bilateral plantar exten-

sor responses (Babinski) occur, due to pyramidal involvement. If pressure is allowed to continue, brainstem involvement soon occurs and the patient exhibits decerebrate rigidity. The nurse should watch for hemiparesis, hemiplegia, decerebration and abnormal posturing and notify the physician immediately of any changes (Fig. 20-5).

The following symptoms which may occur with increased intracranial pressure are classical ones but may not occur until late in the course of illness. Although other criteria may be more useful indicators of a rise in intracranial pressure, the nurse should not overlook these symptoms.

HEADACHE. Headache, which occurs in the presence of increased intracranial pressure, is

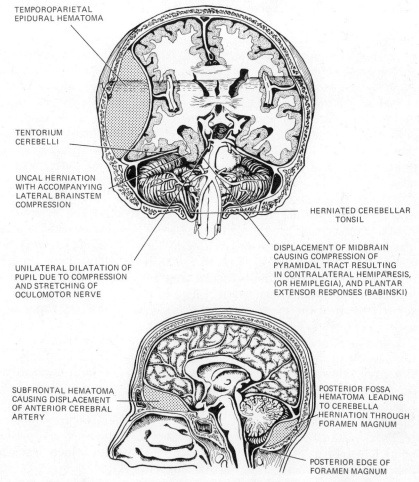

TEMPOROPARIETAL EPIDURAL HEMATOMA

TENTORIUM CEREBELLI

UNCAL HERNIATION WITH ACCOMPANYING LATERAL BRAINSTEM COMPRESSION

HERNIATED CEREBELLAR TONSIL

DISPLACEMENT OF MIDBRAIN CAUSING COMPRESSION OF PYRAMIDAL TRACT RESULTING IN CONTRALATERAL HEMIPARESIS, (OR HEMIPLEGIA), AND PLANTAR EXTENSOR RESPONSES (BABINSKI)

UNILATERAL DILATATION OF PUPIL DUE TO COMPRESSION AND STRETCHING OF OCULOMOTOR NERVE

SUBFRONTAL HEMATOMA CAUSING DISPLACEMENT OF ANTERIOR CEREBRAL ARTERY

POSTERIOR FOSSA HEMATOMA LEADING TO CEREBELLA HERNIATION THROUGH FORAMEN MAGNUM

POSTERIOR EDGE OF FORAMEN MAGNUM

FIGURE 20-5.
The pathophysiology of head injuries.

thought to be caused by tension and displacement of pain-sensitive structures, such as intracerebral vessels (basal arteries, large venous sinuses) and the dura. Coughing, sneezing, straining at bowel movements, stooping, and straining with activities, all increase intracranial pressure, thus intensifying the headache. Patients with brain tumors (and other space-occupying masses) frequently wake up with a morning headache, which is somewhat alleviated by getting up and moving about. Negative pressure exists in the ventricles in the erect position, but pressure in the brain and spinal cord is about the same when lying flat. Therefore, intracranial pressure is greater when the patient lies down. These principles help explain why headaches very often occur upon waking and serve as the rationale for elevating the head of the bed. Elevation also serves to aid venous return. Patients with headache are often more comfortable with the head of the bed elevated and even prefer to sleep this way. Activities which increase the pressure and the headache, such as straining and stooping, should be avoided. Particular attention should be paid to maintaining adequate elimination so that constipation and straining do not occur. With a sudden increase in pressure, the brain may be forced down and herniations through the incisura, or foramen magnum may occur.

Patients with headache due to increasing intracranial pressure are usually uncomfortable. Analgesics (such as aspirin, caffeine, Darvon) may be ordered to help provide relief. Dehydrating drugs and restriction of fluids may also be instituted. Lumbar puncture is usually contraindicated (except when examination of fluid is absolutely vital) in the presence of increased intracranial pressure, and so removal of fluid is not a desirable method of alleviating headache. Performing a lumbar puncture and releasing pressure from below may cause cerebral transtentorial herniation or cerebellar herniation into the foramen magnum with resulting compression of cardiac and respiratory centers.

Providing a comfortable environment should be an integral part of the nursing care for these patients. Quiet, nondisruptive surroundings are most helpful. It is best to produce the least

amount of irritation as possible for the patient. For instance, he should not be placed in a room where building or remodeling are going on nearby or with an overactive, confused patient. He should be helped to assume a position of maximum comfort. He should not be kept waiting for his medication. Above all, he should be consulted as to what specific things are most helpful and provide the most comfort.

PAPILLEDEMA. Papilledema may appear in both the early and latter stages of increased intracranial pressure. With a rise in pressure, the optic disc becomes swollen and is pushed forward above the level of the retina (choked disc). Although observation for papilledema is the responsibility of the physician, the nurse should be alert for any signs of blurring, failing, or double vision. Blurring of vision may be precipitated by coughing, straining, and stooping and should be reported.

VOMITING. Vomiting may be a sign of increasing intracranial pressure. It may or may not be projectile in nature. Vomiting is thought to be due to irritation of the vagal nuclei in the floor of the fourth ventricle. Any vomiting should be immediately reported. If it is severe, oral intake should be stopped and the patient should be given intravenous fluids. Measures to decrease the pressure, either medically or surgically, must be instituted.

The nurse should be aware not only of the signs and symptoms of increased intracranial pressure but also of the complications which ensue if pressure is not relieved. The cranium is a tightly closed structure, and contains only three openings: the foramen magnum, the subfalcial space and the tentorial opening. With an increase in pressure, brain matter is displaced toward the lines of least resistance. Consequently, herniations can occur such as uncal herniation, an intracranial shift due to increasing intracranial pressure. Herniations may occur across the intracranial cavity under the falx, the sickle-shaped fold of dura mater between the cerebral hemispheres, causing compression of major blood vessels, particularly the internal cerebral vein, which leads to cerebral ischemia (Fig. 20-6).

With posterior fossa lesions, there may be

FIGURE 20-6.
Intracranial shifts with supratentorial lesions. (*1*) Herniation of the cingulate gyrus under the falx. (*2*) Herniation of the temporal lobe into the tentorial notch. (*3*) Downward displacement of the brainstem through the tentorial notch. Source: Plum, F. and Posner, J.: Diagnosis of Stupor and Coma. Contemporary Neurology Series. Philadelphia, F. A. Davis, 1966. Modified from a drawing by Miles. *In* W. Blackwood, T. C. Dodds, and J. C. Somerville: An Atlas of Neuropathology. 1949. Courtesy of E. and S. Livingstone, Ltd., Edinburgh. Used by permission.

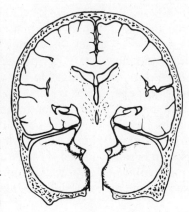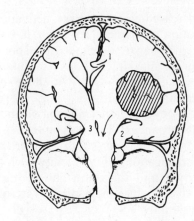

herniation of the cerebellum through the foramen magnum (see Fig. 20-5). Signs which may occur include suboccipital headache, stiff neck, cranial nerve involvement (particularly the lower bulb), and respiratory difficulty. Cardiovascular and respiratory collapse may occur suddenly and without warning. Since there is such a danger of pressure conus in patients with posterior fossa lesions, elevation of the head of the bed is often contraindicated. In this case, the patient is kept in a supine position. Straining of any sort should be avoided, since a rise in intrathoracic pressure disturbs the venous return from the brain and raises the intracranial pressure. Herniation of the cerebellum may also occur upward through the tentorial notch which affects the midbrain structures.

Increased intracranial pressure is a dangerous condition in and of itself. (An exception is pseudotumor cerebri, whereby brain bulk is increased and pressure raised, but there is no blockage of cerebrospinal fluid or displacement of intracranial structures.) Death can occur with increased intracranial pressure (600 mm) without herniation. With such high pressure, cerebral circulation is diminished to such a state that the brain cannot survive. Therefore, both medical and surgical means may be employed by the physician to reduce the pressure. The most reliable and rapid medical therapy used is intravenous urea. Jackson points out that dosage of 1 to 1½ Gm per kg at intervals of 12 to 24 hours causes the brain to shrink rapidly, the effect becoming maximal in 30 to 90 mintues and disappearing in about 6 hours.[17] This osmotic diuresis produces a great outpouring of urine (2,000 to 4,000 ml). Unless this fluid loss is replaced, the patient becomes acutely dehydrated, even to the point of hypovolemic shock. *It is a nursing responsibility to keep an accurate and specific record of the patient's intake and output.* Replacement therapy may be needed, in which case the nurse must regulate IV flow to maintain the ordered amount of intravenous fluids. Both dehydration and water intoxication produce cerebral signs and symptoms, such as unconsciousness, coma, and increased intracranial pressure, and should be prevented. Jackson also indicates that dehydration, once recommended in the hope of reducing cerebral edema, reduces blood volume, stimulates aldosterone secretion, and increases salt retention, thus increasing the hypernatremia induced by dehydration. Therefore, the results of dehydration may be injurious.

Corticosteroids are also being used successfully to reduce cerebral edema. The effect is less rapid, but appears to be more prolonged. Steroids may be given intravenously in large amounts at first and then either intramuscularly or by mouth. A number of adverse reactions are known to occur with steroid therapy such as Cushing's syndrome, negative nitrogen balance, increased blood pressure, activation and complication of peptic ulcer (such as GI bleeding and hemorrhage), osteoporosis, spontaneous fractures, masking of signs of infection and decreased resistance to it, fluid and electroyte imbalance with edema, corneal ulcers, leukocytosis, thromboembolism, and psychic disturbances. These symptoms should be observed by the nurse (see Chapter 18). In addition, complications of immobility such as skin breakdown and infection should be particularly avoided, since the patient on steroids is prone to these.

In severe situations and with rapid deterioration of the patient, surgical intervention may be necessary in order to reduce the increased intracranial pressure. Multiple burr holes may be made for exploration. If they fail to reveal a lesion or to reduce the pressure, surgical decompression can be lifesaving. Subtemporal decompression may be performed on one side, or in severe cases bilaterally. A large opening is made in the temporal region to allow for expansion of compressed edematous brain tissue. In extreme cases, requiring even greater decompression, the anterior 5 cm of the temporal lobe on the nondominant side may be removed.[18]

SUMMARY

The nurse is responsible for observing changes in the patient's neurologic status. Observation for signs and symptoms of increased intracranial pressure is vital when caring for the patient with cerebral dysfunction resulting from injury or disease. The level of consciousness, vital signs, and motor and pupillary signs are important indicators of increasing intracranial pressure. However, it must be emphasized that no two patients are alike, and, therefore, patients may demonstrate varying clinical pictures. The nurse must also be aware that there is no exact course with increased intracranial pressure. While one patient may deteriorate rapidly, another may be relatively lucid with no apparent change in vital signs until very late in the process. Therefore, the nurse must be alert to *subtle* changes in the patient. This requires having baseline information and adequate assessment of each patient.

The nurse should realize that often behavioral changes, such as not eating or feeding oneself, lack or change in interaction with family and staff, irritability, incontinence, restlessness, changes in pattern of activities, often may indicate a worsening of the patient's condition prior to any noticeable changes in vital signs. The nurse is best able to look for these changes if knowledge of the patient as an individual is obtained through a nursing history, and if day-by-day contact and descriptive nursing progress notes are maintained.

Neurologic Problems and Dysfunction

BULBAR INVOLVEMENT

Caring for the patient with bulbar involvement poses a tremendous responsibility and challenge for the nurse and is a serious problem for all concerned. Involvement of the cranial nerves of the lower brain stem, particularly cranial nerves IX and X, occurs with many neurologic disorders. Bulbar involvement may be present in myasthenia gravis, progressive bulbar palsy, amyotrophic lateral sclerosis, Werdnig-Hoffmann paralysis of early infancy and childhood, Guillain-Barré syndrome (ascending polyneuritis), poliomyelitis, tetanus, botulism, diphtheritic palsy, bulbar neoplasms, syringobulbia, and epidemic encephalitis. Although the causes of these illnesses are different, they all affect the lower brain stem to some extent, resulting in bulbar palsy.

Patients with bulbar palsy due to glossopharyngeal, hypoglossal, and vagal involvement may have difficulty in swallowing (dysphagia), decreased gag reflex, nasal and hoarse voice, dysarthria, or even anarthria, drooling, and increased salivation with pooling of secretions in the oropharynx, nasal reflux of fluids and foods, choking, as well as having danger of aspiration, difficulty in breathing, paralysis, and atrophy of the tongue. Therefore, the patient may have difficulty maintaining a patent airway and respiring, maintaining adequate nutrition, and communicating to others. Nursing intervention for patients with bulbar involvement should include the following goals:

1. Helping the patient maintain a patent airway.
2. Helping to provide the patient with adequate nutrition.
3. Preventing complications.
4. Maintaining communication with the patient (if dysarthric).

In assisting the patient to maintain a patent airway, the head of the bed should be elevated and the patient should be put in a lateral position to promote drainage of secretions, lessen obstruction to the air passages, and prevent the tongue from falling back (many of these patients have hypoglossal paralysis). The nurse should observe the patient for respiratory changes. Frequent suctioning and mouth care are necessary, due to pooling of secretions. One of the greatest causes of deaths in patients with bulbar involvement is aspiration pneumonia, due to aspiration of *water, food, vomitus, and their own secretions*. Any signs of dyspnea, tachypnea, cyanosis, and so on should be reported immediately. Many of these patients, particularly if they have an acute process such as Guillain-Barré syndrome or myasthenia gravis, are tracheostomized. In this case, suctioning and care of the tracheostomy tube is necessary to maintain a patent airway.

The bulbar diet has been specifically designed to help provide nutrition for patients with bulbar involvement. The bulbar diet requires:

1. No milk or milk products, such as eggnogs and milkshakes, since they produce increased mucous formation in the mouth and throat.
2. No sticky foods such as potatoes, macaroni and cheese and other carbohydrate foods, due to difficulty in swallowing such foods.
3. Soft, smooth-grain foods; fruit, vegetable and meat purees; and most liquids are allowed.

Since the patient has such difficulty swallowing, the diet is best given in small, frequent feedings (usually five or six a day). Nursing personnel should remain with the patient while he is eating or drinking, due to the danger of choking and aspiration. A suction machine should be at the bedside to deal with this danger if it arises. Although a side-lying position facilitates drainage of oral secretions, and poses less danger of an obstructed airway, some patients find eating in this position extremely difficult and prefer to have their meals in a sitting position. Regardless of the position used (as long as it is not supine), the nurse should allow at least 30 minutes for feeding. Many patients take much longer to eat. They are extremely frightened of choking to death. The once simple act of eating is no longer pleasant for them. The patient simply cannot be hurried and the nurse should allow him to determine when he is ready to eat. All intake of food and fluids should be recorded. If dysphagia is so severe that oral intake is inadequate, a nasogastric or gastrostomy tube may be necessary.

Some patients have trouble swallowing fluids, because they regurgitate easily through the nose. Thicker fluids such as thick soups and consommés are often tolerated better than other liquids. Also, patients appear to be able to take their fluids better with a cup or spoon rather than from a straw. If a spoon is used in feeding, a whole teaspoon should be given rather than a smaller portion, since a sizable bolus is needed to aid in swallowing. The patient with bulbar involvement may find it difficult to swallow medications. If so, pills can be crushed and given with his food.

It is very helpful for the nurse to consult with the dietitian in planning nutrition for the patient. Each patient has his own preferences in eating and it is best not to make generalizations or rules of thumb.

Dysarthria often occurs with bulbar involvement, compounding the patient's difficulties, for he is unable to speak clearly and intelligibly. (Nursing intervention for the dysarthric patient is discussed on pp. 697-698.)

These patients are often very apprehensive and do not want to be left alone. Many of them have additional neurologic involvement, such as weakness of extremities, and feel totally helpless. The nurse should be aware of these fears and provide as much support as possible. It is usually best if the patient is placed under intensive care so that he can be observed around the clock. Many patients with bulbar involvement have "strange" sensations and feelings. For instance, one patient described her inability to move her tongue and her difficulty in swallowing to be like a giant spider in her mouth. She would wake up and feel as if the "spider" were coming down her throat and choking her. Another patient focused on his secretions and felt that his mouth was never clean, no matter how thoroughly or often he had mouth care. After he recovered from Guillain-Barré syndrome, he stated, "One of the most frustrating things is to feel secretions running down your face and not be able to do anything about it." The nurse should show understanding and provide skillful and compassionate care, for bulbar palsy is, as one patient put it, "The most horrid feeling of strangulation a person can ever know."

SEIZURES

Local or generalized seizures may occur in the neurologic patient for a variety of reasons. Irritation in the cranium, due to edema, tumor, hematoma, or some other space-occupying mass, may cause seizures. Other etiological factors include infection (such as meningitis, or encephalitis), poisoning and electrolyte disturbances (such as hyponatremia), all of which may produce single convulsive seizures or status epilepticus.

The primary function of the nurse is to *prevent* the patient from injuring himself and to observe and record the nature of the seizure. Restraints of any sort should not be used because injury to the patient may result—the patient with arms or legs restrained may incur fractures and other injuries should he have a seizure. Padded side rails are helpful in preventing injury. (Pillows should not be used for padding, since there is danger of suffocating the patient.) Constricting clothing should be loosened, particularly around the neck. If clothing is tight when the neck becomes turgid and swollen, the resistance to the return of blood is increased, and extravasations into the skin or conjunctiva are more probable.[19] Because there is also danger of asphyxiation, the head should be supported and turned to the side to allow the tongue to fall forward and not occlude the airway. The use of a padded tongue blade may or may not help. In most instances, the patient's mouth is clenched tightly closed and attempts to insert a tongue blade may damage his teeth and his gums. The notion that one should place something in a person's mouth when he is

in the midst of a seizure is overemphasized. All too often spoons, handkerchiefs, and other miscellaneous items have been used by uninformed people, to the detriment of the patient. The practice has sometimes resulted in death, due to obstructed airways, gagging, and aspiration. If a properly padded tongue blade cannot be inserted, then one can assist the patient by proper positioning. If it is possible to insert a tongue blade or airway, care should be taken during insertion not to defeat the purpose by pushing the tongue back and occluding the airway.

To observe the seizure is the second responsibility of the nurse. She should remove bedclothes in order to allow for more complete observation of the movements. Accurate observation from the beginning of the seizure is important, since it provides data which assists the physician in localizing a cerebral lesion or obtaining a diagnosis. Some of the important observations to be made and recorded include: onset; deviation of head and eyes; progression; movements and sites involved; incontinence; level of consciousness during all phases; pupillary changes; duration; condition and behavior of a patient afterward; patient's ability to remember anything about the seizure (not obtainable in the comatose patient).

Status epilepticus is a state of continuing or recurring seizures in which the patient does not usually regain consciousness, or recovery is incomplete between attacks. There are many other varieties besides the most familiar grand mal status. These include petit mal status, automatisms, and epileptic confusional states which last for hours and even days. The grand mal status epilepticus it the most severe and demands prompt attention or death rapidly ensues.

An adequate airway is of utmost importance for patients "in status." In many instances, an endotracheal tube may be inserted or a tracheostomy performed. *Since large doses of anticonvulsants are usually given, the patient must be observed for signs of respiratory arrest.* Positive ventilatory assistance may also be required.

Medications used to arrest status epilepticus may include phenobarbital, given intravenously at first and then in subsequent intramuscular injections. Paraldehyde and diazepam (Valium) are also being used. In severe uncontrolled cases, it may be necessary for the patient to undergo general anesthesia. The nurse has a tremendous responsibility in administering the drugs ordered and in regulating the flow of intravenous fluids. Accurate recording of the frequency and patterns of seizures is necessary as are maintaining a safe environment and preventing injury to the patient.

VISUAL-SPATIAL DEFECTS

Visual-spatial defects are often encountered in the patient with central nervous system dysfunction. A newly graduated staff nurse became quite upset when one of her patients seemed to ignore her but interacted with other staff and personnel. The brief patient presentation is as follows:

Mrs. B., a 54-year-old housewife, developed left-sided denial, left homonymous hemianopia, and left hemiplegia following complications of a right carotid arteriogram, which resulted in a right posterior cerebrovascular accident. Following the arteriogram, it was soon noted that she ignored people and objects in the left visual space. She was unaware of the existence of the left side of her body. When asked to comb her hair, she combed only the right side. If asked to touch her left ear, she would touch her right ear. She ignored items such as objects and food that were placed to her left on her overbed table and would not communicate with those talking to her on her left. The patient was right-handed and had no difficulty speaking or understanding the spoken word. But she neglected the left in reading and writing.

The parietal lobe serves in the perception of body image, position in space, and the relationship of different parts of the body to one another, and is the seat of somatic sensation. In lesions of the nondominant parietal lobe (right hemisphere in the right-handed person), there may be disturbance of discriminative sensory functions, such as astereognosis (loss of ability to recognize the form and nature of objects by touch), loss of position sense (inability to recognize limb positions), extinction (when one of two bilateral simultaneous stimulations is not perceived), as well as impairment of pain, temperature, touch, and vibratory sense (inability to perceive vibra-

tions over certain bony prominences when a tuning fork is applied). In addition, lesions of the nondominant parietal lobe are known to cause both spatial and visual disturbances. There may be anosognosia, which is the unawareness or ignorance of an illness, such as hemiplegia or hemianesthesia. The patient may deny that there is anything wrong with him and deny he cannot use the affected extremity in a normal manner. Autotopagnosia, which is a loss of ability to orient different parts of the body, or to identify individual parts and their relation to the body, is also seen with lesions of the minor parietal lobe. Often the patient may believe that someone else's hand or leg is in bed with him, or that someone else put it there. The patient fails to recognize it as his own. Neglect of the left side of the body (agnosia of the body half) and neglect of the visual space to the left of the midline is often present as well. These phenomena occur mostly in lesions of the right posterior parietal lobe, but some cases have been reported in which there is involvement of the left parietal lobe.

The lesion usually producing these visual-spatial disturbances is located in the posterior and inferior portions of the nondominant parietal lobe (the right lobe for most people and even the right hemisphere for many left-handed people) and the areas near the occipital lobe. Since the optic radiations travel through the parietal lobe to the visual cortex, left homonymous hemianopia usually occurs, resulting in blindness in the left half of each visual field which consequently contributes to the patient's visual-spatial neglect. The exact mechanisms responsible for left-sided neglect, left-visual neglect, anosognosia, and autotopagnosia are not completely understood. It seems reasonably certain, however, that the parietal and occipital lobes play an important part in this spatial orientation.

The nature of visual-spatial disturbances has not only baffled medical researchers, but has also posed even more confusion for nurses and students unacquainted with the phenomena. The recognition and understanding of the nature of these disturbances can make a difference in whether a patient improves or regresses to complete dependence upon others. Nursing staff members who have no understanding of the pathophysiology are apt to ignore these patients and even accuse them of being confused, antisocial, uncommunicative, or psychotic. Therefore, it is very important to communicate to all involved in the care of the patient the nature of the illness and specific nursing orders relevant to care.

Above all, it should be recognized that the patient's disturbances are sequelae and due to cerebral insult. When a patient first suffers a cerebrovascular accident resulting in left-sided denial and neglect of the left-visual space, it facilitates matters to place all important personal items on the right and within easy sight and reach of the patient. In most instances, communication and visual attention cannot be easily elicited on the left side, so that interaction with the patient should be carried out at his right side or slightly to the right of the midline. In assisting the patient with activities of daily living, it should be remembered that he may neglect washing, grooming, dressing of the left side and will need assistance in these areas. Since most of these patients are right-handed, they do not require much assistance with eating. However, the patient may ignore food placed on the left. The nurse should see to it that food is within the right-visual space or else call attention to the fact that the food is there. Ambulating is often very difficult if the patient is unaware of his left side, and assistance should be provided. Activities of daily living must be modified in view of the patient's limitations. each patient may manifest varying symptomatology, due to the complexity of the nervous system. The above are only suggestions which can be implemented if appropriate to the individual patient's problems.

In the acute stage, the patient cannot begin extensive visual-spatial therapeutics; therefore, the nurse must accept the patient as he presents himself. This is true of the patient with a disturbance of body image. It does not matter how much one insists that the patient wash his left hand; if he does not believe that it is his or if he is simply unaware of it, he will not wash it. The patient who insists that there is a corpse in bed with him, believes it. Rather than agree that there is a corpse in bed with the patient, or respond emphatically that the arm is his, it is better to show understanding of his perception. A question such as "Does the arm not feel as if it belongs to you?" often produces more optimum results and improvements. In addition, Ullman lists three implications for nursing patients with disorders of body image.[20]

1. By a variety of means, the patient attempts to preserve a state of unawareness of, or unrelatedness to, an existing illness or handicap.

2. When irrational behavior occurs or inappropriate responses are given, they are more apt to be related to the illness than to other aspects of life.

3. Delusional material relating to the illness may exist side by side with appropriate responses in other areas.

The above implications are helpful in providing understanding of the patient's behavior and disability. Disorders of perception resulting from parietal lesions can produce behavior which is so bizarre to the observer as to suggest hysteria, psychosis, and severe confusion. The nurse must have insight and understanding into the patient's difficulties if optimum rehabilitation is to be achieved. All too often, these patients are avoided because personnel do not really know what factors are contributing to the patient's behavior. If it is difficult for staff to care for a patient with unilateral neglect, how difficult it must be for a patient's family to cope with his disabilities!

As the patient recovers, unawareness of the left half of the body and denial of hemiplegia often diminish, along with much of the inappropriate responses to illness. However, neglect of one-half of external space (the left half usually) and homonymous hemianopia usually persist and extensive rehabilitation employing visual-spatial therapeutics should be initiated. The nurse and the patient's family can hasten this phase by reinforcing and informing the patient of his visual neglect. For instance, the patient can be asked to read or name objects. Since he can read only half of the paragraph or name objects only in the right half of the visual field, concrete evidence can be obtained to inform the patient of his visual neglect. The patient first must become aware of his disability, before any attempt at therapeutics is made.

Although specialists, such as neuropsychologists and rehabilitation specialists in this area, are primarily responsible for assisting the patient and his family, the nurse can reinforce some of the visual exercises while caring for the patient. He must be taught to explore the left visual space by turning his head to the left and scanning the left visual space with rapid successive eye movements.[21] This must become a conditioned and permanent habit if rehabilitation is to be successful. Postural adjustments and conditioning activities are difficult, even for the most intelligent person. Reading, writing, object-naming, and visual-verbal exercises, as well as development of new patterns necessary for activities of daily living, must be included in a comprehensive program.

The nurse can play an integral part in the care and rehabilitation of patients with visual-spatial disturbances. It requires knowledge and understanding of his disabilities and deficits and purposeful, intelligent intervention based on his needs and problems. Very little documentation concerning nursing intervention is available. Since the phenomenon is thought to be present in anywhere from 50 to 70 percent of patients with right posterior cerebral lesions, it might well be made the subject for more nursing research.

CEREBELLAR DISTURBANCES

Although the cerebellum is the second largest area of the brain, it is one of the least discussed in nursing literature. Yet symptoms of cerebellar involvement occur in many different conditions which the nurse encounters. Cerebellar symptoms can occur with multiple processes such as congenital abnormalities (platybasia or basilar impression), neoplasms, trauma, chronic, infectious and toxic disorders, tumors of the brain or acoustic neuroma with cerebellar involvement, deficiency states such as beriberi, intracerebellar hemorrhage, vascular lesions, cerebellar atrophy, hereditary cerebellar, and spinocerebellar ataxias. Symptoms of degeneration have also been associated with Dilantin (diphenylhydantoin) intoxication, multiple sclerosis, hyper-

pyrexia, alcoholism, Hodgkin's disease, olivopontocerebellar degeneration, and carcinomatous cerebellar degeneration.

The cerebellum is located infratentorially in an area called the posterior fossa and is separated from the cerebrum by a transverse fold of dura mater called the tentorium cerebelli. It consists mainly of white matter that contains several gray masses called nuclei, the largest being the dentate nucleus. Three paired cerebellar peduncles which contain many afferent and efferent fibers enter and leave the cerebellum and connect it to the rest of the central nervous system. The inferior peduncle forms the connection between the cerebellum, spinal cord, and medullary centers. It contains many afferent fibers such as the posterior spinocerebellar tract from the spinal cord, external arcuate fibers from the nuclei of gracilis and cuneatus, a branch from the vestibular nerve, and the olivocerebellar, reticulocerebellar, and nucleocerebellar pathways. The descending pathways include the cerebellospinal, cerebellovestibular, cerebello-olivary, and fastigiobulbar fibers.

The main connection between the cerebellum and the cerebral cortex is the middle cerebellar peduncle, which contains pontocerebellar pathways. The superior cerebellar peduncle is the major efferent connection and contains many efferent fibers such as dentorubral and dentothalamic.

The cerebellum is not considered a sensory organ, although all sensory modalities carry impulses to it; nor can it be considered a motor organ because of its effect on muscle synergy, coordination, and voluntary movement. It is best thought of as an adjustor or giant computer which detects errors between the performance of muscle groups and the intention of the cortex. For instance, if the intention of the cortex is to have an arm move to a specific point, but the arm begins to surpass the desired point, the cerebellum detects the error and transmits impulses to slow down movement. Inhibitory impulses are sent to the motor cortex to excite antagonist muscles. In this way movement may be stopped at the desired point.

Assessments and calculations of motor activ-

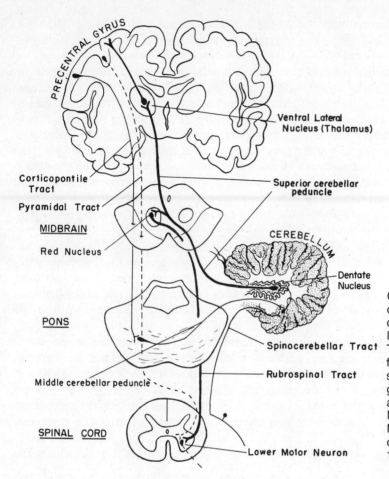

FIGURE 20-7.
Cerebellar circuits. The spino-cerebellas and cortico-ponto-cerebellar pathways to the cerebellum are represented by thin fibers. Thick fibers show efferent paths from the dentate nucleus to the spinal cord and to the precentral gyrus. The pyramidal tract is shown as a dotted line. Source: Gatz, A. J.: Manter's Essentials of Clinical Neuroanatomy and Neurophysiology, ed. 4. Philadelphia, F. A. David, 1970, p. 74. Used by permission.

ity must be performed by the cerebellum with great rapidity and from many sources. It receives information from the motor cortex by way of the corticopontocerebellar pathway. In addition, reports are sent to it through the spinocerebellar tracts, as well as through other afferent pathways carrying tactile, auditory, and visual stimuli. Like a computer or servomechanism, the cerebellum has to analyze and integrate this information, then make any corrections in muscle movement and modifications of muscular activity which may be necessary. Impulses which leave the cerebellum may reach the voluntary motor system to modify or slow down activity by various routes. One of these is the dentatorubrospinal tract whereby fibers from the dentate nucleus synapse in the red nucleus and give rise to the rubrospinal tract. The dentatothalamocor-tical pathway relays impulses to the motor area and influences the activity of the pyramidal system. Impulses to both facilitory and inhibitory reticular nuclei are transmitted by the reticulospinal tracts to the motor neurons[23] (Fig. 20-8).[24]

The cerebellum operates in a similar manner with involuntary movement, the difference being that different pathways are involved (Fig. 20-8).

Another function of the cerebellum is the role it plays in maintaining equilibrium, muscular posture, orientation of the organism in space, and changes in direction of motion. Afferent impulses are received from vestibular centers, labyrinths, the spinal cord and the brain stem. The cerebellum then transmits impulses to lateral vestibular nuclei by way of cerebellovestibular fibers. Fibers from the lateral vestibular nucleus become the vestibulospinal pathway and de-

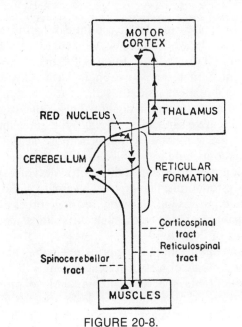

FIGURE 20-8.
Pathways for cerebellar "error" control of voluntary movements. Source: Guyton, A.C.: Textbook of Medical Physiology; ed. 2. Philadelphia, W. B. Saunders, 1961, p. 784. Used by permission.

scend in the cord, helping to maintain and regulate muscle tone and posture.

With cerebellar dysfunction, an individual is no longer able to carry out the simplest of activities such as walking, and eating, without difficulty. The following signs usually accompany cerebellar disturbance: Dysmetria, dysdiadochokinesia, ataxia, nystagmus, tremor, hypotonia. In addition, decomposition of movement may be present whereby an act of several movements which requires synchronous activity is broken down into its separate parts. For instance, when reaching for an object, the joints of the shoulder, wrists, and elbow may move separately rather than move as a synchronized activity. This resembles robotlike and puppetlike movements.

The signs and symptoms of cerebellar disease depend upon the severity and acuteness of the process. In the more acute process, symptoms are more profound. In chronic cerebellar disturbances, progressive worsening of symptoms may be slow and the patient is able to function as he learns to compensate for his deficiency. The

nurse, however, must have knowledge of pathophysiology in order to anticipate problems which occur and to understand the nature of the patient's disabilities. A nurse who has scanty knowledge of cerebellar function cannot appreciate just how frustrating and difficult activities of daily living can be for the patient with cerebellar involvement. One needs only to think how distressing it is to spill things, or no longer be able to play an instrument, drive a car, or care for one's family, in order to appreciate the tremendous adjustments and restrictions these patients often face.

Nursing intervention for patients with cerebellar dysfunction is based on the patient's physiologic problems as well as on his psychosocial needs. Although each patient is different and nursing interventions may vary, similarities occur, particularly in the area of activities of daily living.

If the patient is ataxic, which is often the case, assistance with walking should be provided. The nurse should look for any particular pattern and see whether the patient swerves to either side or forward or backward. Swaying is often lessened by having the patient place his feet farther apart (wide-based gait). Many patients with cerebellar involvement benefit by the use of a walker. Some, on the other hand, prefer walking close to a wall or holding onto objects. Often the nurse can assist by walking next to the unaffected side if there is unilateral involvement. The patient should be encouraged to walk slowly, since difficulties in gait increase when walking rapidly. Physiotherapy has also been utilized to improve walking through exercises. All efforts should be made to preserve the patient's mobility and independence with a maximum of safety, through collaboration with the physician and other members of the health team. As progression of symptoms occurs, the patient may be unable to walk. However, there are degrees of involvement. One 18-year old boy with platybasia* had been ataxic all his life but

*A congenital deformity whereby the basilar and condylar portions of the occipital bone are displaced upward and exert pressure on the cerebellar tonsils, lower cranial nerves, and lower part of the medulla.

was not confined to a wheelchair. Although he could not engage in sports, he managed to participate in school activities well enough to graduate and enter college. Two years ago, he underwent an involved and intricate operation for repair and correction of the maldevelopment. The operation was successful and the young man should have no further progression of his cerebellar symptoms. He will always be ataxic since the damage that was incurred prior to the corrective surgery was permanent, but he will lead a relatively normal life.

Speech disturbances may range from minor slurring to almost completely unintelligible sounds. When speech is totally indiscernible, the patient may have to communicate by other means. The nurse should consult a speech therapist who can evaluate the problem more accurately and provide further suggestions to foster communication.

Activities of daily living can pose many problems which challenge the ingenuity of the nurse and tax the morale of the patient. The nurse, however, is often able to do simple things that help the patient to assist himself to a greater extent. A glass should not be filled to the top, to prevent spilling when lifting and drinking. Since the patient is apt to overshoot or undershoot in reaching for objects, if possible use objects made of plastic rather than of glass. Paper cups are usually too unstable to manage well. If movements are made worse by the presence of an intention tremor, eating, and activities of daily living may prove very frustrating. However, there are several self-help devices and utensils available through occupational therapy and rehabilitation agencies that may prove helpful. One nurse assisted a patient by placing suction cups under his plate and cup so that they would be stationary and easier to manage. A special straw was placed through a hole in the lid of the cup. This patient was able to eat and drink with very little assistance and much less embarrassment. Conferences were held by the nurse with the patient's wife to assist in planning for home care. Individual planning with the family is quite helpful. Family members should be made aware of agencies, facilities, and literature that can assist them and the patient at home.

There are, no doubt, countless techniques and gadgets which can be utilized to help the patient. The important thing is for the nurse to recognize that the situation is far from completely hopeless and that the patient can be helped to maintain his dignity. This is one of the most creative aspects of nursing—the nurse must assist the individual to perform those activities which contribute to health and its recovery. The nursing care of patients with central nervous system dysfunction calls for great ingenuity, creativity, and purposeful planning, for in no other area are patients faced with such disabilities in activities of daily living.

One important nursing principle in the care of the neurologic or neurosurgical patient is that the bedside table, personal items, and so on be placed on the nonaffected or least affected side and within easy reach of the patient. The nurse should remember that the *right* side of the cerebellum controls and influences the *right* side of the body; in other words, there is ipsilateral control. If a patient is admitted with left cerebellar involvement, most of his difficulties and symptoms will be on the left. This *differs* from cerebral lesions (such as strokes, hemorrhage, or tumor), which produce contralateral effects and symptoms. Patients with unilateral cerebellar lesions can often assist themselves to a great extent, provided that the nurse uses foresight in placing things near his unaffected side. The bell cord should be accessible to the patient. In addition, it is often helpful to place the side rails part way up to help provide support in his turning or sitting up in bed. Monkey bars are also helpful for this purpose.

The maintenance of safety and provision of a safe environment should be of utmost concern in the care of the patient with cerebellar involvement. It is well to instruct the patient to perform acts unhurriedly, since walking fast, getting up suddenly from a chair, stopping suddenly increase the possibility of injury from falls. If the patient is unable to walk without falling, assistance should be provided, particularly when he is getting out of bed. This is particularly true at night and the patient should be instructed not to try to walk to the bathroom without help (scalp lacerations due to fall are common occurrences).

An electric razor is much safer to use than a hand razor for personal hygiene. Another important point is that smoking may be very dangerous for the patient who has coordination difficulties. It is a good policy to have someone present with him if he wishes to smoke. In preparing for discharge, the family should be instructed about safety in the home. Such things as hand rails along the wall and in the bathroom, removal of scatter rugs, cords and other such obstructions should be included as part of a safety program. If the home has stairs, it is usually better for the patient to be located on the first floor. There are additional safety suggestions which the family can receive by writing to various foundations and rehabilitation settings.

Finally, the nurse should be aware of the tremendous psychological and psychosocial problems which often occur with the patient with cerebellar disturbance. In most instances, life patterns are affected and complete reorientation to life's goals is necessary. The following case summary of a young man suffering from multiple sclerosis, with cerebellar signs, illustrates psychosocial aspects.

Mr. R., age 24, was admitted as an ambulatory patient to a large teaching hospital. His admitting diagnosis was multiple sclerosis.

Mr. R., a guidance counselor and school band director, for the past year has been developing slowly progressive incoordination and other symptoms of multiple sclerosis. Approximately a year prior to admission he began to experience clumsiness of his lower extremities. The patient stated, "I began to trip over my own feet." He then noticed difficulty in his ability and coordination to play musical instruments. He noticed the calf and thigh muscles of his right leg "stiffen and tighten" a few weeks prior to admission. (The patient cannot walk a straight line and drifts to the left as he walks.)

Mr. R. stated, "I first noticed my difficulty stumbling and tripping, when friends began joking with me saying that I walked as if I were drunk and clowning around." These remarks troubled him so that he withdrew from social situations and was reluctant to engage in them. In addition, because of his difficulty in coordination, he was stopped by the police and accused of drunken driving. When he was tested at the local police station for his ability to drive safely, his driver's license was taken away. Finally the patient stated, "I'm engaged and I have to come here to find out definitely whether I have multiple sclerosis. If it's what my doctor says, then I won't be getting married."

The patient also complained of sensory symptoms and involvement such as numbness and tingling of his fingers and feet. In addition, Mr. R. had his glasses changed three times in the last year for blurring of vision. He also had been having increased frequency and precipitancy of micturation and had to get up once or twice during the night.

Mr. R. has no known allergies or difficulty with respiration. His daily nutrition consists of three large meals with emphasis on meats and starches. He has no difficulty with constipation and has regular bowel movement once each day, usually after breakfast. He does have urinary frequency and nocturia. He presently is taking no drugs or medications. He usually sleeps seven to nine hours each night and takes no sleeping pills or sedatives.

During the interview, the patient appeared easy-going, cooperative and pleasant. He verbalized willingly and did seem very apprehensive about his future, particularly in regard to his job, and his fiancée. Others significant in his life include his parents. He attended graduate school and has an M.A. in music.

Many adjustments and restrictions may exist for the patient with neurologic dysfunction. The nurse as well as professional counselors, vocational rehabilitation experts, the physician, and other health team members must assist the patient in coping with such overwhelming crises. In this particular case, it was decided that the nursing staff would focus on assisting the patient with his activities of daily living and on teaching him particular aspects of self-care and prevention of complications. Collaboration with the physician and physical and occupational therapists was carried out to assist with this purpose. Another nursing goal was to assist the patient in adjusting to his hospitalization. This was Mr. R's first hospital admission and he was extremely apprehensive about the battery of tests, procedures, and stresses he would have to face. It was felt the nursing staff could not adequately handle some of his psychosocial problems in addition to the goals they had already set. Therefore, sessions with a professional counselor were arranged, where the patient could begin to explore his feelings and fears, as well as arrive at possible decisions concerning his future plans. A community health nursing consultation was made to provide further help for the patient after he was discharged from the hospital. In addition, information concerning multiple sclerosis and the Multiple Sclerosis Society was given to the patient and his family when the diagnosis was established.

APHASIA

The most frequent speech problems seen in the neurologic patient are aphasia (milder forms called dysphasia) and dysarthria. Both of these disturbances create many and varied communication problems.

To attempt to classify or define aphasia is a subject which cannot be covered here. However, some amount of classifying and simplification is necessary if the nurse is to have any guide upon which nursing care is to be based. With this in mind, aphasia can be defined as a loss of ability to understand and use the faculty of language, both written and spoken. Aphasia technically denotes a complete functional loss, whereas dysphasia refers to incomplete or partial loss of functions. However, the term dysphasia is rarely used (possibly since it is easily confused with the word dysphagia), and so the word aphasia is used in this text to include both complete and incomplete deficiencies.

In simplified form, aphasia can be divided into three major types: 1) expressive or motor (verbal, executive, or Broca's aphasia); 2) receptive or sensory (Wernicke's aphasia); and 3) global.

GLOBAL APHASIA occurs when there is complete or nearly complete loss of speech function. A lesion or damage to the middle cerebral artery or internal carotid is usually responsible for this type of aphasia. The middle cerebral artery provides nourishment to all the major speech areas. Since the majority of cerebrovascular accidents involve the middle cerebral artery or its branches, aphasia commonly occurs as a result of cerebrovascular accident (usually on the left or dominant side).

The patient with global aphasia is usually speechless. Some can utter a few words which consist mostly of automatisms or emotional speech. They can understand only a few words, if any, that are spoken to them and are unable to read and write. Due to such extensive damage, speech rehabilitation is not very helpful and usually only little recovery is possible.

EXPRESSIVE APHASIA is characterized by the loss of ability to speak, write, or gesture. It can be likened to a verbal apraxia in that there is inability to carry out a motor skill in the absence of paralysis. Although the organs for articulation are intact, the patient is unable to combine or integrate the movements of these organs in order to speak. Expressive or motor aphasia usually occurs in lesions or damage to the lower part of the precentral gyrus of the cortex (Broca's area) or just above this site. (Hence, expressive aphasia is often called Broca's aphasia or cortical motor aphasia.) Since there is great difficulty in speech, it is also termed *nonfluent* aphasia.

The expressive aphasic patient may have difficulty in speaking, writing, or gesturing, but has no difficulty comprehending the written and spoken word well. The patient knows what he wants to say, but simply cannot say it. He usually is not able to talk, repeat what he hears, or read aloud. He has difficulty naming objects, although if asked to pick out a certain coin or object, he can do so correctly.

Agraphia, which is the loss of ability to write effectively, often accompanies expressive aphasia. The patient may have errors in writing, mirror writing, or exclusion of letters and syllables. He may also have a milder form called dysgraphia, in which writing is less difficult and the ability to copy written material correctly is retained. There is a difference of opinion concerning the exact basis for agraphia. Many contend that there is a writing center called Exner's writing center, located in the middle frontal convolution. When this "writing center" is damaged, a person loses his ability to express himself through writing.

The loss of ability to express oneself through gestures may also accompany expressive aphasia. In this case, the patient may lose his ability to use his hands, face, and so on to express himself. Just as speaking and writing are forms of symbols used to communicate, so are gestures a form of symbols. The patient who is unable to gesture may or may not be able to nod his head, shrug his shoulders, use his hands. This may vary from total loss to only minor difficulty.

The patient with expressive aphasia is able to utter some forms of speech. There are basically three levels of speech which occur in man: 1) automatic or emotional speech, the most primitive level, such as cursing, responding to pain by exclamatory speech ("Ouch," "Ah," and may include such words as "Dear"); 2) propositional speech, that is, automatic, casual speech, which may include recitation of the alphabet, prayers, chants, songs, or casual social speech such as "Howdy," or "How do you do?", "Yes" and "No"; 3) volitional speech—the highest level—characterized by speech requiring thought, concentration, and perception.

Volitional speech is the first level to be affected in the aphasic patient and the last to return during recovery. The most automatic and primitive speech is often retained and least affected. The language used early in life or learned first usually returns first in recovery. It is not uncommon for a patient to begin speaking a foreign language first, since many patients learned a native tongue first and learned English at a later age.

With the retaining of some primitive forms of speech, the patient with expressive aphasia may respond to questions, statements, and his environment and family by using many curse words or yelling exclamatory remarks which are completely out of context with the conversation. Propositional speech in the form of prayers, recitations, and social speech may be present. Serial speech, which consists of recitation of things in sequence (such as months, days, counting) may also be common forms of speech for the patient. The nurse should not be misled by the fact that the patient can say, "How are you?" or "I am fine" as responses. This may be the only level of speech remaining and the patient may be incapable of higher forms of speech.

The patient with expressive aphasia may have varied and individual combinations of involvement. It should be emphasized that no two patients are exactly alike. This again points out the necessity for an individual approach to the patient (see Nursing Intervention, pp. 694-696).

RECEPTIVE APHASIA. This is much more complex than expressive aphasia and equally hard to describe. Essentially, it is a loss of the ability to comprehend the spoken language and the written word. A person's speech remains *fluent* but the content and information are poor. Receptive aphasia usually occurs following damage to the posterior part of the temporal cortical convolution and white matter beneath it. Since receptive aphasias are characterized by the loss of ability to comprehend the spoken or written word or to interpret gestures, they are considered to be a type of agnosia (loss of perceptive power or ability).

Visual receptive aphasia (visual sensory aphasia, visual agnosia) occurs when the patient has a loss of power of recognition and interpretation of the visual symbols of language, namely the written or printed word, letters, or syllables. Lesions of the angular gyrus of the dominant hemisphere, which is the center for the recognition and interpretation of symbols used in writing and so on, cause visual receptive aphasia. The patient's vision is intact, but the center for the recognition and interpretation of what he sees is damaged. In the pure form, this is word blindness or alexia. Many levels of visual receptive aphasia occur. Some patients may or may not have agraphia, due to the loss of comprehending visual symbols of writing. Nominal aphasia in which the patient is unable to name objects, but yet knows what they do and are used for, may also be present in receptive aphasia.

Auditory receptive aphasia (auditory sensory aphasia, auditory agnosia) is an inability to comprehend the significance of spoken words in the absence of deafness and in its pure form is known as word deafness. The center for recognition, interpretation and recall of word symbols is located in Wernicke's area. Patients with auditory receptive aphasia have a loss of ability to recall the meaning of the spoken word and are unable to repeat what they hear. The loss of ability to comprehend the spoken word may involve the patient's own words as well, resulting in defects in grammar, use of inappropriate words, ridiculous combinations, and so on (paraphasia or jargon aphasia). Patients with auditory receptive aphasia may be able to read, but often visual receptive aphasia occurs along with auditory agnosia.

Patients with receptive aphasia often have a receptive aphasia for gestures and are unable to comprehend gestures, pantomime, and acts performed by others. In addition, the patient with receptive aphasia may also have variations of involvement, which require individual assessment and evaluation by skilled speech specialists.

Figure 20-9 illustrates the major centers for language, symbolization, and perception.

Nursing Intervention for the Aphasic Patient

In caring for the aphasic patient, the nurse must first realize that she has a role in assisting and rehabilitating the patient. Although the speech therapist is primarily responsible for teaching the aphasic the actual mechanisms of relearning speech, the nurse can assist the patient in coping with his disability and offer encouragement and support to both him and his family. In many institutions, speech therapists are not available while the patient is in the hospital, and so the nurse must rely on her knowledge and skill in assisting with speech therapy.

The first major step in caring for the aphasic patient is to assess his capability of communicating and comprehending through writing, speaking, and gesture forms of expression. To simply say that a patient has expressive aphasia is nonspecific. There are many levels of expressive

and receptive involvement. For instance, a patient with expressive aphasia may not be able to speak or write and may only have few gestures that can be used to communicate. On the other hand, he may be able to speak relatively well with occasional incorrect words and minimal difficulty in word finding. Between these two extremes are many varying levels of involvement, which make for differences in how one interacts and approaches each patient.

In assessing the aphasic patient, the nurse does not have sophisticated methods of testing, and so the procedure must be simple and basic. In addition, it is often difficult to get extensive information, due to the difficulty interacting with the patient. The following guide line is suggested as a tool which can be used in the nursing assessment of the aphasic patient. From this, data can be obtained which are useful for planning nursing intervention.

NURSING ASSESSMENT OF THE
APHASIC PATIENT[25]

1. Is the patient able to speak intelligibly with proper sentences, phrases and words?

2. Can the patient imitate what is spoken to him?

3. Does the patient have automatic emotional speech (such as cursing and so on)?

4. Is propositional speech present (automatic, serial, casual, social speech)?

5. Is the patient capable of using gestures such as facial expressions, nodding the head Yes and No, using his hands?

6. Is the patient able to write? (Even if the

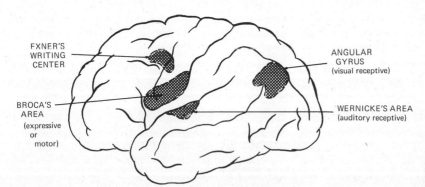

FXNER'S
WRITING
CENTER

ANGULAR
GYRUS
(visual receptive)

BROCA'S
AREA
(expressive
or
motor)

WERNICKE'S AREA
(auditory receptive)

FIGURE 20-9.
Major brain centers for language, symbolization, and perception.

patient has right-sided paralysis, this can be tested by having him use his left hand.)

7. Can the patient read, and how well?

8. Can the patient understand what is said to him? (To test for this, the nurse can ask the patient to do simple tasks such as shake hands, squeeze hands, touch his left ear. The patient should be asked to do more than one thing, for often there may be perseverance or failure on additional questioning.)

9. Is the patient capable of interpreting and understanding gestures?

10. Is the patient able to name objects which he is shown, such as keys, pictures, coins, pen, glasses?

It is extremely important for the nurse to encourage the patient to express himself through any means available. By assessing what the patient is capable of understanding and expressing, the nurse can begin to plan an effective means of communicating with him. With the aphasic patient who is unable to speak or write, the use of gestures may be the only means available to him. If the patient is capable of answering Yes or No by nodding his head, the nurse can communicate effectively by using questions and statements which require simple Yes or No answers. Questions should be short and uncomplicated. The environment should not be distracting or disruptive, since communicating with the aphasic patient necessitates concentration on the part of both the patient and the nurse. The conversation should be geared to the patient's immediate needs and surroundings. For instance, at mealtime, ask the patient what he needs. If he is unable to say the word, then say it for him to help facilitate relearning. Care should be taken not to shout at the patient, and to speak slowly and pause between sentences. Topics of conversation should be changed gradually. If the patient is able to write, he should be encouraged to do so (though often this is not feasible, for the patient's right hand is usually paralyzed). The use of picture books and gestures may be effective with the patient who has auditory receptive aphasia. Whenever using these media, the nurse should speak while showing the pictures (or pantomime) to help relearning of speech. If the patient understands certain words for objects, things, or people, these should be used as much as possible

in conversation. The patient with receptive aphasia has to be approached at his level of receptive language.

If the patient is capable of uttering some forms of speech, he should be encouraged to do so. As long as he is able to use some words, he should not fall into the habit of writing or gesturing. He should be taught to think in positive terms of speech so that his incentive does not waiver. The use of social conversation such as "Thank you," "How do you do?" should be reinforced. These automatic expressions are easily relearned (if not already present) and will help the patient feel more socially and personally adequate. Automatic, emotional responses, such as cursing should be taken in stride without becoming angry at the patient or being amused by his profanity. He is aware of his cursing, and making a fuss over it only serves to upset and frustrate him more. The nurse can help supply the correct word in its place.

The family must be taught not to answer for the patient or speak to the patient as a child. Also, they should not insist that the patient "talk right" or overdo focusing on his speech problems. In most situations, the family is often as tense and inadequate as the patient. The nurse should provide assistance to the family through consultations with them, and refer them to a speech therapist, or other speech specialist, who may be available in the community. When both the family and staff are consistent in their approach to the patient, rehabilitation is hastened.

The aphasic patient is often extremely rigid and compulsive about his environment, as are most patients who have suffered brain damage. He does not like disruption and things to be out of order. This mechanism, no doubt, serves to help the patient exert some control over his physical world and also allows him to operate with a minimum of effort. A routine daily plan is helpful and the same personnel should care for him each day, if possible. His personal items and belongings should be kept in place so as to minimize frustration and contribute to his sense of security. With fewer of these kinds of irritation, the patient is apt to concentrate more readily on overcoming his difficulties.

Concretism is another characteristic of the

patient who has had a stroke and cerebral insult. The aphasic patient cannot see similarities between situations, and thus approaches each situation as unique. He has difficulty remembering names of people and objects from one moment to the next. He is often incapable of broad abstraction and conceptualization and is not interested in material that does not touch upon his own interests. The nurse must speak in specific terms rather than in abstractions and needs to direct the patient from one situation to another.

Withdrawal is another mechanism commonly seen in the aphasic patient. Not only is it an attempt on the part of the patient to create an environment that is not threatening to him, but it also relieves him from having to communicate and, consequently, being subjected to frustration and ridicule. He should be drawn out through various means. If he has a hobby or special interest, the nurse may call attention to this. All efforts should be made to keep the patient in contact with his surroundings and with others. One effective means is simply the consistent presence of the nurse who takes the time to talk and stimulate the patient each day.

In situations where performance seems impossible, the patient may exhibit the catastrophic response which may be manifested by irritability, aggressiveness, evasiveness, vascular changes, motor and sensory loss, thrashing about, and even unconciousness. The responses serve as devices for coping with a situation beset by extreme frustration and too difficult for the patient to perform. The nurse should be alert to this, as must the patient's family. Without knowledge of this mechanism, panic may ensue, thus making matters worse. Whatever activity is causing the catastrophic response should be stopped.

The aphasic patient is in need of strong support not only from the staff, but also from his family. Speech is the most important tool which enables man to relate to his environment and to others. In today's society, where communication is valued at such a high premium, the adult aphasic has a difficult adjustment to make. Relearning speech is a tedious and difficult task for

anyone, and in the presence of hemiplegia and other disabilities, it is extremely overwhelming.

The nurse should see to it that the nursing intervention formulated is made available to all those involved in the care of the patient. For far too long, nursing personnel have been approaching the aphasic patient with mysticism, confusion, feelings of inadequacy, and scanty knowledge about aphasia itself. Understanding the pathophysiology involved and the clinical aspects of aphasia enables the nurse to deal more effectively and intelligently with the patient.

DYSARTHRIA

Dysarthria is a disorder of articulation and differs from aphasia in that word formulation and power of expression by speech are preserved. The dysarthric patient has no difficulty understanding what is said to him and (if literate) is able to read and write. His main difficulty lies in making himself understood by others. Although processes governing word formulation and phonation may be intact, the patient may be unable to utter a single intelligible sound and is said to be inarticulate.

Articulation involves the enunciation of words through contractures of the tongue, lips, larynx, pharynx, palate, and respiratory musculature in a highly complex and coordinated fashion. These organs and muscles used to utter words are innervated by the hypoglossal, vagal, facial, and phrenic nerves. The nuclei of these nerves are controlled chiefly through corticobulbar tracts, but are also influenced by the cerebellum and basal ganglion (extrapyramidal) regulation. Dysarthria can be caused by any involvement of these muscles and organs, the nerves and nuclei of the nerves to them, or their regulation through pyramidal (corticobulbar), cerebellar, and extrapyramidal influences. Thus, it becomes apparent that central nervous system damage in many areas can result in some degree of dysarthria.

There are four general types of dysarthria which frequently occur in the neurologic patient and are encountered by the nurse: cerebellar, that occurring with extrapyramidal involvement, that due to lower motor neuron or myoneural disturbance, and that resulting from supranuclear lesions.

CEREBELLAR DYSARTHRIA. This dysarthria is characteristic of cerebellar disease, but can also be present in Freidreich's ataxia and multiple sclerosis. Coordination of speech is poor and slurring, due to asynergy of muscles. It may be scanning (unnatural separation of syllables), slow, monotonous, explosive or staccatolike.

DYSARTHRIA OCCURRING WITH EXTRAPYRAMIDAL INVOLVEMENT. In lesions of the basal ganglion, speech may be jerky, irregular, and hesitant, due to violent abnormal movements of chorea and athetosis which affect the face, tongue and respiratory muscles. In paralysis agitans or postencephalitic Parkinson's characterized by muscular rigidity, speech is slow, slurring, monotonous, lacks inflections and modulations, and becomes increasingly weaker as the patient talks. Often the speech is hurried at the ends of sentences (festination speech), and the words seem to run into each other. Talking may be less intelligible while walking, or when fatigued or excited. In the presence of tremor, speech may be choppy.

DYSARTHRIA DUE TO LOWER MOTOR NEURON OR MYONEURAL DISTURBANCE. Examples may be seen in bulbar poliomyelitis, myasthenia gravis, progressive bulbar palsy, amyotrophic lateral sclerosis, Bell's palsy causing paralysis of the facial nerve, myopathies, Guillain-Barré syndrome, and hypoglossal nerve palsy. Speech may be slurring and thick, nasal sounding, drawling, slow, hoarse, lisping, whispering, or monotonous. The patient often sounds as if he were talking with a mouth full of mashed potatoes. Most evident is slurred speech with poor enunciation resulting in unintelligible and indistinct speech.

DYSARTHRIA RESULTING FROM SUPRANUCLEAR LESIONS. This usually is caused by vascular, degenerative, neoplastic or inflammatory diseases involving the corticobulbar tracts. Since corticobulbar fibers are both crossed and uncrossed, unilateral cortical lesions do not usually cause disturbance in speech. However, bilateral cortical lesions and bilateral lesions of the pons, upper medulla, and internal capsule can cause pseudobulbar palsy. The accompanying dysarthria resembles that of bulbar palsy (lower motor neuron) except that there is no atrophy of paralyzed muscles.

Nursing Intervention

In caring for the dysarthric patient, the nurse should always keep in mind that communication can be just as difficult for these patients as it is for the aphasic patient. It is often as annoying not to be understood as it is not to be able to express what one wishes to say. When speech is unintelligible, the patient can be encouraged to communicate to others by various means such as pad and pencil, flash cards, picture books, spelling blocks, gestures, and pantomime. Another technique which the nurse may employ with the dysarthric patient is encouraging him to speak slowly and pause frequently to see if he is being understood. Communication is facilitated by the use of short sentences instead of long rambling ones. If speech is too nasal, have the patient open his mouth wider to allow more sounds to come through the mouth instead of the nose. The patient with feeble speech can be taught to speak louder by taking deep breaths before attempting to articulate. In myasthenia gravis, the patient can sometimes be made more intelligible by supporting the jaw when speaking. In cases of paralysis of the soft palate, dysarthria may be less marked when the head is tipped upward and the patient is in a recumbent position. The nurse should remember that taxing the patient with Parkinson's or myasthenia gravis only serves to worsen his speech.

There may be instances when the patient is almost totally incapacitated, due to paralysis, and is unable to write, gesture, or barely move his head about. This often occurs in Guillain-Barré syndrome, commonly known as ascending polyneuritis. In severe cases, the patient may be markedly dysarthric or even anarthric. The nurse then must use great ingenuity to open avenues for communication. One middle-aged man was so severely paralyzed that he could relate to others only by blinking his eyes. In another case, a young college girl was admitted with Guillain-Barré. Only her right foot was spared, so that a bell-system was immediately set up which she could manipulate with her toes. In both instances, the staff utilized any abilities the patient had in order to communicate. It must be emphasized that each patient is different and will require individual approaches according to his deficits, personality, and so on.

In most dysarthric patients, communication can be facilitated through the use of questions requiring simple Yes and No answers. However, one soon tires of being asked nothing but questions. Many patients attempt to articulate regardless of their difficulty. One young man with congenital choreo-athetosis had jerky, irregular speech and abnormal movements, but continued to work toward an advanced college degree. Many personnel avoided talking with this man due to his difficulty, and this probably did more to dehumanize his hospital stay than did all the hospital procedures. One *must* listen, concentrate, and allow no feelings of discomfort, frustration, and impatience to prevent interrelating with these patients. Observation, a quiet environment, and discipline may be necessary to carry on the simplest of conversations. The skill of listening can be improved. The more the nurse listens to and communicates with patients having speech disturbances, the easier and more rewarding it becomes. Nursing assessment, specific nursing goals and orders, and evaluation of nursing actions are required to care for the dysarthric patient effectively. It is extremely important that the staff be aware of what methods are most effective in maintaining and promoting optimum communication and be consistent in their care of these patients.

Summary

In caring for the patient with central nervous system dysfunction, the individual problems and assessment of each patient must be identified and nursing goals and orders (care plan) formulated. Knowledge of the underlying scientific principles and pathophysiology is essential in order for the nurse to plan effective and intelligent care. Collaboration with all members of the health team is necessary for maximum rehabilitation of the patient. In addition, provision for care after discharge may be vital in promoting continuity of care.

The nurse has a tremendous responsibility in the care of the neurologic patient. Observations for neurologic status must be carried out accurately and critically—an action which requires knowledge of the nature of the nervous system, its structure and function. To attempt to care for the neurologic patient without understanding his complex difficulties is to flounder around in confusion.

Nursing is a clinical art and science—by clinical is meant "patient, or pertaining to patient." For far too long, nursing has been procedure-oriented and not patient-oriented. Many of the answers to the care of the neurologic patient lie with the patient himself. Nursing personnel must seek out these answers through engaging in more clinical nursing research, data collection and case recording. Only in this way can she arrive at nursing principles. Neurologic nursing is not a new field but it is the least explored. The challenge is to everyone.

The author expresses her thanks to Dorothy M. Smith, Dean Emeritus of the College of Nursing at the University of Florida, for the opportunity to present the Nursing History Form as a tool which can be used in the nursing assessment and intervention of the neurologic patient; to the Departments of Medicine and Neurology at the Shands Teaching Hospital, University of Florida; to the Department of Neurology and those affiliated with the Spiller Unit at the Hospital of the University of Pennsylvania.

References

1. Henderson, V.: The nature of nursing. Am. J. Nurs. 62-68, Aug. 1964.
2. Smith, D. M.: A clinical nursing tool. Am. J. Nurs. Nov. 1968.
3. Mayers, Marlene Glover: A Systematic Approach to the Nursing Care Plan. New York, Appleton-Century Crofts, 1972.

4. Cogan, D. G.: Neurology of the Ocular Muscles, ed. 2, 5th printing. Springfield, Ill., Charles C Thomas, 1970.

5. Plum, F. and Posner, J. B. (eds.): The Diagnosis of Stupor and Coma. Philadelphia, F. A. Davis, 1966.

6. Delong, R.: The Neurologic Examination. New York, Harper and Row, 1967, p. 949.

7. Guyton, A.: Textbook of Medical Physiology. ed. 2. Philadelphia, W. B. Saunders, 1961, p. 762.

8. Plum and Posner, *op cit.*

9. *Ibid.*

10. *Ibid.*

11. *Ibid.*

12. *Ibid.*

13. *Ibid.*

14. Jackson, F. E.: The treatment of head injuries. Clin. Sympos. 19:4-34, Jan.-Mar. 1967.

15. Adams, R. D., Webster, H. and Asbury, A. K.: Intracranial tumors. *In* T. R. Harrison, et al. (eds.): Principles of Internal Medicine, ed. 6. New York, McGraw-Hill, 1970.

16. *Ibid.*

17. Jackson, *op. cit.*

18. *Ibid.*

19. Gowers, W. R.: Epilepsy (reprint of original publication in 1885). New York, Dover Publication, Inc., 1964.

20. Ulman, M.: Disorders of body image after stroke. Am. J. Nurs. 89-91, Oct. 1964.

21. Pigott, R. and Buckett, F.: Visual neglect. Am. J. Nurs. 101, Jan. 1966.

22. Gatz, A.: Manter's Essentials of Clinical Neuroanatomy and Neurophysiology, ed. 3. Philadelphia, F. A. Davis, 1966.

23. Gatz, *op. cit.*

24. Guyton, *op. cit.,* p. 784.

25. Adams, R. and Mohr, J. P.: Affections of speech approach to clinical problem of aphasia. *In* T. R. Harrison, et al. (eds.): Principles of Internal Medicine, ed. 6. New York, McGraw-Hill, 1970.

Bibliography

Alpers, B. J. and Mancall, E.: Clinical Neurology, ed. 6. Philadelphia, F. A. Davis, 1971.

Barker, R., Wright, B., Myerson, L., and Gonick, M.: Adjustment to Physical Handicap and Illness: A Survey of the Social Psychology of Physique and Disability. New York, Social Science Research Council, 1953.

Beeson, P. B. and McDermott, W.: Cecil-Loeb Textbook of Medicine, ed. 11. Philadelphia, W. B. Saunders, 1963.

Brock, S. and Krieger, H.: The Basis of Clinical Neurology, ed. 4. Baltimore, Williams & Wilkins, 1963.

Brumlik, J.: Disorders of motion. Am. J. Phys. Med. 46:536-43, Feb. 1967.

Cogan, D. G.: Neurology of the Ocular Muscles, ed. 2, 5th Printing. Springfield, Ill., Charles C Thomas, 1970.

Chusid, J. and McDonald, J.: Correlative Neuroanatomy and Functional Neurology, ed. 13. Los Altos, Calif. Lange Medical Publications, 1967.

Collins, D. R.: Illustrated Manual of Neurologic Diagnoses. Philadelphia, J. B. Lippincott, 1962.

Davis, L. and Davis, R.: Principles of Neurologic Surgery. Philadelphia, W. B. Saunders, 1963.

Elliott, F.: Clinical Neurology. Philadelphia, W. B. Saunders, 1964.

Elson, R.: Practical Management of Spinal Injuries for Nurses. Baltimore, Williams & Wilkins, 1965.

Ettlinger, G.: Further study of visual-spatial agnosis. Brain, 335-361, Sept. 1957.

Frost, A.: Handbook for Paraplegics and Quadriplegics. Chicago, The National Paraplegia Foundation, 1964.

Gardner, E.: Fundamentals of Neurology, ed. 4. Philadelphia, W. B. Saunders, 1963.

Garret, J. F. and Levine, E. S.: Psychological Practices with the Physically Disabled. New York, Columbia University Press, 1962.

Goda, S.: Communicating with the aphasic or dysarthric patient. Am. J. Nurs. 7:63, 7:80-84, 1963.

Harrison, T. R. et al.: Principles of Internal Medicine, ed. 6. New York, McGraw-Hill, 1970.

Haymaker, W.: Bing's Local Diagnosis in Neurological Diseases. St. Louis, Mosby Co., 1969.

Horwitz, B.: An open letter to the family of an adult patient with aphasia. Rehab. Lit. 23, 5:141-144, May 1962.

Jackson, F. E.: The pathophysiology of head injuries. Clin. Sympos. 18:67-93, July-Dec. 1966.

Lance, J. W.: A Physiological Approach to Clinical Neurology. New York, Appleton-Century Crofts, 1970.

Lawson, I. R.: Visual-spatial neglect in lesions of the right cerebral hemispheres. Neurology 23, Jan. 1962.

Matheney, R. et al.: Fundamentals of Patient-Centered Nursing, ed. 2. St. Louis, Mosby, 1968.

Merritt, H. H.: Textbook of Neurology, ed. 4. Philadelphia, Lea & Febiger, 1967.

Morgan, W. L. and Engel, G. L.: The Clinical Approach to the Patient. Philadelphia, W. B. Saunders, 1969.

Moser, D.: An understanding approach to the aphasic patient. Am. J. Nurs. 61:52-55, Apr. 1965.

Ranson-Clark, S. L.: Anatomy of the Nervous System, ed. 10. Philadelphia, W. B. Saunders, 1959.

Schmidt, R. P. and Wilder, B. J. (eds.): Epilepsy—A Clinical Textbook. Philadelphia, F. A. Davis, 1968.

Slater, M. C.: Case Presentations Documenting Physiological and Psychological Principles of the Central Nervous System. Unpublished data, 1966.

Smith, D. M. et al.: Manual for the Use of the Nursing History Form. Unpublished. College of Nursing, University of Florida, Gainesville, Florida, Third Revision, March, 1971.

Steegman, A. T.: Examination of the Nervous System, A Student's Guide, ed. 3. Chicago, Yearbook Medical Publishers, 1970.

Stryker, R. P.: Rehabilitative Aspects of Acute and Chronic Nursing Care. Philadelphia, W. B. Saunders, 1972.

Terry, F. et al.: Principles and Techniques of Rehabilitation Nursing. St. Louis, Mosby, 1961.

Toohey, M.: Medicine for Nurses, ed. 8. Edinburgh, E. & S. Livingstone, Ltd., 1968.

Toole, J. F. (ed.): Special Techniques for Neurologic Diagnosis. Philadelphia, F. A. Davis, 1968.

Toole, J. F. and Patel, A: Cerebrovascular Disorders. New York, McGraw-Hill, 1967.

Wepman, J.: Recovery From Aphasia. New York, Ronald Press, 1951.

Weiner, H. L. and Levitt, L. P.: Neurology for the House Officer. New York, Med. Com. Press, 1974.

21

Inflammation and Repair: Nonspecific mechanisms of immunity

DEBORAH LINDELL

Homeostasis • Adaptation • Inflammation • Repair • The Patient with an Inflammatory Response • Factors Affecting Inflammation • Care of the Patient with an Inflammation

Homeostatis

One of the basic characteristics of any organism is the need to preserve its composition within the relatively narrow limits that permit the chemical processes fundamental to life. In the case of the simplest life forms, existence can occur only under specific environmental conditions, and the organism reacts directly with the external environment. In contrast, the more complex and highly integrated organisms have acquired an "internal milieu" of tissue fluids which bathe the cells with a relatively constant environment despite changes in the external world.[1]

Cannon developed the concept of homeostasis in 1932.[2] Langley describes homeostasis as the self-regulating, negative feedback systems which serve to maintain the constancy of the internal environment of all living organisms.[3] In lower life forms, these activities are automatic; in the higher forms of integration, they may also be volitional.[4]

Yet, though man possesses a cerebral cortex which is capable of making decisions and determining courses of action, he remains subject to the powerful persuasions that direct his attention (conscious or unconscious) to the homeostatic drives. Centers in the hindbrain, which appeared early in vertebrate evolution, respond to these basic drives for oxygen, water, food, internal body temperature of 98.6° F. (37° C.), sleep, and elimination of urine and feces. A chemical imbalance in the tissues stimulates the hindbrain centers to send out signals which cause a state of tension or discomfort. When necessary, these signals can dominate all thought and action. As a need is alleviated, the organism may be left with a secondary sense of pleasure.[5]

Evolution has provided man with the unique capability to find new ways to assume the chemical transactions essential to life in the face of competition and environmental change. However, as Theodore Lidz observes, the chemical processes mandatory for the existence of the unicellular organism are no less vital to the most complex forms of life.[6]

Adaptation

To preserve homeostasis, the organism enters into a multitude of activities called adaptations. Myra Levine has defined adaptation as "the process of change whereby the individual retains his integrity—his wholeness—within the realities of his environment."[7]

The mechanism for the control of body temperature exemplifies the many beautifully designed control systems that operate within the human body. The normal surface temperature is 98.6° F. (37° C.) orally and 99.6° F. (37.55° C.) rectally; it rises and falls with the temperature of the environment. In contrast, the core temperature of the interior is regulated very accurately, varying by not more than 1° F. under normal conditions.[8]

The body temperature is controlled almost entirely by nervous feedback systems, most of which operate through a temperature-regulating center in the hypothalamus.[9] Table 21-1 lists the locations and types of temperature detectors. When the core temperature moves above or below 98.6° F. (37° C.), the temperature detectors send signals to the thermostatic center in the preoptic and adjacent areas of the anterior hypothalamus. The thermostatic center controls body temperature by altering both the rate of heat loss from the body and the rate of heat production.[10]

The rate of heat loss is increased by: 1) stimulating the sweat glands to cause evaporative heat loss from the body and 2) inhibiting the sympathetic centers in the posterior hypothalamus with resultant vasodilatation and loss of heat from the skin. When the body temperature is too low, heat is conserved by: 1) intense vasodilatation of the skin; 2) piloerection, which is more effective in animals; and 3) abolition of sweating. Heat production is increased by stimulating the posterior hypothalamic motor center for shivering and by increasing the rate of cellular metabolism.[11]

The mechanism of temperature regulation is just one of the body's adaptive systems which provide for the preservation of homeostasis.

Adaptation is a unique response by an individual organism to a change in its environment. The extent to which adaptation returns the human body to a state of dynamic homeostasis is influenced by physiological, psychological, social, and cultural factors. To illustrate, two persons may suffer what is medically diagnosed as a "right cerebrovascular accident." However, each individual's ability to function in daily life will be determined by variables in each of the four categories noted above. Table 21-2 gives examples of each.

TABLE 21-1
Temperature Detectors in the Human Body

LOCATION	TYPE
Preoptic area—Anterior hypothalamus	Heat sensitive
Hypothalamus	Cold sensitive
Septum	Cold sensitive
Reticular substance of midbrain	Cold sensitive
Skin	Warm and cold sensitive
Internal organs	?

Source: Anderson, W. A.: Synopsis of Pathology. St. Louis, C. V. Mosby, 1972, p. 66.

TABLE 21-2
Variables Affecting Adaptation

PHYSIOLOGICAL
  Areas of brain affected, speech center in particular
  Handedness
  Age
  Concomitant illnesses
  Sex
  Presence or absence of urinary and fecal continence
PSYCHOLOGICAL
  Attitudes toward illness
  Attitudes toward life
  Previous experience with illness and hospitals
  Level of intelligence
  Nature of personality
SOCIAL
  Occupation
  Relationships with family, friends, significant others
  Resources available—family, friends, living
    arrangements
CULTURAL
  Cultural attitudes toward illness, hospitals

While homeostasis has been said to be essential for survival of the organism, the concept itself represents an ideal. The adaptive process may or may not return the organism to the previous state of function. In some cases, the adaptive response is not appropriate—or it may be excessive or misguided, resulting in an injurious or destructive reaction.[12] Selye calls these conditions "diseases of adaptation" and cites Curling's ulcer as an example.[13]

The extent to which adaptation is successful may be viewed on a continuum with endpoints of homeostasis, or health, and illness.[14]

Homeostasis (health) .... Illness

Illness indicates a particular individual's level of adaptation whereas disease connotes a composite of the number of individuals who have responded to certain alterations in their external or internal environments. For example, the "classic" description of the patient with an acute myocardial infarction includes such symptoms as crushing pain involving the central portion of the chest and epigastrium and radiating to the arms in approximately 25 percent of the cases. The pain is often accompanied by nausea, vomiting, a feeling of weakness, and a sense of impending doom. Yet, a minimum of 15 to 20 percent of patients with documented electrocardiographic evidence of an acute myocardial infarction have experienced no pain at all.[15]

Thus, in giving care to a particular patient, the nurse should consider the following questions as part of an initial and ongoing assessment: 1) is the patient in a state of homeostasis? If not, 2) how does his illness compare to a description of the disease? What factors are operative in his attempts to regain homeostasis? 4) To what extent have his adaptation energies been successful (location on the health-illness continuum)?

STRESS AND ADAPTATION. Selye has done considerable investigation into the relationship between levels of corticosteroids and adaptation. He defines stress as "the rate of all wear and tear caused by life"[16] and suggests that an essential feature of adaptation is the delimitation of stress to the smallest area capable of meeting the requirements of a situation. Selye calls this process of delimitation the general adaptation syndrome.

In the first stage, the alarm reaction, the local site of stress cannot immediately respond so the activity must spread to the neighboring tissues; corticoid production is high. In the second stage, the stage of resistance, adaptation is acquired due to optimum development of the most appropriate channel of defense. Spatial concentration of the reaction makes corticoid production unnecessary. If the irritation persists over a long period of time, the directly affected tissues eventually break down from fatigue. Then, during the stage of exhaustion, the reaction must again spread to the neighboring areas, and corticoid levels again rise. (For further information on the corticosteroids, see Chapter 18.)

In summary, Selye's hypothesis is that the goal of adaptation is to limit stress to the smallest area capable of dealing with the situation and that the level of corticosteroids is inversely related to the ability of the local area to cope with the stress applied. Selye describes the role of adaptation well when he states: "In maintaining the independence and individuality of natural units, none of the great forces on inanimate matter are as successful as that alertness and adaptability to change which we designate as life— and the loss of which is death."[18]

Cellular injury is one type of stress to which the body responds with a complex series of events. These events are protective in nature, with the organism seeking to maintain homeostasis by either returning itself to the preinjury conditions or repairing itself after the injury.[19] The process of adaptation to cellular injury, be that injury mechanical, chemical, or self-destructive, occurs by one or both of two types of responses: nonspecific (inflammatory response) or specific (immune response). (For a discussion of the immune response, see Chapters 22 and 23.)

Inflammation

Inflammation is the "reaction of living tissue to injury which comprises the series of changes of the terminal vascular bed, of the blood, and of the connective tissue which tends to eliminate the injurious agent and to repair the damaged tissue.''[20] The basic anatomical features of inflammation are almost always the same, regardless of the type of injurious agent or the site of occurrence.[21] However, the morphology and clinical signs and symptoms will vary widely according to many factors, including the extent of damage, site of injury, and age of the patient. Despite its protective nature, inflammation may result in a temporary or permanent decrease in function of the affected part. For example, in a patient with a third-degree burn, cell death is the direct result of the agent inflicting the burn and the indirect result of the large amounts of fluid which move into the extravascular space and cause decreased blood supply to the affected area.

Agents which injure tissue and/or elicit the inflammatory response may arise from a variety of sources originating either within the body (intrinsic) or outside the body (extrinsic). Table 21-3 gives examples of both types.

INITIATION AND CONTROL OF INFLAMMATION

Severe irritation produces a direct injury to the microcirculation and adjacent tissues. However, indirect, or chemically mediated, injury is probably more common. Many naturally occurring inflammatory reactions seem due, in part, to direct injury and, in part, to chemically mediated vascular injury.[22]

Four substances, or groups of substances, have been identified as chemical mediators of inflammation: histamine, serotonin, the kinin system, and the complement system. Histamine is contained in two types of cells which are found in almost all tissues of the body—the basophilic leukocytes of the blood and the mast cells in the tissues. It is theorized that histamine initiates, but does not sustain, the vascular responses

characteristic of inflammation.[23] In the tissues, histamine is formed by the decarboxylation of histadine which is stored in the granules of mast cells. Its physiologic effects include: contraction of smooth muscle, increased vascular permeability, headache, and increased gastric, nasal, and lacrimal secretions. Histamine is quickly deactivated by histaminases.[24] Serotonin, 5-hydroxytryptamine, has also been considered as a possible mediator of the early inflammatory response. In rats, it is contained in mast cells and causes increased vascular permeability, capillary dilatation, and contraction of smooth muscle.[25]

Bradykinin is the one chemical mediator of inflammation which explains both the vascular and leukocytic responses to tissue injury. Bradykinin and two other vasoactive kinins are the end result of a sequence of enzymatic steps in the plasma or interstitial spaces, similar to those found in the complement or coagulation systems. The system may be activated by the Hageman factor or the interaction of antigen and antibody. In small doses, the kinins cause increased vascular permeability, vasodilatation, decreased blood pressure, contraction of smooth muscle, and pain. In larger doses, the accumulation and migration of leukocytes occurs.[26] Figure 21-1 illustrates the current knowledge of the sequence of steps leading to the formation of the kinins.[27]

Current research has led to the idea that the balance between blood coagulation, through the clotting mechanism, and blood fluidity, through histamine, heparin, and bradykinin, is maintained through the interaction of these systems.[28]

The complement system is the fourth chemical mediator of the inflammatory response. Like the kinin and blood-clotting systems, it involves the interaction of several discrete components; biological activity has been demonstrated at several points along the pathway. The components of complement may be activated by immunologic and nonimmunologic mechanisms.

The normal pathway of the complement system is initiated when antigen-antibody complexes bind to the first component (C1). This component is actually a complex composed of three subunits: $C1_q$, $C1_r$, and $C1_s$. Subunit $C1_s$ is converted to $C1_a$ (C1 esterase) which acts on the

TABLE 21-3
Origins of Inflammatory Agents

INTRINSIC	EXTRINSIC
Neoplastic cells	Organ transplant
Infarcted cells	Microorganism
Thrombosis	Thermal burn
Atherosclerosis	Surgical incision

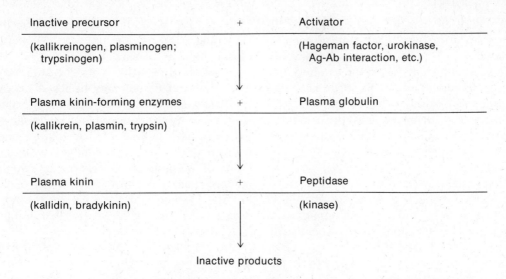

FIGURE 21-1. Kinin formation

fourth (C4) and second (C2) components converting them to a $C42_a$ complex (C3 convertase).[29] No definite biological activity has been found for these first three components of complement.[30]

The $C42_a$ complex acts enzymatically on C3 to split it into fragments. One fragment of C3 reacts with the complex EAC142 to become cell-associated (EAC1423). This complex now becomes biologically active and demonstrates the properties of immune adherence and immune phagocytosis. The C3 fragment that is cleaved off has some of the biological properties of classic anaphylatoxin; it elicits release of histamine from mast cells, thereby compromising vascular integrity which results in increased vascular permeability.[31]

The components C5, C6, and C7 exist in serum as a complex that interacts with EAC1423 to become activated ($C\overline{567}$). The $C\overline{567}$ complex is not bound to the cell surface, but can diffuse through the interstitium to the vascular walls and exert its biological effect. It is chemotactic and causes specific, unidirectional migration of neutrophils toward an attractant such as an antigen-antibody complex. As it interacts with EAC1423, C5 is, like C3, cleaved into biologically active fragments which demonstrate chemotactic activity for neutrophils and stimulate release of histamine from mast cells. It is not clear if the same fragment accounts for both phenomena.[32]

The terminal components of complement, C8 and C9, are responsible for reacting with the previous components to cause structural defects or holes on the cell surface and, thus, lysis of red cells, mast cells, or bacteria.[33]

The components C3 and C5 may be split into biologically active fragments (see previous paragraphs for properties) without going through the entire complement sequence and without the presence of immune complexes. In this alternative process, C3 and C5 act as substrates in a variety of reactions. Ward notes that "the nature and biologic activity of the fragment produced depends upon the reactants: they may have the biologic properties of contraction of smooth muscle, release of histamine from mast cells, or chemotaxis of neutrophils. All have the ability to initiate events that culminate in acute vascular injury and inflammation."[34]

There are two other important aspects of complement: 1) its effect on normal blood coagulation which it exerts by activation of platelets which then set the blood-clotting system in motion, and 2) human diseases which occur as a result of a problem with the complement system, be it an inborn error or an acquired abnormality.[35] In summarizing his discussion of complement, Peter Ward noted that "in the seventy years that complement has been a laboratory curiosity in search of a function, it can be stated with reasonable assurance that complement will be accorded a place high on the list of substances involved in the mediation of the acute inflammatory response."[36]

VASCULAR RESPONSES

As they are stimulated by histamine, the blood vessels local to an injured area undergo an initial transitory vasoconstriction. The vasoconstriction is immediately followed by vasodilatation of the arterioles, the venules, and finally, the capillaries. Vasodilatation is accompanied by an increased filtration pressure and increased permeability of the capillaries; fluid and plasma proteins move from the capillaries into the adjacent tissue spaces.

Early in the vascular response, there is an active increase in the flow of blood through the injured area (hyperemia). The site of inflammation appears reddened relative to surrounding tissues. Later, several factors lead to a slowing of blood flow in the injured tissues: 1) severe injury of the blood-tissue barrier followed by 2) an increase in vascular permeability, 3) rapid exudation of plasma, 4) an increase in viscosity of the blood, and 5) loss of hemoglobin from the red cells.[37]

Sequelae of the slowing of blood flow may include the formation of thrombi in the microcirculation and a throbbing sensation in the inflamed area. To summarize the vascular responses during inflammation, hyperemia (slowing of the blood) and increase in vessel permeability are the result of mild to moderate vascular injury. With more severe damage, thrombosis and hemorrhage may develop.[38]

FLUID EXUDATION

Exudation refers to the extravasation of fluid (plasma) but not of cellular elements; the cause is increased vascular permeability. Three mechanisms could account for, or partly contribute to, increase in vascular permeability and exudation:

1) changes in blood flow, 2) increase in hydrostatic and filtration pressures, and 3) alterations of the blood-tissue barrier.[39]

Robbins notes that "fluid exudation into more compact tissues may be less marked and less easily defined since the amount of exudation is modified by the resistance of the tissue to the extravasation of fluid."[40] The nature and the quantity of the exudate are influenced by the severity of the tissue injury. As the severity of the damage increases, particularly when the capillary itself is damaged, the greater is the capillary permeability and the larger the size of particles which move into the tissue spaces.[41]

In other than very minor injuries, the exudate includes fibrinogen which precipitates to form a network and wall off the damaged tissues. The resultant fixation of the injurious agent enhances the efficiency of phagocytosis by white blood cells and delays the spread of microorganisms. However, the network may also hinder repair by limiting the removal of microorganisms from the tissue and the exposure of the agent to various therapeutic modalities. In addition, certain invasive agents (pneumococcus, *Clostridium welchii,* neoplastic cells) elaborate spreading factors which diminish the viscosity of the exudate and promote the free permeation of the tissues by the agent.

One of the means by which inflammatory processes are classified is according to the character of the exudate. In many inflammations there is a mixed pattern of exudates present at one time or during the course of the process.

SEROUS. A serous exudate is one in which there is an extensive outpouring of a watery, low-protein fluid. Depending upon the site of the inflammation, the serous exudate is derived either from the blood serum or the secretions of serosal mesothelial cells, that is, those of the peritoneal cavity or the joint spaces. Serous exudates are usually associated with minimal damage to the vascular endothelium. In a severe inflammation, the serous exudate may be transferred to one of the other types. The blister which accompanies a second-degree burn is an example of a serous exudate.

FIBRINOUS. A fibrinous exudate is one in

which there is a transfer of large amounts of fibrinogen from the vascular to the interstitial spaces and large masses of fibrin are deposited in the area of the injury. A fibrinous exudate is characteristic of more severe acute inflammation in which marked endothelial damage allows the escape of the large fibrinogen molecule from the blood vessels. Certain types of bacterial infections (e.g., pneumococcal pneumonia) are known to be accompanied by a fibrinous exudate. As it is deposited, fibrin assumes a characteristic threadlike and tangled meshwork appearance.

CATARRHAL. In an inflammation marked by a catarrhal exudate, there are large amounts of mucinous secretions present. This type of exudate occurs only when the inflamed tissues are those capable of secreting mucus, that is, nasopharynx, lungs, gastrointestinal tract, uterus, and mucous-secreting glands. A catarrhal exudate contains faintly basophilic, amorphous, stringy mucoid material plus white blood cells. Ulcerative colitis exemplifies inflammations associated with a catarrhal exudate.

SUPPURATIVE/PURULENT. A purulent exudate contains large amounts of pus. Pus is a thick fluid composed of many numbers of viable and necrotic polymorphonuclear leukocytes and necrotic tissue debris that is liquefied by proteases, peptidases, and lipases liberated by the dead leukocytes. Because it is highly viscous, the evacuation of pus from an inflamed area is difficult. Yet, its removal is essential for satisfactory repair of the injured tissue. Suppurative inflammations are seen with certain organisms (pyogenic) and injury of tissues by selected chemicals. Acute appendicitis is an example of a purulent inflammation.

HEMORRHAGIC. A hemorrhagic exudate occurs when damage to blood vessels is severe and red blood cells enter the tissue spaces.

ACCUMULATION OF INFLAMMATORY CELLS

When the flow of blood in the small vessels is optimal, the white blood cells are carried in the middle of the stream with the red blood cells surrounding them. During an acute inflammation, however, the slowing of the flow of blood causes the red blood cells to adhere together in clumps larger than the single leukocytes. The leukocytes then move to the vascular epithelium and line up or marginate along the wall of the blood vessel. They squeeze through the junctions between the endothelial cells and migrate toward the inflammatory focus by ameboid motion. The direction, but not the speed, of migration may be augmented by a chemical stimulus (positive chemotaxis) which is elaborated by bacteria and products of injured cells.

Several types of cells appear during the inflammatory process: leukocytes (neutrophils, eosinophils, basophils), lymphocytes, plasma cells, mononuclear phagocytes, and erythrocytes. Their characteristics are summarized in Table 21-4. Within 30 to 60 minutes after an injury neutrophilic granulocytes may be seen in the locus of inflammation. By their active phagocytosis, they are the first line of defense against invading microorganisms. Four to five hours into an acute inflammation, mononuclear cells and lymphocytes appear from the blood vessels. The monocytes add further phagocytosis and the lymphocytes convey the immunologic capacity to respond to foreign agents by way of specific humoral and cell-mediated phenomena.

In most instances, the disintegration of leukocytes in the inflamed tissue causes elaboration of a factor which acts on the bone marrow to stimulate leukocytosis. Thus, many inflammations are accompanied by an increased white blood count with a high proportion of immature neutrophils. In certain infections, there may be an absence of leukocytosis or even a leukopenia (typhoid fever, brucellosis, malaria). When leukopenia occurs in the presence of an inflammation usually accompanied by leukocytosis, an overwhelming infection or a toxic effect on the bone marrow may be suspected.

PHAGOCYTOSIS

Phagocytosis is the culmination of the cellular phase of inflammation and is the process of ingestion and immobilization of the irritant. The neutrophilic leukocytes and mononuclear phagocytes (macrophages and monocytes) are the primary cells exhibiting this function. Phagocytic

TABLE 21-4
Cells of Inflammation*

TYPE	CHARACTERISTICS	INFLAMMATORY PROCESS	FUNCTION	ORIGIN
A. PML 1. Neutrophil	Segmented nucleus Granules in cytoplasm	*Acute first and most numerous cell type	1. Motile, ameboid, phagocytic 2. Primary defensive element 3. Appear early after injury 4. disintegrates → substance stimulates leukocytosis	Blood—50–70% PML Ameboid—direction by chemotaxis Increases until irritant overcome if bone marrow can produce
2. Eosinophil	Large reddish granules in cytoplasm	Presence in significant numbers means resolution and healing	1. Obscure function 2. Under control of adrenal cortical hormones (increase in hormones→decrease in eosinophils) 3. Emigrate from blood in increasing numbers when healing in any non-specific inflammatory reaction has begun	Blood—1–2% PML Motile—more sluggish than neutrophil
3. Basophil	Granules in cytoplasm	Acute—anaphylaxis	1. Role in allergy 2. Contain histamine and heparin 3. Damage→chemical mediators	Blood—1% PML
4. Lymphocytes	Smaller than PML Rounded cell Large dark nucleus Scant cytoplasm	*Chronic (Acute—lymph nodes & nervous system)	1. Function uncertain 2. Immunocompetent→antibody 3. Rarely phagocytic. May be transformed→macrophage→phagocytic 4. See chapter 22, The Immune Response	Blood—25–33% PML Found in lymph nodes

				Found in tissues
B. Plasma Cell	Slightly larger than lymphocyte	Chronic	1. Concerned with production of antibody (primary source)	Rarely seen in circulating blood ? derived from stem reticular cells
C. Mononuclear phagocytes	1. Monocyte—granular cytoplasm 2. Macrophage—agranular cytoplasms	Late acute & chronic	1. Phagocytosis 2. Arrive after polys—prepare for repair 3. Persist after polys destroyed by increased acidosis 4. Second line of defense at injury site. 5. Fuse around unsoluble particulate matter→ giant cells (multinucleated)	1. Monocytes—emigrate from blood 2. Macrophages—arise in immediate area of injury from reticuloendothelial cells or lymphocytic elements
D. Erythrocytes		Hemorrhagic exudate characteristic of certain infections; i.e., anthrax	Hemorrhagic exudate	Pass through permeable vessels (diapedisis) or ruptured vessel walls

*Adapted from Robbins, Stanley L. *Pathology*. Philadelphia: W. B. Saunders 1967, pp. 44-49.

cells are motile and the neutrophils respond to positive chemotaxis.

The actual mechanism of ingestion probably depends upon cellular changes in surface tension. It is known that the phagocytosis of some bacteria is aided by the nature of their surfaces while the more highly virulent bacteria tend to resist phagocytosis. Certain substances present in the tissue fluids (opsonins, tropins, and agglutinins) also aid phagocytosis.

Cellular enzymes digest the bacteria, tissue cell fragments, and foreign particles engulfed by the phagocytes. Some bacteria have the ability to resist digestion and continue to live and multiply within the phagocyte (organisms of histoplasmosis, leprosy, and tuberculosis). When a relatively large foreign particle cannot be absorbed by a mononuclear phagocyte, several may surround the material and fuse to form a giant cell.[42]

SIGNS AND SYMPTOMS OF INFLAMMATION

The several phases of the acute inflammatory response lead to certain cardinal signs and symptoms. Their appearance in a particular inflammation will depend upon the nature of the offending agent, the extent and site of damage, and the success of the host response.

HEAT (CALOR). Heat results from an increased blood flow to the affected area and possibly from an increase in the local metabolic activity.

REDNESS (RUBOR). Redness at the site of an inflammation is also due to hyperemia of the affected area.

SWELLING (TUMOR). Swelling is the consequence of accumulation of the inflammatory exudate.

PAIN (DOLOR). In the past, pain was believed to be the outcome of direct stimulation of sensory nerve endings by injury and the pressure of the inflammatory exudate. Recently, however, several research findings have led to the hypothesis that there are one or more chemical mediators which are responsible for the pain, exudation of fluid, and leukocyte migration of inflammation. These observations include: 1) that pain often accompanies the inflammatory

process and may actually become less severe as the response gains speed, and 2) that substances which dilate arterioles and increase capillary permeability can induce pain of varying intensity if they are injected intradermally or applied to a blister base.[43]

LOSS OF FUNCTION (FUNCTIO LAESA). Loss of function occurs as a result of pain and muscle spasm. This is a protective activity designed to allow the walling off process by the fibrin to achieve its optimal effect.

In addition to these local signs of inflammation, the body may also respond in a systemic manner. As previously discussed, Selye theorized that the total body responds to a local injury in the early stages before the inflammatory response reaches its height and later if the local response does not contain the irritant. The generalized manifestations of inflammation may include: fever and its sequelae, weakness, general malaise, anorexia, headache, vomiting or diarrhea, leukocytosis, increased erythrocyte sedimentation rate, and loss of weight.

CLASSIFICATION

Inflammations are classified according to four characteristics: 1) amount and character of exudation, 2) duration, 3) location, and 4) causative or etiological agent.

EXUDATE. The types of exudate include: serous, purulent, hemorrhagic, catarrhal, and fibrinous. (See pp. 706-707 for a detailed discussion of the types of exudates.)

DURATION. The terms "acute," "subacute," and "chronic" are used to indicate the length of time an inflammatory response has existed. Acute inflammations have a clinical picture of a sudden onset with heat, swelling, redness, pain, and loss of function of the affected area. The predominant anatomical changes are vascular and exudative with vascular congestion and exudation of fluids and white blood cells.

When an injurious agent persists for several weeks or months and continues to stimulate an inflammatory response, the process enters into the stage of a chronic inflammation. This is a proliferative response characterized by fibroblastic and vascular cell duplication and the presence of mononuclear cells, particularly the macrophage, lymphocyte, and plasma cell. Inflammations which continue for long periods of time are likely to result in scarring and deformities due to the proliferation of fibroblasts.

The granuloma, a type of chronic inflammation, is a tumorlike mass of granulation tissue composed of actively growing fibroblasts and capillary beds. A chronic granulomatous infection is associated with tuberculosis, syphilis, sarcoid, and leprosy.

The subacute inflammation is a poorly defined entity which is situated between acute and chronic inflammations. It has some elements of an exudative vascular response associated with the proliferation of fibroblasts and infiltration by the eosinophils and mononuclear cells of a chronic process.

LOCATION. The clinical signs and symptoms of an inflammation will vary widely with the tissues and organs involved. The suffix "itis" is used to indicate "inflammation" (e.g., appendicitis, gastritis, endocarditis).

Abscess. An abscess is a localized collection of pus which occurs when suppuration is present in a tissue, organ, or confined space. The most common cause of an abscess is the deep seeding into a tissue of pyogenic bacteria. An abscess can heal only after the suppurative exudate and necrotic debris have been removed. The material may burrow to the surface of the organ or tissue and rupture, the physician may perform a procedure to drain the abscess, or there may be a total proteolytic digestion of the necrotic tissue and debris. The sterile fluid which is left by the digestion is reabsorbed. An abscess is frequently accompanied by the total destruction of local parenchymal and stromal cells, a defect which leads to the formation of scar tissue and permanent deformity of the affected tissues.[44]

Cellulitis. Cellulitis is a spreading, diffuse, edematous, and sometimes suppurative inflammation which occurs within solid tissues. It tends to dissect widely through tissue spaces and is often the result of infection by a highly invasive bacteria such as beta-hemolytic streptococcus.[45]

Ulcer. An ulcer is a local defect of the surface of an organ or tissue which is produced by the sloughing or shredding of inflamed, necrotic tissue. Ulcers tend to occur in three types of situations: 1) a focal inflammatory necrosis of the mucosa of the mouth, stomach, or intestines (e.g., chronic ulcerative colitis); 2) a subcutaneous inflammation of the lower extremities in individuals who have circulatory disturbances that predispose to extensive necrosis (e.g., venous stasis ulcer); and 3) inflammation of the cervix of the uterus.[46]

Pseudomembranous Inflammation. A pseudomembranous inflammation is the formation of a false membrane made of precipitated fibrin, necrotic epithelium, and white blood cells. The process occurs only on mucosal surfaces and results from an acute response to a powerful necrotizing toxin. A pseudomembranous inflammation is diagnostic for diphtheria.[47]

CAUSATIVE AGENT. Any agent which injures tissue cells or acts as a foreign body to them may incite the inflammatory response. The agent may be either extrinsic or intrinsic.

Repair

Repair is the process by which dead or damaged cells are replaced by new healthy cells. The new cells may be derived from either the parenchymal or connective stromal components of the injured tissue. If the repair is characterized by the proliferation of parenchymal cells, the tissue will return to a state of normal or near-normal function. However, when the area of repair is composed primarily of connective tissue cells, scar tissue which is fibrous, permanent, and nonspecialized replaces the parenchymal cells. The ability of the tissue to carry out its function is diminished according to the proportion of functional tissue replaced by connective tissue.

Like its parent phenomenon adaptation, repair may be considered along a continuum as a function of the contribution of parenchymal and connective tissue elements. The quality of the reparative process is governed by many factors including the inherent capacity of the parenchymal cells in question to regenerate or multiply.

RESOLUTION .... COMPLETE FIBROTIC
(normal state)   REPLACEMENT
(parenchymal cells)   (connective tissue cells)

REPAIR BY PARENCHYMAL REGENERATION

Each type of cell in the human body has been described in terms of its ability to regenerate. Three categories have been defined: labile, stable, and permanent cells. Permanent cells are unable to reproduce after birth, whereas labile and stable cells can regenerate, to varying degrees, throughout life.

LABILE CELLS. Because they are constantly being destroyed, labile cells are normally in a state of continual reproduction. The two types of labile cells are epithelial surface cells and cells of the splenic, lymphoid, and hematopoietic tissues. Epithelial surfaces, which include the skin, oral cavity, cervix, alimentary and respiratory tracts, excretory ducts, uterus, tubes and urinary tract, exfoliate continually throughout life. Integrity is maintained by the constant replacement of lost tissues (e.g., menstrual cycle).

When the underlying supporting tissue is intact, but epithelial cells are lost, regeneration of the marginal preserved cells will result in excellent reconstitution. However, if the underlying support tissue is destroyed, the defect must be filled before epithelial regeneration is completed.

The cells of the splenic, lymphoid, and hematopoietic tissues are also labile. They are constantly reproducing and only when the total destruction of the stem cell precursors occurs is the tissue replaced with fibrous nonfunctioning cells.

STABLE CELLS. Normally, stable cells do not multiply to a great extent during adult life. However, with appropriate stimulation, these cells can proliferate, and injury may be replaced with perfect reconstitution. There are two types of stable cells: the parenchymal cells and the mesenchymal derivatives.

Parenchymal cells are located in the glands, including the liver, pancreas, salivary, endocrine, kidney tubular cells, and skin. As in the case of the epithelial cells, the supporting tissue must be present to permit perfect reconstitution. Otherwise, proliferation may be haphazard and

disorganized. Although a rare occurrence in the larger organs, the total destruction of a gland makes regeneration impossible. The smaller glands, for example, in the hair shaft of the skin, are most susceptible to permanent loss of function and replacement by scar tissue.

Mesenchymal derivatives include fibroblasts, osteoblasts, and chondroblasts. Fibroblasts are resistant to injury and can reproduce throughout life. Fibroblasts are involved in the formation of connective tissue scar and are also capable of differentiation into other types of supporting tissue cells, for example, osteoblast, chondroblast, and lipid cell.

PERMANENT CELLS. Permanent cells, the most highly differentiated units, rarely proliferate after birth and, when injured, are replaced by fibrous tissue. The two types of permanent cells are *nerve cells* and *muscle cells*.

A destroyed neuron in the central nervous system is always replaced by a glial cell (supportive element). In the peripheral nerves, destruction of the cell body of origin is accompanied by loss of the total structure. However, when the cell body of origin survives and only the peripheral axon process is injured, regeneration of the axon may occur with integrity of the innervation re-established. Occasionally integrity is not restored due to interference by other tissue (e.g., scar or clot) and the result may be a tangled mass of fibers (amputation neuroma).

Although the striated, cardiac, and smooth muscle cells are permanent, losses may be compensated for, to some extent, by the hypertrophy of preserved marginal cells. Thus, a small number of cells may maintain the previous work output (e.g., myocardium following infarction).

REPAIR BY CONNECTIVE TISSUE

Only in rare circumstances is scar tissue not a component in the reparative process. Perfect regeneration is seen only when a few labile or stable cells are injured and the supporting connective tissue is intact. When scar tissue is part of the process of repair, there will be some element of permanent loss of specialized function. The deposition of scar tissue may follow one of two pathways—healing by primary intention or union and healing by secondary intention or union. The factor which determines the type of healing is whether or not the edges of the injured tissue can be apposed.

PRIMARY UNION. Primary union, or union by first intention, is exemplified by the clean surgical wound, where the edges are apposed by sutures and healing occurs with minimal loss of tissue and without bacterial contamination. In the surgical wound, the acute inflammatory response and the reparative process begin almost simultaneously. Sealing occurs within hours of the formation of a blood clot. At three to four days, the clot has become organized and is composed of a newly formed, highly vascularized connective tissue which includes a component of acute inflammatory exudate (granulation tissue). After seven to eight days, fibroblasts have proliferated and are supported by a considerable amount of collagen. Also at this time re-epithelialization has been completed with the loss of such appendages as hair follicles and sweat glands. In the weeks and months that follow, a pale, avascular scar covered by epithelium is the result of collagenization and blanching.

SECONDARY UNION. Secondary union, or union by second intention, occurs when the injury causes a large tissue defect whose edges cannot be apposed. Examples include: infarction, ulceration, bacterial contamination of a surgical wound. The process is similar to that of primary union except that the necessity for removal of a large amount of dead cells, tissue debris, and exudate requires that the process occur very slowly. Granulation tissue appears as quickly as the debris is cleared away. Secondary union differs from primary union in the following respects:

1. Loss of a greater amount of tissue.
2. Production of necrotic debris and inflammatory exudate requiring removal.
3. Formation of larger amounts of granulation tissue to fill the defect.
4. Slower replacement of the destroyed elements.
5. Production of a large amount of nonfunctional tissue.

Robbins states that "the repair of any injury is governed by the regenerative capacity of the affected cells and the proliferative activity of connective tissue that fills in residual defects left by parenchymal regeneration."[48] The basic mechanisms at the cellular level that stimulate the proliferation of cells are not well understood. The major theories include: 1) the diffusion of trephones, wound hormones derived from the cellular debris, into the marginal cells and stimulation of their reproduction; 2) certain chemicals that stimulate cell reproduction; and 3) the destruction of tissue that causes the release of restraints on tissue growth by the pressure of one cell upon another thus permitting a return to normal growth activity.

In summary, the reparative process may be viewed either as a part of the inflammatory response or as a separate entity. Reconstructive activity is begun soon after the inflammatory response has been initiated. The characteristics of a tissue undergoing repair have been described by Robbins:

1. Removal of the inflammatory exudate by drainage or reabsorption.
2. Regeneration of the parenchymal elements where possible.
3. Concomitant proliferation of fibroblasts and capillaries, creating an actively growing, highly vascularized connective (granulation) tissue. The extent of injury and ability of cells to reproduce will affect the proportion of granulation tissue to parenchymal.
4. When tissue damage is considerable or permanent cells are destroyed, formation of a scar due to proliferation of fibroblasts and deposition of collagen.[49]

The Patient with an Inflammatory Response

As the nurse cares for the patient with an inflammatory response, she is concerned with the three components of the process—adaptation, inflammation, and repair—as they interact to produce the illness. In the course of a particular episode of inflammation, a number of factors cause these components to be modified either positively or negatively. Through application of the nursing process, the professional nurse uses knowledge of the basic physiologic processes of adaptation, inflammation, and repair, together with the factors acting upon them, to assist the patient to attain his level of optimal homeostasis. In the previous discussion, we examined the basic events of the inflammatory response; we will now discuss those broad factors which may determine its course and which are manipulated during nursing intervention.

ADAPTATION

The extent to which an individual is successful in adapting to the countless stress-invoking stimuli he confronts each day is reflected in his position on the health-illness scale. Likewise, the closer the individual is to the health pole of the continuum, the better he is able to cope with situations which require adaptation.

Sr. Collista identified three factors which determine the adaptive level or position on the health-illness continuum: 1) focal stimuli, 2) background stimuli, 3) residual stimuli.[50] Focal stimuli are those which immediately confront the person. Background stimuli are all other stimuli present and may include the patient's age, sex, ability to communicate, intellectual level, and family relationships. Residual stimuli are those beliefs, attitudes, traits, and other factors from past experiences which are relevant to the present situation. Examples of residual stimuli include the patient's cultural heritage, previous experiences with illness and hospitalization, patterns of adaptation, and educational background.

Consider the situation of a woman lying in a hospital room who is nine-months pregnant and in the second stage of labor. She has not received sedation or analgesia. Focal stimuli active in this situation might include the following:

1. Increasingly frequent, lengthy, and painful contractions.
2. Fetal monitoring equipment.
3. Intravenous infusion equipment.
4. Bright lights overhead.
5. Temperature of the room—85°
6. Noise level of animated discussion among nursing and medical staff in English.

Examples of background stimuli would be:

1. Age—18
2. Sex—female
3. Primary language—Spanish, speaks only minimal English.
4. Low IQ (80)—considered mentally retarded.

Lastly, residual stimuli would include:

1. Cultural background—Puerto Rican, came to New York City at age 16 to live with an aunt and uncle.
2. No previous hospitalizations, minimal health care—brought to OB clinic when in third trimester.
3. No formal education.
4. Father of child not known; relatives plan to raise child.
5. Parents live in Puerto Rico.

Review of the above factors reveals that each will exert an influence on the young woman's capacities for adaptation to the process of childbirth. It is difficult to categorize focal stimuli for they vary with the specific situation; however, several types of background and residual stimuli will be discussed in detail.

Age

During each of the seven developmental stages of life, the individual is presented with tasks and problems which affect his capacities for adaptation. The nurse applies her knowledge of growth and development in patient assessment and planning intervention. To illustrate the effect of age on adaptation to illness and possible nursing implications, adolescence and old age will be discussed.

ADOLESCENCE. The world of the adolescent is characterized by transition. He vacillates between the roles of a dependent child and an independent adult. The youth lives in an intense present in which he is trying to locate himself with respect to the past and the immediate future. Both the past, a role to be transcended, and the remote future are viewed negatively.

Illness may be very threatening to the adolescent, for it blocks his activities in confronting the developmental tasks of his age group, draws on the high level of energy needed for these activities, and may have a profound effect on his acute awareness of body image. To the adolescent, the concept of death is unstabilized, as the remote future is weakly structured and devoid of values. Death is actively rejected because it stands diametrically opposed to the youth's developmental tasks—identity, significance, positive values, and membership in social units.

Many adults fear the adolescent because he may be highly unpredictable. The nurse will find that a flexible, honest approach that respects the adolescent as an individual will help in meeting his needs for recognition and independence. Firmness and jointly agreed upon, well-defined limits will help to provide needed structure. Both the youth and his parents or significant others should be involved in developing the plan of care. The nurse should also consider the adolescent's concern with body image, special dietary likes and dislikes, and needs for physical activity. His life in the present and near future calls for emphasis on short-term rather than long-term goals so that the youth may receive frequent positive feedback. (See Chapter 8 for further discussion of adolescent health problems.)

AGING. Cummings found that normal aging involves a withdrawal or disengagement between the aging person and others in the social system to which he belongs.[51] The process is mutually agreed upon and normatively governed (e.g., social security, pensions, mandatory retirement).

Disengagement may begin late in life or as early as middle life, whenever changes in perception occur—particularly changes in relation to the individual's sense of worth to society and the inevitability of death. The male finds that he is no longer needed in his occupation and the female finds that her functions in childrearing are no longer required. In disengagement, there is a sense of the shortness of time and often a shift away from achievement. The individual begins to select and allocate, finding a new set of rewards. When the individual has a decreased ability to communicate which is uncompensated, disengagement may be accelerated. As the process of disengagement is completed, the equilibrium which existed in middle life between the individual and society has given way to a new equilibrium characterized by increased distance and a changed basis for solidarity.

The process of disengagement is particularly acute in the United States and is strongly influenced by our ever-changing, future-oriented society which favors the young and the nuclear family. The elderly person often does not fit in and may be relegated to isolation, an action which only favors disengagement. While disengagement has been characterized as a mutual withdrawal, in the United States, the young may actively withdraw from the elderly because the past has little reality or applicability for them (i.e., early retirement). There is an increased incidence of suicide in men over 65. One factor in this increase is that retirement, with its abrupt change in life style, is frequently difficult to face. (See Chapter 9 concerning health problems of the aging individual.)

Generally, the aged person's adaptation to illness will be influenced by his stage of disengagement (will to live) and the effect of the physiologic aging process on his body.

Cultural Heritage

A patient's cultural heritage will influence his response to illness. The individual and the health care worker must mutually recognize and agree that illness or a need of adaptation exists. Dubos notes that any disease or deficiency which is very widespread in a given social group comes to be considered "normal" or accepted.[52] Paul comments that (community) health workers must understand the nature of sociocultural patterns—their purposes, why they persist, and how they change. He lists four gaps which often impede the realization of program aims: 1) cultural, 2) status, 3) urban adjustment, and 4) research.[53]

The cultural gap is a discrepancy between the cultures of the recipient and the deliverer of health care. The deliverer must understand the beliefs and practices before trying to change them. Medical programs should be shaped to fit the cultural and health profile of the target population (individual), and long-range goals should be combined with measures to meet immediate needs.

In many cases, there is also a marked status gap between the educated elite and the bulk of the population. There may be important differences between the "felt needs" of the two groups. The health team may, in reality, be a hierarchy of command: physician-nurse-patient.

In settings where people leave rural areas to enter cities, they may be confronted with the unhealthful conditions of over-crowding, poor sanitation, and malnutrition which follow their arrival. Migrant workers face unique problems of adjustment.

The research gap should prompt the health care team not only to ask the question of how to induce a response to a particular program, but also to set the question in the larger frame of reference of whether to promote a given program at all.

Paul summarizes his comments on the gaps between health care recipients and health care deliverers by noting that "the approach should be to determine what people want and to aid them to achieve it rather than how they can be best persuaded to do what people in another culture thinks best for them" (really what is best for the dominant culture).[54]

An individual's cultural heritage, itself an example of a background stimulus, will also influence the effects of other background stimuli on adaptation, for example, sex and the ability to communicate (language barriers).

The Oriental patient provides an excellent example of the role culture plays in adaptation. These patients frequently have a very high tolerance for painful stimuli. When caring for an Oriental woman in labor, the nurse's concern would be directed toward various means of support for the patient rather than solely to convince her to have analgesia or anesthesia.

The Individual's Role as a "Patient"

The individual's attitude toward his role as a patient will influence his ability to adapt to the stressful situation at hand. For example, if much of his concentration is directed toward "being a good patient," he cannot focus all his energies on getting well.

Lederer notes that "the experience of illness is a complex psychological situation" and describes three stages of the experience: 1) the transition period from health to illness, 2) the period of "accepted illness" and 3) convalescence.[55] In the initial symptom phase of many illnesses, the nurse may encounter evidence of anxiety, guilt, and shame as well as the many personality defenses against their disagreeable effects. Interestingly, in certain neurotic patients there may be a paradoxically positive acceptance of illness. The persistence, and often the increase of symptoms forces the patient into another psychologically difficult set of experiences—those of diagnosis and the initiation of therapy.

At this time, the former habitual patterns of health care still exert a powerful attraction on the patient, whereas his submission to diagnosis and treatment procdures involves entering an unknown area. But, in order to be rid of the problems presented, he must face this unknown situation. Whenever one enters an unknown or partially understood situation, he exhibits fairly typical responses. Anxiety is aroused again because of fantasized dangers and unfamiliarity with what one may expect.[56]

A strong factor in the orientation of the patient is the behavior of the medical personnel who are responsible for the individual's diagnosis and therapy. Their attitudes should be firm, patient, and understanding. The concept that, in many cases, fear of the unknown is due to a lack of knowledge, is a helpful one to apply. Again, Lederer notes that because of the individual's lack of understanding of medical concepts and technical language, care must be taken that explanations of diagnostic and treatment procedures are presented in a simple and forthright manner.[57] Impersonal contact should be minimized. When taking nursing histories, the nurse will take into consideration that patients' anxiety may lead them to unconsciously distort facts during interviews. The patient deserves assistance in overcoming and accepting the paradox that, to be relieved of discomfort, he must at times submit to a transitory increase in it. Explanations should therefore be concise, unambiguous, and include the purpose for the procedure.

The individual enters the stage of "accepted" illness when he has accepted the diagnosis and initial therapeutic procedures. He now sees himself as ill and abandons pretenses of health. Because society frees him from carrying out his normal duties and obligations, he leads a simpler, more childish, restricted life. He may even regress and become somewhat infantile. This behavior permits the patient to accept help and focus on getting well; it is characterized by 1) egocentricity, 2) constriction of interests, 3) emotional dependency, and 4) hypochondriasis.

The attitudes and behavior of those caring for the patient can limit or extend the emotional regression of the patient. Traditionally, hospitals have encouraged regression of the patient by "doing" for him. All evidence of normal life is removed. Regression could be minimized by allowing only that regressive behavior necessitated by the physical limitations of the patient and by avoiding any unnecessary infantizing. Yet, health care personnel should recognize the purpose of regression in the sick and welcome it rather than punishing patients for their behavior. Some patients have developed personalities that resist regression and feelings of dependency. They may deny the illness, instructions of the health care team, and so on and need assistance in accepting regression and dependency.

The patient enters the convalescent phase of illness when optimal regression and medical treatment have reversed or arrested the pathogenic process. The nurse may assist the patient to move into the convalescent phase by focusing his attention on health rather than illness. In many instances, this may require the nurse to change her focus of attention from episodic care to the broader view of "health care" or wellness.

Factors Affecting Inflammation

The human body, a thrifty organism, uses the inflammatory response to respond to a variety of situations in which cell injury has occurred. Thus, while the fundamental sequence of events remains constant, the extent of tissue damage and the exact morphological patterns of alterations which ultimately develop are modified by many influences pertaining to both the invasive agent and the host. These factors govern the course and eventual outcome of all injuries. For example, one patient is hospitalized for a "simple appendectomy" while another patient dies of peritonitis and septicemia following surgery for a perforated appendix. The nurse uses her knowledge to identify the following factors in the patient (whether focal or background stimuli) and to plan appropriate intervention to modify them.

FACTORS RELATING TO THE ATTACKING AGENT

STRENGTH AND AMOUNT OF THE AGENT, DURATION OF EXPOSURE. The amount of injury produced by a noxious agent is a function of the agent's inherent toxcity and the time during which it exerts its effect. For example, two patients may have second-degree burns over 50 percent of their bodies; one was exposed to high temperatures for seconds (fire) and the other to lower temperatures for minutes (sun lamp). Bacteria, while of varying pathogenecity, will induce an infection based on the number of organisms present.

To alter the strength, amount, and duration of exposure of an agent, the nurse may apply warm soaks (phlebitis, infection), assist the physician with an incision and drainage of a wound, do follow-up care of drains or administer antibiotics, or remove a splinter or decayed tooth.

NATURE OF THE INVASIVE AGENT. In many cases, the inflammatory response will be modified according to the attacking agent. For example, a rickettsial infection is characterized by a hemorrhagic-type inflammation.

INVASIVENESS OF THE ATTACHING AGENT. The inflammatory response will be modified according to the ability of an agent to enter the body and penetrate the tissues. This is particularly true in the case of bacterial infections. The penetrability of a microorganism is indirectly related to the presence of lymphatic blockage and vascular blockage by clots and the elaboration of spreading factors by certain organisms. Spreading factors increase tissue permeability and result in the breakdown of the mechanical integrity of the tissues.

SUSCEPTIBILITY OF ORGANISMS TO PHAGOCYTOSIS AND DIGESTION. As noted previously, some microorganisms resist phagocytosis and/or intracellular digestion. In the latter case, the phagocytic cells may actually carry the live bacteria to other areas of the body.

STATUS OF THE HOST

The ability of the host to resist invading agents

and minimize their damage is affected by both systemic and local factors.

PHYSIOLOGIC CONDITIONS OF THE HOST. It is well known that the age, nutritional status, and physiologic tone of the body can affect the health status of the host. The younger patient, with a more adequate blood supply and physiologic age of tissues, is better able to ward off invaders and resist damage. Optimal nutritional status is a necessity and should be directed toward maintaining a positive nitrogen, fluid, and electrolyte balance, and proper vitamin intake. The advent of parenteral hyperalimentation has had a tremendous impact on the nurse's ability to establish optimal nutritional status in patients who would otherwise be unable to maintain this function. This procedure, in which nursing care plays a critical role, is being used as a temporary measure while preparing for definitive therapy on a long-term basis. It has been used in the treatment of patients with esophageal atresia, ulcerative colitis, bowel obstruction, congenital gastrointestinal defects, and malnutrition. Unlike conventional intravenous therapy, parenteral hyperalimentation supplies all the essential or replacement nutrients needed by a patient— amino acids, vitamins, glucose, electrolytes— while having the advantage of bypassing the gastrointestinal tract.

IMMUNITY. The ability of the host to resist invasion is supplemented by the activities of the immune system which includes the cell-mediated and humoral components. (For a detailed discussion of this system, see Chapters 22 and 23.) A simple example of assisting the immune system is the administration of tetanus antitoxin to the patient who has stepped on a nail.

METABOLIC DISEASE. The adequacy of an inflammatory response is influenced by the presence of an intact and stable metabolic system. The presence of abnormally high levels of corticosteroids seems to depress the rate and adequacy of repair. The diabetic patient with poor microcirculation, abnormal metabolism, and possible biochemical alterations at the cellular level, responds poorly to cellular injury. The nurse intervenes in both cases by assisting the patient to achieve an optimal physiologic status and to prevent cellular injury in the first place.

ADEQUACY OF BLOOD SUPPLY. In general, well-vascularized tissues are more resistant to invasion and are better able to localize and contain the injurious agent than poorly vascularized tissues. In the latter case, exudatic fluid diffuses into the area more slowly and the cellular elements arrive later in the process. Thus, the inflammatory response is delayed and inadequate.

LOCATION OF INJURY. The site of an injury in the body will affect the resultant inflammatory response. Densely compact tissues (liver) resist the spread of infection while loose tissues (lungs) allow the spread of harmful agents. Unlike inflammation of solid and deep tissues (peritoneal/joint spaces), inflammation on the surface of the body (skin, mucous) can discharge necrotic debris and facilitate repair.

An inflammatory response in a restricted area, such as the brain, may cause damage of normal tissue, for there is nowhere for the swelling site to expand. Cerebral edema following a head injury or neurosurgery can be at least as serious as the basic problem which caused it.

REPAIR

The extent to which an inflammatory site is returned to its previous state is modified by the conditions under which the repair must occur. As previously discussed, a major determinant is the nature of the tissue involved. Some decayed cells can be replaced with live, functional cells while others do not duplicate and are replaced with nonfunctional granulation tissue.

SYSTEMIC FACTORS

As with inflammation, the reparative process is influenced by three systemic factors: the physiologic condition of the host, nutritional status, and presence or absence of endocrine secretions. In terms of the physiologic conditions of the host, younger patients generally have a greater capacity for repair of injury. While the rate of cell proliferation remains fairly constant, "proliferation begins earlier, is less likely to be slowed down, and ends sooner in the young." In the older patient, the vascular supply to organs may be diminished and, thus, repair is hindered. Excessive fatigue and poor physiologic tone seem to adversely affect the reparative process. However, the mechanism for this phenomenon has not been described. It may be related to diminished circulation.

Systemic nutrition, especially adequate intake of vitamin C and positive nitrogen balance, is essential for an optimal reparative effort.

The endocrine system influences repair in that the adrenal steroids depress the rate and adequacy of repair.

LOCAL FACTORS

Adequate blood supply to the local site of inflammation is mandatory for an optimal healing process. The vascular system supplies oxygen, defensive cells, and nutritive substances. It removes metabolites and digested debris. The effects of insufficient vascular supply to an area may be seen in the patient with a venous stasis ulcer secondary to varicose veins or an arterial ulcer secondary to diabetic small vessel disease. In addition, the deposition of avascular scar tissue further limits the vascular supply and repair of the site of chronic inflammation.

Inflammation is stimulated and repair is prohibited by the presence of infection or inflammatory exudate or other foreign material. Thus, the process is accelerated when these materials are removed (i.e., splinter removed from a finger, retroperitoneal abscess incised and drained, drains left in following surgery, removal of sutures, debridement of a chemical or surgical burn.)

The mobility of tissues may influence the rate and adequacy of repair. It is well accepted that in the care of injuries to bones, joints, and other tissues of the extremities, immobilization of the proximal and distal joints is desirable. In the case of all injuries, immobilization of the wound margins is a basic principle of wound healing.

The amount of tissue damage and the location and character of the tissue injured are critical factors in the extent of repair.

Care of the Patient with an Inflammation

Based on the factors which are known to modify the inflammatory and healing processes, several principles may be identified as guidelines in the care of such patients. Although the principles will be directed toward management of surface wounds, they may be applied to all inflammatory processes.

1. Damage should be minimized by protecting the wound to prevent bacterial contamination, cleansing wounds which are accessible to procedures such as irrigation to remove foreign debris, contaminants, and devitalized tissue, and immobilization of the injured area. The latter allows more rapid clotting and minimizes disruption of the early granulation tissue.

2. The injury should be contained and further infection and/or tissue destruction prevented by minimal manipulation of the site, drainage of exudate when possible and prompt administration of appropriate antibiotics.

3. Insofar as possible, roadblocks to the reparative process should be removed. Noxious material is removed, bleeding is controlled and excessive clotted blood removed, suture material is applied to serve several functions, and blood supply is facilitated.

4. The patient should be provided with an environment which facilitates wound healing. The affected area is placed at optimal rest to minimize damage and permit metabolic activity. When possible, the involved area is elevated to encourage drainage of the inflammatory edema and venous return. Moderate warmth increases the vascular supply to the area and increases metabolic activity. The patient should be placed in positive nitrogen balance and optimal nutritional status achieved.

The dressing applied to a wound provides an excellent example of how the factors influencing inflammation and repair are applied in practice. The function of a dressing is to interact with the factors—host resistance, status of local environment, and number and types of bacteria present—so that the optimum environment for wound healing is created. Dressings must be individualized according to the type of wound and drainage, location of the wound, and so on. However, all types of dressings can serve one or more of the following functions:

1. Protection from trauma, organisms, temperature changes in the environment, and drainage.
2. Antisepsis. The dressing may contain medication that will kill or inhibit the growth of bacteria.

3. Pressure can minimize the accumulation of fluid in the intercellular tissue spaces. Pressure influences wound tension which promotes healing and minimizes hypertrophic scar formation. Ideally, the more convex a surface the more the pressure effect of a dressing will be enhanced. When a body surface which is to be dressed is not convex, it can be increased with gauze. The pressure dressing also helps to immobilize the injured area.

4. Immobilization decreases pain, prevents disruption of new tissue, minimizes spread of bacteria, limits transudation of fluids, and lessens formation of scar tissue. Plaster and splints are often used to provide immobilization.

5. Debridement may be obtained by a dressing through its capillary action and the intertwining of necrotic debris within its mesh. The extent of the debriding action is directly related to the roughness of the material and the wideness of the mesh.

6. A dressing may aid the reparative process by helping to create a physiologic environment, for example, keeping a dressing warm and moist. The more physiologic the environment the less fluids, proteins, and electrolytes will be lost from the wound.

7. With a bulky absorptive layer, the dressing will act as a wick to draw secretions, drainage, and necrotic debris away from the wound and promote healing. The bulk also protects the wound from further damage.

8. Packing a wound provides for the entrance of antiseptic and debriding agents and the exit of drainage, and so on. It also encourages healing from the inside of the wound out.

9. A dressing may assist in supporting an injured area.

10. Dressings allow the examiner to acquire information about the wound. Unnecessary bulk in a dressing may prohibit this function and actually allow drainage (blood), which should be seen, to be hidden from view.

11. Lastly, dressings serve a social or esthetic function, keeping from view a sight which some patients and visitors would rather not see.

Thus, in caring for the patient with an inflammatory response the nurse should bear in mind that this process is the nonspecific response of the body to injury and that the basic sequence of events is adjusted according to the site of the cellular injury and other previously discussed factors. The nurse uses the nursing process to identify those factors operative in this patient as he passes through the responses of adaptation, inflammation, and repair. The goal of the health team is to assist the patient to attain his optimal level of wellness. As W. A. Altemeir stated: "One cannot speed the healing, but one can control the factors which are capable of denying it."[59] With proper consideration of those factors which can alter adaptation, inflammation, and repair, the positive aspects of these processes can be enhanced and the negative aspects minimized to assist the patient back to his normal level of daily living.

References

1. Lidz, T.: The Person. New York, Basic Books, 1968, pp. 25-26.
2. Cannon, Walter B.: The Wisdom of the Body. New York, Norton, 1932, p. 24.
3. Langley, L.: Homeostasis. New York, Van Nostrand Reinhold Co., 1965, Chapter 1.
4. Lidz, *op. cit.*, p. 26.
5. *Ibid.*, pp. 26-27.
6. *Ibid.*, p. 26.
7. Levine, M.: The pursuit of wholeness. Am. J. Nurs. 69, 1:95, Jan. 1969.
8. Guyton, A.: Textbook of Medical Physiology. Philadelphia, W. B. Saunders, 1971, p. 831.
9. *Ibid.*, p. 837.
10. *Ibid.*, p. 837.
11. *Ibid.*, p. 838-839.
12. Dubos, R.: Man Adapting. New Haven, Yale University Press, 1965, p. 257.
13. Selye, H.: The Stress of Life. New York, McGraw-Hill, 1956, p. 179.
14. Ray, Sister Collista: Adaptation: a conceptual framework of nursing. Nurs. Outlook 18:42-45, March 1970.
15. Wintrobe, M.: Harrison's Principles of Internal Medicine. New York, McGraw-Hill, 1970, pp. 1214-1215.

16. Seyle, *op. cit.*, p. viii.
17. *Ibid.*, pp. 120-121.
18. *Ibid.*, p. 118.
19. Bellanti, J. A.: Immunology. Philadelphia, W. B. Saunders, 1971, p. 175.
20. Movat, H. C.: The acute inflammatory reaction. In H. C. Movat (ed.): Inflammation, Immunity, and Hypersensitivity. New York, Harper and Row, 1971, p. 2.
21. Robbins, S.: Pathological Basis of Disease. Philadelphia, W. B. Saunders, 1974, p. 56.
22. Movat, *op. cit.*, p. 104.
23. Robbins, *op. cit.*, p. 68.
24. Bellanti, *op. cit.*, p. 194.
25. *Ibid.*, p. 194.
26. Robbins, *op. cit.*, p. 69.
27. Robbins, S.: Pathology. Philadelphia, W. B. Saunders, 1967, p. 37.
28. *Ibid.*, p. 37.
29. Schur, P. and Frank A.: Complement in human disease. Annual Rev. Inter. Med. 19, 124: 1, 1968.
30. Ward, P. A.: The role of complement in inflammation and hypersensitivity. In H. C. Movat (ed.): Inflammation, Immunity, and Hypersensitivity. New York, Harper and Row, 1971. p. 462.
31. *Ibid.*, pp. 461-463.
32. *Ibid.*, pp. 464, 466.
33. Schur, *op. cit.*, p. 2.
34. Ward, *op. cit.*, p. 464.
35. Muller-Eberhard, H. et. al: Mediators of the inflammatory response. In I. Leopow and P. Ward (eds.): Inflammation: Mechanism and Control. New York, Academic Press, 1972, pp. 83-93.
36. Ward, *op. cit.*, pp. 473-474.
37. Movat, *op. cit.*, pp. 24.
38. *Ibid.*, p. 25.
39. *Ibid.*, p. 25.
40. Robbins, Pathology, *op. cit.*, (1967) p. 33.
41. Beland, I.: Clinical Nursing. ed. 2. New York, Macmillan, 1970, p. 295.
42. Robbins, Pathological Basis of Disease, *op. cit.*, 1974, p. 80.
43. *Ibid.*, p. 80.
44. Robbins, Pathology, *op. cit.*, p. 56.
45. *Ibid.*, pp. 56-57.
46. Movat, *op. cit.*, pp. 72-78, 90-92.
47. Bellanti, *op. cit.*, p. 176.
48. Robbins, Pathological Basis of Disease, *op. cit.*, pp. 74-76.
49. Robbins, Pathology, *op. cit.*, pp. 44-49.
50. Ray, Sr. Collista, *op. cit.*
51. Cummings E.: New thoughts on the theory of disengagement. In R. Kastenbaum (ed.): New Thoughts on Old Age. New York, Springer Publishing Co., 1964.
52. Dubos, *op. cit.*, Chapter IX.
53. Paul, B. Anthropological perspectives on medicine and public health. In J. Skipper and R. Leonard (eds.): Social Interaction and Patient Care. Philadelphia, J. B. Lippincott, 1965, p. 199.
54. *Ibid.*, p. 202.
55. Lederer, H. C.: How the sick view their world. In J. Skipper and R. Leonard (eds.): Social Interaction and Patient Care. Philadelphia, J. B. Lippincott, 1965, p. 155.
56. *Ibid.*, pp. 157-160.
57. *Ibid.*, pp. 160-163.
59. Noe, J. and Laub, D.: The functions of a dressing: wound healing—a dynamic approach. Hosp. Care. 5, 1: 5-13, Feb. 1974.

22

The Immune Response

KAY KINTZEL and DEBORAH LINDELL

Functions of Immunity • Immunization • Development and Organization of the Immune System • Antigens • Antibodies • Mediators of Immunity • Nonspecific Factors • Humoral and Cellular Immunity • Diseases Mediated by the Immune System • Neoplasia • Autoimmune Disease

The immune response is a powerful weapon in our arsenal of body defenses. Recognition of the immune process as a protective mechanism is reflected in our traditional choice of words to describe immunity—we say that the person who possesses immunity to a given substance has "increased resistance" to it. This increased resistance is but a final result of the complex process which begins when a foreign substance enters the body and is chemically recognized as alien. The appearance of this foreign substance (antigen) stimulates increased production of another substance (antibody) uniquely designed to interact with it and nullify detrimental effects in the host. Since this reaction occurs whenever we come in contact with a new antigen, each of us probably manufactures tens of thousands of antibodies in a lifetime of dealing with unwelcome aliens.

Functions of Immunity

Normal operation of the immune system is necessary for our continuing well-being as individuals and as a species. It renders protection from the damaging consequences of invasion by a host of microorganisms, including bacteria, viruses, and fungi. Further, it is a vital homeostatic mechanism. A fundamental requirement for survival of any complex multicellular organism evolving in a sea of hostile elements is the capacity to distinguish between self and nonself. On a day-to-day basis, the immune system helps maintain homeostasis by overseeing normal cell degradation, removal of damaged cell elements, and general catabolic body functions. Finally, the most recently uncovered defensive role of the immune system is that of recognizing and disposing of the abnormal cell elements which continually arise within the body from a variety of causes. This latter function has been appropriately termed "surveillance."

In health, all these functions of immunity are smoothly fulfilled in tandem. However, like most powerful biological weapons, the mechanism may destroy as well as defend. When immunologic responses are altered in some way, disease frequently ensues. A certain exaggerated immune reaction ushers in allergic symptoms; hypoactivity results in an immune deficiency disease; an aberration of the ability to recognize nonself culminates in an autoimmune disorder; faulty surveillance allows the wanton growth of tumor cells. Consequently, a working understanding of the immune process is of immense value to all whose job is health maintenance or the care and treatment of ill individuals. The discipline of immunology is still in its infancy—it is only within the last thirty years that it has ceased being regarded as a curiosity best probed within laboratory confines. Now immunology is a rapidly growing branch of medical science. Such is the light immunologic knowledge is currently shedding on the causes of disease that Dr. Robert Good has said he likes to think of it as "the new pathology."[1]

Immunization

Although some people may be born with a relative ability to resist certain types of antigenic invasion, most people acquire resistance by actually "fighting off" these invaders, after coming in contact with them. Fortunately, a desired resistance to agents causing human illness may be artifically induced by the process of immunization. The individual is thus spared from suffering an actual infection. When such resistance is brought about by the injection of an antigenic substance, it is called active-acquired immunization. In this case, a person is inoculated with microorganisms or their products which have lost the power to produce illness, but which retain the ability to stimulate antibody formation in the inoculated host. The injection of tetanus toxoid is a familiar example of this method. When resistance is brought about by the transfer of antibody-containing serum from a sensitized donor to a normal recipient, it is called passive-acquired immunization. Here the individual is inoculated with borrowed antibodies which are ready to go to work immediately—as is true with the injection of tetanus antitoxin. Since vaccines were first employed as part of a general health program, millions have been protected against such previously dangerous infections as smallpox, diphtheria, whooping cough, tetanus, and poliomyelitis. Yet, much remains to be learned; when to begin routine immunization of infants and the correct number of doses for certain vaccines are but two of the questions still under discussion. Immunologists continue to refine their conceptions of the nature of the "ideal" vaccine,

and extensive research is needed to solve the remaining problems of induced immunity.

Development and Organization of the Immune System

The cells responsible for the immune process are found in the lymphatic tissues. A number of studies have shown that antibody formation begins in the developing fetus. Although only a few cells are competent to produce antibodies during prenatal life, after birth the microorganisms appearing in the intestinal tract following food intake stimulate maturation of the lympatic tissues. Without the stimulation of an external environment populated by many microorganisms and a diet which contains antigens, the immune system remains immature and the immune response is correspondingly weaker.[2]

We now understand that there are two distinct populations of lymphocytes involved in immunity, each with its own function. One of these groups, "T-lymphocytes," originates in the thymus. The other, "B-lymphocytes," is derived from the bone marrow in animals and the bursa in birds. (Much of the basic research concerning the development of the B-lymphocyte system has been done on the bursa, particularly the bursa of Fabricius in chickens.) The T-lymphocytes and B-lymphocytes are equally vital for adequate operation of the immune system.

Both immunologically competent lymphocyte populations develop from primitive hematopoietic stem cells, which, in turn, differentiate during embryonic development to lymphoid stem cells. These lymphoid stem cells have the capacity to enter either the thymus or the bone marrow. Some enter the thymus and mature there, becoming competent lymphocytes which recirculate between the thymus and the peripheral lymphoid system. These are responsible for cell-mediated immunologic responses, such as delayed allergic reactions and homograft rejection. Stem cells which mature in the bone marrow leave as plasma cells which produce and secrete one or another of the serum immunoglobins.

Antigens

An antigen is usually a protein in a collodial state, or a high-molecular weight polysaccharide. However, all proteins are not equally antigenic, and such nonprotein substances as lipids and synthetic polymers may stimulate antibody production. In addition, there are haptens, low-molecular weight determinant groups which are nonimmunogenic in themselves but which become highly antigenic when combined with larger "carrier" proteins. Thus, an antigen has been defined as any substance capable of initiating an immune response. More recently, however, this broad definition has been associated with the term "immunogen" by some authors, the name antigen being reserved for those substances with the ability to combine with antibody.[2]

The immunogenicity of any molecule is determined by a number of properties, the foremost being genetic dissimilarity to the host. Although the mechanism of recognition of an antigen by the host is not yet clearly understood, the "better" antigen is one which the body easily recognizes as being foreign. Other physical and biological factors which determine antigenicity are well summarized by Bellanti. He includes:

1. Size. Effective antigens have molecular weights of more than 10,000, although minimal responses may be elicited by smaller molecules such as insulin and glucagon. Low-weight haptens can induce strong reactions when coupled to a protein whose weight exceeds 10,000.

2. Solubility. Soluble molecules which are non-immunogenic in monomer form may be highly so in the polymeric state.

3. Shape. All protein shapes (linear, branched, globular) are capable of inducing an immune response, but the antibody formed to suit a certain structure is specific for that shape alone. If the molecule is changed solely with regard to shape, the antibody originally formed will no longer combine with it.

4. Molecular charge. The net charge of the antigen "appears to influence the net charge of the resultant antibody which is produced."

5. Accessibility of reactive sites (determinant groups) on the molecular surface. This can influence whether an immune reaction will take place.

6. Digestibility. The more potent immunogen will usually be one that is capable of being phagocytosed and degraded within the body.

7. Chemical type. As previously mentioned, mostly all antigens in nature are protein—either pure or combined with lipids, carbohydrates, or nucleic acids.

8. A number of biologic factors are implicated in the distinctions of immunogenicity. For example, live attenuated vaccines used for immunization are better able to prevent disease than killed or inactivated preparations. Further, antigenicity will vary from one species to another as well as among individuals of the same species. The ability of a molecule to evoke an allergic response is an important biologic trademark of the antigen. Finally, dose and route of introduction of a substance into the host may influence that nature and extent of the immune response.[3]

Antibodies

Antibodies in humans and in many animals are associated with a complex group of physiochemically diverse, but functionally related, proteins called immunoglobulins. Electrophoretic analyses show that antibody qualities are found scattered in the alpha, beta, and gamma fractions of the serum globulin. Five classes of immunoglobulin have currently been identified in humans—IgG or γG, IgA or γA, IgM or γM, IgE or γE, and IgD or γD. Despite the bewildering variety of antigens which may provoke an immune response, the serum antibodies formed are narrowly specific in action. Thus, though each individual can form an overwhelming number of all five classes of antibodies which will differ from one another in some respects, the basic structure of all these antibodies will be similar, irrespective of immunoglobulin class. As Cohen points out, this arrangement "clearly fulfills the biologic functions of antibodies, allowing the specific recognition of an indefinite number of antigens and yet preserving the properties characteristic of a given class."[4]

The basic chemical structure of the immunoglobulins consists of four polypeptide chains. In each globulin molecule, two of these polypeptide strings are identical light chains (L) and two are identical heavy chains (H). All four chains are held together by covalent disulfide bonds. A chemically different heavy chain exists for each immunoglobulin class, and it is this which accounts for observed antigenic and biological differences between classes. The specificity shown by antibodies is a function of the primary amino acid sequence in the molecule, combination with a particular antigen taking place at an active "antigen-binding" site where the amino acid sequence will permit binding with it. Both heavy and light chains are thought to share the antigen-binding site, which occupies the amino acids at the amino-terminal end of each polypeptide chain.[5] (The molecule is diagrammed in simplified form in Figure 22-1.)

Very little is known about the exact structure and biological action of IgD, but more definite information about the other four immunoglobulin classes has accrued. The class which has been most extensively studied, IgG, comprises about 85 percent of the total immunoglobulins, has a molecular weight of around 150,000, and contains about 3 percent carbohydrate.[6] The total fraction is composed of four subtypes, which have been variously designated by different investigators. This class takes part in a wide variety of immune reactions in the intercellular spaces, where it neutralizes toxic microbial products (see Table 22-1).

The class IgA makes up about 10 to 15 percent of human immunoglobulin. In addition to being present in the serum, it constitutes the major immunoglobulin component of secretions exposed to the external environment, including saliva, tears, gastric juices, large and small bowel secretions, bronchial secretions, and colostrum. In these secretions, it is associated with an antigenically distinct protein fragment (transport or T-factor) which renders it resistant to enzymatic degradation. It is active in protecting body surfaces in contact with the external environment from a variety of bacteria and viruses (see Table 22-1).

The molecular weight of the immunoglobulin fraction IgM is approximately 900,000; it constitutes 5 to 10 percent of electrophoretically sepa-

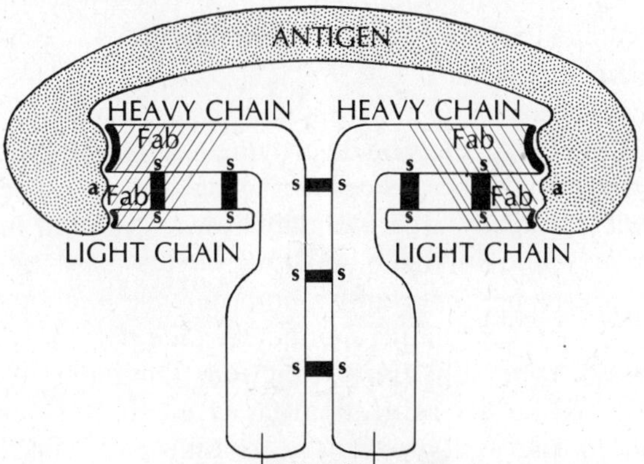

FIGURE 22-1.
Schematic drawing of IgG molecule in T-shaped form showing disulfide bonds (S–S) connecting heavy and light chains. Shaded area (Fab) shows regions of amino acid sequence variability which are associated with antibody specificity. Both heavy and light chains contribute to the two antibody combining sites (a). Flexibility of chains allows bivalent combination with a single antigen.

TABLE 22-1
Some Characteristics of Immunoglobulins

CLASS	MEAN SERUM CONCEN-TRATION (MG/100ML)	APPROXIMATE MOLECULAR WEIGHTS	IMMUNOLOGIC ROLE
G	1,240	150,000	Provides bulk of immunity to most infectious blood-borne agents; fixes complement; crosses placenta.
A	280	170,000	Provides immunity against infectious agents in secretions in contact with external environment; does not fix complement.
M	120	900,000	Agglutinates bacteria and RbC's; of greatest importance in first few days after primary immune response.
D	3	150,000	?
E	.03	200,000	Reaginic antibody; encompassed within external secretory system of AB; responsible for initiation of allergic symptomatology.

rated globulin and about 1 percent of the total serum protein.[7] In human IgM, a number of biologically active proteins have been demonstrated, including cold agglutenins, antibodies to the O antigen of *Salmonella,* and the rheumatoid factor. The IgM fraction is present in higher proportions in the very early stages after antigenic challenge, and is thought to be at least partly designed for rapid protection.

Discovered in 1966, IgE is the class of immunoglobulin now known to be particularly responsible for the production of allergic hypersensitivity. It is normally present in the serum in very low concentration (mean value about .03 mg per 100 ml, but is increased in about half of the patients with allergic disease and in patients with parasitic or helminthic infections. It is encompassed within the secretory system of antibody, being mostly produced in the linings of the gastrointestinal and respiratory tracts. The class IgE appears to unite with antigen to form a complex which reacts with and fixes to cell surfaces to cause release of two chemicals which produce allergic symptoms, histamine and slow-reacting substance (SRS-A).

There is a dearth of proof about the exact mechanism of antibody formation which will account for antibody variability. However, two broad theories have been widely proposed—the instructional, or template, mechanisms and the selection theories. In general, the instructional theory is that an antigen carries a certain pattern of information to the cell and directly or indirectly "impresses" it on the cytoplasmic RNA, determining the kind of globulin to be formed. Though previously popular, this mechanism has been shown to be untenable in the face of modern concepts of protein synthesis, at least in the simple form. The selection theories assume that the host has a variety of cells, each capable of making one kind of globulin, so that, in total, it possesses the cell mechanisms capable of producing all possible globulin types. Cells already committed to production of a particular antibody class may be selectively stimulated by the presence of antigen to proliferate and elaborate their globulin. The fundamental principles of the selection mechanism hold appeal for most im-

munologists, but it remains for future studies to clarify the genetic mechanisms responsible for antibody variability. (A review of current evidence concerning antibody variability and specificity may be found in Nisonoff's exposition on molecules of immunity. See bibliography at the end of this chapter.)

Mediators of Immunity

Apart from antigens and antibodies, an immunologic event encompasses diverse elements, all of which may alter or augment the immune response. For example, in order to serve the total functions of immunity, the lymphoreticular system performs such nonspecific actions as phagocytosis in addition to specific immune reactions. Some lymphoreticular cells are concerned with initial responses to foreign antigens, and others are called into play in repeat encounters. When a foreign substance is presented to the host and recognized as such, a whole group of cellular constituents and soluble serum factors take part in subsequent events. The cellular elements include granulocytes and macrophages, platelets, plasma cells, and lymphocytes; the humoral components comprise a variety of chemical mediator products in addition to complement.

Macrophages and granulocytes are especially adept at ingesting and destroying particulate matter through the process of phagocytosis. The macrophages, large mononuclear cells found in tissues and in the blood (monocytes), are believed to be important in both defense and surveillance. Circulating monocytes take part in delayed hypersensitivity reactions, and are attracted to an injured area by a number of chemotactic factors. The granulocyte most commonly involved in immune reactions is the polymorphonuclear leukocyte (PMN). These PMN's efficiently phagocytize highly virulent bacteria and other particulate material. They gather at an injury site during the inflammatory process in response to chemotactic factors derived from the complement system. (See Chapter 21 for a fuller discussion of phagocytosis and the inflammatory process.) The PMN's also produce the chemical SRS-A, "slow-reacting substance," and a variety of kinins, both of which are important mediators of hypersensitivity responses.

The lymphoid cells, that is, plasma cells and lymphocytes, are of prime importance in immunologic reactions, as they are able to react specifically with antigens. Plasma cells are concerned with antibody synthesis, and have been demonstrated to store and release antibody. Moreover, lymphocytes play the most diversified roles of all cells of the immune system. The lymphocytes are responsible for all cell-mediated immune responses, such as delayed hypersensitivity phenomena. In addition, lymphocytes produce a variety of chemical products which trigger inflammatory reactions and lead to tissue damage. These chemicals include MIF (migration inhibitory factor), a chemotactic substance for PMN's and monocytes; a cytotoxic factor capable of damaging a variety of cell types; interferon; and other factors whose roles are not as yet well defined.

Complement is the principle humoral mediator of biological manifestations of antigen-antibody reactions. The serum complement system comprises a variety of factors which may trigger either protective removal of infective agents or destructive reactions in host tissues. Eleven distinct proteins make up the complement system, and its various activities are generated by an orderly interaction between these components. The majority of complement factors act by triggering the inflammatory response. (See Chapter 21 for a fuller description of the characteristics and action of complement.)

The union of antigen and antibody in vivo is accompanied by the release of chemical mediator products which affect certain cells and tissues. The best known of these products is histamine, a substance found in particularly high concentrations in the mast cells of perivascular connective tissue, where it is bound to a heparin-protein complex. It is released from this bond upon antigen-antibody interaction at the cell surface. Histamine causes contraction of smooth muscle of the bronchioles, uterus, and intestine, dilatation and increased permeability of the capillaries

of the skin and mucous membrane, lowering of the blood pressure, stimulation of secretions of the lacrimal, nasal, salivary, pulmonary and intestinal glands, and production of itching by acting on sensory nerve endings in the skin and mucous membrane.

Other chemicals known to be released in antigen-antibody reactions include serotonin, the kinins, and slow-reacting substance. Serotonin is an amine that is presumably released from target cells simultaneously with histamine. There is as yet no concrete evidence that it contributes to immediate hypersensitivity symptoms in humans. Kinins are polypeptides formed by enzymatic action of the substance kallikrein on plasma kininogen. Kallikrein in the plasma secretes bradykinin while tissue kallikrein yields kallidin which is then degraded to bradykinin enzymatically. Since the first protein which triggers this "kinin cascade" is the plasma Hageman factor, which also initiates the clotting sequence, it remains unclear whether activation is the result of a specific immunologic reaction or a nonspecific tissue injury. In any event, it may aggravate the immune response and contribute to tissue injury by stimulating mucous secretion and increasing capillary permeability.

Slow-reacting substance is a fatty acid whose precise chemical structure has yet to be defined. (It is designated SRS-A to show that it is a product released as a result of antigen-antibody interaction.) Slow-reacting substance has been shown to be released from the human lung on challenge with specific pollen antigen, and renders human bronchiolar smooth muscle extremely sensitive to contraction. Its presence in allergic bronchospasm is thought to be the reason antihistamines are of small benefit in controlling this distressing clinical symptom.

Nonspecific Factors

There are a number of nonspecific factors which may influence antigens, antibodies, or the localization of antigen-antibody complex, thus affecting the nature, rate, and extent of injury to target tissues. However, the approach to assessing the action of these nonspecific factors has been a hesitant one. Samter and Markowitz review some of the questions that exist concerning these factors and their influence on antigen-antibody reactions:

1. Neither the specific role nor the exact nature of chemical mediator products has yet been clearly defined.

2. The ground substance and basement membranes of connective tissues represent a protective barrier which should be able to inactivate chemical mediators before they reach the cell; therefore, perhaps immunological pathology arises from impairment of the integrity of ground substance or from the effects of hormones such as steroids on it.

3. Antigen is taken up at the initial site of contact by macrophage cells. The question is whether these cells might alter the antigen on the way to delivery to the lymph system.

4. Factors which affect protein synthesis also affect synthesis of antibody, and hormones may thus affect both by bringing about modified amino acid transfer, changed secondary or tertiary structure of protein, altered RNA synthesis in general and modified synthesis of activity of messenger RNA coding sites on DNA molecules in particular.

5. Factors which increase or decrease autonomic nervous system responses also affect antigen-antibody reactions, including weather, infections, emotional factors, and various ill-defined components of daily living. Age and metabolism of the host are relevant factors.[8]

Humoral and Cellular Immunity

Antigen-antibody interactions in the body may proceed along three general pathways—the primary, secondary, and tertiary responses. The primary reaction to antigenic challenge consists of phagocytosis and inflammation, the nonspecific immune response. This is fully described in Chapter 21. The immune process may terminate with this response, if the host eliminates the offending antigen. The secondary response, or specific immune reaction, occurs if an antigenic challenge persists. This secondary response may be humoral, in which the antigen interacts with circulating antibody of any of the five immunoglobulin classes, or cell-mediated, in which the reaction is transmitted by lymphoid cells. Most antigens are dealt with successfully at this stage without ill effects on the host, however, if the antigen is still not eliminated, humoral or cellular tertiary responses which may be deleterious to host tissue ensue.

There are basic differences between the humoral and the cellular manifestations of immunity. Humoral reactions frequently occur within minutes (anaphylaxis) although the response may take hours (Arthrus reaction). Cellular events develop more slowly, requiring at least 24 hours to evolve. Hence, the term "immediate" has been employed to designate humoral responses, while cell-mediated responses have been called "delayed." This terminology as a distinguishing characteristic is now limited to discussion of hypersensitivity phenomena.

Another point of differentiation is that transfer of the humoral response to a nonreactive individual may be accomplished with serum alone, since the presence of circulating antibody is the initiating event. Transfer of cellular reactivity can occur only through cells or cell-derived products, as the intact lymphocyte is a prerequisite of the response. The antigens which can trigger the humoral response may be proteins, polysaccharides, lipids, and a variety of other chemicals, while cell-mediated events require a protein or a hapten-protein conjugate to initiate the reaction. Chemical mediators of the two reactions differ also—complement, histamine, the Kinens and SRS-A are effector substances for humoral responses, soluble factors secreted by lymphocytes enhance the cellular response.

Mechanisms of Tissue Injury

Humoral immune reactions in the host may be detected by a number of effects demonstrated on serological assay, including precipitation, agglutination, complement-dependent reactions, neutralization, and cytotropic effects. A discussion of these serological aspects is beyond the scope of this chapter, but a straightforward review may be found in Humphrey and White's *Immunology for Students of Medicine* (see Bibliography). While it should be remembered that immune responses have a protective function that leads to destruction of the inciting antigen, the immune process may initiate tissue damage associated with any or all of the above biological results of antigen-antibody union. There are four distinct pathways by which immune reactions may be deleterious to the individual, three of which are humoral mechanisms. These reactions have been generally classified as follows:

Type I—Immediate hypersensitivity homocytotropic reactions

Type II—Cytotoxic (cytolytic) reactions

Type III—Immune complex reactions

Type IV—Delayed hypersensitivity reactions

Any immunologic disorder may involve mechanisms belonging to one or all of these types of responses.

TYPE I: IMMEDIATE HYPERSENSITIVITY REACTIONS

Immediate hypersensitivity responses are antigen-antibody interactions involving the release of chemical mediator products from target cells to effect local or systemic allergic symptoms. The most rapid and dramatic expression of a Type I reaction is anaphylaxis. Atopic allergies are also products of this type of reaction. (See Chapter 23 for a detailed discussion of hypersensitivity phenomena and anaphylaxis.) The IgE class of immunoglobulins is the antibody mediator of this reaction, which is initiated by the intrusion of an allergen. Events taking place at target cell surfaces are still poorly understood, but it appears that IgE (reaginic) antibody becomes fixed to target tissue cells, ultimately resulting in release of histamine and serotonin from tissue mast cells and slow-reacting substance from PMN's.

TYPE II: CYTOTOXIC REACTIONS

The second variant of humoral immune responses which results in tissue damage is usually effected through IgG. Circulating IgG binds to cell surfaces in response to the presence of their specific antigen. "Coating" of these target cells with antibody renders them more susceptible to lysis. Unlike the Type I hypersensitivity mecha-

nism, this reaction is complement-dependent and antigen-specific. Human pathogenesis incurred by cytotoxic immune responses includes blood transfusion reactions, Rh or ABO hemolytic disease of the newborn, autoimmune hemolytic anemias, immunologic forms of leukopenia and thrombocytopenia, Goodpasture's syndrome, and certain specific aspects of homograft rejection. (See Chapter 17 for a discussion of transplantation immunity.)

TYPE III: IMMUNE COMPLEX MECHANISM

The immune-complex mechanism for initiating tissue damage is typified by Arthrus reaction, in which several hours pass before symptoms fully develop. The reaction is mediated either by IgG of IgM. Antibody combines with antigen in tissue spaces, forming a complex. Complement then fixes to this complex in turn, attracting PMNs which invade the target tissue and release their toxic products, causing a severe inflammatory reaction. In contrast to Arthus's reaction which takes place in the tissues, in experimental serum sickness, the antigen remains in the circulation until antibodies appear and immune complexes are formed which fix complement. These soluble immune complexes tend to localize in the kidney, aorta, and other large vessels, initiating damage. Disorders generated by the deposit of antigen-antibody complexes include systemic lupus erythematosus, poststreptococcal glomerulonephritis, and many features of clinical serum sickness.

TYPE IV: DELAYED HYPERSENSITIVITY REACTIONS

Delayed hypersensitivity reactions are the fourth type of mechanism by which the immune system may cause damage to the human body. Bellanti defines delayed hypersensitivity as that aspect of cellular immunity in which an increased reactivity to specific antigens is mediated not by antibodies, but by cells (sensitized lymphocytes).[9]

It is helpful to clarify the differences between delayed hypersensitivity and cellular immunity. As previously mentioned, cellular immunity "includes those manifestations of the specific immune response expressed by antigen-sensitized lymphocytes derived from the thymic-dependent system. The response is particularly suited for antigens which are cell-bound or in other ways inaccessible to the antibody mechanism."[10] Until recently, these reactions were also labeled as delayed hypersensitivity for they were viewed as "hyper" or undesirable expressions of the immune system. While in some cases this is true (poison ivy contact dermatitis), cellular immunity is now known to be essential to the maintenance of bodily homeostasis and is instrumental in resistance to bacterial and viral infections and surveillance of neoplasia. Cellular immunity is also responsible for the rejection of homografts, a normal immune response which may be considered clinically "undesirable." Aberrations of the cellular response include contact sensitivity, the autoimmune diseases, neoplasia, and overwhelming infections.

The pathogenesis of the delayed hypersensitivity response is not fully understood. Research into the nature of cellular immunity has lagged behind that of the humoral response, which can be more easily defined and measured. Bellanti notes that, while until recently the reaction of a specifically sensitized lymphocyte with its antigen could only be ascertained by in vivo reactions of the delayed type, the reactions of antibody with its antigen can be detected directly or indirectly in a number of ways.[11]

The steps of the delayed hypersensitivity response are essentially the same as those of the cellular response, which is believed to progress as follows:

1. Processing of the antigen—possibly by a macrophage.

2. Recognition of the antigen by a cell surface receptor on a small lymphocyte. The receptor is probably similar to antibody; thus the reactions are highly specific. Recognition may occur at the local site of antigen or the antigen may enter the systemic circulation.

3. Within the lymphatic system, the lymphocyte undergoes blast cell transformation and mitosis thus becoming "sensitized."

4. The lymphocyte becomes capable of elaborating a variety of low molecular weight effector substances which act upon the antigen and other non-specific cells to activate them.

a. Transfer factor—immunologically specific, concerned with the transfer of reactivity to uncommitted lymphocytes; has capacity to transfer delayed hypersensitivity to another individual.

b. Migration Inhibitory Factor (MIF)—macrophage activation and contains macrophages in areas of injury with phagocytosis the end result.

c. Lymphotoxin (LT)—associated with target cell injury: inhibits capacity of cells to divide.

d. Skin Reactive Factor (SRF)—localized cutaneous reaction.

e. Chemotactic Factors—at least two, induce chemotactic migration of monocytes and neutrophils.

f. Mitogenic Factor (recruitment factor)—together with transfer factor may be important in augmenting or amplifying the response by recruiting uncommitted lymphocytes and other cells.

g. Interferon—inhibits replication of viruses.

h. Antibody—may be released following interaction of antigen with specifically sensitized lymphocytes to augment cellular response.

5. A second interaction with the same antigen brings a greatly enhanced response that requires appreciably less time to develop.[12]

A unique feature of the cellular reaction and its variant, delayed hypersensitivity, is that it is manifested through a relatively *small* number of specifically committed lymphocytes. These specific cells produce an array of diverse biologically active substances which then recruit a *large* number of uncommitted, nonspecific cells—macrophages. The cell damage is done by harmful factors released by the committed and noncommitted cells.

Diseases Mediated by the Immune System

The diseases mediated by the immune system are of two basic types: those in which the immune response is hypoactive (immunodeficiency) and those in which it is hyperactive or abnormal and produces clinically undesirable effects. Causes of many of these aberrations of the immune system have been identified; however, there remains a large number of disorders in which the immune system is believed to play a role yet to be specifically defined. The clinical signs and symptoms of the immunologic diseases in which a "hyper" response occurs are the results of one or more of the four mechanisms of tissue injury discussed in the foregoing section.

IMMUNODEFICIENCY SYNDROMES

The immunodeficiency syndromes comprise a heterogeneous group of acquired and inborn defects of the lymphoreticular tissues which, depending upon the specific defect, affect humoral or cellular immunity or both. Patients with immunodeficiency disease are subject to an increased susceptibility to severe, repeated infections, neoplasia (especially lymphoreticular), and possibly autoimmune diseases. The risk of malignancy is markedly increased in the patient with a defect of the thymic-dependent system. Of the two types of immunodeficiency diseases, the primary or inborn syndromes are rare whereas the secondary or acquired syndromes are not uncommon.

Primary Immunodeficiency Diseases

The primary immunodeficiency diseases are the result of an inborn or developmental "failure to produce effectors of the immune response, either antibodies or lymphocytes."[13] In 1952, the first primary immunodeficiency syndrome—infantile, sex-linked agammaglobulinemia—was described.[14] A number of other related disorders were reported during the following years, and, in 1970, a classification system was proposed at a meeeting on the Primary Immunodeficiency Diseases sponsored by the World Health Organization.[15]

Experiments in lower animals have led to the observation that, if the site of differentiation for either the B-cell or T-cell type of immunity is removed at an appropriate time during embryonic life, a profound immunodeficiency is produced. (See discussion of normal development of the immune system.) If the B-cell is eliminated, humoral immunity is affected, and, if the T-cell is removed, cellular immunity is deficient. If both types of cells are eliminated, an essen-

tially absent immune response is the result. Many scientists have drawn comparisons between the various clinical immunodeficiency states and laboratory observations of the normal and experimentally altered development of the immune system. The World Health Organization classification of the specific primary immunodeficiency states is based upon this model (see Table 22-2). It is unfortunate, however, that the specific classification encompasses only a minority of patients with immunodeficiency. At this time, the majority of disorders must be grouped as variable, immunodeficiency syndromes.

The Bruton type of infantile, sex-linked agammaglobulinemia typifies the B-cell type of immunodeficiency disease. "It is probably the result of a genetic defect, perhaps a missing enzyme that interferes with the development of the immunoglobulin producing system after the branching point."[16] The disease is carried by the female and expressed in the male. Children with

TABLE 22-2
Primary Immunodeficiency Syndromes

DISEASE	CELL TYPE
1. Infantile, sex-linked agammaglobulinemia (Bruton Type)	B
2. Selective IgA deficiency	B
3. Transient hypogammaglobulinemia of infancy	B
4. Sex-linked immunodeficiency with ↑ IgM	B
5. Congenital thymic hypoplasia (DiGeorge's syndrome)	T
6. Episodic lymphopenia with lymphocytoxin	T
7. Immunodeficiency with normal or ↑ gamma globulin	T
8. Immunodeficiency with ataxia-telangiectasia	S
9. Immunodeficiency with thrombocytopenia and eczema (Wiskott-Aldrich syndrome)	S
10. Immunodeficiency with thyoma	S
11. Immunodeficiency with short-limbed dwarfism	S
12. Immunodeficiency with generalized hematopoietic hypoplasia	S
13. Severe combined immunodeficiencies	
a. Autosomal recessive	S
b. Sex-linked	S
c. Sporadic	S
14. Variable immunodeficiency (common, largely unclassified)	?

Source: Adapted from Good, R. A. and Fisher, D. W. (eds.): Immunology. Stamford, Conn., Sinaver Associates, 1971, p. 12.

the disorder are normal with respect to thymic-dependent processes; however, they have virtually no ability to form plasma cells and gamma globulin. Signs and symptoms (pyogenic infections) usually do not appear until the ninth month of age when the immune protection of the mother has dissipated. Patients with agammaglobulinemia are given monthly injections of gamma globulin and whole plasma is also given to add the IgA and IgM which appear in only trace amounts in gamma globulin preparations. A significant observation concerning these patients is that they tend to develop a variety of autoimmune diseases. The relationship will be discussed later in this chapter.

Congenital thymic aplasia (DiGeorge's syndrome) is an example of a disease characterized by a lack of cellular immunity. In 1968, DiGeorge reported a congenital anomaly that results from a failure of embryogenesis of entodermal derivatives of the third and fourth pharyngeal pouches—aplasia of the parathyroid and thymus glands. The disorder appears to be the result of some intrauterine accident and not a hereditary problem; the patients have a tendency to present with other congenital defects, particularly cardiovascular and facial anomalies, as well as hypocalcemic tetany. Infants with thymic aplasia who survive have all aspects of humoral immunity intact; however, they do not mount an adequate rejection of skin allografts and are highly susceptible to viral, bacterial, and fungal infections. Two children with this syndrome have shown dramatic reversals of all defects in lymphocytic function following transplants of fetal thymic tissue. There have been several reports of an incomplete form of this syndrome which results in a clinically less severe course with death often the result of the concurrent congenital defects.[17]

The first type of combined defect to be reported was hereditary thymic dysplasia (severe combined immunodeficiency). The defect appears to occur at the point where the stem cells normally differentiate to lymphoid cells. Three different modes of inheritance have been observed; however, they each present in a similar manner in terms of clinical and anatomical abnormalities. Infants with this disease are prey to all types of viral, fungal, bacterial, and protozoan infections and death invariably occurs before the second year. The bone marrow is deficient in plasma cells, lymphocytes, and lymphoblasts. None of the in vitro or in vivo parameters of humoral or cellular immunity can be elicited. Transplants of a variety of lymphoreticular cells and tissues have failed; in most cases, destruction is due to a graft versus host reaction. Very recently, attempts at administering completely histocompatible bone marrow cells have been followed by promising results in three or four cases.[18]

Unfortunately, there is a big gap between the ability to diagnose immunologic deficiency disorders and the ability to treat these problems. In the words of immunologist Paul J. Edelson: ''I don't think there is any single immunologic deficiency syndrome where we can be even 75% sure we have an effective and safe long-term therapy, let alone an effective and safe cure. Even the patient who is given gamma globulin doesn't always fare well. The best we can hope for is that we can ameliorate their life-threatening infections and keep them doing relatively well until somebody comes up with something a little better than what we have right now.''[19]

Since few children with combined immunologic defects live to their second birthday, and those with single defects frequently die before reaching maturity, the family must be helped to face a devastating situation. It is best if they can receive emotional support from health team members who have been involved in their care from the beginning. Continuous support is needed from diagnosis and referral through genetic counseling and decision making at every step (see Chapter 6). Supportive care is required on a week to week, even day to day, basis for these chronically ill children who are plagued by life-threatening infections. According to Dr. Edelson, the health care worker, in a sense, becomes a cosufferer with the parents; he is there to help them in their time of grief if they lose a child.[20]

Secondary Immunodeficiency Diseases

The secondary immunodeficiency syndromes are also a diverse group of disorders which are characterized by a less than optimal immune response (humoral and/or cellular). The syndromes are of an acquired origin and appear in association with, or subsequent to, other diseases or therapies which have had an adverse effect on the immune system. Hodgkin's disease will be discussed as an example of the classic type of secondary immunodeficiency; others are presented in Table 22-3. The autoimmune diseases and neoplasia are aberrations of the immune system in which immunodeficiency has been proposed as a causative factor; they are discussed elsewhere in this chapter.

Hodgkin's disease is "an acquired disorder of the lymphoid system characterized by progressive glandular enlargement without the appearance of characteristic cells in the blood. The diagnosis is made by biopsy, usually of a peripheral lymph node. In the absence of treatment or when therapy is not effective, the condition is fatal within a highly variable number of years. The disease may be localized at the beginning, but it eventually becomes a systemic disorder with symptoms including fever, chills, sweats, itching, weight loss, and anemia.

Hodgkin's disease is accompanied by a progressive immune deficiency. This component of the disease may produce complications which are at least as difficult to manage as the lymphoma itself. The deficiency is characterized by a depression of those immune responses which are cell-mediated in nature; the patients may suffer frequent and bizarre infections. In general, the ability to form plasma cells and antibody is intact, although some subtle alterations in the humoral mechanism have been reported.

The anergy of Hodgkin's disease (except for that of patients with advanced disease) is unrelated to the debility or to obliteration of the lymphoid system by anatomically verifiable disease. A variety of evidence suggests that the absence of cellular immunity is mediated through the peripheral small lymphocytes. Further, it seems likely that a systemic circulating factor of unknown origin leads to functional impairment of the entire lymphoid system.

TABLE 22-3
Secondary Immunodeficiency Syndromes

DEFECT	MECHANISM AFFECTED	EXAMPLE
1. Lymphoreticular malignancy		
a. ↓Cellular immunity	Cellular	Hodgkin's disease
b. ↓Ig synthesis	Humoral	2° to lymphoreticular malignancy
c. ↑Synthesis pathological Ig	Humoral	multiple myeloma, macroglobulinemia
2. Infection or granuloma	Cellular	Leprosy a. Nonspecific defect of cellular immunity b. ? defects genetically controlled or result from damage to host by M. Leprae, or combination of factors
3. Obstruction to lymph flow	Cellular	Intestinal lymphangiectasia a. Obstruction to normal lymphocyte circulation b. Can result in peripheral blood lymphopenia with a loss of cellular immunity
4. Increased Ig catabolism	Humoral	2° to nephrotic syndrome or myotonic dystrophy
5. Increased Ig loss	Humoral	2° to exudative enteropathy or burns
6. Autoimmune diseases	Humoral, cellular	Systemic lupus erythematosus
7. Neoplasia	Cellular	
8. Extrinsic immunosuppression	Humoral, cellular	Immunosuppressive agents

Source: Adapted from Samter, M. A., et al. (eds.): Immunological Diseases, ed. 2, Vol. I. Boston, Little, Brown, 1971, pp. 498, 634, 511.

Neoplasia

The interaction of genetic and environmental factors is believed to be responsible for the development of neoplastic cells. These cells are constantly appearing in the human body, and, normally, the immune system recognizes them as foreign and destroys them through its nonspecific and specific responses. Current evidence establishes the immune lymphocyte as the major responder to tumor antigens, but a role for circulating antibody cannot be excluded.[21]

It is theorized that by carrying out this surveillance function, the immune system protects against or retards the progress of cancer. Evidence pointing to this model includes the following:

1. Studies of cancer systems in lower animals and in humans have demonstrated antigens that are "tumor specific."(TSA)

2. There have been reports of spontaneous tumor regressions; only the immune system can readily account for such activities.

3. Studies indicate that immunocompetent patients with cancer do much better than those who have decreased or absent immune mechanisms.

4. A dramatic increase over the normal incidence of neoplasms has been observed in patients whose immune systems are deficient—either due to inborn or acquired defects. The patient with an immunodeficiency of the cellular type is particularly susceptible.[22]

Today, clinical tumors are viewed as the result of several factors working together, one of which is impaired immunocompetence. Proposed mechanisms for this immunodeficiency include:

defect	*origin*
1. The immune system may be influenced by a number of outside factors so that periods of relative immunosuppression occur and mutant cells reproduce unchecked to the point where even a normal immune response is unable to contain them.	secondary
2. The fact that the immune system becomes increasingly disorganized with age may account for the higher incidence of cancer and autoimmune diseases in elderly patients. In effect, the body lowers its guard.	secondary
3. The TSA may combine with "enhancing Ab" which promotes the growth of malignant cells rather than blocking them.	primary/secondary
4. Various serum complexes, or blocking factors, may cover the tumor cells and prevent their destruction by a sensitized lymphocyte.	primary/secondary
5. The TSA may not be recognized as foreign early enough in the course of tumor growth to be controlled.[23]	primary/secondary

In the light of the evidence supporting the role of immunodeficiency in the pathogenesis of tumors, a recent mode of treatment, particularly in skin cancer, has been immunotherapy. The immunologic system is manipulated in an attempt to bolster its ability to respond to the neoplasm after the cell mass has been reduced by such modalities as surgery, radiotherapy, and chemotherapy. Immunotherapy may include one or more of the following approaches:

1. Active—cancer specific antigens are used to stimulate a specific host response.

2. Passive—tumor specific antibody, sensitized cells, or immune RNA or transfer factor are made outside the host and injected into him.

3. Non-specific, non-cancer agents are used to stimulate the host's immune system in a non-specific way.[24]

Autoimmune Disease

The observation that the immune system is capable of recognizing and responding to foreign antigens, but not to its own, is well known in immunology. However, it is only recently that the mechanisms for this phenomenon have been partially understood. As happens with many areas of clinical research, early study of the tolerance of self-tissue centered around individuals who did not exhibit this unique quality. This state, in which injury occurs caused by an apparent immunologic reaction of the host with his own tissue has been called "horror autotoxicus" (or autoimmune disease25). Today, we recognize a wide variety of disorders of unknown etiology in which autoimmune phenomena are thought to contribute to, or be associated with, the pathogenesis. But in none of these is it actually known that the primary cause is immunologic.

It is important that the distinction between the autoimmune response or phenomenon and autoimmune disease (AID) be made clear. The autoimmune response refers to the appearance of antibody or sensitized lymphocytes in humans directed against a self-antigen. It has been hypothesized that in AID, the tissue damage results from the activities of autoantibody or sensitized lymphocytes; however, it is not known for sure whether the autoimmune response is a cause, consequence, or concomitant finding in AID.[26] It appears that the pathology of the autoimmune response may reflect any one of the four mechanisms of tissue injury discussed earlier in this chapter. Thus, both the humoral and cellular types of immunity are involved.

Many theories have been put forth concerning the mechanism of origin of autoantibodies. Holman summarizes these well in his discussion of systemic lupus erythematosus in Samter's *Immunological Diseases:*

    1. The autoantibodies may arise from an abnormal response of immunocompetent cells and therefore by the consequence of an underlying immunological aberration in patients.

    2. From the opposite point of view, autoantibodies may represent a response by normal immunocompetent cells to altered tissue antigen.

    3. Autoantibodies may arise as a result of antigenic stimulation by foreign materials such as bacteria or viruses which possess structural similarities to components of mammalian tissue. The resultant antibodies cross-react with the host's tissues (e.g., rheumatic heart disease).[26]

The first theory is particularly interesting in light of the previously mentioned observation that the incidence of neoplasia and autoimmune disease is dramatically increased in patients with an immunodeficiency. For example, this has been reported in patients who receive immunosuppressive drugs to prevent the rejection of therapeutic transplants.

Witebsky stated that if a disease is to be called "autoimmune" it should be possible to demonstrate either circulating or cell-bound antibodies in the serum of victims; to characterize and, if possible, isolate the antigen against which the antibody is directed; to produce antibodies against the same antigen in experimental animals; and to observe changes in corresponding tissues of a sensitized animal that are similar or identical to those seen in humans.[27] (These are termed "Witebsky's Postulates.") These standards are quite difficult to fulfill clinically, demonstrating that although the entity of autoimmunity is known to exist, it is not yet clearly understood. Some disorders which are presently thought to have marked immunologic manifestations are listed in Table 22-4; comments include a summary of evidence warranting their characterization as autoimmune diseases. Systemic lupus erythematosus (SLE) will be discussed in detail as an example of an autoimmune disease.

Of all of the collagen-based autoimmune diseases, SLE is the prototype. Its most significant feature is the tendency of the affected patient to form antibodies to a variety of his own tissue constituents, particularly nuclear components. The abnormalities of SLE are currently better understood than those of any of the other collagen diseases.

The exact etiology of SLE is unknown. However, several observations have led to the contention that the syndrome is genetically determined but dependent upon the subsequent intervention of environmental factors for full expression to occur. These observations include the following:

1. In susceptible individuals, SLE can be drug-induced, particularly by: procainamide, hydralazine, isoniazid, and several anticonvulsants, including Dilantin. These are thought to alter

TABLE 22-4
Autoimmune Diseases

CONDITION	COMMENTS REGARDING EVIDENCE FOR ASSOCIATION WITH AUTOIMMUNE PATHOLOGY
COLLAGEN DISEASE Rheumatoid arthritis	Certain clinical and pathological analogies between serum sickness (a proven immunologic phenomenon) and the connective tissue syndromes, including rheumatoid arthritis.
	Autoimmune phenomena are operative in most patients with rheumatoid disease, although there is no direct evidence that RF mediates the pathogenesis of the disease.
	In rheumatoid arthritis there may be some unrecognized chronic antigenic stimulus.
	In some patients a respiratory infection or grippelike illness occurs as a prodrome to the development of arthritis.
	Hypergammaglobulinemia, commonly associated with rheumatoid arthritis, could be cited as evidence for an immunologic process.
	Synovial structures and subcutaneous nodules in chronic rheumatoid arthritis contain plasma and lymph cells in clumps that resemble lymphoid follicles.
	Studies of rheumatoid synovial fluid demonstrate low-complement levels and materials that resemble immune aggregates.
Systemic lupus erythematosus	Presence of many types of autoantibodies in the sera and Y-globulin localized in the lesions of the kidney, spleen, and skin.
	A curious skin reactivity to autologous tissue constituents which resemble the skin response of delayed hypersensitivity.
	Low levels of circulating complement.
	Presence of hypergammaglobulinemia and possibly an increased incidence of rheumatic disease in relatives of patients with SLE.
	(? genetic predisposition to SLE)
Polyarteritis nodosa	Sum of evidence, particularly that gained from experimental studies in animals, states that hypersensitivity can cause arteritis. However, these observations do not tell us whether or not most cases of polyarteritis are caused by hypersensitivity.
	Clinical evidence fragmentary and less convincing.
Polymyositis and dermatomyositis	No firm conclusions at this time on the etiology of these human nyopathies.
	The animal models, either naturally occurring or experimentally induced, and clinical and pathological observations strongly suggest at least delayed hypersensitivity and possibly circulating Ab are involved.
Scleroderma	There has been an impressive collection of clinical and serological evidence of immunologic abnormalities in a high percentage of patients with this sclerosing connective disorder.
OCULAR DISORDERS Sjogren's syndrome	Autoimmune pathology is strongly implicated in this triad of keratoconjunctivitis and oral dryness in conjunction with rheumatoid arthritis or one of the other collagen disorders already mentioned.

TABLE 22-4
Autoimmune Diseases (continued)

CONDITION	COMMENTS REGARDING EVIDENCE FOR ASSOCIATION WITH AUTOIMMUNE PATHOLOGY
Various types of endogenous uveitis, including sympathetic ophthalmia C.	The pathogenesis in sympathetic ophthalmia is presumed to be due to the production of autoantibodies against the patient's own uveal tissue (hypersensitivity to the uveal tissue). The exact mechanism which triggers the hypersensitive response is not yet clearly defined.
HEMATOLOGICAL DISORDERS	Multiple blood disorders have been characterized as autoimmune at one time or another. Although the acquired hemolytic anemias do not fulfill all of Witebsky's postulates, characterizing them as abnormal Ab response has gained much acceptance in recent years. Idiopathic thrombocytopenic purpura, thrombotic thrombocytopenic purpura, and pernicious anemia have also been implicated.
GASTROINTESTINAL DISORDERS Infectious hepatitis Biliary and portal cirrhosis Drug-induced hepatotoxicity Lupoid hepatitis	In all of these liver diseases, autoimmune pathology is suspected. Hypergammaglobulinemia and abnormal Ab responses frequently accompany the clinical illness.
Ulcerative colitis	In addition to hypergammaglobulinemia and the presence of cross-reacting antibodies, this disorder has been noted to occur frequently in conjunction with disorders ascribed to hypersensitivity reactions. Further, it is a familial disease and histologic observations are suggestive of immune response.
DEMYELINATING DISORDERS Allergic encephalomyelitis Acute hemorrhagic encephalopathy	Experimental allergic encephalomyelitis (EAE). Available data suggest that immunological forces are implicated in the pathogenesis of demyelinating disease.
Multiple sclerosis	Injections of nervous tissue into humans or animals induce an acute encephalomyelitis with perivascular demyelination and circulating antibrain Ab. Sera from animals with EAE and sera of patients with MS exert an injurious effect on glial cells and myelinated nerve fibers of brain cultures. ? whether any of the Ab or serum factors uncovered have a role in causing neurological disease or merely represent parallel and unrelated immunologic responses.
MYASTHENIA GRAVIS	Since 1960, immunologic abnormalities have been reported to be associated with myasthenia gravis. Autoimmune etiology may be postulated on the basis of the nature and progression of clinical symptoms, the changes in serum complement activity, which correlate with remissions and exacerbations of the syndrome and a presumed immunologic function of the thymus gland, particularly in producing the thymoma that is a frequent correlate of the disease.

TABLE 22-4
Autoimmune Diseases (continued)

CONDITION	COMMENTS REGARDING EVIDENCE FOR ASSOCIATION WITH AUTOIMMUNE PATHOLOGY
ENDOCRINE DISORDERS Thyroiditis Adrenalitis Aspermatogenesis Orchitis Infertility is possible to tentatively	Here the most prominent example of autoimmune pathogenesis is Hashimoto's disease, a goiterous thyroiditis with the usual consequence of myxedema. Hashimoto's disease satisfies Witebsky's postulates and, therefore, it conclude that it does involve auto-allergic mechanisms. 1. Autoantibodies are present and titers correlate to some extent with severity and chronicity of the disease. 2. Autoantibodies have been detected to several organ-specific Ag's in the thyroid. 3. Injections of homologous and autologous thyroglobulin or thyroid extract into animals produce an immunologic response and disease (EIT) similar to Hashimoto's. 4. The pathological picture of certain examples of EIT is very similar to Hashimoto's. 5. Hashimoto's disease has apparently not been passively transferred with Ab which pass the placenta; EIT has been passively transferred with cells and serum. 6. EIT—experimental immunologic thyroiditis.

Source: Adapted from Samter, M. A. et al. (eds.): Immunological Diseases. Boston, Little, Brown, 1971.

nuclear antigens in patients with underlying lupus diatheses. Other agents may also initiate lupoid manifestations by first giving rise to hypersensitive reactions. Included in this group are: penicillin, sulfonamide, and less often oral contraceptive agents, propylthiouracil, phenylbutazone, and reserpine.

2. The disease is familial and commonly occurs in identical twins. Immediate relatives of SLE patients have an increased frequency of elevated immunoglobulin levels.

3. The disease can be developed genetically. An inbred strain of New Zealand black mice exhibit a syndrome remarkably similar to human SLE with glomerulonephritis.

4. Preliminary investigation suggests that viral agents may also be a factor in the etiology of SLE.

Figure 22-2 summarizes the possible roles of genetics, infectious processes, and the environment in the cause and pathogenesis of SLE.

Although the pathological changes in SLE are less evident than the clinical manifestations, current observations on them include the following:

1. There are hematoxylin bodies found in a variety of tissues. They are made up of DNA-IgG complexes and appear to be the tissue counterpart of the LE cell.

2. Other histological changes are suggestive but not specific for SLE, for example, endocarditis, glomerular capsule thickening, fibrosis of penicillary arteries of the spleen (onionskin lesions), deposit of fibrinoid material in a variety of organs.

3. It is not possible to distinguish between the pathology of the skin lesions of discoid lupus and SLE, although many observations support the idea that the skin lesions are antibody-generated, since immune reactants are found in them.

4. The renal lesion in SLE also includes deposits highly suggestive of immune complex type processes. They appear to be due to the deposition of circulating immune complexes along glomerular basement membranes.

5. Blood vessels throughout the body frequently show deposits of immune reactants.

6. The LE cell is one of the most specific tests for SLE, but even this is not pathognomonic as it also occurs in rheumatoid arthritis, chronic liver

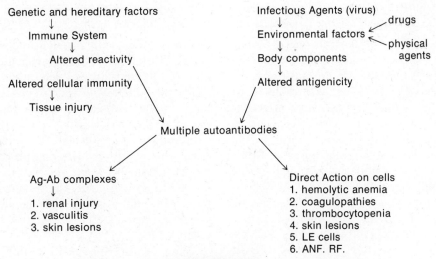

Genetic and hereditary factors
↓
Immune System
↓
Altered reactivity
↓
Altered cellular immunity
↓
Tissue injury

Infectious Agents (virus)
↓
Environmental factors ⟵ drugs
↓   ⟵ physical agents
Body components
↓
Altered antigenicity

Multiple autoantibodies

Ag-Ab complexes
↓
1. renal injury
2. vasculitis
3. skin lesions

Direct Action on cells
1. hemolytic anemia
2. coagulopathies
3. thrombocytopenia
4. skin lesions
5. LE cells
6. ANF. RF.

FIGURE 22-2.
The roles of genetics, infectious diseases and environment in the pathogenesis and cause of SLE.
Source: Adapted from Freedman, S. L.: Clinical Immunology. New York, Harper & Row, 1971.

disease, chronic ulcerative colitis, and leprosy. The LE cell is a poly that has phagocytized fragmented nuclear material which has previously reacted with antinuclear antibody.

7. Hypergamma globulinemia occurs along with the presence of circulating Ab-anti DNA and Ab-anti nucleoprotein.

From the wide variety of pathological changes, as one would expect, the clinical manifestations of SLE are protean. Symptoms usually appear in the second to fourth decades, but may appear at any age; they are more common in females.

Constitutional symptoms. These are common to many acute and chronic illnesses and include fever, malaise, weakness, weight loss, and anorexia.

Systemic Symptoms. The system affected initially usually remains the most seriously involved throughout the course of the disease.

Renal disease. When present, renal disease is the major contributor to morbidity and mortality. Acute or subacute glomerulonephritis (lupus nephritis)→nephrotic syndrome→progressive renal failure. Systemic lupus erythematosus causes 5 to 10 percent of all cases of nephrotic syndrome.

Skin. Erythematous eruptions occur in the skin; butterfly pattern in exposed areas occurs in certain individuals and is exacerbated by sunlight. Other skin manifestations include alopecia, urticaria, and scleroderma.

Polyserositis. This is a nonsuppurative inflammatory reaction in serous tissues. The pericardium and pleura are the most frequently involved sites.

Articular lesions. These appear in the majority of patients with SLE. Although at times the histological changes are identical to those of rheumatoid arthritis, destructive bony changes do not occur.

Hematologic abnormalities. These include coagulation defects, autoimmune hemolytic anemia, lymphadenopathy and splenomegaly which occur more often in children than adults.

Cardiovascular lesions, including Raynaud's syndrome, thrombophlebitis, thrombotic occlusion of arteries and arterioles, arrhythmias and conduction disturbances.

Pulmonary lesions occur in more than 50 percent of SLE patients. These include dyspnea, impaired diffusion capacity, impaired vital capacity, pneumonitis, pulmonary fibrosis and/or vaculitis.

Neurological lesions. Central nervous system involvement is frequent (up to 75 percent); SLE rarely affects the peripheral areas (8 percent in one study). Convulsive disorders and disturbances of mental function are the most common manifestations—the signs are referrable to the function of the cranial nerves. Other effects on the nervous system include hemiparesis and peripheral neuropathies (sensory or motor).

Gastrointestinal lesions including disturbed esophageal motility, nonspecific colitis, sometimes, "lupoid" hepatitis.

Eye lesions occur frequently, for example, retinopathy, and corneal involvement.

Since the advent of steroid therapy, the mean duration of SLE is six to eleven years. The disease is not considered nearly as serious or fatal as it used to be, probably because of earlier diagnosis and more effective therapy. The prognosis of the syndrome becomes increasingly poor according to the following:

1. Adults without renal disease.
2. Adults with renal disease.
3. Children without renal disease.
4. Children with renal disease.

There are several methods of treatment for patients with SLE who have severe involvement:

1. Corticosteroids. Prednisone may be given in moderate (10 to 15 mg per/day to 40 to 60 mg per/day) to massive doses (100 to 500 mg per/day). The largest doses are used to control severe convulsions.
2. Immunosuppressive agents. Azothioprine, either alone or with prednisone, may be given, in which case the dose of the steroid component may be decreased.
3. Avoidance of factors known to exacerbate SLE:
    a. infection
    b. physical stress
    c. emotional stress
    d. sunlight
    e. pregnancy—usually considered inadvisable; may be considered if patient is known SLE for at least three years and controlled on less than 15 mg corticosteroids daily.
    f. avoidance of drugs which initiate lupus syndrome in susceptible individuals.

NURSING MEASURES

Systemic lupus erythematosus is a long-term illness marked by acute physical and psychological crises. Therefore, nursing management can be of paramount importance in determining the quality of life the patient will lead. As is true for all the autoimmune diseases, the implications for nursing intervention for patients with SLE can be extrapolated largely from the clinical signs and symptoms. Thus, the nursing process, particularly assessment, becomes the mandatory approach to patient care. The nursing assessment should be multisystemic and detailed, covering physical, mental, emotional, and demographic components.

The nursing measures which follow are examples of areas of patient care which might be considered for the patient with SLE. Again, each patient's plan of care will depend upon the symptom complex presented by him at any given time.

1. Prophylaxis and health maintenance.
    a. Increased index of suspicion in high-risk groups.
    b. Avoidance of exacerbating factors.
    c. Patient teaching of measures on how best to attain and maintain optimal health status.
2. Patients whose major problem is renal dysfunction.
    a. Measures for conservative nursing management of renal insufficiency or failure secondary to SLE.
    b. Measures for the patient who undergoes peritoneal dialysis or hemodialysis.
    c. Nursing care of the patient who has a renal biopsy.
    d. See Chapter 17 on the patient with renal disease.
3. Measures to promote integrity of the skin.
    a. Patient education to avoid light if exposure aggravates pruritis.
    b. Use of agents such as Alpha-Keri to prevent dryness of skin.
    c. Cotton next to the skin.
    d. No extreme temperatures.
    e. Avoidance of soaps.
4. Measures for the patient who has a problem with the respiratory tract.

a. Goal: alleviate dyspnea, minimize respiratory insufficiency, prevent secondary infections.

b. Recognition of optimal activity levels.

c. Pulmonary toilette, positioning, respiratory therapy.

d. Education of the patient to prevent secondary infectious processes and to recognize and seek early management for those which do occur.

5. Measures concerned with the management of coagulation diatheses.

a. Conduct patient education.

1. Gentle mouth care and blowing of nose.

2. Care in use of sharp implements.

3. Avoidance of accidents—measures to prevent falls.

b. Minimize trauma associated with giving patient care.

1. Keep environment free of clutter.

2. Handle body parts with care.

3. Limit intramuscular and intravenous injections and carry out these techniques with caution.

4. Apply pressure to puncture sites for 3 to 5 minutes to prevent a hemotoma.

c. Observe for evidence of invisible bleeding.

1. Altered vital signs.

2. Evidence of blood in urine or stool.

3. Limit narcotics at times of suspected active bleeding.

6. Measures to prevent intracurrent infection of any type.

a. Patient teaching concerning meticulous hygiene, signs of infections.

b. Patient taught how to avoid being a carrier.

c. Early reporting of infections.

7. Measures related to problems with the gastrointestinal tract.

a. Anorexia—consider patient's preferences, small frequent meals, food from home.

b. Steroid ulcers—bland diet.

8. Care of the patient with CNS dysfunction.

a. Consider the patient's mental status when doing teaching—set realistic goals.

b. Let the patient set the pace in conversations—remain calm with him.

c. Consider both sensory and motor dysfunction when applying heat and cold.

d. Follow prophylactic measures including positioning, active and passive exercises, skin care to pressure sites, comfort devices.

e. Institute nursing measures with impending and actual convulsions.

9. Promotion of optimal cardiovascular status.

a. Close surveillance of vital signs.

1. Baseline data.

2. Consider quality.

b. Observe and institute appropriate measures for:

1. Congestive heart failure.

2. Thrombophlebitis.

3. Cellulitis post intravenous therapy and/or intramuscular injections.

4. Hypertension.

10. Nursing measures related to drug therapy.

a. All precautions for patients receiving steroid therapy and chemotherapy (See Chapter 18)

b. Individualized according to agents being given and patient's mental status.

11. Consider emotional lability and problems in other spheres of the patient's life when planning and giving care.

In carrying out the nursing process with the patient who has SLE, the professional nurse must bear in mind that the patient has a life-threatening problem that may be acute and/or chronic. One study done with adult patients cared for in a Philadelphia medical clinic revealed that they had five types of needs:

1. a trusting relationship
2. a skilled understanding of their behavior
3. a patient agent or advocate
4. medical technologies
5. medications

Of new patients, 91 percent needed medical technologies, so their needs fit well into the traditional medical roles of diagnosis and treatment. But, of returning patients, only 22 percent needed medical technologies, whereas almost four out of five patients had needs which fell into the sphere of nursing—concern with the total patient based on his individual problems.

Because autoimmune disease often assumes a chronic nature, the goal of nursing intervention is to assist the patient in achieving and maintaining a level of health which is optimal for him. This is not an easy task, for the nurse must be concerned with health problems resulting from a tremendous variety of inflammatory reactions. Thus, successful nursing care of the patient with an autoimmune disorder calls for an approach which is problem-oriented in nature and encompasses expertise in technical skills, health teaching, and development of supportive interactions. This is a venture which demands cooperative planning among the nurse, patient, family, and other members of the health team.

Conclusion

Immunology is presently occupying a position of tremendous influence upon health care, and it is an influence which is likely to be further enhanced in the forseeable future. What directions will immunology take in the next few decades? In general, it appears that there will be continued effort to find ways to selectively enhance or diminish the immune response. For example, in the presence of infectious diseases or tumors, effective therapy would depend upon enhancing the immune reaction, while in the case of autoimmune disease or allergy, a diminished response would be sought. Either type of therapeutic intervention would need to be selective in order to avoid abolishing useful and protective mechanisms of the immune process along with those that are undesirable. This is an extremely difficult feat; it becomes more and more evident that the development of the human immune process during the long course of evolution has resulted in "a complex interplay of different forms of immune responses that simultaneously deal with a wide variety of needs."[28] To manipulate these responses "requires a much more precise understanding of how they occur and what controls them than we now have."[29] We need to know much more about how the cells of higher organisms become specialized for their varied functions and how they interact with each other and their environment.

Immunology has come a long way in a relatively short period of time, and we have still arrived only at the beginning of understandings which will shed light on clinical problems. Continued research is certainly necessary. In this respect, Dr. Robert Good recounts an apt quote from a letter written by William Harvey in 1657:

> Nature is nowhere accustomed more openly to display her secret mysteries than in cases where she shows traces of her workings apart from the beaten path; nor is there any better way to advance the proper practice of medicine than to give our minds to the discovery of the usual law of nature, by the careful investigation of cases of rarer forms of disease. For it has been found in almost all things that what they contain of the useful or of the applicable is hardly perceived unless we are deprived of them, or they become deranged in some way.

References

1. Good, R. A.: Cancer therapy: antigens, antibodies, and beyond. Med. Dimensions Dec. 1972.
2. Bellanti, J. A.: Immunology. Philadelphia, W. B. Saunders, 1971, p. 92.
3. *Ibid.*, pp. 93–96, 99.
4. Cohen, S.: Structure and biological properties of antibodies. *In* M. A. Samter, et al. (eds): Immunological Diseases, ed. 2, Vol. 1. Boston, Little, Brown, 1971.
5. Bellante, *op. cit.*, p. 106.
6. *Ibid.*, p. 107.
7. *Ibid.*, p.108.
8. Samter, M. A., et al. (eds.): Immunological Diseases, ed. 2., Vol. I. Boston, Little, Brown, 1971.
9. Bellanti, *op. cit.*, p. 217.
10. *Ibid.*, p. 156.
11. *Ibid.*, p. 217.
12. *Ibid.*, pp. 150–157
13. Good, R. A. and Fisher, D. W. (eds.): Immunology. Stanford, Conn., Sinauer Associates, 1971, p. 12.
14. *Ibid.*, p. 13.
15. Samter, *op. cit.*, p. 511.
16. Good and Fisher, *op. cit.*, p. 12.
17. Samter, *op. cit.*, pp. 506–507.

18. *Ibid.*, pp. 506–510; and Good and Fisher, *op. cit.*, pp. 13–14.
19. Edelson, P. J.: Children Without Defenses. Emer. Med. Sept. 1972, p. 130.
20. *Ibid.*, p. 130.
21. Good and Fisher, *op. cit.*, p. 211.
22. Silverstein, M. and Morton, D.: Cancer immunotherapy Am. J. Nurs. 73, 7:1179, July 1973; and Bellanti, *op. cit.*, p. 323.
23. Silverstein, *op. cit.*, p. 1179; Good and Fisher, *op. cit.*, p. 15.
24. Bellanti, *op. cit.*, p. 331; Good and Fisher, *op. cit.*, p. 218; Silverstein, *op. cit.*, pp. 1179–1181.
25. Bellanti, *op. cit.*, p. 395.
26. Holman, H. R. *In* Samter, *op. cit.*, pp. 998–999.
27. Vaughn, J. *In* Samtee, *op. cit.*, p. 992.
28. Good, *op. cit.*
29. Humphrey, J. H.: What the future holds. World Health, June 1971, p. 26.

Bibliography

Amos, B., (ed): Progress in Immunology. New York, Academic Press, 1971.

Becker, E. L. and Austen, K. F.: Mechanisms of immunologic injury of rat peritoneal mast cells (I). J. Exp. Med. 124:369–395, 1966.

Humphrey, J. H. and White, R. G.: Immunology for Students of Medicine. Philadelphia, F. A. Davis, 1970 Chapter 9.

Ishizaka, K., Ishizaka, T., and Hornbrook, M. M.: Physicochemical properties of reaginic antibody. V. Correlation of reaginic activity with E-globulin antibody. J. Immunol. 97:840–853, 1966.

Ishizaka, K. and Ishizaka, T.: Biological function of E antibodies and mechanisms of reaginic hypersensitivity. Clin. Exp. Immunol. 6:25–42, 1970.

Ishizaka, T., Ishizaka, K., Orange R. P. and Austen, K. F.: The capacity of human immunoglobulin E to mediate the release of histamine and slow-reacting substance of anaphylaxis from monkey lung. J. Immuno. 104:335–343, 1970.

Nisonoff, A.: Molecules of immunity. *In* R. A. Good and D. W. Fisher (eds.): Immunobiology. Stamford, Conn., Sinauer Associates, 1971, Chapter 7.

Orange, R. P., Stechschulte, D. J. and Austen, K. F.: Immunochemical and biologic properties of rat IgE. II. Capacity to mediate the immunologic release of histamine and SRS-A. J. Immunol. 105:1087–1095, 1970.

Piper, P. J. and Vane, J. R.: The release of prostaglandins from lung and other tissues. Ann. NY Acad. Sci. 180:363–385, 1973.

Toward cancer control. Time, 19 March 1973.

23

Nursing Intervention for Patients with Allergic Disorders

KAY CORMAN KINTZEL

Immunologic Basis of Hypersensitivity • Substances which Act as Allergens • Anaphylaxis • Serum Sickness • Atopy • Infective Allergic Reactions • Objectives of Nursing Intervention for Allergic Patients

Allergy is perhaps the most variable of all diseases. It can appear and disappear like a magician's silk. It can change form like a chameleon, appearing in any organ system in any number of ways. It can masquerade as a cold, as bronchitis, as a stomachache, as a headache, as a skin rash, or a dozen other things. It may yield to one treatment and not to another. It may even disappear suddenly without treatment, only to reappear inexplicably months or years later under a different guise.
—Howard Rappaport
** Shirley Kinde**

Though protective immunity and allergy are products of the same biological process, those results of antigen-antibody interaction which benefit the individual are considered manifestations of immunity, while those which are harmful are considered manifestations of allergy. Accounts of maladies now recognized as allergic disorders have long been recorded in medical history, but little understanding of their nature took place until the rudiments of immunology appeared in the late 19th century. In 1906, Von Pirquet introduced the term allergy, taken from the Greek "allos" or other and "ergon" or action. He used the new word to signify an altered reaction of tissues to repeated contacts with infectious agents like bacteria and viruses and antigenic agents like tuberculin.[1] Since that time, the term has come to refer to a whole spectrum of hypersensitivity responses in which the tissues of an individual react to contact with some foreign agent (antigen) in a way that is definitely different from the way the tissues of most persons react. Thus, a person is said to be allergic or hypersensitive to chocolate if the ingestion of a small amount of it gives him unusual symptoms not experienced by the majority of people who eat chocolate. In this instance, chocolate is acting as an allergen, a term reserved for antigens which cause allergic symptoms.

Immunologic Basis of Hypersensitivity

Altered body tissue reactions may be local or systemic, and are mediated by either humoral or cellular agents. (For a discussion of the nature and distinctions of these immune mechanisms, see Chapter 22.) When referring to allergic manifestations, it is conventional to classify humoral immune phenomena as "immediate hypersensitivity" and cell-mediated events as "delayed hypersensitivity." This conveniently distinguishes reactions which may occur within minutes of exposure to an allergen from those which do not become manifest for 24 hours or more. These terms, immediate and delayed, do not alter a more important distinction between the two reactions—in the immediate type, passive transfer of hypersensitivity may be accomplished by means of serum alone, since antigen reacts with an antibody present in the circulation or fixed to tissue; in the delayed variety, sensitivity can be transferred only by means of lymphoid cells or cellular material.

The passive transfer of immediate hypersensitivity is aptly illustrated by the P-K reaction, first demonstrated in 1921 by Prausnitz and Küstner's classic experiment with each other. One of them had a clinical sensitivity to fish and a positive skin test to fish extract. When a small amount of his serum was injected into the skin of his colleague and this site plus several other skin sites were challenged with fish extract, a local inflammatory response occurred only where the serum had been injected.[2] Clinical manifestations of immediate hypersensitivity include anaphylactic reactions and all the atopic disorders.

Immediate hypersensitivity reactions correspond to those humoral immune responses classified as Type I, homocytotropic reactions. (See Chapter 22 for a detailed exposition of the types of immune responses which cause tissue damage.) There is little doubt that these reactions are mediated by reagins, now known to be immunoglobulin E, IgE. Minute amounts of IgE (0.03 ml per 100 ml) are found in the sera of normal individuals but the sera of atopic persons may contain up to six times the amount present in normal subjects. Evidence from various studies indicates that IgE is produced primarily in plasma cells located in the gastrointestinal mucosa and in tissues of the respiratory tract, including tonsils, adenoids, bronchial lymph nodes, and the respiratory mucosa.[3] It has been suggested that this accounts for the fact that many IgE-mediated allergic symptoms occur in these organ-systems. Although it is not yet clear just how IgE operates at the cellular level, it is thought that the combination of mast cell-bound IgE with a specific allergen initiates a change in the IgE molecular structure, which in turn causes a reaction at the surface of the mast cell. This surface reaction activates an enzyme system responsible for the release of histamine and other chemical mediators of allergic inflammation from the cell.

The prototype of delayed hypersensitivity is the tuberculin reaction, used extensively for diagnostic purposes. A person injected intracutaneously with a minute amount of growth products of the tubercle bacillus shows a typical local erythema, induration, and swelling in 48 hours if he is currently producing, or has ever produced, antibodies against the tubercle organism. Sensitivities of this type are developed in a wide variety of other infections, including some viral and fungal infestations, and, hence, may be detected by skin testing. Clinically, the nurse usually sees patients who manifest delayed hypersensitivity in the form of a contact dermatitis. Some food and drug reactions may also be due to delayed hypersensitivity, and the mechanism is pre-eminent in many autoimmune disorders.

Substances Which Act as Allergens

A formidable array of substances may prove to be antigenic to an allergic individual when inhaled, ingested, injected, or merely touched. Plant pollens are the principal offenders of antigens that cause allergic disease when inhaled. Philip Norman indicates that ragweed, widespread from late July to early September and a prolific producer of pollen containing a potent antigen, is the most common cause of hay fever in the United States.[4] He estimates that one single plant produces a billion grains of pollen and that one square mile of ragweed is reputed to produce 16 tons of it. Grasses are the second most common etiological agents in hay fever in the United States and the most frequent offenders in Europe where there is no ragweed. Tree pollens are less often the culprits in respiratory disease.

Plant pollens must share notoriety with molds, fungi, spores, animal danders, and parts of insects, all of which may be inhaled and cause respiratory allergy. House dust is a particular problem for many allergic persons. House dust extract is a mixture of epidermal products of man and animals, bacteria, molds, and degenerative products of fibrous material plants, food, and insects. Despite this wealth of suspects, the search for the antigenic factor(s) in house dust yielded small reward in the past. However, a study by Mitchell et al. at Ohio State University showed that the excretions and remains of disintegrated bodies of the common house mite *(D. farinae)* was the antigenic factor in the great majority of patients in the Central Ohio area who were clinically sensitive to house dust.[5] It is interesting to note that in this area the mite was usually found in mattresses or furniture stuffed with cotton fiber and used frequently by humans—daybeds were specifically cited.

Ingested allergens have not been subjected to as much biochemical study as inhaled antigens. Cow's milk is the most frequently suspected food allergy, and is known to contain at least 16 different antigens that will react with rabbit antiserum. In humans, about four of these are equally implicated, with a pattern of reaction that appears variable from person to person. Egg whites frequently cause allergic reactions, and urticarial responses may follow the ingestion of fish, shellfish, nuts, and fruit. In addition to antigens which may cause clinical allergic symptoms when inhaled or ingested, a veritable host of drugs and physical, or chemical, agents is capable of producing hypersensitivity reactions via injection or contact. Primary skin irritants include such common items as soaps, mineral oils,

and solvents, along with numerous industrial chemicals.

Anaphylaxis

The most dramatic and well-known expression of the immediate type of allergic response is anaphylaxis. This is essentially an "allergic shock" occurring in a sensitized individual, secondary to the precipitate release of large amounts of histamine. In humans the reaction produces urticaria, bronchiolar constriction, facial and laryngeal edema, and hypovolemia with peripheral circulatory collapse. Any of these features may predominate—the response may vary from mild to severe and involve one or many organ-systems. In severe cases, death has occurred within minutes as a consequence of asphyxia or circulatory collapse.

Prompt and vigorous intervention is necessary to prevent death in severe anaphylaxis, and in this situation the nurse should obtain medical help immediately. The nurse should be prepared to work with the physician in order to:

1. Maintain ventilation. Measures may include maintenance of a patent airway (particularly if the patient vomits or becomes unconscious), administration of oxygen, resuscitation, and the performance of an emergency tracheostomy if laryngeal edema is present and does not respond promptly to drug therapy.

2. Ameliorate hypovolemia and shock. This calls for the administration of an intravenous solution (usually 5 percent dextrose in water) to combat depressed blood volume and act as a vehicle for medications, and the intravenous administration of vasopressor agents. Concomitantly, close attention to vital signs is mandatory, and the usual supportive measures for shock are instituted.

3. Combat the allergic response. Epinephrine, which directly antagonizes the action of histamine, is given via the intravenous or intramuscular routes or both. Intravenous hydrocortisone has proved to be valuable as supportive therapy, and antihistaminic drugs may also be administered. Here again, it goes without saying that frequent checking of vital signs is

necessary to evaluate the patient's blood pressure and cardiorespiratory responses to these drugs.

Anaphylactic reactions may occur in response to insect stings or drug injections, including the commonly used penicillin, sulfonamides, hydantoin compounds, and intravenous contrast media containing iodides. Classically, the response is precipitated by the injection of foreign serum, as in antitoxin derived from horse serum. The administration of large amounts of horse serum compounds is preceded by skin or conjunctival sensitivity testing, a precautionary measure that warns of the possibility of the occurrence of a severe reaction. In addition, some reactions may be prevented by obtaining an allergic history before injecting a potentially hazardous antigen. Since persons who have a history of hyersensitivity reactions are more prone to develop anaphylaxis, extreme caution should be observed in administering these substances to them. It is unfortunate that there exists no rapid and reliable method for predicting penicillin sensitivity, considering the potential for sensitivity reactions to it. In the overwhelming majority of cases, it is generally agreed to be more prudent for the physician to administer a different class of antibiotic if there is a suspicion of penicillin sensitivity. (More detailed discussion of the medical and nursing management of anaphylaxis may be found in the bibliography following this chapter.)

Serum Sickness

Serum sickness is a hypersensitivity reaction which occurs several days after the first injection of a foreign serum into a sensitive person. It is considerably less common today than it was prior to the advent of routine immunization programs, and the widespread use of antibiotics and human antitetanus immunoglobulin. The usual etiological agent is tetanus antitoxin derived from horse serum, but antisera for botulism, gas gangrene, snakebite, and rabies may also produce the reaction. There is also a considerable number of serum sicknesslike reactions to various nonprotein drugs, especially penicillin. Primary serum sickness occurs from seven to ten days following serum injection and is characterized by fever, arthralgias, urticaria and other skin eruptions, and lymph node enlargement. If the reaction is severe, a variety of complications may ensue, inlcuding carditis, optic neuritis, brachial neuritis, nephritis, Guillain-Barré syndrome and periarteritis nodosa, while laboratory findings may reveal albuminuria, urinary casts, eosinophilia, and several types of circulating antibodies. Clinical management is symptomatic —epinephrine, antihistaminics, aspirin, antipruritics, and corticosteroids are the drugs most frequently indicated. As in anaphylaxis, the most effective treatment is prophylactic. For example, routine active tetanus immunization by means of tetanus toxoid makes the administration of antitoxin unnecessary.

Atopy

A large group of human allergies commonly encountered in clinical nursing practice is the result of an immediate hypersensitivity response and depends upon a common genetic predisposition. These allergies include bronchial asthma, hay fever, allergic rhinitis, atopic eczema, urticaria and angioedema—collectively known as the "atopic allergies." Atopy is also a convenient classification for denoting an immune mechanism frequently characterized by the presence of skin-sensitizing antibody inducing the Prausnitz Küstner reaction, and by immediate urticarial reactions to application of antigens to the skin.

HEREDITARY INFLUENCES
Those afflicted with atopic allergies do not inherit the disorder as such, but they do inherit the predisposition to develop hypersensitivity reactions. Sensitization may then manifest itself differently in each family member. Sheldon et al. indicate that there is currently no clear intimation of the factors that determine which tissue— nasal mucosa, bronchioles, skin, and so on—will respond to antigens in a given atopic individual.[6] However, it has been shown that about 50 percent of patients with asthma, hay fever, or other

atopy have a family history of allergic disease, as opposed to only 15 percent of the remaining population. Sherman reports that most investigators believe susceptibility to atopy to be determined by a single pair of genes, being manifested in the homozygous state.[7] Some heterozygotes also become atopic, but not all—the degree of penetration has been placed anywhere from 20 to 45 percent by various investigators. The mechanism of inheritance of atopy is not yet clear. Many or most atopic individuals are clinically sensitive to more than one agent, and the extent of sensitization varies from one time and situation to another. Also, although heredity plays a major role in atopic sensitization, the particular allergies developed depend on the antigens to which the individual is exposed and the intensity of this exposure. Thus determination of specific causes of allergic atopic disease presents a considerable challenge even to experts.

BASIC PATHOLOGY

The basic pathology encountered in this group of hypersensitive individuals is that of vasodilatation and increased capillary permeability, resulting in erythema and edema of the affected tissue. In bronchial asthma, hay fever, and allergic rhinitis there is also increased secretion of mucus, and in asthma, spasm of the smooth muscle of the bronchioles occurs. Consequently, in hay fever, for example, inhalation of seasonal pollens to which the patient has become sensitized, produces the familiar misery of repetitive sneezing, watery nasal discharge, excessive tearing, nasal obstruction, and perhaps itching of the orophyaryngeal mucosa. Understandably, this distressing pathology often produces the more general symptoms of malaise and irritability. Many of the symptoms of atopic allergy have been shown to be related to the presence of histamine, and in bronchial asthma to the release of slow-reacting substance as well (see Chapter 22).

The nurse should understand that allergy sufferers are prey to a variety of secondary factors which, together with a shared immunologic basis, produce clinical illness. This is the "total allergenic load" concept. As outlined in 1946 by Feinberg, this concept states that any individual reaction stems from immunologic causes which depend upon heredity, the individual's state of sensitization, and the current and cumulative effects of allergen exposure. However, many "precipitating elements" must be added to these—weather, infection, irritants, psychic state (tension, worry), endocrine factors, fatigue, exertion, and local trauma.[8] The symptoms of bronchial asthma, for example, frequently first become manifest after an acute respiratory infection, which apparently triggers a previously latent sensitization. (Table 23-1 gives a compilation of initiating, aggravating, and perpetuating factors in bronchial asthma.) It is not difficult to see why the manifestations of allergy are protean, varying considerably from individual to individual with puberty, menstruation, pregnancy, and menopause, as well as with life style and conditions of the external environment.

Infective Allergic Reactions

Among allergic patients there are many persons in whom reactions to external allergens cannot be demonstrated. These reactions ("intrinsic" reactions) are rather associated with various infections. They are frequently recurrent and usually affect the sinuses, oral cavity, or respiratory tract. Aspirin intolerance, often manifested by severe and intractable asthma occurring in nonatopic persons, is thought to be one of this group of reactions (see Table 23-1).

Most investigation has centered around the characteristics of intrinsic or infective bronchial asthma as opposed to those of atopic asthma. The infective form of asthma appears to be distinct from the atopic variety in a number of ways. The age of onset is often over 35 years, associated hay fever is uncommon, skin tests for sensitivity are negative except to bacterial antigens, skin-sensitizing antibody is absent, there is no response to antiallergic therapy, the patient's sputum often contains bacteria and leukocytes in addition to eosinophils, respiratory infection is primary rather than secondary to the disease, and the asthma is more commonly intractable and a cause of death. Although the association of respiratory infection with asthma symptoms is

TABLE 23-1
Initiating, Aggravating, and Perpetuating Factors in Bronchial Asthma

MECHANISM-ASSOCIATION	SETTING	DIAGNOSTIC STUDY	TREATMENT
Immunologic			
Immediate hypersensitivity (reagin-mediated)	Exposure to inhalant, ingestant or injected allergens precipitates asthmatic episode. Frequently associated rhinoconjunctivitis, urticaria, or anaphylaxis	Wheat-flare skin tests Inhalation/ingestion challenge	Avoidance of allergen Hyposensitization Symptomatic
Humoral antibody-mediated	Microbial colonization or organic dust contamination of the bronchial tree	Sputum smear/culture Serum precipitins Inhalation challenge	Antimicrobial Corticosteroid Avoidance of allergen
Infection			
Sinusitis	Obstruction of sinus drainage by inflammatory, allergic, or vasomotor reaction, or a combination of these	Transillumination Sinus x-rays Culture of aspirate	Drainage Antimicrobial
Upper-respiratory tract infection	Relapse of asthma coincides/follows "head cold"	Nose-pharynx examination Viral culture Viral serology	Symptomatic
Purulent sputum	Relapse of asthma coincides/follows change of sputum production/color	Sputum/transtracheal Smears, cultures	Antimicrobial Symptomatic
Postviral onset	"Flulike" syndrome evolves into persistent cough, then asthma	Viral serology	Symptomatic
Aspirin intolerance	Severe asthmatic episode follows ingestion of aspirin Frequently associated nasal polyps and sinusitis	If history negative, cautious aspirin challenge	Avoidance of aspirin Corticosteroids
Isoproterenol abuse syndrome	Increased use (frequency and dose) of nebulizer with decreased symptom relief	Isoproterenol inhalation challenge	Discontinue isoproterenol
Irritant inhalation	Smoke or other irritant exposure	History	Avoidance Symptomatic
Exercise	Increased physical activity	Treadmill exercise provocation	Exercise modification Symptomatic
Atmospheric change	Temperature, humidity or barometric pressure change	History	Symptomatic
Emotional	Emotional upset precedes relapse of asthma (not vice versa)	History	Symptomatic Psychotherapy
Associated disease			
Chronic bronchitis and emphysema	Acute bronchitis Precipitation of respiratory failure	Pulmonary function (irreversible airways obstruction, loss of elastic recoil)	As indicated
Cardiac disease ("cardiac asthma")	Cardiac failure	As indicated	As indicated
Esophageal disorder	Motility disturbance, acid reflux	As indicated	As indicated
Carcinoid tumor	Bronchial or systemic release of serotonin	Urinary 5-hydroxyindoleacetic acid	Surgery Symptomatic
Bronchial obstruction	Localized bronchial obstruction (foreign body, neoplasm)	Bronchoscopy	Surgery
Pulmonary embolus	Venous stasis/thrombosis	As indicated	As indicated
Unknown	Not recognized	Any of above if indicated	Symptomatic

Source: Mathison, D. A., et. al.: clinical profiles of bronchial asthma. JAMA 224:1135, May 21, 1973.

the hallmark of the problem, the role of infection in terms of etiology is not clear. There is controversy over whether the bacterial infective agent per se induces the allergic reaction or whether the infection is a nonspecific, secondary factor which increases the severity of the reaction by increasing the obstruction of bronchioles and the volume and tenacity of sputum. It is still uncertain whether bacterial allergy can induce asthma. But since the clinical signs and symptoms of the two types of asthma are indistinguishable, a common chemical mediator is presumed (see Table 23-1).

Objectives of Nursing Intervention for Allergic Patients

Allergic responses exhibited by individual patients are many and varied. Nevertheless, the adolescent who greets each spring with a dripping nose and an endless cascade of watery sneezes, the businessman plagued by an itchy rash a few hours after enjoying a good fish dinner, and the asthmatic housewife who wheezes and temporarily endures near suffocation each time she empties the vacuum cleaner bag, all share the same immunologic mechanism of altered sensitivity. The nurse is thus able to consider prevention and treatment for all allergic patients in terms of this mechanism, no matter how the problem is manifested in any particular patient. Nursing intervention involves instituting care and working in collaboration with the physician and other health team members to:

1. Help the patient separate himself from actual or potential offending antigens whenever possible.
2. Relieve the effects produced when the patient and offending antigens have not been, or cannot be, effectively separated.
3. Help the patient increase his resistance to offending antigens.

ENVIRONMENTAL CONTROL MEASURES

Perhaps the most important and challenging role the nurse has in caring for the allergic patient is that of exploring with him ways and means of increasing his comfort by reducing encounters with irritating environmental factors. It has been said that man is the only animal who is able to consciously tailor his environment to suit himself. For the individual afflicted with multiple allergies, however, such environmental engineering is not so easily accomplished. For example, many nurses have heard patients with allergic asthma recite the minor skirmishes and major battles they and their families wage daily with the environment—''I haven't been out of the house all summer—the pollens, you know,'' or ''I know it's my wife's favorite perfume, but the smell irritates me so much I can hardly stand it.''

Much like the diabetic patient, the allergic patient must learn to live as constructively as possible with his problems. There is no room for mystery. He should be encouraged to learn as much as possible about the vagaries of his disorder, so that he can manage each situation as it arises without undue dismay or panic. The knowledgeable and supportive nurse can be an invaluable health team member in efforts to help the patient develop a healthy consciousness of the factors in his particular life style which may precipitate allergic attacks. This must be a cooperative venture between health personnel and patient. A rigid program resulting in barracks-style living is to be avoided, since it will probably result in frustration and the eventual creation of bigger problems than those it was intended to circumvent.

Hospital Care

When the allergic patient is hospitalized, the nurse often has the responsibility for maintaining his immediate surroundings in as allergen–free a state as possible. This is not always easily accomplished. Simply having the patient in a private room bare of excess furnishings, where temperature and humidity are regulated, may not even begin to provide an optimum environment. For example, Mrs. B., a 35-year-old housewife who was recovering from an acute bronchial asthma attack was placed in such a room by her physician to ''minimize irritating factors.'' However, when the author visited Mrs. B. she discovered that the patient was actually surrounded by allergens. Mrs. B. volunteered that she had first noted asthma symptoms when working in her garden. Misguided friends, knowing of her hobby, had sent many growing plants and flowers to cheer her. These she kept at the far end of the room "where I can see them but where they won't bother me so much." She also kept a variety of cosmetics in plain sight—including an open box of face powder and a host of perfumes. House-keeping personnel had just completed dusting the venetian blinds with a dry cloth, effecting a visible shower of dust particles throughout the room. Mrs. B. said that this had just caused a "coughing spell," so the housekeeper had opened the window to give her some fresh air. Thus easy access for pollens was provided. Finally, although the patient's chart revealed that she was allergic to feathers, observation of the "tight" plastic covering on her feather pillow disclosed a large rip along the seam.

Once these allergenic factors were recognized, the nursing team, in collaboration with Mrs. B.'s physician and other personnel, found that they could be eliminated rather easily. It was arranged to damp dust all items in her room while she was absent, an intact plastic cover was secured for her mattress, arrangements were made to have her husband bring the nonallergenic pillow she used at home, and efforts were made to minimize noise and limit the numerous visitors, which, the patient frankly stated, she found to be "bothersome." Nurses also observed Mrs. B. closely after administering ordered medications, in order to evaluate her response, in light of previous known reactions, to a number of drugs. When the patient became more comfortable, she readily complied with suggestions that she put away the cosmetics and remove the plants with which she had hated to part. It was decided to replace the latter with bouquets of bright paper flowers, much to Mrs. B.'s pleasure. Full cooperation of the patient is often better secured if reasonable attempts are made to apply easier control measures first. Also, as pointed out by Landrum, in removing the patient from the irritant, the nurse tries to help the patient find satisfaction in acceptable substitutes.[9]

Home Care

The nurse might now begin to think about helping a patient like Mrs. B. to be more comfortable in her home when she leaves the hospital. In developing a structured teaching program for a particular patient concerning environmental control, the nurse must consider the patient's present readiness and desire to learn, the extent and correctness of his previous knowledge, his habits, and the family constellation involved. If the patient is a young child, the teaching approach to the parents must be carefully considered on an individual basis. Observant, informed parents can often best determine the cause of the child's allergic reactions, and, once the offending substances have been removed, they are able to do the most to ensure the success of any treatment regimen. Discussion with the patient's physician should include talking about his experiences with the patient, his knowledge of the extent of the patient's allergies, and his plans for medical management. All this is obviously an involved undertaking, and one that cannot be profitably accomplished in a short space of time. However, after organizing a plan and enlisting the aid of appropriate personnel, many opportunities are available for the busy nurse to introduce segments of teaching within the context of meeting the patient's daily physical needs.

If collection of data is needed to establish cause-effect relationships between any environmental agent and the patient's symptoms, the patient may be asked to list factors he knows or thinks may cause trouble, and a reasonable means of avoiding or mitigating these can be discussed. Frequently, more attention to removing allergens from the patient's bedroom at home is the primary requirement for comfortable living, and elimination measures in the remainder of the home need not be so stringent. Dacron bed pillows are recommended, since foam rubber pillows may grow molds within the pores as they age. The patient should avoid using bed pads, comforters, woolen blankets, chenille bedspreads, and the mattress and box springs (unless composed of nonallergenic materials) should be enclosed in airtight plastic covers. Washable throw rugs and decorative vinyl shades or lightweight washable curtains should be substituted for wall to wall carpeting and heavy draperies. The patient should indulge elsewhere any fondness for numerous items of furniture (especially the overstuffed variety) and knicknacks. Keeping the bedroom window open at night is not a healthy practice for the pollen- and spore-sensitive individual, regardless of its benefits to others.

Temperature

Some patients have identified the heating and cooling systems within their homes as sources of difficulty. Forced-air systems are the worst offenders for those allergic to house dust, since the convection currents keep dust particles constantly in motion. If such a system is present, outlets or registers might be covered with a filter. If finances permit, central electronic precipitator-filters are available and may be added to the heating system for a few hundred dollars. The use of air-conditioning for allergic individuals does not provide a panacea, since it may also act to circulate considerable dust. However, Feinberg[22] has aptly pointed out that air-conditioning in the broad sense of mechanical maintenance of optimum temperature, water and particle content, electrical charge, and barometric pressure of the air we breathe, offers special benefits for allergic patients.[10] Rapid changes in room temperature or too high or too low humidity, both of which often result in allergic flareups, can be avoided through proper air-conditioning.

Animals

Since animal danders are a common source of allergens, hypersensitive patients should be warned against acquiring pets, if they do not already have them. If sensitivity to a pet is suspected, patients may be urged to "farm out" the animal for awhile, or at least keep the pet strictly out of doors. If is often difficult to separate an allergic patient and a beloved pet. In some instances, tropical fish, turtles, or domestic animals to which the patient is not allergic may be satisfactorily substituted. (Although, as one young asthmatic told his mother, "It's hard to love turtles."[23])

Smoking

Smoking is intolerable for many allergic patients, and is particularly undesirable for those with bronchial asthma, because it causes considerable irritation of the respiratory tract. Sheldon et al. aptly state that "In smoking, one voluntarily creates for himself far more air pollution than he would be exposed to from outside sources."[11] It must also be remembered that although allergic individuals may not smoke, they often live with family members who do. The husband of Mrs. S., an allergic wife, deeply resented her habit of watching him carefully as he smoked, then immediately rushing to dispose of ashes as soon as he stubbed the offending cigarette. The tension created in this situation aggravated her allergies quite as effectively as did the inhalation of tobacco smoke and ash particles.

Other Irritants

If the nurse is a sympathetic listener, problems of employment, family or marital life may be unburdened. Sometimes airing and sharing the problem is all that is needed in order to see irritations in proper perspective, and to find ways to approach and alleviate frustrating situations. Mr. T., for example, who was sensitive to the odor of glue and paint, revealed somewhat bitterly that his family was unhappy with him because he had forbidden his young son to pursue a favorite hobby of building model airplanes. After talking about this, Mr. T. himself suggested that perhaps the family had not explored sufficient alternatives to simple elimination, and mused that maybe a workshop could be set up for the boy in the loft of the family garage. In caring for the allergic patient in whom emotional factors predominate, the nurse must, of course, recognize appropriate limits in nursing function. The most helpful course may be to recognize when specific psychotherapeutic intervention is indicated and find proper ways to initiate such help.

The allergic child with asthma may encounter problems in his school environment as well as in the home, so the school nurse should be apprised of his particular problem. If the nurse is aware of stimuli which usually generate an adverse reaction in a particular child, she is able to work closely with the child and his teachers to avoid attacks, minimize symptoms, and act appropriately if an emergency arises. For example, it has been pointed out that class projects involving oil paints and turpentine could prove irritating. In such cases, acrylics or watercolors might be substituted. In addition, the school nurse may be an appropriate monitor with regard to physical education, advising gymnastics teachers and providing support and counseling for the child who finds lengthy periods of exercise too demanding.

PSYCHOLOGICAL COMPONENTS OF ALLERGY

Much has been written about the psychological components of allergic disease, with particular stress being placed on the role of these factors in bronchial asthma. Hippocrates, in his early writings, said that "the asthmatic must guard against anger," and Osler stated that asthma was a "neurotic affection."[12] Although a few psychiatrists and allergists may maintain that asthma is primarily a psychosomatic illness, most have now come to recognize the importance of the immunologic basis of the disorder. While psychic stresses have a definite role in triggering asthmatic symptoms, psychological components are not regarded as the prime etiological agent in producing the disease.

Generally, allergic patients might be classified according to placement along a hypothetical continuum, in which emotional factors exert little influence in the disease process in those at one end of the spectrum, and assume a great deal of importance in those at the opposite end. Such a classification should not be regarded as static—a given patient might move in either direction along the continuum from one point to another and from one life situation to another. This concept corresponds well with the "total allergenic load" theory described earlier in this chapter.

McGovern and Knight point out that ". . . external stresses most frequently incriminated in allergic disease have been those of parental rejection (usually maternal), overprotection (usually maternal), and emotional instability of the entire family or in the immediate environment."[13] Perhaps the most classic example of the role of maternal rejection in precipitating asthma attacks is found in the report of French and Alexander in 1941.[14] They studied 27 asthmatic patients with demonstrated allergic hypersensitivity and found that these patients exhibited a common pattern of fear of physical separation from the mother, as well as fear of loss of maternal love and approval, due to possession of impulses which the patients felt would repulse or shock her. French and Alexander believed that these patients showed a strong urge to confess their thoughts, cry, and obtain forgiveness, but were blocked from doing so because the sinful nature of these thoughts might precipitate the rejection that was feared in the first place. Thus these investigators felt that the anxiety-provoked urge to confess and cry was blocked by an equal anxiety that the confession would be rejected, and that the asthmatic wheeze represented the suppressed cry for the mother. Since this hypothesis was formulated, numerous attempts have been made to correlate a specific personality constellation with asthmatic symptoms. Unfortunately, the situation is not so simple; although certain general connections have been confirmed in different studies, attempts to correlate specific personality patterns with particular allergic manifestations have led to little agreement among investigators.

Certainly any chronic illness can place excessive strain on the family unit. In the case of the asthmatic child, the parents' attitudes toward the child are conditioned by his illness and the additional burden involved in caring for him. The mother may consciously or unconsciously resent this dependent and insecure child, and the resentment and rejection may be sensed by the child and cause continued wheezing. Fontana suggests that parents should be taught to adopt a casual attitude toward the child, to avoid discussing his condition in his presence, and to allow his activities to be as unrestricted as possible, while supporting him when he feels distressed at not being able to keep up with others.[15] However, the asthmatic child needs extra rest and protection from excessive activity forced on him by siblings or classmates. The parents should recognize the importance of extra daily rest and be assisted by the physician and nurse in scheduling it. Empathy and understanding on the part of all health team members form the cornerstone of successful management.

FOOD

Almost any food may cause an allergic reaction of some kind, although foods such as nuts, berries, seafood, cereals, milk, eggs, and chocolate are prominent offenders. The keeping of a "diet diary" of foods eaten and exact times at which symptoms occur may be recommended by the patient's allergist. The allergist may also place some patients on elimination diets. There are a number of ways to effect such a diet, but two common approaches include either eliminating all commonly allergenic foods, and having the patient observe his reactions as he adds one previously restricted food at a time to his regimen, or eliminating one food at a time from the usual diet and instructing the patient to observe his reactions for a period after each eliminatory measure. The key to success in any dietary regimen lies primarily in the hands of the patient and his family. If the patient is merely handed a diet list and sent on his way without thorough supportive instruction, the procedure is likely to be carried out incorrectly, necessitating a complete repeat of the whole process. The physician, nurse, dietitian, patient, and the patient's family must work together to avoid undue frustration and to insure success.

According to Mathews, experience with evaluation of food allergy has yielded the following observations:

1. Patient's food likes and dislikes do not correlate well with clinical sensitivity.
2. Patient's food suspects may be correct but are also often influenced by suggestion.
3. Skin tests are not, on the whole, good indicators of clinical sensitivity to food.
4. Diet diaries are an aid for determining foods causing intermittent urticaria, but frequently fail in determining food factors in atopic respiratory disease.
5. Success in using elimination diets depends on the timing of the procedure, so that other variables are minimized, in addition to the proper manipulation of foods.
6. The longer the time required for symptomatic improvement from an elimination diet, the more likely it is that the improvement is due to other factors or to a natural remission of the disease.
7. The longer the period of time between reintroduction of a food and the appearance of symptoms, the more likely it is that the symptoms are not due to ingestion of the food.[16]

The nurse should remember that it is not always easy for the allergic patient to avoid certain foods, even when he is quite aware of his sensitivity to them. For example, Mr. R., a man conscious of his hypersensitivity to nuts and nut products, unexpectedly experienced swelling of the oropharyngeal mucosa after eating a fried fish dinner at a seafood restaurant. Unknown to him, the chef at the establishment always used peanut oil for frying the fish. Individuals like Mr. R. do well to cultivate the habit of discreet inquiry as to the nature of foods served to them, both in restaurants and by hostesses who may be unaware of the existence of their guests' allergies to certain food ingredients. Likewise, these patients and their family members should be aware of the need to scan the list of ingredients contained in packaged foods purchased at the supermarket.

ATOPIC ECZEMA

Infantile eczema is a frequent manifestation of atopy. The most common sensitizations are to foods, such as milk, eggs, wheat, and fish liver oils, although the atopic infant may also become sensitive to any of the innumerable pollens, molds, spores, or dusts to which he is normally exposed. The baby with eczema may follow a variety of pathways during his lifetime with respect to his atopy—the eczema may clear spontaneously or as a result of dietary changes; the eczema may persist into adulthood as atopic dermatitis; or respiratory allergies (asthma and hay fever) may develop, either alone or simultaneously with cutaneous manifestations. Although sensitization does not follow exposure in a regular fashion, many authorities recommend that infants with a strong family history of atopy or a known tendency to atopic disorders be kept from contact with potential allergens. This course of action is based on the thought that intensity of exposure to antigens is an important factor in determining the likelihood of clinical sensitization, especially in individuals of heterozygous genetic makeup.

To illustrate such a preventive regimen, the author will describe her experience with her

an aerosol containing epinephrine or iso-proterenol. The nurse may render invaluable assistance to these patients by teaching proper use of the hand nebulizer. If used promptly when "wheezing" begins, the inhaler often prevents development of asthmatic paroxysms. Hence, use of the nebulizer should not be considered a last-ditch reserve, patient-initiated treatment. Nor should it be viewed as a nearly constant support, so that the patient becomes inhaler-dependent. Indeed there is evidence that excessive use of isoproterenol aerosol over a prolonged period may precipitate airway obstruction that is similar to the very asthmatic attacks for which it would commonly be prescribed as therapy. According to Fontana, side effects of excessive use of bronchodilator nebulizers include psychological dependency, progressively shortened duration of drug effectiveness, toxicity involving tachycardia and arrhythmias, development of a refractory state to other forms of antiasthmatic medication, irritative bronchitis and excessive drying of respiratory mucosa, and a "rebound effect" of transient bronchodilation followed by bronchoconstriction.[22]

The nebulizer must be used properly to avoid loss of medication in the atmosphere or by precipitation on the oral mucosa. The patient's lips should be enclosed around the mouthpiece of the inhaler, which in turn should be pointed neither upward nor downward. The inhaler should then be activated, releasing the medicated mist *as* the patient inhales deeply.

The nurse may also be responsible for teaching some patients, as well as a family member to inject epinephrine preparation subcutaneously in order to cope with acute attacks. In this case, the nurse should remember to give the learner opportunity to practice such procedures often enough to ensure sufficient competence to carry them out, even in the face of anxiety-producing dyspnea or severe allergic symptoms. The patient and family members should be given the opportunity to express opinions, fears, and superstitions with respect to oral or injectable medications received by the patient. McGovern and Knight feel that in their experience the most "feared" medication is epinephrine. Because the

patient may experience an increased pulse rate, precordial throbbing, or transient facial pallor after administration, either he or his family may come to fear that damage to the heart is occurring. These authors aptly point out that ". . . it is unfortunately true that many times family members will adjust dosages, substitute medication and alter the therapeutic regimen in other ways because of private convictions, stubbornly and secretly maintained, and often at the expense of the atopic subject."[23]

Corticosteroid drugs are now widely used for allergic dermatitis, hay fever, acute and chronic bronchial asthma, and drug reactions. The mechanism by which these medications help the allergic patient is not clearly understood, but their dramatic effectiveness in bringing status asthmaticus to an end when other measures fail, and their alleviation of many chronic allergic symptoms is not questioned. In general, the physician must carefully weigh possible benefits of steroid therapy against the well-known dangers engendered by continued use of these drugs. (The challenges and difficulties of the nurse's role in aiding patients receiving corticosteroids are discussed in Chapter 18.) Rodman and Smith mention that aerosol steroid treatment may be used in order to attain a high local concentration in the lungs, with the result that patients so treated seem to require less oral systemic steroid preparation.[24]

Cromolyn sodium, a drug obtained from the seeds of an Eastern Mediterranean plant (ammi visnaga) and synthesized into a compound that is distinct from the bronchodilators, the antihistamines, and the corticosteroids, has recently been shown to be effective in the treatment of bronchial asthma. Taken on a daily basis (even when the patient feels well) it inhibits the release of histamine and SRS-A in the lung and acts to prevent acute asthmatic attacks. It does not alleviate an acute attack of asthma in progress. The drug is administered via a special inhaler, designed to puncture a capsule that releases a fine mist of white powder which the patient inhales.

Cromolyn has been particularly helpful in allowing decreased long-term maintenance requirements of steroids. It is now marketed under the names Aarane and Intal and is proving a useful adjunct in the treatment of asthma, especially the seasonal childhood variety of the disease.[25]

While drugs are an invaluable aid in the treatment of sensitivity reactions, these very reactions may in fact be precipitated by drugs. Allergic manifestations secondary to drugs differ from drug toxicity reactions in a number of ways. The hallmarks of the allergic drug reaction are pointed out by Parker and are summarized here. Drug reactions due to hypersensitivity may be characterized by:

1. Having no linear relationship to drug dosage, often being precipitated by small amounts of drug.
2. Requiring an induction period on primary exposure but not upon being administered a second time.
3. Occurring in a minority of patients receiving the drug, with few exceptions.
4. Having no correlation with known pharmacological properties of the drug.
5. Usually reappearing on readministration of the drug in smaller amounts than were previously given.
6. Frequently including as clinical manifestations of the reaction such features as anaphylaxis, serum sickness, urticaria, contact dermatitis, and asthma.[26]

The clinical syndromes of drug allergy are legion. In addition to the features mentioned in item six above, the following have been reported as drug sensitivity reactions: erythema nodosum and multiforme, photosensitivity, thrombocytopenia, agranulocytosis, aplastic anemia, hemolytic anemia, acute and chronic vasculitis, syndromes resembling systemic lupus erythematosus, hepatic damage, fevers, acute interstitial nephritis, lymphadenopathy, and cardiopathy of various types. The nurse must be particularly alert in observing known atopic patients for the appearance of allergic drug reactions.

ACUTE BRONCHIAL ASTHMA

Moody has presented the pathophysiology of status asthmaticus in relation to the changes which occur in lung mechanics, arterial blood gases and ventilation/perfusion ratios. Salient points are summarized here.

1. Lung Mechanics
   a. Marked increase in expiratory flow resistance results from airway obstruction.
   b. Decreased FEV^1 occurs secondary to (a). (There is a severe reduction in the amount of air that can be forcefully and rapidly expelled in one second.)
   c. Increased functional residue capacity (FRC) becomes evident as a result of (b). The amount of gas in the lungs at the end of a normal quiet inspiration is appreciably greater than normal.
   d. Increased dynamic compliance of the lungs occurs secondary to bronchial constriction. More pressure is required to distend the alveoli to the same volume; concomitant loss of alveolar wall elasticity results in slower emptying.
   e. Increased oxygen requirement comes about because of extreme expiratory effort. Vital capacity and forced expiratory volume are decreased; tidal volume may be reduced and the total amount of air reaching the alveoli decreased, resulting in inefficient O_2-CO_2 exchange (see Chapter 16).
2. Arterial blood gases
   a. Arterial Pco_2 may be normal (35 to 45 mm Hg) or somewhat reduced early in the acute attack. As status asthmaticus proceeds, hyperventilation may result in respiratory alkalosis (arterial pH above 7.45); hypoventilation secondary to mucus plugging and airway obstruction will result in respiratory acidosis (arterial pH less than 7.35). (See Chapter 16 for an extended discussion of acid-base anomalies and arterial blood gas changes.)
   b. Hypoxemia may occur. Minor effects become evident with an arterial Po_2 less than 70 mm Hg at sea level; marked effects occur when the Po_2 falls below 45 mm Hg.
3. Ventilation/Perfusion Ratio
   a. Ventilation may be decreased in relation to perfusion, ushering in hypoxemia and hypercapnia. The situation is reflected in an alteration of the Va/Qc ratio, in which the

normal ratio of ventilation (alveolar air flow) to perfusion (blood flow through the plulmonary capillaries) is 5.1 to 6.0 liters or 0.8 to 08.5. This occurs secondary to increased airway resistance and altered dynamic compliance.

b. Depletion of surfactant may become evident if the Va/Qc ratio is not corrected. Atelectatic areas ensue throughout the lungs.[27]

Prompt, vigorous treatment by medical and nursing personnel is mandatory for the acutely ill asthmatic patient who arrives at the hospital in a state of status asthmaticus. In fact, in this case the patient is sufficiently ill that he will probably have difficulty simply getting to the hospital. Asthmatics who live alone or who have no easy access to a car should be provided with the telephone number of the nearest ambulance or rescue squad. The nurse usually finds that such a patient is pale, perspiring, and fully engaged with the formidable task of breathing through an airway strictured by smooth muscle spasm and occluded by thick, tenacious sputum. His audible wheezing is more marked during expiration, which is prolonged and often incomplete. Often he is unable to talk because of severe coughing spasms. This is a distraught, agitated, and frequently exhausted patient, and real relief cannot be expected until he is both mentally and physically at ease. The reassuring and confident attitudes of ministering personnel are all-important in helping the anxious patient secure the rest he needs. Many of these patients arrive at the hospital emergency room in the middle of the night, after repeated efforts to obtain enough relief from symptoms to allow sleep have proven fruitless. The nurse, by decreasing the patient's anxiety, may lessen the physiological severity of the attack. Anxiety which causes overbreathing leads to increased air resistance and greater use of accessory muscles of respiration; shallow, rapid respiration likewise results in an increased arterial carbon dioxide tension. Mild sedation or tranquilizing medication is often necessary, but it does not supplant the equal necessity for continued calm reassurance as various care measures are instituted. Any sedation ordered by the physician to be given "as necessary" should be administered by the nurse only when judged to be essential for providing rest and calm, since respiratory depression must be avoided. Allergists feel that overmedication of any sort should be avoided, since often before entering the hospital, the patient either has taken antiasthmatic medication himself or has been given a variety of drugs by a physician. In many cases, simply discontinuing these drugs will result in symptomatic improvement.

A nurse should remain with the patient until severe symptoms are under control. If continuous surveillance is impossible, the nurse should provide an easy means for the patient to call and observe him at frequent intervals even when he does not call. Mounting fear occasioned by breathlessness tends to trigger new paroxysms. In observing the patient, the nurse should be aware that what may superficially appear to be a lessening of agitation or relaxed somnolence might actually represent quietness stemming from exhaustion and anoxia. This dangerous combination sometimes results in sudden death, just as the patient appears to be improving. Also, night duty personnel should always observe the patient with the lights turned on, since developing or deepening cyanosis cannot be seen by flashlight. The patient secures most effective rest in a sitting position. In fact, it has been said that no one suffering a true attack of asthma voluntarily lies down, unless completely exhausted. The nurse can help the patient to assume a comfortable orthopneic position, leaning slightly forward over an overbed table topped with a foam pillow. This position allows fullest utilization of the accessory muscles of respiration.

ADEQUATE HYDRATION

Statistics indicate that the most common immediate cause of death in acute bronchial asthma is suffocation from dry, hard bronchial mucous plugs. Therefore, measures to liquify the sputum are often lifesaving. Adequate hydration is one way to combat the problem. These patients are frequently extremely dehydrated, secondary to curtailment of eating, drinking, loss of water in perspiration, and exhaled air. Further, electrolyte imbalances and acidosis may be present.

The nurse is responsible for accurate administration of ordered parenteral fluids and intelligent monitoring of intake and output, in light of the patient's overall condition. (See Chapter 16 for a detailed discussion of the nursing measures related to problems of fluid-electrolyte imbalance and the administration of parenteral fluids.) The patient may be too dyspneic to take large amounts of fluid by mouth, but judiciously spaced sips of liquid are often encouraged. Iced fluid is generally avoided, since it may cause reflex bronchospasm.

Expectorants and mucolytic agents, such as potassium iodide or glyceryl guaiacolate, are given the patient as an adjuvant to hydration, in order to thin secretions and help him cough productively. Bronchodilating agents are employed after the problem of secretions has been dealt with. Sheldon et al. reiterate that status asthmaticus patients fail to repond to epinephrine, and that, therefore, aminophylline, either intravenously or via retention enema, is usually required.[28] Hydrocortisone or ACTH via the intravenous or intramuscular route may be administered if the patient fails to respond to other measures, and may dramatically improve the patient's condition in a short time. Here again, the effectiveness of the treatment with parenteral aminophylline or steroid depends upon careful monitoring of the rate of administration and alert observation of the patient's reactions. Further illustration of all these principles may be found in Moody's discussion of the medical and nursing history of a patient with asthma, and in Mathison, et al., "Clinical Profiles of Bronchial Asthma."[29]

OTHER SUPPORTIVE MEASURES

Other supportive measures for the patient in status asthmaticus may include:
1. Maintenance of environmental control, as previously described.
2. Control and elimination of infection. Febrile patients with purulent sputum are often given broad spectrum antibiotics, while the results of sputum culture are awaited. Penicillin is frequently avoided, because of the potential for severe sensitivity reactions to it. Prevention of infection, and prompt alleviation of infection already present, is especially important. There is some evidence that asthma uncomplicated by a significant infectious component does not lead to deterioration of breathing mechanics or to pulmonary emphysema. If the patient frequently experiences asthma attacks following upper respiratory infections, the physician may use tetracycline or another broad spectrum antibiotic without waiting for the development of fever, leukocytosis, purulent sputum, and the other usual indications for antibiotic therapy. The patient should be taught to avoid unnecessary exposure and chilling, and to seek prompt treatment from his physician if even a minor cold occurs.
3. Administration of oxygen with controlled humidity to help combat anoxemia. The nurse should be thoroughly familiar with use of the intermittent positive pressure breathing apparatus and other oxygen delivery equipment, since the patient often displays nervousness about using it if he feels that personnel caring for him do not completely understand how to operate such machinery. (A detailed discussion of management of the patient receiving oxygen therapy is found in Chapter 14.) Intermittent positive pressure breathing treatments with inhalation of a solution of isoproterenol and alevaire, usually given for about 10 to 20 minutes four times daily, often greatly facilitate relief of bronchospasm and expectoration of tenacious sputum. (However, it should be remembered that the anxious patient in the most acute throes of status asthmaticus frequently does not accept or tolerate intermittent positive pressure treatments.) If the patient is cyanotic, continuous oxygen may be given between positive pressure treatments. The nurse should also be alert to the danger of carbon dioxide retention in the acutely ill asthmatic patient with a significant degree of superimposed chronic emphysema, particularly if he is receiving high concentrations of oxygen via mask or tent. (See Chapter 14 for discussion of hypoxic respiratory drive in chronic lung disease.)
4. Other measures to maintain ventilation. In extreme cases, a tracheostomy may be necessary to maintain a patent airway. Bronchoscopy may

also be performed to remove thick, inspissated secretions. In some instances, general anesthesia must be administered to panicky patients, so that the work of breathing may be effectively and automatically carried out by a respirator.

5. Breathing exercises and postural drainage. Patients with long-standing asthma, who have a superimposed emphysematous component, may benefit from exercises to encourage complete emptying of the lungs in the expiratory phase of respiration, and to facilitate use of the diaphragm and abdominal muscles of respiration. Following postural drainage, percussion and vibration, deep breathing or coughing therapy, auscultation of the patient's chest will reveal if the treatment has been effective. Rales and rhonchi should be decreased, breath sounds improved in quality. (See Chapter 12 for a discussion of chest auscultation.)

6. Teaching. The asthmatic who is recovering from a severe attack will need teaching if he is to manage his continued care at home. Such teaching should, of course, be tailored to the individual's particular needs and include detailed information regarding his use of drugs, oxygen therapy, or nebulizers, as well as environmental engineering measures to help prevent or abort future attacks. The importance of follow-up care should be emphasized.

DESENSITIZATION

The final major goal for the nurse's consideration in caring for the allergic patient is that of helping him to increase his resistance to offending antigens. The procedure of desensitization helps to accomplish this by administration of small but increasing doses of a specific antigen over a period of time. This was described by Noon in 1911, and has been used by allergists since then with varying success.[30] Several studies have shown that the treatment leads to statistically significant symptomatic improvement of ragweed hay fever in adults.[31] Controlled studies of such immunotherapy for bronchial asthma and allergens other than ragweed are meager. "Since 1955 it has been recognized that treatment of allergic individuals with a series of injections of the offending allergens leads to the formation of an additional humoral antibody, termed blocking antibody, capable of neutralizing the allergen."[32] The effectiveness of this therapy is thought to be due to the blocking effect of this antibody, now known to be IgG, with reaginic antibody. Richardson points out that desensitization therapy continues "to be more art than science, although science is gaining."[33] The state of immunotherapy for allergic disease is not such that allergists speak of cures. According to Dr. Philip Norman, "the fact is that you don't cure, but immunotherapy makes it better for the patient; he's more comfortable and less sick, even though he is still allergic. And, we know that during treatment the basophils are less and less sensitive to allergic attack. Each year, the spikes in IgE that usually accompany exposure to a particular allergen or allergens grow smaller and eventually serum IgE directed toward the allergen declines. In the months following cessation of therapy, we have also found that IgE antibody levels decline and the clinical situation begins to revert."[34]

Though the exact mechanism of protection afforded by the injection of repeated and progressive doses of antigen is still indefinite, it is known that the schedule of doses must be adjusted by the allergist to the degree of sensitivity of the particular patient. "Too large a dose may cause a serious and even fatal reaction, too small a dose cannot be expected to produce the desired reduction in sensitivity."[35]

Desensitization is preceded by skin testing, in which the detection of the presence of a particular atopic reagin in the patient's skin is afforded by introduction of an aqueous solution of antigen into the dermis. This is usually done in the skin over the patient's back by:

1. The prick or scratch method, in which a needle is used to scratch the skin through a drop of the antigen-containing solution.

2. The intracutaneous method, in which a small amount of allergen solution is injected superficially into the epidermis.

A positive reaction, indicating, that the patient has antibodies for the allergen in his skin, is indicated either by a reddened, flushed area or a blanched wheal at the test site. A panel of these skin tests is usually "read" by the allergist within 20 minutes. The intracutaneous method is both the more sensitive and the more dangerous, and thus may require some precautions. Sheldon et al., recommend that when the intracutaneous method is used, or the dose of allergen to be given is a concentrated one, the skin of the forearm should be used and a tourniquet made available for application proximal to the test site to help prevent systemic reactions.[36] Severe anaphylactic-type reactions are also countered by the administration of systemic epinephrine and antihistamines, as well as intravenous hydrocortisone if necessary.

When desensitization is begun, Landrum has pointed out, the nurse involved in the care of a patient during this process must be sure that the rationale for treatment is understood, explaining specifically how "a weak solution of an irritant to which the patient is sensitive can be introduced into his body, causing him to gradually become desensitized to this irritant."[37] As the patient becomes less sensitive to the irritant, relief of symptoms should occur. The patient should be instructed to observe his condition closely after each injection, since the length of total treatment, frequency of injections and dosage of each injection all depend upon the degree to which his symptoms are alleviated. The nurse should be aware, most of all, of the need to bolster the patient's flagging spirits over the considerable period of time it may take to achieve concrete results, if, in fact, the desired results occur at all. Nurses who work in special units or clinics for allergic patients, or those who practice in allergists' offices, are often responsible for carrying out series of desensitization injections or for performing skin testing under the supervision of an allergist.

Summary

In summary, the nurse caring for the allergic patient finds considerable challenge in helping to effectively separate patient and antigen, dealing with the adverse effects produced by contact of patient with antigen, and helping to increase the resistance of patient to antigen. Allergic patients present nursing problems calling for the exercise of technical skills, as well as expertise in developing and maintaining interpersonal relationships. Most of all, successful nursing intervention for these patients depends upon the nurse's ability to teach and to provide supportive reassurance. These are the nursing actions which frequently determine how well the patient is able to live with his allergy.

References

1. Sherman, W. B.: Hypersensitivity—Mechanisms and Management. Philadephia, W. B. Saunders, 1968.
2. Asthma—new ideas about an old disease. UCLA Conference, Annals Intern. Med. 78:405–419,1973.
3. Friedman, S. O.: Clinical Immunology. New York, Harper & Row, 1971, p.84.
4. Norman, P.: Immunological diseases. *In* M. A. Samter, et al. (eds.): Immunological Diseases. Boston, Little, Brown, 1972.
5. Mitchell, W. F., et al.: House dust, mites and insects. Ann. Allerg. 27, 3:93–99, Mar. 1969.
6. Sheldon, H., Lovell, R. G. and Mathews, K. P.: A Manual of Clinical Allergy. Philadelphia, W. B. Saunders, 1968.
7. Sherman, W. B.: The atopic diseases—introduction. *In* Samter and Alexander, *op. cit.,* Chapter 43.
8. Feinberg, S. M.: Allergy in Practice. Chicago, Yearbook Medical Publishers, 1946.
9. Landrum, F. L.: Nursing in an allergist's office. Am. J. Nurs., 58, May 1958.
10. Feinberg, S.: Allergies and air conditioning. Am. J. Nurs. 66:1333–1336, June 1966.
11. Sheldon, H., et al, *op. cit.,* p.
12. Fontana, V.: Allergy and emotions. Med. Insight Feb. 1971.
13. McGovern, J. P. and Knight, J. A.: Allergy and Human Emotions. Springfield, Ill., Charles C Thomas, 1968.
14. French, T. M. and Alexander, F.: Psychogenic factors in bronchial asthma. Psychosomatic Medicine Monographs 4. Washington, D.C., Washington National Research Council, 1941.

15. Fontana, *op. cit.,* p. 17.
16. Mathews, K. P. *In* Sheldon, et al., *op. cit.*
17. Sherman, W. B.: The atopic diseases—introduction. *In* Samter, et al., *op. cit,* pp. 771–772.
18. Managing four common skin disorders in children. Patient Care, 76–78, March 15, 1971.
19. Rostenberg, A., Jr. and Solomon, L.: Atopic dermatitus and infantile eczema. *In* Samter et al., *op cit.,* chapter 53.
20. *Ibid.*
21. Rodman, M. W., and Smith, D. W.: Pharmacology and Drug Therapy in Nursing. Philadelphia, J. B. Lippincott, 1973.
22. Fontana, V.: Status asthmaticus. Hosp. Med. 84–87, Jan. 1972.
23. McGovern and Knight, *op. cit.*
24. Rodman and Smith, *op. cit.*
25. Collins-Williams C. et al.: Treatment of bronchial asthma with disodium cromoglycate in children. Ann. Allerg. 29:613–620, Dec. 1971. Cohen, E. P.: New asthma treatment, p. 20, Today's Health, Sept. 1973.
26. Samter, *op. cit.,* Chap. 59, 127.
27. Moody, L.: Asthma-physiology and patient care. Am. J. Nurs. 1212–1217, July 1973.
28. Sheldon, et al., *op. cit.*
29. Moody, *op. cit.* and Mathison, et al., *op. cit.*
30. Richardson, H. B.: *In* Allergy as science, art and magic. Current Med. Digest 227–236, Mar. 1973.
31. *Ibid.*
32. Friedman, *op. cit.*
33. Richardson, *op. cit.*
34. Norman, *op. cit.*
35. Sherman, *op. cit.*
36. Sheldon, et al., *op. cit.*
37. Landrum, *op. cit.*

Bibliography

Amos, B. (ed): Progress in Immunology. New York, Academic Press, 1971

Asthma. Med. World News, March 12, 1971.

Asthma, myths and realities. Med. World News, May 19, 1972.

Augustin, R. and Chandradasa, K. D.: IgE levels and allergic skin reactions in cancer and non-cancer patients. Int. Arch. Allergy. Appl. Immunol. 41:141–143, 1971.

Austen, K. F.: and Humphrey, J. H.: In vitro studies of the mechanism of anaphylaxis. Adv. Immunol. 3:1–96, 1963.

Beland, I.: Clinical Nursing, ed 2. London, Macmillan, 1970, pp. 165–180.

Buckley, R. H., Wray, B. B. and Belmaker, E. Z.: Extreme hyperimmunoglobulinemia E and undue susceptibility to infection. Pediatrics 49:59–70, 1972.

Chan-Yeung, M. M. W., Vyas, M. N. and Grzybowski, S.: Exercise-induced asthma. Am. Rev. Resp. Dis. 104:915–923, 1971.

Coca, A. F. and Cooke, R. A.: On the classification of the phenomena of hypersensitiveness. J. Immunol. 8:163–182, 1923.

Dollery, C. T.: Aerosol inhalers—how safe are they? Consultant May, 1972.

Freeman, E. H., et al.: Psychological variables in allergic disorders: a review. Psychosom. Med. 26:543, 1964.

Gazioglu, K., Condemi, J. J. and Hyde, R. W., et al.: Effect of isoproterenol on gas exchange during air and oxygen breathing in patients with asthma. Am. J. Med. 50:185–190, 1971.

Ishizaka, K., and Ishizaka T.: Human reaginic antibodies and immunoglobulin E. J. Allergy 42:330–363, 1968.

———: Immunoglobulin E and homocytotropic properties. *In* B. Amos (ed.): Progress in Immunology. New York, Academic Press, 1971, pp. 859–874.

Itkin, I. H.: Fundamentals of the treatment of asthma. Prac. Therapeutics, Aug. 1971.

———: The pros and cons of exercise for the person with asthma. Am. J. Nurs. 66:1584–87, July 1966.

Katz, R. M., Whipp, B. J., and Heimlich, E. M., et al.: Exercise-induced bronchospasm, ventilation, and blood gas in asthmatic children. J. Allergy 47:148–158, 1971.

Kumar, L., Newcomb, R. W. and Ishizaka, K., et al.: IgE levels in sera of children with asthma. Pediatrics 47:848–856, 1971.

Lanser, T. and Pencoast, A.: Caring for the asthmatic

at home, in school and on the job. Nurs. 73, 62–65, Nov. 1973.

Luparello, T. J., Leist, N., and Lourie, C. H., et al.: The interaction of psychologic stimuli and pharmacologic agents on airway reactivity in asthmatic subjects. Psychosom. Med. 32:509–513, 1970.

Meisner, P., and Hugh-Jones, P.: Pulmonary function in bronchial asthma. Brit. Med. J. 1:470–475, 1968.

Orange, R. P. and Austen, K. F.: Slow-reacting substance of anaphylaxis. Adv. Immunol. 10:106–145, 1969.

Reed, C. E.: Beta adrenergic blockade, bronchial asthma and atopy. J. Allergy 42:238–242, 1968.

Rosendahl, R.: Allergy hospital in Finland. Am. J. Nurs. 7:1445–46, July 1967.

Smith, J. M.: A 5 year prospective survey of rural children with asthma and hay fever. J. Allergy 47:23–30, Jan. 1971.

Vassallo, C. L., Lee, J. B. L., and Domm, B. M.: Exercise-induced asthma; observations regarding hypocapnia and acidosis. Am. Rev. Resp. Dis. 105:42–49, 1972.

Index